PRIMARY CARE MANAGEMENT

OF

HEART DISEASE

Visit our website at **www.mosby.com**

PRIMARY CARE
MANAGEMENT
OF
HEART DISEASE

GEORGE J. TAYLOR, MD
Associate Professor of Medicine
Medical University of South Carolina
Charleston, South Carolina

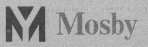 Mosby

St. Louis   Baltimore   Boston   Carlsbad   Chicago   Minneapolis   New York   Philadelphia   Portland
London   Milan   Sydney   Tokyo   Toronto

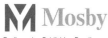

Editor: Elizabeth M. Fathman
Senior Developmental Editor: Ellen Baker Geisel
Project Manager: Patricia Tannian
Project Specialist: John Casey
Design Manager: Gail Morey Hudson
Cover Design: Teresa Breckwoldt

NOTICE

Pharmacology is an ever-changing field. Standard safety precautions must be followed, but as new research and clinical experience broaden our knowledge, changes in treatment and drug therapy may become necessary or appropriate. Readers are advised to check the most current product information provided by the manufacturer of each drug to be administered to verify the recommended dose, the method and duration of administration, and contraindications. It is the responsibility of the treating physician, relying on experience and knowledge of the patient, to determine dosages and the best treatment for each individual patient. Neither the publisher nor the editor assumes any liability for any injury and/or damage to persons or property arising from this publication.

Mosby, Inc.
A Harcourt Health Sciences Company
11830 Westline Industrial Drive
St. Louis, Missouri 63146

Printed in the United States of America

Library of Congress Cataloging-in-Publication Data
Primary care management of heart disease / [edited by] George J. Taylor.
    p.   cm.
    Includes bibliographical references and index.
    ISBN 0-323-00256-0
    1. Cardiology. 2. Heart—Diseases. 3. Primary care (Medicine) I. Taylor, George Jesse.
    [DNLM: 1. Heart Diseases—therapy. 2. Heart Diseases—diagnosis. 3. Primary Health Care. WG 210 P952 2000]
    RC669 .P668 2000
    616.1'2 21—dc21
                                                    99-042879

99 00 01 02 03 GW/KPT 9 8 7 6 5 4 3 2 1

Contributors

CHAD ALFORD, MD
Department of Medicine
Medical University of South Carolina
Charleston, South Carolina

MICHAEL E. ASSEY, MD
Professor of Medicine
Director, Adult Cardiac Catheterization Laboratories
Director, Division of Cardiology
Medical University of South Carolina
Charleston, South Carolina

RICHARD T. BILINSKY, MD
Clinical Associate, Department of Medicine
Southern Illinois University School of Medicine
Springfield, Illinois

GERALD E. BOYD, MD
Professor, Department of Family Medicine
University of Illinois College of Medicine
Rockford, Illinois

ALAN S. BROWN, MD
Director, Lipid Clinic and Preventative Cardiology
Midwest Heart Specialists
Naperville, Illinois;
Clinical Associate Professor of Medicine
Stritch School of Medicine, Loyola University
Maywood, Illinois

ELISHA L. BROWNFIELD, MD
Assistant Professor of Medicine
Medical University of South Carolina
Charleston, South Carolina

WALTER A. BRZEZINSKI, MD
Associate Professor, Department of Internal Medicine
Medical University of South Carolina
Charleston, South Carolina

ROBERT C. BUSSING, MD
Assistant Professor of Medicine
Chief, Division of General Internal Medicine
Department of Medicine
Southern Illinois University School of Medicine
Springfield, Illinois

ANGELA J. CALDIERARO-BENTLEY, RN, MS, CCRN
Adult Critical Care Nursing Educator
Intensive Care Unit, St. John's Hospital
Springfield, Illinois

BLASE A. CARABELLO, MD
Professor of Medicine
Baylor University College of Medicine
Houston, Texas

TIMOTHY D. CARTER, MD
Associate Professor of Neurology
Medical University of South Carolina
Charleston, South Carolina

LYNN COFER, MSN
Clinical Director, Lipid Clinic
Midwest Heart Specialists
Naperville, Illinois

DENNIS COPE, MD
Professor of Medicine
Director, Division of General Internal Medicine
VA Medical Center
Charleston, South Carolina

JEROME J. EPPLIN, MD
Clinical Associate Professor, Family Medicine
Southern Illinois University School of Medicine
Springfield, Illinois;
Litchfield Family Practice Center
Litchfield, Illinois

MARCEY R. ERVIN, AS
Research Associate
Prairie Education and Research Cooperative
Springfield, Illinois

MARY B. FRANKIS, MD, PhD
Assistant Professor of Medicine
Director, Coronary Care Unit
Medical University of South Carolina
Charleston, South Carolina

ROGER L. FULTON, MD
Chairman, Department of Medicine
St. Joseph's Hospital
Highland, Illinois

WILLS C. GEILS, MD
Department of Internal Medicine
Medical University of South Carolina
Charleston, South Carolina

DONALD R. GRAHAM, MD
Clinical Associate Professor of Medicine
Southern Illinois University School of Medicine;
Chief, Department of Infectious Diseases
Springfield Clinic
Springfield, Illinois

MARK E. HANSEN, MD
Clinical Associate Professor of Medicine
Southern Illinois University School of Medicine
Sangamon Medical Associates
Springfield, Illinois

JOSEPH R. HARTMANN, MD
Associate Professor of Medicine
Stritch School of Medicine, Loyola University
Maywood, Illinois;
Midwest Heart Specialists
Director of Cardiology, Good Samaritan Hospital
Downers Grove, Illinois

ELAINE G. HEARNEY, MD
Assistant Professor of Medicine
Assistant Director of Clinical Research
Department of Medicine
Northport VAMC/SUNY at Stony Brook
Northport, New York

MICHAEL G. HUBER, MD
Assistant Professor of Medicine
Instructor, Department of Psychiatry and Behavioral Sciences
Medical University of South Carolina
Charleston, South Carolina

STEPHEN H. JENNISON, MD
Clinical Associate Professor of Medicine
Southern Illinois University College of Medicine;
Medical Director, Heart Transplantation and Heart Failure
    Clinics
Prairie Cardiovascular Consultants
Springfield, Illinois

SARITA KANSAL, MD
Assistant Professor of Medicine
Department of Internal Medicine
Southern Illinois University School of Medicine
Springfield, Illinois

RICHARD E. KATHOLI, MD
Professor, Department of Pharmacology and Medicine
Southern Illinois University School of Medicine;
Department of Cardiology, St. John's Hospital
Prairie Heart Institute
Springfield, Illinois

BERT KELLER, DMin
Associate Professor, Department of Family Medicine
Medical University of South Carolina
Charleston, South Carolina

MARK KOHNLE, MS
Exercise Physiologist
Cardiopulmonary Rehabilitation Program
Prairie Heart Institute/St. John's Hospital
Springfield, Illinois

ROBERT KUSHNER, MD
Professor of Medicine, Northwestern University;
Medical Director, Wellness Institute
Department of Medicine, Northwestern Memorial Hospital
Chicago, Illinois

JULIE D. LAWRENCE, PharmD, BCPS
Clinical Assistant Professor
Department of Pharmacy Practice
Medical University of South Carolina
Charleston, South Carolina

ROBERT B. LEMAN, MD
Professor of Medicine
Director, Adult Electrophysiology
Director, Pacemaker Surveillance
Department of Adult Cardiology
Medical University of South Carolina
Charleston, South Carolina

LEONARD S. LICHTENSTEIN, MD
Assistant Professor of Medicine
Department of Internal Medicine
Medical University of South Carolina
Charleston, South Carolina

ALEX LICKERMAN, MD
Assistant Professor of Internal Medicine
University of Chicago
Chicago, Illinois

J. ANTONIO G. LOPEZ, MD
Clinical Associate Professor of Internal Medicine
Southern Illinois University School of Medicine;
Director, Prairie Lipid Clinic
Prairie Cardiovascular Consultants, Ltd.;
Director, Preventive Cardiology, Prairie Heart Institute
Springfield, Illinois

CHARLES L. LUCORE, MD
Clinical Assistant Professor of Medicine
Southern Illinois University School of Medicine;
Interventional Cardiologist
Prairie Cardiovascular Consultants, Inc.
Springfield, Illinois

DAVID P. MALONE, MD
Clinical Assistant Professor of Medicine
Medical University of South Carolina
Charleston, South Carolina

ANSEL R. McFADDIN III, MD
Clinical Assistant Professor of Medicine
Medical University of South Carolina
Charleston, South Carolina

RENEÉ P. MEYER, MD
Assistant Professor of Medicine
Medical University of South Carolina;
Medical Director, Geriatric Evaluation and Management
Department of Geriatrics and Extended Care
VA Medical Center
Charleston, South Carolina

H. WESTON MOSES, MD
Clinical Associate Professor of Medicine
Southern Illinois University School of Medicine;
Prairie Cardiovascular Consultants, Ltd.
Springfield, Illinois

BARBARA A. MULCH, MD
Department of Internal Medicine
Springfield Clinic
Hillsboro, Illinois

CHRISTOPHER D. NIELSEN, MD
Assistant Professor of Medicine, Division of Cardiology
Medical University of South Carolina
Charleston, South Carolina

TERRENCE X. O'BRIEN, MD
Assistant Professor of Medicine
Research Associate, Department of Medicine
Cardiology Division Office of Research Development
Ralph H. Johnson Veterans Affairs Medical Center
Medical University of South Carolina
Charleston, South Carolina

STEVEN D. O'MARRO, MD
Clinical Assistant Professor of Medicine
Southern Illinois University School of Medicine;
Staff, Department of Infectious Diseases
Springfield Clinic
Springfield, Illinois

SARA CREVELING PAUL, RN, MSN
Nurse Practitioner, Heart Failure Clinic;
Clinical Assistant Professor, College of Nursing
Medical University of South Carolina
Charleston, South Carolina

LESLYE C. PENNYPACKER, MD
Associate Chief of Staff
Geriatric and Extended Care
VA Medical Center;
Assistant Professor of Medicine
Department of Geriatrics
Medical University of South Carolina
Charleston, South Carolina

BRENT G. PETTY, MD
Associate Professor of Medicine
Division of General Internal Medicine
The Johns Hopkins University
Baltimore, Maryland

QUENTIN A. PLETSCH, PhD, MD
Clinical Associate Professor of Anesthesiology
Southern Illinois University School of Medicine
Springfield, Illinois

KIMBERLY D. RAKES, MD
Assistant Professor of Medicine
Medical University of South Carolina
Charleston, South Carolina

HOWARD ROTH, MD
Interventional Radiologist
Midwest Heart Specialists
Downers Grove, Illinois

JOEL A. SCHNEIDER, MD
Clinical Associate Professor, Department of Surgery
Southern Illinois University School of Medicine;
President, Prairie Cardiovascular Center, Ltd.
Springfield, Illinois

WILLIAM M. SIMPSON, Jr., MD
Professor, Department of Family Medicine
Medical University of South Carolina
Charleston, South Carolina

SARAH E. STAPLETON, MD
Clinical Assistant Professor of Medicine
Department of General Medicine, Carolina Family Care
Medical University of South Carolina
Charleston, South Carolina

GEORGE J. TAYLOR, MD
Associate Professor of Medicine
Division of Cardiology
Medical University of South Carolina
Charleston, South Carolina

C. CAROLYN THIEDKE, MD
Assistant Professor, Department of Family Medicine
Medical University of South Carolina
Charleston, South Carolina

DOUGLAS J. THOMPSON, MD
Lowcountry Medical Group
Beaufort, South Carolina

JERRY T. THOMPSON, PhD
Research Associate, Laboratory of Molecular Toxicology
Pennsylvania State University
University Park, Pennsylvania

ROBERT TRASK, MD
Clinical Assistant Professor of Medicine
Southern Illinois University School of Medicine;
Prairie Cardiovascular Consultants
Springfield, Illinois

BRUCE W. USHER, Jr., MD
Fellow, Department of Medicine
Division of Cardiology
Medical University of South Carolina
Charleston, South Carolina

ADRIAN B. VAN BAKEL, MD, PhD
Associate Professor of Medicine
Division of Cardiology
Medical University of South Carolina
Charleston, South Carolina

KIRK W. WALKER, MD
Medical Director, Salem Hospital Heart Failure Program
Salem Cardiology Associates
Salem, Oregon

W. THOMAS WOODS, PhD
President, Clinical Investigators Pact Ltd.
Adjunct Professor, Department of Pharmacology
Southern Illinois University School of Medicine
Springfield, Illinois

For

Matt, Jesse, and Luke

all scholarly fellows

Preface

Your practice is changing. Primary care doctors working in the managed care setting are expected to rely less on subspecialists yet still provide state-of-the-art care. At the same time, drastic changes have occurred over the past two decades in the treatment of hyperlipidemia, coronary heart disease, hypertension, heart failure, and cardiac arrhythmias. This text is designed for the busy primary care practitioner who needs rapid access to new information and a clear and concise description of the pathophysiology, natural history, and treatment of cardiac and vascular illness.

The book is comprehensive. Most of the heart-related conditions you will encounter in adult patients are reviewed. On the other hand, we have worked hard to keep it from being exhaustive (and exhausting). This differentiates it from some of the excellent, more encyclopedic cardiology texts.

Although this text is not encyclopedic, we do not ignore the literature and are particularly sensitive to your need for an evidence-based rationale for treatment. Evidence-based therapies are highlighted, and we have provided practice guidelines where they are available. We have attempted to be selective. Many of the cited references consist of current review articles that we found especially helpful.

A special feature of this text is that each chapter was written by a team comprising a primary care practitioner and a cardiologist. We believe this approach helped us to focus on what is practical and to describe the science clearly and succinctly. Tables and boxes have been used to condense the data when possible. Our primary care co-authors had us address a number of management issues that are encountered in practice and are often shortchanged in specialty texts. For example, there are chapters on counseling patients who need to apply for cardiac disability, the palliation of end-stage heart disease, women's health issues, and geriatric cardiology.

Other chapters plainly introduce high-tech cardiology so that primary care doctors (especially those of us long out of training), house officers, medical students, nurses, and nurse practitioners will find it more understandable. Individual chapters review electrocardiography, nuclear cardiology, echocardiography, the catheterization laboratory, and intensive care unit technology.

We are grateful to Gordon Grindy and his colleagues at Marquette Electronics, Inc., for the high quality of ECG reproduction. My thanks to Lisa Murray who did the artwork. My gratitude to the team at Mosby that has worked diligently on this project, Liz Fathman, Patricia Tannian, John Casey, Gail Hudson, and especially my gifted developmental editor, Ellen Baker Geisel, who is largely responsible for getting this project finished.

Marilyn Taylor is a patient woman, and I appreciate her forbearance during this writing adventure.

George J. Taylor

Contents

PART ONE

General Principles

1 Biology of the Circulation, 3
   W. Thomas Woods and George J. Taylor

2 Cardiac and Vascular Anatomy and Useful
   Physiologic Concepts, 8
   George J. Taylor and W. Thomas Woods

3 Cardiac History, 24
   George J. Taylor and Gerald E. Boyd

4 Physical Examination, 36
   George J. Taylor and Dennis Cope

5 Electrocardiogram, 54
   George J. Taylor and Brent G. Petty

6 Treadmill Testing, 69
   H. Weston Moses and Steven D. O'Marro

7 Chest X-ray and Vascular Studies, 77
   Terrence X. O'Brien and Sara Creveling Paul

8 Echocardiogram, 85
   Mary B. Frankis and Elaine G. Hearney

9 Nuclear Cardiology, 97
   Robert Trask and Jerome J. Epplin

10 Cardiac Catheterization, 103
    Michael E. Assey and Ansel R. McFaddin III

PART TWO

Illnesses

SECTION 1 *Atherosclerotic Disease*

11 Atherosclerotic Cardiovascular Disease: an
    Overview, 115
    George J. Taylor and William M. Simpson, Jr.

12 Practical Management of Dyslipidemia, 121
    Alan S. Brown and Lynn Cofer

13 Angina Pectoris, 135
    George J. Taylor and Robert C. Bussing

14 Acute Myocardial Infarction, 168
    George J. Taylor and C. Carolyn Thiedke

15 Reperfusion Therapy for Acute Myocardial
    Infarction, 181
    George J. Taylor and Jerome J. Epplin

16 Complications of Myocardial Infarction, 194
    George J. Taylor and Sarah E. Stapleton

17 Long-Term Treatment after Myocardial
    Infarction, 206
    George J. Taylor, Mark Kohnle, and Leslye C. Pennypacker

SECTION 2 *Valvular Heart Disease*

18 Mitral Valve Disease, 217
    Blase A. Carabello and Donald R. Graham

19 Aortic Valve Disease, 230
    Blase A. Carabello

20 Tricuspid and Pulmonic Valve Disease, 240
    Blase A. Carabello

21 Endocarditis, 244
    Donald R. Graham and Blase A. Carabello

SECTION 3 *Heart Failure*

22 Congestive Heart Failure: Systolic
    Dysfunction, 259
    Adrian B. Van Bakel and Reneé P. Meyer

23 Diastolic Heart Failure, 276
    Kirk W. Walker and Douglas J. Thompson

24 Cardiomyopathy and Cardiac Muscle
    Disease, 288
    Stephen H. Jennison and Barbara A. Mulch

SECTION 4 *Arrhythmias*

25 Atrial Arrhythmias, 296
    Walter A. Brzezinski and Robert B. Leman

26 Ventricular Arrhythmias, 307
    Elisha L. Brownfield and Robert B. Leman

27 Bradyarrhythmias and Evaluation of
    Syncope, 320
    Leonard S. Lichtenstein and Robert B. Leman

28 Pacemaker Therapy, 331
H. Weston Moses and Roger L. Fulton

SECTION 5 *Other Cardiac Conditions*

29 Pericardial Disease, 342
Mary B. Frankis and Kimberly D. Rakes

30 Congenital Heart Disease in Adults, 347
George J. Taylor and Chad Alford

SECTION 6 *Vascular Disease*

31 Hypertension, 359
Richard E. Katholi, George J. Taylor, and Marcey R. Ervin

32 Diseases of the Aorta, 378
Kimberly D. Rakes and George J. Taylor

33 Peripheral Arterial Disease, 384
Joseph R. Hartmann and Howard Roth

34 Cerebrovascular Disease, 392
Timothy D. Carter and Adrian B. Van Bakel

SECTION 7 *Noncardiac Illnesses and Special Conditions That Affect the Heart*

35 Pulmonary Heart Disease, 404
Christopher D. Nielsen and David P. Malone

36 Endocrine Disorders and Cardiovascular Disease, 414
Robert C. Bussing and George J. Taylor

37 Cardiac Manifestations of Connective Tissue Disease, 422
William M. Simpson, Jr., and George J. Taylor

38 Neoplastic Disease and the Heart, 428
Wills C. Geils and George J. Taylor

39 Neuromuscular and Neurologic Disorders, 433
Jerome J. Epplin and George J. Taylor

40 Pregnancy and Heart Disease, 441
Sarita Kansal and George J. Taylor

41 Women and Heart Disease, 450
Sarah E. Stapleton and George J. Taylor

42 Infections in Patients with Heart Disease, 456
Steven D. O'Marro and Adrian B. Van Bakel

43 Nutritional Disorders, Obesity, and Alcoholism, 463
Robert Kushner and Alex Lickerman

44 Effects of Renal Disease on the Heart, 477
Richard E. Katholi, J. Antonio G. Lopez, and Richard T. Bilinsky

45 Cardiovascular Genetic Diseases, 481
Jerry T. Thompson and Terrence X. O'Brien

46 Psychologic Disorders, Stress, Drugs, and Drug Abuse, 489
Michael G. Huber and George J. Taylor

47 Advanced Age and Heart Disease, 500
Leslye C. Pennypacker and George J. Taylor

SECTION 8 *Management Issues*

48 Cardiac Risks of Noncardiac Surgery and Perioperative Management, 507
Quentin A. Pletsch and George J. Taylor

49 Insurance, Disability, and Other Legal Issues, 519
Charles L. Lucore and Mark E. Hansen

50 Cardiac Emergencies Including Cardiac Arrest, Resuscitation, and Trauma, 526
Bruce W. Usher, Jr., and George J. Taylor

51 Technical Aspects of ICU-CCU Care, 536
Angela J. Caldieraro-Bentley and George J. Taylor

52 Heart Surgery, 542
Joel A. Schneider and George J. Taylor

53 Palliative Care and End-of-Life Decisions, 550
George J. Taylor, Bert Keller, and Leslye C. Pennypacker

PART THREE
Cardiology Drug Reference, 559
Compiled by Julie D. Lawrence and George J. Taylor

PART ONE

General Principles

1

Biology of the Circulation

W. Thomas Woods
George J. Taylor

THE FUTURE OF PREVENTION AND TREATMENT

A text that appears at the turn of the century properly begins with an essay describing the latest developments. It is curious that current research in cardiovascular medicine seldom involves classic physiology and hemodynamics. Instead, the modern researcher studies "noncardiac" subjects including thrombosis and platelet function, lipid biochemistry, membrane receptor and ion channel physiology, and molecular genetics. Some of these subjects are discussed in the following chapters. This chapter provides a sampling of what the future holds.

ANTICOAGULATION AND ANTIPLATELET STRATEGIES FOR CORONARY ARTERY DISEASE

Acute coronary syndromes usually are caused by coronary artery thrombosis. The roles of platelets and coagulation in the pathogenesis of acute coronary syndromes underscore the therapeutic importance of aspirin and heparin. However, both agents have drawbacks. Platelet activation by thrombin does not use the thromboxane A2 pathways, so aspirin cannot block it. Thrombosis can be resistant to heparin, because heparin is neutralized by platelet factor 4, which is released from platelets and activated at sites of plaque disruption; antithrombin complexes interact with heparin and prevent it from inactivating thrombin bound to fibrin clots. New antithrombotic agents are being designed to overcome the limitations of aspirin and heparin.

Until recently, it was thought that treatment with the new thrombolytic agents in combination with conventional anticoagulants might be sufficient to remove life-threatening clots from blood vessels. However, recent experimental evidence has indicated that the failure of this strategy can be attributed to the character of the clot itself. Clots contain the enzyme thrombin, bound within their structure and protected from inactivation by antithrombin III (ATIII). Thrombolytic therapy or breakdown of the clot by the body's own natural plas-

minogen activators releases this thrombin, which is then able to begin the clotting process again. Therefore in many cases the clot is being built up or extended as quickly as it is being removed.

The current therapeutic strategy is systemic treatment with heparin or warfarin. Treatment with these agents (and those under development, such as hirudin) often causes bleeding at other sites.

Recent understanding that the clot itself is the focus of clot extension has prompted the design of a novel anticoagulant that acts precisely where thrombin is being released, that is, at the site of the clot. Targeted anticoagulant that works only at the site of clot may avoid the overdosing that causes bleeding complications.

Role of Thrombin in Coagulation

Thrombin is activated at the site of plaque rupture or vascular damage by a process involving the interaction of platelets and coagulation factors. It is an enzyme with two key actions that promote the formation and extension of thrombi: (1) conversion of fibrinogen into fibrin and (2) activation of platelets. These two actions result in an activated prothrombinase complex that leads to the generation of more thrombin to continue the cycle.

Problems with Conventional Anticoagulants

Although thrombin has been earmarked for years as an obvious target in the treatment of thrombotic diseases, the two most widely used drugs, warfarin and heparin, inhibit thrombin only indirectly. Furthermore, the efficacy of warfarin and heparin depends on the *systemic* inhibition of multiple coagulation factors. Evidence is growing that the progression of thrombosis depends on the potent procoagulant activity associated with clots and their ability to activate prothrombin and induce *local activation* of the coagulation system and platelets.

New Agents

Antagonists of the platelet glycoprotein IIb/IIIa receptor (GPIIb/IIIa) and the direct thrombin inhibitors, hirudin and hirulog, have been introduced recently. By blocking the final common pathway of platelet aggregation, GPIIb/IIIa antagonists prevent platelet aggregation

3

by all agonists, including thrombin. Hirudin and hirulog have potential advantages over heparin because they are not neutralized by platelet release products and, unlike heparin, can inactivate thrombin bound to fibrin.

Chimeric-7E3 (c7E3) (ReoPro), a humanized monoclonal antibody against GPIIb/IIIa, has been shown to reduce recurrent ischemic events in patients undergoing coronary angioplasty both at 30 days and at 6 months. Thus c7E3 is the first agent to produce a clinically meaningful reduction in long-term ischemic outcomes in a large-scale randomized clinical trial. To date, the results with synthetic GPIIb/IIIa antagonists have been less promising, with early benefits diminishing over time. This may reflect their shorter half-life compared to c7E3. Hirudin and hirulog appear to be superior to heparin at preventing recurrent ischemic events early after coronary angioplasty, but this effect is transient, indicating ongoing thrombin generation at the site of vascular injury.

Further studies will define the role of these new agents in the treatment of acute ischemic conditions including unstable angina, acute myocardial infarction (MI), transient ischemic attack, and stroke.

Hormone Replacement Therapy for Prevention of Coronary Artery Disease

Advocates of estrogen replacement or hormone replacement therapy appreciate the anticancer effects of co-administered synthetic progestins despite the vasoconstrictive and prothrombic risks associated with progestins. Natural progesterone is a far less potent vasoconstrictor and is being tested in a vaginally delivered preparation. Early results suggest women who have received the drug acquired improved exercise tolerance and reduced myocardial ischemia.

CARDIOVASCULAR AND AUTONOMIC RECEPTORS
Cardiac Natriuretic Peptides

Elevated circulating levels of cardiac natriuretic peptides have important prognostic and therapeutic implications. They are not like the vasoconstrictors activated in left ventricular (LV) dysfunction—norepinephrine, the renin-angiotensin system, and arginine vasopressin—all favoring progression of ventricular dysfunction and thus having a pathogenetic role in the progression of ventricular dysfunction and heart failure. Instead, cardiac natriuretic peptides promote systemic arterial dilation, natriuresis, diuresis, and renin inhibition.

Atrial natriuretic peptide (ANP) is a 28-amino acid peptide synthesized and secreted by the atria. It is now well established that circulating ANP is increased in chronic congestive heart failure in proportion to the severity of the disease and elevated in asymptomatic LV

dysfunction. Atrial wall stress and stretch, rather than atrial pressure, are the predominant stimuli for ANP release. ANP is secreted in increased amounts from ventricle and atrium in heart failure. Infusion of ANP in patients with heart failure results in decreased right atrial and pulmonary artery wedge pressures, decreased systemic vascular resistance, increased stroke volume, enhanced natriuresis and diuresis, and inhibition of both the renin-angiotensin system and the sympathetic nervous system.

Brain natriuretic peptide (BNP) is a 32-amino acid peptide similar to ANP and shares the same guanylate cyclase receptors on endothelial cells. BNP is secreted predominantly from atria and ventricles in response to dilation. Circulating BNP level is increased in patients with heart failure in proportion to the severity of the disease. Infusion of BNP in patients with heart failure results in decreased preload and afterload, increased stroke volume, enhanced natriuresis and diuresis, and a reduction in aldosterone. Unlike ANP, BNP does not reduce norepinephrine levels but may actually increase norepinephrine through baroreceptor-mediated sympathetic discharge. Because ANP and BNP share common guanylate cyclase receptors, large amounts of intravenously administered BNP compete with ANP for these receptors and may increase circulating ANP levels despite the reduction in right and left atrial pressures. ANP and BNP together represent a potentially important natriuretic system with important compensatory actions in patients with heart failure. They also hold promise as new therapies for LV dysfunction and congestive heart failure.

Adenosine Receptors

Adenosine receptors (A_1, A_{2A}, A_{2B}, A_3) are ubiquitous throughout the cardiovascular system and mediate a large number of physiologic responses to adenosine. The ubiquity of the four adenosine receptor subtypes makes them difficult to study as individual receptors. However, potent, specific, selective agonists and antagonists are emerging, and we may expect to encounter them as therapeutic agents in the next century.

LOWERING LIPOPROTEIN RISK FACTORS FOR CORONARY ARTERY DISEASE

Increased levels of plasma cholesterol and triglyceride and decreased levels of HDL cholesterol have all been shown to predispose to the development of premature coronary artery disease (CAD). Indeed, most victims of CAD have some form of plasma lipid abnormality.

Premature CAD will not develop in every person with elevated total cholesterol (or elevated LDL cholesterol), nor will everyone with low LDL cholesterol levels remain immune from premature CAD. However, long-term observations in the Framingham Study and somewhat shorter-term observations in large numbers of subjects in the MRFIT Study indicate that coronary risk increases appreciably with total cholesterol values over about 5 mmol/L (roughly above 220 mg/dL). In patients with established CAD, abnormalities in lipids and lipoproteins remain highly predictive of future CAD and death.

Elevated triglycerides generally have been predictive of increased CHD, but this remains controversial, partly because many subjects with increased triglycerides also have low concentrations of HDL cholesterol. Patients with increased triglycerides and reduced HDL cholesterol may have a different form of LDL, regardless of whether LDL cholesterol concentration is elevated. This so-called B-LDL pattern is characterized by LDL particles that are smaller and denser than normal. This pattern has been shown to be atherogenic and may be present in around 80% of subjects with triglycerides > 2.3 mmol/L. Small, dense LDL also are more subject to oxidative damage. Elevated triglycerides, reduced HDL cholesterol, and small, dense LDL may form part of a syndrome containing many other atherogenic features; this grouping of findings is designated as the *syndrome of insulin resistance* or the *metabolic syndrome*. A major contributing feature in the development of this syndrome is central or visceral obesity.

Other lipid and lipoprotein factors have been implicated in the genesis of coronary heart disease (CHD), including elevations in lipoprotein(a). Observations in this area are inadequate. No definitive intervention studies have been conducted.

Controlled trials of plasma lipid modification by diet or by drugs have been under way since the 1970s. Although a reduction in LDL cholesterol generally has led to a decrease in CAD events, only recently was definitive evidence obtained that LDL reduction prolongs life in patients with established CAD or no CAD. Randomized intervention studies that specifically target triglyceride-lowering or HDL-raising have yet to be conducted.

The same pattern of risk factor relationships operate in women as in men. Although women have been underrepresented in intervention studies, they have obtained similar benefit to men. The risk factor relationships between LDL cholesterol and atherosclerosis appear to be attenuated in the elderly. Subjects older than 60 years of age benefited in intervention studies, but few data are available for those older than 70 years.

Current Lipid Wisdom   (see Chapter 12 for treatment guidelines)

1. Plasma lipid and lipoprotein concentrations are key factors in the development of premature CAD.

2. Elevated levels of LDL cholesterol and reduced levels of HDL cholesterol are each independent predictors of premature CAD.
3. Intervention trials have established that lowering of LDL cholesterol levels is safe and leads to fewer CAD events and, in high-risk subjects, to a prolongation of life.
4. Measures that increase HDL cholesterol also decrease CAD risk, although it remains to be proven in human subjects that the benefit is a direct result of the increase in HDL level.
5. Plasma cholesterol, triglyceride, and HDL cholesterol levels should be measured in all high-risk patients.

ENDOTHELIAL CELL FUNCTION

Vascular endothelium is the interface between tissue and blood. It protects against vascular injury and maintains blood fluidity. Normal endothelium releases prostacyclin and nitric oxide (NO), potent vasodilators and inhibitors of platelet and monocyte activation. The normal endothelial surface contains a binding site for thrombin, secretes tissue plasminogen activator and von Willebrand factor, and produces endothelium-derived relaxation factor (EDRF), which is believed to be NO. Injury to endothelium is accompanied by loss of protective molecules and expression of adhesive molecules, procoagulant activities, and mitogenic factors. The result is thrombosis, smooth muscle cell migration and proliferation, and atherosclerosis.

Risk factors associated with the development of coronary artery disease all affect the coronary artery endothelium. Many of these adverse effects are the result of reduced NO, an endogenous vasorelaxant produced by healthy vascular endothelial cells. Clinical correlates of vascular endothelial dysfunction may include manifestations of myocardial ischemia, including angina.

Atherosclerosis is a prominent cause of the defects in the vascular endothelium marked by diminished NO activity. One goal of reversing the atherosclerotic process is restoration of normal endothelial function. Treatments that reduce LDL or total cholesterol have been shown in several small clinical trials to have a beneficial effect on some measures of endothelial-dependent arterial vasomotion in patients with one- or two-vessel CAD or hypercholesterolemia without CAD. Preliminary evidence demonstrates that such treatments will be beneficial in patients with more severe CAD. L-arginine, the precursor for NO synthesis in the endothelial cell, has been shown in preliminary clinical studies to exert positive effects on vasodilation and platelet aggregation.

Accumulating evidence indicates that disorders of NO production (from L-arginine) through NO synthetase (NOS) might play a role in several cardiovascular disorders. In hypercholesterolemia, atherosclerosis, ischemia-reperfusion, transplant vasculopathy, restenosis, tobacco use, and pulmonary hypertension, dysfunction of the NOS pathway can be overcome by supplemental L-arginine. The administration of L-arginine also reverses endothelial vasodilator dysfunction in hypercholesterolemia, some forms of systemic hypertension, CAD, transplant vasculopathy, and restenosis and can slow or even reverse atherogenesis in animal models. NO also is known to suppress the proliferation of vascular smooth muscle cells. Further elucidation of these disturbances in NOS may lead to new therapeutic strategies for a wide variety of cardiovascular disorders.

MOLECULAR BIOLOGY AND GENE THERAPY

We have reached the point at which DNA may be thought of as a drug. Gene augmentation strategies involving plasmid, electromechanical transfection, or viral vectors already have been used to alter the function of cardiovascular cells. Likewise, antigene strategies (involving antisense oligonucleotides) have been shown to modify cardiovascular cell function. Perhaps the most exciting prospect in the twenty-first century is molecular therapeutics using DNA (and RNA) for cardiovascular disease. The following examples are the tip of the iceberg.

Vascular Endothelial Growth Factor

Genes can be delivered into cells by biologic carriers known as plasmids or by electromechanical injection. The simplicity of using injections of naked plasmid DNA into skeletal muscle tissue as an effective means to deliver a potent angiogenesis factor into ischemic peripheral vascular beds is both an exciting and encouraging finding. Plasmid DNA tends to be an inefficient gene transfer system, but it is comparatively simple to prepare and relatively free of serious side effects. It works especially well in skeletal muscle.

In the United States over 150,000 patients annually require lower limb amputation for ischemic peripheral vascular disease. Recent reports suggest DNA for angiogenesis factors can be incorporated into ischemic tissue which may express factors like vascular endothelial growth factor (VEGF). VEGF is one of the best candidates. It promotes new vessel formation in areas of normal perfusion, and the expression of both the cytokine and its receptors is enhanced by tissue ischemia, thus rendering ischemic areas responsive to even low concentrations of VEGF. The delivery of a vector containing DNA encoding VEGF to targeted cells in ischemic limbs resembles gene therapy strategies being developed for many other clinical problems and therefore shares the requirement of demonstrating efficient gene transfer.

However, circulating VEGF levels may trigger initiation of latent tumor growth or exacerbate diabetic retinopathy. Whether the VEGF plasmid DNA delivery strategy will achieve success in other settings must await further study.

Factor IX

Electroporation involves the application of very brief, carefully controlled pulses of electric fields to cells, causing pores to open in the cell membrane and allowing a functional gene to pass into the cell where it expresses its product (protein) long after the pore closes. The treated cells can then be put back into the patient to synthesize a missing protein. Gene therapy by electroporation does not use virus DNA sequences or proteins to gain access to the cell interior and therefore is free of potentially harmful side effects related to virus-mediated gene therapy approaches.

Experiments with gene therapy via electroporation already have been carried out with factor IX–deficient cells. Cultured human bone marrow stromal cells, which are normally factor IX negative, were successfully electrotransfected with the human factor IX gene. These genetically engineered cells were then injected into the bloodstream of a strain of mouse that does not reject human cells to evaluate their persistence and expression of the factor IX gene. Three weeks after injection, six out of seven mice produced the human clotting factor, which remained detectable in their blood for up to 2 months. More important, the mice tolerated the procedure well. These observations have raised hopes that clotting factor defects may be correctable by gene therapy in the future.

Nitric Oxide

Several molecular therapies are currently being evaluated for the treatment of restenosis after revascularization procedures. Preliminary evidence suggests that NO donor agents may prevent restenosis. In animal studies, transfection of antisense nucleotides directed against the expression of cell cycle regulatory genes have inhibited neointima formation in vein grafts. Targeting the critical steps in vascular disease progression at the molecular level will bring about the development of many therapeutic agents. Ongoing research will further define the role of these agents in the treatment of atherosclerosis and cardiovascular disease.

Ion Channels
Long-QT Syndrome

A more detailed understanding of cardiac arrhythmias is emerging as the workings of most of the types of ion channels underlying cardiac action potentials are elucidated. The various long-QT syndromes are the first genetically determined arrhythmias known to be caused at the molecular level by defects in myocardial ion channels.

The congenital long-QT syndrome has an estimated incidence of 1 in 10,000 to 1 in 15,000. A person with long-QT syndrome may have unexplained syncope, seizures, or sudden death. Most are asymptomatic and are identified during electrocardiographic screening or routine evaluation (see Chapter 5). In patients with long-QT syndrome, the T-wave morphology often is abnormal, and heart rhythm can degenerate into a polymorphic ventricular tachycardia, usually torsade de pointes (see Chapter 5).

The prolonged QT interval as measured on the electrocardiogram results from a prolonged cardiac action potential. The ventricular action potential begins when sodium and calcium channels open and inward sodium and calcium currents initiate the action potential upstroke. Inward current quickly subsides (as sodium channels close), allowing outward currents through potassium channels to create the plateau phase of the action potential. The plateau lasts about 300 msec and is maintained by competition between outward-moving potassium currents and inward-moving calcium currents (phase 2). Progressive closing of calcium channels and openings of potassium channels terminate all inward current and restore the cell to the resting state.

Long-QT syndrome has several subtypes, and the genetic bases for some are known. For example, a mutated sodium channel gene causes slow channel closure in a subtype characterized by prolonged action potential. Another subtype with prolonged action potential contains a mutated potassium channel gene that causes delayed opening of the potassium channels that terminate the action potential. Correction of these defects by gene therapy would return action potential duration to normal and eliminate long-QT.

BIBLIOGRAPHY

Ackermann MJ, Clapham DE: Ion channels: basic science and clinical disease, *N Engl J Med* 336:1575, 1997.

Celermajer DS: Endothelial dysfunction: Does it matter? Is it reversible? *J Am Coll Cardiol* 30:325, 1997.

Dzau VJ, Gibbons GH, Mann M, et al: Future horizons in cardiovascular molecular therapeutics, *Am J Cardiol* 80:33, 1997.

Folkman J: Angiogenic therapy of the human heart, *Circulation* 97:628, 1998.

Shryock JC, Belardinelli L: Adenosine and adenosine receptors in the cardiovascular system: biochemistry, physiology, and pharmacology, *Am J Cardiol* 79:2, 1997.

Yeh ETH: Life and death of the cell, *Hosp Prac* Aug 1998, p 85.

2

Cardiac and Vascular Anatomy and Useful Physiologic Concepts

George J. Taylor
W. Thomas Woods

VASCULAR SYSTEM

The vascular system comprises two circuits, pulmonary and systemic, that normally are in contact only at the level of the heart (Fig. 2-1). The pulmonary circuit is the low pressure system, with normal pulmonary artery systolic pressure at about 30 mm Hg. For this reason, the right ventricle (RV), which is the pulmonary circuit pump, is thin walled. The pulmonary vein, which returns blood to the left side of the heart, is the only vein that carries red, oxygenated blood. The systemic system is the high pressure system, and its pump, the left ventricle (LV), has more muscle mass and is thicker. Long-term elevated pressure in either of these vascular circuits leads to an increase in muscle mass of the ventricle that fills it.

The intestinal-portal circulation is unique because it has two capillary beds (intestinal and liver) in series. Elsewhere, capillary beds empty into veins that transport blood to the right heart. Blood flows through the intestinal capillary bed, to the portal vein, into the liver's capillary bed, and finally to the hepatic vein and right heart. Nutrients and drugs absorbed from the gut are processed by the liver before being circulated to the rest of the body. Disruption of the liver's capillary bed (most commonly by cirrhosis) raises portal venous pressure and hydrostatic pressure in the intestinal capillary bed, driving fluid into the interstitial space and causing ascites. Obstruction of the hepatic vein or the inferior vena cava (Budd-Chiari syndrome) first causes hepatic congestion and then portal hypertension and ascites. Right heart failure may do the same thing.

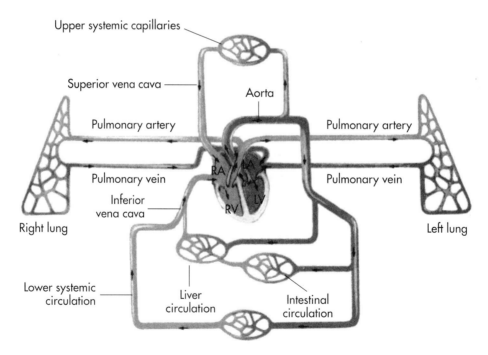

FIG. 2-1

Schematic of the arterial and venous circulations. The pulmonary and systemic circuits are in parallel, meeting at the level of the heart. The intestinal and liver capillary beds are in series, connected by the portal vein.

From Canobbio MM: *Cardiovascular disorders,* St Louis, 1990, Mosby.

Veins empty into atria: the vena cavae into the right atrium (RA) and the pulmonary veins into the left atrium (LA). There are no valves at these entrances to the heart. Both RA and LA pressures are reflected back into the veins throughout the cardiac cycle. For this reason, a catheter pushed out into the pulmonary artery until it "wedges" faces an open, unobstructed conduit through the pulmonary capillary bed and pulmonary veins all the way to the LA. Measuring the pulmonary wedge pressure is the same as measuring LA pressure. Similarly, jugular venous pressure is a measure of RA pressure after correcting for effects of distance and gravity.

Major Arteries and Veins

Figures 2-2 and 2-3 illustrate the largest branches of the arterial and venous systems. Although generally these

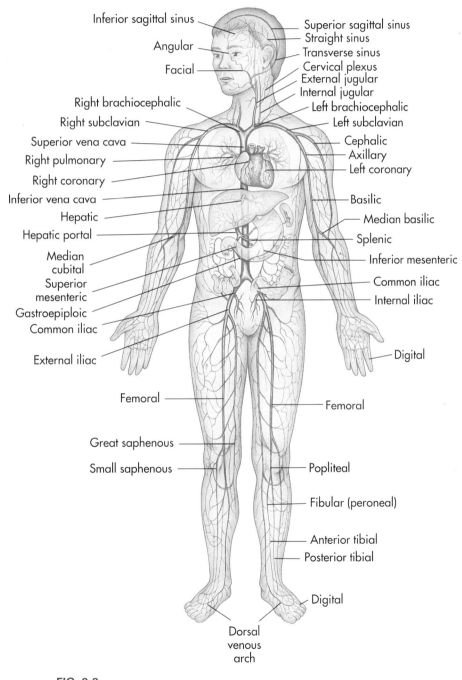

FIG. 2-2
Veins.
From Canobbio MM: *Cardiovascular disorders,* St Louis, 1990, Mosby.

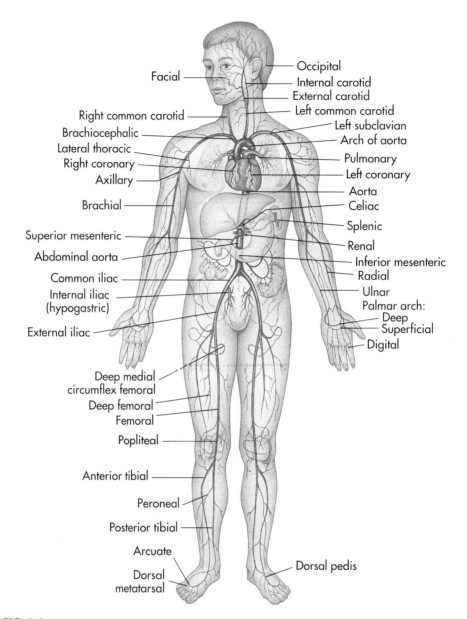

Facial — Occipital
— Internal carotid
— External carotid
Right common carotid — — Left common carotid
Brachiocephalic — — Left subclavian
Lateral thoracic — — Arch of aorta
Right coronary — — Pulmonary
Axillary — — Left coronary
— Aorta
Brachial — — Celiac
— Splenic
Superior mesenteric — — Renal
Abdominal aorta — — Inferior mesenteric
Common iliac — — Radial
Internal iliac — Ulnar
(hypogastric) — Palmar arch:
— Deep
— Superficial
External iliac — — Digital

Deep medial — circumflex femoral
Deep femoral —
Femoral —
Popliteal —
Anterior tibial —
Peroneal —
Posterior tibial —
Arcuate — — Dorsal pedis
Dorsal metatarsal —

FIG. 2-3
Arteries. The brachiocephalic is also called the *innominate.* The major branch of the femoral artery is also called the *superficial femoral.*
From Canobbio MM: *Cardiovascular disorders,* St Louis, 1990, Mosby.

are symmetrical, the origin of the carotid arteries is an exception, with the left coming from the aortic arch and the right from the innominate artery (also called the *brachiocephalic*). The iliac artery divides into three branches, the largest of them referred to as either the *femoral* or *superficial femoral* artery.

One-Way Flow of Blood

Flow is pulsatile, with greater flow during systole than during diastole. The force driving blood forward and through the capillary beds is the pressure gradient, or the difference between arterial and venous pressures. (The term *gradient* is used frequently to discuss the hydraulics of the circulation; blood flows "downhill" from regions of high pressure to those with lower pressure.) Only a small pressure drop (or gradient) occurs between the venous system and the right atrium, so forward flow depends on one-way venous valves (Fig. 2-4). Injury to venous valves, which is a potential consequence of severe or untreated deep venous thrombosis (DVT), leads to chronic venous insufficiency characterized by edema and skin ulcers in the region drained by the vein.

I emphasize the regional character of venous and arterial disease. Heart failure also may cause edema, but it is bilat-

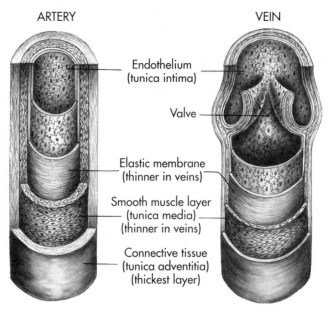

FIG. 2-4
Structure of arteries and veins.
From Canobbio MM: *Cardiovascular disorders,* St Louis, 1990, Mosby.

eral and symmetrical. Venous disease is more often unilateral and asymmetrical, that is, regional.

Veins

Veins, which are thin walled and distensible, are capacitance vessels and influence preload. They may be called "capacitance" vessels, because dilation and venous pooling increase the capacity of the venous reservoir, essentially removing volume from the central circulation. As an example, nitroglycerine causes venodilation. Peripheral pooling lowers blood return to the heart, and this lowered "preload" reduces cardiac work. With less work, heart muscle demands less oxygen, relieving angina. In similar fashion, tourniquets on legs and arms reduce blood return to the heart and provide some relief from pulmonary congestion. This old-fashioned treatment for pulmonary edema has been replaced by more effective preload-reducing agents (e.g., intravenous nitrates and powerful diuretics).

Arteries

Arteries are thick walled and stiffer than veins. They are not capacitance vessels, and arterial volume varies less than venous volume. When arteries dilate, there is usually an abrupt fall in blood pressure and organ perfusion. Arteries stiffen with age; *hardening of the arteries* is an accurate term. This further reduction in compliance (Box 2-1) makes arteries even more dependent on adequate filling (volume) to maintain pressure and flow. Because of increased stiffness (decreased compliance), arterial pressure normally increases with age. Therapeu-

tic reduction of blood pressure to levels appropriate for a 40-year-old may cause postural hypotension in a 70-year-old.

Arterial stiffness increases with chronic pressure overload as well. Hypertension leads to an increase in arterial thickness. Pulmonary hypertension, when prolonged, also causes structural changes in pulmonary arteries. These changes in arterial walls eventually reach a point of irreversibility.

Vascular Tone and Blood Pressure

Arterial pressure is determined by a number of balancing factors, including compliance of the arterial wall just discussed. The renin-angiotensin system has a role, as angiotensin II has a direct vasoconstrictor effect. The effects of the autonomic nervous system on arterial muscle tone are summarized in Table 2-1. Pressure also is influenced by blood flow, or cardiac output, the hydraulic equivalent of Ohm's law (Box 2-2). Systemic blood pressure is the final result of the balance among these competing vasoconstrictor and vasodilator stimuli, vascular volume, cardiac output, and arterial compliance.

Local factors play a minor role in regulating peripheral resistance but are influential in governing arterial flow to the brain and the heart. These beds are said to be "autoregulated." Vasodilators and vasoconstrictors produced by endothelial cells have been the subject of intense study over the past decade (see Chapter 13 for a discussion of endothelial dysfunction and coronary artery disease).

BOX 2-1
COMPLIANCE

Definition: *Compliance* refers to the distensibility of any fluid- or air-containing structure (blood vessel, cardiac chamber, airway, loop of bowel, bile duct, and the like). Increased compliance indicates more give in the vessel wall as volume is added. That is, *volume* increases with little change in *pressure*. The opposite of *compliant* is *stiff*.

Compliance Curves: The relation of pressure and volume defines the compliance of a vessel. Consider the pressure-volume curves of two different blood vessels, A and B:

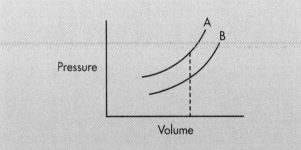

Pressure increases as volume is added to each of the above vessels. The pressure is higher at a given volume in vessel A; it is less compliant than vessel B (vessel A is stiffer). A shift of the pressure-volume curve to the left indicates a loss of compliance.

BOX 2-2
OHM'S LAW APPLIED TO HYDRAULIC SYSTEMS

Resistance = (Difference in pressure across a vascular bed) / (Flow)

Thus, *Systemic vascular resistance (SVR):*

SVR = Mean arterial pressure - Mean right atrial pressure / Cardiac output

And, *Pulmonary arteriolar resistance (PAR):*

PAR = Mean pulmonary artery (PA) pressure - Mean left atrial pressure / Cardiac output

Total pulmonary resistance = Mean PA pressure / Cardiac output

In practice, the pulmonary capillary wedge pressure is substituted for left atrial pressure. Mean right atrial pressure is quite low compared with arterial pressure, and usually it is ignored when calculating SVR.

The implications of the formula are interesting. If peripheral vascular resistance is lowered by 20% and cardiac output increases 20%, blood pressure does not change. This is the rationale for afterload reduction therapy using vasodilators in patients with borderline low blood pressure.

THE HEART
Cardiac Chambers
Atria

Blood entering the heart first reaches the atria—oxygenated blood from the lungs to the left atrium and desaturated blood from the periphery to the right atrium. The atria fill during ventricular systole; when the ventricles have emptied, a reservoir of blood is ready to recharge them. Ventricular pressure falls below atrial pressure and the atrioventricular (AV) valves open (Fig. 2-5). During the first part of diastole there is rapid, "passive" filling of the ventricles. At the end of diastole the atria contract, "actively" providing the final 10% to 20% increment of ventricular filling, which often is referred to as the "atrial kick."

The right atrium is anterior to the left atrium. The left atrium is more posterior and is adjacent to the esophagus. The transesophageal echocardiogram provides a good view of the atria, the left atrial appendage, and mitral valve.

Ventricles

The left ventricle (LV) is thicker than the right (RV). It works against a much higher pressure load; its "afterload" is higher. Weight lifting builds muscle mass. What is true for the weight lifter's arms is true for heart muscle as well. As aortic pressure is much higher than pulmonary artery pressure, the LV works harder and is thicker than the RV. Raising afterload increases the muscle mass of either of the ventricles, and lowering it allows a reduction in muscle mass.

The labels *right* and *left* ventricle do not describe the position of the heart in the chest. Actually, the RV is positioned in front of (anterior to) the LV, and the plane of the interventricular septum is almost parallel to the

Table 2-1	*Effects of the Autonomic Nervous System on the Heart and Peripheral Circulation*

	Agonist(+)/Antagonist(-)	Action
SYMPATHETIC NERVOUS SYSTEM	(+)Epinephrine (E), norepi- nephrine (NE), and dobuta- mine	General: raises blood pressure, heart rate, and contractility (the fight-or-flight response)
Alpha$_1$ receptor	(+) E and NE (-) Prazosin	Vasoconstriction (increasing blood pressure), intestinal relaxation, pupillary dilation
Alpha$_2$ receptor	(+) Clonidine (-) Yohimbine	Blocks the presynaptic release of NE from adrenergic (sympathetic) nerves; has a sympathetic blocking action in the brainstem.
Beta$_1$ receptor	(+) E and NE (-) Metoprolol and the like (see Chapter 13)	Cardiac stimulation (increase in heart rate and contractility) and lipolysis
Beta$_2$ receptor	(+) E > NE (-)"Nonselective" beta- blockers	Vasodilation, bronchodilation
Dopamine$_1$ receptor	(+) Dopamine (-)Phenothiazines and thio- xanthenes	Vasodilation of renal, coronary, and cerebral vascular beds
Dopamine$_2$ receptor	(+) Dopamine (-) Haloperidol	Inhibits transmission in the sympathetic ganglia and NE release from sympathetic nerve endings
PARASYMPATHETIC NERVOUS SYSTEM	(+)Acetylcholine (ACh), bethanechol, and cholinesterase inhibitors (physostigmine, edropho- nium, neostigmine, some insecticides)

(-)Atropine, scopolamine | *Cardiac effects* (through the vagus nerve): ACh slows the heart rate and slows conduction through the atrioventricular node. There are few cholinergic fibers to the ventricular myocardium or peripheral blood vessels (thus little direct regulation of contractility or peripheral vascular resistance). *Noncardiac effects:* Increased gastrointestinal and genitourinary motility and relaxed sphincters; bronchoconstriction and increased bronchial secretions |

chest wall. This is readily demonstrated by an echocardiogram, in which the RV is the chamber closest to the chest wall and transducer (see Chapter 8). The RV impulse, when palpable, is felt along the left parasternal border, and the RV is the first chamber punctured with an intracardiac injection.

Normally, the interventricular septum acts as a part of the LV. The septum has to "choose sides," since it is anatomically a part of both ventricles. It chooses the side that is working hardest, normally the LV. On the echocardiogram (or with other imaging studies that show the heart in motion), the septum moves toward the posterior wall of the LV during systole and away from the free wall of the RV. Conditions that produce RV overload or failure may lead to a reversal of this normal pattern, with the septum moving toward the RV and away from the LV during systole. On the echocardiogram, this "paradoxical septal motion" is one sign of RV volume overload (e.g., it is seen with atrial septal defect).

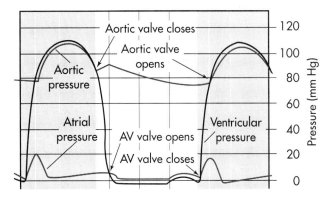

FIG. 2-5
Events of the cardiac cycle, with pressure measurements from the aorta, left ventricle (LV), and left atrium (LA). The valves are passive structures, working like swinging doors in response to changes in chamber pressures. At the end of ventricular systole, LV pressure falls below LA pressure, and the AV (mitral) valve swings open. Rapid ventricular filling begins. At the end of diastole, a bump occurs in atrial and ventricular pressure as a result of atrial contraction. The ventricle then contracts, and when LV pressure rises above LA pressure, the mitral valve is pushed to the closed position. As soon as LV pressure exceeds aortic pressure, the aortic valve opens.

Cardiac Output and Ventricular Function

Ultimately, what the body wants from the heart is blood flow. The heart is just a pump. Output is the product of heart rate and the volume ejected from the LV with each stroke, or heartbeat. The units of measurement are fairly simple (Box 2-3). Three things influence ventricular stroke volume: preload, afterload, and contractility.

Preload. This is the "load," or volume, in the ventricle *before* it contracts. It is, more precisely, the length of each muscle fiber before contraction; think of it as the load that "stretches" the fiber before contraction. A direct relation exists between muscle fiber length and the strength of contraction. When a strip of muscle is stimulated, it twitches and generates tension that can be measured. Within physiologic limits (i.e., the muscle is not overstretched to the point of injury), increasing the resting length produces a stronger contraction (Fig. 2-6). A century ago, E. H. Starling showed in intact animals that this is as true for the working heart as it is for pieces of skeletal muscle. In the intact heart, muscle fiber length is directly related to ventricular volume. Thus increased ventricular filling during diastole is the same as increased preload and leads to more forceful contraction (and increased stroke volume) when the ventricle is stimulated. That is why fluid retention is one of the basic compensatory mechanisms in heart failure. Increased vascular volume means increased venous return to both ventricles, an increase in ventricular diastolic volume. This increase in preload produces higher stroke volume.

BOX 2-3
DETERMINANTS OF CARDIAC OUTPUT

Cardiac output (ml/min) = Heart rate (beats/min)
x Stroke volume (ml/beat)

Stroke volume is augmented (+) or depressed (-) by three factors:
1. (+) Preload—the ventricular load or volume at the end of diastole (higher preload augments stroke volume)
2. (-) Afterload—the load or resistance against which the ventricle empties during systole (higher afterload impedes the ventricle's ability to empty, lowering stroke volume)
3. (+) Contractility—the basic state of ventricular muscle (its innate ability to contract independent of loading conditions; increased contractility results in greater ventricular emptying and greater stroke volume)

Preload thus describes the state of the ventricle at the end of diastole, before ventricular stimulation and contraction.

When considering ventricular "function," it is natural to think primarily of the contractile process. There often is confusion about *diastolic function* and *ventricular compliance.* These terms relate to how easily the ventricle fills during diastole, when it is relaxed, and have nothing to do with ventricular contraction. However, diastolic properties are closely related to stroke volume (Fig. 2-6). A compliant ventricle fills easily, allowing adequate preloading of the ventricle (stretching of muscle fibers) to generate stroke volume. A stiff ventricle may not accommodate an adequate blood volume, so stroke volume suffers. Abnormal stiffness, or diastolic dysfunction, may result from hypertrophy, infiltrative cardiomyopathy, or ischemia.

Think again about the contribution of atrial kick. Contraction of the atria at the end of diastole provides the last increment of ventricular filling, increasing preload and stroke volume (Fig. 2-7). When atrial contraction is lost, as with atrial fibrillation or ventricular pacing, preload, stroke volume, and cardiac output fall. For a person with normal diastolic function, loss of atrial contraction causes a 10% to 15% drop in cardiac output. On the other hand, a patient with diastolic dysfunction relies more on atrial contraction to fill the ventricle. Reduced compliance, or "give," makes the stiff ventricle resistant to passive filling during diastole, and atrial contraction provides a larger than normal proportion of filling. Loss of the atrial kick may cause cardiac output to fall more than 25%. Patients with stiff ventri-

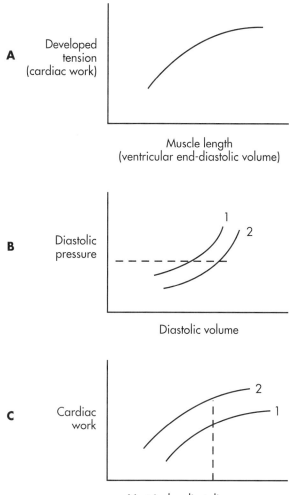

A

Developed tension (cardiac work)

Muscle length (ventricular end-diastolic volume)

B

Diastolic pressure

Diastolic volume

C

Cardiac work

Ventricular diastolic pressure

FIG. 2-6

A, The basis for Starling's law of the heart. Increased resting muscle length *before* stimulation leads to increased strength of contraction and developed tension once the muscle is stimulated. In the intact heart, ventricular volume may be substituted for muscle fiber length, and a measure of cardiac work for developed tension. (Rough measures of cardiac work would include ventricular stroke volume, cardiac output, and ejection fraction.) **B,** Influence of ventricular compliance on diastolic volume. Compliance of the ventricle during diastole influences ventricular filling. At a given ventricular diastolic pressure, patient 1 has a lower ventricular volume (and therefore muscle fiber length) than patient 2. Patient 1 has a stiffer, less compliant ventricle. **C,** Ventricular function curve, substituting diastolic pressure for volume. In practice, it is easier to measure ventricular diastolic pressure than volume. As the two are roughly proportional, pressure is substituted for volume on the ventricular function curve. Altered diastolic compliance may cause an apparent shift in the curve. Patient 1 appears to have worse ventricular function than patient 2, and that would be the case if diastolic compliance is the same for both. However, if patient 1 has a stiffer ventricle (as in **B**), end-diastolic volume may be lower than it is for patient 2. In this case, at equal ventricular volumes, the two could have identical systolic function and therefore identical ventricular function curves. This illustrates the potential problem of substituting diastolic pressure for diastolic volume (or fiber length).

cles are said to be "preload dependent," and are especially susceptible to volume depletion or loss of atrial contraction. It explains why a patient with aortic valve stenosis and LV hypertrophy has a fall in blood pressure with the development of atrial fibrillation.

Afterload. This is the load the ventricle works against when it contracts during systole. Aortic or pulmonic valve stenosis impedes flow and raises afterload, and both induce ventricular hypertrophy. In the absence of outflow tract obstruction, blood pressure is a rough approximation of afterload, but this can be an oversimplification. Afterload may be reduced with no apparent change in blood pressure. Ohm's law shows why a vasodilator drug that lowers resistance by 20% but that allows cardiac output (flow) to increase by 20% causes no change in blood pressure. On the ventricular function curve, a reduction in afterload produces a shift up and to the left (Fig. 2-8).

Hypertrophy, Wall Tension, and Myocardial Oxygen Demand. The heart responds to increased afterload with an increase in contractility and, eventually, with hypertrophy. Myocardial oxygen demand (MVO_2) is proportional to wall tension, and tension is determined by the interplay of ventricular pressure and size as described by Laplace's law (Box 2-4). A dilated ventricle thus has higher wall tension than a smaller one and requires more oxygen. (A dilated aorta, loop of bowel, pulmonary bleb, or uterus all have increased wall tension and are thus more prone to rupture; Laplace's law applies to many areas of medicine.)

Contractility. The third determinant of stroke volume is defined as an increase in the force of contraction when both preload and afterload are constant (see Fig. 2-4). Another name for contractility is the *inotropic state.* At the cellular level, the force of contraction is increased by enhanced movement of calcium ions across the cell membrane through calcium channels. Calcium ions interact with the contractile proteins. Increased calcium influx upon excitation leads to greater contractility (as with digitalis or catecholamines), and reduced calcium influx depresses contractility (as with the calcium channel blockers, verapamil, and beta-adrenergic blockers).

On the ventricular function curve, an increase in contractility appears as an increase in stroke volume for a given preload (see Fig. 2-8).

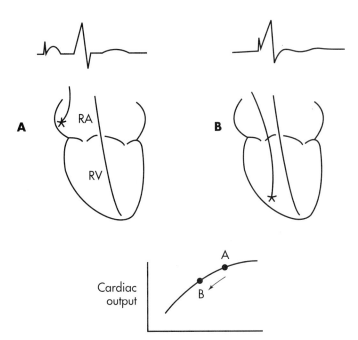

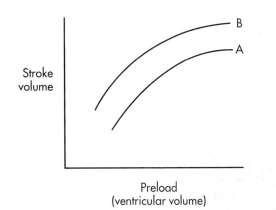

Ventricular end-diastolic pressure

FIG. 2-7
This simple study is often repeated in the cardiac catheterization laboratory. The heart is paced at a rate just above its baseline and cardiac output is measured. **A,** When the pacemaker is in the right atrium *(RA),* atrial contraction is preserved (a P wave follows the pacer spike). **B,** Pacing from the right ventricle *(RV)* leads to a loss of the P wave and atrial contraction. Ventricular diastolic pressure and volume decline—a drop in preload—and cardiac output falls.

Preload
(ventricular volume)

FIG. 2-8
Effects of contractility and afterload. Increased contractility shifts the curve up and to the left, from *A* to *B,* so ventricular work (e.g., stroke volume) is higher at a given preload. Lowering afterload has the same effect.

Ejection Fraction. Another common measure of ventricular function is ejection fraction (EF), or that portion of blood ejected from the ventricle during systole. Thus, if the LV contains 150 ml at the end of diastole and 50 ml at the end of systole, the LVEF is 67%

and the stroke volume is 100 ml. It can be calculated by measuring the volume of the LV at end-diastole and end-systole using either the LV angiogram or echocardiogram. It also can be measured with radionuclide techniques, measuring counts at end-diastole and systole (see Chapter 9). However, this method would not provide ventricular volumes, including stroke volume.

EF is a measure of muscle shortening. Contractility increases EF, but it is important to recognize that EF is not a measure of just contractility. Ventricular loading conditions also have an effect on LV emptying and shortening; increased afterload depresses LVEF, and increased preload raises it (see Fig. 2-8). Stroke volume and EF cannot be equated. A dilated LV with a diastolic volume of 210 ml and ejection fraction of 33% has a stroke volume of 70 ml. So does a smaller ventricle of 140 ml and EF of 50%.

Heart Valves

The atrioventricular valves are the tricuspid in the right side and mitral in the left (Fig. 2-9). These valves close at the beginning of ventricular systole. The mitral valve must withstand the largest pressure load of all the

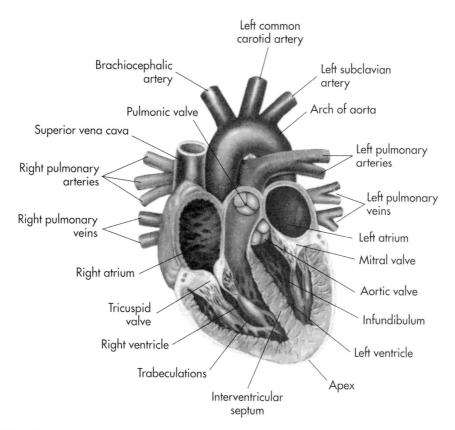

FIG. 2-9
Frontal section of the heart. In this typical schematic, it appears that the right ventricle is on the right, the left on the left, and that we are looking at the interventricular septum on-end. However, that is not the position of the heart in the chest. Instead it is rotated to the patient's left ("clockwise" when viewed from the patient's feet), so the right ventricle is anterior to the left ventricle, the left atrium is the most posterior structure, and the plane of the interventricular septum is almost parallel to the chest wall.

heart valves, since it remains closed against LV systolic pressure. Its tissue leaflets are supported by cords that attach along the free edges of the leaflets and then to the papillary muscles, which are a part of the ventricular wall. When ventricular pressure rises and the valve closes, contraction of the papillary muscles tethers the valve leaflets. Dysfunction of the papillary muscles, which may occur with ischemic injury, leads to incompetence of the valve and mitral regurgitation (see Chapter 18). The regurgitant jet of blood may not be perpendicular to the plane of the valve ring or go through the center of the valve. Instead, one leaflet or the other prolapses back into the atrium, and the opposite leaflet works as a bevel. If the posterior leaflet prolapses, then the jet is aimed anteriorly at the interventricular septum. When the anterior leaflet prolapses, the jet aims at the posterolateral wall. The location and direction of radiation of the murmur caused by papillary muscle dysfunction vary with the direction of the regurgitant jet (Fig. 2-10).

Contraction of the papillary muscles contributes to LV ejection. An advantage of mitral valve repair over re-placement is continued papillary muscle contraction. When repair is possible, overall LV function, measured as the LV ejection fraction, is better after surgery.

One of the causes of mitral regurgitation is dilation of the LV. Some enlargement of the valve ring may contribute to the leak, but distortion of normal papillary muscle geometry plays a role as well.

The aortic and pulmonic valves are tricuspid and "semilunar." There is no external support structure. Although the aortic valve does not have as high a pressure load as the mitral valve, it experiences the highest flow velocity, and therefore turbulence, of the four valves.

Note the proximity of the aortic and mitral valves (Fig. 2-9). When open, the anterior leaflet of the mitral valve lies in the aortic outflow tract. Outflow tract obstruction caused by hypertrophic subaortic stenosis causes an increase in flow velocity in the outflow tract. This creates suction, the Venturi effect, that pulls the anterior leaflet of the mitral valve and causes mitral regurgitation.

Valves, Chamber Size, and Overload. In the evaluation of a patient with valvular disease, it helps to focus on which cardiac chamber is primarily affected and to

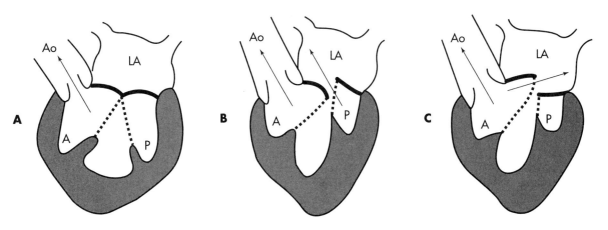

FIG. 2-10
Mitral regurgitation (MR) and orientation of the regurgitant jet during ventricular systole. The dashed lines represent the papillary muscles and cordae tendineae. **A,** No MR; all flow from the LV during systole is through the aortic valve. **B,** Dysfunction of the posterolateral mitral leaflet's support; the leaflet prolapses back into the left atrium (LA) and works as a baffle sending the jet medially. **C,** The jet is oriented laterally when the medial leaflet prolapses. Note how the direction of the regurgitant jet may affect the location of the murmur.

Table 2-2	*Effect of Common Valvular Lesions on Cardiac Chambers*

Valvular Lesion	Effect
Mitral stenosis (MS)	Left atrial (LA) dilation; in response to pressure overload, atria dilate rather than hypertrophy. The valve "protects" the left ventricle (LV), so the LV is small and normal. Back pressure leads to pulmonary congestion.
Mitral regurgitation (MR)	LA dilation is the first change. If the regurgitant volume is large, the LV must handle this extra volume, and it dilates. With no pressure overload, LV thickness is normal. Failure of the LV leads to pulmonary congestion.
Aortic stenosis (AS)	LV pressure overload causes concentric hypertrophy (LVH). LV chamber size remains normal. Persistently high LV diastolic pressure caused by LVH may lead to LA dilation, but not to the extent seen with mitral regurgitation. Back pressure leads to pulmonary congestion.
Aortic regurgitation (AR)	Volume overload of the LV that is dilated but not thickened. Note that overall LV muscle mass is increased. Failure of the LV leads to pulmonary congestion.
Tricuspid regurgitation (TR)	Similar to MR, but on the right side. Initially there is RA dilation followed by RV dilation. Eventual RV failure leads to systemic congestion (peripheral edema, distended neck veins).
Pulmonic stenosis (PS)	Similar to AS, but on the right side. Initially there is RVH, then RA dilation and systemic congestion

consider the nature of the overload (Table 2-2). It is simple and intuitive, but I am surprised at how often doctors fail to consider basic physiology. For example, an echocardiogram report indicates "mitral regurgitation (MR)." The key issue is whether it is severe or mild, and that is where thinking about chamber size comes in. It is obvious from the anatomy that the first chamber affected is the left atrium (see *LA*, Fig. 2-10). If MR is chronic, volume overload causes dilation of the LA. With extra volume back and forth across the valve, the

LV is volume overloaded as well. LA and LV chamber size are the first things to look for on the echo report; if normal, the MR must be mild.

Chamber size and the nature of the load (pressure vs. volume overload) produce key physical findings as well (see Chapter 4), including gallops, changes in the jugular venous and peripheral arterial pulses, and abnormalities of the apical impulse. Hearing a murmur may indicate that a valve is not working properly, but these other physical findings indicate chamber size and function, reflecting the severity of the problem. Their detection and correct interpretation separate the sophisticated examiner from the novice.

Cardiac Nervous System
Innervation of the Heart

The autonomic nervous system regulates cardiac function, matching heart rate and contractility to the body's needs (see Table 2-1). The autonomic system has two divisions—sympathetic and parasympathetic. Sympathetic (also known as *adrenergic*) nerve signals traveling to the heart exit the spine and terminate in the right and left stellate ganglia. Postganglionic fibers leave the ganglia, enter the heart, and, when stimulated, release the neurotransmitter, norepinephrine. Norepinephrine has a number of effects: an increase in the rate of depolarization of the sinoatrial (SA) node leading to increased heart rate, shortened atrioventricular (AV) nodal conduction time and refractoriness, increased ventricular contractility, and shortened refractoriness of ventricular myocardium. (The *refractory period* is the time after depolarization that the tissue is refractory to repeat stimulation.)

The sympathetic system receptors have partitioned functions. Alpha-adrenergic receptors cause peripheral vasoconstriction and bronchodilation with relatively little cardiac effect (see Table 2-1). The beta-adrenergic receptors have direct cardiac effects and cause peripheral vasodilation and bronchodilation. The beta receptors are further partitioned: beta$_1$ receptors are cardiospecific and have less effect on the lung and peripheral vasculature, and beta$_2$ receptors have less cardiac effect and are bronchodilators and peripheral vasodilators.

The parasympathetic receptors (muscarinic in cardiac cells, cholinergic in ganglia) respond to stimulation of the vagus nerve, which releases acetylcholine (ACh). Acetylcholine slows the rate of spontaneous depolarization of the SA node pacemaker cells and therefore slows heart rate. It also causes prolongation of AV nodal conduction time and refractoriness. There are fewer parasympathetic than sympathetic nerve endings in the ventricular myocardium, although vagal stimulation causes a small decrease in contractility and prolongation of refractoriness. Similarly, there is too little parasympathetic innervation of arteries to exert a major effect on peripheral vascular resistance and blood pressure.

The parasympathetic and adrenergic systems are constantly discharging. They balance each other. A need for increased cardiac output leads to both increased sympathetic and decreased vagal discharge; the balance shifts toward increased heart rate and contractility. The vagal system has a faster response time than the sympathetic nerves. Rapid onset and termination of response to vagal impulses allows a beat-to-beat variation in heart rate and AV node conduction. For this reason, sinus arrhythmia, the variation of cardiac cycle length with respiration, is largely the result of periodic vagal bursting.

There is regional variation in the density of innervation. The SA and AV nodes have a rich supply of postganglionic sympathetic and parasympathetic fibers. The right stellate ganglion (the origin of sympathetic fibers) and right vagal nerve send fibers mainly to the SA node, and the left-sided sympathetic and vagal fibers have greater input to the AV node, although some crossover occurs with each. Thus right stellate ganglion stimulation causes sinus tachycardia, with little effect on AV nodal conduction.

Heterogeneity of innervation also exists at the level of the ventricle. For example, the ventricular content of norepinephrine is higher at the base of the heart than at the apex. This is clinically relevant, since heterogeneity of repolarization (and refractoriness) contributes to reentry and the genesis of arrhythmias (see Chapters 25 and 26). In addition, afferent vagal activity is greatest in the posterior region of the left ventricle, which may explain the high vagal tone observed with inferior myocardial infarction. (*Afferent* nerves conduct impulses to the central nervous system, and *efferent* nerves conduct impulses from the central nervous system to end-organs.)

Cardiac pain sensation is transmitted through cardiac afferent nerves that travel in both the vagus and sympathetic nerves. Autonomic neuropathy, a common problem for patients with diabetes, may include dysfunction of these sensory tracts and lead to painless, or silent, ischemia. Prolonged ischemia also can injure sensory nerves, cause "nociceptive dysfunction," and set the stage for silent ischemia, or reinfarction after reperfusion therapy for myocardial infarction (see Chapters 15 and 16).

Cardiac Nerves

The sinoatrial node is located at the junction of the right atrium and superior vena cava (Fig. 2-11). It is cigar shaped, measuring 15 mm by 3 mm. There is rich sympathetic and parasympathetic innervation, and its acetylcholine content is much higher than that of surrounding atrial myocardium. A variety of specialized cells include impulse-forming cells, the actual pacemaker, and transitional cells that are the functional pathway for the transmission of the impulse to the atrial myocardium. The pacemaker cells depolarize spontaneously until reaching an excitatory threshold, at which time the pacemaker discharges. The rate of spontaneous depolarization determines heart rate.

Parasympathetic discharge slows the rate of spontaneous depolarization, slowing the heart rate. It also slows conduction within the node and at times may lead to SA exit block. An increase in background sympathetic tone increases the discharge rate of the SA node.

There are no identifiable nerve tracts in the body of the atria connecting the SA and AV nodes. Although preferred routes of impulse transmission have been described, I think of atrial activation as a broad wave of depolarization moving through the two chambers simultaneously.

The AV node lies just below the right atrial endocardium, directly above the insertion of the septal leaflet of the tricuspid valve. To record electrical activity in the region of the AV node, a catheter with two electrodes is positioned across the tricuspid valve.

A fibrous barrier insulates the atria from the ventricles. Current passing through the atria is funneled into the ventricles through the AV node. The critical function of the AV node is to slow passage of this current to the ventricles until contraction of the atria has occurred. Mechanical activity (contraction) is much slower than electrical activity. Conduction time through the AV node is slowed by vagal activation and accelerated by sympathetic discharge. Beta-adrenergic blockers, some calcium channel blockers (verapamil and diltiazem), and digitalis also slow AV node conduction.

Cells in the lower portion of the AV node, at its junction with the bundle of His, exhibit spontaneous depolarization, much like cells of the SA node. Their rate of depolarization is slower than the SA rate. Because of its

more rapid spontaneous discharge rate, the SA node is the primary pacemaker. If it fails, the AV node can take over, with a baseline heart rate near 45 beats per minute. This rate may increase with atropine, which blocks the Ach receptor, or with beta-adrenergic stimulation.

Unlike conduction through the atria, infranodal conduction to the two ventricles occurs through well-defined cardiac bundles (see Fig. 2-11). Discharge of the bundle of His, immediately below the AV node, produces measurable current. The AV node itself does not. The bundle of His electrogram is recorded using a bipolar catheter positioned across the tricuspid valve and therefore next to the AV node. The distance between the beginning of the P wave and the bundle of His spike (the A-H interval; see Chapter 27) gives an estimate of conduction time through the AV node, whereas the time between the His spike and the beginning of the QRS (H-V interval) is the conduction time below the bundle of His. The His spike thus partitions the PR interval of the electrocardiogram into AV nodal and infranodal conduction times.

The conduction system trifurcates below the bundle of His. The right bundle branch and the left anterior fascicle of the left bundle branch lie close to each other in the interventricular septum. This explains the common association of right bundle branch block and left anterior fascicular block. Each of these fascicles is a thin and relatively fragile structure. For this reason, left anterior fascicular block is much more common than posterior fascicular block. The right bundle branch seems the most fragile of the infranodal trunks, the weakest link in the chain. For this reason, aberrant conduction of a beat that originates in the atrium often has a right bundle branch block pattern. For example, an atrial tachy-

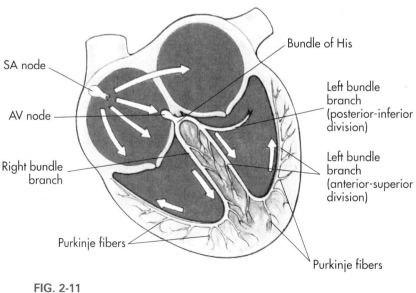

FIG. 2-11
Cardiac conduction.

From Canobbio MM: *Cardiovascular disorders,* St Louis, 1990, Mosby.

arrhythmia may be fast enough to stress the infranodal conduction system. The right bundle is typically the first to go, and the aberrantly conducted beats have a right bundle branch block pattern on the electrocardiogram. The bundle branches have terminal connections with *Purkinje fibers,* relatively large cardiac cells that form interweaving networks on the endocardial surfaces of both ventricles. They have branches that penetrate the inner third of the myocardium. These fibers appear to be more resistant to ischemic injury than myocardial tissue.

Distal to the Purkinje cells the wave of depolarization moves directly from cell to cell. The membranes of adjacent cells have junctions called *intercalated discs,* which have multiple functions. One is strong cell-to-cell adhesion that allows the transfer of mechanical energy during contraction. Another is electrical conduction. The "gap junction" within the intercalated disc is a bridge that provides low resistance electrical coupling between cells. This connection allows the multicellular heart to function as a unified and interconnected electrical unit. Even in the absence of nerve fibers, movement of the "wave of depolarization" through myocardium is an orderly process. For example, conduction velocity is faster and resistance is lower along the long axis of the fiber than it is across its transverse axis. The result is the organization of the sequence of activation of the two ventricles so that there is optimal mechanical efficiency.

Coronary Arteries

At a rate of 70 beats per minute, the heart contracts more than 100,000 times each day. It pumps roughly a box car load of blood each day, and it never rests. This huge mechanical load requires an especially good fuel and oxygen supply. About 20% of the cardiac output is routed to the myocardium through the large epicardial coronary arteries (Fig. 2-12).

These arteries are the first branches of the aorta, and the two coronary ostia lie in the cusps (or sinuses of Valsalva) of two of the three aortic valve leaflets. There are three major coronary branches, two of which originate from the left main coronary artery (LMCA). The three branches divide the ventricular myocardium into three vascular regions.

The anterior wall of the LV is supplied by the left anterior descending (LAD) artery. This vessel runs along the interventricular groove, over the interventricular septum separating the RV and LV. It sends perforating branches into the septum and diagonal branches across the anterior wall of the LV. It reaches the LV apex, often wrapping around it. In fact, this is one way to identify the LAD on an angiogram: find the vessel that reaches the apex and work back.

Two arteries encircle the heart in the atrioventricular groove. On the left side, the circumflex artery branches off the LMCA. It sends branches to the lateral wall of the LV and usually terminates before reaching the base of the heart. The right coronary artery (RCA) originates from the right coronary cusp and encircles the heart in the AV groove on the right side. Branches from the midvessel supply the RV. This artery continues in the AV groove to the base of the heart. The largest terminal branch leaves the AV groove and travels along the base of the heart in the interventricular groove, the posterior descending artery (PDA). Branches of the PDA supply the inferior wall of the LV and the lower portion of the interventricular septum. A small branch of the right coronary artery, just at the origin of the PDA, supplies the AV node. This is one reason that AV nodal block is

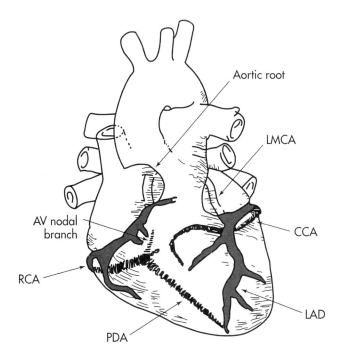

FIG. 2-12
Coronary artery anatomy. *LMCA,* Left main coronary artery; *LAD,* left anterior descending; *CCA,* circumflex coronary artery; *RCA,* right coronary artery; *PDA,* posterior descending artery. The CCA and RCA encircle the heart in the atrioventricular groove, the CCA on the left side and the RCA on the right. Branches of the CCA (marginal branches) provide flow to the lateral wall, and the major branch of the RCA, the PDA, supplies the inferior wall. The LAD and PDA encircle the heart along its long axis in the interventricular groove. The interventricular groove also defines the edges of the interventricular septum. Thus the LAD is positioned on the anterior edge of the interventricular septum, and the PDA is along its inferior edge. Both the LAD and PDA supply septal perforating branches. Note that the dominant right coronary artery is the origin of the branch to the atrioventricular node (AV node).

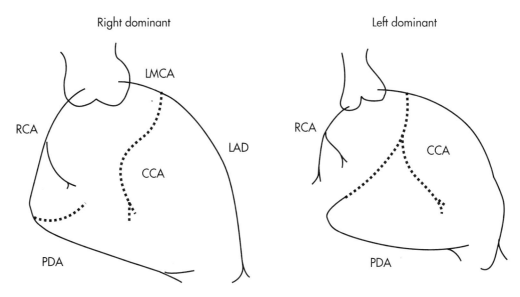

Right dominant

Left dominant

FIG. 2-13
Right and left dominant coronary circulations. Right dominance is more common (85% of patients); in this case the right coronary artery *(RCA)* reaches the base of the atrioventricular groove and is the origin of the PDA and the artery to the AV node (not shown in this diagram; see Fig. 2-12). The left dominant circulation has the circumflex coronary artery *(CCA)* continue in the AV groove to the base of the heart, where it is the origin of the PDA and artery to the AV node.

common with inferior myocardial infarction. Right ventricular failure also may be a consequence of occlusion of the RCA.

There is a fair amount of biologic variation in coronary anatomy. The left dominant circulation is a common variation. The *dominance* of the circulation is defined as the vessel that supplies the PDA (inferior wall circulation). For 85% of people, that is the RCA, and they are said to have right dominant coronary circulations. The other 15% who are left dominant have a small RCA that does not reach the base of the heart. Instead they have a large circumflex artery that continues in the AV groove to the base and is the source of the PDA (Fig. 2-13). The dominant vessel also is the origin of the artery to the AV node.

Intramyocardial Vessels

The coronary arteries are on the epicardial surface of the heart and send perforating branches through the ventricular muscle, ending in a subendocardial plexus of vessels. The subendocardial region is farthest from the epicardial arterial supply source. A large pressure drop occurs across the intramyocardial arterial branches and arterioles; for this reason they are called *resistance vessels,* whereas the epicardial trunks are referred to as *capacitance,* or *conductance, vessels.* The arterioles terminate in a dense network of capillaries, as many as 4000/mm^2. Capillary density is reduced with left ventricular hypertrophy.

Animal studies have shown a subendocardial to subepicardial flow ratio of slightly above 1.0 in the absence of coronary stenosis. This ratio falls to less than 0.4 when a coronary artery stenosis reduces flow by 60%. Thus the subendocardial region is the first to suffer if a mismatch occurs between myocardial oxygen supply and demand (producing characteristic depression of the ST segment on the electrocardiogram; see Chapter 5).

Other important factors influence the distribution of coronary flow. During ventricular systole, contracting muscle compresses the perforating branches and the subendocardial plexus, limiting flow. Because of this throttling effect, most coronary flow takes place during diastole. Pressure overload conditions, such as aortic stenosis or hypertension, lead to higher systolic intraventricular pressures, augmenting the throttling effect. Tachycardia also leads to reduced coronary flow. Rapid heart rate shortens diastole more than systole, so the proportion of time spent in diastole falls and coronary blood flow drops. Increased heart rate generates increasing calcium influx into heart muscle cells, raising contractility. This has a couple of consequences that may induce ischemia: (1) stronger contraction increases myocardial oxygen demand, and (2) higher wall tension during systole aggravates the compression of intramyocardial arteries.

Coronary blood flow may be influenced by the autonomic nervous system. There is constant background of alpha-adrenergic tone, which has a vasoconstrictive effect. Stimulation of the baroreceptors in the carotid sinus blocks alpha discharge, causing coronary and peripheral artery dilation. Interestingly, alpha-mediated constriction of epicardial arteries leads to an increase in perfusion pressure that *augments* flow through the intramural vessels during exercise. Vagal stimulation causes coronary and systemic vasodilation. Chemoreceptors responsible for the Bezold-Jarisch reflex have both afferent and efferent limbs that are part of the vagus nerve.

In addition to autonomic influences, coronary blood flow is autoregulated. Increasing myocardial oxygen demand above current oxygen supply (ischemia) leads to the release of vasodilator hormones from vascular endothelial cells that have a powerful and immediate influence on intramural resistance vessels (see Chapters 1 and 13).

3 Cardiac History

George J. Taylor
Gerald E. Boyd

The initial evaluation, especially talking with the patient and family about symptoms, usually is the most productive clinical encounter. When I take the history myself, as opposed to relying on information gathered by another, I always feel that I know more about the patient. It is a useful exercise, even when I do not know much about the patient's illness, as is so often the case in the practice of medicine. The beauty of the Oslerian history and physical examination protocol is that it allows even the most inexperienced practitioner to gather helpful information and begin the process of evaluation and treatment, even when knowing nothing about the illness. Perhaps the best advice for the inexperienced clinician is to stick with that protocol (Box 3-1).

This is true not only for gathering and recording the information, but also for presenting it to a colleague. Be as meticulous with your formal (and informal) presentations as you are with the workup that goes into the medical record. After all, this is when your colleagues directly evaluate your clinical skills. The most common error when presenting a case is *not following the outline.* When the presenter's opening statement includes the words, "chief complaint," and is followed by the use of each of the terms in Box 3-1, the presentation has a chance of being organized, complete, and succinct. A failure to follow the outline, to "say the words," invariably leads to a rambling and redundant presentation.

Good history taking and physical diagnosis and confident, well-organized presentations are marks of a sophisticated clinician. Does training in cardiology and other subspecialties deemphasize these traditional, physician-like skills? Does modern training focus too much on the technical and procedural? If so, the art of practicing medicine at the bedside and in the clinic may rest with those in primary care. Be meticulous with your initial bedside evaluation of a clinical problem. This first contact is also the time that your patient will evaluate your skill.

COMMON MISTAKES WHEN TAKING A HISTORY

1. *The leading question.* As a student, one of my teachers observed me asking a woman if her chest discomfort felt "like an elephant standing on your chest." Of course she agreed, but it would not do for me to use that description for all my patients with angina. Patients often come up with surprisingly graphic—and entertaining—descriptions and metaphors. One man with angina told me that "it is like that feeling you got when you were a kid and felt like you were going to cry, but didn't—a strangling kind of feeling."

2. *Failure to use the outline (Box 3-1).* During chart reviews for clinical studies, it is amazing to find that experienced doctors sometimes omit the family history or fail to mention coronary risk factors.

3. *Failure to elicit detail.* More is learned about symptoms when asking the patient to describe an episode in detail. What brings it on? (That is not a bad first question.) Give me a "for instance." (That is often a better question.)

4. *Not getting a clear idea of functional ability.* Functional class often is related to prognosis in patients with heart disease, and the New York and Canadian classifications are helpful both for establishing severity of illness and for following its progress (Table 3-1).

5. *Not taking time to formulate an "impression" at the end of the workup.* "Chest pain of unknown cause" is not an impression, but a restatement of the chief complaint.

Reflecting for a moment or two on the data you have collected and then formulating an impression—this is a valuable time for your patient. A wonderful quartet of photographs of William Osler at the bedside shows him performing a series of important clinical tasks. They are entitled *inspection, palpation, auscultation, contemplation.* Do not leave out contemplation; laboratory work and imaging studies are no substitute.

COMMON SYMPTOMS OF HEART DISEASE
Chest Pain

Myocardial ischemia is the leading cause of death in the developed world, and angina pectoris is its common manifestation. Primary care physicians evaluate chest discomfort almost daily. Causes of chest pain are summarized in Table 3-2. Although the usual features of angina are easily recited by most clinicians, it is difficult to differentiate cardiac from noncardiac pain on the basis of the history alone. Most clinicians agree that their best guess about the cause of pain is wrong at least one third of the time. I have learned not to be surprised when the patient describing classical angina has no heart disease, or when the patient with strange symptoms has them reproduced on the treadmill. With this disclaimer in mind, let us review some features of chest pain that point to or away from a cardiac origin.

Location and Radiation

Ischemic discomfort (angina pectoris) is usually midline (Fig. 3-1). It is exertional. When a patient points to a spot under the left nipple ("over my heart)" the pain usually is not cardiac. It may be epigastric. In addition, the pain may be localized to the jaw, neck, any place on the arm (such as the wrist, including the hand), or the upper back. Lower back pain and pain below the epigastrium probably are not of cardiac origin.

Radiation of the discomfort is common but not invariable. Radiation to the jaw or neck suggests a cardiac

---

BOX 3-1

INITIAL PATIENT EVALUATION: HISTORY AND PHYSICAL EXAMINATION

History
  Chief complaint
  Present illness
  Past medical history
  Family history
  Social history
  Review of systems

Physical examination

Impression

Plan

| Table 3-1 | *Two Systems for Classifying Functional Limitations of Patients with Heart Disease* |

	Canadian Cardiovascular Society Functional Class	New York Heart Association Functional Class
Comment	This system applies to angina pectoris and not to other cardiac conditions.	This system can be used to classify patients with any cardiac condition.
Class I	No angina with normal physical activity, including stair climbing. Angina develops with strenuous or prolonged work.	The patient is known to have heart disease, but there are no symptoms with physical activity.
Class II	Slight limitation of activity. Angina occurs after walking more than two blocks, or up a flight of stairs, or uphill, or into cold wind, or during stress.	Slight limitation of activity and no symptoms at rest. Ordinary activity may cause symptoms.
Class III	Marked limitation of activity. Angina develops after walking one to two blocks on level ground or after climbing one flight of stairs.	No symptoms at rest, but marked limitation of physical activity. Minimal activity causes symptoms.
Class IV	Angina may occur at rest. The patient is unable to do any physical activity without angina developing.	Symptoms at rest. Any physical activity provokes symptoms.

Table 3-2	*Chest Pain Syndromes*

Syndrome	Patient's Description	Provocation	Duration	Location	Radiation	Relief
Chronic stable, effort angina	Pressure, tight, heavy, squeezing, dull, burning, and so forth; "not a pain"	Exercise, emotional stress. A predictable level of exertion provokes symptoms.	5-15 minutes	Midsternal, midchest; can be epigastric	Arm, jaw, back, neck, both sides of the chest	Rest, nitroglycerin
Unstable angina	As above; an acceleration of symptoms, or new-onset angina.	Spontaneous, at rest as well as with exertion, often nocturnal	5-15 minutes or maybe longer	As above	As above	Nitroglycerin
Aortic dissection	Severe, "tearing"	None	Prolonged	Midchest	Back	No relief with nitroglycerin
Esophageal reflux	Can mimic angina	Recumbency, eating	10-60 minutes	Substernal, epigastric	A sour taste, may radiate like angina	Antacids
Esophageal spasm	As above	Recumbency, cold liquids, eating	As above	As above	Mimics angina	Nitroglycerin, antacids
Chest wall	Superficial pain, sharp, knifelike, stabbing, variable	Movement, deep palpation	Variable, but often lasts hours	Anywhere in the chest, shoulders, neck; may vary	Variable	Analgesics, antiinflammatory drugs, rest, and time
Cutaneous (herpes zoster)	Superficial, intense; rash may develop after pain	Touch	Lasts for hours	Typical distribution (dermatome)	Localized	Analgesics, time, antiviral therapy
Pericardial	Sharp, severe	Inspiration, "pleuritic"; may be worse with swallowing	Minutes to hours	Mid to left chest	Shoulder, back, neck	Antiinflammatory drugs
Peptic ulcer disease	Burning, boring, gnawing	Lack of food	Hours	Epigastric, substernal	Back (with perforation)	Food, antacids
Biliary disease	Deep, aching, waxes and wanes ("colicky")	Spontaneous, food	Hours	Epigastric, right upper quadrant tenderness	Back	Analgesics, time
Bronchospasm	Tight, associated dyspnea and wheezing	Spontaneous	>30 minutes	Substernal		Bronchodilators
Mitral valve prolapse	Superficial pain, stabbing, fleeting; variable	Spontaneous, no pattern	Minutes to hours; usually prolonged	Left chest, but may be substernal	Variable	Time
Hyperventilation	Tight	With anxiety, not exertional	<10 minutes	Midsternal	Also dyspnea, circumoral paresthesia, tingling in the hands, faintness	Rest and time

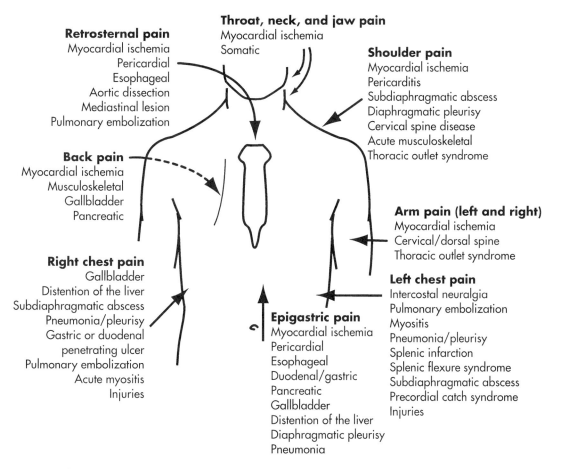

Throat, neck, and jaw pain
Myocardial ischemia
Somatic

Retrosternal pain
Myocardial ischemia
Pericardial
Esophageal
Aortic dissection
Mediastinal lesion
Pulmonary embolization

Shoulder pain
Myocardial ischemia
Pericarditis
Subdiaphragmatic abscess
Diaphragmatic pleurisy
Cervical spine disease
Acute musculoskeletal
Thoracic outlet syndrome

Back pain
Myocardial ischemia
Musculoskeletal
Gallbladder
Pancreatic

Right chest pain
Gallbladder
Distention of the liver
Subdiaphragmatic abscess
Pneumonia/pleurisy
Gastric or duodenal
penetrating ulcer
Pulmonary embolization
Acute myositis
Injuries

Arm pain (left and right)
Myocardial ischemia
Cervical/dorsal spine
Thoracic outlet syndrome

Left chest pain
Intercostal neuralgia
Pulmonary embolization
Myositis
Pneumonia/pleurisy
Splenic infarction
Splenic flexure syndrome
Subdiaphragmatic abscess
Precordial catch syndrome
Injuries

Epigastric pain
Myocardial ischemia
Pericardial
Esophageal
Duodenal/gastric
Pancreatic
Gallbladder
Distention of the liver
Diaphragmatic pleurisy
Pneumonia

FIG. 3-1
Common causes of chest pain based on where the pain begins. Pain that is isolated to either the left or right chest usually is not caused by myocardial ischemia.
Redrawn from Miller AJ: *Diagnosis of chest pain,* New York, 1988, Raven.

origin. Radiation to the arm may as well, although this pattern seems less predictive to me. Movement of pain to a location below the epigastrium and headache usually are noncardiac.

Quality of Pain

Patients typically describe angina with terms like *heavy, squeezing, pressure, constricting,* or *strangling* or related metaphors (*viselike, like an elephant,* and so forth). Many people with coronary disease describe it as a burning pain; "burning" does not indicate a gastric origin. Sharp or stabbing pain usually is not angina, nor is pain aggravated by deep inspiration (pleuritic pain).

Angina may be missed because the examiner specifically asks about chest *pain*. Patients frequently emphasize that "it is not a *pain*." Ask about *discomfort* or *any unusual or funny sensation*. The patient may then describe "heaviness while walking," a symptom that had been minimized (or denied). Patients commonly believe that discomfort originating in the heart must be severe. Despite the symptom not being a severe pain,

most who have angina stop when they get it. Few "walk through" the pain. Cardiac discomfort often provokes a sense of uneasiness. This emotional response to angina has been called "fear of death"; there appears to be a connection between the heart and brain that lets the patient know that, while not excruciating, cardiac pain is serious.

Duration

Angina occurs in brief episodes, rarely longer than 10 minutes. When active myocardial ischemia is prolonged, the patient is having myocardial infarction; in this case pain can last 24 hours or more. A *chronic* chest pain syndrome with multiple episodes of pain that last for hours usually is noncardiac in origin. Chronic and recurrent pain that "lasts all day" is not angina.

Factors That Provoke Angina

Exercise is the most common factor that provokes angina.. Stress, anger, and excitement may as well. Many report that angina is more common with exercise after a meal. On the other hand, eating, without exercise, rarely causes angina but may provoke gastroesophageal reflux and pain. Physical work in the cold, particularly walking into a cold wind or shoveling snow, commonly provokes angina. Myocardial ischemia with angina at rest is unstable and possibly preinfarctional. The unstable angina syndrome is discussed at length in Chapter 13.

Discomfort Often Confused with Angina

Figure 3-1 and Table 3-2 survey the many conditions that cause chest pain. Two of them are especially common as causes of chronic and recurrent symptoms: gastroesophageal reflux and chest wall pain.

An esophageal cause is suggested when discomfort is aggravated by eating (which provokes acid secretion), recumbent posture (which promotes reflux), and a sour taste. It is not predictably exertional. It may develop after retiring, with recumbency. It may be epigastric with radiation upward, but cardiac pain may have a similar distribution. Esophageal spasm in response to irritation of mucosa may be the mechanism of discomfort, and this causes pain that is indistinguishable from angina pectoris. Spasm may be relieved by nitroglycerin. For this reason, a favorable response to nitroglycerin is not diagnostic for angina pectoris. The response of esophageal pain to calcium channel blockers is variable. They may relieve esophageal spasm, but they may further relax lower esophageal sphincter tone and aggravate reflux.

Chest wall pain often is not midline in location. There may be associated chest wall tenderness, with deep palpation reproducing the discomfort. It is aggravated by changes in position, reaching, twisting, or doing arm work. Angina also may be provoked by arm exertion, but with chest wall syndromes there is the sense that a specific task or position taken while doing work is responsible for the pain. Patients often have a prior history of back, neck, or shoulder pain. Many of them tell me that they know it is musculoskeletal, and they are right. However, denial is common with coronary heart disease, and the examiner must resist being drawn into that process.

Dyspnea

Breathlessness is the cardinal symptom of left ventricular failure and of pulmonary disease. A differential diagnosis of dyspnea is provided in Table 3-3. As a symptom of heart failure, a series of symptoms indicates progressively more severe pulmonary congestion.

Dyspnea with exertion is the earliest symptom of left heart failure. As a student I believed that dyspnea was caused by fluid in the lungs and hypoxemia. It turns out that most individuals with early heart failure and exertional dyspnea have normal PaO$_2$. The same is true for patients with asthma and severe dyspnea. In both asthma and heart failure, an increase in the *work* of breathing is the cause of dyspnea. Early heart failure produces interstitial, not alveolar, edema. This has little effect on air exchange, but the soggy, heavy lungs are hard to move.

Orthopnea, dyspnea with recumbency, could be considered a symptom of more severe pulmonary congestion. When the patient lies down, blood volume shifts from the legs to the chest, aggravating congestion. To avoid this, the patient sleeps on two or three pillows. Clinicians may quantify the severity of dyspnea with the number of pillows required, a crude but possibly useful method; four-pillow would be worse than two-pillow orthopnea.

Paroxysmal nocturnal dyspnea (PND) is the next level in severity of congestion. In addition to interstitial edema, there may be intraalveolar edema. It usually develops a couple hours after retiring. The patient is roused from sleep by severe breathlessness with diaphoresis (sweating) and possible wheezing or cough and either sits on the edge of the bed or leaves the bed and stands in front of an open window or a fan. Relief comes in 15 to 30 minutes. Advanced lung disease may also cause nocturnal dyspnea. Unlike the PND of heart failure, coughing or wheezing are the initial and dominant symptoms, with shortness of breath less prominent.

Pulmonary edema is the final stage in the progression of heart failure and pulmonary congestion. The fluid is definitely intraalveolar, and the patient may cough up pink, frothy sputum. Arterial hypoxemia often is present. This dramatic clinical event will be discussed in detail when considering congestive heart failure.

To get an idea of what patients with airway obstruction or heart failure experience, try breathing through a drinking straw for 5 minutes. (I do this with medical students, usually with a bet, and have never had to pay.) "Air hunger" is an apt description.

A common issue leading to cardiology consultation is distinguishing between heart and lung disease. The physical examination helps, but an answer often is derived from the echocardiogram. Normal left ventricular size, thickness, and function and the absence of valvular disease exclude heart disease, and pulmonary function testing confirms lung disease. An exception to this is exertional dyspnea as an *anginal equivalent*. This is the uncommon patient with severe coronary disease who is unable to sense cardiac pain. During ischemia there is no discomfort, but there is left ventricular dysfunction, transient pulmonary congestion, and dyspnea. The echocardiogram shows normal left ventricular function at rest. An exercise echocardiogram is necessary to demonstrate dysfunction during provoked ischemia.

Acute dyspnea at rest merits special mention. It is an especially alarming symptom in hospitalized patients.

Table 3-3	*Frequent Causes of Dyspnea*

Illness	Pathophysiology	Laboratory Findings
CONGESTIVE HEART FAILURE *Valvular heart disease:* usually aortic and mitral valve disease	Low cardiac output causes high left atrial and pulmonary capillary pressures and then transudation of fluid into the interstitial space. Wet lungs are stiff ("noncompliant"), and the work of breathing is increased. It is a restrictive ventilatory defect.	High diastolic pressures in the left atrium, low cardiac output, decreased vital capacity and force vital capacity, decreased maximum oxygen consumption (VO_2 max), plus the findings of the specific cardiac condition
Myocardial disease Primary: idiopathic cardiomyopathy Secondary: ischemic cardiomyopathy, hemachromatosis, other infiltrative cardiomyopathies	As above	As above, plus findings of the specific cardiac condition (low left ventricular ejection fraction, diastolic dysfunction, coronary obstructive disease, and the like)
Coronary heart disease (in the absence of resting or baseline left ventricular dysfunction)	Transient ischemia can cause transient left ventricular dysfunction and pulmonary congestion, an "anginal equivalent."	Normal left ventricular function at rest, with dysfunction appearing during exercise (the stress echocardiogram)
LUNG DISEASE **Restrictive Lung Disease** *Pulmonary fibrosis:* idiopathic, pneumoconiosis, sarcoidosis, drug or radiation induced	Similar to heart disease, as there is difficulty moving the lungs. The increased work of breathing causes dyspnea.	Decrease in lung volumes (total lung capacity and vital capacity)
Chest wall disease: kyphoscoliosis, obesity, ankylosing spondylitis *Neuromuscular:* myasthenia gravis, Guillain-Barré syndrome, muscular dystrophy, cervical spine injury, advanced malnutrition and debility		
Space-occupying lesions (tumor, infiltrates)	Alteration of mechanics plus intrapulmonary shunting	Low PaO_2, reduced lung volumes
Obstructive lung disease: asthma, chronic obstructive lung disease (emphysema and bronchitis), bronchiectasis, cystic fibrosis, bronchiolitis	Increased airway resistance causes a decrease in flow rates. Dyspnea is caused by the increased work of breathing.	Normal or increased lung volumes, reduced forced expiratory volume FEV_1)

Continued

Table 3-3	Frequent Causes of Dyspnea—cont'd

Illness	Pathophysiology	Laboratory Findings
LUNG DISEASE—cont'd		
Restrictive Lung Disease—cont'd		
Pulmonary embolus	Lung mechanics are not altered, but there is a mismatch between ventilation and perfusion causing intrapulmonary shunting and hypoxemia. Dyspnea is the result of low PaO_2.	Low PaO_2
OTHER CONDITIONS		
Deconditioning	Inactivity; this may contribute to other causes of dyspnea	Low VO_2 max; pulse inappropriately high for the level of activity
Conditions that may aggravate dyspnea	Anemia, peripheral vascular disease, hyperthyroidism, fever, muscle wasting, and advanced debility	

Pulmonary congestion can be quickly diagnosed or excluded using physical examination and chest x-ray. Think of *pulmonary embolus*, which is a diagnosis often overlooked unless it is considered, since the patient's symptoms may be vague and physical findings are few. Unexplained dyspnea or an abrupt change in mental status reflecting hypoxia are symptoms that should trigger the consideration of pulmonary embolus.

Cough

In the absence of dyspnea, cough usually is a symptom of lung disease. It may accompany the dyspnea of heart failure, but with heart failure shortness of breath tends to be the dominant symptom. Rare cardiovascular conditions can cause cough without pulmonary congestion. For example, dilated structures may stretch the recurrent laryngeal nerve (aortic aneurysm) or press on the tracheobronchial tree (aneurysm or a dilated left atrium with mitral stenosis).

Hemoptysis

Hemoptysis can be a symptom of heart disease. Self-limited hemoptysis can occur early in the course of *mitral stenosis*. Massive hemoptysis may be the terminal event, with rupture of an *aortic aneurysm*. Blood-streaked sputum may occur with pulmonary infarction. Hemoptysis may complicate *Eisenmenger syndrome*. However, these are relatively uncommon illnesses. A more common cardiovascular cause of hemoptysis, particularly in bedridden or elderly patients, is *pulmonary embolus*.

Wheezing

Bronchospasm is the usual cause of wheezing. Some patients wheeze with heart failure and pulmonary congestion, so-called *cardiac asthma*. They usually have dyspnea as well, although some patients do not. The physical examination, electrocardiogram, and chest x-ray help to sort this out. Again, when there is doubt about heart failure, an echocardiogram provides specific information about cardiac structure and function, and pulmonary function studies confirm or exclude lung disease.

It is unnecessary for every patient with a pulmonary symptom to have an echocardiogram, which is a test properly reserved for uncertain cases or for confirming a suspected cardiac cause. A patient who comes to you with typical bronchitis or asthma and no other cardiac history or symptoms and has a normal cardiac examination, electrocardiogram, and chest x-ray probably has lung disease and does not require an expensive cardiac workup.

Edema

Edema occurs with a variety of illnesses (Table 3-4). Cardiac edema, a result of low cardiac output and elevated right atrial pressure *(right heart failure)*, usually is dependent. Pericardial constriction and effusion may block venous return to the heart and thus limit cardiac output. The resulting pattern of edema is similar to that caused by heart failure. In an ambulatory patient, edema of the ankles, feet, and legs is common. In a bedridden person the edema shifts to the sacral region,

| Table 3-4 | *Location and Character of Edema and Possible Causes* |

Location and Character	Possible Causes
Bilateral, lower extremity, and pitting edema	Congestive heart failure, constrictive pericarditis, bilateral venous insufficiency, inferior vena cava obstruction
Sacral edema in a bedridden patient	Congestive heart failure
Unilateral leg edema	Venous insufficiency, lymphatic obstruction
Lower extremity edema plus ascites	Hepatic cirrhosis (ascites precedes the edema and seems disproportionately severe); congestive heart failure (edema precedes ascites and is more severe)
Edema of face, around the eyes	Nephrotic syndrome, acute glomerulonephritis, angioneurotic edema, hypoproteinemia, myxedema (hypothyroidism)
Edema limited to face, neck, and upper arms	Superior vena cava obstruction (lung cancer, aortic archaneurysm, lymphoma)
Edema of one arm	Venous thrombosis, lymphatic obstruction
Generalized edema (anasarca)	Severe congestive heart failure, nephrotic syndrome, hepatic cirrhosis
Generalized edema that does not "pit," is "doughy," and is not dependent	Myxedema (hypothyroidism)

as it tends to be "dependent" and follows the law of gravity. A patient initially may complain of tight-fitting shoes. When there is swelling in the hands and fingers, but no dependent edema, it is probably not cardiac in origin. High right atrial pressure causes edema in both legs, and unilateral edema suggests venous insufficiency or blocked lymphatics of the affected limb. Bilateral venous insufficiency is possible, although uncommon. When the diagnosis is uncertain, venous Doppler studies may uncover the cause of swelling.

Elevated right heart pressure impedes venous return from the splanchnic bed. Hepatic edema may cause nausea and anorexia. This may contribute to the "cardiac cachexia" experienced by some with advanced heart failure. Similarly, since the pleural space is drained by the systemic venous circulation and not the pulmonary veins, patients with right heart failure and peripheral edema also may have pleural effusion, which may cause or aggravate dyspnea.

Cirrhosis of the liver causes ascites. Ascites may complicate right heart failure, and it may be difficult to distinguish heart from liver disease. With cirrhosis, ascites usually develops before peripheral edema and is the dominant finding. With heart failure, peripheral edema tends to occur earlier than ascites. Although patients with recent onset of heart failure and passive congestion of the liver may have hepatomegaly and ascites, they usually do not have the peripheral findings of cirrhosis (palmar erythema, spider angioma, gynecomastia, and testicular atrophy). However, chronic right heart failure may cause cirrhosis with all its manifestations.

Mass lesions may block veins or lymphatics, causing localized edema. An aortic aneurysm, for example, can obstruct the superior vena cava. However, most cases of lymphatic or venous obstruction involve neoplastic disease.

Low serum protein with low plasma oncotic pressure causes generalized, nondependent edema. Nephrotic syndrome is responsible for the most dramatic cases. Other protein-wasting conditions, including malnutrition, also can cause edema. This may contribute to the edema of patients with advanced heart failure.

Fatigue

Fatigue is such a vague and nonspecific symptom that it rarely points to a definitive diagnosis. Stress and anxiety are common causes. It may be an important symptom of heart disease. A sense of tiredness or fatigue can be a symptom of low cardiac output. Most patients with heart failure have dyspnea (left heart failure) or edema (right heart failure), but only rarely is fatigue the initial symptom.

Chronic fatigue usually is not a symptom of ischemic heart disease. Myocardial ischemia causes chest discomfort. On the other hand, I have heard enough patients describe excessive fatigue in the weeks preceding myocardial infarction that I am convinced it can be a prodromal symptom. Fatigue is a common side effect of treating angina pectoris or hypertension with beta-adrenergic blockers. Rapid or overly aggressive diuresis may aggravate or cause fatigue. Hypokalemia or hypomagnesemia following diuretic therapy is the mechanism in some cases.

Syncope

Syncope is defined as a sudden loss of consciousness. An abrupt drop in cardiac output caused by cardiac arrhythmia is the cause of greatest concern in adults (Table 3-5). The abnormal rhythm may be slow or fast. A minority of patients are aware of an irregular or rapid heartbeat, or *palpitations*, before losing consciousness. Most have no warning and suffer a "drop attack."

The most common cause of loss of consciousness is the common faint—vasovagal or vasodepressor syncope (Table 3-6). This is distinguished from cardiac syncope by a clearly described prodrome. The patient feels strange, possibly nauseated, and usually dizzy before fainting. There may be diaphoresis. Because they have some warning, patients rarely fall or are injured. The period of unconsciousness is brief. Hypotension is relieved by recumbency, and recovery begins as soon as the person is down.

Postural hypotension, another common cause of syncope, usually occurs after a change to upright posture. Often this does not immediately precede dizziness and loss of consciousness; the patient may have been upright for 2 to 5 minutes before symptoms begin. It is a common problem among older people and may be aggravated by commonly used medicines. Syncope may

Table 3-5	Cardiac Causes of Syncope
Mechanism	**Conditions and Comments**
Slow cardiac rhythm with low cardiac output	Heart block (Stokes-Adams attacks), asystole, atrial fibrillation with slow ventricular response (all most common in elderly patients); aggravated by digitalis, beta-adrenergic blockers, verapamil, and diltiazem
Rapid ventricular rhythms	Ventricular tachycardia and fibrillation, the usual cause of sudden cardiac death; an early symptom of acute myocardial infarction; common with poor left ventricular systolic function (of any cause) and hypertrophic cardiomyopathy; syncope may be of sudden onset, without warning; note aggravating conditions, drugs (Fig. 2-8)
Rapid atrial (supraventricular) rhythms	Supraventricular tachycardia including preexcitation syndromes; in most cases patients are aware of palpitations or at least feel badly and have some warning before syncope occurs
Low cardiac output related to "mechanical" problems	*Left heart:* Most common: aortic stenosis, hypertrophic cardiomyopathy (subaortic stenosis), atrial myxoma, prosthetic valve malfunction. Less common: mitral stenosis and aortic regurgitation (syncope occurs only with advanced disease) *Right heart:* pulmonary embolism, primary pulmonary hypertension, pulmonic stenosis, Eisenmenger syndrome, tetralogy of Fallot; pericardial tamponade (reduced cardiac filling)
Pacemaker related	Pacemaker failure with bradycardia, pacemaker-induced tachyarrhythmia, "pacemaker syndrome" (the abrupt drop in cardiac output that some patients have when the ventricular pacemaker turns on and there is loss of atrial contraction)
Neurocardiogenic syncope	A common illness. The reflex loop includes LV baroreceptors and both catecholamine release and vagal stimultation (see Chapter 27).

develop abruptly, and patients often sustain injury. It is important to consider syncope when evaluating an elderly patient who has fallen.

Because of the change in consciousness, it is logical to think of neurologic disease as a possible cause of syncope; however, this is rarely the case. An occasional patient with a seizure will lose consciousness, but seizure disorders usually include other features such as convulsions, preseizure aura, and incontinence. Stroke and transient ischemic attacks (TIAs) usually cause unilateral neurologic symptoms, not syncope. About 6% of strokes or TIAs have syncope as an associated symptom. Almost all these are caused by vertebrobasilar artery occlusion (most often embolic), and patients have related symptoms such as ataxia, vertigo, diplopia, paresthesia, or dysarthria (see Table 3-6).

Palpitations

A palpitation is the awareness of a forceful, irregular, or rapid heartbeat. An isolated atrial or ventricular premature beat causes a "skip, thump, or flip-flop." The patient does not sense the premature beat itself, but instead feels the pause after the ectopic beat or the more forceful normal beat that follows it.

Sustained palpitations indicate a sustained arrhythmia such as atrial fibrillation, supraventricular tachycardia, or ventricular tachycardia. With heart rates exceeding 150 beats/min, time for ventricular filling (between beats) may be inadequate, and cardiac output falls. This may cause syncope, hypotension, or fatigue, or it may precipitate or aggravate heart failure.

Slow cardiac rhythms, such as complete heart block, usually are regular rhythms. Low cardiac output may cause fatigue, postural hypotension, or syncope. Bradyarrhythmias are less commonly accompanied by a sense of palpitations, although some describe an abnormally slow pulse.

Table 3-7 summarizes conditions and drugs that may aggravate palpitations. These should be considered when reviewing systems.

Table 3-6	*Noncardiac Causes of Syncope*
Syndrome	**Description and Comment**
Vasodepressor or vasovagal syncope	The common faint. Follows anxiety, pain, "the sight of blood." Common during surgical, vascular, or endoscopic procedures. Vagal discharge leads to bradycardia or vasodilation and a fall in blood pressure. Prodrome: sweats, pallor, nausea, blurred vision.
Orthostatic syncope	Follows a change in posture, but there may be a 5-minute delay. May be aggravated by vasodilator drugs, diuretics, antidepressants, phenothiazines, and tranquilizers.
Cerebrovascular disease	A symptom of 6% of strokes or transient ischemic attacks. The cause is vertebrobasilar insufficiency; other neurological symptoms are the rule (vertigo, diplopia, dysarthria, paresthesia, or ataxia).
Subclavian steal	Follows upper extremity exertion. There is stenosis or occlusion of the subclavian artery; with arm exertion, blood flow is "stolen" from the vertebral artery, causing vertebrobasilar insufficiency. Look for a pulse deficit on the stenosed side and a bruit.
Carotid sinus syncope	Common in the elderly; 25% report symptoms with stimulation of the carotid sinus (sudden turns, shaving, a tight collar). Many have hypertension or coronary artery disease. A few have other pathologic conditions of the neck (e.g., tumor, a history of radiation, enlarged lymph nodes).
Situational syncope	Micturition, cough or sneeze, defecation, swallowing, and Valsalva syncope
Migraine syndromes	Other features of migraine usually present
Metabolic	Hypoglycemia, hypoxia, hyperventilation
Hysterical syncope	

Table 3-7	Conditions That Provoke or Aggravate Palpitations (Cardiac Arrhythmias)
Arrhythmia	**Aggravating Conditions and Agents**
Atrial premature beats, supraventricular tachyarrhythmias	Hyperthyroidism, hypoxia, low potassium or magnesium (common with diuretic therapy), hypercapnia, digitalis, aminophylline, alcohol, sympathomimetics (caffeine, ephedrine, and bronchodilators), and sympathetic discharge (excitement or exercise)
Atrial fibrillation	Hyperthyroidism, alcohol (the holiday heart syndrome), common after cardiac surgery, low magnesium or potassium
Ventricular premature beats, ventricular tachycardia, ventricular fibrillation	Myocardial ischemia, acute myocardial infarction (the arrhythmia may be an early or presenting symptom); hypoxia, antiarrhythmic drugs (the paradoxical "proarrhythmic" effect), other drugs that prolong the QT interval (phenothiazines, some antihistamines, tricyclics), digitalis, aminophylline, ephedrine and other sympathomimetics, low magnesium or potassium (a common complication of diuretic therapy)

Table 3-8	Other Symptoms of Heart Disease
Symptom	**Possible Cardiac Illness and Comments**
Anorexia	A result of splanchnic and hepatic edema in patients with right heart failure; also consider digitalis toxicity
Cachexia	A symptom of advanced heart failure (other symptoms of heart failure usually are present)
Nausea and vomiting	Another symptom of splanchnic edema; consider digitalis intoxication
Hoarseness	Compression of the recurrent laryngeal nerve by an aortic aneurysm
Fever and chills	Bacterial endocarditis
Polyuria	With new atrial tachycardia, fibrillation, or flutter
Nocturia	An early symptom of heart failure (as well as prostatism, diabetes)
Cyanosis of the fingers	Raynaud's phenomenon
Central cyanosis	Decrease in arterial oxygen saturation; right-to-left intracardiac shunting or pulmonary dysfunction
Joint pain	Most forms of arthritis may be associated with heart disease; as a primary manifestation of heart disease, consider rheumatic fever
Abdominal pain	Aortic aneurysm, mesenteric ischemia, swollen liver
Headache	Hypertension does not, as a rule, cause headache. Angina may radiate to the jaw, teeth, or ear. Typical headache is not a symptom of heart disease.
Pain in the extremities	Occlusive vascular disease (arterial or venous), Raynaud's phenomenon

Table 3-8	*Other Symptoms of Heart Disease—cont'd*
Symptom	**Possible Cardiac Illness and Comments**
Recurrent bronchitis	Common with high pulmonary venous pressures (mitral stenosis) and left-to-right shunting (high pulmonary blood flow)
Squatting	Tetralogy of Fallot
Epistaxis	Hypertension
Dysphagia	Aortic arch aneurysm, enlarged left atrium
Jaundice	Mild jaundice may occur with right heart failure; if severe, consider cirrhosis or pulmonary infarction. Hemolysis may cause jaundice with aortic stenosis or prosthetic valve malfunction.
Insomnia	Heart failure and pulmonary congestion (before developing nocturnal dyspnea)
Cheyne-Stokes respiration	Heart failure
Hiccups	Inferior myocardial infarction
Seizure, convulsion	Not a primary symptom of heart disease, but a common immediate complication of cardiac arrest. (Always check pulse, blood pressure, and respirations when evaluating a patient with seizure; CPR may be needed rather than intravenous diazepam.)
Coma	Not a primary symptom of heart disease, but a common outcome after cardiac arrest

Other Symptoms

When I was a house officer, one of my mentors surprised me by stating that practicing cardiology is "simple." It is, in the sense that we encounter a limited number of symptoms and conditions routinely. Those catalogued above represent the bulk of adult cardiology. A variety of other symptoms that are seen less frequently is summarized in Table 3-8.

4 Physical Examination

George J. Taylor
Dennis Cope

GENERAL EXAMINATION
Vital Signs
Pulse

Normal sinus rhythm ranges between 60 and 100 beats/min; above that is tachycardia, and below it is bradycardia (see Chapter 5). Resting tachycardia is a particularly important physical finding because it may reflect low stroke volume. Recall that cardiac output = (Stroke volume) (Heart rate). An increase in heart rate is an important compensatory mechanism for poor function and reduced stroke volume. A person with heart failure or one who has had a recent myocardial infarction and has a resting pulse >100/min is in trouble.

Inexperienced examiners often are unaware of the importance of resting tachycardia. They are busy looking for physical findings that are more difficult to detect. However, resting tachycardia usually indicates real and potentially serious illness including cardiac decompensation, thyrotoxicosis, anemia, hyperadrenergic states, or fever.

Bradycardia, on the other hand, usually is an indicator of cardiac health (excepting bradyarrhythmias; see Chapter 27). Likewise, a normal heart rate with mild respiratory variation, *sinus arrhythmia*, also accompanies normal cardiac function. A grossly irregular pulse usually indicates an underlying arrhythmia, either atrial fibrillation or frequent ectopic beats (see Chapters 25 and 26).

Pulse Quality. Subtle changes in the quality and contour of the pulse wave may be more evident in the carotid than brachial pulse. Nevertheless, we are reluctant to routinely press hard on the carotid artery, especially in older patients. Overzealous physical examinations performed by medical students have caused stroke. Instead, we examine the brachial pulse as a part of the cardiac examination. If findings indicate a need for better evaluation of pulse quality, we examine the carotids, but gently.

Some pulse abnormalities and related conditions are summarized in Table 4-1. Most of them are detected by prolonged observation and by the examiner looking for the specific finding. For example, when feeling the pulse, if you ask yourself, "Is there a double peak?," you are more likely to detect pulsus bisferiens.

Blood Pressure

The difference between the systolic and diastolic pressures is called the *pulse pressure*. It is "widened" (increased) in conditions with peripheral vasodilation and low peripheral vascular resistance (e.g., thyrotoxicosis, anemia, fever, anxiety states, and pregnancy). Aortic regurgitation is the cardiac condition most commonly associated with widened pulse pressure. Narrowed pulse pressure accompanies a low cardiac output.

Cuff Size. Accurate measurement of blood pressure requires a proper match of cuff size to the patient's arm. If the cuff is too small, higher cuff pressure is required to occlude the artery, leading to an overestimation of arterial pressure (a falsely elevated blood pressure in an obese person). The opposite is true as well. Using a normal size cuff on a small child's arm leads to underestimation of blood pressure.

Leg Pressure. Lower extremity pressure can be measured using a large cuff at midthigh and listening over the popliteal artery or by using a normal arm cuff over the calf and palpating the posterior tibial artery. Although it has been suggested, we have not had much luck auscultating over the posterior tibial.

Normally, the systolic pressure is as much as 15 to 20 mm Hg higher in the leg than the arm, whereas the diastolic pressure is the same. If the diastolic leg pressure exceeds arm pressure, the size of the leg cuff is probably too small. When the leg systolic pressure is more than 20 mm Hg higher than arm pressure, consider aortic regurgitation (Hill's sign).

Reduced blood pressure in the legs is the key physical finding of coarctation of the aorta. This is a correctable cause of hypertension, and it is a diagnosis you do not want to miss. For this reason, measurement of leg pressure is a necessary component of the hypertension workup. Leg pressure also may be low with peripheral arterial disease. This is seldom confused with coarctation, because the pulses are asymmetrical and other signs and symptoms of limb ischemia are present.

Pulsus Paradoxus. With inspiration, blood pressure falls slightly (<10 mm Hg). Pulsus paradoxus is an inspiratory fall in pressure that exceeds 10 mm Hg. This important physical finding is always present with peri-

| Table 4-1 | *Abnormal Patterns of the Arterial Pulse* |

Pulse	Associated Condition	Description, Mechanism
Pulsus tardus	Aortic stenosis	Slow upstroke, often with a "shudder" due to delayed emptying. Low pulse volume also may be present (pulsus parvus et tardus).
Water hammer pulse (Corrigan's pulse)	Aortic regurgitation	Abrupt upstroke of the pulse wave, with rapid collapse (Other peripheral pulse findings of severe aortic regurgitation are reviewed in Chapter 19.)
Bounding pulses	Thyrotoxicosis, anemia, anxiety states, fever, pregnancy, arteriovenous fistula	All conditions that include a hyperkinetic heart and widened pulse pressure
Pulsus bisferiens	1. Aortic regurgitation or 2. Hypertrophic obstructive cardiomyopathy	Two systolic peaks in the pressure wave: 1. Large stroke volume ejected rapidly. 2. With obstructive cardiomyopathy, obstruction peaks in midsystole. Early ejection is normal; the midsystolic dip is caused by maximum obstruction, and this is followed by a reflected wave. Note this difference in the initial portion of the pulse compared with valvular aortic stenosis, which causes pulsus tardus.
Pulsus alternans	Severe heart failure	Alternating pulses are strong and weak. Intensity of heart sounds and Korotkoff sounds also may alternate. The rhythm usually is regular. Irregular rhythms, with variation in ventricular filling time, also may cause variation in pulse volume (and this is not pulsus alternans).
Pulsus paradoxus	Pericardial tamponade (usually present); pericardial constriction (about half the cases); obstructive lung disease, obesity, shock, pregnancy, pulmonary embolus	An exaggerated fall in pulse strength, or systolic blood pressure, during inspiration. Normally, pressure falls less than 10 mm Hg. When the pulsus exceeds 20 mm Hg, you may detect it by feeling the pulse. When it less than 20 mm Hg, it is picked up by carefully recording systolic pressure during expiration and inspiration (see text).
Pulse deficit in lower extremities	1. Coarctation of the aorta 2. Peripheral artery disease	1. Above the diaphragm, pulses are bounding. Below, they are weak and have delayed upstroke. Record upper and lower extremity pressure. There may be a continuous or systolic murmur over the back. (This is a correctable cause of hypertension.) 2. Abnormal pulses often are asymmetrical, and there are other findings of peripheral ischemia

cardial tamponade, and it accompanies constrictive pericarditis about half the time. Excluding pulsus paradoxus rules out the hemodynamics of tamponade even when the patient has a pericardial effusion. Severe obstructive lung disease also can cause pulsus paradoxus.

There is a trick to measuring the systolic pressures during inspiration and expiration. Having the patient inhale and hold the breath while measuring pressure and then exhale and hold the breath does not work.

Pressure must be measured while breathing normally at rest. The best method is to sit at the bedside and have the patient breathe normally. Inflate the blood pressure cuff and then allow it to *deflate very slowly.* You will initially hear the Korotkoff sounds during expiration but not during inspiration; record that blood pressure as the "expiratory pressure." As the cuff continues to deflate slowly, at some point you will begin to hear the sounds during inspiration as well as expiration (throughout the respiratory cycle); record that pressure measurement as the "inspiratory pressure." The difference between these first and second pressure measurements quantifies the pulsus paradoxus.

Respiration

Heart failure may increase respiratory rate. Severe pulmonary congestion increases the work of breathing, which is evident during casual inspection. Rapid, deep respiration, *Kussmaul breathing*, accompanies metabolic acidosis (a compensatory mechanism to "blow off" CO_2). *Cheyne-Stokes respiration*, a cyclical breathing pattern with progressively deeper breaths followed by a brief period of apnea, occurs with advanced heart failure. It is caused, in part, by decreased sensitivity of the respiratory center of the brain to CO_2 and is more likely to develop in patients with cerebral disease. It is aggravated by anything that further depresses the respiratory center, including sleep, narcotics, and some sedatives (particularly barbiturates).

General Appearance, Skin, and Extremities

A number of "cardiac" findings are derived from careful inspection, including examination of the skin, mouth, and extremities (Table 4-2). In addition to those reviewed in Table 4-2, a number of congenital syndromes include a characteristic appearance and are reviewed in pediatric texts.

Does the Fire of Life Burn Brightly?

In the examination of an adult patient, an important initial task is the overall assessment of the state of health or level of vigor. When presented with a potentially tough case, an experienced surgeon I know often asks, "How brightly does the fire of life burn in this patient?" Experienced clinicians know what he is talking about. Frailty is not a nebulous physical finding, and its presence indicates a poor cardiac prognosis.

Cardiac cachexia is a diagnosis of exclusion. When a patient with chronic heart failure starts to lose weight, you must first exclude other causes. For example, occult bacterial endocarditis can cause weight loss in a patient with valvular disease. The pathophysiology of cachexia caused by heart failure is multifactorial. Anorexia is a common symptom of right heart failure because of splanchnic and hepatic congestion. Rarely, right heart failure may cause protein-losing enteropathy. Severe salt restriction may aggravate anorexia, since food does not taste as good. Digitalis toxicity may contribute to anorexia, and this can be a factor when the digoxin level is in a therapeutic range. There may also be increased caloric needs. Both increased cardiac work (e.g., aortic stenosis or regurgitation) and the increased work of breathing associated with chronic pulmonary congestion raise caloric expenditure. More recently, patients with chronic heart failure have been found to have higher levels of the proinflammatory cytokine, tumor necrosis factor, and this may contribute to cachexia.[1]

Important physical findings include bitemporal and thenar wasting.

Cyanosis. Reduced hemoglobin is blue. When the *absolute* amount of reduced hemoglobin in subcutaneous capillaries exceeds 5 g/dL, the skin looks blue. Patients with normal hemoglobin levels develop cyanosis when arterial oxygen saturation is below 85% (or 75% in dark-skinned patients). The *relative* amount of reduced hemoglobin is not the determinant of cyanosis. Thus patients with severe anemia may not have enough reduced hemoglobin to produce cyanosis, even with marked oxygen desaturation.

Using the same argument, cyanosis may develop at higher arterial oxygen saturations in patients with polycythemia; the critical level of reduced hemoglobin (5 g/dL) is reached when O_2 saturation is above 85%. This contributes to the cyanosis of patients with Eisenmenger's syndrome, in whom polycythemia develops to compensate for chronic O_2 desaturation. Cyanosis must be differentiated from the red, florid skin of polycythemia, as well as the cherry-colored flush caused by carboxyhemoglobin.

Peripheral cyanosis is caused by slow blood flow, which leads to greater oxygen extraction. Congestive heart failure, limb ischemia, shock, and cold (with vasoconstriction) are potential causes. Mucous membranes of the mouth may be spared. These patients rarely have clubbing of digits. *Central* cyanosis, caused by an excess of reduced hemoglobin, affects mucous membranes as well. Whether caused by heart disease or chronic lung disease, clubbing of digits is commonly associated.

Clubbing without cyanosis suggests infective endocarditis or ulcerative colitis. It occurs with some occupations (e.g., jackhammer operation). It also may be idiopathic, with no other associated disease.

When cyanosis cannot be explained by heart or lung disease, consider abnormal hemoglobins with a low affinity for oxygen. A number of drugs and toxins cause the oxidation of hemoglobin to methemoglobin (e.g., nitrates, nitrites, nitroprusside, aniline dyes, sulfonamides, lidocaine, procaine, and others). Methemoglobin in small quantities may cause cyanosis. Significant cyanosis may develop in a patient with a deficiency of methemoglobin reductase (an inherited disorder with the heterozygous state usually occult) after exposure to one of these oxidants. Oxidant drugs also can change hemoglobin to sulfhemoglobin, with results similar to those of methemoglobinemia.

Jugular Venous Pulse

Evaluation of the jugular venous pulse comprises three parts: estimation of venous pressure, testing for ab-

Table 4-2	*General Examination*

Finding	Condition	Associated Findings, Comment
HABITUS		
Tall and thin	Marfan syndrome	Arm span > height, arachnodactyly, long legs (pubis to foot > pubis to head), high-arched palate. Aorta and aortic valve disease (see Chapters 19 and 32), mitral valve prolapse
Obesity	Pickwickian syndrome	Sleep apnea, snoring, pulmonary hypertension, heart failure, and arrhythmias
Isolated abdominal obesity	Coronary artery disease, adult onset diabetes	Waist diameter / hip diameter >.85
Birdlike movements	Thyrotoxicosis	Atrial fibrillation common (see Chapter 36)
HEAD		
Bobbing	1 Aortic regurgitation 2. Tricuspid regurgitation	1. de Musset's sign, to-and-fro bobbing (the "yes-yes" sign) 2. Side-to-side bobbing (the "no-no" sign)
Dull, expressionless	Myxedema	Loss of lateral eyebrow, dry, sparse hair, large tongue, periorbital puffiness
Malar flush	Mitral stenosis	Looks like rouge over the cheeks; stenosis usually is severe
Violaceous hue	Carcinoid syndrome	Deep purple or reddish pink over the cheeks and face (this "rash" indicates metastasis of carcinoid tumor to the liver)
EYES AND MOUTH		
Conjunctival or mucous membrane hemorrhages	Bacterial endocarditis	Carefully examine nail beds for splinter hemorrhages and eyes for Roth spots (fluffy with exudate and surrounding erythema)
Blue sclerae	Osteogenesis imperfecta	Aortic regurgitation or dissection, mitral prolapse
Exophthalmos, lid lag, and stare	Hyperthyroidism	May also occur with advanced pulmonary hypertension and heart failure
Pulsatile eyes and earlobes	Tricuspid regurgitation	"Pulsatile exophthalmos"
Hypertensive retinopathy	Hypertension (the presence of these findings supports the diagnosis of hypertension, but their absence does not exclude it)	Grades: 1. Mild narrowing (A/V $\leq$ 1/2) 2. General narrowing (copper wire changes; A/V $\leq$ 1/3). 3. Silver wire changes (A/V $\leq$ 1/4), plus hemorrhages 4. Tiny arterioles, hemorrhages, papilledema
Diabetic retinopathy	Diabetes and associated vascular conditions (see Chapter 36)	The severity of retinopathy may not parallel the severity of diabetes or vascular disease but does suggest concomitant nephropathy.
Roth's spots	Bacterial endocarditis	Hemorrhage with a white center near the optic disc

Continued

Table 4-2	*General Examination—cont'd*

Finding	Condition	Associated Findings, Comment
SKIN AND EXTREMITIES		
Central cyanosis	Intracardiac or intrapulmonary right-to-left shunting	Involves the entire body, including conjunctiva and mucous membranes. Clubbing is common.
Peripheral cyanosis	Reduced peripheral blood flow (with heart failure or peripheral vascular disease)	Cyanosis is restricted to areas of poor blood flow (e.g., ends of extremities in a patient with low cardiac output).
Differential cyanosis	Patent ductus arteriosus with pulmonary hypertension	Hands and fingers are pink (especially on the right), and cyanosis is limited to feet and toes.
Clubbing of fingers and toes	Cyanotic congenital heart disease (see Chapter 30); pulmonary disease with hypoxemia; also may complicate bacterial endocarditis and ulcerative colitis.	Usually follows central cyanosis by 2 to 3 years; may develop within weeks of endocarditis.
Jaundice	Right heart failure, often advanced; also may occur with pulmonary infarction.	Consider *constrictive pericarditis* when evaluation "cryptogenic" liver disease.
Xanthoma	Hyperlipidemia (see Chapter 12)	The pattern may point to the lipid pattern: tendons, high cholesterol; eruptive, high triglycerides.
Osler's nodes	Bacterial endocarditis	Tender, purplish, or erythematous, often at the tips of digits; infected microemboli
Janeway lesions	Bacterial endocarditis	Nontender, raised hemorrhagic lesions, palms of hands and feet
Petechiae and splinter hemorrhages	Bacterial endocarditis	Microemboli; when petechiae occur in nailbeds, they are called *splinter hemorrhages.* Seek them in conjunctiva and mucous membranes as well.
Telangiectasia, hereditary hemorrhagic	Also called Osler-Weber-Rendu disease	Lesions look like the spider angioma of cirrhosis. When present in the lung they represent pulmonary arteriovenous fistula and may cause central cyanosis.

dominojugular reflux, and assessment of the venous waveform.

Venous Pressure

The sternal angle, or angle of Lewis, is 5 cm above the level of the right atrium, regardless of the patient's position. If the top of the distended vein is 3 cm above the sternal angle, right atrial pressure is 8 cm H_2O. Pressure greater than 7 to 8 cm H_2O is abnormal (i.e., a central venous column that is more than 2 to 3 cm above the angle). The patient may be examined in any position, and the optimal angle of inclination depends on the venous pressure. With high pressure, the top of the venous column may not be visible unless the patient is sitting upright. With low pressure, it may be necessary to have the patient lie almost flat to see a distended vein.

To be precise, the venous pressure that reflects right ventricular filling pressure is not at the peak of the venous pulse wave, but at about the midpoint of its total excursion. It thus excludes the bulk of the A wave, created by atrial contraction. In practice, this may be hard to gauge, and the small correction that it represents rarely makes the difference between a normal and an elevated pressure.

In most cases, high venous pressure indicates high right atrial pressure. However, superior vena cava obstruction also causes distention of neck veins. In this case, there is no venous pulsation, as the veins are isolated from the heart. Furthermore, the vein fills from above and not from below.

Abdominal-Jugular Test. With the patient breathing normally (and not holding the breath), push down in the periumbilical area for 10 seconds. In normal individuals, the venous pressure rises less than 3 cm and only transiently. A greater and more sustained rise occurs with *both right and left heart failure* and with tricuspid regurgitation. Although classically proposed as a test for *right heart* failure, an abnormal abdominal-jugular test (AJT) may indicate elevated pulmonary artery wedge pressure in patients with left ventricular dysfunction. A group of patients who had a positive AJT result were found to have elevation of both pulmonary wedge and right atrial pressures[2] (probably because right heart failure usually is caused by left heart failure).

The AJT is especially useful in determining the cause of peripheral edema in the absence of jugular venous distention. If the AJT is negative, heart failure is excluded. The edema must be from some other cause (calcium blocker therapy, venoocclusive disease, low albumen, or lymphatic obstruction).

Jugular Venous Pulse Waveform

No valve separates the right atrium from the superior vena cava and jugular veins. Thus the pressure of atrial contraction is reflected back to the veins, as well as forward through the open tricuspid valve. Venous pressure waves are conveniently labeled: the A wave is generated by atrial contraction, and the V wave by ventricular contraction (Fig. 4-1).

How To Examine the Venous Pulse. I ask the patient to breathe normally while in a position where I can see venous pulsation through the sternocleidomastoid muscle (the internal jugular pulse) or pulsation of the more easily seen external jugular vein. I feel the brachial pulse while watching the vein to distinguish systole from diastole. *If the dominant venous pulse is before the brachial pulse (arterial systole), it is an A wave. If the dominant pulse is simultaneous with the arterial pulse wave, it is a V wave.* On the chart I state what I have observed: "A > V" (a normal examination), or "V < A" (an abnormal finding).

The A wave is the dominant pulse wave in normal individuals (Fig. 4-1). However, in a normal person the A wave may be of such low amplitude that it is not vis-

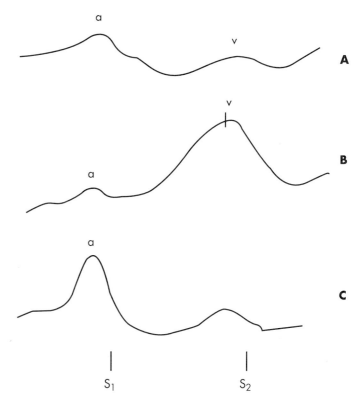

FIG. 4-1
Jugular venous pulse tracings from three patients. **A,** Normal, with A > V. The dominant wave is presystolic, before the brachial pulse. The most obvious finding may be the collapse of the vein after the A wave and simultaneous with ventricular systole (the X descent). **B,** Tricuspid regurgitation, V > A. The dominant wave is systolic (almost simultaneous with the brachial pulse), not presystolic (before the brachial pulse). **C,** Pulmonary hypertension, a giant A wave.

ible. Instead, the most obvious event may be the collapse of the venous column after atrial contraction, at a time of rapid filling of the now-empty atrium. This prominent X descent occurs early during ventricular systole and is a normal finding.

The V wave is created by ventricular systole, by either backward bulging of the tricuspid valve leaflets or slight backward movement of the valve ring during ventricular contraction. The wave is normally quite small.

Tall V Waves and Tricuspid Regurgitation. The diagnosis of tricuspid regurgitation (TR), and distinguishing its holosystolic murmur from the similar murmur of mitral regurgitation, is a particularly important use of the jugular vein examination. With an incompetent tricuspid valve the ventricle is no longer isolated from the atrium and veins during systole, and ventricular systolic pressure is transmitted back to the neck veins (a big V wave; see Fig. 4-1). It is not a subtle finding; it is necessary only to document that the dominant venous pulse wave is systolic (simultaneous with the arterial pulse).

Giant A Waves. Giant A waves are indicators of high right ventricular diastolic pressures (see Fig. 4-1). This may occur with pulmonary hypertension (e.g., the Eisenmenger syndrome, primary pulmonary hypertension, or recurrent pulmonary emboli) or with pulmonic valve stenosis. Tricuspid valve stenosis or atresia is a potential cause, but obstructive disease of the tricuspid valve is rare.

Respiratory Variation and Kussmaul's sign. Venous pressure follows intrathoracic pressure. Thus with inspiration and negative intrathoracic pressure, venous pressure falls. Think of it as blood being sucked into the chest. If there is an increase in right ventricular stiffness (the same as saying "a fall in compliance"), there may be a *rise* in venous pressure during inspiration. This is Kussmaul's sign, and it is present in about half of those with constrictive pericarditis. It usually is not seen with pericardial tamponade.

Right ventricular infarction is another cause of decreased ventricular compliance. An occasional patient has Kussmaul's sign, and many more have no apparent drop in venous pressure with inspiration. Right ventricular infarction should be considered in a patient with inferior infarction who has jugular venous distention with no pulmonary congestion. Pulsus paradoxus above 10 mm Hg also may be present. (Note how similar this may be to pericardial constriction or tamponade.)

Cannon A Waves. *Atrioventricular dissociation* means that atrial contraction may occur at the same time as ventricular contraction. If the atrium contracts when the tricuspid valve is closed, more of the pulse wave is reflected back to the neck veins, creating an unusually tall A wave. The cannon A wave is presystolic (not simultaneous with the arterial pulse) and seems to occur randomly, not with every heartbeat. For example, cannon A waves may indicate ventricular tachycardia in a patient with wide complex tachycardia of uncertain cause.

The Chest and Abdomen

Lungs

Inspection of the chest reveals obvious abnormalities of configuration that may point to underlying heart disease. Advanced obstructive lung disease leads to barrel-shaped deformity and possibly to cor pulmonale. Kyphoscoliosis also may cause cor pulmonale.

Increased respiratory rate and greater effort of breathing may accompany severe pulmonary congestion and obstructive lung disease. Patients with emphysema and hyperexpansion may not have audible rales with congestion; a chest x-ray is necessary for establishing or excluding a diagnosis.

Pleural effusion may be a sign of either right heart or left heart congestion. The pleural space is drained by both the systemic and pulmonary circulations. Physical findings include deviation of the trachea away from the effusion, absence of fremitus (palpable breath sounds),

dullness to percussion, and softer or absent breath sounds. Heart failure is the most common cause of effusion; when it is unilateral, it usually occurs on the right side. An isolated left-sided effusion suggests a noncardiac cause.

Rales, or crackles, may be caused by heart or lung disease. It is common to hear them described as either moist (cardiac) or dry (pulmonary) rales. Concerning fine crackles, I am unconvinced that you can distinguish between the two based only on the quality of the sounds. Perhaps more reliable is the *timing* of rales. With heart failure and early pulmonary congestion, the fine crackles occur late in inspiration ("end-inspiratory rales"), and they are best heard at the bases of the lungs. Pulmonary fibrosis also causes fine crackles, but these rales usually are heard throughout inspiration ("pan-inspiratory rales"). The rales of pulmonary fibrosis may be isolated to the apices of the lungs.

The rales of heart failure are caused by the opening of collapsed airways. In the absence of congestion, there is little airway closure during expiration (Fig. 4-2). Lungs soggy with interstitial congestion have closure of small airways at a higher lung volume than is usual, just because of the weight of the lungs. Thus the airways close during normal expiration. (To use the pulmonary physiology term, there is "elevated closing volume.") With

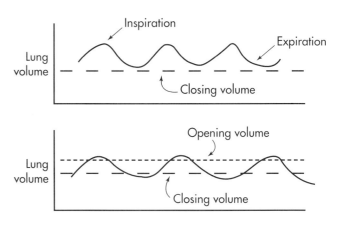

FIG. 4-2

A mechanism for rales in congestive heart failure. In the normal state *(top panel)*, the lung volume at which airways start to collapse, the "closing volume," is not reached during normal expiration. (Perhaps airway closure would occur with marked, forced expiration.) Pulmonary congestion changes this *(bottom panel)*. The water-logged lungs weigh heavily on the airways, and they collapse at a higher lung volume; that is, more airway volume or pressure is needed to keep the airways inflated. Because the threshold for airway collapse has risen, the small airways close during normal expiration. Even greater volume is needed to pop the collapsed airways open, and that happens nearer the end of inspiration. For this reason, the inspiratory crackles of *interstitial* congestion occur at *end*-inspiration.

subsequent inspiration, an even higher lung volume is needed to pop open the collapsed units, and the rales are thus end-inspiratory. Note that the rales are not caused by fluid (or bubbles) in the airways themselves; until gross pulmonary edema occurs, the fluid is interstitial.

Wheezing usually is a sign of airway obstruction. It may develop in a patient with pulmonary congestion ("cardiac asthma"). Occasionally, an acutely ill older patient with wheezing and severe dyspnea may not have audible rales. The absence of a history of asthma points to the cardiac diagnosis, and a chest x-ray readily confirms pulmonary edema.

Abdomen

Like peripheral edema, hepatomegaly is a sign of right heart failure. In acute cases the liver is tender; with chronic congestion, the tenderness resolves. A pulsatile liver is a sign of tricuspid regurgitation. Ascites may develop with chronic congestion, especially when caused by either tricuspid regurgitation or constrictive pericarditis. In such cases splenomegaly also may be present. An abdominal aneurysm is easily palpated in a nonobese patient. At the other end of the spectrum, absence of aortic pulsation may be a sign of coarctation.

CARDIAC EXAMINATION
Apical Impulse

The location of the point of maximum impulse (PMI) must be determined with the patient flat. Its normal location is the midclavicular line and fifth intercostal space. It is tapping in quality and occupies a space no greater than 2 cm. Left ventricular hypertrophy may not displace the PMI, but it becomes more forceful, like a fist hitting your hand. Left ventricular volume overload and dilation cause displacement of the PMI toward the anterior axillary line and enlargement of the apex beat so that it may be felt in more than one interspace. The volume overload apical impulse is diffuse and rocking in quality.

Noninvasive cardiology in the 1970s included recording of the apex cardiogram. Although that test is seldom done in the age of the echocardiogram, evaluation of the apex contour provides valuable physiologic information (and identifies you as a sophisticated bedside examiner). The contour of the apex impulse mirrors that of the ventricular pressure tracing (Fig. 4-3). The most useful finding, and one that can be detected at the bedside with a little practice, is the apical A wave. When the magnitude of the A wave is at least 15% of the total excursion of the PMI, it is palpable. You feel it as a shudder or glitch on the upstroke of the PMI. This corresponds to elevation of the left ventricular end-diastolic pressure and is a more specific finding for abnormal ventricular compliance than the S_4 gallop. You might think of the A wave as a palpable S_4. To demon-

strate this finding to students, hold the end of a drinking straw or pencil against the apex beat. The free end of the straw moves with the apex, amplifying it, and the early systolic shudder is visible. Another method for visualizing the A wave is to draw an "X" on the PMI and then watch its motion with light shining across it.

Detecting an A wave is of more than academic interest. Recently I saw a 48-year-old diabetic man who had no history of hypertension or chest pain. The ECG showed minor T wave changes. There was an equivocal S_4 gallop but a definite apical A wave when he was examined in the left lateral decubitus position. An exercise perfusion scan subsequently was positive, confirming silent ischemia. The apical A wave in the absence of left ventricular hypertrophy was the indication for that study.

Right Ventricular Lift

The right ventricular (RV) lift is felt along the left parasternal area as anterior systolic movement. Both

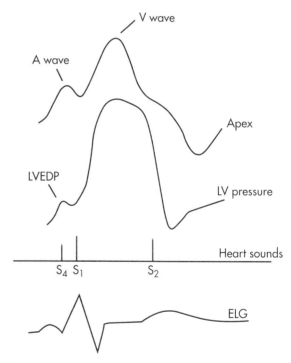

FIG. 4-3
The contour of the apical impulse mirrors the left ventricular pressure tracing. Just before ventricular systole, atrial contraction causes a small rise in left ventricular (LV) pressure, which is measured as the LV end-diastolic pressure (LVEDP). This is elevated in conditions that increase LV stiffness (e.g., ventricular hypertrophy, infiltrative cardiomyopathy, and ischemia). It makes sense; the atrium is kicking into a ventricle that has higher pressure during diastole (it is stiff when it should be relaxed). When the apical A wave is greater than 15% of the total apical excursion, it is palpable as a shudder or glitch on the upstroke of the impulse. This is a reliable indicator of elevated LVEDP and is audible as the S_4 gallop.

pressure overload (pulmonary hypertension or pulmonic stenosis) and volume overload of the RV (right ventricular failure, atrial septal defect, or tricuspid regurgitation) can cause it. When the lift is forceful and sustained, it suggests pressure overload. Volume overload causes a lift that is not sustained through systole.

The parasternal lift may be augmented by left atrial enlargement. The atrium is behind the right ventricle and pushes it forward when enlarged. It is for this reason that a rare patient with severe mitral regurgitation and left atrial enlargement may have a late-systolic parasternal lift in the absence of right ventricular enlargement.

Emphysema changes the position of the heart in the chest. Clockwise rotation occurs, and the left ventricle is more posterior. The heart hangs vertically, a rather dramatic finding on a chest x-ray. The PMI that is felt in the subxiphoid region comes from the right ventricle, not the left. A forceful and sustained apex beat in this position may reflect right ventricular hypertrophy as a result of pulmonary hypertension (cor pulmonale).

Heart Sounds

S_1, the First Heart Sound

The first heart sound is caused by closure of the mitral and tricuspid valves. At the end of diastole, the atria

Table 4-3	Changes in the First Heart Sound (S_1)

Condition	Comment
LOUD FIRST HEART SOUND	
Short PR interval	The valve is wide open at the onset of ventricular contraction (see text); increased excursion to the closed position creates more sound.
Mitral stenosis	A physical finding that appears early in the course of the illness, before the murmur or opening snap
Hyperdynamic states	Hyperthyroidism, fever, anemia, exercise, pregnancy
Thin chest wall	The stethoscope is closer to the valves.
SOFT FIRST HEART SOUND	
Long PR interval	The valve has drifted toward the closed position by the onset of ventricular contraction (see text).
Low flow across the valves	Low cardiac output (heart failure, cardiomyopathy, large myocardial infarction with low output)
Acute aortic regurgitation	High left ventricular end-diastolic pressure causes premature closure of the valve.
Loss of valve mobility; the valve cannot close	Fibrosis or calcification of the valve (the scarred and immobile "fishmouth" valve of advanced mitral stenosis)
Problems of sound transmission	Emphysema, obesity, pericardial effusion, large breasts, thick chest wall
VARIABLE FIRST HEART SOUND	
Atrial fibrillation	
AV dissociation	Varying PR interval
WIDELY SPLIT FIRST HEART SOUND	
Right bundle branch block	
Atrial septal defect	Do not confuse this with fixed splitting of the second sound
Ebstein's abnormality	

contract, producing the last increment of ventricular filling. Ventricular contraction begins, and as soon as ventricular pressure exceeds atrial pressure, the valves close.

Abnormalities of S_1 are outlined in Table 4-3. The intensity of S_1 is determined by the position of the valve leaflets at the onset of ventricular contraction. This explains the effect of the PR interval on S_1. With a short PR, ventricular contraction begins shortly after atrial contraction, and the valve leaflets are wide open. They have a long way to move back into the closed position, and that produces a louder sound. When the PR is long, atrial contraction is well over, and the valves have drifted toward the closed position at the time of ventricular systole. There is less excursion and a softer closing sound.

Diminished excursion of the valve leaflets with low flow (low cardiac output) also explains softer sounds with cardiomyopathy. This is dramatically illustrated on the M-mode echocardiogram; the valves barely seem to open.

Acute aortic regurgitation causes a rise in left ventricular end-diastolic pressure. The pressure may be so high that the mitral valve closes before ventricular systole, and this premature closure leads to a soft or absent S_1. Chronic aortic regurgitation does not cause this elevation of ventricular diastolic pressure and does not change the first heart sound.

Minimal splitting of S_1 is normal. Wide splitting usually is abnormal and may be caused by delayed electrical activation of the right ventricle (right bundle branch block). In atrial septal defect, closure of the tricuspid valve may be delayed as a result of the increased volume of flow through the right atrium and ventricle.

S_2, the Second Heart Sound

Physiologic Splitting. S_2 comes from closure of the aortic and pulmonic valves. During expiration, the aortic and pulmonic components (A_2 and P_2) are simultaneous. With inspiration, negative intrathoracic pressure sucks blood and air into the chest. Blood return to the right ventricle increases. RV ejection time is longer, and pulmonic valve closure is delayed; that is, P_2 moves away from A_2 (Fig. 4-4). In addition, negative intrathoracic pressure tends to pull blood from the RV into the pulmonic bed even after RV contraction (the so-called "hangout" of flow into the pulmonary bed beyond RV contraction). This contributes to the delay in RV emptying.

Conditions that further delay RV emptying or that promote earlier aortic valve closure may cause wider inspiratory splitting of S_2 (Table 4-4).

Fixed Splitting of S_2. Wide splitting of S_2 during both inspiration and expiration is the classical finding of atrial septal defect. Two mechanisms are responsible:

1. Increased pulmonic blood flow further increases pulmonic vascular capacitance, which accentuates the "hangout" of flow beyond RV contraction, fur-

ther delaying P_2. Because capacitance is so increased, there is little incremental increase with inspiration.
2. The increase in flow to the RV from shunted blood delays P_2 so much that the small increase in RV filling with inspiration is masked. In fact, P_2 may move away from A_2 with inspiration, but it is minimal, and the two components of S_2 remain widely split during expiration.

Paradoxical Splitting of S_2. Expiratory splitting of S_2, with a single S_2 during inspiration, is caused by delayed emptying of the left ventricle. The aortic second sound is late (see Fig. 4-4). Timing and movement of P_2 are normal. Because of the late A_2, P_2 moves toward rather

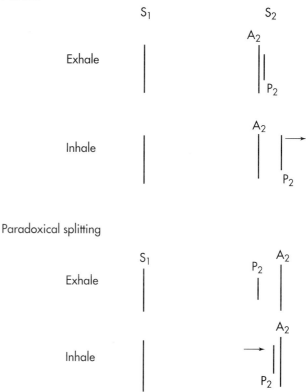

FIG. 4-4
Top panel, Normal splitting of S_2 during inspiration occurs when P_2 moves away from A_2. Increased venous return to the chest with inspiration increases right ventricular (RV) filling, and RV emptying takes longer. *Bottom panel,* A number of conditions delay left ventricular (LV) emptying, including left bundle branch block, valvular aortic stenosis, and hypertrophic subaortic stenosis. When LV emptying is delayed, a delay also occurs in A_2, which is farther from S_1. The position of P_2 relative to S_1 is normal. During inspiration, P_2 moves normally, but now it is going toward A_2 rather than away from it. This expiratory splitting of S_2 is termed *paradoxical.*

| Table 4-4 | *Altered Splitting of S₁* |

Abnormality	Mechanisms	Conditions
Wider inspiratory splitting	1. Delayed onset of right ventricular systole 2. Delayed emptying of right ventricle (RV) 3. Earlier A2	1. Right bundle branch block 2. RV failure, pulmonic stenosis, idiopathic dilation of the pulmonary artery 3. Mitral regurgitation of ventricular septal defect; the "unloaded" ventricle empties earlier
Fixed splitting	Persistent delay of P2 caused by increased capacitance of the pulmonary vascular bed	Atrial septal defect
Paradoxical (expiratory) splitting	Delayed emptying of the left ventricle (LV)	Left bundle branch block (delayed onset of LV systole); outflow tract obstruction from valvular or subaortic stenosis; rarely with severe LV ischemic injury

than away from it with inspiration (see Fig. 4-4). A late A₂ may result from delayed activation of the left ventricle (e.g., left bundle branch block, pacing from the right ventricle, or an ectopic beat originating in the RV) or from prolongation of LV emptying (e.g., aortic stenosis, hypertrophic subaortic stenosis, a rare patient with coronary disease and severe LV injury). We have seen a patient with paradoxical splitting of S₂ during an episode of chest pain; the ECG documented transient left bundle branch block.

Intensity of A₂ and P₂. The aortic second sound usually is louder than P₂, which is normally heard only over the pulmonic area (Fig. 4-5). When P₂ is audible to the right of the sternum, it is abnormally loud. A loud P₂ may indicate pulmonary hypertension, which also may cause loss of normal inspiratory splitting of S₂.

A₂ may be louder with systemic hypertension or with dilation of the aortic root. An especially useful finding is the soft or absent A₂ that occurs with calcific aortic stenosis in elderly patients. The rigid valve eventually stops moving, and A₂ disappears. To elicit this finding, listen in both the pulmonic and aortic areas. P₂ is audible at the left sternal border, but no second sound can be heard at the right base. An absent A₂ indicates a significant reduction in valve area.

"Extra" Heart Sounds

Extra sounds may occur during systole or diastole (Fig. 4-6).

Gallops. Gallops are low-pitched sounds. The best way to hear a soft gallop is to concentrate on the segment of the cardiac cycle where it should be found. For example, to hear an S₃, listen to the space just after S₂, ignoring all other cardiac sounds. Ask yourself, "Is there

anything there?" If there is, you probably are hearing a gallop. If you are convinced there is no sound in that space, then there is no gallop.

Both of the left ventricular gallops are best heard at the apex. They are soft and may be more audible while the patient is on his or her left side. The room must be quiet; hearing gallops requires optimal conditions. Since the sounds are low pitched, use the bell of the stethoscope, taking care not to press too firmly (which would, by tensing the underlying skin, make it work like the diaphragm). The S₃ may be localized, and you must carefully survey the apex and areas close to it. It may be difficult to hear gallops in a patient with a thick chest wall. In such cases, the S₄ may be easier to hear over the sternum (bone conduction providing an aid). The timing of gallops is easier to ascertain by placing a hand on the brachial pulse to identify systole. The S₄ is a presystolic sound, and the S₃ an early diastolic ("protodiastolic") sound.

Think for a moment about the significance of gallops and the quality of the apical impulse. They are physical findings that provide direct information about the state of the ventricles. Murmurs receive a lot of attention, but they indicate little about the severity of disease. The gallops do just that: they tell us about ventricular size, function, and compliance.

S₃ Gallop: Big, Flabby Ventricle ("Volume" Overload). Low-pitched vibration in early diastole comes from the rapid filling wave in early diastole hitting a dilated ventricle. The mechanism is related to (1) high volume flow and (2) the recipient ventricle being dilated and compliant. Any condition that causes ventricular dilation and low cardiac output (with compensatory volume overload) may cause an S₃. It is the hallmark finding of

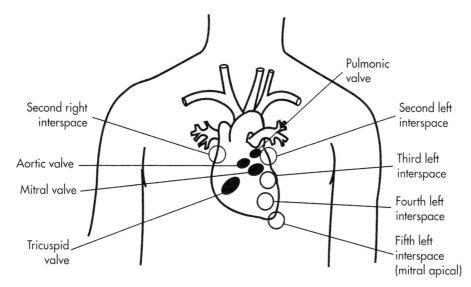

FIG. 4-5
Position of the heart valves and auscultatory regions. Although positioned behind the sternum, forward flow across the aortic valve is "aimed" at the right side of the sternum, and the "aortic area" is the second right interspace. Conversely, the jet of aortic regurgitation is "aimed" at the apex of the heart and is best heard at the mid and lower left sternal border. Pulmonic valve sounds and murmurs are heard in the second left interspace at the left sternal border, the "pulmonic area." Mitral valve sounds and murmurs usually are loudest at the apex. The tricuspid regurgitant murmur is heard near the lower left sternal border.

From Canobbio MM: *Cardiovascular disorders*, St Louis, 1990, Mosby.

cardiomyopathy. When an S_3 develops after myocardial infarction, it indicates substantial injury and worse prognosis.

S_4 Gallop: Stiff, Noncompliant Ventricle ("Pressure" Overload). This gallop at the end of diastole corresponds to elevation of ventricular end-diastolic pressure and the A wave of the precordial impulse (see Fig. 4-3). It may be called the "atrial gallop," since atrial contraction pushing the last increment of blood into a stiff ventricle generates the sound. The S_4 is absent when there is no atrial kick (e.g., atrial fibrillation, ventricular pacing, nodal or ventricular rhythms, or complete heart block). Any increase in ventricular stiffness may cause an S_4, including ventricular hypertrophy, infiltrative disease, and ischemia.

As an example of how gallops may clarify pathophysiology, consider the case of mitral regurgitation (MR). *Chronic* MR causes left ventricular dilation; that, plus volume overload, produces an S_3 gallop. *Acute* MR caused by papillary muscle injury causes LV volume overload, but ventricular dilation has had no time to develop. The increased volume pushed into a relatively stiff, inelastic ventricle (relative to the volume load) produces an S_4 and an apical A wave. Which gallop is

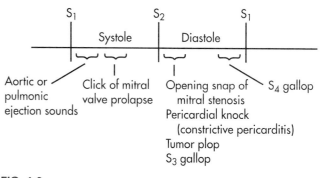

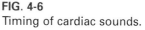

FIG. 4-6
Timing of cardiac sounds.

present indicates the size of the ventricle and thus the duration of valvular dysfunction.

Note that I have referred to "ventricular" rather than "left ventricular." Right ventricular disease may produce gallop sounds, best heard over the left parasternal area. They may be subxiphoid in a patient with obstructive lung disease. RV gallops are augmented by inspiration (increased venous return and flow to the RV). I have had little luck hearing the right-side S_3 gallop; look for it with tricuspid regurgitation and isolated right heart failure. The right-side S_4 that accompanies pulmonary hypertension is easier to hear.

When the heart rate is fast, it may be impossible to determine whether the gallop occurs early or late in diastole. An occasional patient with ventricular dilation also may have increased stiffness and thus have both S_3 and S_4 gallops that are fused when heart rate is elevated. In both cases the patient is said to have a "summation" gallop. A "gallop rhythm" refers to this combination of sounds when the rate is high (it sounds like a galloping horse).

Opening Snap. The opening snap (OS) of mitral stenosis is high pitched, best heard with the diaphragm over the lower left sternal border. Because of its pitch it is rarely confused with the S_3. It bears a fixed relation to S_2 throughout the respiratory cycle, and inspiratory splitting of S_2 heard over the pulmonic area differentiates the OS from P_2. This opening sound indicates that the mitral valve is still mobile; it disappears with advanced calcification and fusion. It accompanies the other findings of mitral stenosis: a loud, snapping S_1 and the diastolic murmur.

The distance between S_2 and the OS is inversely proportional to the severity of stenosis. An S_2-OS interval ≤ 0.10 second indicates severe stenosis. You can estimate this interval with surprising accuracy using an old-fashioned diagnostic trick. The interval between the letters "b" and "t" in "butter" is 0.14 second; between the "b" and "l" in "blah" about 0.10 second. This relationship between the S_2-OS interval and mitral valve area falls apart in elderly patients with systolic hypertension; they have elevated LV systolic pressure that takes longer to fall below left atrial pressure, and opening of the mitral valve is delayed even in the presence of high LA pressure.

Other Diastolic Sounds. Atrial myxoma may produce a sound as it moves on its pedicle through the AV valve. The tumor plop occurs when it comes to a halt on reaching the end of its tether.

A pericardial knock is audible in about half of those with constrictive pericarditis but not with pericardial tamponade. It occurs about 0.12 second after S_2, slightly later than the OS of tight mitral stenosis and slightly earlier than the S_3 gallop, which is 0.14 to 0.16 second after S_2. It is higher pitched than S_3 and usually is audible over the entire precordium. It may get louder with inspiration. It is caused by the sudden halt to cardiac filling that is caused by the rigid pericardium (the column of blood "hits the wall").

Diastolic sounds may be produced by hardware. Mechanical valves in the mitral or tricuspid positions have opening clicks. The movement of the tricuspid valve across a pacemaker lead may cause diastolic clicks or lower frequency sounds that occur at any time during diastole.

Systolic Clicks. Ejection clicks usually are caused by the opening of an abnormal aortic or pulmonic valve and occur just after S_1. Aortic ejection clicks are heard widely over the precordium. Pulmonic clicks are higher pitched and are more localized over the pulmonic area (see Fig. 4-5). An ejection click, even in the absence of a murmur, indicates a need for echocardiography. If the valve is abnormal (e.g., a bicuspid aortic valve), antibiotic prophylaxis for dental procedures is warranted.

Ejection clicks do not always indicate structural abnormalities of the valve. Dilation of either the aorta or pulmonary artery can lead to a click. Hyperdynamic states including thyrotoxicosis, anemia, and pregnancy also can cause aortic ejection clicks.

Midsystolic clicks occur with mitral or tricuspid valve prolapse, are best heard at the apex or lower left sternal border, and may be single or multiple. They are midsystolic or late systolic and therefore are not easily mistaken for ejection clicks. A systolic murmur often follows the click. Although a click may be loud and audible over a wide area, it is more common for the sound to be localized and heard only after a careful search.

Heart Murmurs

Systolic Murmurs

Aortic Stenosis. Valvular aortic stenosis (AS) produces the diamond-shaped ejection murmur that begins after S_1 and ends before S_2 (Table 4-5). As severity of stenosis increases, the length and intensity of the murmur increase, and it may lose its crescendo-decrescendo shape (but it still ends before A_2). The murmur radiates to the carotids, the key finding that distinguishes it from mitral or tricuspid regurgitation. When loud, the AS murmur is audible over the entire precordium. When it radiates to the apex, higher-pitched sounds may predominate, giving it a musical quality (the Gallavardin phenomenon). Because of the different quality of sound, this may be mistaken as a separate murmur.

Peak systolic pressure in the ventricle may vary with cycle length; a longer diastolic filling period increases contractility and stroke volume, as governed by the Starling mechanism (see Chapter 2). Increased venous return has the same effect, and both increase the intensity of the AS murmur (Table 4-6). The pressure generated in the ventricle has less effect on the amount of regurgitation across the mitral valve because the left atrium is a low-pressure chamber; varying cycle length thus has less effect on the murmur of MR. Physiologic maneuvers that change venous return, ventricular size, afterload, and contractility are summarized in Table 4-6.

Recognizing the murmur as AS usually is straightforward. The more difficult task is distinguishing mild from severe AS, and this is what the cardiologist is often asked to do. It is not that difficult with the physical examination: a loud murmur, late peaking, and a palpable

Table 4-5 *Valvular Lesions, Heart Murmurs, and Key Physical Findings*

Conditions	Murmur	Other Physical Findings
SYSTOLIC MURMURS		
Aortic stenosis	*Mild:* crescendo-decrescendo, ends before S2 *Advanced:* later peak, louder, associated thrill; audible at URSB* and radiates to neck	Forceful, pressure overload PMI, S_4 gallop, and palpable apical A wave; delayed carotid upstroke; soft or absent A2 with valve calcification; paradoxical splitting of S_2; ejection click if valve is mobile
Hypertrophic subaortic stenosis	Crescendo-decrescendo; heard at the apex and LLSB; may not radiate to the neck	Pressure overload PMI, S_4 gallop, and apical A wave; increases with lower ventricular volume (strain phase of Valsalva and standing after squatting); paradoxical splitting of S_2 more common than with AS; pulsus bisferiens (two systolic peaks)
Pulmonic stenosis	Crescendo-decrescendo; at the ULSB	Ejection click; murmur increases with inspiration; right ventricular lift; right-side S_4 (that appears or intensifies with inspiration)
Mitral regurgitation	Holosystolic; at the apex and radiating to the axilla or the LSB or base	*Chronic MR:* volume overload, rocking and displaced PMI, S_3 gallop *Acute MR:* nondisplaced PMI, S_4 gallop
Mitral valve prolapse	Mid to late systolic; follows the click; apex or LSB	Young woman or tall, thin patient ("loose jointed"); rest of cardiac examination normal
Tricuspid regurgitation	Holosystolic; at the LLSB	Increases with inspiration (murmur may disappear with expiration); right ventricular lift; right-side S_3 gallop (louder or heard only in inspiration); large V wave on jugular pulse and increased jugular venous pressure; pulsatile liver
DIASTOLIC MURMURS		
Aortic regurgitation (AR)	Early diastolic and decrescendo; at the LSB (a RSB location indicates a dilated aortic root suggesting Marfan syndrome or luetic aortitis)	*Chronic AR:* displaced, volume overload PMI, S_3 gallop; wide pulse pressure, water-hammer pulse, pulsus bisferiens, systolic flushing of nail beds (Quincke's sign), Duroziez's sign (to-and-fro bruit with the stethoscope pressing on the femoral artery) *Acute AR:* peripheral signs of AR but a normal PMI, soft S_1 and S_4 gallop (the LV has not had time to dilate)
Pulmonary regurgitation (Graham Steell's murmur)	Early diastolic, decrescendo; at the LSB	Occurs with pulmonary hypertension; right ventricular lift, loud P2 may be present; classic finding of mitral stenosis and pulmonary hypertension
Mitral stenosis (MS)	Early to mid-diastolic, following the opening snap (OS); a longer murmur = more severe stenosis; low-pitched, soft, and at the apex.	PMI is tapping and in the normal position (left ventricular size is normal); no gallop; opening snap is 0.08-0.12 second after S_2; S_2-OS interval <0.10 second indicates severe stenosis
Austin Flint murmur	Presystolic flow murmur across the mitral valve; low pitched and at the apex	Occurs with AR (backward filling of the LV during diastole pushes the mitral leaflets to a semiclosed position; atrial contraction creates the flow murmur)
Tricuspid stenosis (TS)	Diamond shaped and late diastolic (occurs during right atrial contraction); at the LSB	Murmur increases with inspiration

*Common shorthand for the location of murmurs or sounds: *SB,* Sternal border; *L,* left; *R,* right; *LL,* lower left; *LR,* lower right; *UL,* upper left; *UR,* upper right.

| Table 4-6 | *Effect of Physiologic Maneuvers on Heart Sounds and Murmurs* |

Maneuver	Action	Change in Cardiac Examination
Inspiration	1. Increased venous return to the heart 2. Increased right ventricular stroke volume	*1. *Increase:* murmur of tricuspid stenosis, right-sided S_3 and S_4 2. *Increase:* murmurs of TR (Carvallo's sign) and PS and the pulmonic ejection click (but not an aortic ejection click)
Passive leg raising	Increased venous return; within three to five beats, ventricular size and both RV and LV stroke volume increase	*Increase:* murmurs of TS, TR, and PS and AS. *Decrease:* murmur of hypertrophic subaortic stenosis
Squatting	1. Increased venous return (compression of veins and legs and abdomen). 2. Increased arterial resistance (afterload).	*1. Changes similar to passive leg raising 2. *Increase:* the murmur of AR
Standing after squatting	1. Decreased venous return 2. Decrease LV volume 3. Decreased stroke volume.	*Increase:* murmur of hypertrophic subaortic stenosis (2)*. *Decrease:* murmur of valvular AS, PS (3*). Both S_3 and S_4 may soften (1*). The murmur of PDA may disappear with standing. *Mitral prolapse:* earlier click and longer murmur (2*). The murmur may intensify and change quality.
Strain phase of the Valsalva maneuver	Decrease in venous return LV size, and stroke volume (similar to standing after squatting)	*Increase:* murmur of hypertrophic subaortic stenosis. *Decrease:* murmurs of PS, AS as well as innocent murmurs (that are due to pulmonic flow).
Isometric hand grip (for 40-50 seconds)	Increases in (1) blood pressure, (2) LV systolic pressure, (3) LV filling pressure, and (4) LV volume	*Increase:* murmur of AR (2*), murmurs of MR and VSD (2*), left-sided S_3 and S_4 (3*) *Decrease:* murmur of hypertrophic subaortic stenosis (4*)
The pause after a premature beat	Increased contractility of the beat after the pause	*Increase:* murmurs of valvular AS and PS and the murmur of hypertrophic subaortic stenosis. *No change:* murmurs of MR or TR.

*This specific change is the result of that action with the same number in column two.

thrill indicate severe AS. When severe, AS causes left ventricular hypertrophy and its associated physical signs (the pressure overload apical impulse, palpable A wave, and S_4 gallop). A heavily calcified valve is less mobile; A_2 softens, then disappears. Late closure of the aortic valve may cause paradoxical splitting of S_2, and delayed emptying of the LV causes slow upstroke of the carotid pulse. On the other hand, an ejection click early in systole usually means that the valve is still mobile and is not a sign of advanced stenosis.

A patient with a soft ejection murmur that radiates to the neck, normal A_2, and no evidence of LVH on examination may be said to have "aortic valve sclerosis" rather than stenosis.

Hypertrophic Cardiomyopathy with Subaortic Stenosis. Asymmetric septal hypertrophy (ASH) obstructs flow through the outflow tract of the left ventricle, before the aortic valve. It is also known as *idiopathic hypertrophic subaortic stenosis* (IHSS) and *hypertrophic obstructive cardiomyopathy* (HOCM). The murmur of ASH is diamond shaped. It is heard at the apex and lower left sternal border but does not radiate to the neck. It may radiate to the axilla (a component of the murmur is caused by mitral regurgitation). Because of the pattern of radiation, it is more common to confuse the murmur of subaortic stenosis with MR than with AS. Associated physical findings are important in differentiating the two (see Table 4-5). Paradoxical splitting of S_2 is of particular importance, since it is more common with subaortic stenosis than with valvular AS.

Physiologic maneuvers often are the key to the diagnosis. Obstruction is caused by the thick septum crowding into the outflow tract. Anything that reduces ventricular size aggravates the crowding (see Table 4-6) and intensifies the murmur. The two preload-reducing maneuvers I use routinely are the Valsalva and standing after squatting. Venodilators (amyl nitrite or nitroglycerine) lower venous return in an upright patient and intensify the murmur. Increasing contractility (exercise, isoproterenol, postextrasystolic potentiation) also increases the murmur. Raising afterload (alpha-adrenergic stimulation, handgrip, squatting) lowers the systolic pressure difference between the left ventricle and the aorta and decreases the murmurs of both subaortic and valvular stenosis.

Pulmonic Stenosis. An ejection click may be heard, as well as the diamond-shaped systolic murmur over the pulmonic area. The murmur intensifies with increased venous return during inspiration. With advanced disease and failure of the right ventricle, inspiratory augmentation of the murmur may disappear.

Pulmonic flow murmurs are common in the absence of valvular stenosis. The pulmonary artery and valve are the most anterior of cardiac structures and are thus close to the stethoscope. Flow across the pulmonic valve may be audible in children or those with a thin chest wall or chest wall deformities (pectus excavatum). Hyperdynamic circulatory states (e.g., thyrotoxicosis, anemia, fever, and pregnancy) may produce audible flow. Increased flow and a pulmonary ejection murmur are characteristic of atrial septal defect and anomalous pulmonary venous return.

Innocent Systolic Murmurs. Common in children and occasionally heard in thin adults, innocent systolic murmurs usually are caused by flow across the pulmonic valve. The absence of an ejection click excludes valvular PS, and normal splitting of S_2 excludes ASD. The innocent murmur usually is soft and is early to midsystolic.

Infundibular Pulmonic Stenosis. Stenosis of the pulmonary outflow tract occurs with tetralogy of Fallot. There is no pulmonic valve ejection click, and P_2 is soft or absent. As outflow tract stenosis becomes severe, more blood is shunted across the ventricular septal defect, causing cyanotic spells. Increased ventricular size reduces infundibular stenosis, much like it does on the left side with hypertrophic subaortic stenosis. In fact, both conditions are treated with beta-blockers that reduce contractility and increase ventricular size.

Mitral Regurgitation. Chronic mitral regurgitation (MR) causes a holosystolic murmur, beginning with the first heart sound and ending with A_2. There is left ventricular volume overload and dilation, producing the

characteristic apical impulse and S_3 gallop. The murmur of rheumatic MR is heard at the apex and radiates to the axilla; the fused mitral leaflets form a fish-mouth-shaped structure that is aimed at the axilla. MR caused by papillary muscle dysfunction may not have this classic pattern of radiation. When the posterior leaflet prolapses, it functions as a baffle, and the regurgitant jet is aimed at the septum. The murmur radiates along the left sternal border and possibly to the base of the heart. As papillary dysfunction worsens with peak contractility, the murmur may even have a diamond shape and can be mistaken for AS. It does not, however, radiate to the neck, and the remainder of the physical examination is inconsistent with pressure overload (e.g., forceful PMI, apical A wave, S_4 gallop) or delayed LV emptying (e.g., slow carotid upstroke and paradoxical splitting of S_2).

Acute MR may present an even more confusing picture. The murmur may not radiate to the axilla (again, the baffle effect of a dysfunctional leaflet). Because MR is acute, the ventricle has not had time to dilate, so there may not be an S_3 gallop. Instead, the larger volume of blood pushed into a relatively nondistensible ventricle by atrial contraction may cause an S_4. The high pressure in the normal-sized and nondistensible left atrium may cause the murmur to soften at the end of systole so that it ends before S_2. Valvular AS is excluded because the murmur does not radiate to the neck and the PMI is less forceful. IHSS is excluded by the absence of paradoxical splitting of S_2 and by the use of physiologic maneuvers (see Tables 4-5 and 4-6).

Mitral Valve Prolapse. Midsystolic and late systolic murmurs are caused by mitral and, less commonly, tricuspid valve prolapse. They usually are soft and are heard at the apex or lower left sternal border. There may or may not be an associated midsystolic click just before the murmur. Maneuvers that reduce ventricular size accentuate the degree of mitral and tricuspid prolapse; this moves the click closer to S_1 and lengthens the murmur, although it may be softer. The murmur of tricuspid valve prolapse increases in intensity with inspiration, but it may be shorter as the RV is larger.

An occasional patient with mitral or tricuspid prolapse has a loud, musical, whooping or honking murmur. The timing of the murmur is the same (mid or late systolic), and the musical quality may vary from one day to the next. Most musical sounds that are mid or late systolic are caused by prolapse (think of it as vibrating strings).

Tricuspid Regurgitation. Tricuspid regurgitation (TR) is heard at the lower left sternal border, and it may radiate to the right sternal border. The key to differentiating it from the murmur of MR is its increase with inspiration and the presence of associated physical findings (e.g., peripheral edema, swollen liver, jugular venous V wave, and RV lift; see Table 4-5). Drug addicts with tricuspid endocarditis may not have an audible murmur during expiration. Listen carefully throughout the respiratory cycle when you suspect TR. When TR is acute, an S_4 gallop may occur during inspiration (analogous to the S_4 of acute MR). I have had poor luck hearing an inspiratory S_3 with chronic TR, although it is described by physical diagnosis texts.

Ventricular Septal Defect. When small, the velocity of flow across a ventricular septal defect (VSD) is high, the murmur is loud, and there is an associated thrill ("maladie de Roger"). The actual shunt volume is small. A larger VSD has a bigger shunt volume but a lower flow velocity and therefore a softer murmur. Increased flow through the pulmonary bed provokes an increase in vascular resistance until left-to-right shunting stops (Eisenmenger's syndrome). The VSD no longer makes noise, and the soft pulmonic flow murmur of pulmonary hypertension may be present.

Diastolic Murmurs

Mitral Stenosis. The murmur is soft, located at the apex, and may be heard only with the patient in the lateral decubitus position. Because of its low pitch, listen with the bell of the stethoscope using a light touch. The opening snap (OS) of the rigid valve occurs early after S_2, and the murmur begins at that time. When stenosis is severe and there is a high pressure gradient between the left atrium and ventricle, the murmur is long, ending with S_1. It is useful to note the length of the murmur in a patient with atrial fibrillation and variable cycle length. A murmur that lasts to S_1 even during long cycles indicates severe stenosis. Presystolic accentuation of the murmur is caused by atrial contraction in those who are in sinus rhythm.

Tricuspid Stenosis. Tricuspid stenosis (TS) usually occurs in patients with mitral stenosis and is uncommon. Its murmur is distinguished from that caused by MS by location (right sternal border rather than apex) and by inspiratory increase (see Table 4-6).

Aortic Regurgitation. The murmur begins at A_2 and has a decrescendo, blowing quality. The jet is aimed at the left sternal border, which is where soft AR murmurs are best heard. Have the patient sit up, lean forward, exhale, and stop breathing. This brings the aortic valve close to the stethoscope and makes it possible to hear the soft, decrescendo blow. More severe AR causes a longer and louder murmur.

The murmur is usually blowing in quality. A musical quality, the cooing dove diastolic murmur, indicates perforation or rupture of a valve leaflet. The common causes are endocarditis or trauma.

The location of the murmur is useful in defining pathophysiology. When the murmur is well heard at the *right* sternal border, the aortic root and coronary sinuses are dilated (Harvey's sign). This is the classical finding

of AR caused by Marfan's syndrome, but it also may develop with a number of other conditions that cause dilation of the aortic root (see Chapter 19).

Acute AR caused by acute bacterial endocarditis or dissection sounds and feels different, primarily because the previously normal left ventricle has not had time to dilate. LV stiffness and diastolic pressure are high relative to the large volume of blood it must handle, causing an S_4 gallop (rather than the S_3 you would expect with the dilated, compliant LV of chronic volume overload). In many cases the valve is essentially destroyed, and nothing separates the aorta and LV during diastole; diastolic pressures are equal. Equalization of the pressures occurs early in diastole, and at that point backward flow across the valve stops. *The murmur may be short or nonexistent.* As noted earlier, high LV diastolic pressure pushes the mitral leaflets together, closing them before the end of diastole; S_1 disappears.

Thus the findings that may indicate acute AR include wide pulse pressure, absent S_1, hemodynamic instability, or pulmonary edema and a relatively normal heart size—*but no murmur.* The clinical setting is important (endocarditis, trauma, dissection of the aorta).

Austin Flint Murmur. This diastolic flow murmur across the mitral valve occurs in patients with moderate to severe aortic regurgitation. Dr. Flint described it as "blubbering" in quality. It is usually low pitched and presystolic (during atrial contraction) and is heard only at the apex. This, like many other cardiac findings, usually is missed because the examiner does not look for it. Listen for it in the patient with AR, and you will impress your colleagues.

The mitral valve is structurally normal. Backward filling of the left ventricle from the aorta during diastole pushes the mitral leaflets to a semiclosed position. Atrial systole generates increased flow across the semiclosed valve and creates the noise.

Pulmonic Regurgitation. This is also known as the *Graham Steell murmur.* It occurs with pulmonary hypertension and has quality, location, and timing similar to that of mild AR (early diastolic, decrescendo blowing murmur at the upper left sternal border). The association with pulmonary hypertension helps with the diagnosis, but an echocardiogram often is needed to be sure.

Continuous Murmurs

Continuous murmurs have a variety of causes (Table 4-7). Most of the murmurs end in diastole, before S_1. A murmur is considered "continuous" if it begins in systole and continues through S_2 and into diastole. They must be differentiated from "to-and-fro" murmurs; the most common of these is the combination of aortic stenosis and regurgitation, in which there is a clear break in the murmur at S_2.

Table 4-7	*Continuous Murmurs*
Condition	**Comment**
Patent ductus arteriosus (PDA)	Murmur at the ULSB; pitch varies with the caliber of the defect; it peaks at around S_2 (which it envelops) and tails off in diastole; a rough or machinery-like quality; diastolic component augmented by handgrip (increased blood pressure)
Arteriovenous (AV) fistula	A variety of locations: coronary AV fistula, anomalous origin of coronary artery from the pulmonary artery, coronary artery to right atrium or ventricle shunt, pulmonary AV fistula, AV shunts created for dialysis
Rupture of a congenital aneurysm of a sinus of Valsalva (the cusps or "sinuses" formed at the base of the aorta by the valve leaflets)	The aneurysm usually involves the right coronary sinus; rupture creates an AV fistula between the aorta and the RV (5%-15% are from the posterior cusp to the RA); murmur along the left or right lower sternal border with accentuation in diastole; often a thrill; chest pain may mark the time of the dissection
Coarctation of the aorta	Murmur may be continuous with high-grade stenosis; possible intercostal thrills or bruits (collateral vessel flow), and development of the upper body > lower body
Venous murmurs (hums)	Caused by increased flow and disappear with local pressure; louder in hyperdynamic states (anemia, thyrotoxicosis, fever, pregnancy, and so on)

Since continuous murmurs are not broken up by the cardiac cycle, it makes sense that they originate in blood vessels rather than the heart. A venous hum is caused by high flow rather than stenosis of the vein and may disappear with local pressure (over the neck with a cervical hum, over the epigastric area with an hepatic venous hum, or in other areas with increased pressure with the stethoscope).

The murmur of patent ductus arteriosus usually is heard over the pulmonic area. When it is lower, in the third interspace, it may be confused with the murmur of coronary arteriovenous fistula. A small ductus causes a high-pitched murmur; with larger defects, the pitch is lower. The murmur may have a "machinery-like" quality.

Pericardial Friction Rub

The typical rub has three phases: mid-diastolic, presystolic, and midsystolic. The diagnosis is obvious when you hear three components, although many patients have a rub that is heard only during systole. The presystolic phase is created by atrial contraction and disappears with atrial fibrillation. The sound is scratchy and superficial, "close to the stethoscope." It may vary with position, often louder with the patient leaning forward and during exhalation, or even while on elbows and knees. The rub caused by movement of visceral against parietal pericardium may disappear with the accumulation of fluid that separates them. Thus the absence of a rub does not exclude pericarditis.

A pericardial rub is common after heart surgery. It must be distinguished from Hamman's sign, a crunch-like sound caused by air in the mediastinum (which also may be caused by esophageal rupture).

REFERENCES

1. Levine B, Kalman J, Mayer L, et al: Elevated levels of tumor necrosis factor in severe chronic heart failure, *N Engl J Med* 323:236, 1990.
2. Butman SM, Ewy GA, Standen JR, et al: Bedside cardiovascular exam in patients with severe chronic heart failure: importance of resting or inducible jugular venous distension, *J Am Coll Cardiol* 22:968, 1993.

BIBLIOGRAPHY

Seidel HM, Ball JW, Dains JE, Benedict GW: *Mosby's guide to physical examination*, St Louis, 1995, Mosby. A good review with excellent graphics that help with understanding the pathophysiology of physical findings.

Shapiro LM, Fox KM: *Color atlas of physical signs in cardiovascular disease*, London, 1989, Mosby. In addition to good photographs of skin and retinal lesions, there is a great collection of phonocardiograms and apex, arterial, and jugular venous pulse tracings (a good source of teaching materials).

5 Electrocardiogram

George J. Taylor
Brent G. Petty

BASIC PRINCIPLES
Voltage, Time, and Sequence of Cardiac Activation

The electrocardiogram (ECG) is a voltmeter that measures the small electrical current generated by depolarization of heart muscle. More voltage is generated when a thick portion of muscle is depolarized (the ventricle) than when a thinner, smaller segment is depolarized (the atrium). The vertical, or y axis, on the ECG tracing is voltage, and each millimeter (mm) of paper equals 0.1 millivolt (mV) when recorded at normal standard (10 mm/mV). In daily use, we often refer to the amplitude, or height, of an ECG complex in millimeters of paper rather than in millivolts.

Voltage may have a negative (below the baseline) or positive (above the baseline) value. While the wave of depolarization moves through the heart in three dimensions, each ECG lead records it in just one dimension, between two poles. Having 12 leads grouped in frontal and horizontal planes allows us to conceive of the electrical events in three dimensions (Fig. 5-1). Think of it as looking at the wave of depolarization from 12 different angles.

When the wave of depolarization is moving toward the positive pole of a lead, the deflection is upright, or positive. Moving away from the positive pole causes a downward, or negative, deflection. The general direction of the wave of depolarization, the orientation of its vector in space, is referred to as the *electrical axis*. Methods for rapidly estimating axis are reviewed in all of the basic ECG manuals.

The ECG records the voltage generated by depolarization of the different regions of the heart in sequence and through time. The sequence of cardiac activation is summarized in Figure 5-2. The horizontal axis (x axis) of the ECG is time. Each millimeter of paper equals 0.04 second, and each large square, or 5 mm, equals 0.2 second when the ECG is recorded at the usual paper speed of 25 mm/sec. One way to calculate heart rate is to measure the distance (that is, the time) between two R waves. This *RR interval* is the time of one complete cardiac cycle, or heartbeat. If the RR interval is 5 large squares, or 1 second, then the rate is 60 beats/min. If the RR interval is 4 squares, or 0.8 second, then the rate is 60 beats/min divided by 0.8 sec/beat, or 75 beats/min. A rough estimate of heart rate is 300 / RR interval in number of large squares (3 squares = 100/min; 4 squares = 75; 5 squares = 60, and so on).

Intervals

Drugs and conditions that affect intervals are summarized in Table 5-1.

PR interval (Normal Range, 0.12 to 0.22 Second)

The PR interval (Fig. 5-2) includes atrial activation, or the P wave, plus the delay of the wave of depolarization in the AV node before ventricular activation. It is prolonged if there is slowed conduction in the AV node. It also may be long if there is slow conduction in the His-Purkinje system below the AV node. A delay of atrial activation, with a broad P wave, could conceivably lengthen the PR interval, but this is not recognized in clinical practice.

QRS Duration (Normal, <0.12 Second)

The QRS duration is the time it takes to depolarize the two ventricles. Normally, when current exits the AV node and the bundle of His, it moves simultaneously through the infranodal bundle branches (see Figs. 5-2 and 5-10). The ventricles are activated at the same time. When impaired conduction causes a delay in activating one of the ventricles, the QRS duration is longer.

QT Interval

Repolarization, or the return of muscle to its resting state, spontaneously follows depolarization of heart muscle. Repolarization of the thin-walled atria produces no apparent deflection on the surface ECG; the current generated is buried in the QRS complex. Repolarization of the thicker ventricles produces the T wave. It generally has the same axis as the QRS complex. That is, when the QRS complex is upright (positive) in a given ECG limb lead, usually the T wave also is upright.

Repolarization of an individual muscle cell takes just a few milliseconds, but the T wave is broad be-

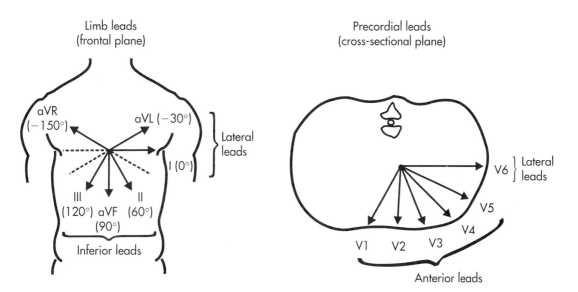

FIG. 5-1

Orientation of the 12 ECG leads, organized in frontal and cross-sectional planes. The positive pole of each lead is indicated by the arrowhead. The general direction of the wave of depolarization through the myocardium is called the *electrical axis;* the ECG deflection would be strongly positive in the limb leads that are aligned in the same direction. Thus a wave moving at 60 degrees below horizontal would be most strongly positive in lead II (negative in aVR and possibly isoelectric in aVL). The limb lead where the QRS is most positive provides a rough estimate of the QRS axis in the frontal plane.

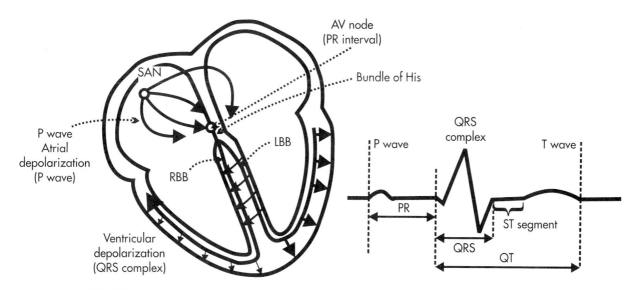

FIG. 5-2

Sequence of cardiac activation and components of the normal ECG complex. (The sequence of activation is reviewed in Chapter 2.) The sinoatrial node *(SAN)* is the usual cardiac pacemaker. Depolarization of the atria is rapid. The current is delayed in the atrioventricular *(AV)* node, accounting for most of the PR interval of the ECG. The wave of excitation then moves through the two bundle branches (*RBB* and *LBB*), and the left and right ventricles depolarize simultaneously.

Table 5-1	Alterations in Intervals	
Interval	**Cardiac and Noncardiac Conditions**	**Metabolic Abnormality or Drug**
Prolonged PR (>0.22 sec*)	First degree (1°) AV block, inferior myocardial infarction, increased vagal tone	Digoxin, beta-blockers, calcium channel blockers (verapamil and diltiazem; see Table 13-11), adenosine, and dipyridamole
Short PR (<0.12 sec)	Preexcitation syndromes	
Prolonged QRS (>0.12 sec*)	Bundle branch block and other ventricular conduction abnormalities, preexcitation	Flecainide, propafenone, quinidine, and other antiarrhythmics; hyperkalemia
QT QTc (≥0.45 sec*)	Long QT syndrome, myocardial ischemia, hypothermia, intracranial bleeding	Quinidine, procainamide, disopyramide, sotalol, amiodarone, phenothiazine and its derivatives, erythromycin; hypokalemia, hypomagnesemia, hypocalcemia

*Top normal value.

cause it reflects repolarization of the large population of cardiac cells, some of which repolarize early and others much later. The T wave looks like a bell-shaped curve (see Fig. 5-2); in some ways it is, with the average cell repolarizing at the peak of the T wave. A broader T wave indicates temporal dispersion of repolarization ("temporal dispersion" is electrophysiology technospeak for "takes longer"). A broader wave just means that time, measured along the x axis of the ECG, is longer.

All this is clinically important, since increased heterogeneity of repolarization underlies the pathogenesis of serious cardiac arrhythmias (see Chapters 26 and 27). A long QT interval may identify the patient at risk for ventricular arrhythmias and sudden death. The normal duration of the QT interval varies with heart rate. The corrected QT (QTc) is calculated using Bazett's formula:

$$QTc = \frac{QT}{\sqrt{R\text{-}R}}$$

Thus when the RR interval is 1 second (and the heart rate is 60 beats/min), the QTc = QT. At higher heart rates, when the RR is less than 1 second, the QTc > QT. ECG manuals may provide a table that gives the normal QT for a given heart rate, based on Bazett's formula. The top-normal QTc varies with age and sex, but in general, QTc is <0.45 second.

There is a quick and easy way to estimate whether the QT interval is normal. When the interval is less than half the RR interval, it is probably normal for that heart rate. At higher heart rates, this method of estimation is less reliable (as is Bazett's formula), and there is a tendency to overdiagnose QT prolongation.

A second hump, called the U wave, may occur after the T wave. This is a part of ventricular repolarization, and it may be a normal finding. Hypokalemia, especially in combination with hypomagnesemia, can increase U wave amplitude and prolong the QTU interval, but easily discernible U waves may be present as a normal variant without any electrolyte abnormality.

Where To Measure Intervals

A common question is which lead to use. It is preferable to use limb leads, since the normal ranges for intervals were determined using the limb leads. The sensitivity of particular leads for recording P, QRS, or T waves may vary slightly, and the lead that is most sensitive varies from patient to patient. Use the limb lead that records whatever wave that you are measuring most clearly and in which the interval is the longest. For example, if the PR interval is obviously prolonged in a couple of leads but is not as well seen or looks shorter in others, you have still identified prolonged AV conduction.

THE CARDIAC RHYTHM

Normal sinus rhythm is a regular rhythm between 60 and 100 beats/min, with a P wave before each QRS complex and a QRS after each P wave. A faster rate defines *tachycardia*, and a slower rate, *bradycardia*. The term *sinus* indicates that the rhythm originates in the sinoatrial (SA) node, that there is atrial depolarization (with a P wave before each QRS), and that atrial contraction precedes ventricular contraction. Disturbances in the normal cardiac rhythm are reviewed in Chapters 25 to 27.

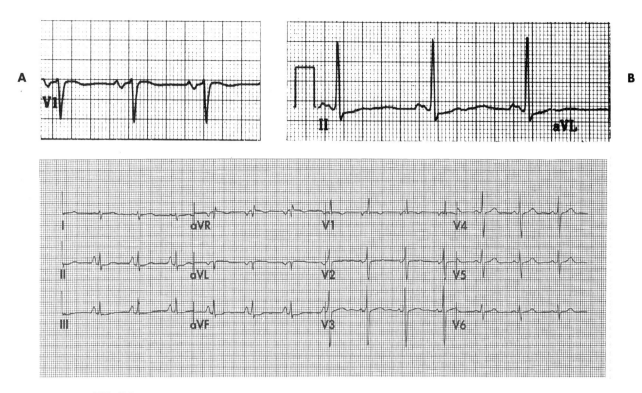

FIG. 5-3
Top panels, Two patterns of left atrial abnormality (LAA). **A,** A biphasic P wave in V₁.
B, Broad, notched P waves in one of the limb leads, usually II, III, or aVF as the P wave
vector is "aimed" in the direction of the inferior leads. *Bottom panel,* Right atrial abnormality (RAA). Tall, peaked P waves in inferior leads (at least 2.5 mm in one of
these leads).

Table 5-2	*Atrial Abnormalities*	
	Common Clinical Conditions	**ECG Morphology**
Left atrial abnormality (LAA)	Hypertensive heart disease, aortic stenosis, hypertropic subaortic stenosis, other causes of left ventricular hypertrophy, mitral stenosis, mitral regurgitation	Either (1) biphasic P wave in V₁, with the terminal, negative deflection at least one box wide and one box deep, or (2) broad, notched P wave in a limb lead, usually lead II. This "P" mitrale pattern is common with mitral disease.
Right atrial abnormality (RAA)	Pulmonary hypertension, pulmonic stenosis, Eisenmenger's syndrome, cor pulmonale	Tall, peaked P waves in limb leads, usually II, II, or aVF (P amplitude ≥2.5 mm)

MORPHOLOGIC CHANGES IN P, QRS, AND ST
Atrial (P Wave) Abnormalities
Left Atrial Abnormality

Left atrial abnormality (LAA) usually occurs with conditions that increase the left ventricular diastolic pressure (recall that the left atrium and ventricle are in open communication during ventricular diastole, when the mitral valve is open). It is common in patients with hypertension and may be the earliest evidence of hypertensive heart disease. Mitral valve stenosis is an example of a condition that may cause LAA without affecting the left ventricle, as the stenosed valve "isolates" the atrium from the ventricle during diastole. The ECG appearance of LAA and associated clinical conditions are summarized in Figure 5-3 and Table 5-2.

Right Atrial Abnormality

Right atrial abnormality (RAA) is the result of conditions that raise right ventricular pressure, most commonly pulmonary artery hypertension (e.g., congenital heart disease or advanced lung disease, so-called P pulmonale). The ECG appearance is reviewed in Figure 5-3 and Table 5-2.

Intraventricular Conduction Abnormalities

Bundle Branch Block

When the wave of depolarization exits the bundle of His, it normally moves down the right and left bundle branches and activates the two ventricles simultaneously. If one of the bundle branches fails to conduct normally, the blocked ventricular region is stimulated *late* by current that has spread from an adjacent ventricular region. Late activation creates a deflection at the terminal end of the QRS complex, making the overall QRS complex wider. A QRS duration of 0.12 second or more (3 mm) is the first diagnostic criterion for bundle branch block.

Right bundle branch block (*RBBB*, Fig. 5-4) results in late activation of the right ventricle, producing a terminal S wave in leads I and V_6 and a terminal R wave in V_1. Early activation of the interventricular septum and left ventricle is unaffected.

Many patients with RBBB have normal left ventricular size and function. In fact, the echocardiogram often shows no structural heart disease despite RBBB.

Left bundle branch block (*LBBB*, Fig. 5-5), in contrast, commonly indicates underlying left ventricular dysfunction. Since the left bundle is a broad structure within the septum and ventricle, it takes more than a small area of injury or fibrosis to impair conduction.

Incomplete RBBB

Incomplete RBBB is diagnosed by an RSR pattern in V_1, just like RBBB, but the QRS duration is shorter (<0.12 second, Fig. 5-6). It may be a normal variant but also may reflect right ventricular (RV) volume overload or hypertrophy. For example, IRBBB is a usual finding with atrial septal defect (ASD), in which the RV may pump two or three times as much blood as the left ventricle. Most people with ASD are asymptomatic, so this finding on a routine ECG should at least provoke a careful physical examination to look for signs of ASD (see Chapter 30).

Hemiblocks

The left bundle has a thin anterior branch, or fascicle, that is located in the ventricular septum close to the right bundle. Blocked conduction causes extreme left axis deviation (axis to the left of −45 degrees). Block of the broader posterior fascicle causes right axis deviation (to the right of +105 degrees). Block of one of the fas-cicles may accompany RBBB (usually the anterior because of its proximity), and this is referred to as *bifascicular block*. By definition, LBBB also is a bifascicular block, because two of the three branches below the common bundle of His are blocked. In common use, however, *bifascicular block* is meant to indicate RBBB plus block of one of the fascicles of the left bundle. It is diagnosed when RBBB is associated with marked axis deviation.

Ventricular Hypertrophy, R Wave Progression, and QRS Voltage

QRS nomenclature is reviewed in Figure 5-7.

Pressure overload in a ventricle is caused by outflow tract obstruction (aortic or pulmonic valve stenosis or subvalvular stenosis) or by increased vascular resistance (systemic or pulmonary artery hypertension). The ventricle responds to pressure overload by adding muscle, just as you would add muscle to your arms with weight lifting. Increased muscle thickness on one side of the heart or the other causes a shift in QRS axis toward the hypertrophied side and an increase in voltage (thicker muscle, more voltage).

The large coronary arteries are located on the epicardial surface of the heart, and they send blood to underlying muscle through small perforating branches. Increased ventricle thickness increases the distance from the epicardial artery to the endocardium. Capillary density is reduced in the subendocardial region when there is hypertrophy. ST depression and T wave inversion develop with hypertrophy, and it is tempting to attribute these changes to "perpetual ischemia," the myocardium "outgrowing its blood supply." That apparently is too simplistic, although relative coronary insufficiency plays some role. The final changes caused by high ventricular diastolic pressures are atrial (P wave) abnormalities.

Left Ventricular Hypertrophy

The Estes criteria for left ventricular hypertrophy (LVH) are summarized in Table 5-3. All of these findings may not be present, and the diagnosis can be made when just some of these features are present (Fig. 5-8). Using multiple diagnostic criteria rather than QRS voltage alone provides better specificity (fewer false positives, less overdiagnosis). The sensitivity of the ECG in detecting LVH is poor; with the Estes point system, echocardiographic and anatomic correlation studies have shown that only about half of the cases of LVH meet ECG diagnostic criteria. Relaxing the criteria by using voltage alone increases sensitivity, but it also increases the number of false positives.

This choice between sensitivity and specificity is common when reading ECGs. We would prefer to avoid overdiagnosis. Young people often have high QRS volt-

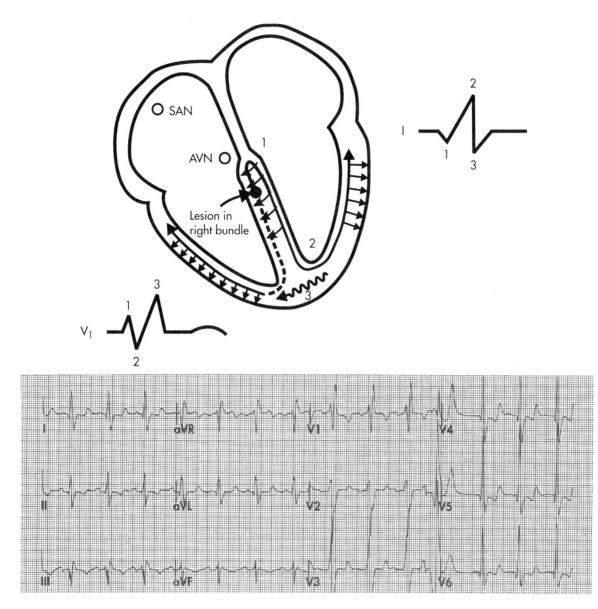

FIG. 5-4

Right bundle branch block (RBBB). The sequence of ventricular activation. *1,* Normal septal activation from left to right. *2,* Normal left ventricular (LV) activation but blocked conduction through the right bundle. *3,* Late activation of the right ventricle (RV), by current that works its way over from the LV. The tail end of the QRS is slurred because of late depolarization of the RV, producing a terminal R wave in V_1 (the lead that overlies the RV). Pattern recognition: wide QRS plus RSR in V_1.

age, and assignment of a diagnosis of LVH may create problems when applying for a job or health insurance. It seems better to adhere to strict diagnostic criteria, recognizing the insensitivity of the ECG.

The intrinsicoid deflection (see Table 5-3) is the time from the beginning of the QRS to its peak and is an approximation of the time it takes to activate the ventricle. This activation takes longer with increased muscle mass.

Right Ventricular Hypertrophy

Normally, most of the voltage in the QRS complex is generated by the left ventricle. This makes the QRS complex in the right-sided precordial leads, V_{1-2}, negative. In left-sided leads, V_{4-6}, the QRS complex is positive. However, the QRS complex changes with right ventricular hypertrophy (RVH), in which right axis deviation is combined with an increase in voltage in the right chest leads and with unusual persistence of S

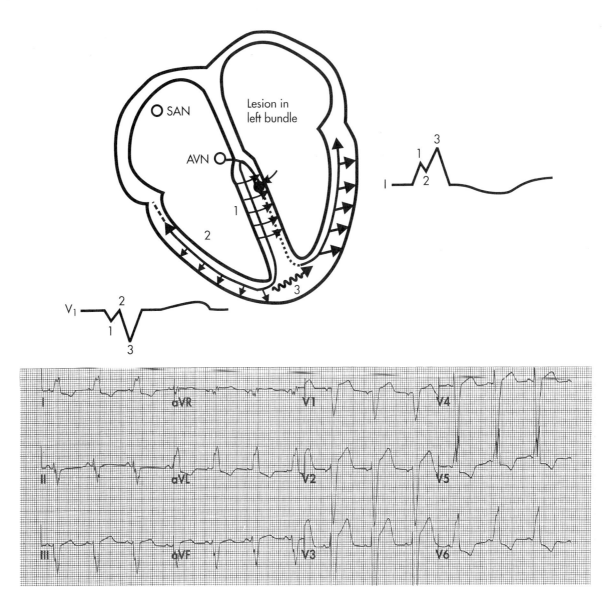

FIG. 5-5
Left bundle branch block (LBBB). The sequence of ventricular activation. *1,* The normal left-to-right activation of the septum is blocked, and the septum is activated from right-to-left. *2,* Depolarization of the thin-walled RV produces little current. *3,* The LV is activated late by current from the RV, and terminal QRS forces are oriented toward the left. Pattern recognition: broad positive complex, possibly notched, in left side leads (I and aVL). Because of the gross distortion of LV activation, it is not possible to diagnose myocardial infarction or left ventricular hypertrophy when there is LBBB.

waves in V_{5-6} (Box 5-1, Fig. 5-9). A tall R in V_1 is the most specific finding for RVH; a deep S in V_6 without a tall R in V_1 is not as reliable.

Delay in R Wave Progression

The QRS normally becomes positive (R waves are taller than S waves) by lead V_4. A persistently negative QRS beyond V_4 is called "poor R wave progression (PRWP)" or "delayed transition" (Fig. 5-10). There are a number of causes.

1. Obstructive lung disease is such a common cause that our computer is programmed to call "PRWP" a "pulmonary pattern." It is probably caused by the position of the heart in the hyperexpanded thorax. On chest x-ray the heart appears to be hanging more vertically, and on physical examination the apical impulse is felt in the subxiphoid region. With this shift in position, the heart rotates clockwise, to the left, so the LV is more posterior and to the left than usual. This causes a delay in R wave transition.

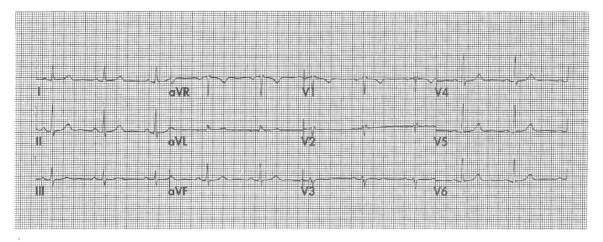

FIG. 5-6
Incomplete right bundle branch block. There is an RSR pattern in V_1, but QRS duration is normal.

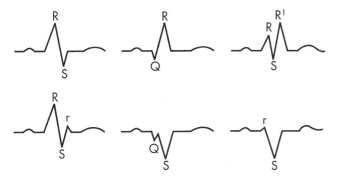

FIG. 5-7
QRS nomenclature. All positive deflections are R waves. A negative deflection at the beginning of the QRS is a Q wave. A negative deflection after an R wave is an S wave. Low voltage deflection may be designated using lower case letters. A second R wave may be called R' (R-prime).

Table 5-3	*The Estes Criteria for Left Ventricular Hypertrophy (LVH)*	

High QRS voltage (any of the following):
    R in V_5 or V_6 ≥30 mm
    S in V_1 or V_2 ≥30 mm
    R or S wave in a limb lead
    ≥20 mm
		3 points

T wave inversion in lateral leads (often with ST depression)
    No digitalis therapy
    On digitalis therapy
		3 points
		1 point

Left axis deviation (at least −30°)		2 points
Left atrial abnormality		3 points
QRS duration ≥ 0.09 second		1 point
Intrinsicoid deflection in V_5 and V_6 ≥0.05 second		1 point
LVH = more than 5 points Probable LVH = 4 points		

2. Left ventricular dilatation, as seen with volume overload (e.g., mitral or aortic regurgitation), also may displace the mass of the LV to the left. The precordial leads may not overlie the body of the LV until position V_5 or V_6, causing a delay in R progression.
3. Anterior MI and a loss of positive forces in anterior leads
4. Left anterior fascicular block (extreme left axis deviation)
5. Misplacement of the chest leads, with V_{1-2} positioned over the left chest

Low QRS Voltage

The diagnostic criterion of low QRS voltage is QRS amplitude < 5 mm in all of the limb (frontal) leads. When this occurs, the amplitude of the QRS in each of the precordial leads usually is less than 10 mm, but this is not necessary for the diagnosis.

Like PRWP, low voltage is a description rather than a diagnosis. Although perhaps a normal finding, low QRS voltage may be seen with dilated or infiltrative cardiomyopathy, pericardial effusion, constrictive pericarditis, hypothyroidism, Addison's disease, emphysema, and obesity. It is nonspecific enough that it is not a diagnostic criterion for any of these conditions, but

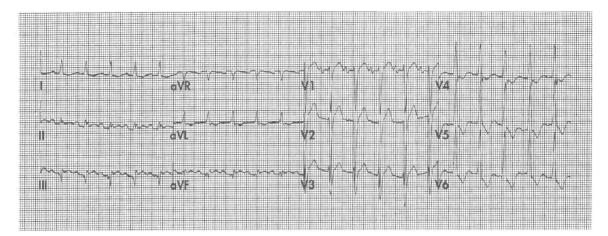

FIG. 5-8

Left ventricular hypertrophy. The S in V_2 is > 30 mm and the QRS axis is −30 degrees (left axis deviation). In addition, there is LAA, the QRS is wide, and there is T inversion in V_{4-6}. That adds up to 12 points on the Estes scale (Table 5-3).

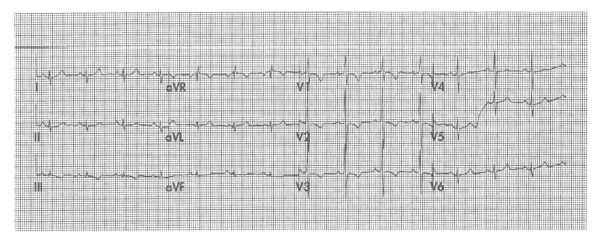

FIG. 5-9

Right ventricular hypertrophy. A tall R in V_1 is present (not quite 7 mm, but R/S is >1, and the sum of the R in V_1 plus the S in V_5 is >11 mm). Supporting the diagnosis are RAA and right axis deviation.

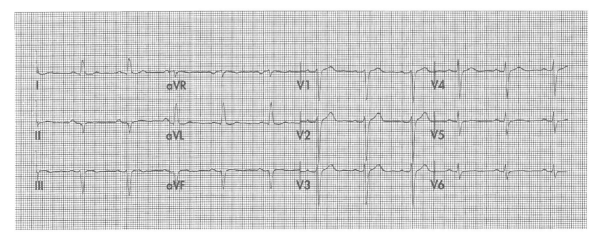

FIG. 5-10

Poor R wave progression. The QRS remains negative in lead V_4. "Transition" from a net negative to a positive complex normally occurs between leads V_3 and V_4.

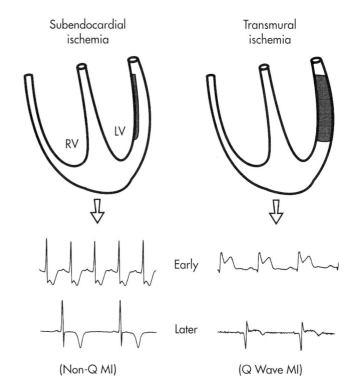

FIG. 5-11
Patterns of myocardial ischemia. The epicardium is the outside surface of the heart, and the endocardium is the surface adjacent to the ventricular cavity. Subendocardial, nontransmural ischemia causes ST segment depression. This resolves with resolution of chest pain. If ischemia persists and injury occurs, T wave inversion develops. Symmetrical T wave inversion is the pattern of nontransmural, or non–Q wave infarction. ST segment elevation occurs promptly with transmural ischemia caused by coronary artery occlusion. Note that ischemia does not equal infarction. If the artery is opened after a brief period of ischemia (relief of spasm or perhaps thrombolysis), the ST elevation resolves before onset of permanent muscle injury. This would be considered an episode of angina pectoris with transmural ischemia. Infarction, or myocardial cell death, occurs if coronary occlusion and ischemia persist. In that case, the evolutionary changes of Q wave infarction develop (also called *transmural infarction*, Table 5-5).

should bring this differential diagnosis to the clinician's attention.

ST Segment and T Wave Changes, Q Waves: Patterns of Ischemia and Infarction

Myocardial ischemia is a regional event (Fig. 5-11). Only one of the major coronary arteries is likely to cause ischemia or infarction at a time. Rarely do multiple branches simultaneously develop stenoses and cause active ischemia. Thus ECG evidence of ischemia is regional (Fig. 5-12). For most patients the anterior descending artery is responsible for anterior changes (the precordial, or V, leads), the circumflex artery for lateral changes (leads I, aVL, and V_6), and the right coronary artery for inferior changes (leads II, III, and aVF).

Anatomic differences among people account for occasional variations in this pattern; also some overlap of vascular regions may occur. Thus occlusion of an unusually large right coronary artery that sends branches to the lateral and the inferior wall might cause "inferolateral" infarction, with ECG changes in the inferior leads plus one or more of the lateral leads. A large anterior descending artery also might have branches to the lateral wall resulting in "anterolateral" ischemia (changes in anterior leads plus one or more of the lateral leads).

ECG changes that are global, involving all the vascular regions, are rarely caused by ischemia. Pericarditis, for example, affects the entire heart and causes ST segment and T wave changes that are global (present in anterior, inferior, and lateral leads).

ST Segment Depression. Patterns of ischemia are illustrated in Figure 5-11. Subendocardial ischemia causes ST segment depression, which is typical for exercise-induced angina (Table 5-4, Fig. 5-13). The ST segments have a check-mark or hockey-stick appearance, and the segments are either horizontal or downsloping (Fig. 5-14). A depressed but upsloping ST segment is not as specific for ischemia. In this case the J point, the junction between the QRS and ST segment, is depressed below the baseline but moves rapidly upward.

Poor specificity is a problem with the diagnosis of subendocardial ischemia based on ST depression. Many conditions may cause it (LVH, digitalis, and hypokalemia among others). It is a common finding in

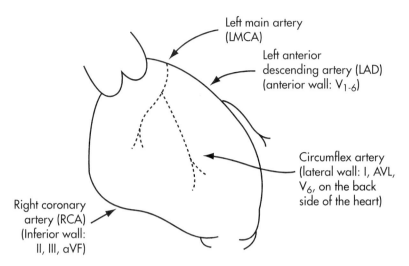

FIG. 5-12
Schematic of the three major coronary branches. The circumflex is drawn as a dashed line, as it circles around the back of the heart. In this view, the LAD and RCA are seen in profile. Occlusion of one of the three branches is responsible for myocardial infarction, and injury is localized to one of the three vascular regions: anterior wall, lateral wall, or inferior wall. An exception to this would be occlusion of the LMCA, resulting in ischemia of both the anterior and lateral walls. That is too much myocardium to lose at once, and few survive LMCA infarction. (See also Figs. 2-12 and 2-13.)

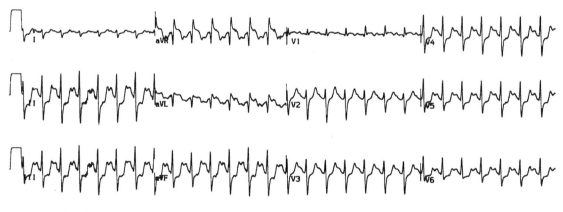

FIG. 5-13
A positive stress ECG. During treadmill exercise, ST depression developed in inferior and lateral leads, and within 2 minutes the patient had typical angina pectoris.

older patients both with and without a history of ischemic heart disease. ST depression on a routine ECG does not necessarily indicate the presence of coronary artery stenosis, and in the absence of any clinical history you should consider it a "nonspecific" finding. Associated T wave flattening and inversion are common; their presence does not change the fact that the findings are nonspecific. Do not be frustrated by an interpretation of "nonspecific ST-T wave changes" (NSSTTWCs). In a clinical context these "nonspecific" findings may become "specific." For example, ST segment depression that is documented by an ECG during chest pain may make

the diagnosis of angina pectoris. The absence of ST changes during pain makes ischemia less likely.

ST Segment Elevation. Total occlusion of an artery causes transmural ischemia with ST segment elevation (Fig. 5-11). This is the usual pattern with coronary artery spasm as well as with acute, transmural infarction. Elevation of ST segment is more specific for ischemia than ST depression. ST elevation also may be caused by pericarditis, but the changes are global rather than regional.

Another nonischemic cause of ST elevation is *early repolarization.* The cause is uncertain, but it is believed that

Table 5-4	ECG Changes with Syndromes of Myocardial Ischemia		
Condition	**ECG Changes**	**Timing**	**Comment**
Angina pectoris with fixed stenosis	ST depression	ST depression during pain; often exercise induced	Antegrade flow is present but is inadequate to meet increased oxygen demands—the pattern of "subendocardial ischemia."
Angina due to coronary spasm	ST elevation	ST elevation during pain, which may occur at rest	The pattern of "transmural ischemia"; the artery often is totally occluded.
Non–Q wave MI	ST depression (may be trivial or nonexistent)	During pain	Tightly stenosed artery, but angiography usually shows some antegrade flow; subendocardial ischemia, then necrosis.
	Symmetrical T wave inversion	Develops with pain, may be permanent	
Q wave MI	ST elevation	Develops immediately with occlusion of the artery and persists for days. (If permanent, consider LV aneurysm.)	Total occlusion of the artery and transmural ischemia. ST elevation does not indicate necrosis; if coronary occlusion is transient, ST elevation may resolve without infarction.
	Q wave	Minutes to hours after the onset of MI; permanent	Indicates some tissue necrosis
	T wave inversion	Minutes to hours after the onset of MI; usually resolves	T waves invert while there is still ST segment elevation.

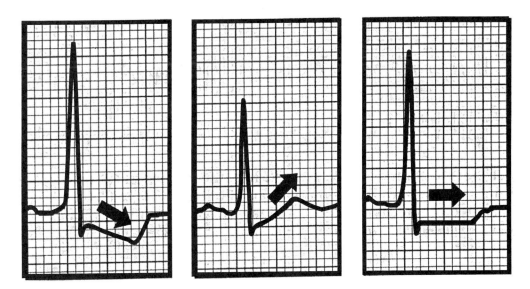

FIG. 5-14

Three examples of ST segment depression. The J point is the junction between the QRS and the ST segment. *Middle panel,* J point depression with an upsloping ST segment. This pattern is not as specific for ischemia as downsloping *(left panel)* or horizontal *(right panel)* ST depression.

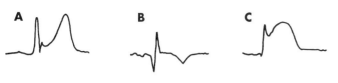

FIG. 5-15

Three examples of ST elevation. **A,** The ST segment is still upwardly concave, the normal pattern. This may be seen with transmural ischemia but it also is the pattern that occurs with pericarditis. Early repolarization also may cause this kind of ST elevation, although the ST segments usually are not as high as in this example. In both nonischemic cases, the ST elevation involves leads reflecting multiple vascular distributions (global involvement). **B,** Simultaneous ST elevation and T inversion. This combination indicates infarction. Pericarditis may cause T inversion, but the STs usually become isoelectric before the T waves turn over. **C,** Marked ST elevation with upward convexity. This pattern indicates transmural ischemia and is the earliest ECG abnormality of transmural infarction. Of course the ST changes would resolve with prompt relief of ischemia; however, most patients with this pattern have acute transmural infarction.

some portion of the ventricle repolarizes before the obvious onset of the T wave, spilling over into the ST segment and raising it. This change may be global, and, if so, must be differentiated from pericarditis (based on clinical findings). However, it may affect just a couple leads, raising confusion about possible ischemia. With early repolarization and pericarditis, the shape of the ST segment may help. Usually there is normal upward concavity with both conditions, whereas ischemia often causes upward convexity (Fig. 5-15) . The clinical setting also helps; early repolarization is common in young, healthy people, and the pattern varies little from day to day. Comparison with old tracings helps. Patterns of ischemia evolve with time.

Q Waves and Evolution of Myocardial Infarction

In the absence of reperfusion therapy, the ECG pattern of myocardial infarction (MI) evolves over a few days (Table 5-4, Fig. 5-16). Coronary occlusion causes transmural ischemia and injury, or *Q-wave MI.* ST segment elevation occurs almost immediately after occlusion. It may rarely be associated with tall, peaked T waves ("hyperacute" T waves). Q waves appear within hours of the onset of MI, and T waves may invert at about the same time (or a bit later). The diagnosis of MI is most certain when these evolutionary changes are recorded by serial ECGs. ST elevation without evolutionary changes raises the possibility of a nonischemic cause. The location of the infarction is determined by the group of leads with the above changes (Fig. 5-12).

For Q waves to be significant, they must be a millimeter (0.04 second) wide and a millimeter (0.1 mV) deep. Narrow Q waves are a common finding and are not indicators of myocardial scar. In addition, it is common to see an isolated Q wave or T wave inversion in either of leads III or V_1. For the diagnosis of inferior MI, a Q wave or T wave inversion must be present in at least one of the other inferior leads. Similarly, the diagnosis of anterior MI requires Q waves or T inversion in at least one lead other than V_1.

ST segment elevation and T wave inversion may resolve during the weeks after acute MI. Q waves persist in 70% to 90% of patients. Although Q waves may disappear or shrink after a small inferior MI, they tend to be permanent after a large MI.

Acute reperfusion therapy for MI hastens the evolution of ECG changes. As soon as the occluded infarct artery is opened, the ST segment elevation either resolves or improves. Q waves develop rapidly with reperfusion, possibly within minutes. Experience with reperfusion also has provided new insights into the significance of Q waves. Previously, Q waves were thought to indicate transmural scar with loss of all muscle in the zone of infarction. Now we know that deep Q waves may develop when there is early reperfusion and only partial injury to muscle in the infarct zone. Q waves do not reliably define a left ventricular segment as irreversibly damaged.

Non-Q infarction develops differently. Acute angiography shows that the infarct artery usually is not occluded, but instead is tightly stenosed with a trickle of antegrade flow. The ECG may have ST segment depression initially, with T wave inversion developing with persistence of ischemia (Figs. 5-11 and 5-17). Injury tends to be limited to the subendocardial region rather than the full thickness of muscle, and the extent of myocardial injury is less than with Q wave MI. Since the infarct artery is tightly stenosed and injury is not complete, recurrent ischemia is an obvious danger (see Chapter 14).

T wave inversion also may occur with prolonged angina (see Chapter 13). The diagnosis of angina rather than non-Q MI usually is made by the prompt reversal of ECG change with resolution of chest pain. However, it is not uncommon for a patient with prolonged angina and no elevation of cardiac enzymes to have persistent T wave inversion.

Silent MI. It is common to find Q waves or T inversion on a "routine" ECG of a patient with no history of MI. As many as 10% of MIs are clinically silent, and the incidence of silent MI is higher in patients with diabetes and autonomic neuropathy. Unexplained Q waves may be sorted out by studying regional wall motion. Transmural MI causes akinesis of the infarcted segment, readily detected with an echocardiogram or radionuclide angiogram. This should be done before the diagnosis of

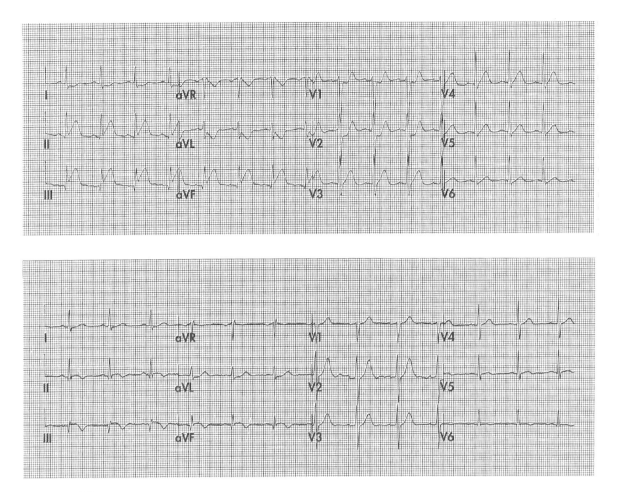

FIG. 5-16
Evolution of transmural, inferior myocardial infarction. *Top panel,* Limb leads showing ST segment elevation in leads II, III, and aVF. There is "reciprocal" ST depression in aVL. *Bottom panel,* The next day there is less ST elevation, and the reciprocal ST depression has resolved. The T waves have inverted in the inferior leads, and deeper Q waves have developed.

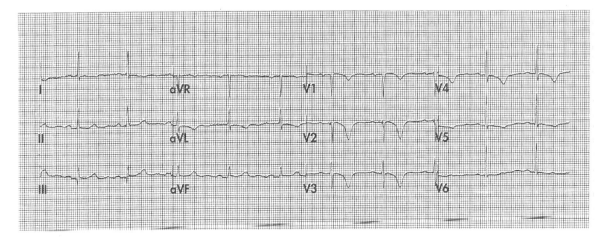

FIG. 5-17
Anterior, non–Q wave myocardial infarction. There is symmetrical T wave inversion in anterior precordial leads (with minimal ST depression as well). This ECG was obtained 2 days after a long episode of chest pain.

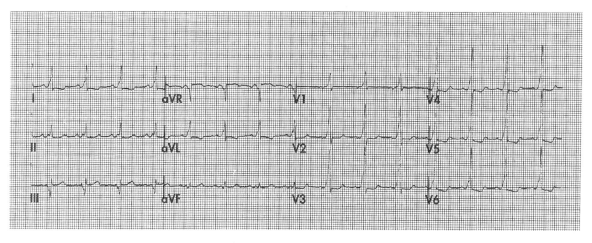

FIG. 5-18
Q waves in lead III and a tall R in V_1, raising the possibility of inferoposterior myocardial infarction. However, the PR interval is short, and a delta wave is present in the anterior precordial leads. The inferior *Qs* are delta waves. The preexcitation syndrome (Chapter 25) is one of the conditions that may cause a "pseudoinfarction" pattern. It also may be mistaken for a ventricular conduction abnormality (Fig. 25-4).

MI is assigned to a patient with no history of chest pain or infarction.

Pseudoinfarction. It is possible to have false-positive Q waves. Poor R wave progression is often misinterpreted as anterior MI. Q waves may occur with hypertrophic cardiomyopathy (see Chapter 23). The delta wave of the preexcitation syndrome may be a Q wave (Fig. 5-18; see Chapter 25). Uncertainty about the significance of Q waves in patients with no history of MI is clarified by the assessment of regional wall motion (an echocardiogram).

BIBLIOGRAPHY

Taylor GJ: *150 practice ECGs: interpretation and board review,* Cambridge, Mass, 1997, Blackwell Science. Short on text, although adequate, and long on practice. There is a good description of electrical axis measurement.

6

Treadmill Testing

H. Weston Moses
Steven D. O'Marro

PHYSIOLOGY OF EXERCISE

Cardiac output (CO) gradually increases during exercise as a result of increased heart rate and myocardial contractility, along with decreased peripheral vascular resistance (PVR). The Masters Two-Step was the first of the exercise test protocols and had one significant limitation: many people were unable to achieve maximal heart rate because the exertion required did not increase with time. Unlike the Masters protocol, graded exercise tests, such as the widely used Bruce protocol, start at a low level of exercise but then increase the speed and elevation of the treadmill every 3 minutes until even the most physically fit individuals reach exhaustion and their maximal ability to exercise. Even marathon runners become exhausted after about 20 minutes on the Bruce protocol.

Exercise physiology can be understood, in part, using this simple formula:

$$\text{Blood pressure} = \text{PVR} \times \text{CO}$$

With exercise, resting cardiac output can be raised from 4 to 5 L/min to 25 L/min. An increase in heart rate accounts for some of this, but a fall in peripheral vascular resistance also must occur. If it did not, blood pressure would be sky high (blood pressure does rise, but not several times over baseline). This relationship is useful for understanding how vasodilators help patients with heart failure. They commonly have elevated peripheral vascular resistance. Lowering peripheral vascular resistance with a vasodilator raises cardiac output.

Several terms and concepts used by exercise physiologists are helpful in understanding treadmill testing and interpretation.

VO₂ Max

VO2 max refers to an individual's maximal oxygen uptake and is the gold standard for measuring physical fitness. Using the Bruce protocol, the person with the highest VO_2 max is, in general, the most physically fit. World class distance athletes often have VO_2 max above 70 ml O_2/kg/min. At the other end of the spectrum, a patient with severe heart failure and VO_2 max of 14 ml O_2/kg/min or less is a candidate for a heart transplant.

It is possible to measure VO_2 max directly during exercise testing by using the so-called metabolic stress test. For most patients, however, the number of minutes walked on the treadmill using the Bruce protocol is roughly proportional to VO_2 max. A marathon runner may last 20 minutes; the average, physically fit middle-aged man may walk for about 9 to 10 minutes. Individuals with severe heart or lung disease usually have a low VO_2 max and are able to walk for just a short time. For this reason, the total time on the treadmill is a rough indicator of prognosis in patients with heart disease.

Bruce Protocol

Using a standard protocol allows comparison of patients' levels of fitness. The most commonly used protocol is the Bruce protocol, which defines the treadmill speed (miles per hour) and elevation (percent grade) for each 3-minute exercise stage. Stage 1 is 3 minutes at 1.7 miles per hour and 10% grade, regardless of where or when the test is done. There is a considerable increment in exercise level between stages in the Bruce protocol. Other protocols, such as the Naughton, have smaller increments and are more suitable for unfit individuals.

Mets

Mets, or "metabolic equivalent," is a physiologic description of the level of exercise. One Met is equal to the energy expenditure of an individual at rest in a sitting position, about 3.5 ml O_2/kg/min. Multiples of Mets can be used to describe levels of different types of activity and allows comparison of physical fitness among patients using different treadmill protocols. For example, completion of stage 1 of the Bruce protocol requires about 5 Mets; stage 3, about 9 or 10 Mets.

Mild activity such as sitting and writing requires about 1.7 Mets, and golfing with the use of a golf cart uses about 2.5 Mets. A moderate activity, golfing without use of a cart and not carrying a bag, requires about 5 Mets, and a modest walk about 3.3 Mets. Jogging at 10 min/mile requires about 10 Mets.

Maximal Predicted Heart Rate

Heart rate increases with exercise. Before starting the treadmill, the technician generally writes down a predicted maximal heart rate, usually taken from standard tables and based on age. As a rough guide, the maximal rate is the patient's age subtracted from 212. The predicted maximal heart rate provides the physician with an estimate of when the patient should be at VO₂ max (which is close to exhaustion) while exercising. It needs to be emphasized that this is an approximation.

Predicted maximal heart rate varies with age. The standard deviation in normal patients is quite large. Most diagnostic studies use 85% of the maximal heart rate as a goal. In addition to monitoring heart rate, it is important to gauge exercise time by "perceived exertion." This is accomplished by watching patients as they exercise, talking with them, and getting a sense of whether they are truly exhausted. A patient who is malingering and claims exhaustion despite a low heart rate would raise suspicion; this also would be confirmed by the patient's general appearance. The maximal heart rate also depends on physical conditioning (physically fit athletes have lower resting and, occasionally, maximal heart rates) and the effort the patient makes.

The predicated maximal heart rate becomes even more variable and less useful in elderly patients and in patients taking medications (e.g., beta-blockers, verapamil, and diltiazem) that blunt the usual heart rate response to exercise.

Predicted maximal heart rate has significant clinical relevance when the treadmill test is combined with a nuclear scan. If the patient exercises to maximal ability but does not reach 85% of the predicted maximal heart rate, the nuclear scan is less sensitive and specific. We tend to watch for that on our nuclear treadmill tests. If the patient clearly will not reach the target rate, the test is stopped and the scan is taken using "pharmacologic stress" (e.g., dipyridamole or adenosine; see Chapter 9). At times the patient cannot push up to target levels, and the technician has to settle for a lower maximal heart rate, realizing sensitivity is somewhat sacrificed.

The increase in heart rate in a normal patient correlates with a rise in oxygen uptake (VO₂, Fig. 6-1). The patient's heart rate increases with increasing work load on the treadmill. With sinus rhythm, heart rate increases as VO₂ increases, which also correlates with a longer time on the treadmill test. This relationship also exists in patients taking beta-blockers.

It is possible to measure VO₂ directly using the "metabolic treadmill test." Most cardiovascular centers have that option. The following is a comparison of VO₂ max of normal people with those of world class distance athletes, at one end of the spectrum, and with patients with advanced heart failure, at the other:

VO₂ Max (ml O₂/kg/min)	Status
14	Heart transplant candidate
30 to 40	Normal
> 70	World class distance athlete

When VO₂ max is measured directly, multiple measurements are made, including the "anaerobic threshold," at which the patient passes from aerobic exercise to anaerobic exercise. This type of measurement is used

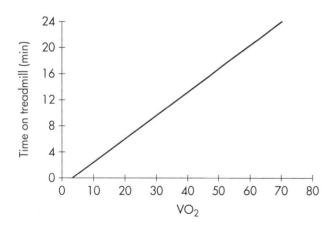

FIG. 6-1
Exercise time using a graded protocol is proportional to oxygen uptake (VO₂). VO₂ max correlates roughly with time spent on a treadmill. An unusually well-trained distance athlete is able to go as long as 24 minutes in the Bruce protocol (stage 8!) and at that level is using more than 70 ml O₂/kg/min. One definition of remarkable fitness is the ability to process large quantities of oxygen.

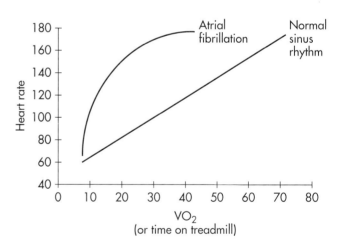

FIG. 6-2
Heart rate and VO₂ are proportional. The slope of this curve is another way to think of fitness or conditioning. The deconditioned person has a steep curve, with maximal heart rate reached at a relatively low VO₂ (and a brief time on the treadmill); this person has a low ability to "process oxygen." With training, the slope of the curve flattens, and the time on the treadmill to reach maximal heart rate increases. That is the *training effect.* This relationship between heart rate and VO₂ falls apart with atrial fibrillation.

only in specialized settings, for example, in the evaluation of a patient for a cardiac transplantation.

In a patient with atrial fibrillation, heart rate tends to increase earlier, and the linear relationship of VO_2 and time on the treadmill is lost (Fig. 6-2). Figure 6-3 demonstrates other treadmill performance examples.

Double Product

Another term used when defining exercise performance is *double product*, which is simply the product of peak systolic blood pressure and maximal heart rate. It is proportional to myocardial oxygen demand: the heart is pumping faster and also is pumping against increasing systolic pressure. That number has been particularly useful for research. It would be helpful, for instance, in a patient with a blunted heart rate response but with a very high blood pressure response to exercise.

INDICATIONS AND CONTRAINDICATIONS TO TREADMILL TESTING

General indications for exercise testing are listed in Box 6-1, and Box 6-2 summarizes contraindications. Box 6-3 outlines possible complications of exercise testing. The American Heart Association and the American College of Cardiology have published practice guidelines that parallel Boxes 6-1 and 6-2.[1] Although unnecessary for our purposes, it would be important to be familiar with these if you routinely perform treadmill testing. Further discussion of the application of exercise testing accompanies chapters related to specific conditions.

One basic factor in deciding whether to have a patient undergo an exercise test is the understanding of Bayesian analysis (Box 6-4): the posttest likelihood of disease being present and of a positive result being a "true positive" are related to the pretest likelihood of disease. For example, if a primary care physician tests middle-aged and elderly patients who have multiple risk factors (including smoking, diabetes, and chest pain), most of the abnormal (positive) tests will be associated with disease. Conversely, if a physician routinely tests all his or her patients, including young patients with no risk factors, particularly young women who are more prone to false positives, then many if

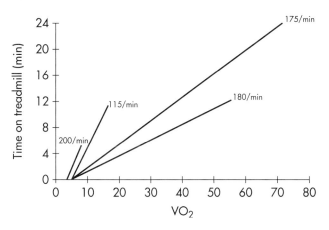

FIG. 6-3
Exercise performance of four different individuals. The man whose heart rate reached 175/min after 23 minutes on the treadmill is a marathon runner. VO_2 max near 70 places him in the "world class" category. The woman whose heart rate peaked at 180 has better than average exercise tolerance; she was on the treadmill 12 minutes before reaching that peak. The man who stopped exercise at heart rate 115/min could be a malingerer, but probably not. He exercised for 12 minutes and appeared exhausted. His blunted heart rate response was caused by use of beta-blockers. The patient whose heart rate reached 200/min after just 5 minutes of exercise had severe heart failure and was being evaluated for heart transplantation.

BOX 6-1

GENERAL INDICATIONS FOR EXERCISE TESTING

To assist in the diagnosis of coronary artery disease in symptomatic individuals

To assess functional capacity of and prognosis for patients with known coronary artery disease

To evaluate prognosis and exercise prescription for patients after uncomplicated myocardial infarction

To obtain serial follow-up of patients after coronary revascularization

To evaluate asymptomatic individuals (men older than 40 years of age, postmenopausal women)
  Special occupations
  Significant risk factors
  Before initiation of vigorous exercise program

To evaluate recurrent, exercise-induced cardiac arrhythmias

To evaluate functional capacity of selected patients with valvular heart disease

---

BOX 6-2

CONTRAINDICATIONS TO EXERCISE TESTING

Unstable coronary syndromes (chest pain within 48 hours)

Severe symptomatic left ventricular function

Potentially life-threatening cardiac arrhythmias

Severe aortic or subaortic stenosis

Uncontrolled hypertension (>200/115)

Active endocarditis or myocarditis

Acute pulmonary embolus

Aortic dissection

Acute systemic illness (e.g., pneumonia)

BOX 6-3

COMPLICATIONS OF EXERCISE TESTING

Up to 10 myocardial infarctions or deaths/10,000 tests

In patients with coronary artery disease, an adverse event is 60 to 100 times more likely to occur during an exercise test than during usual activity.

Risk is greatest in patients who have had an infarction and in those being evaluated for malignant arrhythmias.

BOX 6-4

BAYESIAN ANALYSIS

The posttest likelihood of disease actually being present (i.e., correctly being diagnosed) after a positive (abnormal) test is related to the pretest likelihood that the disease is present in the individual.

The pretest likelihood is determined by the prevalence of disease
 Age
 Risk factors
 Nature of symptoms (typical angina, atypical chest pain, no chest pain)

BOX 6-5

POSSIBLE CAUSES OF FALSE-POSITIVE OR INDETERMINATE RESULTS IN EXERCISE TESTING FOR CORONARY ARTERY DISEASE

Female gender

Hyperventilation

Mitral valve prolapse

Left ventricular hypertrophy

Drugs (digoxin, beta-blockers)

Electrolytes (hypokalemia)

Conduction disorders (left bundle branch block, Wolff-Parkinson-White syndrome, pacemaker)

---

not most of the abnormal treadmill tests will be false positives. Treadmill testing is thus less useful for patient populations with a low incidence of disease. This is a simple but important concept to keep in mind when determining which patients warrant treadmill testing.

Box 6-5 reviews possible causes of false-positive or indeterminate results in exercise treadmill testing.

Who Should Perform Stress Tests

It is beyond the scope of this chapter to teach the primary care physician how to do treadmill testing. On

---

BOX 6-6

STRESS ECHOCARDIOGRAPHY

Rapid interpretation

Additional information
Left ventricle size, ejection fraction
Regional wall motion abnormalities
Valvular heart disease
Pericardial disease

Intravenous contrast agents enhance endocardial border definition

Can only be performed by a cardiologist

About half the cost of nuclear stress testing

---

the other hand, this procedure can be performed by any competent and interested primary care physician. We encourage primary care physicians who work with our group to learn treadmill testing if they have the interest and have a patient population that warrants the time and trouble involved. Some primary care groups encourage one or two of their members to become skilled at treadmill testing. Those doing treadmill tests should know the indications and contraindications of exercise testing, as well as how to identify low- and high-risk subjects. They should understand the alternative diagnostic procedures to routine exercise testing (discussed below). They should have competence in CPR, ACLS, interpreting 12-lead ECGs, and managing arrhythmias. They should understand basic cardiology and exercise physiology. They should understand how Bayes theorem affects the interpretation of test results and the selection of patients for undergoing treadmill testing. The American College of Physicians/American College of Cardiology/American Heart Association Task Force has made recommendations about clinical competency and credentialing.[2] This summary gives a more detailed review of the skills needed to perform treadmill testing and could be used in approaching a hospital credentials committee. In our practice we offer a treadmill testing course to primary care physicians with the option of proctoring for a number of treadmill tests.

Even if the primary care physician does not perform treadmill testing, it helps the physician providing that service if the patient has been screened as a proper candidate for treadmill testing and that the best possible stress testing method has been chosen.

Ancillary Studies and Alternatives to Exercise Testing

The most common alternative to exercise testing is to add nuclear stress testing. Perfusion imaging is performed using sestamibi or thallium or a combination of the two. Myocardial blood flow imaging increases the sensitivity and specificity of stress testing in general. Patients in whom this is considered include those with significant conduction abnormalities on the baseline ECG (including those with pacemakers), those with preexisting ST segment abnormalities, and patients taking digoxin, which predisposes to ST segment depression.

Nuclear imaging and pharmacologic stress testing is discussed in detail in Chapter 9, including indications and costs. This option has greatly expanded our ability to evaluate for coronary artery disease noninvasively. Patients with medical problems that would not allow them to achieve target heart rate and work load on the treadmill can now have accurate, noninvasive testing.

Patients with left bundle branch block represent a special situation. In theory, a routine nuclear stress test with exercise would solve the problem of the conduction defect. However, for uncertain reasons they often develop a false positive septal perfusion defect with exercise. This becomes less of a problem with *pharmacologic stress* testing (the rate of false positives drops from 46% to 10%).

When the heart is stressed with exercise or dobutamine, another imaging option is echocardiography. The purpose is to demonstrate wall motion abnormalities in relation to exercise, presumably due to ischemia (see Chapter 8). Although it is a useful and valuable technique, it is especially operator dependent and requires special skills of the echocardiographer and the cardiologist interpreting it. The primary care physician has to have confidence in the center performing the study. This also is true of radionuclide interpretation; currently this is a more widely used test, and experienced interpreters usually are available. The pros and cons of stress echocardiography are summarized in Box 6-6.

ECG CHANGES DURING EXERCISE AND STRESS TEST INTERPRETATION

Much of the information obtained from treadmill testing relates to physical fitness. Prognosis is related to exercise tolerance. If a patient can walk for more than 7 minutes on a Bruce protocol, the prognosis is reasonably good, even if the stress ECG is positive (but especially if it is negative). (See Table 13-4 for a summary of markers of poor prognosis for patients with coronary

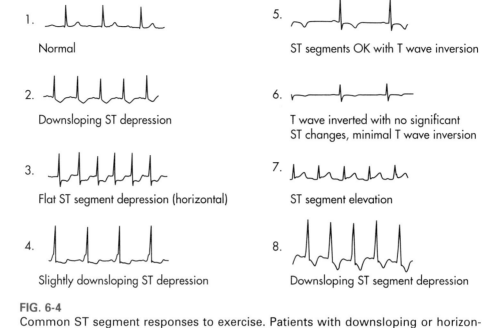

1. Normal

2. Downsloping ST depression

3. Flat ST segment depression (horizontal)

4. Slightly downsloping ST depression

5. ST segments OK with T wave inversion

6. T wave inverted with no significant ST changes, minimal T wave inversion

7. ST segment elevation

8. Downsloping ST segment depression

FIG. 6-4
Common ST segment responses to exercise. Patients with downsloping or horizontal ST segment depression have a higher probability of ischemia (examples *2, 3, 4,* and *8*). Isolated T wave inversion (example *5*), normalization of inverted T waves, and ST segment elevation (example *7*) may or may not indicate ischemia.

artery disease, including stress test, nuclear, and echocardiograph findings.) ST segment interpretation is, of course, very important but must be considered within the total clinical picture.

Figure 6-4 illustrates various ST segment responses (see also Figs. 5-13 and 5-14). The normal finding is no ST depression. "J point" depression is depression at the end of the QRS complex at the "junction" of the QRS and the ST segment. A mild amount of J point depression can be normal. More than 1 to 2 mm of upsloping J point depression suggests cardiac ischemia. Flat ST segment depression is more specific for cardiac ischemia. The greater the level of ST depression, the greater the likelihood of cardiac ischemia. Downsloping ST segment depression is most diagnostic for cardiac ischemia, and the magnitude of depression correlates statistically with the likelihood of cardiac ischemia.

These changes are not diagnostic by themselves. Numerous factors affect the ECG response to exercise. Hundreds of papers have been written in an attempt to increase the sensitivity and specificity of the interpretation of ECG response to exercise. However, focusing on smaller ECG changes in an effort to increase sensitivity brings about more false-positive results and lower specificity. Conversely, requiring more stringent criteria for ST segment depression and for diagnosing coronary artery disease brings about fewer false-positive but more

false-negative results. There is not one perfect solution to this, and the clinician must understand that ECG interpretation leads to both false-positive and false-negative results.

Even with nuclear stress testing, false-positive and false-negative results are possible. In fact, programs that are new to nuclear stress testing have a fairly high incidence of false positives because they overread diaphragmatic attenuation in the inferior wall and soft tissue attenuation in other views. There is a "learning curve." Even a nuclear treadmill test can be normal despite the presence of significant coronary artery disease, and it is important to point this out to patients. Remember that all the exercise study methods test for flow-restricting stenoses. They do not detect early or borderline plaque that is not hemodynamically significant. Fortunately, most serious coronary events are caused by tight stenoses, but it is possible for a 40% to 50% lesion to erode, clot, and occlude (see Chapter 14).

The terms *positive* and *negative* should be avoided when describing treadmill results. More appropriate terminology includes "low probability of cardiac ischemia," "high probability of cardiac ischemia," or something in between. Treadmill testing yields probabilities, not unequivocal diagnoses. This is an important distinction to make when discussing test results with colleagues, and even more important when describing

The patient was exercised using the _____ protocol.

The patient was able to walk for _____ minutes.

The maximum heart rate was _____ (if the maximal heart rate was particularly low you may make such comments as "The patient has been taking a beta-blocker," "The patient has been taking verapamil," "This did appear to be a maximal effort despite the blunted heart rate response," or "The maximum heart rate was not reached and the patient did not appear to be making a good effort on this test").

The maximum blood pressure was _____ (or blood pressure response was appropriate).

The patient quit due to _____.
                             or
The test was stopped due to _____.

The ECG demonstrated _____.

At this point, you may make miscellaneous comments such as "frequent PVCs," "nonsustained ventricular tachycardia," "transient SVT," "This was a submaximal test due to hip discomfort," or "This was a submaximal test due to poor patient effort."

Conclusion

1. Low probability of cardiac ischemia
   Indeterminant test
   High probability of high cardiac ischemia

2. Discuss physical fitness level

3. Other comments such as unusual blood pressure response, arrhythmias, and so forth

FIG. 6-5
Dictating the treadmill report.

them to patients. When telling a patient about a "negative" test, we cover the following points:

The test looked good, with no evidence of a blood flow problem to your heart. This means that the chance of you having a heart problem is low, *although the risk of problems is not zero.* For example, the test detects only tight, flow-restricting blockages, not borderline blockages that may rarely cause problems. At any rate, this result indicates that you are in a low-risk group for major problems like heart attack. With this result, no further testing is needed at this time.

SUMMARY OF THE TREADMILL REPORT

Figure 6-5 provides a format for a treadmill test report. It describes the protocol that was used, the patient's exercise effort, physiologic response, and any ECG changes. Recall that total time on the treadmill correlates with VO$_2$ max. If the same protocol is used, the time walked allows the physician to compare one patient's fitness level with another's. If different protocols were used, the maximal exercise capacity can be converted to Mets using a table, allowing patients to be compared.

It is important to indicate why exercise was stopped (Box 6-7). An experienced clinician's eyewitness description of symptoms that limit exercise ability often provides the critical insight into the patient's problem. Blood pressure should rise continually. A significant drop in blood pressure from one stage to the next is an ominous sign that could indicate left main coronary disease, triple vessel disease, or cardiomyopathy. It is one of the most important reasons to stop a treadmill test. Patients frequently quit as a result of general fatigue. True angina usually is a reason to stop a treadmill test unless it is being done for a very specific assessment of known anatomy. If a patient has atypical pain, but no ECG changes, exercise may be continued. Stopping the test for atypical

---

BOX 6-7

REASONS TO STOP A TREADMILL TEST

Greater than 20 mm Hg drop in blood pressure from one stage to the next

General fatigue, dyspnea, or patient distress

Anginal chest pain (often, if atypical pain occurs, the treadmill is not stopped)

Asymptomatic ST depression greater than 2 to 3 mm

Ominous arrhythmias, particularly if ischemia is evident

Orthopedic or other clinical problems

Claudication

Systolic blood pressure greater than 250 to 260

Target heart rate and work load achieved, no ECG changes (a diagnostic, "negative" test). Despite the patient having achieved the target heart rate, many physicians push on until symptoms necessitate stopping.

---

pain and below the target rate results in an inconclusive study .

The most common reason for stopping exercise is the patient's reaching of the target work load and heart rate (a "negative" study). Frequently, deconditioned individuals reach the target heart rate after 5 or 6 minutes on the treadmill. If there is no discomfort or distress, we continue exercise beyond the 7 minute mark. An ability to walk for more than 7 minutes in the Bruce protocol places a patient in a good prognostic group.

REFERENCES

1. Task Force on Practice Guidelines, Committee on Exercise Testing. American College of Cardiology: American Heart Association practice guidelines for exercise testing, *J Am Coll Cardiol* 30:260, 1997.
2. Task Force on Clinical Privileges in Cardiology. Clinical competence in exercise testing; a statement for physicians from the American College of Physicians, American College of Cardiology, American Heart Association Task Force on Clinical Privileges in Cardiology, *J Am Coll Cardiol* 16:1061, 1990.

7

Chest X-Ray and Vascular Studies

Terrence X. O'Brien
Sara Creveling Paul

CHEST X-RAY: OVERVIEW AND COST EFFECTIVENESS

In this era of high technology, newer and more expensive imaging techniques continue to be developed, and the conventional radiographic means of diagnosing cardiovascular disease is often overlooked. However, standard radiographic interpretation of heart disease is a cornerstone of clinical cardiology, and costly workups can be avoided by first obtaining a standard chest x-ray (CXR). Furthermore, the CXR can be interpreted by a nonradiologist and is easily accessible, with the results providing an immediate image of a patient's physiologic status. In the current climate of managed care, expense is often a factor included in clinical evaluations.

INDICATIONS FOR OBTAINING A CHEST X-RAY

Although a plain chest film rarely provides the specific diagnosis of a cardiac abnormality, it often indicates the nature of a functional derangement and its severity.[1,2] Usually a CXR is used in conjunction with other tests and may direct medical personnel to other, more specific testing. Many times the diagnoses *ruled out* by a CXR are critical in selecting a clinical pathway for patients. A chest film may be indicated in the following situations.

Congestive Heart Failure

The CXR is a standard diagnostic tool in the evaluation of patients with shortness of breath and also can be used to monitor response to therapy (see also Chapter 22). For example, a chest film can support the diagnosis of congestive heart failure by revealing cardiomegaly, pulmonary edema, pleural effusions, or left ventricular aneurysm.

Myocardial Infarction

A CXR usually is obtained in patients with suspected myocardial infarction to search for diagnostic signs such as pulmonary edema and increased cardiac or aortic size. It also rules out other sources of chest pain, particularly in the emergency department or other primary care setting (see Chapter 14).

Other cardiac causes of chest pain detectable by CXR include calcified valvular, pericardial, and coronary disease, cardiac masses, pericardial effusions, and dissecting aortic aneurysms. Implantable devices such as pacemakers and automatic defibrillators, as well as their associated wires and hardware, can be evaluated for position and type. Some types of congenital heart disease can be assessed (see below and Chapter 30). Mechanical prosthetic valves also can be viewed for position and, to some degree, type.

CHEST X-RAY INTERPRETATION
Cardiac
Size

The average normal value of the cardiothoracic ratio is ≤ 0.50 in most adults. In general, enlarged hearts are abnormal; however, when the cardiac size is within normal limits, the heart may or may not be normal.[2] Gross cardiomegaly can be caused by left-sided or right-sided heart failure or may be the result of a myriad of causes entirely unrelated to heart failure. The combination of alveolar pulmonary edema and an enlarged heart is the hallmark of acute left-sided heart failure.

Chambers

The cardiac contour on a CXR is formed by the cardiac chambers, aorta, and pulmonary arteries (Fig 7-1). In the posteroanterior view the left heart border is formed by the left ventricle, left atrial appendage, pulmonary artery, and aorta. The right heart border is formed by the right ventricle, right atrium, pulmonary artery, ascending aorta, and superior vena cava. The left ventricle also forms the lower posterior border in the lateral view.[3] Left ventricular enlargement from left ventricular hypertrophy tends to create a rounding of the cardiac apex, whereas dilation is more likely to elongate the cardiac apex to the left or to the left and downwards in the frontal view. For example, hypertension, coarctation, aortic valve disease, and congenital aortic obstruction can produce pressure overload and hypertrophy of the left ventricle. Likewise, mitral or aortic regurgitation, a left-to-right shunt, ischemia, or other cause of cardiomyopathy can lead to volume overload.

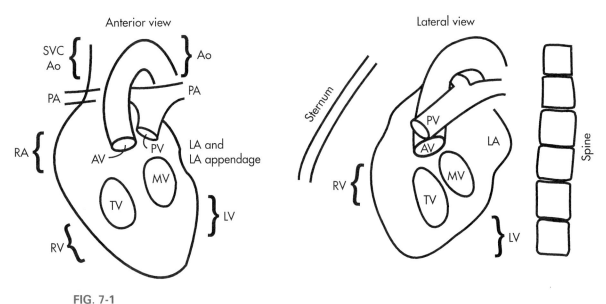

FIG. 7-1
Relative positions of cardiac structures on a chest x-ray. *Ao,* Aorta; *SVC,* superior vena cava; *PA,* pulmonary artery; *RA,* right atrium; *LA,* left atrium; *LV,* left ventricle; *RV,* right ventricle; *AV,* aortic valve; *PV,* pulmonic valve; *TV,* tricuspid valve; *MV,* mitral valve.

In the frontal CXR view, the right ventricle appears triangular. It forms most of the front of the heart in the lateral view. In the lateral view, right ventricular enlargement may be recognized by a forward bulging of the front of the heart, increasing the area of contact with the sternum. Right ventricular enlargement may result from pulmonary hypertension, pulmonary incompetence, tricuspid valve disease, or left-to-right shunts.

The left atrium has an oval shape when viewed from the front and is flat when viewed from the side. When the esophagus is opacified with barium, it marks the posterior wall of the left atrium. Left atrial enlargement is most commonly associated with mitral valve disease (see Chapter 18) or any pathologic condition causing pressure or volume overload to be transmitted to the left atrium. Also, the vast majority of atrial myxomas occur in the left atrium. The appearance of a myxoma may vary from a normal CXR to an enlarged left atrium and atrial appendage.

If the right atrium is enlarged, the right heart border protrudes to the right and its radius of curvature increases as the diameter of the chamber increases. Right atrial enlargement can occur in relation to both stenosis and incompetence in acquired tricuspid valve disease and in congenital anomalies of the tricuspid valve, most notably Ebstein's anomaly. The right atrium also can be enlarged if it is exposed to high flow, as in atrial septal defect or any prominent left-to-right shunt (see Chapter 30).

Pericardium

The pericardium contains the heart and proximal great vessels. A sufficient amount of fluid in the pericardium enlarges the heart shadow on the CXR and must always be considered in the differential diagnosis of cardiomegaly. One of the striking characteristics of a pericardial effusion is a large heart with clear lungs, unlike the congestion seen in heart disease. Serial films demonstrating rapid changes in heart size also suggest accumulation or dispersal of fluid in the pericardium.

Calcification

Abnormally increased densities may be found within the heart on CXR. Large cardiac calcifications are seen particularly well in the lateral and oblique views. Any radiologically detectable calcification in the heart is of clinical importance. Calcification occurring within the left atrium and left atrial appendage may suggest rheumatic heart disease that may be associated with mitral valve dysfunction. The radiographic presence of calcification within a cardiac valve often represents hemodynamically significant stenosis. As a rule, the extent of valvular calcification usually is proportional to the severity of the valve stenosis.[1] Mitral valve calcification can indicate long-standing and severe mitral valve disease and is best seen in the lateral view. Mitral annular calcification in the valve rings is a degenerative process that occurs with aging and is commonly found in individuals over age 40, especially women.[1] Clinical findings associated with aortic annular calcification include atrial fibrillation, conduction abnormalities, endocarditis, and mitral valve incompetence.[1]

Calcification also can be present in a number of other structures and may mark the evolution of atherosclerosis in the coronary arteries due to calcium deposits found early in plaque formation. Aortic calcifications are commonly found in individuals over the age of 50 years, particularly in the region of the arch. However, when the calcification is deep to the aortic border, dissection may be present. Pericardial calcification is most often associated with previous acute or chronic pericarditis, constrictive heart disease, tuberculosis, or trauma. As an aside, the presence of sternotomy wires in an older adult indicates previous surgery, usually for coronary or valvular disease (or both).

If calcification is considered a possibility, order a repeat CXR with "overpenetration."

Valves

The plain film signs of valvular disease are usually those of selective chamber enlargement, which may vary from trivial to gross. For instance, left atrial enlargement suggests congestive heart failure or mitral valve disease, whereas right atrial enlargement is associated with tricuspid valve disease. Aortic stenosis may be seen as left ventricular hypertrophy, poststenotic dilation of the ascending aorta, and calcification of the aortic valve. In severe aortic stenosis, the left atrium and the left ventricle decompensate and enlarge. Longstanding aortic regurgitation may be seen as left ventricular enlargement; however, acute aortic incompetence may reveal congestive cardiac failure despite a virtually normal size heart.

The CXR also may reveal information about implanted prosthetic cardiac valves. The structures of mechanical valves, such as the caged-ball, tilting disc, and bileaflet valves, are seen on CXR. Tissue valves also may be evaluated on CXR, in that abnormalities are revealed by signs of valve stenosis or insufficiency. Although irregularities in the structure or function of a mechanical valve may be seen on CXR, often they are better evaluated with direct fluoroscopy.

Congenital Heart Disease

Coarctation of the aorta in adult patients manifests as localized postductal narrowing of the aorta or rib notching (i.e., enlarged intercostal vessels erode the lower rib edge). The most useful radiographic sign is an abnormal contour of the aortic arch, which may appear as a double bulge above and below the usual site of the aortic knob, the "figure 3" sign. *Ostium secundum atrial septal defect* is the most common left-to-right shunt diagnosed in adults. The chest radiograph may be normal in a patient with a small shunt, but with a hemodynamically significant shunt the main pulmonary artery and branches, the right atrium, and the right ventricular borders are enlarged. *Tetralogy of Fallot* is the most common cyanotic congenital heart defect in adults and children. Most adults have had this defect surgically corrected but may still demonstrate mild to moderate pulmonary hypovascularity or a boot-shaped heart on

CXR. *Situs inversus* is readily identified by the mirror image reversal (dextrocardia) of the heart.

Pitfalls

The patient's body build determines the position of the heart in relation to the midline of the thorax. In asthenic patients, the heart shadow is positioned midline, projecting only slightly to the left. In stockier builds, the heart shadow is a little more to the left of midline. With most portable chest x-rays, in which anteroposterior imaging magnifies the heart, assessing cardiac size by relating it to the cardiothoracic ratio may be problematic if not impossible. In addition, the size and contour of the heart may vary from one examination to another as a result of the influence of systole and diastole. The cardiac size and contour also may change from the height of the hemidiaphragm, intrathoracic pressure, and body position (e.g., when a patient is recumbent, the heart is broader than when erect). Of course, the quality of the film, especially in relation to previous chest x-rays, is key to interpreting abnormalities.

Vessels

On the CXR the aorta lies just above the middle of the heart shadow in both frontal and lateral views. The ascending aorta bulges to the right when dilated, as commonly happens in old age or hypertension. General significant dilation of the aorta is a hallmark of severe aortic insufficiency, whereas selective proximal poststenotic dilation of the ascending aorta suggests aortic stenosis. The pulmonary arterial trunk is quite large relative to the aortic knob in atrial septal defects, severe mitral stenosis, and in other causes of pulmonary hypertension or left-to-right shunts.

In a patient with dissecting aortic aneurysm, radiographs of the chest may reveal widening of the mediastinum, localized dilation of the aortic knob and upper descending aorta, or displacement of the trachea. A helpful diagnostic clue may be gained by comparing the current film to a previous one (see Chapter 32).

Lungs

Careful evaluation of pulmonary vasculature helps to narrow down the differential diagnosis to a manageable level. The appearance of the pulmonary veins correlates with left atrial pressure and volume status. In cases of isolated right-sided heart failure, the lungs become unusually radiolucent due to decreased pulmonary blood flow. Left-sided failure is characterized by pulmonary edema (i.e., loss of lower lobe vascular distinctness with progressive alveolar edema as severity increases). When right-sided failure occurs as a result of left-sided failure, pulmonary congestion may improve because of decreased pulmonary blood flow.

The CXR plays a vital role in diagnosing pulmonary congestion in patients with obstructive lung disease.

For example, pulmonary rales may be inaudible when the lungs are hyperexpanded.

Pleura

Left-sided heart failure often is associated with a right pleural effusion, whereas bilateral hydrothorax suggests bilateral heart failure or a noncardiac cause of the effusion. Of course, the noncardiac causes of pleural effusions are numerous.[5]

Bony Configurations

Fractures and abnormalities of the bony structures of the chest that are not always suspected may be seen and subsequently direct patient evaluation.

Devices

Central intravenous lines, pacemakers, and automatic implantable cardioverter/defibrillators and their leads, as well as endotracheal tube placements, may all be seen and at least partially evaluated on CXR.

FLUOROSCOPY

Direct real-time fluoroscopy is reserved for specific indications. Unlike the chest film, which is a stop-motion exposure, cardiac fluoroscopy demonstrates the dynamic features of the heart that are discernible only during motion. Cardiac fluoroscopy can be used to detect small calcifications and evaluate cardiac valve mechanical prostheses, pacemakers, and radiopaque foreign bodies. Fluoroscopic analysis of mechanical valve components compares favorably with echocardiography because metallic or highly calcified structures are not obscured by ultrasonic shadowing. Fluoroscopy involves more radiation exposure than a two-view chest x-ray, so it should be used selectively and be accomplished as quickly possible.

A cautionary note: Certain x-ray findings are rarely by themselves diagnostic of a disease but often indirectly suggest a specific diagnosis or a particular physiologic state. Radiographic findings should always be correlated with clinical information and laboratory results before any final conclusions are drawn.

DIAGNOSTIC TESTING FOR EVALUATION OF PERIPHERAL ARTERIAL DISEASE

Recent advances in surgical and percutaneous techniques have made revascularization possible in the treatment of increasingly complex peripheral vascular diseases (see Chapter 33). Also, as a result of advances in diagnostic testing, critical anatomic and physiologic information is now available, providing greater accuracy and earlier disease detection. If peripheral vascular disease is suspected, further diagnostic evaluation almost

always is essential. As such, a primary care provider should have a working knowledge of the common types of vascular testing available, how they are best used, and what to do with the information garnered. Keep in mind that specialized testing is always a supplement to a thorough history and physical examination.

Laboratory Tests

Initial laboratory screening should include lipid fractionation and glucose testing, since atherosclerosis and diabetes (plus tobacco smoking) are the most common risk factors for peripheral arterial disease. If considering a coagulation abnormality, you should obtain a prothrombin time, partial thromboplastin time, and complete blood count with platelets. Additional laboratory studies are ordered based on clinical suspicion such as unexplained thrombosis, evidence for microemboli, signs of connective tissue disease (many of which have an associated arteritis), or certain rare diseases that may have vascular manifestations (Table 7-1).

Electrocardiography and Echocardiography

Peripheral embolism usually comes from the heart. An electrocardiogram is part of a routine evaluation, particularly if an arrhythmia (especially atrial fibrillation) or evidence of a previous or current myocardial infarction is found, since these are common sources of arterial thrombi. Echocardiography, either thoracic or transesophageal, may reveal a cardiac or thoracic aortic source of emboli, for example, from the left atrial appendage, the left ventricle, or a cardiac valve (vegetation) (see Chapter 8).

Noninvasive Diagnostic Imaging

Several noninvasive tests substantiate and quantify the diagnosis of arterial and venous disease. A basic understanding of these tests and what they can provide for patients is important for primary care providers as the ones responsible for ordering the tests and usually for interpreting the results clinically.

Doppler Stethoscope and Blood Pressure Cuff: the Ankle Brachial Index

A hand-held continuous wave Doppler stethoscope (5 to 10 MHz) is a fast, inexpensive way to audibly detect peripheral pulses. Listening for a pulse with a blood pressure cuff allows a straightforward measurement of the ratio of the brachial and ankle systolic blood pressures, the *ankle brachial index* (ABI). A blood pressure cuff is placed above the ankle, and a Doppler probe is used to detect the dorsalis pedis or posterior tibial pressure (the systolic pressure is where the Doppler signal is no longer heard). The ankle pressure is normally higher than the brachial, but with arterial insufficiency ankle pressure is decreased, depending on occlusion severity.

Table 7-1	*Laboratory Testing for Diseases That May Have Associated Peripheral Vascular Manifestations*

UNEXPLAINED THROMBOSIS	
Protein S, C, or antithrombin III deficiency	Directly measure, hereditary
Heparin induced	May be preceded by thrombocytopenia
Fibrin D-dimer	Reflects fibrin turnover and activated coagulation
Other	Laboratory evidence of inflammatory bowel disease, myeloproliferation, neoplasm, Kawasaki's disease or Bachet's disease
Microembolic events	Suggested by an elevated sedimentation rate, C-reactive protein, anemia, leukocytosis, azotemia, or an abnormal urinary sediment
Myxedema	Thyroid function tests
Raynaud's disease	Search for secondary causes, protein electrophoresis, cryoglobulin, cryofibrinogen, and cold agglutinins
CONNECTIVE TISSUE DISEASES	
Systemic lupus erythematosus	Circulating anticoagulant, antinuclear antibody (ANA), anti-DNA antibody, other lupus-associated antibodies
Rheumatoid arthritis	Rheumatoid factor
LESS COMMONLY ASSOCIATED	
Pheochromocytoma	Serum and urinary catecholamine levels
Thrombotic thrombocytopenic purpura	Hemolysis, thrombocytopenia, fragmented RBCs, renal and neurologic involvement
Polycythemia vera	CBC, elevated red cell mass, splenomegaly, thrombocytosis

The ABI is obtained by dividing the ankle systolic pressure by the brachial systolic pressure and will be >0.95 with normal flow, >0.80 with mild insufficiency, <0.80 with moderate disease, and <0.50 with severe disease.[6] Most patients with claudication commonly have ABI ratios between 0.50 and 0.80 and those with ulcers or gangrene <0.50. Exercise may enhance the ABI abnormality (thereby demonstrating functional impairment), with <0.50 indicating moderate and <0.15 severe insufficiency in both men and women.

The ABI may falsely underestimate disease severity in patients with diabetes and end-stage renal disease because of tibial artery calcification. In these cases, transcutaneous oximetry may be ordered to help document tissue ischemia. For example, transcutaneous oxygen tension less than 10 mm Hg often means that a distal lesion may not be capable of healing. Since an arterial occlusion must be proximal to its associated decrement in systolic pressure (and, when present, the symptomatic area), measuring blood pressure at several levels helps to approximate the level of the occlusion, although measurements may be inaccurate when there is multilevel disease. Another major limitation of ABI is its inability to locate precisely the anatomic site(s) of occlusion. Therefore more accurate ultrasonic techniques are now the mainstay of primary care evaluations.

Duplex Ultrasound Scanning

Piezoelectric crystals generate and receive reflected sound waves and are the basic component of an ultrasound transducer. When each reflectance is rapidly updated, a real-time two-dimensional image can be produced. Similarly, Doppler ultrasound is based on frequency shifts in the ultrasound echoes returning from moving red blood cells. Just as the sound of a train whistle or jet plane engine has a higher pitch as it is coming toward you as opposed to going away from you, so is Doppler flow imaging a processed rendition of intravascular blood flow, turbulence, and velocity. The combination in one probe of real-time B-mode ultrasonography (i.e., gray-scale imaging) and Doppler flow signal interrogation is termed *duplex scanning*.[7] This provides a two-dimensional picture of a blood vessel and an index of blood flow. Duplex scanning yields highly accurate, relatively inexpensive anatomic and physiologic information that can be used to diagnose or serially follow patients. This contrasts with arteriography, which provides anatomic detail but less information about physiologic significance. Duplex scanning can be used on all accessible vascular beds including the peripheral, cerebrovascular, visceral, and venous circulations. Other common uses include detecting aneurysms (e.g., iliac, femoral, and popliteal) and pseudoaneurysms (e.g., postcardiac catheterization), monitoring vein bypass grafts, and selecting patients for percutaneous intravascular procedures.

Doppler interrogation allows for identification and grading of arterial stenosis. Basically, although blood cell velocities upstream of an occlusion may be normal, velocities are increased at the point of stenosis in proportion to the degree of obstruction (like putting your thumb over a garden hose). For example, a hemodynamically significant stenosis, say of 50%, may demonstrate a 100% increase in peak systolic velocity within the narrowed segment. Distal to a high-grade stenosis, Doppler signals are likely to reflect a low flow state because of a reduction in blood velocity and low resistance. The use of velocity ratios to calculate stenoses has the advantage of being independent of distal or proximal vessel tone or cardiac output. For example, the ratio of a stenotic vessel's blood velocity to normal ratio of 4:1 or greater corresponds to >75% narrowing, and a ratio of 7:1 to >90% narrowing. Likewise, large arteriovenous fistulas can be seen by their high, arterial-type profiles in the involved vein and distal low flow resistance in the involved artery.

Gray-scale images of blood vessels can demonstrate atherosclerotic plaque or thrombus, and the structure of a plaque, such as hemorrhagic involvement or an ulcerated appearance, also may be seen. Echolucent masses near a vessel or bypass can be identified as a hematoma, seroma, or abscess. Wave form analysis uses characteristic Doppler flow patterns to further identify the severity of a lesion. An increased (perturbed) range of recorded velocities is termed *spectral broadening* and is proportional to the degree of stenosis.

Duplex scanning is limited by obstructive lesions at either extreme (i.e., severe obstruction or little obstruc-

tion with or without vessel wall plaque), as well by the expertise or experience of the operator. Technical quality worsens with morbid obesity or marked peripheral edema.

Color flow Doppler interrogation processes the Doppler-derived images of flowing blood into more easily interpretable color pictures that can rapidly identify vessels with disturbed flow. This greatly expedites examinations of the lengthy vasculatures of extremities. Color flow imaging compares favorably with arteriography, with a sensitivity for identifying occluded arterial segments of 92% and for normal segments of 97%. The diagnosis of an occluded arterial conduit or other occlusion may be made by an absence of color flow and Doppler signal.

Exercise testing may be diagnostic in some patients who do not have hemodynamically significant blood flow abnormalities at rest but do so after exercise (such as treadmill walking, see Chapter 6). This is often suggested by a history of claudication.

Arteriography

Contrast arteriography has clinically been the diagnostic gold standard since the mid-1960s. It is not without risk, such as puncture site and contrast-related complications, which, it should be noted, are usually managed by the primary care physician. Any history of allergy to contrast material, iodine, or shellfish must be known, and renal function must be optimized. Arteriography is not suited for serial studies, does not commonly provide physiologic information, and has a significantly higher cost. Arteriography does anatomically define the location of arterial disease and the condition of the proximal vessel and the degree of distal runoff, which are all important surgical considerations. Digital subtraction angiography improves images by using computer technology to digitally subtract out a precontrast image of the vessel. Since noninvasive studies can be used to follow patients serially, arteriography is generally reserved for when revascularization is being considered. Possible exceptions include unusual presentations and less common diagnoses (e.g., for multiple segmental occlusions in small and medium-sized arteries that might be seen in thromboangiitis obliterans [Buerger's disease]).

Magnetic Resonance Angiography and Computed Tomography

The physics of magnetic resonance angiography (MRA) is well suited to noninvasive imaging of flowing blood, and the technology is rapidly developing in the evaluation of peripheral vascular disease, including preoperative assessment in lieu of arteriography. MRA also may view the venous system and is particularly useful in obtaining information about intrathoracic veins (e.g., inferior and superior vena cava and pelvic veins). Another promising approach, computed tomographic (CT) angiography, has been reported to have results comparable to digital subtraction angiography and also is a rapidly developing technology.

Individualized Approach

In all these evaluations involving ever-changing technology, you must always individualize your workup according to each patient's level of symptoms and co-morbid diseases. This also depends on which techniques and expertise are available locally.

DIAGNOSTIC TESTING FOR EVALUATION OF PERIPHERAL VENOUS DISEASE

Venous diseases are challenging to diagnose, and significant deep venous thrombosis (DVT) may be clinically subtle. Superficial phlebitis, trauma, cellulitic changes, and peripheral edema from other causes such as congestive heart failure may be difficult to sort out from DVT during the physical examination. Consequently, objective testing often is necessary, and all tests must be correlated within their clinical context.

Impedance Plethysmography

Impedance plethysmography has been used for many years to diagnose DVT. It relies on indirect detection of venous obstruction by detecting abnormalities in the normal fluctuations in leg volume that occur with venous occlusion. With a large acute DVT, the leg veins are already filled and the volume tracing does not change significantly with inflation of a blood pressure cuff. Plethysmography is an indirect test that yields many false-positive results as a result of other causes of venous obstruction, as well as false-negative results due to nonocclusive thrombi.

Duplex Ultrasound Scanning

Duplex ultrasound is now the usual initial screen for DVT. Proximal DVT may be detected either by visualizing the thrombus, vein compressibility (the lack thereof is a very sensitive method), or Doppler flow analysis to determine vein patency. Fresh thrombus can be discriminated, since it is relatively echolucent. Duplex scanning has a sensitivity of 83% and a specificity of 92%. Color Doppler imaging is particularly sensitive below the groin. Plethysmography and duplex Doppler may be up to 95% sensitive at the thigh level, but less so below and above the groin and below the knee. Therefore a combination of techniques can prove diagnostically useful. Chronic venous insufficiency may be suggested by duplex Doppler by finding venous valvular

reflux. The combination of techniques also may help distinguish edema caused by heart failure from that caused by venous insufficiency.

Venography (Phlebography)

Contrast venography of the distal lower extremities or pelvic veins remains the gold standard for diagnosing DVT. Venography also can be used to guide venous catheter placement, balloon dilation, and vein suitability for conduit harvest. Limitations include cost, puncture complications, and the possibility of contrast-induced endothelial injury or postphlebography thrombosis.[11]

Isotope Venography

Radiolabeled I^{125} fibrinogen scanning is particularly sensitive for detecting venous clots below the knee. However, this nuclear technique is limited by the inability to distinguish clot that is internal to a vein from that which is external. Also, peripheral edema, cellulitis, or arthritis may give false-positive results.

DIRECTED VASCULAR TESTING

The main manifestations of peripheral arterial disease are chronic obstruction, acute occlusion, aneurysm, and arteriovenous fistula. Accordingly, vascular diagnostic testing must be tailored to clinical suspicion.

Chronic occlusive peripheral arterial disease usually is evaluated initially with ABI or duplex scanning. Arteriography or other imaging techniques are pursued if revascularization is being considered.

Acute peripheral arterial disease may present dramatically with severe extremity pain, pulselessness, paresthesias, pallor, or paralysis. Likewise, the disease may present more subtly with any degree or combination of these symptoms. Clinical manifestations depend on the location of the occlusion and the status of collateral and distal arteries. Angiography is used to plan repair, especially if there is preexisting occlusive or aneurysmal disease or if the cause is unclear. Serial noninvasive monitoring is often necessary.

Thrombotic

History and diagnostic testing may reveal peripheral vascular disease, arteritis, trauma, dissection, myeloproliferative disease, or popliteal or femoral aneurysm.

Embolic

Besides peripheral diagnostic studies, perform echocardiography if you suspect cardiac disease. Cardiac sources are especially common with a history of atrial fibrillation, recent myocardial infarction, or left ventricular dysfunction. Transesophageal echocardiography is often the best way to define a cardiac embolic source because of its superior image quality, especially of the left atrial appendage (see Chapter 8).

Traumatic

Injury is usually apparent, but some situations require the skilled use of diagnostic testing. For example, complications arising from percutaneous procedures can be diagnosed noninvasively and, in the case of pseudoaneurysms, can often be treated directly by ultrasound-guided compression. Duplex imaging may show echolucent areas adjacent to or involving a traumatized artery. Doppler imaging can confirm flow in the abnormality, yielding a high diagnostic accuracy of its cause.[18] Arteriography also may be used to define sites of trauma and to plan surgical repair.

Cartoid Artery Disease

Carotid artery disease usually is screened by carotid duplex scanning as the noninvasive method of choice. In some cases this may be adequate to plan revascularization without cerebral arteriography or MRA. B-mode ultrasound scanning also identifies carotid stenoses and plaque characteristics. Doppler flow can assess physiologic significance, with peak velocities relating the degree of stenosis. Caution is required in determining lesions of >95%, since velocities may be decreased because of the marked fall off in blood flow. However, detection is aided in the marked spectral broadening throughout systole and the lack of color flow distally. Indirect oculoplethysmography (a measure of ocular arterial pressure) has been used in some institutions. Although carotid arteriography is considered the gold standard, it carries a small risk of stroke. A brain CT or MRI scan usually is also performed to exclude other causes of symptoms. Transcranial ultrasound is often used to monitor middle cerebral artery flow preoperatively or intraoperatively.

Abdominal Aortic Aneurysm

Abdominal aortic aneurysm (AAA) diagnosis relies on demonstrating aortic dilation by abdominal ultrasound, often by comparing serial tests. The size and extent may then be studied by CT with contrast or MRA. Contrast aortography may also be required to evaluate the size and extent of the AAA and its relationship to the surrounding vessels and other abdominal structures. Recently, helical CT has been used to preoperatively image AAAs.

Peripheral Bypass Grafts

Vein-bypass graft monitoring is important, since arterial bypass graft obstructions ideally must be identified before becoming thrombosed. Serial ABI and duplex scan measurements are used to follow graft patency. Although traditionally monitored by serial ABIs with, for example, a drop of >0. 15 being significant, Doppler ultrasonography appears more sensitive in predicting graft dysfunction.

Preoperative Assessment

Preoperative assessment is commonplace as PVD patients carry a lifelong risk of coronary disease, which is often the most significant consideration before noncardiac surgery.[9] For elective surgery, screening for coronary disease and left ventricular dysfunction is routine. Cardiac catheterization may be necessary.

REFERENCES

1. Raphael M, Donaldson R: The normal heart: methods of examination. In Sutton D, editor: *A textbook of radiology and imaging*, ed 5, Edinburgh, 1993, Churchill Livingstone.
2. Chen J: *Essentials of cardiac roentgenology*, Boston, 1987, Little, Brown.
3. Boxt L: Plain film examination of the chest. In Topal E, editor: *Textbook of cardiovascular medicine*, Philadelphia, 1998, Lippincott-Raven.
4. VanHouten F, Adams D, Abrams H: Radiology of valvular heart disease. In Sonnenblick E, Lesch M, editors: *Valvular heart disease*, New York, 1974, Grune & Stratton.
5. Fraser R, Pare J, Genereux G: *Diagnosis of diseases of the chest*, ed 3, Philadelphia, 1988, WB Saunders.
6. Spittell JA Jr: Peripheral arterial disease, *Disease-a-Month* 40:643, 1994.
7. Barnes BW: Noninvasive diagnostic assessment of peripheral vascular disease, *Circulation* 83:20, 1991.
8. Hallett JW, Brewster DC, Darling RC Jr: *Handbook of patient care in vascular surgery*, ed 3, Boston, 1995, Little, Brown.
9. Gersh BJ, Rihal CS, Rooke TW, Ballard DJ: Evaluation and management of patients with both peripheral vascular and coronary artery disease, *J Am Coll Cardiol* 18:203, 1991.

8 Echocardiogram

Mary B. Frankis
Elaine G. Hearney

Transthoracic echocardiography (TTE) is a versatile noninvasive diagnostic tool for evaluation and management of many cardiovascular disorders. Although the use of high frequency ultrasound in cardiac examinations can be traced as far back as the 1950s, widespread use began in the 1960s with the evaluation of pericardial effusion.[1] M-mode technology was employed, producing a one-dimensional, or "ice pick," view of the heart along a single sector. Two-dimensional scanning began in the mid-1970s, and Doppler imaging of valves in the late 1970s. Most recently, imaging probes on flexible endoscopes have allowed enhanced visualization of the heart from the transesophageal echocardiographic (TEE) approach. Technology continues to be developed rapidly, including three-dimensional reconstruction and the testing of injectable agents to improve visualization of blood-tissue interface and to define regional tissue perfusion.

The echocardiogram accurately measures chamber dimensions and ventricular wall thickness (Table 8-1 and Fig. 8-1). Normal fractional shortening of the left ventricle (LV) is greater than 25%, and this corresponds to left ventricular ejection fraction (LVEF) greater than 50%.

The Doppler device measures blood flow velocity on the basis of the principle that sound frequency increases as the source (in this case red blood cells) moves toward the echo transducer and decreases as the source moves away from the transducer. These frequency shifts can be translated to blood flow velocity. The frequency shifts, their direction relative to the transducer, and the extent of turbulence also can be color coded and superimposed on two-dimensional echo images. Blood flow away from the transducer is coded in shades of blue, and toward the transducer in shades of red. Since both regurgitant and stenotic lesions lead to turbulent blood flow, characteristic Doppler color flow imaging is created (Fig. 8-2).

The modified Bernoulli equation is used to convert Doppler-derived velocity measurements to estimates of a pressure gradient across a valve or shunt. This equation is explained exhaustively in textbooks on echocardiography.[2]

Echocardiography has become an invaluable technology in clinical medicine. For example, timing of surgery for valvular regurgitant lesions is governed by the size of the left ventricle and ventricular function, which is easily monitored with serial echocardiograms (see Chapters 18 and 19). On the other hand, echocardiography is routinely ordered despite the lack of outcome data to support its use. It becomes the duty of the primary care doctor and the subspecialist to ensure that this powerful but expensive technology is applied appropriately. From a financial perspective, a complete echo-Doppler examination costs between $700 to $900, a transesophageal echocardiogram, $700 to $800, and a stress echocardiogram, $500 to $600.

Transthoracic echocardiography is a noninvasive, painless test that requires no special patient preparation and can be performed in approximately 45 minutes. On the other hand, TEE requires esophageal intubation and can cause patient discomfort. The patient should be kept fasting for 4 to 6 hours before the procedure. To maximize patient comfort, a local anesthetic is applied to the posterior pharynx, and intravenous sedation is routinely employed. The test usually takes 30 to 45 minutes to complete. Since it is an invasive procedure it carries a small risk (e.g., arrhythmia, esophageal damage, bleeding). Patients with some pathologic conditions of the esophagus should be excluded.

EVALUATION OF LEFT VENTRICULAR FUNCTION AND CONGESTIVE HEART FAILURE

The most frequent indication for an echocardiogram is to evaluate LV function; this accounts for approximately 25% of studies in our laboratory. LV dimensions, wall thickness, LV mass, and LVEF are accurately measured. The echocardiogram is sensitive and specific for regional wall motion abnormalities. If the study is technically difficult, precise measurement of chamber size may not be possible, but a qualitative assessment of LVEF is commonly reported.

Echocardiographic assessment of contractile performance is useful in patients with a clinical diagnosis of heart failure or suspected cardiomyopathy. Signs and symptoms of congestive heart failure can occur as a result of systolic dysfunction, but also with preserved systolic performance and abnormal diastolic performance. Heart failure caused by diastolic dysfunction may require pharmacotherapy that is different from that for systolic dys-

Table 8-1	*Normal Reference Values*	
	Normal Range	**Normalized to BSA**
Left ventricular end-diastolic diameter	3.6 to 5.6 cm	2.0 to 2.8 cm/m²
Left ventricular end-systolic diameter	2.3 to 4.1 cm	1.3 to 2.2 cm/m²
Ejection fraction	≥ 50%	
Left atrial dimension	1.9 to 4.0 cm	1.1 to 2.2 cm/m²
Wall thickness end-diastole	0.6 to 1.1 cm	

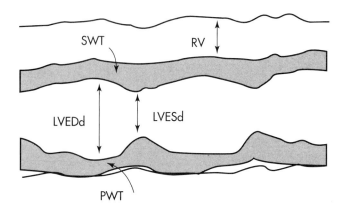

FIG. 8-1
Schematic of an M-mode echocardiogram from the parasternal long axis view. The abbreviations refer to measurements: *LVEDd,* Left ventricular end-diastolic dimension; *LVESd,* LV end-systolic dimension; *PWT,* LV posterior wall thickness; *SWT,* interventricular septal wall thickness; *RV,* right ventricular dimension.

function. In fact, echocardiographic studies in the evaluation of heart failure have been reported to change management in over half of the patients studied.[3]

Many echocardiographic techniques have been used to evaluate diastolic function. Spectral Doppler assessment of left ventricular filling velocity pattern—the E and A waves—can reflect the abnormalities of compliance and relaxation that constitute diastolic function. In the absence of systolic dysfunction and in the presence of clinical signs and symptoms of heart failure, it is reasonable to assume diastolic dysfunction. This is especially true if LV hypertrophy coexists.

Whether dyspnea is caused by cardiac or noncardiac disease is a common clinical issue. The Doppler/two-dimensional echocardiogram accurately distinguishes dilated cardiomyopathy, diastolic dysfunction, hypertrophic cardiomyopathy, and the less common restrictive cardiomyopathies as causes of congestion or low output syndromes. A normal left ventricle and the absence of valvular disease on an echocardiogram indicates that dyspnea is not caused by heart disease.

EVALUATION OF CORONARY ARTERY DISEASE AND CHEST PAIN

Chest pain is a common complaint, and misdiagnosis can carry a high risk of morbidity or mortality. The standard echocardiographic test, with two-dimensional and Doppler interpretation, usually does not provide a diagnosis for an unselected population of patients with chest pain. However, if the history, physical examination, and ECG suggest valvular heart disease, pericardial

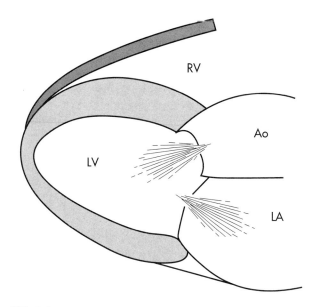

FIG. 8-2
Schematic of a two-dimensional echocardiogram. This patient has both aortic and mitral valve regurgitation, and in the color flow Doppler study the regurgitant jets (seen during diastole and systole, respectively) would be colored differently from antegrade flow. *Ao,* Aorta; *LV,* left ventricle; *RV,* right ventricle; *LA,* left atrium.

disease, or prior infarction, then the resting echocardiogram can add valuable information.

We are beginning to obtain an extensive database of both exercise and pharmacologic echo-stress testing in stable patients with known or suspected coronary artery disease. The theory behind the interpretation of echo-stress testing is based on fundamental physiologic concepts. Ischemia depresses regional contractility, leading to reduced wall thickening and motion during systole. The stress portion of the examination is carried out in the usual fashion with echocardiographic images obtained both before the treadmill test and as soon as the patient steps off the treadmill. It is especially helpful for patients with conduction abnormalities and other ECG abnormalities that are associated with false-positive tests.

The pharmacologic stress test is used when a patient cannot exercise. Since accuracy is similar, whether a nuclear study or an echocardiogram is chosen depends on local expertise, cost, and availability. As extensively described in the literature, typical symptoms and exercise ECG changes have an overall sensitivity in the range of 65% and a specificity of 85%. The addition of echocardiographic imaging of changes in wall motion appears to improve the overall sensitivity of the exercise test to 90%, with specificity remaining in the 80% to 85% range.[3]

The heart is imaged in four major views, typically subdivided into 16 sections, thus allowing for visualization of the territory supplied by each of the three major coronary arteries (Fig. 8-3). Digital recording and computer manipulation increase the accuracy of stress echocardiography; once an ideal image is captured, a single cardiac cycle can be replayed continuously (a "loop" recording). Digital imaging also helps to overcome the technical limitation imposed by interference from hyperventilation and allows display of resting, exercise, and recovery images side by side in the same view. The sections are then graded for contractile function, and wall motion is assessed *as normal, hypokinetic, akinetic, dyskinetic,* or *aneurysmal.* The American Society of Echocardiography has proposed a scheme to designate wall motion with a numeric score.[4] In this scheme, a normal segment is assigned a value of "1." Hypokinetic segments are assigned a value of "2," akinetic are "3," dyskinetic are "4," and aneurysmal are "5." For an individual test, the wall motion scores can be summed and indexed to normal, thus allowing for generation of a severity score that includes a reflection of the number of abnormal segments, as well as the degree of wall motion abnormalities.

The method of stress chosen depends on the ability of the patient to exercise and the expertise of the particular laboratory. Treadmill testing has been the most popular form of exercise in the United States. However, bicycle ergometry is both a viable and attractive alternative, since imaging can be performed during exercise. Unfortunately, it is common for patients to achieve a lower metabolic equivalent with bicycle testing than with treadmill testing. In treadmill testing the "peak"

exercise images must be obtained immediately after exercise, after the patient is properly maneuvered to the left lateral supine position for standard imaging. If too much time elapses before this maneuver, sensitivity may be diminished, since wall motion recovers in the post-exercise phase. However, it is reassuring that the reported sensitivities and specificities of treadmill exercise echocardiography are similar to that of treadmill nuclear perfusion imaging.[5]

For patients who cannot exercise, pharmacologic stress testing is a popular alternative. The adrenergic agonist, dobutamine, is the most commonly employed agent in pharmacologic stress echocardiography. This drug exerts inotropic and weak chronotropic actions on the heart. It is given in incremental doses, up to a maximum of 40 to 50 μg/kg/min. In many protocols, intravenous atropine is given to augment heart rate response. Arbutamine is a newer adrenergic agent being used in stress testing and has the advantage of having a greater chronotropic effect than dobutamine. However, it is more expensive, and, as mentioned above, atropine can be given to augment inadequate chronotropic response to dobutamine infusion. In addition, a low dose dobutamine infusion of 5 to 10 μg/kg/min has been used to assess for viability in segments of myocardium with baseline wall motion abnormalities. Viable tissue usually is able to exhibit augmented contractility at low dose inotropic stimulation. Dipyridamole and adenosine also have been used in the evaluation of ischemia and are proposed to work by creating a shunting of blood away from a fixed obstructive lesion. However, ischemia must be produced by this "steal phenomenon" so that wall motion abnormalities can be visualized, and some studies suggest a lower sensitivity versus the adrenergic-stimulating agent.[5]

The final interpretation of stress test results and the subsequent clinical application cannot be performed accurately unless the pretest likelihood of the disorder is first considered (Bayes Theorem, Chapter 6). In patients with a low pretest likelihood (e.g., those with chest pain that clinically is interpreted as nonanginal and with no significant risk factors for obstructive lesions), a positive stress echocardiogram is often a false-positive test. In patients who have an intermediate pretest likelihood of coronary disease, stress echocardiography would be expected to have the greatest effect on posttest likelihood of coronary artery disease. Subsets of patients with intermediate pretest likelihood of obstructive coronary disease include those with significant risk factors and atypical angina, abnormal ECG pattern at baseline, and premenopausal women with typical angina. The sensitivity of the test also is influenced by the severity of the underlying coronary disease and is higher in patients with multivessel versus single vessel disease and in

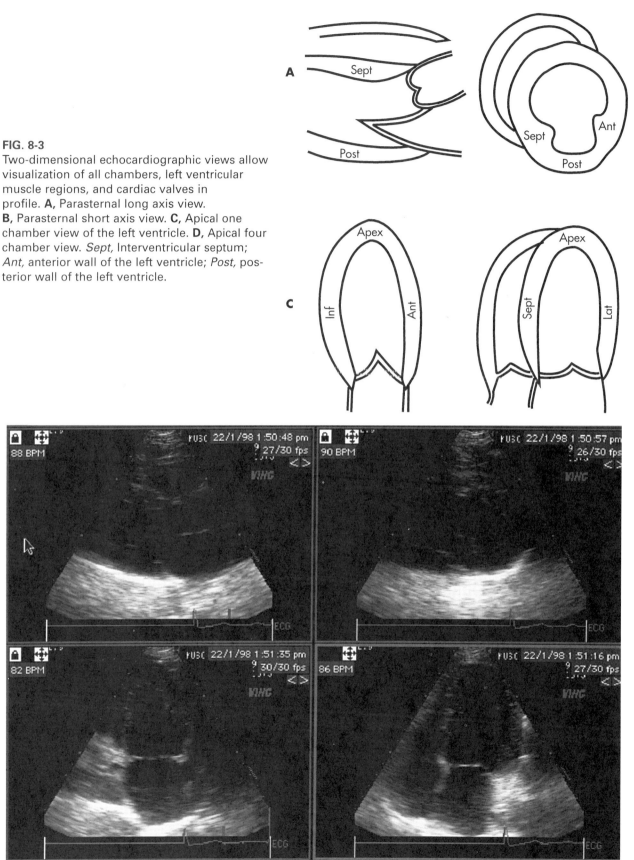

FIG. 8-3

Two-dimensional echocardiographic views allow visualization of all chambers, left ventricular muscle regions, and cardiac valves in profile. **A,** Parasternal long axis view. **B,** Parasternal short axis view. **C,** Apical one chamber view of the left ventricle. **D,** Apical four chamber view. *Sept,* Interventricular septum; *Ant,* anterior wall of the left ventricle; *Post,* posterior wall of the left ventricle.

those with greater than 70% stenosis. Considering all these factors, a negative stress echocardiogram (clinically negative with normal wall motion scores) still portends a low cardiovascular event rate during follow-up. If the stress test results in a positive ECG response but normal wall motion on the echocardiogram, the cardiovascular event rate is still very low but higher than a completely normal test.[6]

After myocardial infarction, the echocardiogram is useful for evaluation of LV function and any complications resulting from the infarction. Ejection fraction is the most commonly reported index of systolic performance. Resting postinfarction LVEF has profound correlation with long-term prognosis. The more extensive tissue damage results in reduced ejection performance and is accompanied by an increased risk of early and late complications such as recurrent infarction, congestive heart failure, ventricular and atrial arrhythmias, heart block, and sudden death. Management and pharmacotherapy may thus be tailored according to systolic performance. For instance, ACE inhibitors have been shown to have beneficial effects, preventing subsequent development of congestive symptoms in patients with asymptomatic LV dysfunction (EF <40%). In addition, as with routine stress testing and nuclear imaging techniques, stress echocardiography can provide information regarding prognosis. Resting wall motion abnormalities may be a result of prior irreversible myocardia necrosis but also may be a result of stunned or hibernating myocardium. Improvement in regional wall motion during low dose dobutamine stress testing indicates viable myocardium that may recover with revascularization. Results from stress echocardiography can then help guide medical therapy, help triage to invasive strategies such as catheterization, and risk stratify for noncardiac surgical procedures.

Other functional and mechanical complications may occur after infarction. In the setting of an inferior MI with hypotension and clear lung fields on physical examination, right ventricular infarction should be considered in the differential diagnosis. Echocardiography can identify abnormal motion of the right ventricular free wall and right ventricular dilation. Significant mitral regurgitation may be identified after infarction and is associated with worsened prognosis and congestive symptoms. The Doppler echocardiogram identifies the degree of insufficiency. Causes of the regurgitation may be apparent on two-dimensional imaging and may be secondary to annular dilation, papillary muscle dysfunction, scarring and fibrosis, or chordal rupture. Cardiogenic shock or death may result from acute rupture of the papillary muscle head.

If a new murmur is heard in the setting of myocardial infarction and hemodynamic instability, Doppler echocardiography is the preferred method for distinguishing between papillary muscle disruption and ventricular septal rupture (see Chapter 16). For septal rupture, Doppler echocardiography can localize the defect and demonstrate left-to-right shunting.

Free wall rupture also can occur after infarction and usually is fatal, but a few patients survive with the development of pseudoaneurysm (i.e., a rupture contained within a barrier formed by clot and pericardium). Doppler echocardiography can identify the flow of blood from the ventricle to the pericardial space. Pseudoaneurysm is distinguished from true aneurysm by the smaller width of the neck of a pseudoaneurysm. This distinction made by echocardiography is clinically important because of the continued risk of rupture of a pseudoaneurysm. It is an indication for surgery.

Left ventricular thrombus formation is common after large anterior and apical infarctions. Echocardiography is the diagnostic test of choice for detecting intracardiac thrombus and thus for detecting an increased risk of systemic or cerebral embolism. Since echocardiography is an effective screening test and effective anticoagulant therapy is available, we believe it is a cost-effective test after large anterior or apical infarctions. If a follow-up echo is performed in 6 months and no thrombus is visualized, no aneurysm has formed, and the EF is >30%, then anticoagulation treatment can be discontinued.

VALVULAR HEART DISEASE AND MURMURS

Echocardiography is invaluable in the assessment of native valvular pathologic conditions (e.g., regurgitation or stenosis), prosthetic valve function, endocarditis, and pathologic murmurs. Echocardiographic interrogation of the valves can provide detailed anatomic information, such as the presence of valvular fibrosis, calcification, immobility, prolapse, and vegetations. Doppler measurements can so precisely define the degree of stenosis and regurgitation that further invasive evaluation by catheterization may not be needed.

A murmur identified on cardiac auscultation is thought to be caused by turbulent blood flow and can reflect abnormal shunts or stenotic or regurgitant lesions. However, the most common murmur found on cardiac auscultation is the "innocent" or "functional" systolic murmur and is not associated with any known clinical significance. If all patients with heart murmur identified on auscultation were referred for echocardiography, the financial burden to the health care system would be overwhelming. Therefore it becomes imperative for primary care physicians and cardiologists to screen patients with a careful physical examination and to effectively distinguish functional from pathologic murmurs before referring patients for further testing. Functional murmurs are usually systolic, short in duration, seldom louder than grade III, most intense at the left upper sternal border, are associated with a normal S_2, do not increase in intensity with the Valsalva maneuver, and may decrease in intensity in the upright position. If the clinical findings are inconclusive, if the patient with a murmur has associated cardiorespiratory symptoms, or if the clinical features indicate a moderate probability of structural heart disease, then Doppler echocardiography is a reasonable examination.

Mitral Valve Prolapse

Mitral valve prolapse (MVP) is estimated to be a common finding in the population and deserves special mention because of several misconceptions. The advent of echocardiography likely resulted in the *overdiagnosis* of this malady, especially in studies performed in the 1980s. Currently, more rigid diagnostic criteria have reduced the number of false-positive echocardiograms. The physical

examination is a good method for diagnosing MVP, and the most recent ACC/AHA guidelines state that echocardiography is not useful in the absence of physical findings unless other evidence of structural heart disease or a family history of myxomatous valvular degeneration exists.[3] If MVP is suspected on clinical grounds or by physical examination findings, then the echocardiogram is helpful in the assessment of leaflet and subvalvular morphology, hemodynamic severity of associated mitral regurgitation, and ventricular size and function. Mitral valve prolapse with mitral regurgitation or markedly redundant leaflets on echocardiogram should be considered for bacterial endocarditis prophylaxis.[7]

Valvular Stenosis

As blood flows through a narrowed orifice, flow velocity increases proportional to the tightness of the stenosis. Using a modification of Bernoulli's equation, the pres-

Table 8-2	*Echocardiographic-Doppler Assessment of Valvular Heart Disease*

Lesion	Doppler Findings (Hemodynamic Profile)	Supportive Echocardiographic Findings
Mitral stenosis (MS)	1. PHT: Mild MS >110-140 msec Severe MS >220 msec 2. Mean gradient ≥12 mm Hg	1. M-mode: abnormal leaflet excursion during diastole 2. Two-dimensional echo: domed, thickened valve; reduced opening 3. Large LA, small LV
Aortic stenosis (AS)	1. Mean gradient ≥50 mm Hg 2. Flow velocity of the AS jet: Mild AS >3 m/sec Severe AS >4.5 m/sec 3. Severe AS: valve area ≤ 0.75 cm²	1. Calcified, immobile valve with reduced opening 2 Concentric left ventricular hypertrophy, usually with normal LVEF (although LVEF may be depressed with advanced AS) 3. Normal LV dimension
Mitral regurgitation (MR)	Severe MR: a large regurgitant jet (area of the MR jet/area of the LA >40%)	1. Abnormal valve (mitral prolapse, flail leaflet, rheumatic valve) 2. Dilated LA and LV (Table 8-3); with acute MR, chamber size may be normal 3. Reduced LVEF and increased LV systolic dimension indicate LV decompensation (and a need for surgery)
Aortic regurgitation (AR)	Severe AR: a large regurgitant jet (area of the AR jet/area of the LV >60%); PHT <250 msec	1. Abnormal valve or aortic root 2. Dilated LV, usually normal LV thickness 3. Reduced LVEF and increased LVESd indicate LV decompensation (these are the key measurements that indicate a need for surgery)
Tricuspid regurgitation	Possible elevation of pulmonary artery pressure (a Doppler calculation)	1. Possibly an abnormal-appearing valve (prolapse, vegetation, flail leaflet) 2. Dilated right atrium and ventricle

*Rheumatic MS: the anterior leaflet of the valve fails to drift toward the closed position in mid-diastole, then to reopen with atrial contraction. *PHT*, Pressure half-time, or the time required for peak flow velocity to decrease to half its initial level. With valve stenosis, the PHT is increased; with regurgitation it is decreased. *LVEF*, Left ventricular ejection fraction; *LVESd*, LV end-systolic diameter (Table 8-1); *LA*, left atrium; *PAP*, pulmonary artery pressure.

sure gradient across a stenosed mitral or aortic valve can be determined by measuring flow velocity downstream from the valve. For the aortic valve, flow velocity in the ascending aorta is proportional to degree of stenosis, and for the mitral valve, flow velocity in the left ventricle next to the valve is proportional the gradient. In addition, with mitral stenosis there is a diminished rate of decline of flow in early diastole. This results in an increase in the "pressure half-time," or the time it takes for the velocity to decrease by 50%. The pressure half-time measurement is used to calculate mitral valve area (Table 8-2). Mitral valve area less than 1 cm² is considered to represent severe mitral stenosis. Measurements derived from the Doppler examination have been correlated with both autopsy and surgical measurements, as well as with cardiac catheterization data.

Aortic stenosis, most frequently the result of calcific degenerative disease or an inherited bicuspid valve, is effectively evaluated by echocardiography. Doppler flow velocity (in meters/sec) is converted to peak instantaneous and mean transvalvular pressure gradients. As a rule, a flow velocity less than 3 meters/sec indicates mild stenosis. A mean systolic gradient ≥50 mm Hg generally suggests severe aortic stenosis. The continuity equation can be used to calculate an aortic valve area; less than 0.75 cm² represents severe stenosis (Fig. 8-4). In the presence of depressed systolic function and low cardiac output, the pressure gradients may be lower, even in the face of severe aortic stenosis. In this setting it may be helpful to administer an inotropic agent such as dobutamine or to rely on aortic valve resistance measurements. If a patient has mild to moderate aortic stenosis, follow-up echocardiography is indicated for progressive symptoms or signs of congestive failure.

In addition to hemodynamic measurements derived from the Doppler study, it is usually possible to view the mitral and aortic valves in cross section and directly visualize the orifice when the valve is open.

Valvular Regurgitation

Regurgitant valvular lesions are frequently identified on Doppler echocardiography, but the accurate delineation of the degree of severity is more problematic. Since Doppler signals are generated from frequency shifts of ultrasound waves, they are converted to spectral patterns representing *velocity*, not volume. Since the hemodynamic significance of regurgitation depends on the volume of regurgitation (or regurgitant fraction), it is the task of the echocardiographer to interpret two-dimensional Doppler velocity and color flow Doppler patterns and convert these to estimates of regurgitant volume or degree of severity. It is important for the clinician to realize that the echocardiographic interpretation of valvular regurgitation is more subjective than the interpretation of valvular stenosis. This means

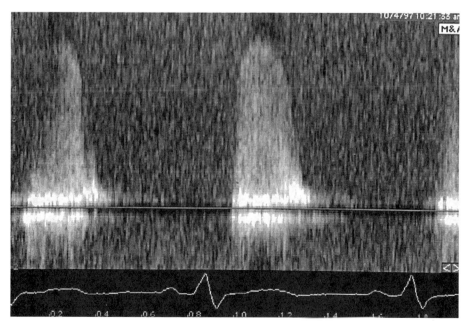

FIG. 8-4
Continuous wave Doppler tracing of a patient with aortic stenosis. In this example, the peak velocity is 6 m/sec (the calibration numbers are not visible on the tracing). Using the modified Bernoulli equation, Pressure (mm Hg) = $4 \times V_2$, so the calculated peak instantaneous gradient across the valve is 144 mm Hg. Another calculation allows determination of the valve area.

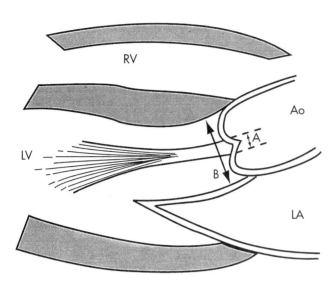

FIG. 8-5
Schematic of an echocardiographic Doppler study in a patient with aortic regurgitation. The ratio of the width of the regurgitant jet (A) and the width of the left ventricular outflow tract (B) is used to calculate the severity of regurgitation.

that both intraobserver variability and a chance of error are greater.

One of the most common methods for assessing the degree of mitral regurgitation is to estimate the two-dimensional area of the abnormal systolic color flow jet in the left atrium and then calculate a ratio to the total two-dimensional area of the left atrium in that same view. With this method, a ratio of 20% or less has been correlated with angiographically confirmed mild regurgitation, 20% to 40% with moderate regurgitation, and greater than 40% with severe mitral regurgitation.

These measurements are subject to several technical limitations. For instance, the area of the regurgitant jet depends on color flow gain settings and field depth of the two-dimensional image. In addition, eccentric jets, directed toward the wall of the left atrium rather than centrally, are frequently underestimated by this method. An additional complicating factor is that regurgitant volumes, and therefore estimated severity of the lesion, can vary with different loading conditions. Therefore factors such as blood pressure and intravascular volume may greatly influence study-to-study variation even if other technical factors are rigorously controlled.

Several quantitative approaches have been espoused to limit some of the subjectivity of interpretation. Since all these are time consuming and their accuracy is user dependent, they are seldom used in busy laboratories. Studies in the literature report the "PISA," or "proximal isovolumic surface area," for the determination of regurgitant volume and effective regurgitant orifice. In the right hands, this is an accurate Doppler and color flow mea-

surement of mitral regurgitation. However, it is an order of magnitude more complicated than other estimates and is used primarily by research-oriented laboratories.[2]

The evaluation of aortic insufficiency suffers from many of the above technical limitations described for mitral regurgitation. Similar to those used in mitral regurgitation, methods include assessment of regurgitant jet characteristics, such as area and width. Most commonly, the area and width of the color flow jet is calculated as a ratio to the area or width (i.e., diameter) of the left ventricular outflow tract at the plane of the aortic valve (Fig. 8-5). In general, if such ratios are greater than 60%, the aortic insufficiency is severe; if less than 30%, the aortic insufficiency is mild. Another Doppler feature used in the assessment of aortic insufficiency is the pressure half-time (PHT) of the aortic insufficiency signal. This measurement is based on the concept that the Doppler velocity measurements are proportional to the instantaneous pressure gradient at any particular moment in diastole. Therefore, if aortic insufficiency is severe, the pressure gradient across the aortic valve dissipates more quickly, and the measured Doppler velocities decrease faster. A rapid fall off in measured velocity results in a steeper slope and a short PHT measurement. In aortic insufficiency, a PHT less than 250 msec suggests severe regurgitation and greater than 400 msec indicates mild regurgitation (see Table 8-2).

Other echocardiographically derived data can support the presence of significant aortic insufficiency. If there is holodiastolic reversal of flow in the descending aorta, the insufficiency likely will be severe. In a similar fashion to mitral regurgitation, regurgitant volumes and fractions can be estimated and related to severity, but this estimation is more technically challenging. As with mitral regurgitation, the calculated degree of aortic insufficiency depends on loading conditions regardless of the method used. The length of the aortic insufficiency jet, that is, how far it reaches toward the apex of the left ventricle, has not been shown to correlate with severity, since it is highly afterload dependent.

Since it is a noninvasive test, TTE is ideal for the serial follow-up of patients in whom significant valvular regurgitation has been previously identified. Hemodynamically significant regurgitant lesions result in abnormal ventricular loading and stress and thus can eventually result in irreversible left ventricular dysfunction. If this occurs, even if valvular regurgitation is successfully corrected by surgical intervention, increased postoperative morbidity and mortality rates persist. For mitral regurgitation, ejection fractions less than 60% and left ventricular end-systolic dimension greater than 45 mm have been correlated with poor long-term postsurgical outcomes. Even if a patient with mitral regurgitation is asymptomatic, surgery should be contemplated if the measurements from the echocardiogram approach these proposed "cut-off" values. For aortic insufficiency,

Table 8-3	Indications for Surgery in Valvular Regurgitation	
	Mitral Regurgitation	**Aortic Insufficiency**
Ejection fraction	<60%	<50%
Left ventricular end-systolic diameter	≥45 mm	≥55 mm
Left ventricular end-diastolic volume	>160 ml/m²	>220 ml/m²

similar suboptimal postoperative outcomes have been observed when surgery is delayed until LVEF has fallen below 50% or left ventricular end-systolic diameter is greater than 55 mm (see Table 8-3).

Mild valvular regurgitation also can occur in normal individuals, that is, in those who have no appreciable murmur on auscultation and in whom the noted regurgitation has no apparent hemodynamic significance. Such "physiologic" regurgitation is frequent at the tricuspid and pulmonic valves and becomes more frequent with advancing age. With continuous technologic improvements in echocardiographic instrumentation, improved Doppler sensitivity has demonstrated trivial to mild mitral regurgitation in more and more patients. Since the finding of clinically inapparent regurgitation in an asymptomatic patient carries no known significance, the ACC/AHA guidelines discourage routine reevaluation of asymptomatic patients with mild valvular insufficiency and normal LV size and function.[3] Many investigators believe that any degree of aortic insufficiency is pathologic, but it is a fairly common finding in patients with long-standing hypertension. The observation that regurgitation may be an anatomic variant in normal subjects should be kept in mind, especially in light of recent revelations that certain weight loss medications may cause symptomatic pathologic conditions of the valves. Obviously, mass screening by echocardiography of all individuals exposed to these agents would result in identifying a large number of people with previously undiagnosed, but echocardiographically apparent, valvular regurgitation. The significance of such findings currently is unknown.

ENDOCARDITIS: NATIVE AND PROSTHETIC VALVES

Echocardiography is in a unique position to add to the clinical management of patients with suspected endocarditis, with ability to image lesions suspicious for vegetations and to characterize the hemodynamic conse-

quences of infection. Associated abnormalities such as abscess formation, shunts, ruptured chordae, and ventricular dysfunction also can be detected. The classic or strict criteria for the diagnosis of endocarditis relied only on major and minor clinical variables. However, a more recent reevaluation proposed new criteria that include a positive echocardiogram as one of the major features used in the diagnosis.[8] It concludes that echocardiography should be used in all patients with suspected endocarditis and further notes that TEE is more sensitive. Transesophageal echocardiography would not be necessary in cases in which the transthoracic echocardiography is clearly positive.

Many other clinical studies have confirmed that TEE is more sensitive than TTE in detecting vegetations (90% or greater vs. 40% to 60%). This makes it difficult to decide on the appropriate, least invasive, and most cost efficient test to order for our patients. Obviously not everyone with a fever of uncertain cause can be screened in a cost effective manner by TEE. Furthermore, despite its excellent sensitivity and specificity, even a normal TEE cannot exclude the diagnosis. Since even the best technique in echocardiography is not 100% sensitive or specific, clinical and microbiologic findings must always be the cornerstone of diagnosis.

A few clinical situations seem to justify the use of echocardiographic examination, including bacteremia of uncertain source, fever plus a murmur, and suspicion of endocarditis despite negative blood cultures. Even if endocarditis has been diagnosed without the help of an echocardiogram, an echocardiogram can still help to characterize the valvular lesion, assess the hemodynamic consequence, and detect associated abnormalities. It may be appropriate to repeat the initial study if clinical status changes (e.g., persistent bacteremia or fever) and to reevaluate the hemodynamic significance and effect of severe regurgitant lesions on ventricular performance.

TTE remains the best technique for initial evaluation in most cases. However, TEE is especially well suited for the initial evaluation of suspected prosthetic valve endocarditis, because this technique helps overcome (but does not eliminate) imaging artifacts, such as reverberations and attenuation caused by prosthetic material. Such artifacts can effectively "shadow" or "drop out" areas of the valve and remaining cardiac structures, and TEE usually improves visualization owing to its superior image quality and posterior transducer position. If there are preexistent valvular abnormalities such as aortic sclerosis or mitral annular calcification, TEE can better delineate superimposed infection or vegetation. Certainly, TEE can be used to overcome poor quality TTE in the setting of inadequate transthoracic echocardiographic window. If a fever persists despite appropriate antibiotic therapy, TEE may identify abscess formation of the aortic root and annulofibrosis.

PERICARDIAL DISEASE AND CARDIAC MASSES

One of the first clinical applications of echocardiography was in the diagnosis of pericardial effusion. It provides a semiquantitative assessment of effusion and its location and distribution. This information is valuable if pericardiocentesis is contemplated. It is often possible to note thickening of the pericardium; however, pericardial thickness is better evaluated with magnetic resonance imaging.

If enlarging pericardial effusions result in elevated intrapericardial pressure, cardiac tamponade can ensue. Echocardiographic signs of tamponade include right atrial collapse during ventricular systole, right ventricular diastolic collapse, distention without respiratory variation of the inferior vena cava, respiratory variations in ventricular inflow Doppler velocity measurements, and alterations in venous flow patterns. All these signs have imperfect predictive values and can be mimicked by conditions other than tamponade. In most echocardiographic laboratories, the sensitivity and specificity of these findings are suboptimal, so the diagnosis of tamponade should be made on established clinical criteria.

In a similar fashion to tamponade, echocardiographic features are associated with constrictive pericarditis. Multiple echocardiographic abnormalities usually are present, but no single sign is pathognomonic. Unfortunately, as with tamponade, the predictive accuracy of echocardiographic measurements in most laboratories is not high, since the measurements are tedious and require a familiarity and accuracy that develop only with frequent use. Most nonreferral centers do not have the expertise to make this diagnosis consistently, but certainly some combination of echo-derived data along with other imaging modalities or heart catheterization can help make the diagnosis in the appropriate clinical context.

Intracardiac masses are often identified by TTE or TEE. Atrial myxoma is the most common primary tumor of the heart and can be easily identified by two-dimensional/Doppler echocardiograms. Metastatic tumors also can be visualized, with melanoma, breast cancer, lung cancer, and renal cell cancer having a predilection for the heart or pericardium.

DISEASES OF THE AORTA

Acute aortic dissection requires early diagnosis. Although TTE can identify dissection flaps, it lacks needed sensitivity. However, TEE has sensitivity that rivals other available techniques such as spiral CT, MRI, and aortography. Echocardiography has the advantage of allowing bedside imaging and complete interrogation of cardiac valves, wall motion, overall left ventricular function and coexistent pericardial effusions. TEE also can detect atheromatous disease of the aorta, including mobile plaques and clots that are prone to producing embolic occlusions. Aneurysms of the proximal ascending aorta can be characterized by TTE, and Doppler imaging can be used to characterize rupture of aneurysms of the sinus of Valsalva and communication into cardiac chambers.

SYSTEMIC HYPERTENSION

Echocardiography is an excellent tool for the measurement of LV wall thickness and estimation of LV mass. It is much more sensitive than the 12-lead ECG, which may miss left ventricular hypertrophy (LVH) in as many as 50%. Since LVH is associated with increased cardiovascular morbidity and mortality, it is tempting to use echocardiography to help risk stratify patients with hypertension and thereby tailor the aggressiveness of antihypertensive therapy. However, clear guidelines exist for the management of hypertension on the basis of systolic and diastolic measures, and no convincing data exist suggesting that echocardiographic endpoints add to patient care. On the other hand, if a patient has borderline hypertension or blood pressure readings taken in the physician's office may not reflect the patient's norm, then hypertrophy detected on a goal-directed two-dimensional/M-mode echocardiogram may prompt treatment (this study need not include a Doppler evaluation). The development of signs and symptoms of congestive heart failure in a hypertensive patient should prompt echocardiographic evaluation in an effort to distinguish systolic from diastolic dysfunction.

CARDIOEMBOLIC DISEASE

Roughly 20% of acute neurologic events stem from a cardioembolic source. Although many patients with embolic events have a potential cardiac source of embolus, proving cause and effect is more difficult. Atrial fibrillation, prosthetic heart valves, rheumatic heart disease, and akinetic left ventricular segments have long been known to predispose to embolic events as a result of a predilection for thrombus formation. Recent studies have found a greater neurologic event rate in patients with other cardiovascular abnormalities noted on echocardiogram, such as mitral valve prolapse, atrial septal aneurysm, spontaneous echo contrast, aortic atheroma, and patent foramen ovale. Although these findings are more common in patients who have had a cerebrovascular accident, a cause and effect relationship is unproved, and it is uncertain that specific therapies (e.g., antiplatelet versus anticoagulant) are effective in preventing recurrence. Since TEE is more sensitive than TTE in recognizing the above abnormalities, some investigators have suggested that TEE is a first-line study in patients with a suspected cardioembolic event. In contrast, many studies have revealed that TTE is a low-yield examination in patients with no clinically apparent cardiac abnormality,[9] is unlikely to alter management, and is therefore not cost effective. A young patient (e.g., 45 years old) with no apparent intrinsic cerebrovascular disease and a high clinical suspicion for embolic event should have an echocardiogram, and TEE can be considered a first-line study. Ongoing clinical trials will further define the role of TEE in the management of potential cardioembolic events.

ARRHYTHMIAS, PALPITATIONS, AND SYNCOPE

Arrhythmias can be a primary abnormality of the electrical system of the heart but also can be associated with other structural heart disease. If arrhythmias occur in a patient with clinical suspicion of heart disease or in a patient with a family history of potentially inheritable forms of heart disease prone to arrhythmias, then an echocardiogram may be helpful. An echocardiogram is rarely indicated for patients with palpitations without underlying arrhythmia or signs of cardiac disease or in patients with isolated premature ventricular contractions for which there is no clinical suspicion of heart disease. Sustained and nonsustained ventricular tachycardias are most commonly associated with depressed left ventricular function and with underlying ischemia or structural heart disease. An echocardiogram is a key part of the workup.

Atrial fibrillation is a common rhythm disorder seen in the primary care setting. The echocardiogram can help stratify patients according to embolic risk and identify underlying pathologic conditions that may influence treatment choices. Valvular heart disease, ventricular hypertrophy or dilatation, or other structural heart disease have been found in approximately 10% of patients with no clinically suspected disease and in up to 60% of patients with equivocal clinical markers.[10] Because of this high yield of information, TTE is warranted for newly diagnosed atrial fibrillation. Intracardiac thrombus or spontaneous echo contrast (that looks like "smoke" in the atrium or ventricle) indicates a high-risk for thromboemboli. However, the left atrial appendage, a frequent site for thrombus formation in patients with atrial fibrillation, is poorly seen on TTE.

With the advent of multiplane TEE, it became possible to reliably image the atrial appendage in almost every study. Since the LA appendage is a frequent area of thrombus formation, it has been postulated that TEE can be used to risk stratify patients before attempts at cardioversion. This has not yet been tested. Currently, for atrial fibrillation >48 hours in duration the stan-

dard of care includes the establishment of a therapeutic level of anticoagulation for 3 to 4 weeks before and after cardioversion. Preliminary studies have suggested that the exclusion of thrombus by TEE may eliminate the need for prolonged anticoagulation before cardioversion. However, because the tendency toward formation of intraatrial thrombus persists for a significant time after successful conversion to sinus rhythm, periconversion and postconversion anticoagulation is indicated. In other words, TEE may be able to shorten the required period of anticoagulation by obviating the need for prolonged precardioversion anticoagulation, but anticoagulation is necessary both during and after the procedure to reduce the risk of thromboembolism. The final recommendation for use of TEE in cardioversion of atrial fibrillation awaits the results of ongoing trials that are examining the safety, efficacy, and cost effectiveness of this approach.

Syncope has a lifetime incidence of approximately 3% and is therefore frequently encountered in clinical practice. The echocardiogram can identify obstructive lesions and abnormalities of ventricular function or wall motion that provide a substrate for ventricular arrhythmias and thereby predispose to syncope. Retrospective studies of syncope that have attempted to ascertain the diagnostic yield of echocardiography in unselected populations have been inconclusive. Obviously, the diagnostic yield is likely to improve if echocardiography is used in patients with exertional syncope, in those with clinical markers for heart disease, or in the elderly. Conversely, echocardiography is unlikely to be helpful in the evaluation of a young person with no clinical indicators of heart disease.

EMERGING TECHNIQUES AND FUTURE TRENDS

Echocardiography has been further refined and expanded since its initial application in clinical medicine. Advances in this field have been rapidly incorporated into clinical practice. For instance, TEE examinations are now considered invaluable in the intraoperative assessment of valvular repair and replacement, in the evaluation of left ventricular performance in high-risk patients, and in the assessment of congenital heart disease. As mentioned previously, this technique has gained wide acceptance in assessing prosthetic valves and native valvular pathology. In addition, both TEE and TTE have been used in severely injured patients and in the critically ill when hemodynamic instability (or suspected aortic pathology) makes bedside evaluation attractive.

Intravascular ultrasound, which consists of placing a miniature ultrasonic transducer on a small catheter and passing it directly into a blood vessel, enables cardiologists to view the lumen and wall of vessels, thereby providing information about plaque morphology that is not possible to obtain with contrast angiography. However, as with any new technique, the expense can outweigh the possible benefit if significant additional information is not obtained, and the clinical role of intravascular echocardiography continues to evolve.

Contrast echocardiography is an especially exciting application of ultrasound. This technology is based on the fact that almost any liquid injected into the intravascular space causes microbubbles, which appear as "echo densities" on imaging systems. The simplest agent employed is agitated saline solution, which is injected directly into a peripheral vein. This results in opacification of the right-sided chambers of the heart and can greatly enhance the detection of right-to-left and left-to-right shunts. These microbubbles are effectively cleared from the circulation in the pulmonary circuit, and therefore opacification of the left-sided chambers cannot usually be obtained. However, commercial agents are available, such as sonicated albumin, that traverse the pulmonary capillaries and opacify the left-sided chambers. Newer generations of contrast agents are being developed that will opacify the myocardial tissue and thereby allow determination of regional blood flow in the myocardium. The application of this technique in cardiac catheterization laboratories has generated enthusiasm concerning the ability to quickly assess the success or failure of revascularization techniques and thrombolytics. Further refinements in technology, such as the physical principles of "second harmonics" and "spectral backscatter," may make it possible to use echocardiography to detect diastolic function and relaxation accurately, to distinguish thrombus from myocardial tissue reliably, and to identify rejection episodes of the transplanted heart.

Much work has been done and continues toward the application of echocardiography for three-dimensional reconstructions. Investigational work suggests that such imagery can enhance detection of valvular pathology and aortic diseases.

LIMITATIONS AND ADVANTAGES OF ECHOCARDIOGRAPHY

Compared with other noninvasive diagnostic techniques, TTE is painless and avoids ionizing radiation. Higher energy ultrasound may carry a small risk, and this should be kept in mind as new ultrasound techniques are developed. It is not an issue with current techniques. Contrast agents currently used to enhance the quality of the echocardiographic image do not increase the risk.

The most significant limitation of echocardiography is related to the expertise of the technician and the physician who is interpreting the study. These are operator-dependent techniques, and laboratories that do large volumes generally conduct higher quality studies. This is a critical issue with exercise echocardiography, in which inexperience or inadequate training commonly results in false-positive or false-negative studies.

REFERENCES

1. Feigenbaum H: *Echocardiography,* ed 5, Philadelphia, 1991, Lea & Febiger.
2. Oh JK, Seward JB, Tajik AJ: *The echo manual,* Boston, 1994, Little, Brown.
3. Cheitlin MD, Alpert JS, Armstrong WF, et al: ACC/AHA Guidelines for the Clinical Application of Echocardiography: a report of the American College of Cardiology/ American Heart Association Task Force on Practice Guidelines (Committee on Clinical Application of Echocardiography). Developed in collaboration with the American Society of Echocardiography, *Circulation* 95:1686, 1997.
4. Broderick TM, Bourdillon PD, Ryan T, et al: Comparison of regional and global left ventricular function by serial echocardiograms after reperfusion in acute myocardial infarction, *J Am Soc Echocardiogr* 2:315, 1989.
5. Marwick T, Willemart B, D'Hondt AM, et al: Selection of the optimal nonexercise stress for the evaluation of ischemic regional myocardial dysfunction and malperfusion: comparison of dobutamine and adenosine using echocardiography and 99mTc-MIBI single photon emission computed tomography, *Circulation* 87:345, 1993.
6. Sawada SG, Ryan T, Conley MJ, et al: Prognostic value of a normal exercise echocardiogram, *Am Heart J* 120:49, 1990.
7. Dajani AS, Taubert KA, Wilson W, et al: Prevention of bacterial endocarditis: recommendations by the American Heart Association, *Circulation* 96:358, 1997.
8. Durack DT, Lukes AS, Bright DK: New criteria for diagnosis of infective endocarditis: utilization of specific echocardiographic findings, *Am J Med* 96:200, 1994.
9. Lovett JL, Sandok BA, Giuliani ER, Nasser FN: Two-dimensional echocardiography in patients with focal cerebral ischemia, *Ann Intern Med* 95:1, 1981.
10. Godtfredsen J, Egeblad H, Berning J: Echocardiography in lone atrial fibrillation, *Acta Med Scand* 213:111, 1983.

9

Nuclear Cardiology

Robert Trask
Jerome J. Epplin

NUCLEAR TECHNOLOGY

Radiopharmaceuticals, predominantly thallium 201 and technetium 99m–based compounds, are injected intravenously during nuclear imaging. They are either taken up by myocardial cells (perfusion imaging) or remain in the cardiac blood pool (radionuclide angiocardiography, or RNA). The isotopes emit gamma rays that are absorbed by a sodium iodide crystal in the gamma camera. The crystal produces photons that are converted to electrical signals. With electronic integration of an array of photo multiplier tubes, a two-dimensional image of the heart is constructed.

In planar cardiac imaging the gamma camera is positioned to obtain several views, typically the left anterior oblique, anterior, and lateral. The physician interpreting the images must correlate the multiple two-dimensional images with the three-dimensional cardiac structure. Planar imaging is predominantly used for RNA and currently is used less commonly in perfusion imaging because of the availability of single-photon emission computed tomography (SPECT).

SPECT images are reconstructed using computer techniques. The images are presented similar to the presentation of CT or MRI images, that is, as slices at different depths through the heart in short axis, horizontal, and vertical long axis views. This allows both better anatomic delineation of perfusion defects and improved image contrast. Additional advances in SPECT imaging have included multiple detector heads, typically consisting of two gamma cameras set at 90-degree angles. This allows a more rapid acquisition with increased counts, which may improve image quality and shorten the duration of the imaging, thereby improving patient comfort.

Radiation Exposure

Radiation exposure is a common concern expressed by patients. The exposure is comparable to the radiation dose associated with an upper GI series and significantly less than that with coronary angiography. A good rule of thumb for patient explanation is that the radiation dose is similar to the accumulated background radiation exposure for a person living 1 mile above sea level for 5 years.

MYOCARDIAL PERFUSION IMAGING

Myocardial perfusion imaging is used to noninvasively identify stenotic coronary arteries and is by far the most important use of nuclear cardiac imaging. Thallium 201 and technetium 99m–based radiopharmaceuticals are used to determine myocardial perfusion. Thallium 201 is a potassium analog that is extracted from the blood by the myocardial cells. The uptake of thallium is proportional to myocardial blood flow (perfusion). Thus a "cold spot" on the thallium scan indicates reduced perfusion (Fig. 9-1). The heart is scanned at rest and again during stress (exercise or pharmacologic). The resting and stress images are then compared. A perfusion defect during stress identifies a coronary stenosis that narrows the vessel by at least 70%.

Redistribution and Assessment of Myocardial Viability

Thallium has a unique property called *late redistribution.* Thallium is taken into ischemic myocardium slowly over time, even in regions that are ischemic or poorly perfused as a result of coronary stenoses. For this to be effective, the myocardial tissue must be viable (i.e., living myocardial cells with an active Na^+- K^+- ATPase pump).

Late redistribution into a region that had no uptake of thallium during stress indicates ischemic muscle that is still viable. On the other hand, a cold spot during stress that shows no redistribution (remains a cold spot) on the later scan indicates myocardial scar.

Choice of Imaging Agent

Although thallium has many excellent imaging properties, it has some drawbacks. The photon emitted by thallium is low energy (65 to 79 keV), which, in combination with its longer physical half-life, limits the dose to 3 to 4 microcuries. Technetium-based compounds have been developed to take advantage of the higher energy (140 keV) photon emitted by this agent, thus achieving better imaging resolution. In addition, because of the shorter physical half-life and favorable dosimetry of technetium 99m–based compounds, higher doses in the range of 30 to 45 microcuries are used.

Technetium-based radiopharmaceuticals such as sestamibi (Cardiolyte) are similar to thallium; the uptake

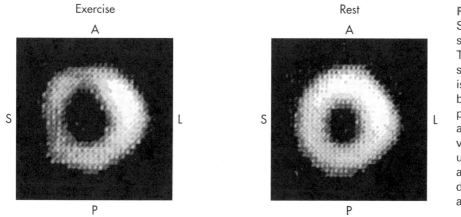

Exercise

Rest

FIG. 9-1
Sestamibi perfusion scans, cross-sectional view of the left ventricle. The scan obtained during exercise shows relatively less uptake of the isotope by the septal (S) and possibly anterior (A) walls. Lateral and posterior wall perfusion is similar at rest and exercise. At rest, all left ventricular regions show uniform uptake. Angiography documented a tight stenosis of the left anterior descending artery (see Figs. 2-12 and 2-13).

in the myocardium is proportional to regional myocardial perfusion of blood flow. In contrast to thallium these agents do not have significant redistribution, and therefore the scan is a "snapshot" of myocardial blood flow, regardless of when the scan is obtained. This makes imaging time more flexible, up to several hours after the injection. On the other hand, since technetium-based agents do not redistribute, late scanning cannot be performed to assess myocardial viability.

The major drawback of technetium-based agents is significant hepatic accumulation with slow clearance from the biliary tract. This gut uptake may overlap portions of the heart and produce imaging artifacts. Newer agents that have better hepatic clearance are being developed to overcome this problem. Tetrofosmin (Myoview) was recently approved by the U.S. Food and Drug Administration for perfusion imaging. Although tetrofosmin does have improved hepatic clearance, overlapping gut uptake can still occur.

The currently available technetium-based radiopharmaceuticals require injections at both rest and stress (exercise or pharmacologic). The injections and imaging can be performed as a 2-day protocol or as a 1-day protocol, which is a lengthy procedure (taking a half day). In our laboratory we use dual isotope sestamibi-thallium imaging. This protocol involves a rest thallium injection with SPECT imaging. Subsequently the patient has exercise or pharmacologic stress with technetium 99m sestamibi injection and SPECT imaging. With this approach the total procedure time is reduced to $1\frac{1}{2}$ to 2 hours. The stress technetium 99m sestamibi injection allows for optimal imaging characteristics of the technetium-based agent with higher resolution and the additional benefit of gating of the images for assessment of left ventricular function and perfusion. The rest thallium portion of the study allows for better assessment of viability of myocardium over rest sestamibi imaging.

A Typical Scan

Figure 9-1 illustrates the standard display of a normal SPECT perfusion study. The ideal presentation for SPECT

or planar imaging consists of comparing the stress images with similarly positioned slices from the rest images in each of the standard views. An overlay technique allows direct comparison to determine the presence, location, and reversibility of a perfusion defect.

Artifact

One of the drawbacks of myocardial perfusion imaging is imaging artifact caused by adjacent structures. Typically, anterior wall attenuation defects are caused by breast or chest wall tissue and can sometimes be confused with left anterior descending artery distribution stenoses or infarction. Alternatively, inferior wall defects can be related to diaphragmatic overlap and may mimic right coronary artery disease. Experienced nuclear cardiologists develop an ability to distinguish perfusion abnormalities from artifact. The difference is subtle, and for this reason perfusion imaging remains an operator-dependent technique; accuracy and reliability are proportional to the laboratory's experience.

Indications for Myocardial Perfusion Scanning

Myocardial perfusion imaging can be used to diagnose coronary disease and to assess prognosis for patients with known coronary artery disease. Table 9-1 lists the typical indications for stress perfusion imaging.

Table 9-2 indicates sensitivities and specificities for myocardial perfusion imaging and stress echocardiography and includes information on costs. Multiple studies have demonstrated an incremental value of myocardial perfusion imaging in assessment of prognosis when compared with clinical information, standard exercise ECG testing, and even cardiac catheterization.

The Value of a Normal Scan

Many studies have demonstrated a very low 1-year event rate in patients having a normal SPECT perfusion study (<1% risk of myocardial infarction or cardiac death). This includes perfusion scanning performed as part of a treadmill study and scanning after the use of pharmacologic agents, either adenosine or dipyrimadole. The event rates after a normal stress echocardiogram have not been shown to be as low as those after myocardial perfusion imaging; the 1-year risk of nonfatal infarction after a normal stress echocardiogram is 4%.

Because of the low event rate associated with a normal study, stress perfusion imaging has become in some respects a gold standard. That is, patients are no longer referred for catheterization with a normal study. For this reason, there is a potential for an apparent alteration of the diagnostic accuracy of perfusion scanning in future studies: if those with a negative scan do not have catheterization, false negatives will be missed, increasing the relative number of false positives.

Pharmacologic Perfusion Scanning

Box 9-1 describes the indications for pharmacologic stress testing. Table 9-3 lists the cost of pharmacologic agents used for nuclear and echocardiographic studies; drug cost is added to the cost of the imaging study (see

Table 9-1	*Indications for Myocardial Perfusion Imaging*
Indication	**Examples and Comments**
Abnormal resting ECG (increasing the risk of a false-positive stress ECG)	Left ventricular hypertrophy Digitalis Left bundle branch block Pacemaker Resting ST and T wave abnormalities Wolff-Parkinson-White syndrome
Abnormal stress ECG	Myocardial perfusion imaging or stress echocardiography are used if a false-positive result is strongly suspected or if further prognostic information is needed.
Risk stratification in selected patients before noncardiac surgery	Pharmacologic perfusion imaging and dobutamine echocardiography have been shown to be helpful in identifying selected high-risk patients (see Chapter 48).
Assessment of extent and location of coronary artery disease	Guide in determining prognosis and therapy (e.g., revascularization versus medical therapy)
Risk stratification after myocardial infarction	Guide in determining prognosis and therapy
Before PTCA	Identify culprit lesions causing myocardial ischemia when there is uncertainty
Identification of restenosis after PTCA in symptomatic patients or after bypass surgery	
Assessment of selective asymptomatic patients after PTCA/stent therapy considered to be at high risk	Decreased left ventricular function Multivessel coronary disease Proximal left anterior descending artery disease Previous sudden death Diabetes mellitus Hazardous occupations Suboptimal PTCA results
Abnormal ultrafast CT result	Stress perfusion imaging is helpful to exclude a hemodynamically significant stenosis in patients with a significantly abnormal ultrafast CT identifying coronary calcification.
Assessment of myocardial viability in patients with left ventricular dysfunction	Thallium scanning is preferred.

Table 9-2	Accuracy and Cost of Myocardial Perfusion Imaging and Stress Echocardiography		
	Sensitivity	Specificity	Costs*
Exercise ECG	68%	77%	$326
Cardiac perfusion imaging	91%	73%	$1468
			(Gated assessment, add $208)
Stress echocardiography	71% to 97%	64% to 100%	$770
			(Echo contrast, add $240)

*Information from 1997 PMIC for 75th percentile of national average fees (including technical and professional fees, but not including the cost of the isotope, about $100 for thallium).

BOX 9-1

INDICATIONS FOR PHARMACOLOGIC STRESS TESTING

Inability to walk to target work loads on the treadmill
    Inadequate motivation
    Elderly or frail patient
    Peripheral vascular disease
    Orthopedic illness

Early noninvasive risk assessment after acute myocardial infarction

Left bundle branch block pattern (where it is superior to exercise imaging)

Preoperative risk stratification for noncardiac surgery (see Chapter 48).

Table 9-3	Pharmacologic Stress Agents	
Agent	Cost*	Increase in Coronary Blood Flow
Adenosine	$350	4-5 ×
Dipyridamole	$100 to $150	4-5 ×
Dobutamine	$27	2-3 ×
Arbutamine	$125 to $150	2-3 ×

*This cost is added to other fees for the imaging study.

Table 9-2). Cardiac imaging with either myocardial SPECT perfusion imaging or echocardiography needs to be used during any pharmacologic stress test, since the sensitivity of the echocardiogram is low during pharmacologic stress testing.

A pharmacologic study is indicated if during the treadmill exercise a patient fails to reach target heart rate and work loads. The reported accuracy of exercise scanning is based on a patient achieving 85% of the maximal predicted heart rate. Perfusion scanning may not be as sensitive in detecting disease when exercise stress is inadequate. In our laboratory, if it appears that the patient will not be able to reach the target work load, we stop the treadmill and, after a short rest, proceed with a pharmacologic study. It is too expensive to tolerate a potentially nondiagnostic study.

The vasodilator agents, adenosine and dipyridamole, work through a common mechanism. Dipyridamole raises extracellular adenosine levels. Adenosine is a potent coronary vasodilator, increasing flow in a normal coronary artery four- to fivefold. If a flow-limiting stenosis is present, flow does not increase as much after administration of the vasodilator. Thus there is heterogeneity of flow when comparing normal and stenosed vessels. The myocardial perfusion scan detects this heterogeneity in flow, with relatively less uptake of isotope in muscle supplied by the stenosed artery. Unlike other forms of stress testing, vasodilators are not designed to provoke ischemia. Instead, they identify a difference in vasodilator reserve when comparing normal and stenosed vessels. It is interesting that a small minority of patients develop ischemia, with angina and ST segment depression, after vasodilator "stress." A possible mechanism is "coronary steal."

Typical contraindications to adenosine and dipyridamole stress testing include a history of bronchospasm (adenosine is a bronchoconstrictor), hypotension, bradycardia, and heart block. These side effects may occur during the study, soon after giving the vasodilator.

Intravenous theophylline reverses these effects. (For this same reason, both theophylline and caffeine must be held before the study.)

Dobutamine and arbutamine are agents more commonly used with echocardiography, but also can be employed with myocardial perfusion imaging. They mimic the effects of exercise, increasing heart rate, contractility, and coronary flow.

RADIONUCLIDE ANGIOCARDIOGRAPHY

Nuclear cardiac imaging techniques are used to assess cardiac function. Gated SPECT acquisition can be used to assess left ventricular ejection fraction (LVEF) as a part of a standard myocardial perfusion study. In addition, cardiac blood pool imaging allows a "radionuclide angiogram" using two different techniques. The first and more widely employed RNA method is the equilibrium-gated technique, the MUGA scan. In this study red blood cells are labeled with radioisotope; the isotope thus remains in the cardiac blood pool.

The photons, or "counts," from many hundreds of heart beats are needed to provide an image of the cardiac chamber. Because the ventricular chamber is in motion, the image is a blur, an average of systole and diastole. This is solved by a computer technique that divides the cardiac cycle into 16 to 32 time compartments, beginning with the peak of the R wave of the ECG. (The cardiac cycle is "gated" from the peak of the R wave.) Counts from each of these time-compartments are saved in separate computer files until each file has enough counts to form an image of the heart, after an adjustment for background activity. Ejection fraction (EF) is calculated from the number of photon-counts in a file timed at peak systole (just beyond the peak of the R wave), and the number of counts from another file timed at end-diastole (just before the onset of the QRS complex); if the left ventricle (LV) emits 1000 counts at end-diastole and 400 counts at peak-systole, the LVEF = 60%. Unlike the echocardiogram or contrast ventricular angiogram, this technique for measuring LVEF does not depend on geometric formulae and thus is not distorted by changes in ventricular shape.

A series of LV images, from each of the time-compartment computer files, can be lined up and played in motion (an endless loop recording), showing the LV in motion. This allows evaluation of regional wall motion. A scarred, infarcted segment of muscle is noncontractile, or "akinetic," and viable but ischemic muscle may be hypokinetic.

The second nuclear blood pool technique is called *first-pass* radionuclide angiography. It requires rapid analysis of a radionuclide bolus as it passes through the central circulation. This technique can be used to assess right ventricular function and left ventricular systolic function including assessment of regional wall motion. It also can be used to assess cardiac shunts in congenital heart disease, although echocardiography is more widely

| Table 9-4 | Indications for Both First-Pass and Equilibrium-Gated Radionuclide Angiocardiography (RNA) | |

Indication	Comment
Diagnosis and follow-up of patient with cardiomyopathy	
Assessment of left ventricular function after transplantation	
Follow-up of patients with valvular heart disease	Changes in resting left ventricular volume and ejection fraction can help with timing of surgery
Following of patients receiving potentially cardiotoxic chemotherapeutic agents such as adriamycin	
Assessment of diastolic dysfunction	Echocardiography is a more commonly used technique
Assessment of intracardiac shunts using first-pass techniques	Echocardiography is a more commonly used technique
Assessment of ischemia and function in patients with coronary artery disease	Stress RNA

used for this purpose. Both first-pass and equilibrium techniques can be used with stress testing. A fall in ejection fraction with exercise of greater than 5% indicates severe coronary artery disease with an attendant poor prognosis. Table 9-4 outlines indications for both first-pass and equilibrium-gated radionuclide angiocardiography.

BIBLIOGRAPHY

Berman DS, Hachamovitch R, Kiat H, et al: Incremental value of prognostic testing in patients with known or suspected ischemic heart disease: a basis for optimal utilization of exercise technetium-99m sestamibi myocardial perfusion single-photon emission computed tomography, *J Am Coll Cardiol* 26:639, 1995.

Berman DS, Kiat H, Friedman JD, et al: Seperate acquisitions rest thallium-201/stress technetium-99m sestamibi dual-isotope myocardial perfusion single-photon emission computed tomography: a clinical validation study, *J Am Coll Cardiol* 22:1455. 1993.

Bonow, RO: Diagnosis and risk stratification in coronary artery disease: nuclear cardiology versus stress echocardiography, *Nucl Cardiol* 4:172, 1997.

Borges-Neto S: Perfusion and function assessment by nuclear cardiology techniques, *Curr Opin Cardiol* 12:581, 1997.

Butler RR Jr, Wilf LH: Radionuclide imaging in the evaluation of heart disease, *Am Fam Physician* 55:221, 1997.

Deedwania PC, Amsterdam BA, Vagelos RH: Evidence-based, cost-effective risk stratification and management after myocardial infarction. California Cardiology Working Group on Post-MI Management, *Arch Intern Med* 157:273, 1997.

Division of Cardiovascular Diseases, Mayo Clinic: Cardiovascular stress testing: a description of the various types of stress tests and indications for their use. Mayo Clinic Cardiovascular Working Group on Stress Testing, *Mayo Clin Proc* 71:43, 1996.

Gibbons RJ: Role of nuclear cardiology for determining management of patients with stable coronary artery disease, *J Nucl Cardiol* 1:118, 1994.

Gibbons RJ, chair: ACC/AHA guidelines for exercise testing, *J Am Coll Cardiol* 30:260, 1997.

Hachamovitch R, Berman DS, Shaw LJ, et al: Incremental prognostic value of myocardial perfusion single photon emission computed tomography for the prediction of cardiac death, *Circulation* 97:535, 1998.

Iskandrian AS: *Nuclear cardiac imaging: principles and applications*, ed 2, Philadelphia, 1996, FA Davis.

Kim SC, Adams SL, Hendel RC: Role of nuclear cardiology in the evaluation of acute coronary syndromes. *Ann Emerg Med* 30:210, 1997.

Ritchie JL, chair: ACC/AHA Task force guidelines for clinical cardiac radionuclide imaging, *J Am Coll Cardiol* 25:521, 1995.

Taylor AM, Pennell DJ: Recent advances in cardiac magnetic resonance imaging, *Curr Opin Cardiol* 11:635, 1996.

Tillkemeier PL, Katz AS, Parisi AF: The role of noninvasive testing in evaluation patients for coronary artery disease, *Curr Opin Cardiol* 11:409, 1996.

Weyman AE: *Principles and practice of echocardiography*, ed 2, Philadelphia, 1994, Lea & Febiger.

10 Cardiac Catheterization

Michael E. Assey
Ansel R. McFaddin III

RISKS OF CARDIAC CATHETERIZATION

Despite impressive technological advances, complications (including myocardial infarction and death) do occur during diagnostic and therapeutic heart catheterizations. The actual complication rate varies depending on the skill and experience of the operator, catheterization volume in the laboratory, and, most important, the medical status of the patient. For stable patients undergoing diagnostic cardiac catheterization, the risk of death and myocardial infarction is approximately 1 in 1000.[1] The risk of stroke greatly depends on the extent of the patient's aortic atherosclerosis. Accordingly, stroke occurs in elderly patients and those with diffuse aortic atherosclerosis. Embolic stroke can occur if the catheter dislodges a thrombus within the left ventricle.

Complication frequency does not vary with the femoral versus brachial approach, provided the operator is experienced in the approach taken. The risk of death or myocardial infarction during catheterization of patients with valvular heart disease is slightly higher (0.15% to 0.25%), with an increased risk of neurologic events, primarily related to embolization. Patients with left ventricular systolic dysfunction, left main coronary artery disease, and diffuse atherosclerosis have two to three times the usual risk for death, myocardial infarction, or stroke (about 0.3%).

A comment should be made about pseudocomplications. A pseudocomplication is a spontaneous event that occurs in hospitalized patients and is unrelated to the procedure. Patients having diagnostic and therapeutic cardiac catheterization commonly have severe heart disease. An example of a pseudocomplication might be an elderly patient who goes into cardiogenic shock after a myocardial infarction. Emergent cardiac catheterization and successful angioplasty may open the vessel, but the patient still has an in-hospital mortality of 40% to 50%. Death is caused by the myocardial infarction, not the procedure. However, outcome managers may attribute the death to a complication of cardiac catheterization (diagnostic or therapeutic) simply because the patient underwent the procedure while hospitalized. Such an approach may ultimately deny severely ill patients potentially lifesaving, albeit high-risk, interventions.

CATHETERIZATION FOR SPECIFIC CONDITIONS

Coronary Artery Disease

Diagnostic Cardiac Catheterization

The coronary angiogram is the key procedure, but other assessments include left ventricular (LV) systolic function (ejection fraction, regional LV wall motion), LV filling pressures, and in some patients pulmonary artery pressures with cardiac output measurements (right heart catheterization).

Typically, *left heart catheterization* begins with insertion of an arterial catheter into the femoral or brachial artery. Rarely, a "cut-down" is performed with placement of the catheter into the exposed brachial artery. The catheter is advanced to the central aorta, and pressure is recorded.

Figure 10-1 shows a typical central aortic pressure tracing. The central aortic pressure wave form may give important information about a patient's underlying cardiac physiology. Figure 10-2 shows how ventricular ectopy can affect blood pressure and pulse pressure. After a normal beat, a premature ventricular contraction occurs, producing an early wave form that is significantly reduced in systolic pressure and has a narrow pulse pressure. The beat after demonstrates "post-extrasystolic potentiation" with an overshoot of systolic blood pressure and a widening of pulse pressure. Clearly, a run of premature ventricular contractions (ventricular tachycardia) could produce serious hemodynamic compromise in this patient.

Figure 10-3 shows a central aortic pressure wave form with *pulsus alternans*. A regular variation in systolic blood pressure occurs every other beat. Physical examination almost always reveals an S_3 gallop. This phenomenon usually occurs in patients with significant systolic dysfunction (the patient in Fig. 10-3 had a global LV ejection fraction of 25%). Pulsus alternans also may be seen during and after a run of supraventricular tachycardia (also present in this patient, as seen on the electrocardiograms at the top of the figure). A most unusual form of pulsus alternans is demonstrated in Figure 10-4. Catheterization of the right heart, using a Swan-Ganz catheter, revealed pulsus alternans in the pul-

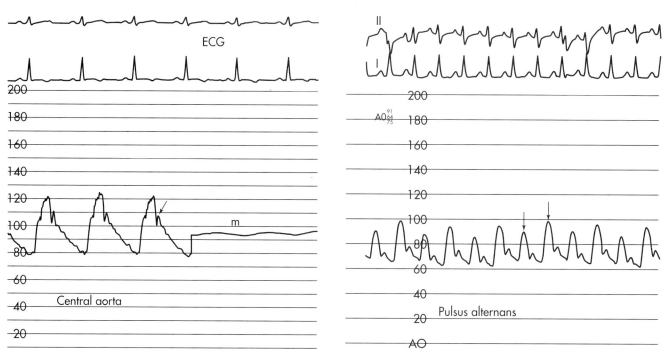

FIG. 10-1
Central aortic pressure tracing. There is a brisk upstroke, well-defined dicrotic notch *(solid black arrow)*, and normal mean *(m)* pressure. *ECG,* Electrocardiogram.

FIG. 10-3
Central aortic pressure wave showing pulsus alternans. See text for detail. Solid black arrows demonstrate beat-to-beat variation in systolic blood pressure.

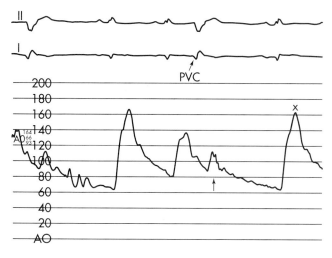

FIG. 10-2
Central aortic pressure wave form influenced by ventricular ectopy (see text for detail). *PVC,* Premature ventricular contraction; *X,* post-extrasystolic potentiation of blood pressure.

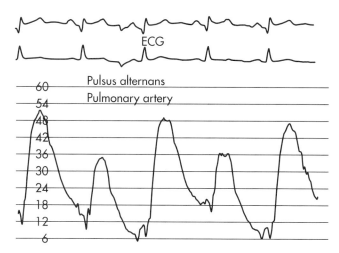

FIG. 10-4
Pulmonary artery pressure wave form demonstrating pulsus alternans. Note beat-to-beat variation in pulmonary artery systolic pressure.

monary artery with peak systolic pulmonary artery pressure varying from 50 to 35 mm Hg on alternating beats. This was caused by right-sided congestive heart failure. Interestingly, central aortic and LV systolic pressures did not show the pulsus alternans.

After recording of central aortic pressure, the catheter is passed across the aortic valve into the left ventricle,

and LV pressures are measured. If there is no aortic stenosis, the LV systolic pressure will equal the central aortic systolic pressure. Many times the LV end-diastolic pressure (LVEDP) will be elevated, often because of a prominent A wave (Fig. 10-5). (see Chapters 2 and 4) This indicates atrial contraction "against" a stiff ventricular and is seen in patients with LV diastolic dysfunc-

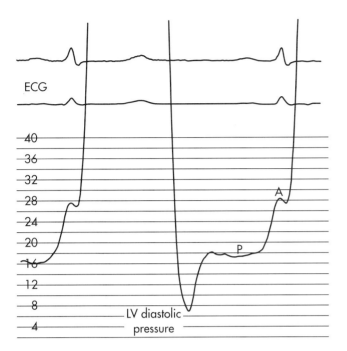

FIG. 10-5
Left ventricular wave form showing left ventricular diastolic pressures. *P,* Pre A pressure, which would correspond to pulmonary capillary wedge measurement. *A,* A wave generated by atrial contraction.

tion, including those patients with hypertension and LV hypertrophy.

After making the baseline hemodynamic measurements, a left ventriculogram may be performed. This is generally done in a single (30 degree right anterior oblique) projection or with biplane imaging. LV volumes, ejection fraction, and regional LV wall motion can be determined. If mitral insufficiency is present, dye refluxes into the left atrium. Today, we often defer the ventriculogram, since this information can be obtained noninvasively from nuclear techniques or echocardiographic imaging. The patient who has a very high LV filling pressure due to congestive heart failure or renal insufficiency may not tolerate the 30 to 50 ml of contrast required for good opacification of the left ventricle.

Coronary Angiography

Coronary disease (*stenosis, lesions, obstructions* are frequently used synonyms) is assessed in multiple views so that eccentric lesions or those hidden by vessel overlap are not overlooked. Physicians are occasionally perplexed when a patient with a normal or near-normal coronary angiogram is found at autopsy to have "severe epicardial obstructive disease." This discrepancy can be explained by considering the difference in what the angiographer sees compared with what the pathologist views.[2,3] Coronary angiography assesses the blood vessel lumen (*luminogram* is as good a term as *angiogram*).

Also, blood vessel caliber is angiographically assessed relative to the adjacent "normal" artery. If both the stenotic segment and "normal" segment are diseased, angiography underestimates the degree of coronary disease. Furthermore, significant atherosclerotic plaque can involve the vessel wall without producing luminal narrowing. Pathologic sectioning of the vessel wall might reveal thickening and disease, yielding a measurement of cross-sectional area that is significantly reduced despite a "normal"-appearing angiogram.

Therapeutic Coronary Intervention

We now have the ability to revascularize the myocardium in the catheterization laboratory. This has made us more aggressive with cardiac catheterization, even for patients whose comorbidity or advanced age previously kept us from recommending catheterization because the patient would "never be a surgical candidate."

Box 10-1 lists many indications for diagnostic cardiac catheterization and coronary angiography and parallels the practice guidelines summarized in Chapter 13. Our usual indications for catheter-based revascularization (using balloons, stents, or atherectomy) as opposed to surgery are summarized in Table 10-1 (see Chapter 13).[4] The recommendations in Table 10-1 assume that coronary anatomy is suitable for either surgery or catheter revascularization. The presence of extremely long lesions, the involvement of large branches at the stenosis site, and the presence of distal disease all affect the applicability of both catheter revascularization and bypass surgery. Comparative data are available for bypass surgery, angioplasty, and medical therapy. The ultimate effect of the newest techniques, particularly stents, has not been studied, but we are finding that lesions not suitable for balloon angioplasty alone can now be approached with confidence using these techniques. Equally important is the "local experience"; that is, specific hospital and operator outcomes must supplement evidence-based medicine. It should not be assumed that the results of a large cooperative trial, generated from medical centers with extensive experience, are applicable to a small community hospital laboratory and staff. In general, hospitals with high volume coronary intervention and high volume cardiac surgery have better results than low volume operators and surgeons.

The multiple trials of surgery, angioplasty, and medical therapy can be summarized as follows. For left main coronary artery disease and triple vessel disease, surgery is recommended if distal vessels are suitable for bypass. For single vessel disease, treatment consists of angioplasty or medical therapy alone. A patient with two vessel coronary artery disease produces controversy. Clinical trials, such as BARI (Bypass Angioplasty Revascularization Investigation), show no difference in overall mortality or the combined end point of death and nonfatal myocardial infarction with follow-up exceed-

---

BOX 10-1
INDICATIONS FOR DIAGNOSTIC CARDIAC CATHETERIZATION

1. Coronary artery disease
   a. Medically refractory angina when angioplasty or surgery is considered
   b. Unstable angina (crescendo angina, rest angina, angina with ST elevation)
   c. Minimally symptomatic or even asymptomatic patient with strongly positive treadmill exercise result (suggesting need for revascularization to lessen mortality)
   d. "Need-to-know" coronary anatomy (high-risk occupation such as commercial airline pilot with positive stress test or recurrent admissions to hospital with atypical chest pain)
   e. Unexplained congestive heart failure (may be secondary to coronary artery disease)
   f. After myocardial infarction with positive stress test suggesting residual ischemia and left ventricular systolic dysfunction or demonstrating complex arrhythmias
   g. Myocardial infarction in a young person
   h. After thrombolytic therapy with recurrent angina or ischemia
   i. Evolving (not completed) myocardial infarction with contraindication to thrombolytic therapy
   j. After postcardiac transplantation (done annually in search of transplant arteriopathy)
   k. Done after aborted sudden death (survivor of cardiac arrest)
2. Valvular heart disease
   a. Before surgery when noninvasive data are inadequate or conflicting
   b. Before surgery when coronary anatomy needs definition for suspected associated coronary atherosclerosis
   c. Before (and often at the same setting) valvuloplasty
3. Congenital heart disease
   a. Before corrective surgery, particularly when noninvasive techniques are inadequate or conflicting
4. Others
   a. Diseases of the aorta including dissection and aneurysm
   b. Endomyocardial biopsy for unexplained heart failure or to evaluate for transplant rejection
   c. Before electrophysiologic studies in a patient with ventricular arrhythmias or a survivor of aborted sudden cardiac death
   d. Chronic pericardial disease (constriction, effuso-constricted disease)
   e. Acute pericardial tamponade in concert with pericardiocentesis

---

ing 3 years.[5] The rate of repeat revascularization after balloon angioplasty, however, is significantly higher than for bypass surgery. The use of intracoronary stents, not studied in the randomized trials to date, may change these results in favor of angioplasty by decreasing the rate of angioplasty restenosis.

Individual patient characteristics also affect the recommendations listed in Table 10-1. *For example, most of the multicenter trials have demonstrated that diabetic patients with multivessel CAD have a lower mortality with surgery than with angioplasty.*

Figure 10-6 is an example of catheter-based myocardial revascularization using angioplasty and stent. A totally occluded right coronary artery is visualized after injection through the guiding catheter. A guide wire is advanced across the obstruction, and an angioplasty balloon is inflated at the site of the obstruction. This opens the vessel but leaves a long area of stenosis in the mid right coronary artery. Placement of two intracoronary stents results in an angiographically normal-appearing right coronary artery.

What will be the long-term impact of advanced stent technology? Evidence-based data to date suggest that stents will reduce but not eliminate restenosis, which is the Achilles heel of angioplasty.[6,7] In those trials, in fact, stents were placed in vessels with very discrete, noncalcified lesions, unlike examples shown in Figure 10-6, which involved a totally occluded vessel. Long-term results may not be as good in these types of complex lesions as in the discrete lesions studied in the clinical trials.

Although Table 10-1 cites angioplasty as the preferred treatment for single vessel disease, medical therapy alone is a viable option for this subset. The ACME Trial (Angioplasty Compared with Medical Therapy)[8] and the MASS Trial (Medicine, Angioplasty, or Surgery Study)[9] failed to demonstrate a difference in long-term mortal-

| Table 10-1 | Surgery versus Angioplasty* |

Condition	Preferred Technique
Left main coronary artery obstruction exceeding 50%	Coronary artery bypass surgery
Triple vessel disease with left ventricular systolic dysfunction	Coronary artery bypass surgery
Triple vessel disease with normal LV systolic function	Coronary artery bypass surgery or angioplasty
Two vessel coronary artery disease, including LAD	Coronary artery bypass surgery or angioplasty
Two vessel disease with normal LV systolic function excluding LAD	Angioplasty
Single vessel LAD disease	Coronary artery bypass surgery or angioplasty
Single vessel disease excluding LAD	Angioplasty
Multivessel disease and diabetes	Coronary artery bypass surgery

*Angioplasty, including all catheter revascularization techniques (balloon dilation, atherectomy, and stenting). *LAD*, Left anterior descending coronary stenosis.

ity between medical therapy and revascularization. In these studies, all patients had single vessel disease with normal LV systolic function, in which case the prognosis is favorable regardless of the type of treatment.

Even these trials must be interpreted in light of advanced technology, since stents were not available in the angioplasty arms of the trial and may or may not have affected outcome. It is clear from these medical versus revascularization trials, however, that there is relief of angina and improved quality of life for those who have angioplasty. A similar message was reported from by the ACIP (Asymptomatic Cardiac Ischemia Pilot) Trial, in which case medical therapy, even when guided by the results of Holter monitoring demonstrating silent ischemia, failed to match total event outcome of revascularization by angioplasty or coronary bypass surgery.[10]

The clinician must integrate this evidence-based data with what the patient needs and expects from treatment. Many older patients are appropriately symptom-oriented in their selection of treatment. Younger patients, working and supporting a family, may be more interested in quality of life and whether

the procedure can reduce the chances of a subsequent intervention. Table 10-1 should be viewed in this regard—a guide but not an absolute indication for treatment in a given patient.

Restenosis after Angioplasty

Intimal hyperplasia and restenosis develop in roughly one third of patients within 6 months of having balloon angioplasty, and angina redevelops in about 20%. Explaining restenosis to patients, we describe it as hyperactive scarring after the plaque and arterial wall have been "injured" by the balloon (albeit controlled injury). It occurs with all angioplasty techniques, although less commonly with stenting. The bigger the lumen at the end of dilation, the less the chance of restenosis, and that may explain the apparent benefit of stenting (see Fig. 10-6). A bigger vessel lumen has more room to accommodate the lump of scar, so there is less chance of flow-restricting stenosis.

No drug interventions have prevented restenosis. Trials of local radiation therapy to blunt the tissue response to barotrauma are in progress.

The risk of restenosis falls off after 6 months. For that reason, 6 months after dilation is a good time to use exercise testing to screen for restenosis. Patients must be instructed to return promptly with any recurrence of angina after angioplasty or stenting.

Valvular Heart Disease

Cardiac catheterization provides critical information about patients with valvular heart disease and traditionally has been the final test before valve surgery.[11,12] Echocardiography has improved enough that much of this information is now available before the patient reaches the catheterization laboratory (see Chapter 8) Catheterization data are confirmatory, clear up uncertainties when the clinical presentation and echocardiogram are inconclusive or conflicting, and outline the status of the coronary arteries.

Table 10-2 summarizes the specific measurements that are made for common valve lesions. All patients with valvular disease need evaluation of LV function, both with angiography (measuring LV volume and ejection fraction, see Chapter 2) and pressure measurements. The LV end-diastolic pressure (LVEDP) is the pressure just before the beginning of ventricular systole. Elevated LVEDP develops when the LV fails and the patient is operating high on the ventricular function curve (see Chapter 2). It also may indicate "diastolic dysfunction," an increase in ventricular diastolic stiffness caused by hypertrophy, ischemia, or infiltrative cardiomyopathy.

To quantify valve stenosis, pressures are measured above and below the valve; the "gradient," or pressure difference, across the valve when it is open is proportional to the degree of obstruction (Figs. 10-7 and 10-8).

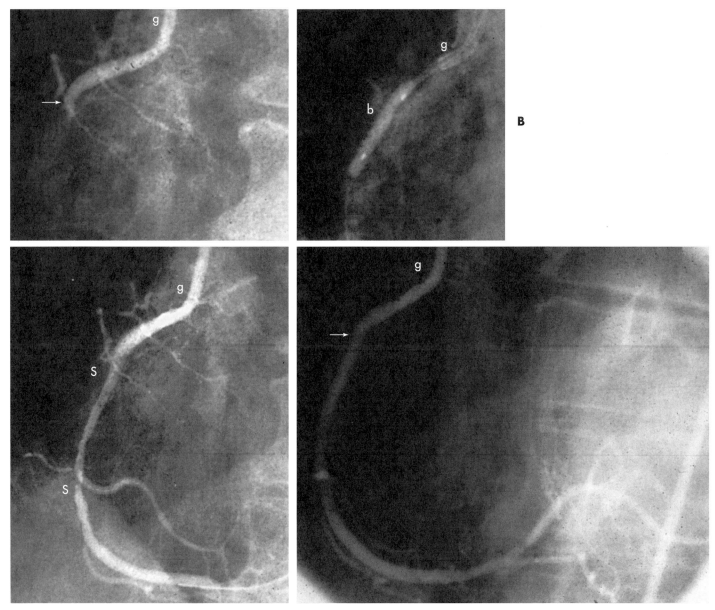

FIG. 10-6
A, Arrow points to totally occluded right coronary artery. *g,* Guiding catheter. **B,** A guide wire has been advanced across the lesion through the guiding catheter *(g).* A balloon angioplasty catheter *(b)* is inflated across the lesion. **C,** The right coronary artery is now open, but a long, residual stenosis *(S)* persists in the midportion of the vessel. **D,** After insertion of 3.0 mm stents and high pressure balloon inflation. The site of previous occlusion *(arrow)* now appears normal.

Combining the pressure gradient and cardiac output (the flow across the valve) allows calculation of the valve area using Gorlin's formula. The hydraulic principle is similar to a garden hose with a nozzle: the force of the jet (or gradient at the muzzle) is governed both by the tightness (area) of the nozzle and total flow. A tight valve lesion may have a small pressure gradient during low flow (cardiac output), and with increased cardiac output, even a modest gradient may indicate tight stenosis.

It is possible, but difficult, to measure left atrial (LA) pressure. For this reason the pulmonary capillary wedge pressure is substituted for LA pressure when assessing mitral stenosis. Regurgitant lesions are evaluated by inject-

Table 10-2	Catheterization Laboratory Evaluation of Valve Disease	
Lesion	**Measurements**	**Comments**
Aortic stenosis (AS)	Simultaneous aortic (Ao) and LV pressure to measure the systolic gradient. Cardiac output (CO), LV diastolic pressure, pulmonary artery (PA) pressure, LV ejection fraction (EF), coronary angiogram. Valve area is calculated using the gradient and CO (the Gorlin formula).	Significant AS = Ao valve area <1.0 sq cm (usually a gradient >40 mm Hg, Fig. 10-7). High LV end-diastolic pressure (LVEDP) is found with left ventricular hypertrophy. Low EF does not contraindicate surgery (see Chapter 19).
Subvalvular AS	All the above, plus a careful "pullback" pressure measurement starting at the LV apex and moving back to the aortic valve to locate the site of obstruction.	Hypertrophic subaortic stenosis usually causes marked elevation of LVEDP. Mitral regurgitation (MR) may be demonstrated on the LV angiogram.
Aortic regurgitation (AR)	Injection of contrast dye into the Ao root, above the valve. Plus LVEF, CO, LVEDP, PA pressure, and coronary arteriogram.	Visual grading of AR (1+ to 4+), admittedly crude but effective if the operator has experience. Marked elevation of LVEDP is seen with acute not chronic AR.
Mitral stenosis (MS)	Simultaneous pulmonary capillary wedge pressure (PCWP, identical to LA pressure) and LV diastolic pressure (Fig. 10-8). Plus CO, PA pressure, LV function, and coronary arteriogram. The diastolic gradient across the mitral valve and CO are used to calculate valve area (the Gorlin formula).	Coronary study (and catheterization) occasionally avoided for a young patient with low CAD risk. Significant MS = mitral valve area <1.0 sq cm/sq M of body surface area (usually a pressure gradient >10-12 mm Hg). The gradient may increase with exercise, confirming significant stenosis in a symptomatic patient.
Mitral regurgitation (MR)	Injection of contrast dye into the LF. Plus LV volume and LVEF, CO, PA pressure, and PCWP, and coronary arteriogram.	Visual grading of the amount of reflux of dye into the LA. Reduced LVEF is a sign of LV failure (as is high end-systolic volume). A tall V wave on the PCWP tracing is typical of acute MR.

ing contrast above the valve and visually estimating the quantity of dye that refluxes back across the leaky valve. Typically, aortic and mitral regurgitation (AR and MR) produce volume overload of the left ventricle, and the critical measurement is LV volume and ejection fraction.

Measurement of pulmonary artery (PA) pressure, right heart catheterization, is important, since pulmonary hypertension may complicate mitral and aortic valve disease. This is usually done with a balloon-tipped catheter. When the balloon is inflated in a PA branch and occludes it, there is an open conduit from the catheter tip beyond the balloon, through the capillary bed and pulmonary veins, and to the left atrium. That is

why this pulmonary "wedge" pressure is identical to LA pressure. It is difficult to reach the LA with a catheter. For this reason pulmonary wedge pressure is substituted for LA pressure when assessing mitral stenosis (see Fig. 10-8). The PA catheters also come with a thermodilution device that allows measurement of cardiac output.

GENERAL CARE OF THE PATIENT WHO IS TO HAVE CATHETERIZATION

The cardiologist performing the catheterization is responsible for the patient's safety and must be relied on to properly manage clinical problems such as diabetes

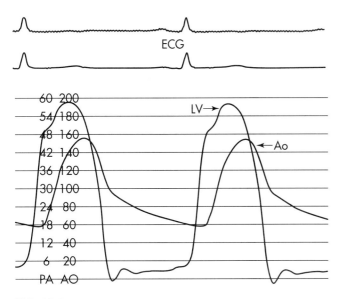

FIG. 10-7
Simultaneous left ventricular *(SLV)* systolic and aortic *(Ao)* systolic pressure in a patient with valvular aortic stenosis. There is a systolic peak-to-peak gradient between the left ventricular and systemic pressures of approximately 40 mm Hg.

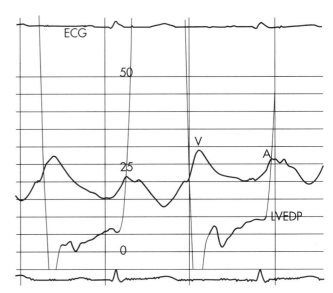

FIG. 10-8
Hemodynamic tracing of mitral stenosis. There is a 17 mm gradient at the end of diastole between the pulmonary capillary wedge A wave and the left ventricular end-diastolic pressure *(LVEDP)*. The A wave is not seen on the left ventricular pressure tracing.

and heart failure immediately before and after the procedure. However, the primary care physician should recognize and begin to manage a number of clinical issues before the patient is transferred for the procedure. In some cases the cardiologist does not meet the patient until the morning of catheterization, and that may be too late to make changes required for safety. The procedure is thus delayed.

Table 10-3 summarizes the most common of these issues and outlines our usual approach. Contrast nephropathy merits special mention, since the use iodinated contrast agents is the most common cause of renal insufficiency that develops in hospitalized patients. When mild, it resolves within several days, but this leads to increased length of stay in the hospital. It may be avoided by recognizing the patient at high risk and administering prophylactic treatment (Table 10-3). This includes adequate hydration, minimizing the contrast load, and using nonionic, low osmolar contrast agents.

A potential breakthrough is the discovery of the role of adenosine in the pathogenesis of contrast nephropathy.[13] Exposure to a high osmolar load stimulates the renal production of adenosine. This causes glomerular hypoperfusion by constricting afferent arterioles (while dilating the efferent arterioles). The measured increase in renal adenosine production is proportional to the worsening of creatinine clearance after contrast administration. Blocking the adenosine receptor with theo-

phylline (Theo-Dur) blunts the worsening of creatinine clearance.[13] Low-dose theophylline is effective (Table 10-3), so the risk of theophylline toxicity is minuscule. We pretreat those at risk for nephropathy with Theo-Dur beginning 3 hours before catheterization. If the procedure must be performed urgently, intravenous aminophylline may be used. It probably is ineffective if given after contrast administration. The theophylline antagonist, dipyridamole (Persantine), may aggravate the effects of contrast on the kidney and should be stopped at least 1 day before catheterization.[13]

Management of the Patient after Catheterization

Reactions to contrast agents are immediate, and a few dangerous complications can develop after hospital discharge. For example, infarction or stroke caused by catheter tip thrombus or injury of the vessel wall usually happens while the patient is still in the catheterization laboratory. Peripheral artery occlusion is apparent within hours of catheterization because of a loss of the peripheral pulse, and patients are rarely discharged with it. (A patient with a cool and pulseless extremity should be sent to the cardiologist promptly.) Nephropathy is an early complication; elevation of serum creatinine develops the day after catheterization and returns to baseline within a week. The drugs that may be given during catheterization (lidocaine, nitroglycerine, anticoagulants, beta-blockers) also have no late or persistent ef-

Table 10-3	*Management Issues Faced by the Primary Care Physician When Sending a Patient for Cardiac Catheterization*

Clinical Problem	Issue	Treatment and Comment
Diabetes	1. Insulin dose	1. Give half the usual dose in the morning and infuse dextrose during the catheterization. Sliding-scale insulin just after catheterization, and the usual dose of insulin the next day.
	2. Oral agents	2. Hold the morning of catheterization; sliding-scale insulin later that day.
	3. Metformin (a special case)	3. Discontinue it for 48 hours before catheterization (may cause lactic acidosis, especially when there is renal dysfunction).
	4. Renal function	4. Contrast nephropathy is more common in those with diabetes. Consider nephropathy prophylaxis even if the creatine is normal (optional and not of proven benefit).
Anticoagulation	1. Warfarin	1. Most operators want the prothrombin time <16 sec. Give the last warfarin dose 3 days before catheterization. Cover with heparin if the need is great (e.g., prosthetic valve, previous thromboemboli). May consider vitamin K if the need for catheterization is urgent, but want to avoid this with prosthetic valves.
	2. Aspirin	2. No modification in treatment necessary.
	3. Heparin	3. Catheterization may be performed while taking heparin (since it can be reversed promptly). If the need for heparin is not great, discontinue it 12 hours before catheterization.
Renal insufficiency	Higher risk: Creatine ≥1.5, diabetes, heart failure and hypotension, dehydration, exposure to contrast within 72 hours	Prophylaxis: 1. Hydration: give normal saline at 100 ml/hour, starting 12 hours before catheterization (with heart failure, the dose may be reduced; proceed with caution; optimal hydration can be tricky). 2. Theophylline: long-acting theophylline (Theo-Dur) 200 mg twice daily started at least 3 hours before catheterization and continued through the next day. 3. Use low-osmolar, nonionic contrast 4. Minimize the contrast load (e.g., defer the LV injection)
Congestive heart failure	Orthopnea	The patient must be able to lie flat during and after catheterization. This may be impossible with severe pulmonary congestion, and diuresis is needed. A delicate balance may exist between volume overload (congestion) and depletion (with higher risk of nephropathy). Fine tuning may best be accomplished with the patient in the hospital a few days before catheterization.
Contrast allergy	Nausea, transient hypotension, or an arrhythmia with dye exposure are not true allergic reactions, although patients may identify them as such. For a true allergy (laryngeal edema, asthma, rash or anaphylactic shock)	1. Avoid catheterization unless necessary 2. Prednisone 20-40 mg every 8 hours beginning 24 hours before catheterization 3. Diphenhydramine the day of catheterization 4. H_2 blockers (e.g., cimetidine)
Iodine or shellfish allergy	Iodine is found in contrast agents and shellfish	If the allergic reaction was "real, " pretreat as described above. Note that dye, particularly ionic, high-osmolar agents, often causes flushing. This must be distinguished from an allergic rash.

fects. One exception is thrombocytopenia, which may develop after brief exposure to heparin.

The most common management problem after catheterization is groin hematoma. Most patients have local induration, but large bruises develop in some patients. This is more common when anticoagulation is required during and after the procedure, when large catheters are used, or when the arterial catheter is left in place overnight after catheterization. These conditions are common after angioplasty for unstable angina or acute infarction, and hematoma may be unavoidable. We tell patients that we at times are faced with a "choice between a bruise in the groin and a blood clot in the coronary artery."[11]

Most small and large hematoma resolve without intervention. Do not let a general surgical colleague drain the hematoma just because of its size. As long as there is a steady reduction in size, surgical treatment is unnecessary. Most patients benefit from warm, moist soaks or soaking in a hot tub (20 minutes, twice a day). If the hematoma is large, mark its boundaries and see the patient at 2-3 day intervals a couple times. Resolution of large hematoma may take a couple of months, and a small, hard knot at the site may persist even longer. Patients need reassurance that this is not a dangerous finding.

*If a large hematoma is pulsatile or becoming larger, have the patient evaluated promptly by the cardiologist who performed the catheterization.*Rarely, a pseudoaneurysm develops, with open communication between the hole in the artery (which has failed to close) and the surrounding hematoma. This requires surgical repair or compression under ultrasound guidance.

Carefully evaluate a patient's description of an "allergic reaction" during the catheterization. A true allergy manifested by rash, laryngeal edema, asthma, or anaphylaxis indicates a risk of an allergic reaction with future contrast exposure. On the other hand, nonallergic reactions to contrast, such as nausea, flushing, arrhythmias, transient hypotension, and even transient renal dysfunction, may not increase the risk of repeat catheterization. Furthermore, prophylaxis for nonallergic dye reactions would be different from treatment to block an allergic response to contrast (Table 10-3). Patients (and doctors) should know with certainty if they are allergic to contrast.

REFERENCES

1. Hildner FJ: Complications of cardiac catheterization and strategies to reduce risks. In Pepine CJ, Hill JA, Lambert CR, editors: Diagnostic and therapeutic cardiac catheterization, ed 2, Baltimore, 1994, Williams & Wilkins.
2. Glagov S, Weisenberg E, Zarins CK, et al: Compensatory enlargement of human atherosclerotic coronary arteries, *N Engl J Med* 316:1371, 1987.
3. Birnbaum Y, Fishbein MC, Luo H, et al: Regional remodeling of atherosclerotic arteries: a major determinant of clinical manifestations of disease, *J Am Coll Cardiol* 30:1149, 1997.
4. Faxon DP: Myocardial revascularization in 1997: angioplasty versus bypass surgery, *Am Fam Physician* 56:1409, 1997.
5. The Bypass Angioplasty Revascularization Investigation (BARI) Investigators: Comparison of coronary artery bypass surgery with angioplasty in patients with multivessel disease, *N Engl J Med* 335:217, 1996.
6. Fischman DL, Leon MB, Baim DS, et al: A randomized comparison of coronary stent placement and balloon angioplasty in the treatment of coronary artery disease, *N Engl J Med* 331:496, 1994.
7. Macay AC, Serruys PW, Ruygrok P, et al: Continued benefit of coronary stenting versus balloon angioplasty: one-year clinical follow-up of Benestent Trial, *J Am Coll Cardiol* 27:255, 1996.
8. Parisi AF, Folland ED, Hartigan P, et al: A comparison of angioplasty with medical therapy in the treatment of single-vessel coronary artery disease, *N Engl J Med* 326:10, 1992.
9. Hueb WA, Bellotti G, Almeida S, et al: The Medicine, Angioplasty, or Surgery Study (MASS): a prospective, randomized trial of medical therapy, balloon angioplasty, or bypass surgery for single proximal left anterior descending artery stenosis, *J Am Coll Cardiol* 26:1600, 1995.
10. Davies RF, Goldberg AD, Forman S, et al: Asymptomatic Cardiac Ischemia Pilot (ACIP) Study two-year follow-up: outcomes of patients randomized to initial strategies of medical therapy versus revascularization, *Circulation* 95:2037, 1995.
11. Assey ME, Usher BW, Carabello BA: The patient with valvular heart disease. In Pepine CJ, Hill JA, Lambert CR, editors: Diagnostic and therapeutic cardiac catheterization, ed 3, Baltimore, 1999, Williams & Wilkins.
12. Carabello BA, Crawford FA: Valvular heart disease, *N Engl J Med* 337:32, 1997.
13. Katholi RE, Taylor GJ, McCann WP, et al: Nephrotoxicity from contrast media: attenuation with theophylline, *Radiology* 195:17, 1995.

PART TWO

Illnesses

11 Atherosclerotic Cardiovascular Disease: an Overview

George J. Taylor
William M. Simpson, Jr.

EPIDEMIOLOGY, ETIOLOGY, AND NATURAL HISTORY

Since the first decade of the twentieth century, heart disease has been the most common cause of death in the United States. The number of cardiac deaths over the past decade has been relatively constant at 750,000 per year, and coronary artery disease (CAD) is responsible for 60% of them.[1] CAD is a disease of both middle and old age. About 45% of myocardial infarctions occur in people younger than 65 years old; almost 40% of men and 30% of women who die of CAD are younger than 55.[1] The economic burden is huge; in 1996, the estimated direct cost of cardiovascular disease in the United States was $259 billion.[2]

Coronary artery disease has been misconceived as being a disease that predominantly affects men. Although CAD tends to develop in women a decade later than in men, the overall risk of death from CAD is similar for women and men, and it is the leading cause of death for both (see Chapter 41). As a rule, all ethnic groups that share a diet rich in animal fats are at risk.

Risk Factors

The Framingham Study reported its 6-year follow-up in 1961, and established the concept of risk factors for premature atherosclerotic cardiovascular disease (ASCVD).[3] A risk factor is a trait that identifies individuals with a greater chance of developing disease. The trait may be a cause of the disease. Causality is best proven when a clinical trial shows that modification of a risk factor prevents disease *(primary prevention)* or halts the progression of already established disease *(secondary prevention)*. Both known and suspected risk factors for ASCVD are summarized in Table 11-1.

Risk Factor Modification

Risk factor modification is a cornerstone for treatment of all atherosclerotic conditions and applies to patients with CAD, peripheral vascular disease, or cerebrovascular disease. Management of hypertension (see Chapter 31), dyslipidemia (see Chapter 12), diabetes (see Chapter 36), and stress (see Chapter 46) is reviewed elsewhere in this book.

Exercise therapy improves outcome for patients with established CAD, and it is most effective for those starting from a sedentary baseline (see Chapter 17). Female gender offers protection from premature CAD; estrogen lowers LDL and raises HDL cholesterol. After menopause, ASCVD develops in women as frequently as in men, but this may be prevented or at least delayed by estrogen replacement therapy (see Chapter 41). Stress, mood, and personality type may be risk factors. It is a difficult area of study, and results have been mixed (see Chapter 46).[16]

Braunwald[2] reviewed the more recently described risk factors[4-15] (Table 11-1) and suggested that future therapy may include folate (to reduce homocysteine levels), niacin (to lower fibrinogen, LDL cholesterol, and lipoprotein (a) levels, and to raise HDL cholesterol), aspirin (specifically to reduce the risk of MI in those with elevated C-reactive protein), and antibiotic therapy for those with chlamydial infection.

Cigarette Smoking

The Problem

"Carnage" is a reasonable term. Roughly 18% of the 1.2 billion living in developed nations will die of the effects of tobacco smoke. Those who die of smoking-related illness in middle age lose an average of 23 years of life, and cardiovascular disease accounts for about 38% of those deaths.[17] Half of all smokers die of smoking-related causes.[18] Continued smoking after myocardial infarction roughly halves life expectancy.[18] More American teenagers are smoking now than in 1970.

Tobacco has been unequivocally linked to premature atherosclerosis. For every 10 cigarettes smoked per day, cardiovascular mortality increases by 18% in men and 31% in women.[19] Low tar cigarettes have been studied and do not appear to lower the risk of ASCVD.[20] Smokeless tobacco products also have been found to increase the risk of vascular disease, although not as much as smoking. Smoking less than 15 cigarettes per day increases the relative risk of disease by a factor of 1.8 (i.e.,

Table 11-1	*Risk Factors for Atherosclerotic Cardiovascular Disease (ASCVD)*

Risk Factor	Current Evidence*
Hypertension	SHEP showed that control of systolic pressure lowers the risk of (1) fatal and nonfatal stroke, (2) nonfatal myocardial infarction (MI) plus coronary death, and (3) combined ASCVD outcomes.[4] A meta-analysis of 14 trials showed that lowering blood pressure 6 mm Hg decreased the CAD event rate 14%.[5]
Dyslipidemia	Lowering cholesterol by 1% reduces the incidence of CAD by 2%. Raising HDL also reduces the incidence of CAD. Trials of intervention show efficacy for both primary and secondary prevention[6] (see Chapter 12).
Diabetes mellitus (DM)	A risk factor for all but with a greater effect on women. In addition to increasing ASCVD, it also increases the risk of heart failure. Treatment may reduce complications of ASCVD, but the effect is not dramatic, and focus should remain on treatment of other conditions (e.g., smoking).[7] DM also indicates a worse prognosis for those with ASCVD (see Chapter 36).
Obesity	Abdominal and truncal obesity are related to insulin resistance, hyperlipidemia, and hypertension—a constellation referred to as *syndrome X*.[8] The Framingham study identified obesity as an independent predictor of ASCVD[9] (see Chapter 43).
Cigarette smoking	There is a "dose response" curve, with the number of cigarettes per day proportional to the incidence of multiple ASCVD endpoints (CAD, stroke, PVD, and death).[9]
Left ventricular hypertrophy	An independent predictor of CAD, particularly for older people.[10] Also indicates poor prognosis for those with CAD.
Physical inactivity	In the MRFIT study those who exercised had a 27% lower CAD mortality rate.[11]
Family history	After stratifying for other risk factors, a positive family history increased risk twofold to fourfold for various ASCVD endpoints.[12]
Gender	CAD morbidity is twice as high in men between the ages 35 and 84.[13] The onset of disease is about 10 years later in women. (CAD is still the leading cause of death in women.)
Age	About four fifths of fatal MI occur in those ≥65 years old.[1]
Stress, mood, and personality type	Proposed risk factors include "negative affectivity," social inhibition, and type A personality. The evidence is mixed. Anger is associated with onset of myocardial infarction, and both infarction and sudden death are most common on Monday morning (see Chapter 46). Depression predicts a poor outcome after infarction. We have been referring patients to our mind-body clinic, which teaches meditation, and other "holistic" techniques. Evidence for efficacy is soft; two randomized trials failed to show survival benefits of nonspecific interventions for general distress after MI.[14]
Homocysteine	Related to deficiency of vitamins B_6 and B_{12} and folic acid (see Chapter 12). About 20% to 30% of patients with ASCVD have elevated homocysteine, compared with 2% in control populations. It may be as important as hypercholesterolemia, and it is more easily treated (a developing story in the treatment of ASCVD).[15]
Hemostatic factors	Fibrinogen, coagulation factor VII, and plasminogen activator inhibitor 1 (PAI-1) have all been reported increased in patients with CAD, as has reduced fibrinolytic activity.[2]
Inflammation	C-reactive protein; elevated levels indicate increased risk for acute coronary syndromes.
Chlamydia pneumoniae	Infection possibly related to atherogenesis and plaque instability.[16]

*Many studies have been conducted; the following are not inclusive, but instead provide examples of available data.

the risk is increased by 80%); dipping snuff increases it by 1.4.[21] Passive, or "second hand," smoking increases the relative risk of CAD by a factor of 1.2 and of lung cancer by 1.3.[17]

Smoking has multiple actions than may promote early ASCVD. It lowers HDL cholesterol, adversely affects endothelial function (see Chapter 13), promotes vasospasm, raises fibrinogen levels, and enhances platelet aggregation. In addition, the carbon monoxide from burning cigarettes raises carboxyhemoglobin levels, reduces the oxygen-carrying capacity of blood, and thus reduces the level of exercise necessary to provoke angina (the angina threshold).

Treatment of Nicotine Dependence

Despite a wide understanding of the dangers of smoking, the number of smokers has increased steadily. Clinical guidelines have been developed for the treatment of nicotine dependence, and a general approach is provided in Table 11-2.[22] Do not underestimate the importance of the practitioner's role. Multiple studies have shown that repeated mention of smoking by the doctor may double the chance of a patient quitting.

Consider making smoking status a "vital sign" that is recorded at each clinic visit.

Nicotine replacement also doubles the chance of a successful quit attempt.[18] Supplemental nicotine does not appear to be dangerous. When a 14 mg nicotine patch was substituted for smoking, patients with effort angina had increased exercise duration and a smaller exercise-induced perfusion abnormality.[23] (This probably is because smoking a burning cigarette carries the additional burden of carbon monoxide inhalation.) Furthermore, supplemental nicotine does not appear to have adverse cardiac effects, *even in patients who continue to smoke.*[24] (Our standard recommendation, however, is that patients not use supplements and cigarettes concurrently.)

A relationship exists between smoking and depression, and depression is a common symptom of abstinence. Antidepressant drug therapy has been helpful; nortriptyline doubled the rate of smoking cessation.[25] A trial of sustained-release bupropion (Zyban 150 mg bid) reported a 44% success rate compared with 19% for placebo.[26] Patients treated with bupropion had *less weight gain* as well.

Currently an optimal smoking cessation effort consists of aggressive behavioral modification in a smoking-cessation clinic, bupropion, and nicotine replacement. Using this approach, you may expect sustained

Table 11-2	The Treatment of Nicotine Dependence

Treatment Approach	Comment
Behavioral modification	Works at multiple levels: 1. The practitioner should mention tobacco at every visit (one survey reported that 50% of doctors failed to comment on continued smoking). 2. Smoking cessation clinic: this intense approach focuses on *skills building* (teaching the patient how to resist smoking, to use substitute behaviors, to make the home-car-office smoke free, and to avoid alcohol while stopping). 3. Social support: enlist family, friends, and the medical team to help with *positive* reinforcement (threatening a bad outcome is less successful).
Nicotine replacement	Patients usually have a preference for gum, nasal spray, or patch. Consider starting with a "kit" containing all three and encourage the patient to experiment (although staying within the recommended dose range).[17] Start replacement the day of the last cigarette. I usually suggest no reduction in the nicotine dose until the new behavior (nonsmoking) is well entrenched. Advise the patient not to smoke while on replacement therapy.
Antidepressant therapy—Zyban	Sustained-release bupropion, Zyban, 150 mg twice daily. (Start with 150 mg once daily for 3 days and then increase the dose.) Begin therapy 1 week before the patient stops smoking, since 1 week is needed to reach a steady-state blood level. Have the patient set a date to stop smoking. Continue therapy for 7 to 12 weeks (if still smoking at 7 weeks, this will not be a successful quit-attempt, and you may as well stop the drug).

(6 months) abstinence in 20% to 40% of patients, depending on the effectiveness of behavioral therapy.

PATHOPHYSIOLOGY

The pathophysiology of various CAD syndromes is reviewed in subsequent chapters. Atherosclerotic plaque is the common denominator of these illnesses.

Response-to-Injury Hypothesis of Atherogenesis

The intimal surface of the artery is lined with endothelial cells that form a barrier between elements of the blood and the arterial wall. The *first step* in atherogenesis appears to be endothelial injury that leads to increased permeability of this barrier. The nature of injury is uncertain, and multiple factors may interact. Shear stress is a possibility, as plaque tends to develop at branch points where there is increased turbulence. Infection has been proposed, since both viral elements and *Chlamydia* have been isolated from plaque (although their presence does not prove causality). Oxidized LDL is cytotoxic and may initiate endothelial injury.

After disruption of the endothelial barrier, the next step is the complex interaction of a number of different cell types that leads to propagation of endothelial injury and infiltration of lipids and other blood elements into deeper layers of the arterial wall (Table 11-3). Circulating monocytes migrate between injured endothelial cells and are transformed into macrophages. These cells scavenge lipid, particularly oxidized LDL, become foam cells, and form the "fatty streak." Activated macrophages produce cytotoxic substances that further endothelial injury. They also produce *growth factors* that stimulate proliferation and migration of smooth muscle cells into the early plaque. In turn, smooth muscle cells secrete growth factors and cytokines and produce connective tissue. As the plaque matures, the fibroproliferative process dominates, with proliferation of smooth muscle cells, attraction of fibroblasts, and production of connective tissue. The core of the mature plaque is rich in lipid, with a combination of fibrous tissue and necrotic debris.

Platelets also have a role in atherogenesis. Platelet adherence and aggregation occur at sites of early endothelial injury, favoring branch points where there is turbulence and stasis. Like other cellular elements, platelets produce growth factors and vasoactive substances. Platelets also have an important role in the progression of plaque and in the genesis of unstable syndromes. A common complication of advanced lesions is the formation of surface cracks and fissures. Platelets immediately adhere to exposed collagen on the injured plaque and form mural thrombi, which may be organized and incorporated into the plaque; this is one mechanism of rapid disease progression and unstable angina. Arterial occlusion by mural thrombus is the usual mechanism for myocardial infarction.

CLINICAL PRESENTATION

Atherosclerotic plaque can cause arterial insufficiency, or "ischemia," in any region of the body. Most commonly affected are the lower extremities (see Chapter

Table 11-3	*Cellular Response to Endothelial Injury: Atherogenesis*

Players	Actions
Endothelial cells	The first step in atherogenesis is endothelial injury with cell-cell separation. Subsequent endothelial dysfunction includes inappropriate vasoconstriction or vasodilation, production of growth factors, procoagulant activity, and loss of the permeability barrier.
Monocytes and macrophages	Monocytes are attracted to the injured endothelium, penetrate to subendothelial regions, and are transformed into macrophages. These secrete growth factors, mitogens for smooth muscle cells, and factors promoting migration of both smooth muscle cells and fibroblasts. They also may secrete oxidized LDL or superoxide anion, which further injures endothelium and other cells in the developing plaque.
Platelets	Platelets are attracted to injured endothelium, adhere, and aggregate. The platelet thrombus releases growth factors (as do the other players).
Smooth muscle cells	In response to growth factors, they migrate from the media into the intima, then proliferate. They may be transformed to foam cells. In cell culture, smooth muscle cells are able to produce growth factors as well as connective tissue.

33), the brain (see Chapter 34), the kidneys (see Chapter 31), and the heart (see Chapters 13 to 17).

Instability

While considering the big picture, think for a moment about the difference between stable and unstable ischemic syndromes. The term, *stable,* suggests no near-term disaster. Although the lesion causes ischemic symptoms, it has little chance of abruptly occluding the vessel and causing ischemic injury. Clinical instability usually is caused by disruption of plaque surface, exposure of connective tissue within the plaque to blood, and initiation of thrombosis. We have little understanding of what disrupts plaque surface, although lowering LDL cholesterol may prevent it. The effectiveness of antiplatelet therapy in preventing instability confirms a prominent role of thrombosis in its genesis.

Chronically Occluded Vessels Are Inherently Stable

Think about it. If an artery is totally blocked, what will happen to it next week or next month? Odds are it still will be blocked. The damage that can be done by abrupt occlusion has already been done. Even when the distal segment of the occluded artery supplies viable tissue, with dependence on collateral blood supply from another vessel, the occluded artery will not create havoc. The collateral branches themselves are reliable. On the other hand, a stenosed vessel presents uncertainty. There is always the chance that it will occlude, with resulting infarction.

MANAGEMENT

A handful of management principles can be applied to all atherosclerotic illnesses.

Risk factor modification (Table 11-1; see Chapter 12) prevents disease and favorably influences prognosis for those who already have it (secondary prevention). Lowering LDL cholesterol to <100 mg/dl is especially effective in slowing or even stopping the progression of the disease. In contrast, continued cigarette smoking may ensure the patient's return with new symptoms. Primary prevention seems mundane when compared with the treatment of disease, but it is a critical element of primary care medicine. We are not doing well. Obesity and teenage smoking have increased, and physical activity has decreased from 1960 to 1990; a majority of people with hypertension or diabetes are unaware of it.[2] It is possible that we will witness a new epidemic of ASCVD in the twenty-first century.

Antiplatelet therapy with aspirin is effective for all patients with ASCVD (barring allergy or other contraindications).

Alcohol intake, in moderation, appears protective. Two drinks per day lowers the risk of CAD, whereas higher consumption increases the risk of myocardial infarction and stroke. Alcohol raises HDL cholesterol and prevents platelet aggregation. Red wine is more cardioprotective as a result of the action of flavonoids, which have antioxidant properties.[27] Dark beer also contains flavonoids.

Chelation therapy has been studied in randomized studies of peripheral artery disease, and it does not work.[28] Since EDTA binds ions in the blood, it was thought that it would bind and remove calcium from atherosclerotic plaque, thus debulking plaque, but it does not. We mention it because chelation clinics still aggressively peddle this expensive technique, and patients occasionally ask about it. The review by Ernst[28] is a good summary of available studies. There is some risk, as intravenous EDTA may cause symptomatic hypocalcemia.

REFERENCES

1. American Heart Association: *Heart and stroke facts: 1999 statistical supplement,* Dallas, 1999, American Heart Association.
2. Braunwald E: Cardiovascular medicine at the turn of the millennium: triumphs, concerns, and opportunities, *N Engl J Med* 337:1360, 1997.
3. Dawber TR, Meadors GF, Moore FE J.: Epidemiologic approaches to heart disease: the Framingham Study, *Am J Public Health* 41:279, 1951.
4. SHEP Cooperative Research Group: Prevention of stroke by antihypertensive drug treatment in older persons with isolated systolic hypertension: final results of the Systolic Hypertension in the Elderly Program (SHEP), *JAMA* 265: 3255, 1991.
5. Collins R, Peto R, MacMahon S, et al: Blood pressure, stroke, and coronary heart disease. II. Short-term reductions in blood pressure: overview of randomised drug trials in their epidemiological context, *Lancet* 335:827, 1990
6. Montague T, Tsuyuki R, Burton J, et al: Prevention and regression of coronary atherosclerosis: is it safe and efficacious therapy? *Chest* 105:718, 1994.
7. Diabetes Control and Complications Trial Research Group: The effect of intensive treatment of diabetes in the development and progression of long-term complications in insulin-dependent diabetes mellitus, *N Engl J Med* 329: 997, 1993.
8. Reaven GM: Role of insulin resistance in human disease (syndrome X): an expanded definition, *Ann Rev Med* 44: 122, 1993.
9. Cupples SA, D'Agostino RB: Some risk factors related to the annual incidence of cardiovascular disease and death using pooled repeated biennial measurements: Framingham Heart Study, a 30-year follow-up. In Kannel WB, Wolf PA, Garrison RJ, editors: *The Framingham Study: an epidemiological investigation of cardiovascular disease,* NIH pub no 87-2703, 1987, National Heart, Lung and Blood Institute.

10. Levy D, Garrison RJ, Savage DD, et al: Prognostic implications of echocardiographically determined left ventricular mass in the Framingham Heart Study, *N Engl J Med* 322:1561,1990.

11. Leon AS, Connet J, for the MRFIT Research Group: Physical activity and 10.5 year mortality in the Multiple Risk Factor Intervention Trial (MRFIT), *Int J Epidemiol* 20:690, 1991.

12. Shea S, Ottman R, Gabrieli C, et al: Family history as an independent risk factor for coronary artery disease, *J Am Coll Cardiol* 4:793, 1984.

13. Lerner DJ, Kannel WB: Patterns of coronary heart disease morbidity and mortality in the sexes: a 26-year follow-up of the Framingham population, *Am Heart J* 111:383, 1986.

14. Carney RM: Psychological risk factors for cardiac events; could there be just one? *Circulation* 97:128, 1998 (editorial).

15. Boushey CJ, Beresford SA, Omenn GS, Motulsky AG: A quantitative assessment of plasma homocysteine as a risk factor for vascular disease: probable benefits of increasing folic acid intake, *JAMA* 274:1049, 1995.

16. Gupta S, Camm AJ: Chronic infection in the etiology of atherosclerosis—the case for *Chlamydia pneumonia*, *Clin Cardiol* 20:829, 1997.

17. Dwyer JH: Exposure to environmental tobacco smoke and coronary risk, *Circulation* 96:1367, 1997 (editorial).

18. Kottke TE: Managing nicotine dependence, *J Am Coll Cardiol* 30:131, 1997 (editorial).

19. Kannel WB, Higgins M: Smoking and hypertension as predictors of cardiovascular risk in population studies, *J Hypertens Suppl* 8:3, 1990.

20. Negri E, Franzosi MG, L Vecchia C, et al: Tar yield of cigarettes and risk of acute myocardial infarction, *Br Med J* 306:1567, 1993.

21. Bolinder G, Alfredsson L, Englund A, de Faire U: Smokeless tobacco use and increased cardiovascular mortality among Swedish construction workers, *Am J Public Health* 84:399, 1994.

22. Smoking Cessation Clinical Practice Guideline Panel: The Agency for Health Care Policy and Research Smoking Cessation Clinical Practice Guideline, *JAMA* 275:1270, 1996.

23. Mahmarian JJ, Moye LA, Nasser GA, et al: Nicotine patch therapy in smoking cessation reduces the extent of exercise-induced myocardial ischemia, *J Am Coll Cardiol* 30:125, 1977.

24. Benowitz NL, Gourlay SG: Cardiovascular toxicity of nicotine: implications for nicotine replacement therapy, *J Am Coll Cardiol* 29:1422, 1997.

25. Benowitz NL: Treating tobacco addiction—nicotine or no nicotine? *N Engl J Med* 337:1230, 1997 (editorial).

26. Hurt RD, Sachs DPL, Glover ED, et al: A comparison of sustained-release bupropion and placebo for smoking cessation, *N Engl J Med* 337:1195, 1997.

27. Constant J: Alcohol, ischemic heart disease, and the French paradox, *Clin Cardiol* 20:420, 1997.

28. Ernst E: Chelation therapy for peripheral arterial occlusive disease: a systematic review, *Circulation* 96:1031, 1997.

12 Practical Management Of Dyslipidemia

Alan S. Brown
Lynn Cofer

Dyslipidemia is one of the most potent risk factors in the development of atherosclerotic vascular disease. Despite this fact, confusion persists regarding the benefits of aggressive therapy, as well as the management of various lipid abnormalities, including hypertriglyceridemia and the low high-density lipoprotein (HDL) syndromes. Because of this confusion, there has been a major shortfall in the treatment of dyslipidemia. In one study as many as 57% of outpatients with coronary disease were not even screened for dyslipidemia.[1] Only 11% of coronary disease patients in the average physician's office have achieved the National Cholesterol Education Program (NCEP) target goals.

The first step in an aggressive—and appropriate—approach to dyslipidemia is to understand the benefits of therapy and to have a rational approach to the choice of therapeutic agents. Always keep in mind that when embarking on "prevention" we must not be intellectually dishonest with our patients. We currently have no way to totally prevent coronary atherosclerosis or vascular events. The control of dyslipidemia and other cardiac risk factors is somewhat analogous to "crossing the street." You can cross the street with the red light or with the green light. If you cross with the red light, you may make it safely to the other side of the street even though the risk of disaster is high. If you cross with the green light, there remains a finite chance of being hit, although the odds are much lower.

Preventive therapy, including lipid management, does not completely alleviate the risk of an event. Therefore the patient and the physician should not be totally disillusioned if a second cardiovascular event occurs despite aggressive therapy. What can be offered is the chance to "cross with the green light," thereby reducing the risk of a morbid or fatal event. An intellectually honest approach regarding the benefits of therapy brings great rewards in terms of improved compliance with preventive strategies and medications.

It is helpful to think of dyslipidemia as a range of illnesses. A normal person can eat indiscriminately and at any weight has a normal fasting lipid profile. On the other end of the spectrum are patients with clearly defined severe genetic dyslipidemias. These patients have abnormal lipid levels no matter what they eat and always require drug therapy. The middle of this range is where most of the population resides. These patients have mild to moderate dyslipidemia and may be able to modify their lipid levels to target levels or almost to target levels with diet and weight loss. Many, however, continue to have significant lipid abnormalities despite following an aggressive diet. These patients have a mild "polygenic dyslipidemia," since a person with a normal genetic makeup does not have dyslipidemia. Understanding that all patients with dyslipidemia have some form of a metabolic disorder makes it easier to consider appropriate drug therapy earlier.

Remember that dietary therapy in itself reduces the risk for cardiac events. The primary goal of prescribing a low-fat, low-cholesterol, high-fiber diet should be to reduce the risk of death or a cardiac event rather than to reduce cholesterol levels. One important effect of dietary therapy is in reducing postprandial lipemia—the rapid rise in triglycerides and other lipid particles soon after eating a fatty meal. This may have only minor effects on the fasting lipid profile. The fasting lipid profile reflects the patient's genetic metabolic abnormalities and is often only slightly affected by diet. However, a low-fat diet seems to significantly reduce the risk of a cardiac event, so it is helpful to consider a low-fat diet for *all patients* to address the cardiac event risk, as well as to focus on drug therapy for all patients with abnormal lipid profiles to correct for their genetic lipid abnormalities. Thus both diet and drug therapy are needed in most patients with dyslipidemia, particularly those with established coronary artery disease (CAD).

THE RATIONALE FOR LIPID MANAGEMENT

The epidemiology of CAD is reviewed in Chapter 11. The risk of the population to be treated is a major determinant of the effectiveness of lipid-lowering drug therapy. Treating a low-risk patient, such as a premenopausal young woman, with an expensive lipid-lowering agent is not cost effective because you would have to treat many thousands of such patients to save one life. However, a middle-aged man with high cholesterol and a family history of coronary disease derives much greater benefit from lipid-lowering therapy. Thus the first issue when selecting treatment is an evaluation of the patient's risk for disease. This risk stratification dramatically reduces the likelihood of making a poor judgment regarding the benefits of therapy.

The guidelines of the Adult Treatment Panel of the NCEP were developed to help practitioners stratify patient risk and develop an appropriate "level of concern" regarding the aggressiveness of therapy in these patients (Table 12-1). The guidelines suggest that all patients who have a low-density lipoprotein (LDL) cholesterol level greater than 190 mg/dL should be treated with lipid-lowering agents early, since with this level of LDL, the risk of having a cardiovascular event with dyslipidemia *alone* is substantial enough to warrant drug therapy. For other patients, you must assess additional risk factors for CAD. Patients with *less than* two risk factors for CAD and no evidence of atherosclerosis should have their LDL level lowered to less than 160 mg/dL. If the patient has two or more risk factors for coronary disease and no atherosclerosis, the goal is to achieve a LDL level less than 130 mg/dL. Finally, if the patient has any atherosclerosis whatsoever, the goal for LDL level is less than 100 mg/dL. These guidelines are conservative enough to warrant aggressive intervention and, if followed, have been cost effective.

In addition to LDL level, recent clinical trial data indicate that all patients with diabetes, whether insulin-dependent or not, should be treated *as if they have atherosclerosis,* with the LDL level reduced below 100 mg/dL (see Chapter 36).

The synergy of dyslipidemia and other CAD risk factors is impressive. Figure 12-1 shows the relative mortality risk based on the presence of cardiac risk factors, such as smoking and hypertension. A high cholesterol level alone in a healthy individual who is normotensive and a nonsmoker increases the mortality per year approximately fourfold. Also, a patient who smokes and has hypertension but normal cholesterol levels has ap-

proximately a fourfold increase in mortality over a healthy individual. A person with hypertension, who has high cholesterol levels, and who smokes has a much higher mortality risk—an increase of approximately 15-fold above normal. It is therefore important to counsel patients with high cholesterol levels and other risk factors that they need special attention and aggressive treatment because of their remarkably increased risk of death, as well as of nonfatal cardiac events.

Clinical Trials—a Nuts and Bolts Summary

For over 3 decades it has been common knowledge that high cholesterol levels predict the risk of a coronary event and of cardiac death. Landmark epidemiologic studies such as the Framingham Study and the MRFIT trials clearly supported the relationship of high cholesterol levels to cardiac events.[2, 3]

Over the past 15 years trials of therapy showed that reducing serum cholesterol levels actually reduces cardiac events. Rather than elaborate on all the studies that have been performed, representative and important clinical studies are discussed as examples, with an attempt to place the value of therapy in perspective.

In general, lipid-lowering trials have been divided into two categories: primary and secondary prevention. *Primary prevention* trials include patients who have risk factors for coronary disease but who have no clinical evidence. *Secondary prevention* trials include patients who have known atherosclerotic heart disease. As you might guess, the risk of a cardiac event is much higher for patients with known atherosclerosis than for those who have risk factors but no clinical history. For example, a woman who already has had a mastectomy for breast cancer is at a much higher risk of dying of breast cancer than a woman who has a family history of breast cancer but who has not yet shown evidence of the disease.

Table 12-1	*National Cholesterol Education Program Guidelines: Emphasis on LDL Cholesterol*

For Individuals with:	Initiate Drug Therapy if LDL Cholesterol is:	LDL Cholesterol Goal
<2 other CHD risk factors and no CHD	≥190 mg/dL after ≥6 months of diet	<160 mg/dL
≥2 other CHD risk factors and no CHD	≥160 mg/dL after ≥6 months of diet	<130 mg/dL
Definite CHD or other atherosclerotic disease	≥130 mg/dL after 6 to 12 weeks of step II diet	<100 mg/dL

LDL cholesterol is the primary target of lipid-lowering therapy.

Expert Panel on Detection, Evaluation, and Treatment of High Blood Cholesterol in Adults: *JAMA,* 269:3015, 1993.

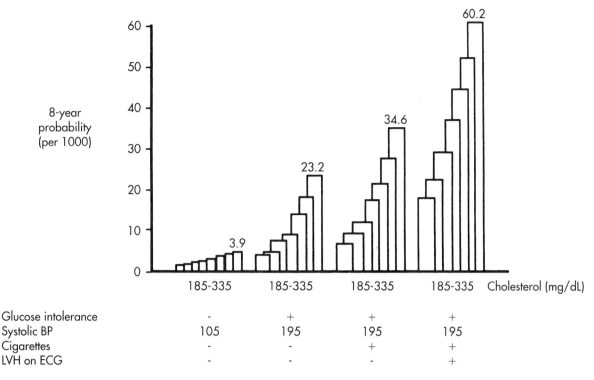

FIG. 12-1
These data from the Framingham Study demonstrate the synergistic effect of risk factors in causing vascular disease. A more aggressive approach to lipid management is warranted for those with multiple risk factors.
From Kannel WB: *Am J Cardiol* 52:9, 1983.

When reviewing clinical studies for lowering lipids, it is important to understand whether the study is a primary or a secondary prevention trial because the benefits of treatment are more substantial for patients in the much higher risk, secondary prevention group.

The best-analyzed and most well-randomized large-scale study of lipid lowering in *primary prevention* is the West of Scotland, Pravastatin Primary Prevention Trial.[4] This study included over 6000 men who had high cholesterol levels and cardiovascular risk factors but no evidence of atherosclerosis. They were randomized to either a low-fat diet or a low-fat diet plus pravastatin at a dose of 40 mg. Over a course of 5 years the pravastatin group's LDL level fell approximately 26%. In this group the combined primary end points of death from cardiac disease and nonfatal cardiac events were reduced by 31%, which was statistically significant. In addition, the risk of nonfatal myocardial infarction was reduced by 31% and death from CAD by 28; noncardiac mortality did not increase because of pravastatin treatment (i.e., there was no increased risk of cancer or any other noncardiac fatal disease). All-cause death was reduced in the pravastatin treatment group by 23%, but the study was too small for this to reach statistical significance.

For the clinician, it is important to understand that a percent reduction in risk does not always tell the story of how many patients one is required to treat to save one event. Careful analysis of the West of Scotland Trial showed that treatment of 1000 men like those in the study with high risk but no coronary disease would result in 20 fewer nonfatal heart attacks and 7 fewer cardiovascular deaths over the period of 5 years. Therefore treatment of approximately 50 patients for 5 years would be required to save a patient from having a heart attack, and treatment of 100 patients for 5 years would result in saving a life. It is unclear how much additional benefit would be achieved if more aggressive LDL lowering had been accomplished.

The best-designed *secondary prevention trial* of cholesterol lowering is the Scandinavian Simvastatin Survival Study (4S Trial).[5] This study included 4444 men and women, ages 35 to 77, recruited in 94 centers in Scandinavia. All patients had known coronary atherosclerosis but had been stable for at least 6 months. After an 8-week diet trial, the patients who had persistently elevated LDL levels were randomized to therapy with simvastatin (20 mg or 40 mg) or placebo. They were then followed for approximately 5.5 years. Simvastatin is a more potent cholesterol-lowering agent than pravastatin, so the average LDL reduction in this trial was 38%, with an average total cholesterol reduction of 28%. HDL levels rose slightly, approximately 8%.

The 4S Trial results were quite remarkable. Over the 5.5-year period of the trial, death from any cause (i.e., total mortality) was 30% lower in the group taking simvastatin compared with those on diet alone. Death due to heart disease was reduced by 42%, and major coronary events, fatal or nonfatal, were reduced by 40%. The risk reduction was highly statistically significant and essentially equal in *both* sexes. The risk of undergoing a repeat bypass surgery or angioplasty was reduced by 37%. There were noncardiac, vascular benefits; simvastatin reduced the risk of stroke by 30%.

From a medical-economic standpoint, there were fewer hospitalizations and fewer hospital days experienced in the simvastatin group. Simvastatin appeared to have no dangerous side effects; there was no increase in noncardiac death and no influence on the incidence of cancer. (Many other long-term trials have confirmed no increase in the risk of cancer with statin therapy for dyslipidemia.)

Based on the 4S Trial, treating 100 patients with known CAD would result in the following benefits over a 6-year period: a savings of 23 out of an expected 86 hospitalizations and a savings of 231 out of an expected 679 hospital days; 6 of 19 revascularization procedures would be prevented.

Diabetes and Coronary Artery Disease

There has been a renewed emphasis on identifying dyslipidemia in all diabetics (see Chapter 36). One of the most striking pieces of evidence from the 4S Trial comes from the subgroup analysis of those with type II (non-insulin-dependent) diabetes.[6] In the control group with stable coronary disease treated with diet rather than with simvastatin, there was a *25% 5-year mortality.* In other words, *one in four* diabetics with CAD who are *clinically stable* will die within the next 5 years unless their lipid levels are controlled. The mortality was reduced to 14% (a 45% reduction) with simvastatin treatment. Treatment of 100 diabetic patients with stable CAD over a 6-year period would save 24 out of 46 expected major cardiac events based on this trial. These data and others have led the American Diabetes Association and several members of the NCEP committee to recommend treating *all diabetics* as if they have atherosclerosis to a LDL goal of 100 mg/dL.[6]

Pathogenesis of Plaque and Benefits of Lowering Lipid Levels

The development of an atherosclerotic plaque is complex and is influenced by many factors, including platelet and endothelial function (see Chapter 11). In brief, normal endothelium tends to protect the intimal and medial layers of the arterial wall from infiltration by cholesterol (Fig. 12-2). With either direct trauma from hemodynamic causes such as hypertension or endothelial damage caused by nicotine or diabetes, the endothelial barrier breaks down. This allows infiltration of LDL cholesterol into the wall of the artery and into the intimal layer. This early atherosclerotic lesion is called a *fatty streak.* These fatty streaks, if unchanged, will not progress and will continue to be relatively benign in terms of posing an atherosclerotic event risk. Unfortunately, the LDL cholesterol in fatty streaks, when oxidized, leads to progression of the atherosclerotic plaque. Oxidized LDL stimulates monocytes in the serum to be recruited and to enter the arterial wall and begin engulfing the oxidized LDL. They become bloated with LDL cholesterol and look foamy under the microscope, so they have been dubbed *foam cells.* The foam cells secrete chemical messengers that recruit more monocytes into the area and increase the inflammation (see Chapter 11).

As part of the process, smooth muscle cells in the arterial wall deposit fibrous tissue, and platelet adhesion to the region of the atherosclerotic plaque increases. The monocytes probably secrete collagenase, an enzyme that breaks down the fibrous cap of the plaque. Fatty plaques with thin fibrous caps are prone to rupture even when they occupy only 20% to 30% of the lumen (hardly a "stenosis"). When the fibrous cap ruptures and the plaque is ulcerated, blood is exposed to the raw surface of the plaque, which is an intense stimulus for acute thrombosis, leading to partial or total arterial occlusion.

Aggressive lowering of serum LDL level reduces the foam cell content within the plaques as well as the amount of cholesterol within the lesion. This leads to a thicker, firmer fibrous cap on the plaque and less

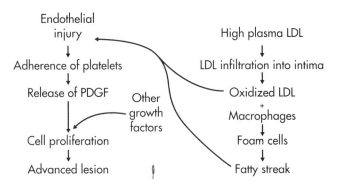

FIG. 12-2

Pathogenesis of atherosclerosis. Postulated linkage between the lipid infiltration hypothesis and the response-to-injury hypothesis. *LDL,* Low-density lipoprotein; *PDGF,* platelet-derived growth factor.

From Steinberg D: *Atherosclerosis Rev* 18:1, 1988.

propensity to plaque rupture. The process of lowering LDL, which leads to a lower propensity for plaque rupture, has been called *plaque stabilization.* Plaque stabilization is thought to be the major reason for the dramatic reduction in clinical event rates in patients treated with cholesterol-lowering agents. The benefits of plaque stabilization seen in clinical trials become evident in the comparison of treatment groups with diet groups after approximately 6 months of treatment and become highly statistically significant after 18 months to 2 years. Several angiographic trials have suggested that with aggressive LDL lowering, the progression of atherosclerotic lesions can be halted in about 60% of patients, with some regression (reduction in the atherosclerotic plaque size) in approximately 30% of patients over a 4- to 5-year period.[7, 8]

Effect of Diet

The effectiveness of a low-fat diet or, at the very least, a diet low in saturated fats, has long been established to reduce the risk of cardiovascular events. In general, the percentage of fat content in the diet of a population predicts its death rate independent of blood cholesterol levels. Yet what is interesting is an apparent dietary "paradox"; that is, a low-fat diet significantly reduces the risk of a cardiovascular event, but aggressive low-fat diets only lower serum cholesterol levels modestly (approximately 10% to 15%). Despite this fact, most discussions on the benefits of dietary fat reduction relate to the attempt to lower fasting serum cholesterol levels (somewhat missing the point).

Another conclusion regarding the paradox is that the prevention of cardiac events attributable to a low-fat diet may be mediated by a mechanism other than the lowering serum cholesterol level. A recent theory includes the concept of "postprandial lipemia." Figure 12-3 illustrates how dietary fat is handled through the exogenous pathway of lipid metabolism, as compared to the liver's production of lipids through the endogenous pathway. When a person eats a high-fat meal, the fats in the intestine are packaged into large particles of primarily triglycerides, called *chylomicrons.* Chylomicrons have approximately 10 triglycerides for every 1 cholesterol particle within their core. These triglyceride-rich particles are then metabolized by an enzyme called *lipoprotein lipase,* which in essence digests the triglycerides out of the particle, leaving a smaller particle that is about 50% triglycerides and 50% cholesterol, referred to as a *chylomicron remnant.*

These cholesterol-rich remnants are then cleared by "remnant receptors" in the liver. Some individuals have very effective remnant receptors and clear them rapidly. They tend to have a lower incidence of heart disease. Others have delayed clearance of chylomicrons and their remnants and have a higher incidence of atherosclerotic events. The increased risk may result from the atherogenicity of the triglyceride-rich particles and remnants or from the increased serum viscosity and thrombosis that may complicate postprandial lipemia. Postprandial lipemia also can alter the regulation of vasomotor tone, leading to increased vasoconstriction.

A low-fat diet reduces postprandial lipemia. These postprandial particles, except in rare genetic dyslipidemias, have been cleared before the measurement of a 14-hour fasting lipid profile. The fasting lipid profile thus reflects endogenous lipid metabolism (Fig. 12-4).

Endogenous Lipid Production

The liver produces a particle called *very low-density lipoprotein* (VLDL) cholesterol, which also is large and triglyceride-rich (see Fig. 12-4). This particle is broken down by the same enzyme, lipoprotein lipase. Triglycerides are removed from the particle to yield a smaller, also atherogenic particle called *intermediate-density lipoprotein* (IDL). These particles are then further metabolized to a small particle containing only cholesterol,

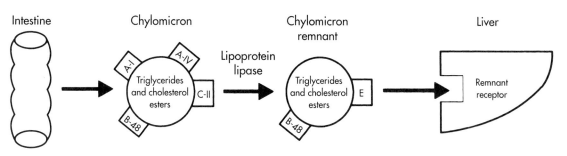

FIG. 12-3

Exogenous fat transport. A-I, A-IV, B-48, C-II, and E are apolipoproteins. C-II functions as a cofactor for the enzyme, lipoprotein lipase, and E interacts with the "remnant receptor" on the hepatocyte.

From Breslow JL: *Cardiol Board Rev* 6:10, 1989.

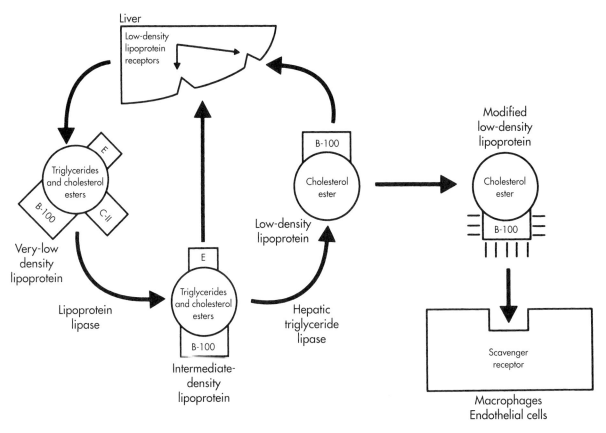

FIG. 12-4
Endogenous fat transport. B-100 and E are apolipoproteins and bind with specific liver receptors. The liver uses large amounts of cholesterol for the manufacture of bile. Any condition or therapy that reduces the liver's supply of cholesterol provokes an increase in the number of LDL receptors, so cholesterol-rich LDL is removed from the circulation, thus meeting the liver's needs.
From Breslow JL: *Cardiol Board Rev* 6:10, 1989.

called LDL. The LDL is cleared by the LDL receptor on the liver. There are multiple genetic abnormalities of this endogenous lipid pathway, including diseases that lead to overproduction of VLDL cholesterol (e.g., familial combined dyslipidemia) and diseases that lead to abnormal function or reduced numbers of LDL receptors (e.g., familial hypercholesterolemia).

The previous discussion emphasizes the importance of recommending a low-fat diet because it reduces postprandial lipemia. The effect of dietary therapy cannot be judged by the 14-hour fasting lipid profile. Although it may be slightly modified by diet, in most patients the lipid panel reflects endogenous lipid metabolism. If abnormal, drug therapy is usually required. When a patient points out that his fasting lipid profile is excellent on his statin medication and asks whether he can eat pizza, he should be told that the statin medication is controlling his genetic dyslipidemia. He should avoid the pizza to reduce postprandial lipemia, which also decreases his risk for subsequent heart attacks, an effect in-

dependent of the lipid profile. This, by the way, is suggested by clinical trials of drug therapy. When considering only patients who receive drug therapy, those who follow a low-fat diet have better long-term results than those who do not.

Physician Performance

Most physicians believe they are well aware of the benefits of lipid-lowering therapy. When asked, physicians believe they are quite aggressive in treating lipid levels, especially in patients with CAD. To evaluate this perception a study called Quality Assurance Program was performed through a grant from Merck Pharmaceutical Company.[1] This study enlisted 1100 cardiology and general practice groups from around the United States. A separate corporation was enlisted to send nurses to each of the 1100 offices. In each office, charts, which were coded for CAD by ICD-9 codes, were pulled to determine whether dyslipidemia had been identified in these patients and whether treatment was initiated. Despite a known diagnosis of CAD, 57% of the charts had no record of an LDL level. Only 11% had achieved the LDL goals outlined by the NCEP guidelines. In addition, only 4% of all charts reviewed showed an LDL level that was at goal without drug therapy, indicating that *90% to 95% of patients who have a known diagnosis of atherosclerosis will require drug therapy to achieve their goal.* Finally, most patients who were on drug therapy were at the starting dose of a statin and had not been appropriately titrated to achieve their LDL goals.

These results indicate a huge treatment gap in patients with coronary atherosclerosis. When compared with other preventive approaches after myocardial infarction, such as beta-blockers and aspirin, a statin seems at least as effective—and possibly more effective—for reducing long-term risk. Despite this fact, many more patients are routinely given aspirin and beta-blockers than are given a statin. It seems imperative that an organized approach to screening patients for dyslipidemia in clinical practice be required, followed by appropriate step-wise titration of therapy to achieve the NCEP goals. While other controversies rage, such as the importance of fibrinogen, serum iron, and homocystine, we still have a serious challenge to appropriately reduce LDL levels in patients with known atherosclerosis.

Triglyceride Levels as a Risk Factor for CAD

There has been a controversy about whether elevated triglyceride level alone is a risk factor for CAD. The role of hypertriglyceridemia in predicting cardiovascular risk has been confusing to most clinicians. An attempt will be made to clarify what is currently known about this issue, recognizing that more information is needed.

The first risk issue regarding hypertriglyceridemia is pancreatitis, not atherosclerosis. Patients with persistent triglyceride levels over 1000 mg/dL are at a significantly increased risk for acute pancreatitis and should be treated aggressively. The therapy of choice is a fibric acid derivative, either gemfibrozil or fenofibrate. After the triglyceride levels have been reduced, preferably to below 500 mg/dL, secondary causes of hypertriglyceridemia should be ruled out, such as hypothyroidism, excessive alcohol and sweet intake, or poorly controlled diabetes mellitus. Occasionally, oral estrogen therapy also can lead to marked hypertriglyceridemia in susceptible patients, and these individuals may be better with an estrogen patch; this route of estrogen delivery bypasses the liver. Other lipid-lowering drugs, particularly the bile acid resins such as cholestyramine, can also aggravate hypertriglyceridemia, and these drugs should be withdrawn on finding markedly elevated triglyceride levels.

With regard to the risk of CAD, not all patients with hypertriglyceridemia appear to be at increased risk. Re-

analysis of the Helsinki Heart Trial found that when the LDL to HDL ratio was less than 5 (i.e., normal lipid profiles with relatively low LDL and relatively high HDL levels), there was no increased cardiovascular risk with triglyceride levels over 200 mg/dL.[9] These usually are patients with moderate alcohol consumption or women taking estrogen. These patients have a decreased rather than an increased incidence of CAD.

However, for patients with low HDL or relatively high LDL levels, with a ratio greater than 5, elevated triglyceride levels (above 200 mg/dL) exponentially increased the risk of a cardiac event. The controversy about treatment revolves around these patients.

Here is the issue: should the major effort be to lower triglyceride level or to lower LDL level? The majority opinion is that the greatest benefit comes from lowering the LDL level to below 100 mg/dL. The next most potent reducer of risk in such patients is raising HDL level. Finally, the third goal of therapy should be to normalize triglycerides. Unfortunately, relatively few studies compare treatment strategies primarily directed toward HDL and triglycerides with those primarily directed toward LDL. This may be wrong, and theoretical reasons support a primary triglyceride strategy. For example, with high triglyceride and low HDL levels, the LDL cholesterol shifts to a smaller and denser (so-called "pattern B") form, which may be much more atherogenic. In the laboratory one can show that lowering the triglyceride level often shifts the LDL particles to a less dense, larger, "fluffy" particle, which, theoretically, should be less atherogenic.

Nevertheless, based on available clinical studies the current strategy for patients with high LDL, low HDL, and high triglyceride levels begins with statin therapy to lower the LDL level to the NCEP goal. Then the addition of a second agent such as niacin to normalize triglyceride and HDL levels should be considered.

Nonpharmacologic attempts to lower triglyceride levels are much more effective than similar attempts to lower LDL levels, so patients with high triglyceride levels should avoid alcohol, reduce sweets, follow a low-fat diet, lose weight, and exercise.

GENETIC DYSLIPIDEMIAS

Several genetic disorders can lead to serious lipoprotein abnormalities. Currently, genetic dyslipidemias are categorized by their metabolic abnormality rather than by the abnormalities in the lipid profile. This helps the practitioner understand the actual causes of the lipid abnormality and therefore choose appropriate strategies for treatment. A simplified approach to understanding genetic dyslipidemias follows, and the lipid disorders are categorized based on whether they are primarily disorders of LDL, of triglycerides, or of HDL.

LDL Disorders

The disorders that virtually only affect the LDL level are familial hypercholesterolemia and familial defective apoB-100.

Familial hypercholesterolemia is an autosomal dominant inherited trait in which the gene that codes for the liver's *LDL receptor* produces an abnormal and ineffective LDL receptor. The most common form of this disease is the heterozygous form, wherein a person inherits a defective LDL receptor gene from one parent and a normal gene from the other parent. These individuals have approximately 50% functioning LDL receptors on their liver. For this reason, LDL clearance is reduced, and patients have high levels of LDL in their blood with normal levels of HDL and triglycerides (see Fig. 12-4). The incidence of this heterozygous familial hypercholesterolemia is approximately 1 in 500. There is a high incidence of premature coronary atherosclerosis. Women with the disorder seem to have a lower risk than men for early atherosclerosis, but develop a high risk after menopause. Importantly, however, if young women with familial hypercholesterolemia also smoke cigarettes, their risk increases dramatically for symptomatic coronary atherosclerosis by age 40 to 45 years. When examining families of patients with familial hypercholesterolemia, one would expect all family members to have *only* LDL elevations, since they have no disorders of triglyceride or HDL metabolism. Classic physical findings are present in about 40% of patients and include tendonous xanthomas of the Achilles tendons and knuckles, as well as corneal arcus. Since familial hypercholesterolemia is an inherited disorder of LDL receptors, the lipid abnormalities can be seen in infants. This is one of the few genetic lipid abnormalities that can be identified virtually at birth.

The second LDL disorder, *familial defective apoB-100*, is essentially indistinguishable from familial hypercholesterolemia. The clinical manifestations of this disorder and the lipid profiles are exactly the same as in familial hypercholesterolemia, but the disorder is caused by a genetic abnormality in the apoB-100 protein, which is the ligand on LDL that binds LDL to the LDL receptor, rather than an abnormality of the LDL receptor.

Finally, extremely rarely a patient inherits both defective LDL receptor genes from parents who each have heterozygous familial hypercholesterolemia. These children have no functioning LDL receptors and suffer what is called *homozygous familial hypercholesterolemia*. They have extremely high cholesterol levels—in the range of 600 to 1000 mg/dL—and often die of atherosclerotic disease in the second decade of life.

Disorders of Triglycerides

Four major disorders lead to elevated triglyceride levels:
1. Familial combined dyslipidemia
2. Chylomicronemia
3. Familial hypertriglyceridemia
4. Type III dyslipidemia

In *familial combined dyslipidemia,* the most common disorder, the liver overproduces apoB-100 apoproteins (see Fig. 12-4). Since each VLDL particle produced by the liver has one apoB-100 protein attached to it, the effect of overproducing apoB-100 causes the production of a large number of small, dense VLDL particles. It is generally thought that the smaller and denser the particle size, the more atherogenic it is. These patients may have varying abilities to handle the small, dense LDL particles, and therefore their lipid profiles can vary widely within different family members. Some family members may have only high LDL levels, and others in the same family may have high triglyceride levels; still others have elevations of both triglyceride and LDL levels. All these patients, however, have an apoB-100 to serum LDL ratio greater than 1. This is in contrast to the previously mentioned familial hypercholesterolemic patients, who also have elevated apoB-100 levels, but their apoB-100 levels are less than or equal to their LDL levels. This is one of the few benefits of ordering an apoB-100 level in clinical practice.

Patients with familial combined hyperlipidemia usually have lower than normal HDL levels also. This relatively common disorder is seen in many patients with CAD. The physical findings associated with this disorder, although not seen in all patients, include corneal arcus and tuberoeruptive xanthomas in patients who have extremely high triglyceride levels.

The second genetic disorder that can manifest high triglyceride levels is *chylomicronemia,* which is caused by either a deficiency in the enzyme lipoprotein lipase, the enzyme that metabolizes triglycerides, or to an abnormal apoC II apoprotein, which is necessary to activate lipoprotein lipase (see Fig. 12-3). Like other high-triglyceride syndromes, these patients can have tuberoeruptive xanthomas and xanthelasma. The ratio of triglycerides to cholesterol in these patients is often 10 to 1.

Another disorder that includes high triglyceride levels is *familial hypertriglyceridemia.* Unlike familial combined dyslipidemia, there is no overproduction of apoB-100. Instead, the liver makes large, abnormal, "fluffy" VLDL particles, but with a normal rather than an increased number of particles. For this reason these patients have normal apoB-100 levels but markedly elevated triglyceride levels, and their LDL to apoB-100 ratios are less than or equal to 1. The importance of diagnosing this disease is that, despite high triglyceride levels, there is only a slightly increased risk for coronary disease over the normal population. This is in contrast to familial combined dyslipidemia, in which patients have a markedly increased risk for coronary atherosclerosis. Therefore in patients with high triglyceride levels the finding of an apoB-100 level less than the LDL level implies a much better prognosis and the diagnosis of familial hypertriglyceridemia, as opposed to a diagnosis of familial combined dyslipidemia. Despite a lower risk of vascular disease, these individuals may have the classic physical findings of hypertriglyceridemia, such as tuberoeruptive xanthomas on the buttocks and elbows.

The last and rarest disorder that elevates triglyceride levels is called *type III dyslipidemia*. Type III dyslipidemia is actually a combination of two genetic disorders: familial combined dyslipidemia (as described earlier) plus an abnormal apoE apoprotein (see Fig. 12-4). These patients have inherited the so-called apoE-2E-2 phenotype. With this phenotype the apoE receptor (the so-called remnant receptor) cannot adequately bind intermediate-density lipoproteins, so these lipoproteins accumulate in the serum. Intermediate-density lipoproteins have a cholesterol to triglyceride ratio of approximately 1:1, so these patients often have roughly equivalent cholesterol and triglyceride levels. They have an increased incidence of coronary atherosclerosis, and their physical findings include orange palmar creases on their hands. These orange palmar creases actually represent deposits of intermediate-density lipoproteins. The importance of diagnosing this rather rare disorder is that these patients are extremely sensitive to dietary therapy and often, inappro-

priately, are given multiple drugs for cholesterol management. A marked reduction in sweets and alcohol along with a low-fat diet often dramatically improves the lipid profiles of these patients without drug therapy. Unfortunately, although apoB-100 levels are greater than LDL levels in these patients, the diagnosis of apoE-2E-2 phenotype is more difficult to make, and this laboratory value must be sent to a reference laboratory. The disease should be suspected, however, in patients with roughly equal cholesterol and triglyceride levels and orange palmar creases.

Disorders of HDL

Unfortunately, HDL metabolism is much more confusing and is less well analyzed than VLDL metabolism (Fig. 12-5). HDL is predominately produced in the intestine and participates in the removal of cholesterol from the peripheral tissue. It is a "garbage collector." HDL also interacts with the VLDL particles to remove triglycerides and "trade off" cholesterol to the VLDL particles in the process of converting VLDL to LDL. *Familial hypoalphalipoproteinemia* is a genetic disorder that leads to decreased production of HDL particles. These patients have isolated low HDL levels on their serum lipid profile and have a markedly increased risk for atherosclerosis.

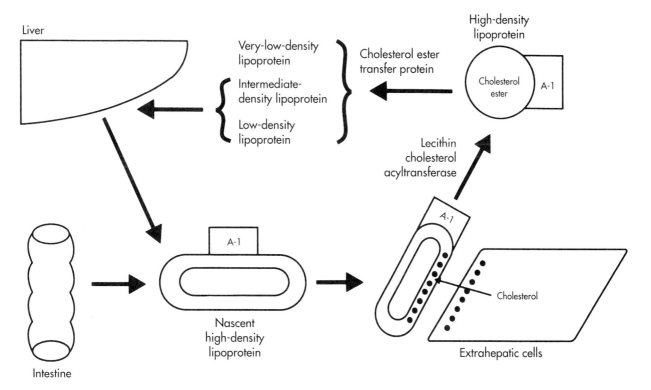

FIG. 12-5
Reverse cholesterol transport. The nascent HDL particle draws cholesterol from extrahepatic cells (including the vascular endothelium) and transfers it to VLDL and then LDL particles, which are then taken up by the liver.
From Breslow JL: *Cardiol Board Rev* 6:10, 1989.

In other situations, however, patients may have low HDL levels and not have an increased risk for coronary atherosclerosis, as with the so-called A1-Milano gene. A family in Milan, Italy, has been identified with low serum HDL levels but active production of an HDL particle that participates aggressively in cholesterol removal from the peripheral tissues. They also have rapid metabolism of their HDL, so serum levels remain low despite a normal or increased production. These patients appear to have a very low incidence of coronary atherosclerosis.

Currently no laboratory study can determine whether a patient with low HDL is at high risk for coronary disease. The appropriate strategy regarding HDL levels therefore is to consider low HDL a risk factor for CAD and aggressively treat LDL levels in patients with low levels of HDL. In a patient with no known atherosclerosis who has only an *isolated low HDL level,* the most important question for the clinician is whether the patient has a *family history* of coronary disease. If rampant coronary atherosclerosis exists in the family, be concerned about familial hypoalphalipoproteinemia and consider attempts to raise the HDL level, perhaps with the use of niacin. If, however, the patient has no family history of atherosclerosis, it is unclear whether raising the HDL level is warranted. The patient should be encouraged to follow a healthy lifestyle.

Current wisdom suggests that the order of treatment of an abnormal lipid profile with regard to the benefits and risk reduction for cardiac events should be (1) treat the LDL, (2) treat the HDL, and (3)treat the triglycerides. Future studies may modify this strategy, but currently this appears to be the appropriate approach.

NEWER, MORE CONTROVERSIAL ATHEROSCLEROTIC RISK FACTORS

Several newer risk factors for CAD have been identified, although most remain controversial with regard to their prognostic implications and, more important, approach to treatment. Such risk factors include elevated serum iron concentration, high fibrinogen levels, elevated homocystine levels, and excess Lp(a). Although several studies have suggested that high serum iron levels and high fibrinogen levels are predictive of increased risk for coronary disease, no treatment trials of lowering either iron or fibrinogen have been performed to date. It will be necessary to show whether these risk factors are direct causes of atherosclerosis or whether lowering of these markers themselves translates into a reduced risk of events.

The same can be said about elevated *homocystine* levels. Elevated homocystine levels in the serum are strongly predictive of an increased risk for cardiovascular events. No study to date, however, has shown that reducing homocystine levels with folic acid, vitamin B_6, or vitamin B_{12} leads to a reduced risk of cardiac events (an approach to treatment is described in Chapter 44). A large study is in progress in Europe that has a limb of patients with high homocystine levels; it should soon provide information concerning the benefits of treating high homocystine levels.

Elevated *Lp(a)* levels have been studied to some extent. Lp(a) is a lipid particle that is genetically determined, and familial elevated Lp(a) is a relatively common autosomal dominant trait. The particle is similar to LDL in that it is often primarily made up of cholesterol and also has an apoB-100 apoprotein on its surface. Levels of this particle are an acute phase reactant, and levels rise with acute inflammation, the significance of which is unclear. In the resting state, however, elevated Lp(a) levels seem to predict the risk of atherosclerotic events as well as early bypass graft closure and restenosis after angioplasty. The higher the level of Lp(a) in the serum, the higher the risk of subsequent events. These "LDL-like" particles also have a protein on their surface called apo a. Lp(a) may be atherogenic because it is relatively easy to oxidize. In addition, the apoprotein on the surface of the particle has an amino acid sequence that is somewhat similar to that of plasminogen. The particle therefore competitively inhibits the conversion of plasminogen to plasmin in the serum, thereby making the patient hypercoagulable. No direct treatment studies have shown that reducing Lp(a) levels in the serum reduces clinical events. However, several small studies have suggested that in patients with elevated Lp(a) levels, the approach to treatment should be to lower LDL level below the currently recommended goals. In the FATS trial, patients who had elevated Lp(a) levels were found to have excessive risks alleviated by lowering serum LDL levels to less than 80 mg/dL. Our current approach for patients with coronary disease and high Lp(a) levels is to push LDL levels to below 80 mg/dL.

Finally, studies using vitamins and antioxidants have been generally disappointing. The concept of antioxidant therapy is quite enticing, because it would seem that blocking the oxidation of LDL particles should interrupt the atherosclerotic process (see Fig. 12-2). Randomized prospective studies performed with vitamin C, beta-carotene, and vitamin E have failed to show benefit with aggressive treatment.[10] A study performed using probucol, which is a very potent antioxidant, showed no reduction in clinical events in humans. One study in patients with bypass surgery, the "CHAOS" trial, suggested that patients who have had previous bypass surgery and who took 400 to 800 IU of vitamin E had a significant reduction in events.[11] Vitamin C and beta-carotene have not been shown to reduce cardiac events. In studies of patients who previously were smokers, beta-carotene has actually increased the risk of carcinoma of the lung; therefore beta-carotene is not recommended.

In our opinion, patients should be told that if they want to take an antioxidant, they should consider vitamin E at levels of 400 to 800 IU per day. Based on the clinical evidence currently available, antioxidant therapy is nowhere near as potent a risk reducer as the proven benefits of lowering LDL with drugs such as statins.

DRUG THERAPY OF DYSLIPIDEMIA

Before a few years ago, the available medications for patients with dyslipidemia were considered expensive, poorly tolerated, and limited in effectiveness. However, several extremely effective and well-tolerated pharmacologic agents recently have been developed. Most have been shown to be effective not only in treating dyslipidemia but also in decreasing clinical cardiac events and, in some cases, total mortality. In addition, virtually none of these agents has adversely increased noncardiac mortality. The dangers of drug treatment for dyslipidemia, which were of concern in the past, have become much less so. The balance of evidence indicates that drug treatment of dyslipidemia not only is safe but also is one of the most effective approaches to decreasing cardiovascular events in patients at risk.

Currently available agents can be categorized loosely into the following categories:
1. Drugs that primarily reduce LDL
2. Drugs that primarily reduce triglycerides
3. Drugs that affect both LDL and triglycerides

A few agents have the added benefit of favorably affecting HDL levels. Drugs that predominately affect LDL include the HMG-CoA reductase inhibitors (the statins) and the bile acid–binding resins. Drugs that predominately lower triglycerides are the fibric acid derivatives and omega-3 fatty acids (fish oils). Drugs that have a significant effect on both triglycerides and LDL cholesterol include nicotinic acid and its derivatives, as well as combination therapy.

LDL-Lowering Drugs

Statins

By far the most effective agents in lowering LDL levels are the HMG-CoA reductase inhibitors, the *statins*. They work by blocking the production of intracellular cholesterol by the hepatocyte, thus inhibiting the rate-limiting enzyme in cholesterol production, HMG-CoA reductase. Hepatocytes require cholesterol to make bile and other substances. They counteract reduced production by *increasing the number of LDL receptors on the surface of the hepatocyte* and thus extract more LDL from the blood (Fig. 12-6), leading to a lowering of the serum LDL level.

When high doses of statins are administered, a secondary benefit may be achieved. Low intrahepatic production of cholesterol also seems to reduce the produc-

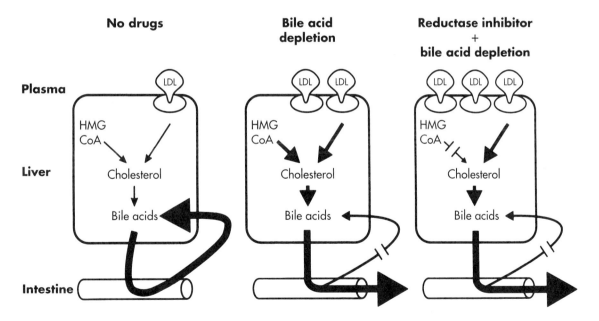

FIG. 12-6
How cholesterol-lowering therapy works. The final common pathway is reduced cholesterol availability to the liver, which increases the number of hepatocyte LDL receptors so that cholesterol can be extracted from the circulation. This happens with a low-cholesterol diet. Bile acid–binding resins block the enterohepatic circulation of bile, a cholesterol-rich substance *(middle panel)*. Reductase inhibitors block cholesterol synthesis in the hepatocyte. The combination of reductase inhibitors with either resins or diet therapy is synergistic.
From Brown MS, Goldstein JL: *Science* 232:34, 1986.

Table 12-2	*Relative Potencies of Available Statins*

Statin	Relative Potency
Fluvastatin	1
Lovastatin	2
Pravastatin	2
Cerivastatin	2
Simvastatin	4
Atorvastatin	8

tion of VLDL cholesterol in the liver. This leads to a modest reduction in triglyceride levels. This effect on triglycerides is more pronounced with high-dose statin therapy and is more predictable in patients whose baseline triglyceride levels are extremely high.

Currently six statin medications are available. The predominant differences in these medications are their LDL-lowering potencies and their cost. Table 12-2 lists the currently available statins and their relative potencies, with the least potent statin being given an arbitrary potency value of 1.

Statins are well-tolerated medications with few side effects. The most common side effects include myalgias, which are diffuse muscle or joint aches not associated with any blood chemistry abnormalities. Other side effects such as headaches, nausea, and insomnia can occur but are less common.

Asymptomatic liver enzyme elevation is quite common with statin therapy, but modest elevation is not an indication for discontinuing the drug. It is unnecessary to discontinue therapy until the enzyme level reaches *three times* the upper limit of normal.

The most dangerous potential toxicity from statins is myositis with secondary rhabdomyolysis. This severe toxicity, which can lead to acute renal failure, is rare with the use of statins alone. When statins are combined with other agents such as fibric acid derivatives, erythromycin-like antibiotics, azole antifungal agents, and certain immunosuppressive drugs, the likelihood increases. These combinations should be avoided unless no other option for treatment is available.

Resins

The second class of agents predominately used for LDL lowering includes the bile acid–binding resins (cholestyramine and colestipol). These agents are often chosen in children because they are not absorbed, and they are not thought to have significant systemic side effects. Their mechanism of action is to bind the bile acids and cause them to be excreted in the stool rather than reabsorbed through the intrahepatic circulation. Since

bile acids are rich in cholesterol, when they are reabsorbed in the intrahepatic circulation, they provide the hepatocytes with a source of cholesterol, thereby reducing the need to remove LDL from the serum. When resins prevent the reabsorption of bile acids, the liver receives less cholesterol from the intrahepatic circulation and must extract more LDL from the serum (again, by increasing the number of LDL receptors on the surface of the hepatocytes). This reduces the serum LDL level.

The combination of statins and bile acid–binding resins is extremely effective in increasing the number of LDL receptors and reducing serum LDL levels. In fact, the combination of statin therapy plus a resin is synergistic, in that their LDL-lowering potency together is greater than the sum of the two separately. The disadvantage of bile acid–binding resins is their gastrointestinal side effects. They frequently cause constipation and bloating and may affect the absorption of other medications. In addition, resins may aggravate mild hypertriglyceridemia.

Resins should be avoided in patients with significant gastrointestinal disease and in those with modest hypertriglyceridemia. They should also be taken several hours before or after dosages of other medications to avoid the possibility of reducing the absorption of these medicines.

Triglyceride-Lowering Drugs

The most effective agents for lowering triglyceride levels are the fibric acid derivatives, including gemfibrozil and fenofibrate. These agents are extremely effective in lowering triglyceride levels and, in patients with modest hypertriglyceridemia, also will raise HDL levels. The predominant mechanism of action of the fibric acid derivatives is to activate lipoprotein lipase in the serum, which is an enzyme critical to the metabolism of triglycerides in the free fatty acids. The fibric acid derivatives increase the breakdown of triglycerides, thereby lowering serum triglyceride levels. Some evidence suggests that fenofibrate also may act within the liver to reduce the production of VLDL. These drugs should be considered for use predominately in patients with markedly elevated triglyceride levels who are at risk for pancreatitis, such as those with persistent triglyceride levels of 500 to 1000 mg/dL or greater and in whom no treatable secondary causes of hypertriglyceridemia are identified.

The side effects of the fibrates are generally gastrointestinal. Long-term use can increase the risk of cholelithiasis. In addition, many patients have increased LDL levels when given a fibric acid derivative. These drugs therefore should not be the first choice in patients with only mild hypertriglyceridemia; rather, the LDL level should be treated to goal with a statin or niacin. Combination therapy with a fibric acid derivative and a statin should generally be avoided because of the increased risk of myositis. However, if no other option except this combination exists, the risk factors for myositis developing during the combination therapy are renal insufficiency, diabetes, and advanced age.

Omega-3 fatty acids also are quite effective in lowering triglyceride levels. Doses of 4 to 8 g of fish oil may be required for the desired effect. Fish oil capsules are somewhat cumbersome to take, since 8 to 16 capsules may be required in divided doses and patients may complain of "smelling like fish" and having a "fishy taste." Fish oil can be a helpful adjunct to statin therapy in diabetic patients, who often have high triglyceride levels, as well as high LDL levels, and who are at higher risk of myositis on the combination of fibric acid therapy and statins. Fish oil does not seem to significantly affect diabetes control but, unfortunately, is high in calories.

Drugs That Affect Triglyceride and LDL Levels

If one were to design an ideal pharmacologic agent for dyslipidemia, it would have the effects of nicotinic acid. Nicotinic acid (niacin) in essence does everything correctly to the lipid profile. It lowers triglyceride levels substantially and, at appropriate doses, will raise HDL and lower LDL levels. It is the single best agent for elevating HDL levels, with the potential to raise these 30% to 35%.

Compliance with niacin has been difficult because of its multiple side effects. First, regular niacin requires three doses per day. In addition, multiple gastrointestinal side effects, such as aggravation of peptic ulcer disease and nausea, can occur. Because of the release of prostaglandins resulting from niacin therapy, patients can experience itching and flushing. Niacin also aggravates glucose intolerance and can markedly worsen glucose levels in patients with diabetes. Other side effects include aggravation of gout and of supraventricular arrhythmias. The long-acting niacin preparations may cause less itching, but these have been avoided because of their increased risk of hepatotoxicity. Newer once-a-day formulations that last about 6 hours and are given once at bedtime appear to be effective and have fewer side effects.

Many niacin side effects can be decreased if the dose is taken on a full stomach and if the patient takes an aspirin approximately 1 hour before the dose to reduce the prostaglandin effects. The dose of niacin required to treat dyslipidemia is 3 g/day.

Combination Drug Therapy

Another approach to the patient with high triglyceride and high LDL levels is combination therapy. The combination of statins and fibric acid derivatives has been discussed and should be avoided unless there are no other alternatives. The increased risk of myositis, especially in patients with other chronic diseases or renal insufficiency, may outweigh the cardiovascular benefits.

Gratifying lipid profile results, however, can be achieved with this combination if given to selected patients who are monitored carefully for signs for toxicity.

In nondiabetic patients the combination of statins plus niacin is extremely effective in treating modest hypertriglyceridemia and low HDL levels, as well as high LDL levels. If one keeps the total daily niacin dose to 2 g or less, the incidence of toxicity is low. However, careful follow-up of liver function is recommended when this combination is used. In patients who cannot tolerate statin therapy, the combination of bile acid–binding resins with fibric acid derivatives also can be effective. The addition of a fibric acid derivative to cholestyramine (Questran) can counteract some of the potential for triglyceride elevation by the resin in susceptible individuals.

Raising HDL Levels

Very few currently available therapies are effective in consistently raising HDL levels. Avoidance of tobacco and regular exercise are the mainstays of therapy, but all of the previously mentioned agents raise HDL level slightly, with niacin being the most potent, followed by fibric acid derivatives in those patients with mild hypertriglyceridemia. The reductase inhibitors across the board generally raise HDL levels only slightly (approximately 8%).

REFERENCES

1. Merck Quality Assurance Program: Fourth International Conference on Preventative Cardiology, Montreal, July 1997.
2. Anderson KM, Castelli WP, Levy D: Cholesterol and mortality: 30 years of follow-up from the Framingham Study, *JAMA* 257:2176, 1987.
3. Stamler J, Wentworth D, Neaton JD for the MRFIT Research Group: Is relationship between serum cholesterol and risk of premature death from coronary heart disease continuous and graded? *JAMA* 256:2823, 1986.
4. Shepherd J, Cobbe SM, Ford I, et al: Prevention of coronary heart disease with pravastatin in men with hypercholesterolemia: The West of Scotland Coronary Prevention Study, *N Engl J Med* 333:1301, 1995.
5. Pederson TR et al: Randomised trial of cholesterol lowering in 4444 patients with coronary heart disease: the Scandinavian Simvastatin Survival Study (4S), *Lancet* 344:1383, 1994.
6. Pyorala K, Pederson TR, Kjekshus J, et al: Cholesterol lowering with simvastatin improves prognosis of diabetic patients with coronary heart disease, *Diabetes Care* 20:614, 1997.
7. Blankenhorn DH, Nessim SA, Johnson RL, et al: Beneficial effects of combined colestipol-niacin therapy on coronary atherosclerosis in coronary venous bypass grafts, *JAMA* 257:3233, 1987.
8. Brown G, Albers JJ, Fisher LD, et al: Regression of coronary artery disease as a result of intensive lipid-lowering therapy in men with high levels of apolipoprotein B, *N Engl J Med* 323:1289, 1990.

9. Manninen V, Tenkanen L, Koskinen P, et al: Joint effects of serum triglyceride and LDL cholesterol and HDL cholesterol concentrations on coronary heart disease risk in the Helsinki heart study, *Circulation* 85:37, 1992.

10. The Alpha-Tocopherol, Beta-Carotene Cancer Prevention Study Group: The effect of vitamin E and beta carotene on the incidence of lung cancer and other cancers in male smokers, *N Engl J Med* 330:1029, 1994.

11. Stephens NG, Parsons A, Schofield PM, et al: Randomised controlled trial of vitamin E in patients with coronary disease: the Cambridge Heart Antioxidant Study (CHAOS), *Lancet* 347:781, 1996.

BIBILIOGRAPHY

Ascherio A, Katin MB, Zock PL, et al: Trans fatty acids and coronary disease, *N Engl J Med* 340:1994, 1999. A review of studies from the 1990s showing the adverse effect of trans-unsaturated fatty acids (found in solid margarines): they lower HDL and raise LDL. Saturated fatty acids also raise LDL but have less effect on HDL. Cis unsaturated fatty acids (in vegetable oils and liquid margarine) are best, lowering LDL and having the least effect on HDL. With oils and liquid margarines, the LDL/HDL ratio is the lowest.

Waters D: Cholesterol lowering: should it continue to be the last thing we do? *Circulation* 99:3215, 1999. A review of data that support immediate initiation of lipid-lowering therapy after acute coronary events. Endothelial function and platelet effects may occur early with lowering of LDL cholesterol. There are no clinical trial data, but the MIRACL study is in progress, with results available in late 2000.

13 Angina Pectoris

George J. Taylor
Robert C. Bussing

Angina behaves like more than one illness. The clinical syndromes included in angina pectoris share pathophysiologic elements, and most cause chest discomfort, but the illnesses have different natural histories and require different management approaches. It is useful to think of them separately, and, when a patient comes to you with chest pain, to decide which of these conditions you are evaluating and treating.

The symptom is discussed in Chapter 3. The term *angina* comes from the Latin term with the same spelling. When used alone, it originally meant an inflammatory affliction of the throat, such as quinsy. *Angina pectoris* is more specific for the discomfort of myocardial ischemia, but we will follow the common practice of using *angina* alone. Etymologically related is "anguish," defined as an agonizing pain of body or mind. The related French word, *angoisse,* means choking, and the Latin word, *angustia,* tightness or narrowness. All of these describe the symptom. Angina is not a superficial, fleeting, or stabbing pain. Rather, it is a deep, choking, tight discomfort with elements of agony and anguish—even though patients commonly say they "have no pain" (Chapter 3).

For years I was ambivalent about the pronunciation. *An gi' na* (with a long *i*) seems to be preferred by patients. *An' gin a* (with a short *i*) sounds better to me, and both are correct.

EVALUATION OF CHEST PAIN: CHEST PAIN OF UNCERTAIN ETIOLOGY

There is no diagnostic code for chest pain of uncertain etiology (CPUE), but I think of it as a clinical entity because its evaluation is such a common exercise. It is slightly different from the evaluation of angina pectoris when the clinician is relatively certain of the diagnosis. Instead, CPUE refers to a patient admitted to the emergency department in the middle of the night with somewhat atypical pain and no electrocardiographic (ECG) changes, or a patient who sees you in the clinic with vague discomfort that is hard to characterize.

Epidemiology, Etiology, and Natural History

New chest discomfort is among the most common clinical encounters. From your own experience, think of the percentage of your patients over age 40 who have men-tioned chest discomfort to you at some time. Is it more than half? (I had to take an antacid last night.) In the United States, more than 3 million people visit emergency departments because of chest pain each year.

Most who practice general medicine become good at the differential diagnosis of chest discomfort (Tables 3-3 and 13-1). An immediate goal is the recognition of cardiac pain, since heart disease is life-threatening. While Tables 3-2 and 13-1 list a number of other serious illnesses that may cause chest discomfort, experience indicates that the most common causes of noncardiac chest pain are gastroesophageal reflux and chest wall syndromes. The initial screening process, including history, physical examination, and simple laboratory studies (Table 13-1), usually is adequate for exclusion of the most serious syndromes.

Clinical Presentation

The characteristics of angina and nonanginal chest discomfort are reviewed in Chapter 3. The onset of angina is gradual, and it mounts in intensity. The location is the midchest area with or without radiation to dermatomes C2 to T12. It may have a vague quality, and rest or nitroglycerine therapy provides relief within minutes. If a patient points with one finger to the left side of the chest, indicating "over my heart," the pain probably is not angina.

However, as you have probably learned from experience, the history may be misleading. Symptoms that indicate a cardiac origin of pain may occur in those without ischemia. Similarly, atypical chest pain may be angina. Although textbooks confidently recite the characteristics of ischemic discomfort, most of us in clinical practice are used to being fooled.

Symptoms that point to noncardiac illnesses may be more reliable and, when they are clear-cut, exclude angina pectoris. Pleuritic chest pain indicates an inflammatory condition, not angina. A typical description of reflux esophagitis—particularly pain with recumbency, an associated sour taste, occurrence after meals and relief by sitting upright—make angina unlikely. A musculoskeletal cause is indicated by discomfort that occurs with movement, reaching, twisting, or use of one limb (e.g., pain when using the right shoulder, but not with other forms of exertion) or reproduction of the

Table 13-1	Chest Pain Syndromes (see also Table 3-2)		
Syndrome	**Associated Conditions**	**Physical Examination**	**Laboratory Evaluation**
Chronic stable angina	Risk factors for coronary disease (see Chapter 11)	Usually normal; S_4 gallop or soft systolic murmur during pain	ECG often normal; new ECG changes during pain; abnormal stress study
Unstable angina	As above	As above	As above
Aortic dissection	Hypertension, other risk factors for coronary disease; connective tissue disease (see Chapter 32)	Unequal or missing pulses; soft diastolic murmur of aortic regurgitation	Chest x-ray (wide mediastinum), echocardiogram, CT or MRI studies, angiography
Esophageal reflux and spasm	Advanced age; possibly smoking and obesity	Normal	Endoscopy, pH monitoring, motility studies, barium studies
Esophageal rupture	Follows severe vomiting	Subcutaneous emphysema	Chest x-ray—air in the mediastinum
Pancreatitis	Alcoholism, gallbladder disease	Epigastric tenderness	Elevated amylase, white count
Peptic ulcer disease	Possibly smoking	Epigastric discomfort	Endoscopy, barium studies
Chest wall pain	Osteoarthritis, chronic back and neck pain	Pain with deep palpation, stretching, or change in position	None—usually a diagnosis of exclusion
Herpes zoster	Advanced age, immunocompromised host (but may develop in healthy, young patients), prior history of shingles	Pain may precede the typical rash by 48-72 hours; rash is maculopapular, then vesicular; lesions usually few in number	Tzanck smear of a lesion, fourfold rise in antibody titer (acute vs. convalescent)
Pericarditis	Often follows a flulike illness in young patients	Friction rub, occasionally fever	High sedimentation rate, white cell count usually normal, echocardiogram (see Chapter 29)
Biliary disease	Middle age, obesity, female > male	Right upper quadrant tenderness	Ultrasound, cholecystogram, high alkaline phosphatase and bilirubin
Bronchospasm	Obstructive lung disease, asthma	Wheezing, prolonged expiratory phase	Abnormal chest x-ray, pulmonary function studies
Pneumonia		Fever, splinting, signs of pulmonary consolidation	Chest x-ray, elevated white blood cell count
Pulmonary embolus	Elderly or bedridden, congestive heart failure, malignancy	Tachycardia, tachypnea, localized wheezes, signs of phlebothrombosis usually absent	Low Pao_2, abnormal lung scan, abnormal venogram
Mitral valve prolapse	Young, female > male, anxiety	Often thin, tall; midsystolic click, late systolic murmur (see Chapter 18)	Echocardiogram
Hyperventilation	Anxiety	Normal examination; during attacks, pallor and tachycardia	Low $Paco_2$ during attack, but blood gases rarely needed to make the diagnosis

pain by pressing on the chest wall. When sure of one of these noncardiac illnesses, I do not pursue an expensive cardiac workup.

Laboratory Evaluation of Chest Pain

Baseline Laboratory Studies

Complete Blood Count. Anemia alone does not cause angina, but it lowers the anginal threshold in the presence of coronary disease. Inflammatory conditions that may affect the heart usually do not raise the white blood cell count. The erythrocyte sedimentation rate is a nonspecific but sensitive indicator of inflammation; when normal, acute pericarditis is unlikely.

Serum Electrolytes. None of the chest pain syndromes is influenced by electrolyte abnormalities. However, an argument can be made for checking magnesium and potassium levels in any patient being treated with diuretics when there are new symptoms.

Screening Chemistry Panel, the Chem-20. The chemistry panel is of little diagnostic benefit, although the liver panel may help diagnose biliary disease, and the panel usually includes cholesterol. I do not order the screening panel as part of the chest pain workup unless there is a specific reason (e.g., a new patient, multiple other medical problems that require monitoring, or a suspicion of gallbladder disease). If the differential diagnosis includes coronary disease, a lipid panel including triglycerides and low-density lipoprotein (LDL) and high-density lipoprotein (HDL) cholesterol is more useful.

Electrocardiogram (ECG). The resting ECG is often normal in patients with coronary artery disease (CAD). Unfortunately, many patients with chest pain are told not to worry because the ECG is normal. Permanent change of the ECG may not occur until there is myocardial infarction.

On the other hand, an ECG obtained during chest pain is quite useful. With ischemia there should be a shift in ST segments, either depression or elevation. The absence of ECG changes during the patient's typical pain is an argument against myocardial ischemia. This is not absolute proof of a noncardiac cause, since some regions of the heart are electrocardiographically "silent." For example, ischemia of a small portion of the lateral wall caused by circumflex artery obstruction may cause little or no change on the ECG. In this case the region of ischemia is small. Ischemia involving large areas of myocardium causes ECG changes. If a patient has a normal ECG during pain, the risk of ischemia is low enough that the workup can be expedited, going directly to stress testing.

Of course, if no previous ECG is available for comparison, the ECG on presentation or during pain is less useful. Establishing a baseline is another good reason for obtaining an ECG for any patient with chest discomfort.

Chest X-ray. This is especially useful when screening for thoracic aortic aneurysm or dissection (see Chapters 7 and 32). A widened aortic silhouette raises suspicion, and this finding is present in more than 80% of patients with dissection. There may be abnormalities with other causes of chest pain, but, with the exception of pneumonia, the chest x-ray provides nonspecific rather than diagnostic information. It is worth doing if lung disease is suspected.

Diagnostic Studies

We perform the following tests to establish a cardiac diagnosis, often to rule out coronary heart disease (Table 13-2).

Stress ECG. Indications, limitations, contraindications, and technical aspects of stress testing are reviewed in Chapter 6. In the evaluation of chest pain of uncertain etiology, stress testing is done to exclude coronary heart disease. A negative study with good exercise tolerance (more than 7 minutes on the treadmill using the Bruce protocol) reliably excludes *flow-restricting* coronary lesions. Patients who exercise for more than 7 minutes with no symptoms or ECG changes have a good prognosis.

In the face of this claim, how do we explain the unusual patient who has a negative stress ECG, is told not to worry, and then has a heart attack the next week? Note that a negative study excludes *flow-restricting* coronary lesions. A plaque that narrows the coronary artery by less than 50% may not restrict flow, even during exercise. However, even a nonstenosing plaque may rupture, develop hematoma or surface thrombus, and occlude. This is the mechanism of acute myocardial infarction with minimal disease, but it accounts for a minority of acute infarctions. For patients with CPUE that does not sound like typical angina and with an adequate and negative stress ECG, the prognosis is good and further cardiac evaluation is unnecessary. I take care to tell the patient that, although fairly reliable, the negative stress test has the limitations just described.

The issue of false-negative and false-positive diagnostic studies is reviewed in Chapter 6. Good *sensitivity* indicates a small number of false negatives; little disease is missed. Good *specificity* means a small number of false positives; there is little overdiagnosis of disease.

The stress ECG is fairly sensitive but has poor specificity. False-positive results are common. A patient with atypical chest discomfort and an abnormal stress test has a 10% to 40% chance of having normal coronary arteries, depending on gender, appearance of the baseline ECG, and quality of symptoms (see Chapter 6). Bayesian analysis teaches us that when the discomfort sounds like angina and the likelihood of coronary disease is higher, the chance of a false-positive study is lower. False positives are still a fact of life, and the

Table 13-2	Techniques for Diagnosing Coronary Artery Disease (CAD)

Technique	Advantages	Disadvantages/Limitations
Stress ECG	Widely available, a primary care procedure	False positives are common (lower specificity than other techniques)
Exercise perfusion imaging	Sensitive and specific; proven for risk stratification; late uptake of Tl^{201} used to test viability of stunned muscle	Operator dependent
Pharmacologic perfusion imaging	As above	Exercise tolerance is not demonstrated; operator dependent
Exercise echocardiogram	Provides left ventricular size and function measurements	Slightly less sensitive than perfusion imaging; utility in risk stratification unproved; operator dependent
Dobutamine echo		Exercise tolerance not demonstrated; operator dependent
Coronary angiography	Only technique that shows nonstenosing plaque (all others require flow restriction); only one that shows a left main coronary lesion; anatomy is related to prognosis; allows definition of plaque morphology (e.g., ulceration) and shows thrombus	Invasive with a small but definite risk of complications (see Chapter 10)

workup is seldom complete with a positive stress ECG. Most patients require confirmatory study.

Perfusion Imaging. Combining the exercise test with thallium or sestamibi scanning using the latest gated tomographic methods adds specificity (see Chapter 9). There are fewer false positives. It may add some sensitivity, but not much. Like the stress ECG, these techniques detect flow-restricting stenoses; the borderline, nonstenosing lesion would not cause a perfusion abnormality. As mentioned earlier, nonstenosing lesions may become unstable. Nevertheless, a negative perfusion scan indicates a good prognosis and usually signals the end of the cardiac workup.

Perfusion imaging is expensive (see Chapter 9). For this reason, it is not a routine test for all patients with CPUE. Specific indications have been outlined (see Chapter 9). Perfusion scanning is used for those who have had a positive stress ECG that is suspected to be false positive. This and other imaging studies may be used as the initial test for others at high risk for having a false-positive stress ECG (e.g., digoxin therapy, left

ventricular hypertrophy, or baseline ST depression), patients with poor exercise tolerance who will not be able to push themselves to maximal heart rates on the treadmill, or those with ECG changes that will make the performance or interpretation of a stress ECG impossible (e.g., atrial fibrillation, left ventricular hypertrophy, diffuse ST segment changes, or conduction abnormalities).

Patients with poor exercise tolerance may have perfusion scans using coronary vasodilators (dipyridamole or adenosine) or pharmacologic stress (dobutamine). These techniques are considered as accurate as exercise scanning. A disadvantage of this approach is that it does not define exercise tolerance, and I prefer exercise studies when feasible.

Exercise Echocardiogram. Normally, the myocardium contracts more forcefully with exercise. When a region of myocardium becomes ischemic, it stops contracting immediately. An ECG done just before and then during stress (either exercise or dobutamine infusion) documents these changes; a positive study shows new regional hypokinesis or akinesis and an overall reduction in left ventricular ejection fraction (LVEF) rather than the normal increase. Sensitivity for the detection of ischemia is similar to that of perfusion imaging (between 80% and 90%, depending on the study).

Exercise Radionuclide Angiogram. This test works like the exercise echocardiogram. It provides an image of the left ventricle in motion plus an accurate measurement of LVEF. A study is positive when the ejection fraction falls and new wall motion abnormalities develop with stress (using either exercise or dobutamine infusion).

Like other stress studies, those using left ventricular function imaging—both echocardiography and radionuclide techniques—detect only flow-restricting coronary lesions and will miss subcritical stenoses.

Accuracy of Stress Imaging Studies. I am adding a warning about the reliability of stress echocardiography, radionuclide angiography, and perfusion imaging in the average hospital setting. These are operator-dependent techniques. The excellent sensitivity and specificity described in the literature are from dedicated laboratories that do large volumes. In addition to greater experience, such programs are staffed by cardiologists and technicians specializing in that specific technique. They do not spend a part of their time doing liver or lung scans. Their impressive results may not be possible in a small community hospital, where a radiologist is doing everything. A general cardiologist trained to read echos, but who does not read exercise echos daily (myself, for example), may not be good at interpreting exercise echos. The same is true for nuclear cardiology. False-positive perfusion scans are more common from small-volume laboratories that are not in the full-time business of nuclear cardiology. Which of these imaging studies you choose to rely on must depend partly on the expertise of your program.

Electron Beam Computed Tomography (EBCT). This is the newest of the noninvasive screening techniques for coronary artery disease (CAD), and experience with it is limited.[2] Unlike stress studies that test for flow-restricting lesions, EBCT tests for plaque. Most atherosclerotic lesions contain minute quantities of calcium, detectable by EBCT. Reported sensitivity for *flow-restricting* lesions is 70% to 90%, with specificity around 45%. The lower specificity—meaning more false positives—is consistent with the ability of EBCT to identify early, nonstenosing plaque. At least one study has shown that the presence of coronary calcification increases the chance of a future coronary event. Since EBCT may detect preclinical disease, it has been promoted as a screening test for asymptomatic individuals with risk factors (or for those with curiosity and cash).

Where EBCT fits into the evaluation of chest pain is uncertain. The high sensitivity figures were obtained from studies of subjects with known CAD. A potential problem is that patients with unstable angina are more likely to have noncalcified coronary lesions than those with chronic angina. This may be especially true for younger patients. Before recommending EBCT as an initial test for CPUE or unstable angina, more experience is needed.

Cardiac Catheterization. This expensive and invasive study is rarely the initial diagnostic test for patients with atypical chest pain or CPUE (Table 13-2 and Chapter 10). It is reserved for a patient with a positive screening study who is suspected of having coronary heart disease. An occasional patient with negative screening studies continues to have chest pain that necessitates repeat hospital admission. Angiography may be recommended to prevent repeated admission to the hospital and possibly to prevent cardiac neurosis. Although not a recognized indication for catheterization, this is a reality in everyday practice.

Management of CPUE

The first step is making a cardiac diagnosis—heart disease or no heart disease. It is both useful for the patient and cost effective if this is done quickly. A patient who is admitted to the hospital with atypical chest pain should, in an ideal world, have a diagnostic study within 24 hours. Many hospitals have started "chest pain centers" where such patients are observed in a holding area and, if stable, have a stress imaging study done after 4 to 8 hours of observation. The major advantage of these programs is the protocol that ensures rapid access to the exercise, nuclear, and echo laboratories.

Patients also benefit from rapid evaluation in an outpatient setting. The ability to discriminate between cardiac and noncardiac pain minimizes the risk of adverse events, including myocardial infarction or sudden death. Exercise testing should be scheduled within a week for those with atypical pain and sooner when the discomfort is more "anginal."

Abnormal studies indicating CAD move the patient out of the CPUE category and into one of the angina pectoris syndromes. Diagnosis of another of the specific causes of chest pain dictates an alternative evaluation and treatment approach (see Table 13-1).

Among our most difficult management dilemmas is the patient with a negative cardiac workup and no other obvious cause for pain. They usually have either chest wall discomfort or gastroesophageal reflux. Esophageal diagnostic studies, in my experience, usually do not help. When the pain sounds esophageal, I recommend a therapeutic trial of antacids, H_2 blockers, elevation of the head of the bed, avoidance of late evening meals, and so forth. If there is no response to this and I still suspect peptic disease, I order esophageal studies.

On the other hand, if the discomfort sounds more musculoskeletal and the pain is reproduced by palpation, I recommend a trial of nonsteroidal antiinflammatory agents and observation. Symptoms persisting beyond 2 weeks would prompt the evaluation of the chest wall using x-ray or other imaging studies. (Who can forget the rare patient with osteosarcoma of the ribs?)

Follow-up and Expected Clinical Course of CPUE

After heart disease and other dangerous conditions have been excluded and the patient is being treated symptomatically on the basis of your best clinical guess, it is important to monitor the response carefully, since "excluded" is a relative term in medicine. Although the exercise test, even with the addition of an imaging study, is sensitive (few false negatives), it is not perfect. Remember that most of these techniques test for flow-restricting coronary lesions and can miss a borderline lesion that could be the nidus for thrombus formation.

Those with noncardiac chest pain tend to improve with time. If they do not, and especially if they get worse, they need reevaluation. Instruct them to return or seek help promptly if they have prolonged pain. When you begin treatment for a patient with chest pain, see him or her back in clinic the next week.

CHRONIC STABLE ANGINA PECTORIS
Epidemiology and Natural History

CAD is the leading cause of morbidity and mortality in the United States, accounting for about one third of all deaths; 700,000 patients are hospitalized with chest pain each year. The illness costs $80 billion annually, 15% of the U.S. health care budget.[3]

There is a gender difference, with 70% of angina pectoris occurring in men. CAD is common in women as well and is the most common cause of death in women over 50 years old. Half of those who die each year of CAD are women. It tends to develop about a decade later in women than in men, and it is a mistake to discount the possibility of CAD in women with chest discomfort (see Chapter 41).

Data from the Framingham study collected before 1970 shows that about one fourth of men with angina had myocardial infarction within 5 years; the mortality was lower for women with angina. Almost one third of patients over 55 years old who had angina died within the 8-year follow-up period. Half the deaths were sudden, and most of the rest followed myocardial infarction. Interestingly, only 23% of myocardial infarctions were preceded by angina. Patients with angina, on the other hand, rarely had silent myocardial infarction.

Information from the Framingham study may be used as a rough guide for prognosis, but it probably overestimates the risk of death or myocardial infarction using current therapies. The incidence of CAD fell by 1% per year from 1960 to 1986, and annual mortality fell about 2% per year. In the decade after 1980 the slope of the declining mortality curve steepened.[4] The 1990 case fatality rate was 34% lower than could have been predicted from the event rates and risk factor levels of 1980. Only one fourth of this decline can be attributed to primary prevention. The major explanation for lower CAD mortality in the last 15 years is improved treatment: a combination of aggressive risk factor and lipid reduction in patients with CAD plus superior medical and revascularization therapies.[4]

Pathophysiology of Angina
Oxygen Supply and Demand

Myocardial ischemia occurs when oxygen supply falls below oxygen demand (MVO_2). Variables in the supply-demand equation are illustrated in Figure 13-1. The typical coronary stenosis causing chronic effort angina is calcified, rigid, and stable. The bulk of the plaque (percent stenosis) dominates the supply side of the equation; spasm and thrombus have little role. The hydraulics of coronary flow thus approximate those of fuel lines in machines, and this is a good way to explain it to patients. When a car has fixed narrowing of a fuel line, it runs normally when idling. Opening the throttle increases the workload of the engine, but fuel flow is limited by the "stenosis," and the engine misses. Because of the fixed nature of the fuel line stenosis, you would expect the engine to begin missing at the same workload (speed or rpms) every time. That is usually the case with

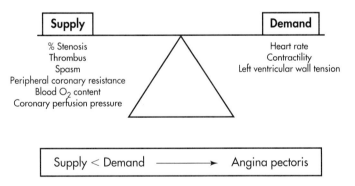

FIG. 13-1
Angina develops when myocardial oxygen demand (MVO_2) exceeds supply. In chronic stable angina, the bulk of the plaque, or percentage of stenosis, places a ceiling on blood supply. Unstable coronary syndromes are characterized by "dynamic stenosis," with variation in its severity caused by either thrombus on the surface of plaque or spasm. A failure of peripheral coronary vasodilation, reduced oxygen-carrying capacity of blood, and low coronary perfusion pressure all may aggravate under-supply. Increased oxygen demand results from conditions that increase heart rate, myocardial contractility, or left ventricular wall tension.

exercise-induced angina. Discomfort and ST segment changes develop at the same cardiac workload. MVO_2 is directly proportional to the product of heart rate and systolic blood pressure at any level of work (see Chapter 6). The heart rate–blood pressure (HR-BP) product at which angina occurs is referred to as the *angina threshold*. Serial exercise testing shows that the angina threshold, or HR-BP product that results in angina, is consistent from day to day in those with stable angina.

Other factors that influence oxygen supply may change the anginal threshold (Fig. 13-1), including anemia and methemoglobinemia, which reduce the oxygen-carrying capacity of blood. Hypotension may reduce coronary perfusion pressure and flow. Tachycardia, by shortening the diastolic phase of the cardiac cycle, also may reduce coronary flow, since most coronary flow occurs during diastole (see Chapter 2).

Variations in Coronary Blood Flow in Stable Angina: Qualifying the Fixed Plaque Model

Qualifications must be added to this simple model of oxygen supply versus demand across a rigid, unchanging stenosis. Even with chronic angina the stenosis may not be "fixed." In an occasional patient the coronary artery can dilate at the level of the stenosis. This usually is caused by an eccentric plaque that leaves a portion of the arterial wall uncovered (Fig. 13-2). The unaffected segment of vessel is compliant and able to relax or contract.

Vascular Tone, Vasodilator Reserve, and Endothelial Function. Anginal symptoms often vary in frequency and severity, producing so-called *variable threshold angina*. Patients tend to have good days and bad days. They may describe a warm-up phenomenon wherein angina occurs with minimal exertion early, but not at all later in the day despite greater exertion. One mechanism

explaining variation is vasospasm or dilation at the site of the lesion. Another is vasodilator reserve.

Flow in a diseased coronary artery is determined not just by resistance at the site of the stenosis, but also by resistance in the remainder of the vascular bed (Fig. 13-3). In animal studies, occlusion of a coronary artery and then release of the occlusion is followed by intense vasodilation and hyperemia, with a fivefold or greater increase in flow compared with the preocclusion baseline. This ability to lower peripheral coronary resistance and increase distal flow is called the *vasodilator* or *coronary flow reserve*.

Coronary blood flow is autoregulated. In response to ischemia, vasodilation is mediated by local factors that include low tissue oxygen tension, adenosine (a product of anaerobic metabolism), and endothelium-derived relaxing factor (EDRF, Box 13-1). EDRF, which is released by normal endothelial cells in response to ischemia, probably is the nitric oxide (NO) radical.[5] The atherosclerotic lesion, as well as many of the risk factors for atherosclerosis, induce endothelial dysfunction, blunting or preventing the normal release of NO in response to ischemia.[5]

Some vasoconstrictors are released by endothelial cells, and normal endothelial function entails maintaining a proper balance between vasoconstriction and dilation. In addition, alpha-adrenergic discharge is a powerful coronary vasoconstrictor. Alpha stimulation due to stress or the cold pressor test causes constriction

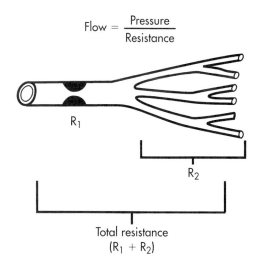

$$Flow = \frac{Pressure}{Resistance}$$

FIG. 13-3
Ohm's law indicates that flow is proportional to perfusion pressure and inversely proportional to vascular resistance. In a patient with angina, total resistance is the combined resistances at the site of stenosis (R_1) as well as downstream (R_2). R_1 may not change with vasodilator therapy, but R_2 may. In addition, angina may worsen with abnormally high R_2, the case with endothelial dysfunction.

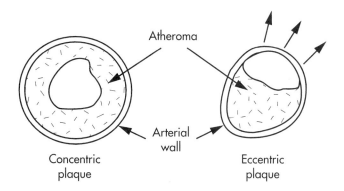

FIG. 13-2
Each of these arteries has 70% stenosis. The artery on the right has eccentric narrowing, and a segment of arterial wall is not covered by atherosclerotic plaque. This unaffected segment may expand or contract, changing luminal size at the level of the plaque. This is not thought to occur when the plaque is concentric.

BOX 13-1

ENDOTHELIAL FUNCTION

Vascular endothelium was previously considered a passive, semipermeable membrane. Now it is recognized as a large endocrine organ, producing substances that regulate vascular resistance, vessel growth, platelet function, and thrombosis.

VASOACTIVE SUBSTANCES RELEASED BY ENDOTHELIAL CELLS

Relaxing Factors
Nitric oxide (endothelium-derived relaxing factor, EDRF)
Prostacyclin
Endothelium-derived hyperpolarizing factor

Contracting Factors
Endothelin-1
Thromboxane
Prostaglandin H2

ANTIATHEROSCLEROTIC FUNCTIONS
Inhibition of platelet aggregation, monocyte adhesion, vascular smooth muscle cell growth and coagulation (components of atherogenesis and plaque rupture)

AGONISTS THAT STIMULATE ENDOTHELIUM-MEDIATED VASODILATION, POSTOCCLUSION VASODILATION, AND HYPEREMIA
Acetylcholine
Serotonin
Bradykinin
Thrombin
Substance P

MEASUREMENT OF ENDOTHELIAL FUNCTION
Quantitative coronary angiography or brachial artery ultrasound in response to agonist infusion

CONDITIONS OR SUBSTANCES ASSOCIATED WITH ENDOTHELIAL DYSFUNCTION
Atherosclerosis
Increased age
Hypercholesterolemia (especially high oxidized LDL)
Hypertension
Cigarette smoking
Diabetes mellitus (especially sustained hyperglycemia)
High-fat diet
Physical inactivity
Family history of CAD

CONSEQUENCES OF ENDOTHELIAL DYSFUNCTION
Peripheral vasoconstriction and reduction of angina threshold
Atherogenesis
Instability of plaque surface

INTERVENTIONS TO IMPROVE ENDOTHELIAL FUNCTION
Lipid-lowering agents
Antioxidants
Smoking cessation
Estrogen replacement
Exercise
Blood pressure reduction
(The response to these interventions is rapid.)

of diseased coronary branches but not of normal coronary branches in the same patient. Normal vessels with normal endothelial function are able to counter the vasoconstrictor effect by autoregulating. The diseased vessel with endothelial dysfunction has lost all or part of its ability to autoregulate (to respond to adenosine infusion or to release NO).

A second possibility with chronic ischemia is that the vascular bed is making use of all its vasodilator reserve. Because of ischemia, adenosine and NO levels may be as high as they can get (since ischemia provokes the release of both). There is nothing left in the system to counter an additional vasoconstricting influence.

This may explain some of the common provocations of angina: walking into a cold wind (the cold pressor response, an alpha stimulator),and isometric exercise, anger, or stress (all alpha-adrenergic stimulators). Spontaneous variation in baseline alpha-adrenergic tone in the face of reduced or absent vasodilator reserve may explain variation in the anginal threshold: bad versus good days and the warm-up phenomenon.

Remission of Angina

The Framingham study found that 32% of men and 50% of women with stable angina had eventual resolution of symptoms. Some of these patients may not have had true angina; not every patient had documentation of ischemia or CAD. Nevertheless, remission of angina is a well-recognized clinical outcome. There are three ways this can happen.

1. *Regression of plaque.* This has been described for about one third of patients treated with aggressive cholesterol-lowering therapies (see Chapter 12). Regression is a combination of debulking the plaque plus remodeling of the artery at the site of plaque so that luminal size is increased. In serial angiographic studies, most patients who had no regression of plaque at least had stabilization of lesions with no progression of stenosis over 3 to 5 years (the usual follow-up interval). This has translated to lower rates of myocardial infarction. The data are promising enough that there have been calls for randomized studies comparing surgery with medical therapy that includes aggressive LDL cholesterol lowering.[5]

2. *Myocardial infarction.* Angina originates from live muscle, not scar. Occlusion of a stenosed artery that causes angina and infarction of that myocardial region often "cure" the angina by eradicating live muscle. Of course, these processes occur at the expense of left ventricular function—not a good thing. Improvement or resolution of angina is a reason for repeating the ECG, looking for new Q waves.

3. *Collateral circulation.* Symptoms may improve or resolve with the development of collateral circula-

tion. The collateral vessels between the large coronary arteries are preformed and do not represent the growth of new vessels. When antegrade flow in one of the coronary arteries is interrupted, there is retrograde flow to the blocked artery through the collateral branches (Fig. 13-4). The size and quality of collaterals are probably genetically determined. Some animal species have such large collateral vessels that it is impossible to induce myocardial infarction by tying off a coronary artery. It is common to find an occluded coronary artery in a person who has never had angina or myocardial infarction. Some people are born with better collateral vessels.

Prolonged ischemia—a long history of angina—appears to promote the development of coronary collateral vessels. At one time, exercise training was thought to increase coronary collateral flow, but serial angiographic studies have not supported this notion. There also was hope that more potent vasodilators would work on collateral beds. Intravenous nitrate therapy does increase collateral flow, while the effects of oral or cutaneous dosing are less impressive. Unfortunately, calcium blockers have no direct effect on collateral function, nor do beta-blockers. Two endogenous substances released by endothelial cells provoke collateral vasodilation: NO and prostacyclin. Inhibiting prostaglandin synthesis with indomethacin or aspirin reduces collateral flow. Patients with endothelial dysfunction have been found to have reduced collateral flow. The final pathway to collateral vessel growth (as opposed to dilation) may be vascular endothelial growth factor (VEGF), an endothelial, cell-specific mitogen. In animal studies, ischemia promotes the release of VEGF by endothelial cells. One of the earliest studies of gene therapy will soon test whether local delivery of the gene encoding for VGEF promotes angio-

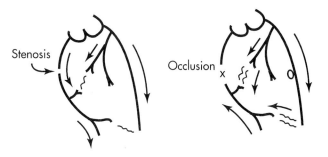

FIG. 13-4
Collateral channels, which are probably present from birth, are small vessels that connect the watershed areas that lie between large vessels. When a large vessel occludes *(right panel)*, there is retrograde filling of the blocked artery through the collateral vessels. With heavy use over time (e.g., chronic ischemia), the collateral vessels enlarge.

genesis, improving collateral flow in patients with lower limb ischemia. If effective, such a pharmacologic approach to revascularization could be revolutionary as well as novel.

Clinical Presentation of Stable Angina

By definition, chronic stable angina is just that; symptoms have not changed over the course of 2 to 3 months. Although most patients with new chest discomfort have it evaluated promptly, some individuals fail to recognize the symptom as serious. How often have you had this conversation:

"Anything else going on?"
"No, just that tight feeling that started last spring."

The symptoms and differential diagnosis of chest discomfort are reviewed in Chapter 3 as well as Table 13-1. After making the clinical diagnosis of angina, the most important thing is to distinguish between stable and unstable angina (see later discussion).

Laboratory Studies

Exercise testing (with and without imaging studies) and cardiac catheterization were described earlier, as well as in Chapters 6 and 8 through 10. The main reason for exercise testing in patients with chronic stable angina is confirmation of the diagnosis. Recall that it is possible for those with a typical history of cardiac discomfort to have noncardiac disease (or no disease). I am never surprised when I am fooled by the history, and I am reluctant to saddle a person with a diagnosis of heart disease without proof. One exception to this is the occasional elderly patient who does not want any laboratory evaluation and who prefers empiric therapy. Even in such cases there often comes a time when I wish I was certain of the diagnosis (e.g., when initial therapy causes side effects).

Making the Diagnosis of CAD

A positive stress ECG supports, but does not make, the diagnosis of CAD with certainty. False-positive studies are too common. This does not mean that the workup must go beyond stress testing. Some patients may reasonably be treated without a definite diagnosis. For example, an elderly patient with a stress test result suggesting low risk (see later discussion) may elect a trial of medical therapy without further study.

The addition of imaging studies—a perfusion scan, radionuclide angiography, or an echocardiogram—increases the sensitivity and specificity of the stress test. False positives are relatively uncommon with each of these techniques (see Chapters 6, 8, and 9). Again, a patient with a study result indicating low risk for future cardiac events may elect a trial of medical therapy.

Coronary angiography remains the gold standard for the diagnosis of coronary atherosclerosis (see Chapter 10). Although angiography has limitations, it is quite reliable for patients with exercise angina. A negative coronary angiogram identifies a good prognosis.

Risk Stratification

A second and equally important role of the laboratory examination is risk stratification. The goal is identification of the patient at risk for a serious "cardiac event," either myocardial infarction or cardiac death, who would benefit from revascularization. It is equally important to recognize the low-risk patient for whom invasive, potentially dangerous, and expensive diagnostic and therapeutic procedures are unnecessary.

Anatomy-Based Strategies. Before the 1980s the risk of CAD was best understood in relation to coronary anatomy (Box 13-2). Stenosis of the left main coronary artery (>70% of luminal diameter) indicates at least a 50% mortality risk during the next year (see Chapter 2). Using medical therapy circa 1980, 1-year mortality was almost 12% with three-vessel CAD compared with 4% for single-vessel disease (it may be lower using current medical therapies). In addition, left ventricular (LV) dysfunction increases the chance of death. Based on such information, angiography could be justified to "rule out left main or three-vessel CAD." This rationale is still invoked by doctors who recommend angiography for patients with stable angina who, by other criteria, are at low risk for myocardial infarction or death. None of the noninvasive studies is able to identify left main or three-vessel coronary disease with certainty.

Risk-Based Strategies. The development of sensitive and specific noninvasive techniques has allowed a shifting away from an anatomy-based strategy. With perfusion imaging particularly, some criteria allow the identification of high-risk patients (Box 13-2). Multiple studies have shown that patients with normal scans have less than a 1% chance of having myocardial infarction or cardiac death[7] (Fig. 13-5). A trial of medical therapy is appropriate, and angiography would be necessary only if symptoms cannot be controlled.

On the other hand, patients with chronic stable angina who have positive exercise studies should have angiography, especially when the scan or exercise ECG meets high-risk criteria.

A Cost-Effective Approach to Evaluation of Chronic Stable Angina. The range of costs of diagnostic procedures influences the workup of chronic coronary syndromes and CPUE. No practice guidelines have been established for chronic stable angina, and I am describing a commonly used approach that I favor. The stress ECG alone is adequate for the initial evaluation of most patients with chest discomfort of uncertain etiology. A negative study with good exercise tolerance (more than 7

BOX 13-2
MARKERS OF POOR PROGNOSIS FOR PATIENTS WITH CORONARY ARTERY DISEASE*

CLINICAL PREDICTORS
Congestive heart failure (or documented left ventricular dysfunction)
Prior MI (indicates increased risk of death with subsequent MI)
Complex ventricular arrhythmia
Diabetes (possibly)
Left ventricular hypertrophy (possibly)

RESTING ECG
New T wave inversion
Diffuse ST segment depression during chest discomfort
ST segment elevation during chest discomfort
New bundle branch block

STRESS ECG
≥2.0 mm ST segment depression
ST depression in exercise stage I
ST depression in multiple leads
ST depression persisting for more than 5 minutes during recovery
Low workload (<4 METS or <6 minutes using the Bruce protocol)
Symptoms developing at heart rate <120 (off beta-blockers)
Angina during exercise
A drop in blood pressure >10 mm Hg with exercise (may indicate left main coronary disease)
Ventricular tachycardia

PERFUSION IMAGING USING THALLIUM 201 OR SESTAMIBI
Perfusion defects in multiple vascular regions (indicating multivessel coronary disease—combined anterior and lateral defects could mean left main coronary disease)
Increased lung thallium 201 uptake (indicating exercise-induced left ventricular dysfunction)
Post-exercise left ventricular cavity dilation

LEFT VENTRICULAR FUNCTION IMAGING WITH STRESS (RADIONUCLIDE ANGIOGRAPHY OR ECHOCARDIOGRAPHY)
Poor left ventricular function at rest
Fall in left ventricular ejection fraction with exercise (≥10 percentage points)
Left ventricular dilation with exercise
Wall motion abnormalities involving multiple vascular distributions

CORONARY AND LEFT VENTRICULAR ANGIOGRAPHY
Left main coronary artery stenosis†—always an indication for revascularization
Three-vessel coronary artery disease—usually an indication for revascularization
Proximal left anterior descending coronary stenosis—when present, upgrades the level of risk (e.g., moves two-vessel disease into a high-risk category)
Ragged plaque surface and associated thrombus (probable)
Depressed left ventricular function—when present, increases the urgency for revascularization for those with active ischemia; a graded effect: the worse the LV, the greater the need for revascularization

*Indicating an increased risk for death or myocardial infarction.
†"Stenosis" and "disease" indicate ≥70% reduction of luminal diameter.

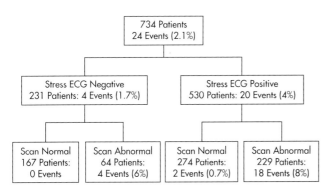

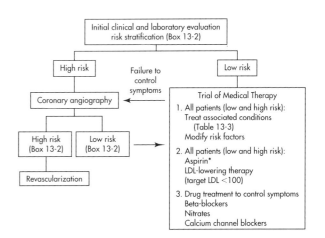

FIG. 13-5

A representative study of the efficiency of the stress ECG and the exercise perfusion scan (in this case using sestamibi) for identifying the risk of future ischemic events, either myocardial infarction or cardiac death. With a negative stress ECG the risk of events is 2%. A negative scan indicates that risk is well below 1%.

Data from Berman DS, Hachamovitch R, Kiat H et al: *J Am Coll Cardiol* 26:639, 1995.

FIG. 13-6
Management of chronic stable angina pectoris.
*Clopidogrel may be given if aspirin cannot.

minutes using the Bruce protocol) excludes flow-restricting disease and identifies a good prognosis. A patient with typical angina and a strongly positive test—both angina and ST segment depression—at low workloads may have cardiac catheterization as the next step. Repeating the stress study with imaging is expensive and unnecessary, unless you think that you are dealing with a false positive stress ECG. A *stress ECG with an equivocal result* may be cleared up with an exercise imaging study. Patients with an *anticipated false positive stress ECG* may have stress imaging studies as the initial test. If the exercise study or exercise imaging study indicates high risk (Box 13-2), angiography is indicated.

Management of Chronic Stable Angina
Medical Therapy

Medical treatment of chronic stable angina lacks evidence-based medical studies. Although many randomized trials of therapy for acute coronary syndromes, myocardial infarction, and unstable angina have been conducted, few have compared different drug therapies for stable angina. (Exceptions include aspirin and drug therapy to lower LDL cholesterol levels.) Recall that the case fatality rate for CAD has fallen steadily, which has been attributed to effective medical and revascularization therapy.[3] Figure 13-6 provides an outline of the treatment strategy.

Treatment of Associated Conditions. These are common illnesses that affect the balance between MVO_2 and oxygen supply (Table 13-3). Consider them when symptoms change.

Risk Factor Modification. The secondary prevention of CAD—that is, the aggressive treatment of risk factors for those who have established CAD—probably has as much to do with improved survival as other available therapies.[3] One obvious reason for this is the favorable

effect on atherogenesis. Another and more immediate benefit relates to the effect of risk factors on endothelial function and coronary blood flow (Table 13-4).

For example, reducing LDL cholesterol level reduces mortality from CAD as early as 6 weeks after treatment begins. This is too soon if inhibition of plaque formation is the only beneficial effect. In addition, serial angiographic studies have shown that, although lipid-lowering therapy stabilizes plaque and in a minority induces minimal regression of plaque, the overall effect on plaque morphology is modest. In contrast, the reduction in coronary events is much more striking.[8] These observations indicate that elevated LDL cholesterol has a direct deleterious effect on the artery apart from atherogenesis. Now we understand that oxidized LDL cholesterol causes endothelial dysfunction and that LDL-lowering therapy improves endothelium-mediated coronary vasodilation.

The response of endothelial function to risk factor modification is prompt. A patient with angina may be modifying lifestyle and risk factors for the relief of symptoms in addition to stopping the progression of disease (see Chapter 11). This is in sharp contrast to what I told patients 10 years ago. At that time, I advised them to change risk factors for the long-term future (progression of disease), but that for short-term benefit the answer is drug therapy. We may be more successful convincing patients to make uncomfortable changes if we emphasize short-term, symptomatic benefits.

Drug Therapy

LDL-Lowering Drugs. The effect of lowering LDL cholesterol levels on endothelial function has been discussed. Multiple trials have shown that pushing LDL levels below 100 mg/dL halts the progression of atherosclerosis for most patients and leads to regression of plaque for some. These serial angiographic studies performed the second, follow-up angiogram 3 or 5 years

Table 13-3	Conditions That May Aggravate Angina

Condition	Mechanism
INCREASED MVO$_2$ (OXYGEN DEMAND)	
Anemia	Peripheral hypoxia creates a need for increased cardiac output, so there is higher MVO$_2$. There is a decrease in oxygen delivery to the myocardium as well because of reduced oxygen content of arterial blood.
Thyrotoxicosis	Increased heart rate and contractility
Fever and infection	Increased heart rate
Marked weight gain	Increased cardiac output needed to maintain normal cardiac index
Sympathomimetic drugs, including amphetamines (diet pills)	Increased heart rate, possibly increased blood pressure
Hypertension	MVO$_2$ is proportional to heart rate and systolic blood pressure.
Congestive heart failure	Cardiac dilation causes increased wall tension (the Laplace relationship), and tension is proportional to MVO$_2$. Plus, there is an increase in heart rate.
Tachyarrhythmias	High heart rates; the patient may not sense palpitations.
REDUCED OXYGEN SUPPLY	
Anemia	Low hemoglobin means reduced oxygen-carrying capacity.
Smoking and air pollution (carbon monoxide)	Carbon monoxide is a component of cigarette smoke, and methemoglobin levels are higher. Note that air pollution with high carbon monoxide levels may lower the angina threshold.
Drugs that provoke coronary spasm	Cocaine and (in a rare patient), beta-blockers; consider spasm if angina worsens after starting beta-blocker therapy.
High altitude	Decreased arterial oxygen content

after the first one. The effect of longer term treatment is uncertain, but it is possible that aggressive LDL reduction may be even more beneficial over 10 to 20 years. Drug therapy is discussed in Chapter 12. In general, treatment may be initiated with a statin, niacin, or resin if LDL exceeds 130 mg/dL. When it is between 100 and 130 mg/dL, a 6-week trial of diet therapy and weight loss is reasonable before committing the patient to long-term drug treatment. (This conservative recommendation has been challenged by recent trials showing benefits with statin therapy for those with mild elevation of LDL cholesterol level and definite CAD; see Chapter 12.)

Aspirin, Other Antiplatelet Agents, and Anticoagulation. Blocking platelet aggregation makes sense for all patients with CAD. Platelet aggregation increases the risk for myocardial infarction, and it has a role in the progression of atherosclerosis (see Chapter 11). This is one of the few areas of treatment of chronic stable angina for which there is evidence-based medicine; small randomized trials of aspirin therapy for stable angina have shown a reduction in the incidence of myocardial infarction, and a meta-analysis confirms prevention of cardiac death and stroke as well.[9]

Most studies indicate that 325 mg of aspirin per day is an adequate dose, and for some indications 75 mg per day is effective. Adult patients find that taking a single adult-sized tablet (325 mg) is convenient. If a patient has gastrointestinal problems with aspirin, a baby aspirin (81 mg) may be taken once daily with food. Although a lower dose therapy has theoretical advantages, no clinical trials have proved its efficacy.

Table 13-4	*Short-Term Benefits of Risk Factor Modification*
Dyslipidemia	Reducing LDL, especially oxidized LDL, stabilizes the endothelial surface; there is less chance of plaque ulceration, thrombus, and occlusion. Lower LDL improves endothelial function.
Low fat diet	Improves endothelial function
Hypertension	Lowering afterload reduces oxygen demand. Control also improves endothelial function. Lowering diastolic left ventricular wall tension improves flow in coronary arteries (which takes place during diastole).
Diabetes	Glucose control favorably improves endothelial function.
Cigarette smoking	Stopping improves endothelial function, and it reduces methemoglobin (improving oxygen capacity of arterial blood; see Box 13-2).
Exercise therapy	Improves endothelial function
Estrogen replacement	Improves endothelial function

The more expensive antiplatelet agents, dipyridamole or sulfinpyrazone, are no more effective than aspirin, nor does combining them with aspirin increase efficacy. In fact, there have been fewer studies of their use with CAD, and they may not work as well as aspirin. Ticlopidine, although an effective antiplatelet agent, has not been studied as treatment for chronic CAD.

Anticoagulation using warfarin (Coumadin) has some benefits after myocardial infarction, but no studies support its use for chronic stable angina.

Nitrates. Nitroglycerin relaxes vascular smooth muscle, even in the presence of endothelial dysfunction. In essence, nitrates provide the transmitter for endothelial-mediated vasodilation. EDRF is the NO radical (see Box 13-1). At the cellular level, medicinal nitrates are converted to NO or S-nitrosothiols, which, like EDRF, activate guanylate cyclase to produce cyclic guanine monophosphate (GMP). This triggers smooth muscle relaxation.

The dominant effect is venous, but nitrates work on systemic and coronary arteries as well. Dilation of veins, the "capacitance vessels," results in venous pooling and reduced blood return to the heart. With lower preload, the heart becomes smaller, and ventricular wall tension is decreased. Myocardial oxygen demand falls and angina is relieved (see Fig. 13-1). As venodilation plays a major role in their action, nitrates work better with the patient in an upright position and are less effective with recumbency. Suggest that your patient sit, and not lie down, after taking nitroglycerin.

Nitrates also work on the coronary arterial circulation, improving coronary blood supply. This appears less important than venodilation for those with effort angina. Nitrates can dilate the artery at the site of the plaque (Fig. 13-2). They also can promote peripheral coronary dilation in patients with endothelial dysfunction (Fig. 13-3).

Various preparations are reviewed in Table 13-5. Short-acting sublingual nitroglycerin is still the drug of choice for relief of an anginal episode. The duration of a sublingual dose is as long as 20 to 30 minutes. For this reason, it may be used prophylactically, 5 to 10 minutes before activities known to provoke angina. The major benefit of the newer nitroglycerin spray is maintenance of potency over time. The tablets lose potency within weeks of exposure to room air and must be kept in their dark glass, airtight container. Loss of potency is more rapid if they are carried about in a metal or plastic pill case. Most patients develop a preference for either the spray or the pills.

Nitrate tolerance is a major issue with long-acting treatment. It develops quickly, as early as 24 hours at a stable nitroglycerin blood level.[10] The mechanism is uncertain. A possible explanation is the accumulation of oxygen free radicals that degrade NO before it can work. Co-administration of an antioxidant (hydralazine) with nitroglycerin has prevented the development of tolerance.[10] Tolerance is avoided with a 10- to 12-hour nitrate-free interval each day, and responsiveness is quickly restored by a 1-day nitrate holiday.

Tolerance may develop with all long-acting nitrates. Instruct your patients to remove the nitroglycerin patch in the early evening and to put on a fresh patch in the morning. Adjust the dosing schedules of oral nitrates.

Table 13-5	*Nitroglycerine Preparations*

Preparation	Dose (Duration of Action)	Cost*	Comment
Sublingual nitro-glycerin	0.4 mg sublingual, prn (15-20 min)	100 0.4 mg tablets: $6 spray: $25 per can	Aerosol spray or tablet; use prophy-lactically 5-10 min before angina-provoking activity
Ointment	0.5-2 inches, bid (3-6 hr)	60 g tube: $16	Eccentric dosing is needed to avoid tolerance.
Transdermal patch	0.4-1.2 mg/hr for 12 hours, then remove (24 hr)	$32-$63	Must remove the patch at night to avoid tolerance (but patients fre-quently forget).
Sustained-release nitroglycerine	9.0-13.5 mg bid (12 hr)		Eccentric dosing needed
Isosorbide dinitrate	10-60 mg bid or tid (4 hr)	$2-$30	Eccentric dosing needed
Isosorbide dinitrate, sustained release	80-120 mg once daily (12 hr)	$6-$12 (a wide range in price)	Tolerance avoided with once-daily dosing or with twice-daily dosing with a 16-18 hr tablet-free interval.
Isosorbide mononi-trate, sustained re-lease	60-240 mg once daily (12 hr)	$30-$90	Tolerance avoided with once-daily dosing.

*Retail cost per month of the lowest-highest maintenance doses (adapted from Section III). The much lower price of older agents such as isosorbide dinitrate reflects the availability of generic preparations.

Isosorbide dinitrate is active for 4 hours; eccentric dos-ing at 7 AM and 2 PM provides an adequate nitrate-free interval. An additional dose may be given at 5 PM, but no later. A late evening dose does not allow the blood nitrate level to fall for the 10 to 12 hours needed to avoid tolerance. Although eccentric dosing works with drugs with intermediate durations of action, how many of your patients will remember to take a pill in the mid-afternoon?

Treatment with longer acting isosorbide mononitrate is somewhat better. With the standard formulation, a 20 or 30 mg dose can be given at 8 AM and 3 PM. Exercise tolerance is improved for up to 5 hours after the second dose. Many patients find a twice-daily oral preparation more convenient than the nitroglycerin patch because they must remember to remove the patch in the evening.

Even more convenient is the sustained-release form of isosorbide mononitrate. The dose may range from 30 to 240 mg/day, and it is given once daily. The duration of action is 12 hours. Clinical trials have shown that the antianginal efficacy of large doses (120 to 240 mg) lasts for 12 hours.[10] No clinical trials have demonstrated the

efficacy of the sustained-release preparations of nitro-glycerine or isosorbide dinitrate.[10]

An obvious problem with interrupting nitrates each day is the possibility of angina during the nitrate-free interval. Nocturnal "patch-off" angina may occur in those with severe angina, and such patients should not be treated with nitrates alone. An evening dose of either a beta-blocker or a calcium channel blocker is one ap-proach. If most of the angina is nocturnal, a nitrate-free interval may be added during the day.

Long-acting nitrate therapy is suitable as monother-apy for less severe, chronic stable angina. Table 13-6 re-views associated conditions that may influence the ini-tial choice of therapy. As preload-lowering agents, nitrates may be especially useful for patients who also have heart failure.

Beta-Adrenergic Blockers. There are two classes of beta-adrenergic receptors (see Chapter 2). The beta$_1$ re-ceptor is cardiac, and the beta$_2$, peripheral. Beta$_2$ stimula-tion causes bronchodilation and peripheral vasodilation.

Beta$_1$ blockade treats angina by lowering heart rate and contractility and, thus, MVO_2 (see Fig. 13-1). It has no beneficial effect on coronary blood flow. Beta block-

Table 13-6	Associated Conditions That Influence the Choice of Treatment for Angina Pectoris

Condition	Comment
Coronary spasm (Prinzmetal's angina)	*Good:* calcium blockers and nitrates *Warning:* beta-blockers may aggravate spasm.
Left ventricular (LV) dysfunction	*Good:* nitrates reduce preload; calcium blockers (pure vasodilators) reduce afterload; possibly improved survival with low-dose beta-blockers. *Warning:* beta-blockers, verapamil, and diltiazem depress contractility.
Complex ventricular arrhythmias	*Good:* beta-blockers lower the risk of sudden cardiac death. *Warning:* complex ventricular arrhythmias often accompany poor LV function; beta-blockers may further depress contractility.
Atrial tachyarrhythmias (including sinus tachycardia)	*Good:* beta-blockers, verapamil, and diltiazem reduce heart rate. *Warning:* pure vasodilators (short-acting nifedipine) may aggravate sinus tachycardia.
Bradycardia, bradyarrhythmias	*Warning:* beta-blockers, verapamil, and diltiazem may aggravate bradycardia and atrioventricular nodal block.
Peripheral vascular disease	*Warning:* beta blockers may provoke peripheral vasospasm.
Bronchospasm	*Warning:* beta-blockers aggravate bronchospasm (even cardioselective agents given at higher doses).
Left ventricular hypertrophy	*Good:* beta-blockers and calcium blockers induce regression of hypertrophy.
Myocardial infarction (MI)	*Good:* beta-blockers improve long-term survival after MI.
Hypertension	*Good:* beta-blockers and calcium blockers are effective antihypertensive agents.
Depression	*Warning:* possibly aggravated by beta-blockers
Sexual dysfunction	*Warning:* beta-blockers may aggravate or precipitate impotence.
Dyslipidemia	*Warning:* increased LDL and lower HDL cholesterol with nonselective beta blockade
Insulin dependent diabetes mellitus	*Warning:* beta blockade may mask the symptoms of hypoglycemia.

ade also reduces mortality and reinfarction when used long-term after myocardial infarction, suppresses ventricular arrhythmias, effectively lowers blood pressure, promotes regression of LV hypertrophy, and, for carefully selected patients, may reduce mortality from heart failure.

There is no evidence-based medicine (randomized trial) showing that any of the medical therapies that prevent or control the symptoms of *chronic stable angina* either lowers mortality or prevents heart attack—it is an issue that has not been studied. But many clinicians, myself included, extrapolate survival data from the conditions described previously to the treatment of effort angina. Beta blockers *may* improve survival, and my preference is to prescribe them when they are tolerable. (There is nothing to lose, possibly something to gain.)

A number of beta-blockers are available (Table 13-7). At equivalent doses, all block the effects of isoproterenol (a cardioselective beta₁ agonist). The unique properties of some of these may influence the choice of agent for patients with other medical problems (Table 13-8). Bronchospasm, diabetes, peripheral vascular disease, and dyslipidemia would direct us to use a beta₁ se-

Table 13-7	Beta-Adrenergic Blockers					
Drug	**Maintenance Dose**	**Cost**	**ISA**	**Beta₁ Selectivity**	**Indications and Uses**	**Comment**
Metoprolol	50-100 mg bid-tid (SR available)	$12-$32*	0	+	HBP, MI, AP	Generic available, a workhorse
Atenolol	50-100 mg qd or divided doses	$4-$6*	0	+	HBP, MI, AP	As above; drug accumulates in renal disease (renal excretion)
Nadolol	40-80 mg qd	$26-$40	0	0	HBP, AP	Accumulates in renal disease; long half-life due to water solubility
Propranolol	60 mg qid (SR available)	$3*	0	0	HBP, MI, AP	Also a membrane stabilizer (a quinidine-like action)
Timolol	20 mg bid	$40	0	0	HBP, MI	Water soluble
Pindolol	5-20 mg bid	$25-$70	0	0	HBP, MI	Membrane stabilizer (not as strong as propranolol)
Acebutolol	200-600 mg bid	$29-$56	+	0	HBP	Accumulates in renal disease
Labetalol	100-600 mg/day	$14-$53	+	+	HBP	
Bisoprolol	5-20 qd	$25-$50	0	0	HBP	Renal accumulation
Betaxolol	5-20 qd	$12-$34	0	+	HBP	Renal accumulation
Penbutolol	20 qd	$32	0	+	HBP	Renal accumulation
Carteolol	2.5-10 mg qd	$31-$61	+	0	HBP	Renal accumulation
Carvedilol	6.25-25 mg bid		+	0	HBP, CHF	Improved survival, exercise tolerance, and left ventricular function in congestive heart failure.
Sotalol	80-240 mg bid	$107-$230	0	0	Ventricular arrhythmias	In addition to beta blockade, it has an amiodarone-like action.

*Retail cost per month of the lowest-highest maintenance doses (adapted from Section III). The remarkably low cost of the older agents reflects availability of generic preparations. *ISA,* Intrinsic sympathetic activity; *HBP,* high blood pressure, *MI,* postmyocardial infarction; *AP,* angina pectoris; *SR,* sustained-release preparation.

lective agent. Neurologic side effects during beta blockade may improve with the use of a water-soluble drug that does not cross the blood-brain barrier. Hypertension may improve with the use of a drug with combined alpha- and beta-adrenergic blocking activity. Resting bradycardia is not aggravated by drugs with intrinsic sympathomimetic activity; during exercise, when sympathetic activity is high, they work like other beta-blockers, limiting the increase in heart rate.

Note that special properties of these agents, such as beta1 selectivity, are lost at high doses. At high doses, they all work like propranolol. The choice of an agent for a par-

ticular patient is based on special properties of the drugs, cost, and the doctor's familiarity with the agent and its side effects. Those approved by the Food and Drug Administration (FDA) for the treatment of angina are atenolol, metoprolol, nadolol, and propranolol (drug companies have initially sought approval for the treatment of hypertension).

Adverse effects are reviewed in Section III, where each drug is described in detail. Some of them are subtle and may not be recognized by the patient as side effects.

1. Neuropsychiatric: depression, nightmares, mood changes

Table 13-8	Beta-Adrenergic Blockers with Special Properties	

Property	Potential Benefit	Drugs
Cardioselective, beta$_1$ blockade	Less bronchospasm (beta$_2$ blockade); less peripheral vasoconstriction, less effect on lipids	Atenolol (Tenormin), metoprolol (Lopressor), acebutolol (Sectral), bisoprolol (Zebeta), betaxolol (Kerlone)
Water soluble	Longer half-life; do not cross the blood-brain barrier; possibly fewer neurologic side effects	Atenolol, nadolol (Corgard), labetalol (Normodyne), acebutolol, carteolol (Cartrol)
Intrinsic sympathetic activity	Less depression of heart rate at rest (at levels of higher sympathetic activity, exercise, they behave like other beta blockers)	Pindolol (Visken), acebutolol, carteolol, penbutolol (Levatol)
Alpha-adrenergic blocker	Increased antihypertensive effect	Labetalol
Class III antiarrhythmic (an amiodarone-like action)	Antiarrhythmic action	Sotalol (Betapace)
Nonselective beta-blockers	Therapy for essential tremor	Propranolol

2. Sexual dysfunction in men
3. Bronchospasm: beta-blockers are contraindicated in those with asthma and obstructive lung disease with associated bronchospasm; use even beta$_1$ selective agents with caution in this setting. If there is a definite history of asthma or wheezing on examination, I do not prescribe them. With an equivocal history or with mild obstructive lung disease without wheezing, a beta$_1$ selective agent may be prescribed at low dose (and with careful monitoring and follow-up).
4. Diabetes: poorly controlled insulin-dependent diabetes plus a history of hypoglycemic attacks are contraindications to beta blockade because it inhibits the sympathetic-mediated symptoms of hypoglycemia (shakiness and diaphoresis). In the absence of this history, patients with well-controlled diabetes who are taking insulin may use a beta-blocker but require careful monitoring and education.
5. Peripheral vasoconstriction: the beta$_2$ receptor has a vasodilating effect in the peripheral circulation. Blocking it leaves alpha-mediated vasoconstriction unopposed. For this reason, beta-blocker therapy may aggravate Raynaud's phenomenon or symptoms of peripheral vascular disease. Some patients describe cold hands.
6. AV nodal blockade: if it is symptomatic, beta-blockers should not be used unless the patient has a pacemaker. You may try beta-blockers in a patient with first-degree AV block, but careful follow-up is required.

Beta-blockers work by slowing the resting heart and blunting the heart rate response to exercise. Monitoring heart rate is a good way to monitor therapy (blood levels are not available), and a sinus rate between 55 and 65 beats/min is a reasonable therapeutic range. The rate may drop to 40 to 50 beats/min during sleep. *That poses no danger and is not an indication to stop beta blockade.*

Caution is needed when stopping beta-blockers after long-term therapy. Years ago there was concern about a rebound, hyper-beta effect with precipitation of myocardial infarction when therapy is interrupted (as may occur during an elective operation). Although rebound has not been confirmed, a small but definite risk exists if beta-blockers are discontinued in a patient with chronic stable angina, since MVO$_2$ rises with increased adrenergic tone. Progression of disease may have been masked by long-term beta blockade, and increased angina or even infarction is possible when it is withdrawn. For this reason, it is safest to withdraw therapy gradually. If that is not possible, add another agent (nitrate or calcium blocker) and carefully instruct your patient about a possible change in symptoms.

For patients with angina who are undergoing surgery and cannot take oral medicines, intravenous metoprolol can be substituted during postoperative recovery. Another approach consists of therapy with cutaneous nitrates. An argument could be made that a patient who has only *effort* angina does not need to continue antianginal treatment while at bed rest after surgery. In such cases, you still must be aware of the potential for unmasking ischemia when antianginal therapy is withdrawn.

Calcium Channel Blockers. When a nerve stimulates smooth or cardiac muscle, calcium ions enter the muscle cell and serve as the switch-on signal for the contractile proteins. Calcium antagonists block the slow-conducting calcium ion channels in the cell membrane. Arterial smooth muscle relaxation and vasodilation in the peripheral circulation reduce afterload, lowering the cardiac workload and MVO_2. In addition, calcium blockers increase blood and oxygen supply in two ways. The first is the prevention of vasospasm at the site of coronary stenosis (Fig. 13-2). The second is peripheral coronary vasodilation (Fig. 13-3 and Box 13-1). *Variable threshold angina* is best explained by a fluctuation in peripheral coronary resistance and endothelial dysfunction, and calcium blocker therapy is effective.

Drugs that work only to reduce myocardial oxygen demand do not change the anginal threshold. That is, the HR-BP product that results in angina does not change even though the length of time walking on the treadmill to reach that HR-BP product is greater. Calcium blockers raise the HR-BP product required to cause angina, indicating an increase in oxygen supply (see Fig. 13-1).

There are three classes of calcium channel blockers, and they have substantially different effects on myocardial contractility, atrioventricular (AV) node conduction, and heart rate (Table 13-9). These differences dictate the choice of drug for many patients. For example, symptomatic bradycardia or conduction disease would obviate the use of verapamil or diltiazem. However, a high resting heart rate and good LV function would make these good choices because lowering heart rate is one of the goals of treating angina. Another example: drugs that depress contractility may aggravate congestive heart failure (CHF). The PRAISE trial has shown that, when combined with other CHF therapy, the vascular selective agent amlodipine had no adverse effect on patients with class III-IV heart failure and a mean left ventricular ejection fraction of 21%. [11]

The calcium blocker scare of the mid-1990s is worth mentioning. Retrospectives studies of short-acting nifedipine found an increased risk of myocardial infarction, death, or cancer. Closer analysis uncovered serious problems with each of these studies, and examination of larger groups disclosed no special risk. [12] Although the studies were flawed, there is concern about short-acting nifedipine. As a pure vasodilator with a rapid onset of action, it may cause blood pressure to drop, followed by reflex tachycardia. [12] Apparently this is not a problem with sustained-release preparations of nifedipine or with longer acting calcium blockers. There is no benefit in using short-acting nifedipine as long-term therapy.

Giving nifedipine sublingually for the abrupt reduction of blood pressure is not an FDA-approved indication, and this practice also carries substantial risk. [13] Absorption of nifedipine through the buccal mucosa is erratic, with unpredictable effects on blood pressure. This practice should be abandoned.

If symptoms are not being controlled by one drug, calcium blockers work well in combination with either nitrates or beta-blockers. Beta blockade blunts the reflex tachycardia caused by dihydropyridines but may aggravate the bradycardia associated with verapamil or diltiazem use. Patients with heart failure may benefit from the combined effects of nitrates (preload reduction) and dihydropyridines (afterload reduction). [11] However, remember that the goal of medical therapy for chronic stable angina is symptom relief. No study has shown a survival benefit with a particular drug or drug combination. For purposes of convenience and expense, it is best to use one drug as long as symptoms are controlled. In fact, when monotherapy is not working well, it also is reasonable to switch to another drug class rather than committing the patient to a two-drug regimen.

Revascularization

Indications. There are three reasons for considering coronary angiography and revascularization therapy for chronic stable angina:

1. High risk for myocardial infarction or cardiac death based on initial clinical and laboratory evaluation (see Box 13-2)
2. Failure of medical therapy to adequately control symptoms
3. Worsening symptoms, with more frequent episodes, angina at lower workloads, or longer spells of pain (in essence, a patient moving toward the unstable angina category)

The high-risk patient has been described (see Box 13-2). Coronary angiography showing left main or multivessel CAD (particularly when it involves the proximal left anterior coronary artery) are indications for revascularization, with solid evidence-based support. [14] Smaller studies have shown that percutaneous transluminal coronary angioplasty (PTCA), particularly with stenting, is better than medical therapy for the control of symptoms, and PTCA also may confer a survival advantage when there is multivessel CAD. [15]

Inadequate symptom control is subjective and is based largely on the patient's expectation. I have rec-

| Table13-9 | Calcium Channel Blockers |

Drug	Maintenance Dose	Cost*	Noteworthy Properties
Class: Phenylalkylamine (L-type channel blockade): Inhibits conduction in the AV node and slows the sinuatrial rate; depresses myocardial contractility.			
Verapamil (Calan, Isoptin)	180-480 mg/day	$34-$68 (for SR)	Contraindicated in symptomatic heart block, bradycardia. (Do not use with a beta-blockers.) May precipitate clinical heart failure.
Class: Benzothiazepine (L-type channel blockade): Actions are intermediate between those of phenylalkylamine and dihydropyridines. There is some depression of SA and AV nodes and contractility, but not as much.			
Diltiazem (Cardizem and Dilacor)	120-240 mg/day	$40-$65 (for SR)	Use with caution in those with heart block or bradycardia and those taking beta-blockers. Rarely precipitates heart failure (monitor carefully).
Class: Dihydropyridine (an L-type channel blocker): Little effect on SA and AV nodes or on contractility. Pure vasodilation causes reflex tachycardia and peripheral edema.			
Nifedipine (Procardia, Adalat)	30-120 mg/day	$28-$80 (for SR)	Reflex tachycardia may be more prominent with short-acting preparations. Limit use to SR forms.
Amlodipine (Norvasc)	5-10 mg/day	$38-$62	Long duration of action (half-life, 36 hours). SR preparations unnecessary for this and the following drugs; safe in heart failure; vascular selective.
Felodipine (Plendil)	5-10 mg/day	$28-$51	Vascular selective. FDA approved for hypertension only.
Isradipine (DynaCirc)	2.5-10 mg/day	$17-$26	Vascular selective. FDA approved for hypertension only.
Nicardipine (Cardene)	60-120 mg/day	$37-$75 (for SR)	FDA approved for angina and hypertension.
Bepridil (Vascor)	200-400 mg/day		A sodium channel blocker used for atrial arrhythmias. Approved for angina. Causes QT interval prolongation and may be arrhythmogenic (torsade de pointes). Other drug interactions. Not an easy drug to use, and expensive.
Class: T-type channel blocker (calcium channels found in arterial wall and conduction tissue but not in myocardium)			
Mibefradil	50-100 mg qd	$83-$118	No myocardial depression, no reflex tachycardia, no peripheral edema; some decrease in heart rate (comparable to diltiazem) and minimal effect on AV node conduction

* Retail cost per month.

SR, Sustained-release preparation, which I recommend for treatment of angina. The short-acting preparations are cheaper, but concerns have been raised over greater reflex tachycardia, especially with short-acting nifedipine. Short-acting drugs also require qid or tid dosing, and most patients have difficulty remembering the midday doses (note Section III).

Table 13-10	Practice Guidelines for Coronary Angiography for Patients with Known or Suspected Coronary Artery Disease (CAD)[16]		
Clinical Setting	**Appropriate**	**Equivocal**	**Not Indicated**
No symptoms but known or suspected CAD	1. High risk with noninvasive tests (Box 13-2) 2. Occupational hazard (heavy or dangerous work) 3. After cardiac arrest	1. Borderline stress ECG, ischemia confirmed with noninvasive study 2. Prior MI, normal LV function, positive but low-risk stress test 3. Before high-risk surgery, after a positive stress test with imaging	1. As a screening test without prior noninvasive testing 2. Positive stress ECG alone, no other adverse circumstances 3. Routine follow-up after revascularization, without evidence for active ischemia
Symptoms (angina) with probable CAD	1. All circumstances listed above 2. Uncontrolled angina 3. Uncontrolled angina after revascularization 4. Unstable angina 5. Prinzmetal's angina	1. All circumstances listed above 2. Worsening exercise tolerance with serial stress ECG 3. Inadequate noninvasive study	1. Mild symptoms (Canadian class I or II, Table 3-2), normal LV function, noninvasive studies indicate low risk 2. Patient is not a candidate for revascularization
Atypical chest pain or CPUE	1. Noninvasive study indicates high risk 2. Probable coronary spasm 3. Associated LV dysfunction	1. Inadequate data from noninvasive study 2. Negative noninvasive study but persistent and severe symptoms (e.g., repeat hospitalization)	Previous normal coronary angiogram; no new objective evidence for ischemia

Does not include indications for angiography soon after myocardial infarction (see Chapter 14). This is a simplification of the guidelines and provides an idea of *when to refer* for angiography. You will rely on your cardiology consultant to understand the guidelines and apply them appropriately

ommended angiography for distance runners who did not wish to give up their sport. On the other hand, many are satisfied with less vigorous activities and are able to live comfortably with a lower anginal threshold. When I discuss revascularization in this fashion and point out that there is no survival benefit for the low-risk patient, most elect to try medical therapy first.

Practice guidelines have been established for coronary angiography (Table 13-10), coronary bypass surgery (Table 13-11), and angioplasty (Table 13-12).[16-18]

An indication for revascularization that merits emphasis is CAD and left ventricular (LV) dysfunction. Depressed LV ejection fraction (LVEF) is the best predictor of late mortality in patients with CAD. Think of LV dysfunction as a "cumulative" problem: every time the pa-

tient loses muscle, LVEF falls a few more percentage points. The overall effect of multiple, small infarctions may be as devastating as the effect of one large myocardial infarction. I tell patients who have had a myocardial infarction that they have "lost all the muscle they can afford to lose" and that a goal of evaluation and treatment is to lower the chance of future injury.

Choice of Revascularization Technique: Surgery versus Angioplasty. These techniques are described in detail in Chapters 10 and 52. Randomized trials have shown comparable survival given proper patient selection (Table 13-13).[19] These selection issues should be discussed with patients who are referred for angiography and possible revascularization. If they are not or if the rationale for the choice of procedure does not make sense, you should raise concerns.

Table 13-11	*Indications for Coronary Artery Bypass Grafting (CABG)*[18]

Clinical Setting	CABG Indicated	Equivocal Indication for CABG	CABG Not Indicated
Asymptomatic patient	1. Noninvasive testing indicates high-risk coronary disease, as does angiography (Box 13-2). 2. As above plus the need for major noncardiac surgery 3. Urgency of CABG increases with worsening LV function	1. Mild or no ischemia shown with noninvasive testing, but angiography shows high risk for disease 2. LV dysfunction would favor CABG, even with low to moderate risk CAD (e.g., two-vessel CAD not involving the LAD)	1. One- or two-vessel CAD, not including the LAD or LMCA, low-risk noninvasive study, normal LV function
Chronic stable angina	1. High-risk coronary anatomy 2. Lower risk coronary anatomy, but a failure of medical treatment to control symptoms	All of the above	Low-risk coronary anatomy and adequate control of symptoms
Unstable angina	All of the above	All of the above	Noninvasive testing indicates low risk plus good control of symptoms

Does not include indications for revascularization soon after myocardial infarction (see Chapters 14 to 16). This table provides the big picture and for some cases may be oversimplified. You must rely on your cardiology consultant to understand the guidelines and apply them appropriately for each patient.

Multivessel CAD is a special challenge for PTCA. *Complete revascularization*, that is, restoring flow to all branches with significant stenosis, is considered an important surgical goal. Some lesions cannot be reached or dilated using catheter techniques. Although no data prove it, a failure to fix these lesions may adversely affect clinical course. Most interventional cardiologists recommend bypass surgery if they believe revascularization will be inadequate with PTCA. In some patients, especially surgical candidates with the highest risk, dilating the "culprit lesion" and settling for incomplete revascularization to palliate symptoms is the sensible approach.

A problem with using randomized trials to make decisions is that they may be out of date by the time of publication. The field of interventional cardiology is changing that rapidly. For example, the BARI trial, an influential study comparing PTCA and surgery for multivessel CAD, was a study of balloon angioplasty alone.[19] BARI did not include arterial stenting or the use of new antiplatelet drugs, both of which have dramatically improved the results of PTCA. Stenting and the use of newer antiplatelet drugs represent the current standard of care, and with them we achieve a better initial result, have an ability to fix more complex lesions, have fewer acute complications such as myocardial infarction, and see less restenosis. In fact, the new technology has made angioplasty safe enough that there are now clinical trials of PTCA for carotid artery disease.

Based on the steady improvement in catheter-based techniques over the past decade, my impression is that we will see more of them and fewer surgical procedures. This is an area of development that will be continuously reviewed in the medical literature.

Problems with PTCA have occurred in patients with diabetes. Randomized studies involving diabetic patients have shown better late survival with bypass surgery.[20] This has been attributed to the use of internal mammary artery (IMA) grafts and the resistance of the IMA to atherosclerosis. In addition, the incidence of restenosis after PTCA with and without stenting is higher in those with diabetes. The pathophysiology of restenosis is poorly understood, and the emergence of effective preventive measures may improve outcomes. At this time, recognition of the special difficulties of diabetic patients is important in the choice of procedure.

Another common patient selection issue is the poor surgical candidate. PTCA offers palliation in this common clinical situation, which includes treatment of

Table 13-12	Practice Guidelines for Percutaneous Transluminal Angioplasty (PTCA)[17]		
Clinical Setting	**PTCA Indicated**	**Equivocal Indication for PTCA**	**PTCA Not Indicated**
1. Single-vessel CAD 2. Mild or no symptoms 3. No medical therapy	1. Noninvasive test is positive and indicates high risk (Box 13-2), or 2. After cardiac arrest, or 3. Needs high-risk noncardiac surgery *and* stenosis of a major coronary artery supplying viable muscle; lesion suitable for PTCA	Lesion in a major artery supplying a large area of viable myocardium, with a positive noninvasive test, and the lesion is a good one for PTCA (low risk, good chance of success)	1. Stenosed artery supplies a nonviable or small area of myocardium 2. Negative noninvasive test for ischemia 3. High-risk lesion 4. Symptoms probably are noncardiac
1. Single-vessel CAD 2. Classes II-IV symptoms (Table 3-2) 3. On medical therapy	Above plus inadequate control of symptoms or inability to tolerate medicines	Definite clinical indication but a complex lesion (e.g., sequential stenoses or a long lesion). Stenting increases probability of success for such cases (and is new since publication of the guidelines)	All of the above
Multivessel CAD, with and without symptoms	All of the above clinical indications for revascularization, plus a high likelihood of success.	Severe angina; not a surgical candidate (PTCA as palliation)	1. Small area of myocardium at risk, mild symptoms, or 2. High-risk PTCA, low chance of success (CABG a good alternative)

Does not include indications for PTCA as therapy during or after acute myocardial infarction (see Chapters 15 and 16). This is a simplification of the guidelines but will allow you to follow your cardiology consultant's reasoning when he or she recommends PTCA.

frail, elderly people with angina. Medical therapy should be tried initially, with PTCA reserved for a failure to control symptoms.

At the other end of the spectrum is the young patient with uncontrolled angina. The risk of progression of CAD is high, and repeat revascularization may be necessary. It is good to avoid multiple operations if possible, so PTCA is a good choice if it is technically feasible.

Expected Clinical Course

As described earlier, it is possible for anginal symptoms to resolve. Most patients with chronic stable angina remain stable. A major concern is the risk of your patient with mild or moderate angina having myocardial infarction or dying. The Coronary Artery Surgery Study (CASS) found that the risk of myocardial infarction was 2.2% per year with medical therapy compared with 2.7% per year after bypass surgery.[21] Note the publication date, 1984. Both surgery and medical therapy have improved; aggressive lowering of LDL cholesterol levels and use of aspirin have lowered rates of infarction and death. Avail-

able trials suggest no increase in mortality when low-risk patients are treated medically (see Box 13-2). In fact, there was a trend toward increased mortality for low-risk patients treated surgically.[22]

Based on angiographic findings, bypass surgery reduces mortality for those with LV dysfunction, left main CAD, or two- and three-vessel CAD when it includes stenosis of the proximal left anterior descending artery. Those with single-vessel disease involving the proximal left anterior descending artery also may possibly benefit. For single- and double-vessel disease without left anterior descending stenosis, surgery offers no survival benefit.[14] (However, note Pitt's new study of aggressive LDL lowering, reviewed in the Bibliography; all of this may be changing.)

Follow-up

It is important to follow patients closely soon after making the diagnosis of stable angina. You want to be certain that symptoms are stable, and risk factor and lifestyle modification requires monitoring and support.

Table 13-13	*Patient Selection Issues: Percutaneous Transluminal Coronary Angioplasty (PTCA) versus Coronary Artery Bypass Grafting (CABG)*

Clinical Issue	Preferred Procedure	Comment
Left main stenosis	CABG	PTCA is contraindicated with "unprotected" left main disease (a rare patient with bypass grafts in place "protecting" some of the downstream branches has PTCA of the left main for relief of symptomatic ischemia of other, ungrafted branches)
LV dysfunction	Both	PTCA occasionally is used for palliation when severe LV dysfunction makes CABG too risky. On the other hand, complete revascularization may be especially important for others with poor LV function, and this may be achievable only with CABG.
Single-vessel CAD	Both, but PTCA the choice of most	Often the best situation for PTCA. Morphology and location of the lesion influence the risk-benefit equation.
Multivessel CAD	Both	Completeness of revascularization may be an issue if lesions are not suitable for PTCA. Random trials show a comparable survival outcome, slightly less morbidity with PTCA, but more repeat procedures.
A stenosis technically unsuited for PTCA	CABG	Some complex lesions may be unsuitable for PTCA (stenosis at a branch point or in a tortuous segment of vessel, a long lesion, an ostial lesion, or one with unstable-appearing plaque surface or thrombus). This is changing rapidly with new technology.
Saphenous vein stenosis	Both	A "lesser-of-two-evils" choice. Redo surgery is tough. Restenosis rates are high after PTCA, even with stenting. The surgeon often encourages an attempt at PTCA before going back to the operating room.
Internal mammary graft stenosis	Both, but PTCA works well	Results with PTCA of internal mammary grafts are better than with saphenous vein grafts.
Poor surgical candidate	PTCA	Uncontrolled symptoms in a patient who is too old, frail, or sick for surgery can be palliated with PTCA. A common indication in current practice.
Diabetes and multivessel CAD	CABG	Randomized trials comparing PTCA and CABG have found that the subset of patients with diabetes has improved survival with surgery.

More aggressive treatment of hypertension, diabetes, or other associated conditions must be pursued. Medicines for angina may need adjustment. About one in five patients treated with nitrates, calcium blockers, or beta-blockers have side effects. Many of them will not tell their families or their doctor unless asked directly. This is especially true of sexual dysfunction, a common problem with beta blockade.

The patient whose condition is stable and who has no other medical problems should be seen at least yearly to monitor therapy, lipids levels, and other risk factors. Many will have dyslipidemia, mandating more frequent follow-up. An argument can be made for repeating the resting ECG at 1- to 2-year intervals (so that a recent baseline is available if prolonged pain develops) or if the patient's condition changes.

Table 13-14	*Clinical Definition of Unstable Angina and the Short-Term Risk of Death or Myocardial Infarction*
Low risk	1. New-onset angina within 2 weeks to 2 months, *or* 2. Worsening of exercise angina (increased frequency, lower angina threshold, slightly longer duration of pain), *plus* 3. No change in the ECG
Intermediate risk	1. Angina lasting ≥20 minutes, at rest, *or* 2. Nocturnal angina, *or* 3. Angina with T wave changes, *or* 4. New-onset angina within 2 weeks, *or* 5. New angina plus Q waves on the ECG ("postinfarction angina"), *or* 6. New angina plus age >65 years
High risk	1. Prolonged and ongoing angina at rest 2. Angina plus heart failure (rales or S_3 gallop) 3. Pulmonary edema possibly caused by ischemia (even without angina) 4. Angina at rest plus ST segment shift ≥1 mm 5. Angina with hypotension 6. Angina with a new or worsening mitral regurgitation murmur

From Braunwald E, Mark DB, Jones RH, et al: Unstable angina: diagnosis and management. Clinical Practice Guideline Number 10, AHCPR pub no 94-0602, Rockville, Md, 1994, Agency For Health Care Policy and Research and the National Heart, Lung and Blood Institute, Public Health Service, US Department of Health and Human Services.

Follow-up exercise testing at specified intervals is unnecessary if symptoms are stable. If symptoms change or if you are uncertain about your patient's symptoms, repeat exercise testing is useful to document a change in exercise tolerance. If symptoms have been stable, no evidence has demonstrated that a "routine stress test" helps to predict the future. That is, a normal or unchanged study does not ensure that the patient's condition will remain stable, although it does indicate good prognosis in a general way. A patient with long-standing angina who has myocardial infarction is as likely to have had a negative stress test in the preceding 6 months as a positive one. Note that my recommendation may be considered at variance with a task force suggestion that yearly exercise testing is a reasonable although unproven strategy.[23] I would emphasize "unproven." Many experienced clinicians (including me) do not routinely order yearly exercise studies for stable patients, and available evidence indicates that they should not be faulted for this.

UNSTABLE ANGINA PECTORIS (USAP)

The term *unstable* is more than descriptive when it is applied to angina pectoris. It indicates a specific syndrome that is associated with a high short-term risk for myocardial infarction and cardiac death. In general usage, angina is unstable when it is of recent onset (<2 months), occurs at rest or nocturnally, is prolonged, or has an accelerating pattern. A more detailed definition and classification by severity of symptoms and laboratory findings is given in Table 13-14.[24]

Epidemiology and Natural History

Since new-onset angina is included in this syndrome, all patients with chronic stable angina were "unstable" at the beginning of their illness. When symptoms are new, it is uncertain whether the angina is a preinfarction syndrome or the start of a chronic illness. Those with chronic stable angina have stood the test of time.

USAP is a common illness, accounting for more than a half million hospital admissions in the United States yearly. In our practice it is the single most common indication for coronary angiography. The mortality risk with unstable angina is intermediate—between that of stable angina and of myocardial infarction. Fewer than 10% of patients have infarction during initial hospitalization, perhaps because of the effectiveness of current treatment. However, the near-term clinical course is rocky. A recent British study of patients with USAP who were on an 8-month waiting list for elective angiography found that 57% had an adverse event (myocardial infarction, new coronary occlusion, or prolonged pain requiring hospital readmission).[25] We also know that a majority of patients with myocardial infarction have a prodrome of USAP, with symptoms often not recognized as angina.

Pathophysiology

Coronary artery stenosis becomes "dynamic" (variable severity of stenosis) with unstable coronary syndromes. Spasm is a potential mechanism (see Fig. 13-1), but it now appears to have a minor role for most patients with USAP. Thrombosis is more important. Angiography and intravascular ultrasound show that the plaque surface is roughened, irregular, or scalloped. Plaque ulceration and thrombus (seen as a filling defect on an angiogram) may be present. Pain at rest may result from intermittent thrombus accumulation, and relief comes with dissolution of the clot. Thrombosis and thrombolysis are in equilibrium.

The cause of thrombosis is disruption of plaque, with exposed collagen activating platelets. What causes plaque disruption? There is uncertainty about the initiating events, but local mechanical factors, including bending of the artery, shear forces, and inflammation, have been suggested. Those with USAP also have been found to have a systemic change in hemostasis, including increased platelet reactivity, increased procoagulant activity, and decreased endogenous fibrinolysis.[26]

The result of spontaneous worsening of coronary stenosis is a primary decline in myocardial oxygen supply (see Fig. 13-1). Studies have supported this finding, showing that chest pain and ST segment depression that develops at rest happens before any change in the HR-BP product. Other studies found that coronary sinus oxygen saturation falls before the onset of angina.

Clinical Presentation and Predictors of High Risk for Myocardial Infarction

Braunwald's classification proposes a hierarchy of risk (see Table 13-14).[24] Those with new-onset angina but no pain during rest have a much lower risk of infarction.

Pain at rest within the last 2 days indicates the highest risk. USAP that develops because of another medical condition is worse than USAP with no aggravating circumstances (Tables 13-3 and 13-14). The amount of treatment also influences the assessment of risk.

Prospective studies of patients with USAP have shown a rough correlation with this classification system and infarct-free survival. Practice Guidelines from the Agency for Health Care Policy and Research (AHCPR) consider the risk of infarction or death (Table 13-15) when suggesting initial treatment.[27]

Laboratory Studies

The resting ECG is especially important, as new T wave inversion identifies a high-risk subgroup. The changes may be similar to those seen with non–Q wave infarction (Fig. 13-7), but finding normal cardiac enzyme levels excludes that diagnosis. At times the distinction between USAP and non–Q wave myocardial infarction is small, and the old-fashioned term *intermediate coronary syndrome* makes sense. T wave changes, extensive ST depression with pain, or both also indicate increased risk.

Myocardial infarction should be excluded using serial cardiac enzyme measurements, and a lipid profile should be obtained if it has not been done recently. The AHCPR Guidelines (Table 13-15) also suggest measurement of LV function, since LV dysfunction identifies a particularly high-risk group. This can be done noninvasively with either an echocardiogram or a radionuclide angiogram (MUGA scan; see Chapter 9). If prior imaging studies have already indicated LV depression, they need not be repeated.

Stress testing with or without imaging studies is safe for lower risk patients whose symptoms have stabilized.

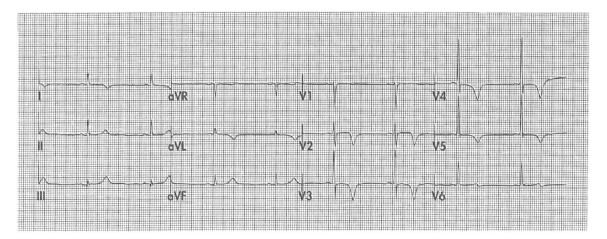

FIG. 13-7
A patient with unstable angina who has symmetrical T wave inversion in anterior precordial leads. This ECG could be interpreted as a non–Q wave myocardial infarction. In such cases, diagnosing infarction rather than unstable angina is based on a rise in cardiac enzyme levels.

The features of the exercise study that stratify risk for those with stable angina also apply to USAP (see Box 13-2 and Fig. 13-5). There is one possible exception to this. The severity of USAP is not always proportional to the tightness of the lesion. Nonstenosing lesions may ulcerate, thrombose, and cause USAP or infarction. For a patient with typical symptoms, multiple risk factors, and new ECG changes, I might question a negative perfusion scan and probably would recommend angiography. A negative exercise study has been shown to indicate good prognosis, but this may be, in part, because exercise studies are used primarily for stable patients, whereas unstable patients often have angiography as their initial evaluation.

Coronary angiography provides information about the state of the plaque surface and percent stenosis. It is the only commonly used technique that does this (intravascular ultrasound and angioscopy are primarily research tools). It is probably safer than exercise testing for high-risk patients.

Table 13-15 | *Practice Guidelines: Management of Unstable Angina*

Early treatment	Medical therapy (to be used in the absence of contraindications) ***Aspirin ***Heparin **Intravenous nitroglycerin if high risk **Beta-blocker, IV if high risk, oral if intermediate or low risk **Calcium channel blocker if symptoms persist while taking nitrates and beta-blockers; avoid with severe LV dysfunction, and use nifedipine only when heart rate is controlled by beta blockade **Newer platelet-inhibiting agents (ticlopidine, IIb-IIIa antagonists) are alternatives to aspirin (and possibly superior)
Ongoing medical treatment	*Switch to oral or topical nitroglycerin when pain-free for 24 hours *Continue heparin 2 to 5 days or until revascularization ***Aspirin daily **Continue beta-blocker
Triage	**High-risk patients to a monitored ICU bed when possible *Intermediate-risk patients to a monitored cardiac bed *Low-risk patients may be managed as outpatients with early follow-up evaluation
Laboratory studies	*Routine protocol to rule out MI plus assessment of LV function within 72 hours *Immediate ECG with any recurrence or worsening of symptoms
Noninvasive tests	**Low-risk patient may have exercise testing within 24 hours **If not having angiography, noninvasive tests should be avoided until pain-free or not in congestive heart failure for at least 48 hours
Immediate coronary angiography	**Failure of chest pain and ECG changes to resolve with 1 hour of starting medical therapy
Coronary angiography	***There is support for both an *early invasive* strategy (in which all hospitalized patients have angiography) and *early conservative* strategy (in which angiography is reserved for those with heart failure, poor LV function, persistent or recurrent ischemia, prior revascularization, or a positive noninvasive test for ischemia)
Revascularization	Tables 13-11 and 13-12.
Treatment after discharge	***Aspirin ***Lipid-altering therapy

From Braunwald E, Mark DB, Jones RH, et al: Unstable angina: diagnosis and management. Clinical Practice Guideline Number 10 (amended), AHCPR pub no 94-0602, Rockville, Md, 1994, Agency For Health Care Policy and Research and the National Heart, Lung and Blood Institute, Public Health Service, US Department of Health and Human Services.
Strength of evidence: ***Supported by randomized clinical trials; **supported by nonrandomized trials; *no clinical trial support but seems reasonable.

Management

The AHCPR Practice Guidelines are practical and provide ample leeway for clinical judgment (Table 13-15).

Triage and Admission to the Hospital

Patients at low risk for myocardial infarction or cardiac death may be evaluated as outpatients (Table 13-14). However, one large prospective study found that only 6% of their patients with USAP met low-risk criteria.[28]

All others should be admitted to the hospital for monitoring and evaluation. Highest risk patients may benefit from intensive care unit (ICU) monitoring, but this is not always possible. Because of bed availability, most of our patients with USAP are admitted to a step-down telemetry unit, not the ICU.

Angiography and Exercise Testing

A comparison of conservative and early invasive strategies in the TIMI-IIIB trial found similar 6-week survival data and rates of nonfatal myocardial infarction.[29] There was more readmission to the hospital in the conservative therapy group. Most of the 63% who had revascularization as part of the invasive group had angioplasty (186 patients had CABG, 278 had PTCA), and stenting was not used. An important feature of the *conservative* strategy is that it used exercise testing for risk stratification, and high-risk patients had angiography. By the time of the 6-week follow-up, 64% of them had had angiography and 50% had revascularization. So even with a conservative initial approach, there was a high degree of intervention.[30] *Taking a conservative approach to USAP, "watchful waiting," can be supported only if you follow the aggressive risk stratification strategy of TIMI-IIIB.28*

Note that the Practice Guidelines indicate equality between early invasive and early conservative strategies (Table 13-15). I favor angiography as the initial study for patients with persistent T wave inversion in anterior precordial leads (Fig. 13-7), significant ST segment depression or elevation during pain, LV dysfunction, and a history of myocardial infarction in addition to other features that indicate a high risk of adverse events (Table 13-14). For lower risk patients, a trial of medical therapy is not an error, but these patients must have further risk stratification with a stress test.[30] A positive stress test would be an indication for angiography.

Drug Therapy

The Practice Guidelines describe medical treatment and specify the level of evidence-based medicine support for use of each agent. Drug classes and agents have been reviewed (Tables 13-5 through 13-9).

Antiplatelet Therapy and Anticoagulation. Aspirin is indicated for all patients with USAP. For those who cannot tolerate aspirin, short-term treatment with ticlopidine may be substituted. Ticlopidine is not ulcerogenic, although 40% of patients have gastrointestinal side effects. It has not been recommended as long-term therapy because of potentially dangerous marrow suppression.

The platelet receptor blockers (e.g., Rheopro) reduce the thrombotic complications of angioplasty and may reduce rates of restenosis as well. They have also been found more effective than heparin in reducing mortality, infarction, and refractory ischemia during USAP.[31]

Heparin. Heparin has been the mainstay of therapy for USAP.[32] When we first learned to use it routinely, we stopped getting calls in the middle of the night about recurrent pain. It may be more than stopgap treatment used as a bridge to angiography for high-risk patients. Those with endstage CAD who are not candidates for revascularization and who develop unstable angina may "cool off" after 4 to 6 days of heparin therapy while in the hospital. Roughened plaque surface can heal with time, and heparin and antiplatelet therapy may provide the time. (Such palliation is as easily accomplished in the community hospital as in the referral center.)

Low-molecular-weight heparin has been more effective than intravenous unfractionated heparin for the treatment of USAP.[33] It has a number of advantages, including twice-daily subcutaneous dosing and no need for monitoring activated partial thromboplastin time.[34] The initial cost is slightly higher, but when the expense of intravenous infusion gear and nursing time (in understaffed hospitals) is considered, low-molecular-weight heparin may be more cost effective.

Intravenous Nitroglycerin. This is another therapy that seemed revolutionary when first introduced. Before we had it, use of the intraaortic balloon pump (IABP) was common. With modern therapy, the IABP is rarely needed.

Beta-Adrenergic Blockade. All the agents approved for the treatment of angina pectoris may be used (Table 13-7). When the possible side effects of beta blockade are of concern, consider intravenous esmolol, which has a half-life of just 9 minutes. (It does not have FDA approval for angina, so this would be an off-label use.) Intravenous therapy using one of the approved drugs is recommended for patients with ongoing pain and those in the highest risk categories.

Calcium Channel Blockers. When spasm was being emphasized as a cause of USAP, we believed that calcium blockers would be important. The current thinking is that the pathophysiology of USAP is more thrombotic than vasospastic. Calcium blockers may be useful for the relief of symptoms, but they are not considered first-line therapy. For the choice of agent, see Tables 13-6 and 13-9.

Revascularization Therapy and Referral Considerations

Recall that 50% to 60% of patients in the TIMI-IIIB trial had revascularization, including those randomized to initial conservative treatment. Revascularization is more often needed by high-risk patients and those with T wave changes on the resting ECG. Lower risk patients are more apt to stabilize with medical therapy.

I would advise early referral of high-risk patients. Unstable angina has a way of becoming even more unstable, often without warning. You may find yourself treating acute myocardial infarction in the middle of the night. A patient who has acute infarction in the cardiac center has immediate access to treatment in the catheterization laboratory.

Treatment of lower risk patients involves an element of choice (Table 13-15). Whether to pursue early interventional or conservative strategies is determined by the patient's wishes and influenced by diagnostic capabilities. If a patient has not had any symptoms for at least 48 hours, exercise testing can be safely done in the community hospital setting.

The choice of revascularization methods is reviewed in Chapters 10 and 52. (Chapter 10 is written by an interventional cardiologist and Chapter 52 by a surgeon; their differing viewpoints are interesting.) Both work well for the appropriate patient. Cardiologists and surgeons, in my experience, reliably state expectations for success and risks of complications. In this era of oversight where everyone's results are monitored, it is unusual for a cardiologist or surgeon to attempt more than can be reasonably accomplished. As a primary care physician, it should be important to you that your patient is treated by a busy operator. The quality of surgery and PTCA is directly related to the volume of work done by the doctor and hospital.

Expected Clinical Course and Follow-up

Using the treatment approach of the TIMI-IIIB trial, 2.5% died within 6 weeks and 5.5% had nonfatal myocardial infarction. Those results may be expected using therapy circa 1993. It is possible that outcomes will be better with more effective anticoagulation/antiplatelet therapy. Coronary artery stenting, which lowers the chance of abrupt closure of unstable arteries during angioplasty, was not used in TIMI-IIIB and also may improve outcome.

Most patients with USAP stabilize after a program of medical therapy. Symptoms may resolve completely, or a pattern of stable angina may evolve. Close follow-up after the initial evaluation is needed to ensure the patient does not become more unstable. Even with an honest effort at patient education, it is common for patients to refuse to return to the doctor with worsening symptoms, "because the doctor said I was ok."

Patients who have had stabilization or resolution of symptoms, and others who have had revascularization, need risk factor modification, long-term aspirin therapy, and treatment to bring LDL cholesterol levels below 100 mg/dL. This and the management of associated conditions also mandate close follow-up.

Low-risk patients who have documented CAD and whose condition has stabilized may benefit from a follow-up exercise test. My argument regarding serial, routine stress testing for stable patients (see p. 159) applies in these cases as well.

Any patient whose condition becomes more unstable or who develops pain at rest, more frequent angina, prolonged pain, or new ECG changes needs angiography.

PRINZMETAL'S VARIANT ANGINA
Epidemiology, Etiology, and Natural History

As originally described by Marvin Prinzmetal, this syndrome includes angina at rest that is not provoked by exercise or stress. During pain there is ST segment elevation, and angiographic studies have shown focal coronary artery spasm as the cause.

Spasm may occur at the site of atherosclerotic plaque, as was the case with Dr. Prinzmetal's initial cases. It also may occur in angiographically normal arteries. Variant angina may appear as part of generalized vasospasm, including both Raynaud's phenomenon and migraine syndromes.

Most patients have no apparent cause. Cigarette smoking may be a risk factor. Cocaine is known to provoke spasm; it blocks the presynaptic uptake of norepinephrine and dopamine, increasing alpha-adrenergic tone and provoking coronary artery spasm. Similarly, beta-adrenergic blockers may aggravate coronary spasm by leaving alpha stimulation unopposed.

Attack frequency may wax and wane, with occasional symptom-free intervals. Coronary spasm also may cause myocardial infarction, which may be complicated by malignant arrhythmias (heart block or ventricular fibrillation).

Clinical Presentation

The quality of anginal discomfort is similar to that of other anginal syndromes. Pain typically occurs at rest and tends to occur at the same time each day. Nocturnal angina is common. Continuous ST segment monitoring has shown that many ischemic episodes are painless, especially when of short duration. Exercise tolerance usually is normal. Many patients are heavy smokers.

Another presentation is syncope. In these cases, ventricular tachycardia or complete heart block develops early during the ischemic episode, so anginal discomfort is a less prominent symptom.

The diagnosis is confirmed when an ECG during chest pain demonstrates ST segment elevation (Fig. 13-7). ST elevation usually is localized to one of the three coronary artery distributions. When ST elevation involves both anterior and inferior leads, indicating extensive ischemia, the risk of sudden death is high.

Laboratory Studies

An ECG during chest pain is the most useful noninvasive test. It is both sensitive and specific. Patients whose typical pain involves no ST segment changes almost certainly do not have coronary artery spasm. In such cases, we do not have an obligation to pursue angiography and ergonovine testing.

Stress testing may be considered as a screen for underlying coronary artery disease, but is of no use for the diagnosis of spasm.

Angina at rest is unstable angina, and many of these patients undergo coronary angiography. This is especially true when there is ST segment elevation during pain, but also when the diagnosis is uncertain. Angiography both confirms the diagnosis of spasm and determines the extent of atherosclerotic CAD.

Provocative testing with ergonovine maleate during angiography is the standard test for spasm. After identifying normal-appearing coronary vessels, the patient is given gradually increasing doses of ergonovine intravenously (from 0.05 to 0.40 mg) and observed. If angina and ST segment elevation develop, the angiogram is repeated. Spasm usually causes occlusion or near-occlusion of the artery. A normal response to ergonovine includes an overall reduction in coronary artery caliber but without focal spasm.

For angina that is provoked in the catheterization laboratory, sublingual or intravenous nitroglycerine is given for relief. An occasional patient requires intracoronary infusion of nitroglycerin. For this reason, the test is done as part of coronary angiography rather than with noninvasive techniques such as echocardiography or perfusion imaging. Safety requires catheter access to the coronary artery ostium.

The ergonovine stress test is sensitive and specific for coronary artery spasm. Those with spasm after the lowest dose of ergonovine tend to have more frequent attacks; there is a rough "dose-response" relationship. If the angiogram looks normal and the ergonovine test is negative, I tell patients that we have done all that we can to exclude ischemia as a cause of chest discomfort.

Management of Variant Angina
Drug therapy

The mainstay of therapy is calcium channel blockade. These agents are so effective that I have come to think of spasm as an "illness of the calcium channel" (realizing that the pathophysiology has not been identified with certainty). All of the long-acting preparations work and are given at maximally tolerated doses. An occasional patient who does not respond to one of them may respond to another from a different class (see Table 13-9). A rare patient needs treatment with two drugs from different classes.

Symptoms may rebound once calcium blockers are stopped, such as during and after surgery. For a patient with frequent symptoms, consider intravenous diltiazem during the perioperative period.

Anginal attacks usually are relieved by nitroglycerin. In this case, it works by relieving coronary spasm. Peripheral venodilation (reducing preload and cardiac work) is not the mechanism of action. Long-acting nitrates may be used to prevent attacks and can be combined with calcium blockers in resistant cases. Remember that nitrate tolerance must be avoided by providing a 10- to 12-hour nitrate-free interval. Patients who have nocturnal episodes need to have nitrates on board overnight rather than during the day.

Spasm may be provoked by alpha-adrenergic discharge (e.g., the cold pressor test). Some patients get relief with prazosin, which should be considered if calcium blockers and nitrates fail.

Two of the standard therapies for CAD and angina may cause *worsening* of symptoms. Beta-adrenergic blockade leaves alpha-adrenergic stimuli unopposed. In patients with hypertension, consider coronary spasm if angina develops after starting beta-blocker therapy. Aspirin inhibits the synthesis of prostacyclin, a coronary vasodilator, and therefore may aggravate coronary spasm. Avoiding aspirin may help the patient with variant angina and no underlying atherosclerosis. With coronary artery plaque as well as spasm, the benefits of aspirin may exceed risks (but monitor symptoms).

Revascularization Therapy

Pure vasospasm, with no underlying atherosclerosis, is a medical condition, not a surgical one. In fact, a failure to recognize that a stenosis is caused by spasm rather than plaque can lead to surgical disaster. The spastic artery often is touchy and may develop spasm at the site of manipulation or graft insertion. Postoperative ST segment elevation, arrhythmias, and infarction may follow. Angioplasty with stenting or bypass surgery may be considered for spasm that develops at the site of a tight atherosclerotic stenosis.

Expected Clinical Course and Follow-up

As noted, spasm may wax and wane. The risk of myocardial infarction and death is highest for those with severe underlying atherosclerosis. Those with angiographically normal coronary arteries (pure vasospasm) have an excellent prognosis, with 5-year survival of about 95% and myocardial infarction risk less than 10%.

Many patients have resolution of symptoms during the 6 months after initial presentation. It is reasonable to taper calcium blocker therapy slowly and possibly to stop medicine. Symptoms may recur and usually respond to the same medical regimen. I would be more concerned about stopping calcium blockers for a patient who initially presented with malignant arrhythmias. One of our patients had right coronary artery spasm and complete heart block and survived out-of-hospital cardiac arrest. Despite control of spasm with felodipine therapy, he had a pacemaker inserted prophylactically.

SYNDROME X: MICROVASCULAR CAD

This syndrome has been defined as angina or angina-like chest pain with normal-appearing epicardial coronary arteries. Many of the patients included in syndrome X have noncardiac pain.

However, some have microcirculatory dysfunction. About 20% have an abnormal stress test, and a smaller percentage have both ST segment changes and increased lactate production (proving ischemia) during provoked angina. In such cases, there is an apparent abnormality of coronary vasodilator reserve, since coronary blood flow does not rise with exercise or dipyridamole infusion. For this minority of patients with syndrome X, calcium blocker or nitrate therapy may help.

Treating *all* patients with chest pain and normal coronary arteries will be frustrating, because most will not respond. Consider a therapeutic trial of calcium blockers or nitrates for those with a positive stress test who have discomfort that sounds like angina. Estrogen replacement has been found helpful in postmenopausal women.

Clinical Course

Most patients with normal coronary arteries and unexplained pain have resolution of symptoms. The risk of myocardial infarction or death is low, and it is important to emphasize the good prognosis when counseling patients and their families. An occasional patient has persistent symptoms, with recurrent hospitalizations and multiple catheterization laboratory procedures. For most, this pattern can be avoided by using exercise imaging studies to evaluate recurrent symptoms.

SILENT ISCHEMIA
Epidemiology and Pathophysiology

One in four patients with myocardial infarction in the Framingham study had no history of the event, and half of these had no symptoms at all. The other half could recall a prolonged episode of heartburn, indigestion, bursitis, or other discomfort that was probably the infarction. Other epidemiologic studies suggest that 2% to 4% of middle-aged men have asymptomatic but flow-restricting coronary stenoses. Patients with angina also may have silent ischemia, since ambulatory monitoring indicates that some episodes of ischemia are not perceived. As a rule, ischemia that is longer or is associated with greater ST segment shift is more likely to cause pain. This is true of variant angina with ST segment elevation, as well as effort angina with ST depression.

Three mechanisms of silent ischemia have been proposed. The first is that a threshold quantity of ischemia must be exceeded before pain occurs. The second relates to variation in pain threshold among patients. Some have a higher threshold, and a subset of patients have been found to produce more endorphins. The third relates to cardiac pain receptors or nociceptive function. Patients with diabetes and neuropathy may have denervation and reduced perception of cardiac pain, as well as foot pain. "Stunned nerves" may cause silent ischemia in as many as 70% of patients who have had successful reperfusion therapy for myocardial infarction.[35] Silent ischemia is common after heart transplantation because of nociceptive dysfunction.

Evaluation

Silent ischemia usually is identified with stress testing. This may present a dilemma, as painless ST segment depression during exercise is one of the features that indicates a false-positive study. It usually is worked out with perfusion or LV function imaging, which will be abnormal during ischemia, even silent ischemia.

Ambulatory ST segment monitoring is accurate when using systems designed for that purpose, but less so with arrhythmia detection monitors. Ischemia monitors are not widely used clinically but have been useful research tools.

Management and Clinical Course

Silent ischemia indicates an increased risk of myocardial infarction or cardiac death. When it occurs at rest, it may be considered as dangerous as other unstable angina syndromes. A special concern with silent ischemia with effort is the failure of the patient to perceive it and to stop working—the absence of a warning system.

Silent ischemia should be managed like symptom-producing ischemia. Nitrates, beta-blockers, and calcium channel blockers have all been effective. Whether the threshold for revascularization should be lower for patients with silent ischemia is uncertain at this time and is the subject of randomized trails that are in progress.

REFERENCES
1. Allen MR, Oh JK, Behrenbeck T: Echo versus nuclear imaging to assess ischemic coronary syndromes, *Contemp Intern Med* 9:27, 1997.

2. Hundley WG, Grayburn PA: Utility of screening for coronary artery calcium, *Am J Cardiol* 78:1266, 1996.

3. American Heart Association: *Heart and stroke facts: 1995 statistical supplement*, Dallas, 1995, American Heart Association.

4. Hunick MGM, Goldman L, Tosteson ANA, et al: The recent decline in mortality from coronary heart disease, 1980-1990, *JAMA* 227:535, 1997.

5. Vogel RA: Coronary risk factors, endothelial function and atherosclerosis: a review, *Clin Cardiol* 20:426, 1997.

6. Forrester JS, Shah PK: Lipid lowering versus revascularization: an idea whose time (for testing) has come, *Circulation* 96:1360, 1997.

7. Berman DS, Hachamovitch R, Kiat H, et al: Incremental prognostic value and cost implications of normal and equivocal exercise Tc-99m sestamibi myocardial perfusion SPECT, *J Am Coll Cardiol* 26:639, 1995.

8. Scandinavian Simvastatin Survival Study Group: Randomised trial of cholesterol lowering in 4444 patients with coronary heart disease: the Scandinavian Simvastatin Survival Study (4S), *Lancet* 344:1383, 1994.

9. Antiplatelet Trialists' Collaboration: Collaborative overview of randomized trials of antiplatelet therapy. I. Prevention of death, myocardial infarction, and stroke by prolonged antiplatelet therapy in various categories of patients, *Br Med J* 308:81, 1994.

10. Parker JD, Parker JO: Nitrate therapy for stable angina pectoris, *N Engl J Med* 338:520, 1998.

11. Packer M, O'Connor CM, Ghali JK, et al for the PRAISE study group: Effect of amlodipine on morbidity and mortality in severe chronic heart failure, *N Engl J Med* 335:1107, 1996.

12. Messerli FH: Safety of calcium antagonists: dissecting the evidence, *Am J Cardiol* 78(suppl 9A):19, 1996.

13. Grossman E, Messerli FH, Grodzicki T, Kowey P: Should a moratorium be placed on sublingual nifedipine capsules given for hypertensive emergencies and pseudoemergencies? *JAMA* 276:1328, 1996.

14. Yusuf S, Zucker D, Peduzzi P, et al: Effect of coronary artery bypass graft surgery on survival: overview of 10-year results from randomized trials by the Coronary Artery Bypass Graft Surgery Trialists Collaboration, *Lancet* 344:563, 1984.

15. Solomon AJ, Gersh BJ: Management of chronic stable angina: medical therapy, percutaneous transluminal coronary angioplasty, and coronary artery bypass surgery: lessons from the randomized trials, *Ann Intern Med* 128:216, 1998.

16. Ross J, Brandenburg RO, Dinsmore RE, et al: Guidelines for coronary angiography. A report of the American College of Cardiology/American Heart Association Task Force on Assessment of Diagnostic and Therapeutic Cardiovascular Procedures (Subcommittee on Coronary Angiography), *J Am Coll Cardiol* 10:935, 1987.

17. Ryan TJ, Bauman WB, Kennedy JW, et al: Guidelines for percutaneous transluminal coronary angioplasty. A report of the American College of Cardiology/American Heart Association Task Force on Assessment of Diagnostic and Therapeutic Cardiovascular Procedures (subcommittee on PTCA), *J Am Coll Cardiol* 22:2033, 1993.

18. Kirklin JW, Akins CW, Blackstone EH, et al: Guidelines and indications for coronary artery bypass graft surgery. A report of the American College of Cardiology/American Heart Association Task Force on Assessment of Diagnostic and Therapeutic Cardiovascular Procedures (Subcommittee on Coronary Artery Bypass Graft Surgery), *J Am Coll Cardiol* 17:543, 1991.

19. The Bypass Angioplasty Revascularization Investigation (BARI) Investigators: Comparison of coronary bypass surgery with angioplasty in patients with multivessel disease, *N Engl J Med* 335:217, 1996.

20. Ellis SG, Narins CR: Problem of angioplasty in diabetics, *Circulation* 96:1707, 1997.

21. CASS Principal Investigators and Their Associates: Myocardial infarction and mortality in the Coronary Artery Surgery Study (CASS) randomized trial, *N Engl J Med* 310:750, 1984.

22. The Veterans Administration Coronary Artery Bypass Surgery Cooperative Study Group: Eleven-year survival in the Veterans Administration randomized trial of coronary bypass surgery for stable angina, *N Engl J Med* 311:1333, 1984.

23. Schlant RC, Blomqvist CG, Brandenburg RO, et al: Guidelines for exercise testing, a report of the American College of Cardiology/American Heart Association Task Force on Assessment of Cardiovascular Procedures (Subcommittee on Exercise Testing), *J Am Coll Cardiol* 8:725, 1986.

24. Braunwald E: Unstable angina: a classification, *Circulation* 80:410, 1989.

25. Chester M, Chen L, Kaski JC: Identification of patients at high risk for adverse coronary events while awaiting routine coronary angioplasty, *Br Heart J* 73:216, 1995.

26. Shah PK: New insights into the pathogenesis and prevention of acute coronary syndromes, *Am J Cardiol* 79(12B):17, 1997.

27. Braunwald E, Mark DB, Jones RH, et al: *Unstable angina: diagnosis and management*, Clinical Practice Guideline Number 10 (amended), pub no 94-0602, Rockville, Md, 1994, Agency for Health Care Policy and Research.

28. Katz DA, Griffith JL, Beshansky JR, Selker HP: The use of empiric clinical data in the evaluation of practice guidelines for unstable angina, *JAMA* 276:1568, 1996.

29. TIMI-IIIB investigators: Effects of tissue-plasminogen activator and a comparison of early invasive and conservative strategies in unstable angina and non-Q wave myocardial infarction: results of the TIMI-IIIB trial, *Circulation* 89:1545, 1994.

30. Hillis WS: The continuing debate: conservative or interventional therapy for unstable coronary artery disease, *Am J Cardiol* 80(5A):51, 1997.

31. The PRISM Study Investigators: A comparison of aspirin plus tirofiban with aspirin plus heparin for unstable angina. The Platelet Receptor Inhibition Syndrome Management (PRISM) Study, *N Engl J Med* 338:1498, 1998.

32. Oler A, Whooley MA, Oler J, Grady D: Adding heparin to aspirin reduces the incidence of myocardial infarction and death in patients with unstable angina: a meta-analysis, *JAMA* 276:811, 1996.

33. Cohen M, Demers C, Gurfinkel EP, et al: A comparison of low molecular weight heparin with unfractionated heparin for unstable coronary artery disease (ESSENCE trial), *N Engl J Med* 337:447, 1997.

34. Weita JI: Low molecular weight heparins, *N Engl J Med* 337:688, 1997.

35. Taylor GJ, Katholi RE, Wokak K, et al: Increased incidence of silent ischemia after acute myocardial infarction, *JAMA* 268:1448, 1992.

BIBLIOGRAPHY

Achenbach S, Moshage W, Bachmann K: Noninvasive coronary angiography by contrast-enhanced electron-beam computed tomography, *Clin Cardiol* 21:323, 1998. A review of studies of EBCT, or "ultrafast CT," for the noninvasive detection of CAD. Sensitivity and specificity are about 90%, with best results with bypass grafts and the left main and left anterior descending arteries.

Adgery AAJ: An overview of the results of clinical trials with glucoprotein IIb/IIIa inhibitors, *Am Heart J* 135:43, 1998.

Antman EM, Handin R: Low-molecular-weight heparins, *Circulation* 98:287, 1998. Review of clinical trials showing that LMW heparin is as effective as unfractionated heparin for non–Q wave MI and unstable angina.

Bennett RM: Emerging concepts in the neurobiology of chronic pain: evidence of abnormal sensory processing in fibromyalgia, *Mayo Clin Proc* 74:385, 1999. Another cause of chest pain, with an interesting review of "nociceptive" function.

Cannon RO: The cardiovascular syndrome X: is it real? *ACC Education Highlights* 14:1, 998. Excellent review. The diagnosis is often bogus; there is a risk of labeling a patient with heart disease when there is none.

Gibbons RJ, Chatterjee K, Daley J, et al: ACC/AHA/ACP-ASIM guidelines for the management of patients with chronic stable angina: a report of the American College of Cardiology/American Heart Association Task Force on Practice Guidelines (Committee on the Management of Patients with Chronic Stable Angina), *J Am Coll Cardiol* 33:2092, 1999. This is a thorough summary of clinical trials evidence for the evaluation and treatment of angina (more than 200 pages and 891 references). The recommendations of Chapter 13, compiled before the release of these guidelines, match them closely. Although the guidelines are authoritative, you should be aware that new studies will influence management choices. For example, the guidelines were written before clinical trials that show that medical therapy with aggressive lipid lowering may match the benefits of angioplasty, even for patients with two-vessel CAD, including anterior descending artery stenosis.

Grundy SM, Balady GJ, Criqui MH, et al: When to start cholesterol-lowering therapy in patients with coronary heart disease: AHA Science Advisory, *Circulation* 95:1683, 1997.

Lewin HC, Berman DS: Achieving sustained improvement in myocardial perfusion: role of isosorbide mononitrate, *Am J Cardiol* 79(12B):31, 1997.

O'Rourke RA: Cost-effective management of chronic stable angina, *Clin Cardiol* 19:497, 1996.

Pitt B, Waters D, Brown WV, et al: Aggressive lipid-lowering therapy compared with angioplasty in stable coronary artery disease, *N Engl J Med* 341:70, 1999. (This study appeared too late to be incorporated into this chapter.) Patients with one- or two-vessel CAD had either angioplasty or Lipitor 80 mg (pushing the LDL to 77 mg/dL). During the 18-month follow-up the Lipitor group had fewer ischemic events. Mortality and MI were similar in the two groups. If confirmed by other trials, this may change our approach to the treatment of stable angina.

Sharis PJ, Cannon CP, Loscalzo J: The antiplatelet effects of ticlopidine and clopidogrel, *Ann Intern Med* 129:394, 1998. Clopidogrel has been approved by the FDA for use after MI. It appears to be a reasonable substitute for aspirin for patients with angina, when aspirin cannot be taken.

Solomon AJ, Gersh BJ: Management of chronic stable angina: medical therapy, percutaneous transluminal coronary angioplasty, and coronary bypass graft surgery—lessons from the randomized trials, *Ann Intern Med* 128:216, 1998.

Thadani U: Management of patients with chronic stable angina at low risk for serious cardiac events, *Am J Cardiol* 79:24, 1997.

14 Acute Myocardial Infarction

George J. Taylor
C. Carolyn Thiedke

EPIDEMIOLOGY, ETIOLOGY, AND NATURAL HISTORY

In 1998, 1.1 million Americans had a new or recurrent myocardial infarction (MI), and about one third of them died.[1] At least 250,000 died within 1 hour of the onset of symptoms, before reaching the hospital. The coronary care unit (CCU) era began in the early 1960s, and since then hospital mortality has fallen dramatically[2-3] (Table 14-1). In addition to the effectiveness of modern therapy, the incidence of MI has declined.[2-3] Interestingly, the incidence of unstable angina has increased, suggesting that patients are coming to the hospital earlier with warning symptoms, instead of later with acute MI.

PATHOPHYSIOLOGY

An abrupt interruption or critical reduction in coronary artery blood flow causes contractile activity to stop within a few heartbeats. All energy is devoted to maintenance of cellular viability. Cell death occurs within minutes to hours, depending on oxygen supply by collateral or residual antegrade flow. Cell membrane deteriorates, and cellular contents, including contractile proteins (the "cardiac enzymes"), leach out of the infarct zone and into circulating blood.

Platelet Function and Onset of MI

Atherosclerotic plaque is the underlying illness, but infarction usually is initiated by thrombosis. For reasons that are unclear, the lipid-rich plaque ruptures, injuring plaque surface. Fissures in the surface expose collagen, which is thrombogenic. Platelets adhere and are activated (see Chapter 11), forming "white clot" at the core of the coronary thrombus. Platelets release vasoactive amines, promoting local spasm. Platelets are also rich in plasminogen activator inhibitor-1 (PAI-1), a potent inhibitor of fibrinolysis. Because of PAI-1, thrombolytic agents have less effect on white clot than they have on fibrin and red cell-rich thrombus (red clot). The continued activation of platelets is one reason that thrombolytic therapy can fail, and better antiplatelet adjunctive therapy may be the key to im-

proving the results of coronary thrombolysis[4] (see Chapter 15).

It is possible for this sequence of plaque injury and thrombus formation to develop on coronary plaques that are not flow restricting; this is the usual mechanism of heart attack in a person with a recent, normal stress ECG. One study of patients with MI who had angiography *months to years earlier* found that many "infarct arteries" (cardiology jargon for the coronary artery branch responsible for MI) had less than 50% stenosis, suggesting a change in the plaque just before MI.[5] Unstable coronary syndromes, including unstable angina and MI, begin with unstable plaque. The degree of stenosis may be dynamic, as thrombi can form, dissolve, and reform. A negative stress ECG is a distinct possibility in a patient with unstable angina, since the unstable plaque may not restrict flow at the time of study. Yet fresh thrombus on the plaque surface may obstruct flow the next day.

On the other hand, a normal stress ECG with good exercise tolerance is said to be a indicator of good prognosis in large populations with stable chest pain. It is not as reliable an indicator of good outcome for those with unstable angina (and therefore unstable plaque surface).

Infarct Size and Cumulative Injury

The prognosis of all patients with coronary artery disease (CAD) is most accurately predicted by left ventricular (LV) function, measured by LV ejection fraction (LVEF). LVEF is the proportion (or fraction) of blood ejected by the LV with each beat. For example, with an end-diastolic LV volume of 150 ml and an end-systolic volume of 75 ml, LVEF = 50%. Normal LVEF is about 55%, with slight variation depending on the technique used to measure it.

The first goal of MI treatment is to minimize the loss of muscle. The lower the LVEF, the worse the prognosis. LVEF after an MI is inversely proportional to the size of the MI, which is determined by the size of the occluded artery and its branches. In the absence of early reperfusion, the amount of creatine kinase (CK) released during MI is proportional to infarct size.

Cardiac injury is cumulative. Damaged muscle is replace by scar and never grows back. I tell patients that

| Table 14-1 | Short-Term (30-Day) Mortality of Patients Hospitalized with Acute Myocardial Infarction (MI) |

Era	Mortality(%)	Treatment and Treatment Advances*
Pre-CCU (pre-1960)	25-30	Supportive care (bed rest, morphine oxygen)
CCU (1960-1970s)	15	ECG monitoring, defibrillation, early ambulation, beta blockade after hospital discharge
Reperfusion (early 1980s)	6.5	Coronary thrombolysis, early intravenous beta blockade, primary angioplasty, more emphasis on antiplatelet therapy, risk stratification for recurrent ischemia and arrhythmia.

*Admittedly, an oversimplification, but these seem to be the major changes in treatment of MI.

losing heart muscle is like losing a finger, which cannot regrow. Thus a person who loses 10 ejection fraction points with a first MI, and later loses another 10, must then live with an ejection fraction of about 35%. When either a large MI or repetitive ischemic injury pushes LVEF below 30%, some exercise tolerance usually is lost, and symptomatic heart failure may develop. (An LVEF <30% is one of the Social Security Administration's criteria for cardiac disability.)

Because damage is cumulative, a major treatment goal *after* MI is the prevention of future ischemic injury. The mortality risk with a second MI is much higher than that of the first. After any heart attack you may tell your patient, "You have lost all the muscle you can afford to lose."

Non-Q vs. Q wave MI

It is useful to think of the spectrum of instability of coronary syndromes. At the most stable end of the spectrum is chronic stable angina (see Chapter 13). The first of the unstable syndromes is unstable angina, which involves unstable plaque surface or at least some change in the plaque.

Non–Q wave MI, also called *nontransmural* or *subendocardial* MI, is the next level of instability (Table 14-2). Early angiographic studies have demonstrated that the infarct artery is usually open, although tightly stenosed. The plaque surface appears ragged, scalloped, or ulcerated, and thrombus may be present, which appears as a filling defect on the angiogram. The appearance of the plaque is similar to that which causes unstable angina. Patients with stable angina generally have smooth plaque surface. A non–Q wave infarction is relatively small: the peak CK may be just two to three times normal, usually below 600 U. LVEF is either normal or minimally depressed. Injury is localized to the subendocardial region of the heart, the portion of myo-

cardium farthest from the epicardial coronary arteries (see Fig. 5-11). This produces the distinctive ECG pattern of symmetrical T wave inversion, possibly with ST depression during pain (see Fig. 5-11 and Table 5-5).

Your initial report to the patient and family is optimistic: this was a small MI. After all, long-term prognosis is determined by LVEF, reflecting cumulative LV injury. On the other hand, non–Q MI must also be considered an "incomplete" infarction. The tightly stenosed and unstable infarct artery is at risk for thrombosis and occlusion, or "completion of the MI." We learned about this in the 1970s, when multiple studies found that patients with non–Q MI had a 1-year prognosis as poor as those with larger Q wave infarction. In-hospital survival was better, but on medical therapy many of them reinfarcted soon after discharge, suffering the consequences of the larger MI. Because of this, you should consider non–Q MI a step more unstable than unstable angina. The patient should be anticoagulated and have angiography before hospital discharge (Table 14-2).

Q wave infarction begins with occlusion of the infarct artery, transmural ischemia, and ST segment elevation on the ECG (Table 14-2; see Fig. 5-11). Later in the course of infarction, Q waves evolve. The infarction is larger with higher CK levels and a substantial fall in LVEF, particularly with anterior MI. The infarction is "complete." That is, the occluded artery damages all of the muscle that is susceptible to injury, and recurrent injury of that myocardial region is not possible.

The distinction between non–Q and Q wave infarction is not completely reliable. Some patients with transmural ischemia do not develop Q waves (usually with lateral wall MI). Conversely, many patients have Q waves but do not have completed, transmural injury. This is common when infarction is interrupted early in its course by either thrombolytic therapy or angioplasty. In fact, rapid evolution of Q waves is characteristic of

Table 14-2 | *Distinction Between Q Wave and Non–Q Wave Myocardial Infarction (MI)*

MI Type (Alternative Terminology)	Status of the Infarct Artery; ECG	Peack CK*; Location of Injury	Implications for Early (1) and Late (2) Therapy
Q wave (transmural MI)	Occluded artery; ST segment elevation, then Q waves†	>1000; full thickness of the myocardium	(1) Open the blocked artery: reperfusion therapy (see Chapter 15) (2) If MI is complete: "risk stratify" and treat using aspirin, beta-blockers and ACE inhibitors, exercise, and angiography (when appropriate; see Chapter 17)
Non–Q wave (nontransmural or subendocardial MI)	Tightly stenosed artery but with antegrade flow; ST depression, T wave inversion†	<500-900; inner one third of the myocardium	(1) Prevent occlusion: aspirin, heparin; possibly vasodilators and beta-blockers (2) Because this is an unstable syndrome with a risk of early reinfarction: early angiography and revascularization when appropriate

*Assuming that the top normal creatine kinase (CK) =150.
†See Fig 5-11.

early reperfusion. Spontaneous thrombolysis may occur early enough to open the infarct artery and save ischemic myocardium. Regardless of whether early thrombolysis is spontaneous or drug induced (see Chapter 15), the patient is left with incomplete injury and is at risk for recurrent thrombosis and reocclusion. This is the usual mechanism of infarct "extension," or a recurrence of chest pain and ST segment elevation with further injury and release of cardiac enzymes that may occur days after the initial MI.

The exceptions to the rule that Q waves indicate completed MI and the absence of Q's indicates incomplete infarction are thus fairly common, especially in the age of reperfusion therapy. It is important to understand these exceptions, and some have argued that the Q/non-Q categories should be abandoned. However, we believe this classification remains useful because it makes us think in terms of complete and incomplete infarction—a distinction that strongly influences evaluation and therapy (Table 14-2).

CLINICAL PRESENTATION
Triggers of the Onset of MI

The peak incidence of MI is between 6 AM and noon, a pattern that coincides with an elevation of plasma catecholamines and cortisol and an increase in platelet aggregability during the morning hours. Interestingly, patients taking beta-blockers and aspirin who have MI do not exhibit this circadian variation in the timing of infarction. There are a number of well-recognized triggers of MI: heavy physical work, particularly when fatigued

or exposed to environmental extremes (especially the cold); stress, anger, and upsetting life events; hypoxemia of any cause; use of ergot preparations, cocaine and other agents that may provoke coronary spasm (including beta-adrenergic blockers and, rarely, cyclophosphamide and 5-fluorouracil); use of short-acting calcium blockers with a precipitant fall in blood pressure; multiple other illnesses (stroke, hypoglycemia, shock, sepsis); and possibly the abrupt withdrawal of beta-blocker or nitrate therapy. Sexual activity can trigger the onset of MI, but this is uncommon, occurring in less that 1% of cases.[6]

MI develops in less than 10% if patients admitted to the hospital with unstable angina, but approximately one third of patients with MI describe prodromal symptoms during the days or weeks before infarction. In retrospect, they had unstable angina.

History and Physical Examination

Abrupt occlusion of a coronary artery usually causes chest pain. The quality and location of pain are "anginal" (see Chapters 3 and 13). Patients who have had angina and then develop MI usually report that the pain is recognizable as cardiac but that it is more severe. Associated with the pain are diaphoresis and a sense of impending doom. Nausea and vomiting are common, regardless of the location of MI, as is dyspnea.

Silent MI (without any symptoms) accounts for at least 10% of all cases.[7] It is more common in those with diabetes or hypertension and in patients with no history of angina before MI. Silent MI is more often followed by silent ischemia (a positive stress ECG without angina).

Table 14-3	*Killip Classification System*

Class	Mortality(%)	Clinical Definition
I	6	No rales ("no heart failure")
II	17	Rales
III	38	Pulmonary edema
IV	81	Cardiogenic shock

From Killip T, Kimball JT: *Am J Cardiol* 20:457, 1967.

The prognosis of silent MI and MI with symptoms is similar.

On physical examination during MI, the patient is in obvious distress and is often restless. An S_4 gallop usually is present. A soft systolic murmur indicates papillary muscle dysfunction and mitral regurgitation and is more common with inferior and lateral MI. The Killip classification is useful for defining prognosis at the time of presentation and is based on clinical evidence of LV dysfunction[8] (Table 14-3). It is thus important to note the presence or absence of rales. Other signs of LV dysfunction include an S_3 gallop and resting tachycardia (especially in the absence of severe pain).

The importance of sinus tachycardia at rest is often missed. This "arrhythmia" indicates a worse long-term prognosis than does successfully treated ventricular fibrillation. It is a marker of poor LV function, and ventricular fibrillation in the first 24 hours of MI is not.

A transient pericardial friction rub indicating pericarditis is common during the first 3 days after transmural infarction. Pericarditis developing more than 10 days after MI indicates Dressler's syndrome (see Chapter 16). Early pericarditis is more common with large MI and with anterior MI. About 70% of patients with a rub also have pleuritic or positional chest pain.

MANAGEMENT
Laboratory Evaluation

The diagnosis of acute MI is based on the triad of chest pain, ECG changes, and a rise in cardiac enzymes. As noted, not all patients have pain, and not all have ECG changes. When drawn at the appropriate time, a characteristic rise in enzymes is necessary for the diagnosis; that is, normal enzymes would make it difficult to diagnose acute MI.

Cardiac Enzymes

The typical rise and fall of creatine kinase (CK) and other enzymes documents MI. The amount of CK released by damaged myocardium, measured as peak CK

or the area under the CK curve, is proportional to the size of infarction. Because of the delay in CK release, there has been interest in muscle components that reach the circulation earlier after the onset of MI (Table 14-4). Smaller, lower molecular weight molecules appear earlier; myoglobin, about one fifth the weight of CK-MB, may be elevated 1 hour after the onset of chest pain (Table 14-4). Although there is interest in developing molecular markers of infarction that help with early diagnosis, we are not there yet. *None of the available markers is elevated at the onset of infarction. A decision about reperfusion therapy must be made on the basis of the history and the ECG.*

The other major issue regarding cardiac enzymes is specificity. CK, cardiac-specific troponins, and LDH_1 are relatively specific for myocardial damage. There is a small amount of CK-MB in skeletal muscle, and for this reason the ratio of CK-MB to total CK is reported (Table 14-4). An occasional patient with a tiny MI will have a normal total CK but elevation of the CK-MB and the CK/CK-MB ratio. This person has a worse prognosis than another who is suspected of having MI but who has a normal CK-MB and ratio.[9] Stated another way, a coronary lesion that produces an enzyme rise is more unstable than one causing just angina.

Measurement of troponin is now common in community hospitals, although false positives are a problem. Early in its use, we have found that many patients with mild elevation are transferred to a referral center for angiography and are found to have no disease. On the other hand, false negatives are rare, and a negative troponin level effectively excludes MI. A pilot study indicated an excellent 30-day prognosis for patients with no shift in ST segments on the ECG and with two negative troponin measurements, the second being measured at least 6 hours after the onset of chest pain.[10] Such patients may be discharged from the emergency room rather than admitted to hospital. Subsequent outpatient evaluation should be timely.

Concerning the frequency of measurement, we currently measure "cardiac enzymes" at the time of presentation and at 6- to 8-hour intervals. If skeletal muscle also is injured, cardiac-specific troponins may be useful.

Other Laboratory Studies

Total and HDL cholesterol levels remain at baseline for 24 hours after MI. After 48 hours, both fall considerably, with HDL falling more than total cholesterol. For this reason, draw a serum lipid profile on admission or during the first day of MI. If it is not possible to obtain lipid studies within 2 days, wait 8 weeks.

The white cell count begins to rise the day of infarction. It peaks at 2 to 3 days, usually around 12,000/mm³, with a shift to the left. It may rise to 20,000/mm³ with large transmural MI. Low-grade fever may be present as

Table 14-4	*Cardiac Enzymes*

Enzyme	Timing* Earliest	Peak	Myocardial Specific	Comment
Total creatine kinase (CK)	4-8 hours	20-24 hours	No	Falls to normal in 2-3 days. False positives with muscle trauma, injections, vigorous exercise, alcohol intoxication, pulmonary embolism. Peak CK and the area under the CK curve provide estimates of infarct size.
CK-MB	4-8 hours	24 hours	Yes	The small amount of MB in skeletal muscle can cause false positives with strenuous exercise. Ratio of CK-MB/total CK >2.5% suggests a cardiac source.
CK-MB2	2-4 hours		Yes	Earlier appearance of this isoform may allow earlier diagnosis (experimental).
Cardiac-specific troponins (cTnI and cTnT)	3-12 hours	24 hours	Yes	Elevation may persist for 7-14 days. Earlier appearance may help with early diagnosis. More sensitive than CK-MB and thus able to diagnose smaller MI.
Myoglobin	1-2 hours	1-4 hours	No	Earliest appearing but nonspecific. Do not use to diagnose MI in absence of ECG changes.
Lactic dehydrogenase-1 (LDH₁)	8-24 hours	3-6 days	Yes	Total LDH is nonspecific. The heart contains LDH₁. Hemolysis may raise LDH₁. A ratio of LDH₁/LDH₂ >1.0 is sensitive and specific for MI.

*The timing of enzyme changes in the absence of reperfusion therapy. Earliest = time from the onset of MI to the first abnormal value. Normal values vary between laboratories.

well. The erythrocyte sedimentation rate is normal the first couple of days, even in the presence of fever and leukocytosis, and then rises and peaks on the fourth or fifth day. It may remain elevated for weeks.

ECG Patterns of MI

The ECG evolution of both Q wave and non–Q wave infarction is reviewed in Chapter 5 (see Fig. 5-11, 5-16, and 5-17 and Table 5-5). Briefly, coronary occlusion causes ST segment elevation and, subsequently, T wave inversion and Q waves. The pattern of non-Q MI, caused by tight coronary artery stenosis rather than occlusion, is symmetrical T wave inversion. There may or may not be ST segment depression during pain.

Anterior MI

Anterior transmural MI usually is the largest infarction, with the greatest rise in CK and depression of LVEF. The simple reason for this is that the left anterior descend-

ing artery, which supplies the anterior wall and the bulk of the interventricular septum, is the coronary branch supplying the most muscle (see Fig. 2-11). Coronary artery size varies from patient to patient, but, as a rule, most of those who have heart failure after a first infarction had an anterior MI.

It is possible to estimate the size of an anterior MI from the initial ECG: the peak CK and depression of LVEF are proportional to the number of leads with ST segment elevation.[9] Thus a patient with ST elevation in leads V₁₋₃ is having a smaller MI than another with elevation in six to eight leads (Fig. 14-1). Most non–Q wave MIs are located anteriorly, with T wave inversion in the precordial leads.

Inferior MI

The initial ECG also provides an estimate of inferior infarct size, but in a manner different from that for an anterior MI.[11] Rather than the number of leads with ST

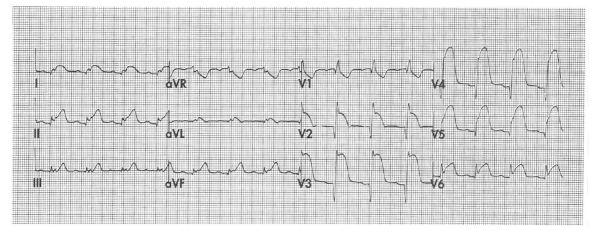

FIG. 14-1
An ECG from a patient with an especially large, acute anterior MI. The number of leads with ST segment elevation is proportional to the size of infarction with anterior MI (as measured by release of CK, or depression of LV ejection fraction). ST segment elevation is present in leads V_{2-6}, as well as in multiple limb leads. The patient died during cardiogenic shock.

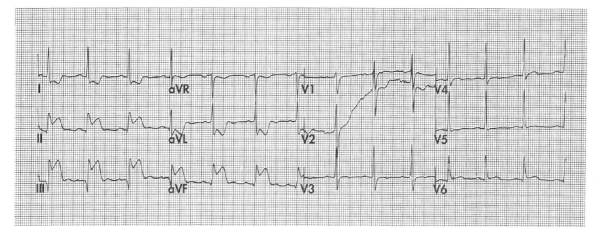

FIG. 14-2
An ECG from a patient with a large inferior MI. With inferior MI, the size of infarction is proportional to the degree of ST segment elevation, and the STs are quite high in this patient's inferior leads. In addition, marked ST segment depression is present in the lateral leads, I and aVL, so-called *reciprocal ST depression*. This is another marker of large inferior MI.

elevation, the sum total of ST elevation in the inferior leads (II, III, and aVF) is proportional to the size of MI. Thus a patient with 3 to 5 mm of ST segment elevation in the three inferior leads is having a much larger MI than another with just 1 to 2 mm of ST elevation (Fig. 14-2).

"Reciprocal" ST segment depression in anterior or lateral leads commonly accompanies inferior ST elevation. The cause of the changes is uncertain. It may be a purely "reciprocal" electrical phenomenon (ST elevation on one side of the heart must lead to depression on the opposite side). "Ischemia at a distance" has been suggested, although patients with these changes commonly have normal blood flow to the anterior and lateral walls. Regardless of the cause, those with reciprocal ST depression tend to have greater CK release and thus larger infarctions.

Right Ventricular Infarction Pattern

The right coronary artery supplies the right ventricular (RV) free wall, as well as the inferior wall of the left ven-

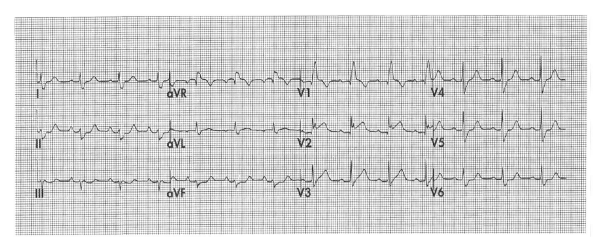

FIG. 14-3
Acute anterior MI plus right bundle branch block. RBBB does not obscure the ST segment elevation seen in leads V₁-₂.

tricle and the base of the interventricular septum. Mild RV dysfunction is common with inferior MI. In some cases it is severe enough to cause RV failure, cardiogenic shock, or both—the RV infarction syndrome. During the acute phase of MI, V leads recorded from the right side of the chest may show ST segment elevation. There may also be mild ST elevation in V_1, but the finding that is both sensitive and specific for RV infarction is ST elevation in V_3R-V_6R. These patients also have ST elevation in the inferior leads.

Lateral MI

The posterolateral wall of the left ventricle tends to be "electrocardiographically silent." Occlusion of a small circumflex artery often does not cause ST segment elevation in lateral leads (see Fig. 5-12). There may be mild ST depression or T wave inversion, which is a pattern more consistent with nontransmural ischemia. Subsequent angiography usually shows circumflex occlusion and akinesis of the lateral wall. The CK usually peaks in the 700 to 1000 range, higher than is usual for non–Q wave infarction. Since there is no ST elevation or Q wave evolution, this technically is a "non–Q wave MI." However, with arterial occlusion and akinesis of the afflicted ventricular segment, these patients have had a "completed" infarction, distinguishing them from those with anterior non–Q wave MI whose infarcts are "incomplete."

Another group of patients have lateral MI but no ECG changes at all. In fact, most patients who have acute MI without ECG changes are having lateral infarction. This is the rationale for observing a patient in the hospital who has *suggestive chest pain but no ECG changes,* at least until serial cardiac enzymes exclude MI.

Anterolateral and Inferolateral Infarction

Acute MI usually affects just one vascular distribution. It would be too great a coincidence for two coronary arter-

ies, supplying two different regions, to occlude simultaneously. When the distribution of infarction spills from the anterior or inferior walls into the lateral wall, it is not because a second artery has occluded; instead, it indicates that the infarct artery, either the right or left anterior descending, is unusually large, with branches to the lateral wall. It reflects variations in coronary anatomy.

Conduction Abnormalities and Patterns of MI

Q waves appear at the beginning of the QRS, and the initial segment of the left ventricle that is depolarized is the interventricular septum. It is possible to discern patterns of infarction when a conduction abnormality develops, as long as it does not disturb septal depolarization. Right bundle branch block (RBBB) affects only the terminal half of the QRS complex and does not influence either the ST segment changes of infarction or the evolution of Q waves (Fig. 14-3).

Left bundle branch block (LBBB) changes the sequence of septal activation, and the usual pattern of ST segment elevation and Q wave formation is altered. New LBBB during acute MI usually indicates occlusion of the left anterior descending artery and a large infarct. The risk of complications is higher than it is for others with anterior MI, and new LBBB is a strong indication for reperfusion therapy.

The best predictor of acute MI in the presence of LBBB is ST segment elevation ≥1 mm in a lead with a positive QRS complex (the vector of the ST segment and the QRS are "concordant"). ST elevation >5 mm in other leads, or ST depression in V_{1-3}, suggests acute MI, but both of these are less specific findings.[12]

TREATMENT

The treatment of patients with acute MI is the subject of the remainder of this, as well as the next three chapters, and the recommendations are consistent with those of the Practice Guidelines of the ACC/AHA Task Force.[13] These guidelines represent a distillation of clinical trials and are thus "evidence based." They are careful to indicate treatment recommendations that are not evidence based and that instead are the consensus of the expert panel.

The most important treatment option soon after the onset of MI is reperfusion therapy. Success depends on the rapidity of its application (see Chapter 15). Having said this, let us review other therapies commonly used during the acute phase of MI.

Prehospital Treatment

About 30% of the deaths from MI occur before the patient reaches the hospital. Ventricular fibrillation (VF) is the usual mechanism, and the risk of VF is highest during the initial 6 hours of infarction. Recognition of symptoms by the patient and early ECG monitoring is the best way to prevent death from early VF. Public education programs that describe the early symptoms of MI are important. In your practice, higher risk patients (those with established CAD or those with multiple risk factors) should be aware of these symptoms. They should be instructed to seek help immediately, even when uncertain about the cause of discomfort.

It is safer for a patient with chest pain to travel to the emergency department (ED) by ambulance, with ECG telemetry, than by family auto. In most locations, the response time is less than 15 to 20 minutes. We are all aware of patients who received successful defibrillation therapy and CPR while in transit. In our community, we believe that the quality of initial resuscitation provided by an Advanced Cardiac Life Support mobile unit is comparable to that of the ED. Generally, reperfusion therapy is begun more rapidly in the ED when patients arrived by ambulance, probably making up for any delay occasioned by waiting for the ambulance to arrive.[14]

Treatment To Start in the Emergency Department (ED) or in the Initial 12 Hours of MI

Oxygen

Little evidence supports the efficacy of oxygen for those who do not have hypoxemia, and it is not identified as a critical therapy in the Practice Guidelines.[13] However, patients often describe improvement in pain with oxygen treatment. Because there is little risk with nasal oxygen 2 to 4 L/min, there is no reason to omit this traditional treatment. It has been common practice to continue oxygen for a couple days or longer. If oximetry shows normal saturation on room air, there is no reason to continue oxygen beyond 12 hours (and stopping it at this time saves money). Another sensible approach would be to stop oxygen as soon as the patient is pain free and has normal arterial oxygen saturation.

Aspirin

Barring a history of drug allergy, one adult aspirin (325 mg) should be given immediately on arrival in the ED. In fact, aspirin is commonly administered by the ambulance team in the field. (If your patient contacts you before calling 911, recommend an aspirin while the ambulance is en route.) Have the patient chew the aspirin so that it is absorbed more rapidly. The ISIS-2 trial reported that one chewed aspirin reduced 30 day mortality by 23%, similar to that achieved with intravenous streptokinase, and mortality was 42% lower when aspirin was given with streptokinase.[15] Its effectiveness highlights the role of platelets in the earliest stage of coronary thrombosis. Continued therapy lowers the risk of rethrombosis after coronary reperfusion, and practice guidelines indicated that 160 g per day is an adequate maintenance dose. In practice, we usually give one adult tablet (325 mg) daily, as enteric-coated aspirin tablets usually are not scored.

Control of Pain

Initial treatment of a patient with a palpable pulse and adequate blood pressure with sublingual nitroglycerin is fine, even before obtaining an ECG. If you are in fact treating angina (with an open but stenosed coronary artery) rather than MI (with an occluded artery), there may be prompt relief of pain. Hypotension after nitroglycerin is easily managed by recumbency. If it persists, elevate the patient's legs.

Morphine is the preferred analgesic, barring a history of allergy. Meperidine is less effective, has similar side effects, and tends to increase heart rate more. Like nitroglycerin, morphine is a venodilator and thus lowers preload. A drop in blood pressure is prevented and treated by placing the patient in a supine position or by raising the legs. The most common error we see with morphine treatment is *inadequate dosing.* Give 4 to 8 mg morphine intravenously and follow this with 2 to 8 mg at 5 to 15 minutes until relief of pain improves. Anxiety and restlessness also may improve, and autonomic output is blunted. Some patients require large doses of morphine for relief, as much as 2 to 3 mg/kg, and such doses usually are tolerated. Patients with cardiac pain or pulmonary edema have a low risk of respiratory depression with morphine. If you are concerned about *morphine toxicity* as a cause of hypotension, severe nausea, or respiratory depression, the effects of morphine are rapidly reversed using naloxone 0.1 to 0.2 mg intravenously and repeated in 10 to 15 minutes if needed.

Beta-Adrenergic Blockers

During the acute phase of MI, patients may respond to intravenous beta-blockers with prompt relief of pain and a reduction in ST segment elevation. Randomized trials have shown a reduction in mortality (by 15%), as well as reinfarction (19%) and cardiac arrest (19%).[16]

The greatest survival benefit is seen during the first day after MI. In contrast, studies of survival after thrombolytic therapy show no improvement in survival in the first 24 hours, with beneficial effects emerging over the next week. There may thus be a complementary role for beta blockade and reperfusion therapy. Lower mortality and less reinfarction have been reported when intravenous metoprolol is given within 2 hours of the onset of MI, compared with starting it in the late hospital phase (day 6). Early treatment also lowered the incidence of intracranial hemorrhage.[17]

An important mechanism of benefit is the reduction of heart rate. In the absence of heart failure, tachycardia during acute MI is a strong indication for beta blockade. The use of beta-blockers in the acute phase of MI is summarized in Table 14-5. If there is concern about the risk or uncertainty about a contraindication, such as a history of bronchospasm, use the short-acting agent, esmolol, 50 to 250 μg/kg/min.

Intravenous Nitroglycerin

During the early phase of acute MI, intravenous nitroglycerin reduces preload, left ventricular wall tension, and therefore myocardial oxygen demand. This limits infarct size and prevents infarct expansion. Intravenous nitroglycerin also may dilate collaterals and improve flow to the infarct zone. The key to therapy, as described by Jugdutt and colleagues,[18] is the titration of intravenous nitroglycerin to specific hemodynamic end points aimed at reducing preload, but without lowering mean arterial pressure below 80 mm Hg (or systolic blood pressure below 105 to 110 mm Hg). If arterial pressure is lowered further, nitroglycerin has no beneficial effect, possibly because of reduced coronary artery perfusion pressure. The goal is preload, not afterload, reduction. Maximal benefit occurs when treatment is begun within 4 hours of the onset of MI. The average dose of nitroglycerin using this protocol was 45 (g/min (range 4 to 192 (μg/min).[18] Hypotension was infrequent with the cautious titration schedule (Table 14-6). Those with inferior MI were more apt to have hypotension and require close monitoring, and intravenous nitroglycerin is *not* recommended for those with the RV infarction syndrome.

Although the study was randomized, it came from a single center and was small.[18] The patients did not have reperfusion therapy, so the applicability of nitroglycerin as adjunctive therapy is untested. Other, larger studies have not confirmed a survival benefit, and the routine use of intravenous nitroglycerin cannot be considered well established. On the other hand, we agree with Rappaport[19] that evidence against efficacy is shaky. The randomized studies showing no benefit were flawed by large numbers of patients in the placebo groups "crossing over" and receiving intravenous nitroglycerin.[18]

The rationale for intravenous nitroglycerin during acute MI seems compelling to us. Using it to improve hemodynamics during acute infarction is sensible *if the doctor and nursing team are able to properly monitor blood pressure and heart rate and titrate the dose.* We especially like it in patients with systolic blood pressure above 120 to 130 mm Hg, where there is "room for maneuver." It is applicable to those with large infarction (where the

---

Table 14-5	**Beta-Adrenergic Blockade During the Acute Phase of Myocardial Infarction (MI)**
Patient selection	Acute MI, <12 hours from the onset of pain
Contraindications	Heart failure (rales >10 above the diaphragm) Heart rate <60 beats/min Heart block (PR >0.24 second) Systolic blood pressure <90 mm Hg Asthma or obstructive lung disease with wheezing
Dose	*Metoprolol* 5 mg IV at 5-min intervals × three doses (no repeat IV dose if the heart rate falls to <60 beats/min or blood pressure <100 mm Hg), then 100 mg po qid for 48 hours, then 100 mg po bid *Atenolol* 5 mg IV infused over 5 min, repeat in 10 min (no second dose if heart rate or blood pressure falls), then 50 mg po 10 minutes later, then 50 mg po bid
Benefits	Blunts catecholamine effects, lowering heart rate, blood pressure, and contractility. This reduces MVO_2 and thus infarct size. Improved survival also may be the result of less ventricular fibrillation and LV rupture (not proven by clinical trials).

risk of infarct expansion is greatest) and for those with congestive heart failure (when beta blockade may be contraindicated). Nitroglycerin does not depress heart rate or contractility, so it can be used with beta-blockers; since both may depress blood pressure, careful monitoring is imperative.

Early ACE Inhibition

Starting ACE inhibitors 3 or more days after MI prevents infarct expansion and improves LV function and survival for patients with large MI (see Chapter 17). Subsequent trials of therapy begun during the first 24 hours have shown an additional survival benefit for patients with large anterior MI (with ST segment elevation, not with the non–Q wave infarct pattern).[19] ACE inhibitors are drugs that depresses blood pressure and therefore must be used with caution in patients who also may have been given intravenous beta-blockers or nitroglycerin (Table 14-7).

Which of these drugs that reduce infarct size should you use? No drug combination protocol has been studied, and there is no established algorithm. Use of medicines with clear evidence of benefit is sensible (Table 14-8). The addition of other agents depends on the patient's condition, particularly heart rate and blood pressure. Heart failure and renal dysfunction also influence the choice of drugs (Table 14-8).

Lidocaine

Prophylactic lidocaine for patients who are in the hospital is no longer recommended. Randomized trials showed that patients given lidocaine had less ventricular fibrillation. However, because they were in the critical care unit and had access to DC cardioversion, there was no survival benefit.[20] Separate studies have shown that the incidence of VF during early infarction may be falling; this is further evidence against lidocaine prophylaxis.[21]

Prophylactic lidocaine is justified in some clinical settings. We use it when CCU care is interrupted, for example, in patients who are being transferred to another hospital during the first 12 hours of MI or in those who are having emergency procedures in the catheterization laboratory. The medicine does work; consider it when defibrillation would be difficult.

The half-life of an initial bolus injection of lidocaine is brief, just minutes. Thus a bolus must be followed by a continuous infusion. On the other hand, if a patient has been taking lidocaine for more than 6 hours and it is then stopped, the half-life is a half day. For this reason, it makes no sense to "wean" a patient from lidocaine. Best to stop it first thing in the morning, with the knowledge that the patient will drift into the subtherapeutic range at midday (when staffing is good and you are not at home asleep).

Frequent or complex ventricular premature beats (VPBs >6/ min, multiform VPBs, triplets, or R on T VPBs) in the early phase of MI indicate an increased short-term risk of ventricular fibrillation and are indications for lidocaine.

Anticoagulation

Full-dose intravenous heparin is included in the Practice Guidelines for those with large anterior MI for the prevention of peripheral embolization, and it may be continued to the time of discharge. If an echocardiogram shows ventricular mural thrombus or a large akinetic segment, warfarin (Coumadin) should be started before discharge. This anticoagulation regimen may be used for patients with dilated and poorly contracting ventricles as well.

Table 14-6	*Intravenous Nitroglycerin During the Acute Phase of Myocardial Infarction (MI)**
Patient selection	Acute MI <12 hours from the onset of pain Large MI including anterior MI and MI with associated heart failure MI with persistent ischemia
Contraindications	Cardiogenic shock, mean arterial pressure <80 mm Hg or systolic pressure <105-110 mm Hg; heart rate >110 beats min; RV infarction syndrome
Dose	Start with 5 μg/min Increase the dose at 10-min intervals to lower mean arterial pressure by 10% in normotensive and 30% in hypertensive patients *Do not lower systolic pressure below 105-110 mm Hg* Decrease the dose if heart rate increases by 10 beats/min, or to >110 beats min
Duration	Continue intravenous nitroglycerin for 48 hours

*Evidence-based support for this therapy is mixed; see text.

Table 14-7	*Angiotensin-Converting Enzyme (ACE) Inhibitor Therapy During the First Day of Myocardial Infarction (MI)*
Patient selection	Patients with anterior transmural MI (with ST segment elevation)
Contraindication	Hypotension, allergy; caution with elevated creatinine or known renovascular disease
Dose	Captopril 6.25 mg po, then 12.5 mg 2 hours later, then 25 mg 10-12 hours later, then 50 bid mg starting the next day
Duration of treatment	Continue after hospital discharge; discontinue if ECG 6-12 weeks later shows good LV function with LVEF >40%

Table 14-8	*Drugs That Improve Survival or Limit Infarction Size When Given in the Early Phase of Acute Myocardial Infarction (MI)*

Drug	Evidence for Efficacy	Patients Who May Benefit	Patients Who May Be Harmed
Coronary thrombolysis	Strong	MI and ST segment elevation or new bundle branch block (see Chapter 15)	Contraindications, see Chapter 16.
Aspirin	Strong	All with suspected MI*	Allergy or contraindication to aspirin
Intravenous beta-blockers	Strong	All with suspected MI,* those with tachycardia	Those with hypotension, bradycardia, heart block, heart failure, bronchospasm
Intravenous nitroglycerin	Equivocal†	Those with anterior MI, ongoing ischemia,* heart failure	Those with hypotension, tachycardia, or RV infarction
Oral ACE inhibitors	Equivocal†	Those with anterior MI and ST segment elevation	Those with hypotension, elevated creatinine.

*If the patient is having unstable angina rather than MI, therapy is still helpful.
†Some but not all clinical trials indicate efficacy.

Low-dose heparin (5000 U every 12 hours) may be given to those at bed rest for the prevention of pulmonary embolus. It usually is possible to stop it at 48 hours. For high-risk patients it should be continued until they are fully ambulatory (high risk: age ≥70, large MI, heart failure, prolonged bed rest, obesity, prior venous disease or pulmonary embolus, physical signs of venous insufficiency).

Calcium Channel Blockers

Most randomized trials found no survival benefit from calcium channel blockade during *transmural (Q wave) infarction.*[19] There was a trend toward increased mortality with nifedipine. In contrast, studies of diltiazem and verapamil showed a trend toward less reinfarction. Nifedipine, a pure vasodilator, causes reflex tachycardia, and the other two drugs depress the sinoatrial node and

slow the heart rate. As a rule, drugs that decrease heart rate appear beneficial after MI.

Diltiazem has been shown to reduce the chance of reinfarction for those with *non–Q wave MI.* The Diltiazem Reinfarction Study treated patients with 360 mg diltiazem per day (in four doses) and delayed angiography for 14 days for study purposes. There was less reinfarction and angina in the treated group than in the placebo group.[22] Patients in this study had angiography after the 2 weeks of observation. There is no reason to delay angiography that long, and this study does not provide a useful treatment model. On the other hand, many patients with non–Q wave MI are not candidates for angiography or revascularization (e.g., those with complicating conditions including excessive frailty). The study shows that diltiazem treatment may lower the short-term reinfarction risk by 50%. It also identifies diltiazem as a useful early therapy to use while the workup is in progress, as when angiography is delayed (e.g., over a holiday weekend).

Hemodynamic Monitoring

Severe or progressive heart failure, hypotension, and cardiogenic shock are the usual indications for right heart catheterization and hemodynamic monitoring. At times, the cause of hypotension is uncertain, and measurement of LV filling pressure distinguishes between LV failure (where it is high) and inadequate LV preload (where is low, as with the RV infarction syndrome). Arterial pressure monitoring is used to monitor patients on vasopressor therapy and those with severe hypotension.

Right heart catheterization is also useful when managing rupture of the interventricular septum or acute papillary muscle dysfunction and severe mitral regurgitation.

The Decision To Transfer a Patient to the Tertiary Care Facility

Recurrent pain, severe congestive heart failure, hypotension or shock, and resistant arrhythmias are good reasons for urgent transfer for interventional treatment (see Chapter 16). Patients who have contraindications to thrombolytic therapy (see Chapter 15) but who are candidates for angioplasty should be transferred immediately, hoping to achieve reperfusion within 6 hours of the onset of MI. Reperfusion as late as 10 to 12 hours also may improve survival.

Development of a new systolic murmur, indicating either ventricular septal defect or mitral regurgitation, necessitates urgent catheterization and hemodynamic monitoring (see Chapter 16).

When a decision is made that a *stable* patient is to have angiography and possible revascularization before hospital discharge, consider transfer sooner rather than later. The day after MI is a good time, since the risk of new arrhythmias is low. There is no good reason to delay transfer, and there is the chance that new problems will develop while waiting (usually in the middle of the night). Considering the logistics of most catheterization and surgical programs, earlier transfer ensures timely study and avoids prolonged hospitalization. This is particularly true when approaching a weekend or holiday.

REFERENCES

1. American Heart Association: *Heart and stroke facts: 1998 statistical supplement,* Dallas, 1998, American Heart Association.
2. Gheorghiade M, Razumma P, Borzak S, et al: Decline in the rate of hospital mortality from acute myocardial infarction: impact of changing management strategies, *Am Heart J* 131:250, 1996.
3. Rogers W, Bowlby L, Chandra N, et al: Treatment of myocardial infarction in the United States (1990 to 1993): observations from the National Registry of Myocardial Infarction, *Circulation* 90:2103, 1994.
4. Topal EJ: Toward a new frontier in myocardial reperfusion therapy: emerging platelet preeminence, *Circulation* 97:211, 1998.
5. Little WC, Constantinescu M, Applegate RJ, et al: Can coronary angiography predict the site of a subsequent myocardial infarction in patients with mild-to-moderate coronary artery disease? *Circulation* 78:1157, 1988.
6. Muller JE, Mittleman MA, Maclure M, et al: Triggering myocardial infarction by sexual activity: low absolute risk and prevention by regular physical exertion. Determinants of Myocardial Infarction Onset Study Investigators, *JAMA* 275:1405, 1996.
7. Sigurdsson E, Thorgeirsson G, Sigvaldason H, et al: Unrecognized myocardial infarction: epidemiology, clinical characteristics, and the prognostic role of angina pectoris: the Reykjavik study, *Ann Intern Med* 122:96, 1995.
8. Killip T, Kimball JT: Treatment of myocardial infarction in a coronary care unit: a 2-year experience with 250 patients, *Am J Cardiol* 20:457, 1967.
9. Yusuf S, Collins R, Lin L, et al: Significance of elevated MB isoenzyme with normal creatine kinase in acute myocardial infarction, *Am J Cardiol* 59:245, 1987.
10. Hamm CW, Goldmann BU, Heeschen C, et al: Emergency room triage of patients with acute chest pain by means of rapid testing for cardiac troponin T or troponin I, *N Engl J Med* 337:1648, 1997.
11. Aldrich HR, Wagner B, Boswick J, et al: Use of initial ST-segment deviation for prediction of final electrocardiographic size of acute myocardial infarct, *Am J Cardiol* 61:749, 1988.
12. Sgarbossa EB, Pinski SL, Barbagelata A, et al: Electrocardiographic diagnosis of evolving acute myocardial infarction in the presence of left bundle branch block, *N Engl J Med* 334:481, 1996.
13. Gunnar RM, Bourdillon PDV, Dixon DW, et al: Guidelines for the early management of patients with acute myocardial infarction. a report of the ACC/AHA Task Force on Assessment of Diagnostic and Therapeutic Cardiovascular Procedures, *J Am Coll Cardiol* 16:249, 1990.
14. Califf RM, Newby LK: How much do we gain by reducing time to reperfusion therapy? *Am J Cardiol* 78(suppl 12A):8, 1996.
15. ISIS-2 Collaborative Group: Randomized trial of intravenous streptokinase, oral aspirin, both, or neither among 17,183 cases of suspected acute myocardial infarction: ISIS-2, *J Am Coll Cardiol* 12:3, 1988.
16. Yusef S, Peto R, Lewis J, et al: Beta blockade during and after myocardial infarction: an overview of the randomized trials, *Prog Cardiovasc Dis* 27:335, 1985.
17. Roberts R, Rogers WJ, Mueller HS, et al: Immediate versus deferred beta-blockade following thrombolytic therapy in patients with acute myocardial infarction: results of the Thrombolysis in Myocardial Infarction (TIMI) II-b Study, *Circulation* 83:422, 1991.

18. Jugdutt BI, Warnica JW: Intravenous nitroglycerin therapy to limit myocardial infarct size, expansion, and complications: effect of timing, dosage, and infarct location, *Circulation* 1988; 78: 906-919.

19. Rapaport E: Pharmacologic therapy for acute myocardial infarction: which agent, how much, how soon, how long? *Postgrad Med* 102:143, 1997.

20. MacMahon S, Collins R, Peto R, et al: Effects of prophylactic lidocaine in suspected acute myocardial infarction: an overview of results from the randomized, controlled trials, *JAMA* 260:1910, 1988.

21. Antman EM, Berlin JA: Declining incidence of ventricular fibrillation in myocardial infarction: implications for the prophylactic use of lidocaine, *Circulation* 86:764, 1992.

22. Gibson RS, Boden WE, Theroux P, et al: Diltiazem and re-infarction in patients with non–Q wave myocardial infarction. *N Engl J Med* 315:423, 1986.

15 Reperfusion Therapy for Acute Myocardial Infarction

George J. Taylor
Jerome J. Epplin

Reperfusion therapy is the standard of care for myocardial infarction (MI) with ST segment elevation. You must be able to use it if you treat patients with acute MI, especially if you are the first doctor to evaluate the patient. Chest pain usually begins within 5 minutes of coronary artery occlusion, and myocardial cell death is progressive beyond that point. With each quarter hour that passes, more heart muscle is lost. Early reperfusion saves more lives than later reperfusion[1] (Fig.15-1). That is the unequivocal message of trials that have carefully studied the effect of time to treatment on both cardiac function and survival. The patient in the emergency department (ED) does not have time to wait for the cardiologist to arrive and make a decision. If you are in the ED with a patient, you must be the treating physician.

THROMBOLYTIC THERAPY FOR ACUTE MI
Lessons From Clinical Trials
Coronary Thrombolysis Saves Lives

The mortality trials that compared intravenous thrombolytic therapy with placebo were conducted in the mid-1980s, with the largest of them testing streptokinase[1] (STK, Fig. 15-1). The survival benefits of treatment are convincing enough that it would be unethical to repeat placebo-controlled survival trials using newer thrombolytic agents. More recent studies are head-to-head comparison trials to determine relative efficacy of newer drugs and drug combinations.

When therapy is begun within 4 hours of the onset of MI with currently used agents and front-loaded dosing, and the addition of modern adjunctive therapy, we estimate a 30% to 50% reduction in 35-day mortality for large MI with ST segment elevation and a hospital mortality rate of 4% to 6%.

Thrombolysis Saves Heart Muscle

Another series of studies compared thrombolytic therapy and placebo and used left ventricular (LV) function as the end point.[2-4] LV ejection fraction (LVEF) was 5 to 8 percentage points higher with thrombolysis. As you would expect, those with the largest MI obtained the greatest benefit. Patients with anterior MI

had an increase in LVEF of 8 to 12 percentage points, and others with inferior MI had an increase of only 2 to 5 percentage points. This pattern of maximal benefit for a patient with large MI holds true with other benefits of thrombolysis, including prevention of death, heart failure, or serious arrhythmia. As a general rule, it is difficult to show a survival benefit with any medical treatment in a population with a low mortality risk.

Earlier Treatment Improves Outcome

Maximal benefit is achieved with early therapy; mortality is barely reduced if treatment is received more than 12 hours after the onset of MI[5,6] (Fig. 15-1 and Table 15-1). Treatment within the first hour of MI is especially effective, since myocardial injury rapidly progresses immediately after arterial occlusion. Many believe that little muscle is saved with reperfusion beyond 4 hours. There may be more effective lysis with early treatment. A fresh thrombus could be easier to lyse than a clot that has had a few more hours to organize.

The importance of early treatment is the rationale for public education programs urging those with chest pain to seek prompt attention. Hospitals are revising ED protocols in an effort to shorten time to therapy to ≤ 30 from the time of arrival, and time to therapy is monitored as a performance indicator.[6,7]

However, the goal is not just to treat the patient quickly, but instead to achieve excellent and complete (TIMI grade 3) flow quickly. The angiography substudy of the GUSTO-I trial found that the short-term survival benefit was limited to patients who had TIMI grade 3 flow (defined as brisk, rapid flow with good run-off) 90 minutes after starting therapy. There was little survival benefit with sluggish or marginal flow (TIMI grades 1 and 2) to the infarct zone.[8] For this reason, research efforts are aimed at developing new drugs and drug combinations that achieve rapid and optimal flow.

An Open Infarct Artery Improves Prognosis

The importance of saving muscle, which happens with early reperfusion, cannot be overemphasized. However, many have shown that an open infarct artery after

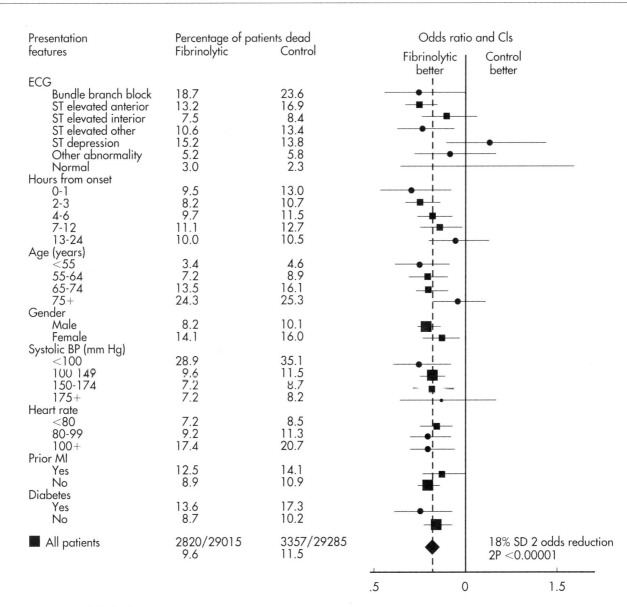

Presentation features	Percentage of patients dead		Odds ratio and Cls
	Fibrinolytic	Control	
ECG			
Bundle branch block	18.7	23.6	
ST elevated anterior	13.2	16.9	
ST elevated interior	7.5	8.4	
ST elevated other	10.6	13.4	
ST depression	15.2	13.8	
Other abnormality	5.2	5.8	
Normal	3.0	2.3	
Hours from onset			
0-1	9.5	13.0	
2-3	8.2	10.7	
4-6	9.7	11.5	
7-12	11.1	12.7	
13-24	10.0	10.5	
Age (years)			
<55	3.4	4.6	
55-64	7.2	8.9	
65-74	13.5	16.1	
75+	24.3	25.3	
Gender			
Male	8.2	10.1	
Female	14.1	16.0	
Systolic BP (mm Hg)			
<100	28.9	35.1	
100-149	9.6	11.5	
150-174	7.2	8.7	
175+	7.2	8.2	
Heart rate			
<80	7.2	8.5	
80-99	9.2	11.3	
100+	17.4	20.7	
Prior MI			
Yes	12.5	14.1	
No	8.9	10.9	
Diabetes			
Yes	13.6	17.3	
No	8.7	10.2	
■ All patients	2820/29015	3357/29285	18% SD 2 odds reduction
	9.6	11.5	2P <0.00001

FIG. 15-1

Proportional effects of thrombolytic therapy on 1-month mortality after acute MI. Pooled data from nine randomized, placebo-controlled trials including 58,600 patients.

From Fibrinolytic Therapy Trialists' (FTT) Collaborative Group: *Lancet* 343:311, 1994.

thrombolytic therapy is an independent predictor of survival, unrelated to LV function and the salvage of muscle. This "open artery hypothesis" suggests that even *late* opening of the infarct artery may promote myocardial healing.[9-10] Flow in the infarct artery may provide "vascular scaffolding," allow more efficient delivery of inflammatory cells, promote scar formation, and prevent infarct expansion. Early treatment would provide both benefits of reperfusion: salvage of muscle plus the effects of the open artery. The explanation for some benefit with late treatment is that there is little or no salvage of muscle, but a small benefit from the open artery.

Mortality Is a Function of Multiple Clinical Risk Factors

Reperfusion therapy lowers the mortality risk for many patients with acute MI, but a patient's chance of dying is primarily determined by age, sex, infarct location, history of prior MI, diabetes, and LV function at the time of MI (see Fig. 15-1) Recognition of these risk factors provides a basis for patient selection.

Pathophysiology of Reperfusion

Reperfusion Injury

Animal studies have shown that transient coronary occlusion followed by abrupt reperfusion of the ischemic

Table 15-1	Time from the Onset of Myocardial Infarction to Thrombolytic Therapy and Survival

Time to Therapy (hr)	Number of Lives Saved per 1000 Patients Treated
0-1	35
2-3	25
4-6	19
7-12	16
12-24	none*

From Fibrinolytic Therapy Trialists' (FTT) Collaborative Group: *Lancet* 343:311, 1994.
*No survival difference comparing thrombolytic therapy with placebo.

region leads to additional myocardial injury. Reperfusion has three possible negative effects.[11] The first is *microvascular damage* that may contribute to the "no-reflow" phenomenon, or a blunting of distal flow despite an open coronary artery. Injured small vessels are leaky, leading to hemorrhagic infarction (although the region of hemorrhagic infarct has not been shown to extend beyond the area of necrosis). Finally, coronary vasodilator reserve is diminished because of ischemic injury to small vessel (see Chapter 2).

A second effect is *stunned myocardium,* the prolonged contractile dysfunction that follows reperfusion. This is attributed to disordered intracellular biochemistry that is further altered by reperfusion.

Reperfusion Arrhythmias

The third negative action of reperfusion is the "electrical storm" that develops immediately with restoration of flow, or *reperfusion arrhythmias.* Accelerated idioventricular ventricular rhythm (AIVR) is common and has been suggested as a marker of reperfusion. It is generally benign and tends not to degenerate to ventricular fibrillation (VF). The mechanism of AIVR is discharge from an automatic focus. VF is caused by reentry, which is a different mechanism. Although it is possible for VF to occur with reperfusion, it is unusual, and prophylactic lidocaine is not recommended. A review of large trials found that thrombolytic therapy does not increase the risk of VF.[12] Bradyarrhythmias with reperfusion may develop in patients with inferior MI, possibly as a result of the Bezold-Jarisch reflex.

The Illusion of Reperfusion

An angiogram showing an open infarct artery soon after thrombolytic therapy suggests but does not prove a benefit to the patient. Some have "no reflow," or poor flow through small vessels at the myocardial level despite flow in the epicardial artery. This manifestation of microvascular injury may appear on an angiogram as slow washout of contrast from the artery and infarct zone.

Others snatch defeat from the jaws of victory by re-occluding the open infarct artery, usually without recurrence of chest pain. Reocclusion of an initially patent infarct artery was reported in 29% of patients in one trial who had repeat angiography 3 months later. Only 20% of them had recurrent chest discomfort.[13] Those with silent reocclusion had a worse clinical course. *Silent ischemia* after thrombolysis is common, as transient ischemia followed by reperfusion stuns cardiac pain receptors, just as it does myocardium.[14]

Inadequate initial flow and reocclusion have led to the suggestion that as few as one third of patients receiving thrombolytic therapy achieve optimal and sustained reperfusion.[25]

Indications for Thrombolytic Therapy

Weighing the benefits and risks forms the basis for patient selection for any treatment—doctors and their patients must play the odds. MI may be fatal, so high-risk therapy may be justified. The chance of dying of some heart attacks is higher than with others. As noted in Figure 15-1, clinical trials have shown that thrombolytic therapy improves survival for those with higher but not lower risk infarction. In fact, patients who have chest pain and suspected MI, but who had either no ECG changes or a pattern of non–Q wave infarction, had an increase in mortality with thrombolytic therapy.

Patient selection is not quite as simple as just interpreting the ECG. Many other clinical features influence mortality during MI, including advanced age, heart failure, female sex, diabetes, and a history of prior infarction. Table 15-2 provides a hierarchy of MI risk plus a list of clinical features that might persuade you to choose reperfusion therapy for a patient with a borderline ECG indication.

Specific Patient Selection Issues
Inferior Myocardial Infarction

Many patients having a first infarction have an inferior MI. As infarction of the inferior wall tends to injure less muscle than anterior MI, the short-term mortality risk is much lower. With low mortality it is difficult to show a survival benefit with reperfusion therapy. The clinical trials demonstrating improved survival with reperfusion did not stratify those with inferior MI into high- and low-risk groups. It is probable that patients in the higher risk category have a survival benefit (this would include patients with large MI, Table 15-2), whereas those in the low-risk group with a mortality risk of less than 4% would not benefit.[16]

Table 15-2	Risk of Death from Myocardial Infarction (MI) and Patient Selection for Reperfusion Therapy

Hierarchy of MI Risk	Clinical Features That Increase Risk of MI and Would Favor Reperfusion Therapy
HIGHEST RISK, DEFINITELY TREAT Anterior MI with ST elevation Large inferior MI* Acute MI with new bundle branch block	Cardiogenic shock (Killip class IV) Pulmonary edema (Killip class III) Rales (Killip class II) History of prior MI History of heart failure Right ventricular infarct syndrome Diabetes
LOWER RISK, consider therapy based on other clinical features Small inferior MI with ST elevation* MI with ST depression or T wave inversion with pain unresponsive to conventional therapy[†]	

*Large inferior MI: marked (as opposed to minimal) ST elevation in inferior leads plus reciprocal ST depression in anterior or lateral leads, or ST elevation in right precordial leads indicating the RV infarction syndrome (see Chapter 13). Small inferior MI: minimal ST elevation in inferior leads, no reciprocal ST depression.
†Including nitrates, chewed aspirin, and beta-blockers given in the acute setting.

Recall that these studies examined short-term mortality. When considering long-term survival, salvage of muscle may be important. Think of the patient's baseline LV function when dealing with a subsequent MI 5 to 10 years later. For this reason, we are biased in favor of treating a young person with a moderately sized inferior MI when it is possible to treat early. If therapy is to be applied late in the course of MI, more than 4 hours after the onset of pain, the risks of thrombolytic therapy for a small inferior MI may exceed benefits.

Inferior Myocardial Infarction and Hypotension

Acute inferior MI is often accompanied by vagal discharge, which causes bradycardia, nausea, and hypotension. This responds to intravenous fluid replacement (normal saline is our first choice) and atropine if the heart rate is low. A vagal reaction during inferior MI does not contraindicate thrombolytic therapy.

Hypotension may also indicate RV failure secondary to RV infarction. The mortality rate with this form of cardiogenic shock is greater than 30%.[16] RV infarction is complicated by high-degree AV block in about half the patients. Other complications of MI also are more common, including ventricular septal rupture, RV thrombus, and pulmonary embolus. Interestingly, most with RV infarction also have significant LV dysfunction. RV infarction has not been the subject of randomized trials because of small numbers of patients, but there is consensus that early reperfusion therapy helps. Recall that the diagnosis is made quickly by right precordial ST segment elevation and is suggested by ST elevation in V_1 (see Chapter 13).

Acute Myocardial Infarction without ST Segment Elevation and Unstable Angina

Studies of reperfusion therapy for non–Q wave MI, or presumed MI with ST and T wave changes, have shown no survival benefit (see Fig. 15-1). This comes as no surprise, since clinical experience has taught us that chest discomfort usually is relieved by aggressive antianginal therapy (nitrates, aspirin, beta blockade) and then heparin. Angiography during the acute phase of non-Q infarction and in those with unstable angina usually shows a patent, though tightly stenosed artery. Thrombolytic therapy is not required to improve flow and interrupt ischemia.

If a patient with symmetrical T wave inversion or ST depression continues to have pain after initial treatment, our first step is to reconsider the diagnosis. If the ST and T wave changes are new, and we are convinced that myocardial ischemia is responsible for the pain, we would consider thrombolysis or angioplasty. If the diagnosis is doubt, angiography and possible angioplasty would be safer than thrombolytic therapy.

Ischemic Chest Pain and No ECG Changes

Lateral MI may not cause ST segment deviation (see Chapter 14). For this reason, a normal ECG does not exclude MI. Fortunately, the small lateral infarctions that present in this manner are low risk. It is doubtful that thrombolytic therapy would favorably influence mortality, and it is not indicated.

Consider other diagnoses. Severe chest discomfort with diaphoresis also can be caused by aortic dissection or esophageal rupture, illnesses in which thrombolysis could be fatal. There is one other thing to do in this situation: *repeat the ECG*. It is common for patients with subtle or no ECG changes to have clear-cut ST elevation on a repeat ECG 15 to 30 minutes later.

Advanced Age

Although patients over the age of 65 have a greater risk of dying of an acute MI, we did not include advanced age as a factor that weighs in favor of thrombolytic therapy (see Table 15-2). The reason for this is that elderly people also have an increased risk of hemorrhagic stroke following thrombolysis. The risk of stroke for those in the GUSTO-I trial who were younger than 65 years old was 0.8%, between 65 and 74 years, 2.1%, and between 75 and 85 years, 3.4%.[17] The chance of other bleeding complications is greater as well.

An increased risk of stroke is not a reason to avoid thrombolytic therapy, but it does indicate a need for meticulous attention to contraindications to therapy and to careful patient selection. Our experience with community hospitals is that most of the elderly who are treated are healthy and active. We see few doctors using this aggressive treatment strategy for debilitated patients living in nursing homes.

The higher risk of stroke justifies thrombolysis only when it will clearly help: early therapy for a large MI in a patient whose health has been good. The chance of treatment doing much good is small if it is started more than 6 hours from the onset of symptoms. However, when used appropriately in elderly patients there is a survival advantage with timely thrombolysis.[17]

Chest Pain Has Resolved but ST Segment Elevation Persists

Symptoms may wax and wane during the initial stage of MI. During the intracoronary streptokinase era we were able to observe the coronary artery while monitoring symptoms and the ECG. We often saw arteries open and then reocclude. Many patients did not have a return of pain with reocclusion despite reelevation of ST segments. In a sense, the patient developed "silent ischemia," possibly because of stunned pain receptors.[14] If a patient is within 6 hours of the onset of MI and still has ST elevation, proceed with thrombolytic therapy. On the other hand, if a patient has had chest pain all night, which resolves the next day, and the STs are still elevated, we would be less inclined to treat, since this sounds more like a completed MI. Patients treated late are more susceptible to myocardial rupture.[18]

Persistent Chest Pain and ST Elevation, but Q Waves Have Evolved

One misconception is that Q waves always indicate completed injury. With reperfusion, and even with transient reperfusion, Q waves may develop in minutes. It is not unusual to see Q waves soon after the onset of MI, early enough in the course of infarction for there still to be viable muscle. Qs do not contraindicate thrombolytic therapy, nor do they reliably indicate that it is too late to save muscle.

Late Treatment

What about the patient who has had pain for 12 hours and still has ST segment elevation? Reperfusion therapy may relieve persistent pain, but do the risks counterbalance any benefit? Clinical trials showed no benefit when thrombolysis is given more than 12 hours after the onset of MI[1] (see Fig. 15-1). The LATE study specifically addressed this issue and showed a small benefit when recombinant tissue plasminogen activator (rt-PA) was given between 6 and 12 hours after the onset of symptoms, but not after 12 hours.

An important clinical issue is the potential increase in myocardial rupture with late thrombolysis (≥ 12 hours from the onset of MI).[18] Rupture may also be more common in those treated with antiinflammatory agents, both steroidal and nonsteroidal. Other complications of thrombolysis occur with similar frequency in patients treated early and late.

In clinical practice we avoid thrombolytic therapy for those having lower risk MI unless it can be given within 6 hours of the onset. For higher risk infarctions, we do not hesitate to treat as late as 12 hours. Beyond 12 hours we might treat a patient with continued pain and ST elevation who is having a high risk MI and who is at low risk for complications. Frankly, it is a judgment call, and in that setting we are careful to explain not only risks and benefits, but also that the indication for therapy is marginal. We would prefer angioplasty to thrombolysis for late reperfusion because of the chance of myocardial rupture.

Contraindications to Thrombolytic Therapy (Box 15-1)

The most important patient selection issue is the risk of bleeding. Many risks are relative. A patient with a high risk MI and a relative contraindication possibly should have thrombolysis, whereas another having a small, first infarction should not. Most bleeding is minor, occurring at vascular puncture sites. As a rule it can be controlled with local pressure.

Intracranial hemorrhage is the worst complication, with an incidence of about 0.75% in the large clinical trials.[20] When the usual contraindications to therapy are followed, especially a history of prior stroke, an indi-

---

BOX 15-1
CONTRAINDICATIONS TO THROMBOLYTIC THERAPY

SYNDROMES MIMICKING MI THAT CARRY A HIGH RISK OF BLEEDING
Peptic esophagitis
Pericarditis
Aortic dissection
Intracranial bleeding with T wave changes

ABSOLUTE CONTRAINDICATIONS
Active internal bleeding
History of cerebrovascular accident
Recent (within 2 mo) intracranial or intraspinal surgery or trauma
Intracranial neoplasm, arteriovenous malformation, or aneurysm
Known bleeding diathesis
Severe uncontrolled hypertension

RELATIVE CONTRAINDICATIONS
Recent (within 10 days) major surgery, e.g., coronary artery bypass graft, obstetric delivery, organ biopsy,
   previous puncture of noncompressible vessels
Cerebrovascular disease
Recent gastrointestinal or genitourinary bleeding (within 10 days)
Recent trauma (within 10 days)
Hypertension: systolic BP $\geq$180 mm Hg and/or diastolic BP $\geq$110 mmHg
High likelihood of left heart thrombus, e.g., mitral stenosis with atrial fibrillation
Acute pericarditis
Subacute bacterial endocarditis
Hemostatic defects including those resulting from severe hepatic or renal disease
Significant liver dysfunction
Pregnancy
Diabetic hemorrhagic retinopathy or other hemorrhagic ophthalmic conditions
Septic thrombophlebitis or occluded atrioventricular cannula at seriously infected site
Advanced age, i.e., over 75 yr
Patients currently receiving oral anticoagulants, e.g., warfarin sodium
Any other condition in which bleeding consitutes a significant hazard or would be particularly difficult to
   manage because of its location

---

vidual's chance of hemorrhagic stroke increases with any of four different risk factors: age >65 years, weight <70 kg, hypertension on presentation (systolic pressure $\geq$170 mm Hg or diastolic pressure $\geq$95 mm Hg), and use of rt-PA rather than streptokinase.[20] The probability of bleeding was related to the number of these risk factors: 0.26% with none, 0.96% with one, 1.32% with two, and 2.17% with three. Thus a small, elderly person with hypertension had an eightfold increase in the risk of hemorrhagic stroke when compared with a young person with no stroke risk factors. Note that these clinical trials excluded patients with contraindications, including "uncontrolled hypertension," which most stud-

ies defined as sustained systolic pressure >200 mm Hg or diastolic pressure >110 mm Hg (Box 15-1). If you mistakenly treat patients with prior stroke or uncontrolled hypertension, a higher incidence of intracranial hemorrhage may be expected.

This analysis of stroke risk is useful but possibly incomplete. For example, stroke risk is continuous with advancing age; an 80-year-old has a 50% higher risk than a 65-year-old.[17] It is likely that severe hypertension with some end-organ disease confers a much higher risk of stroke than mild to moderate hypertension. Guidelines from large trials are helpful, but clinical judgment is still necessary.

Other Contraindications

Invasive Procedures. Recent surgery and percutaneous biopsy of lung, pleura, liver, or kidneys are strong contraindications to thrombolysis. If less than 2 weeks from the procedure, count on bleeding. At 3 to 6 weeks after the procedure the risk of bleeding still is high, and the decision to use thrombolytic therapy should be related to the risk of the MI. Would you consider thrombolysis in a patient with recent cardiac catheterization? Possibly, because bleeding from the groin can be controlled with local pressure. The ability to control bleeding enters into the assessment of risk. Angioplasty as therapy for MI would be preferable for those with an excessive bleeding risk.

Coagulation Disorders. The risk of bleeding appears related to the severity of the disorder. A prior history of bleeding indicates higher risk. A borderline low platelet count is not a contraindication to thrombolysis. Some hospitals still make the mistake of requiring the results of coagulation studies before starting thrombolytic therapy. In the absence of a history of bleeding diathesis, waiting for these laboratory results unnecessarily delays treatment of the MI.

Cardiopulmonary Resuscitation (CPR). Patients with acute MI who have ventricular fibrillation and brief periods of CPR can be treated with thrombolytic agents with reasonable safety. On the other hand, if CPR is prolonged beyond 10 minutes or if obvious chest wall trauma occurs during CPR or intubation, the bleeding risk increases. (Again, weigh the risk of the MI.) Thrombolytic therapy should not be given as a part of a prolonged resuscitation attempt.

Diabetic Retinopathy. Our ophthalmology colleagues believe there is an increased risk of intraocular bleeding with thrombolysis, although the complication has not been mentioned even by the larger studies. Retinopathy remains a relative contraindication, and we would recommend thrombolysis only for those with high-risk MI.

Menstruation. We have treated a few patients in their forties during menstruation, and excessive bleeding has not been a problem. Bleeding can be attenuated with hormonal therapy and could be considered for the menstruating patent with a high-risk MI. We would not consider thrombolysis for pregnant patients or those within 1 month postpartum. Consider angioplasty instead.

Anticoagulation or Prior Thrombolytic Therapy. Warfarin therapy should not contraindicate coronary thrombolysis for those with high-risk MI. It would be one reason to avoid it for low-risk infarction. Aspirin is not a contraindication. Prior treatment with STK leads to antibody formation, and such patients should be treated with rt-PA, which is not antigenic.

Pharmacology of Thrombolytic Therapy

Damage to plaque surface exposes collagen, which, in turn, activates platelets and leads to the formation of a platelet plug. This also triggers the clotting cascade, whose end product is thrombin, a protease that mediates conversion of fibrinogen to fibrin. Fibrin is bound to the platelet plug and is the insoluble, noncellular, fibrous component of thrombus. It is a natural process that allows repair of vascular injury, but it is also the pathologic process that leads to formation of occlusive thrombus on the surface of ulcerated plaque.

Clot formation and dissolution are in dynamic equilibrium. When thrombus forms, its size must be limited; it cannot be allowed to propagate indefinitely. Thrombus that forms in vessels or in ureters must eventually be removed to restore patency. This is the role of the thrombolytic, or fibrinolytic, system; as soon as thrombus forms, the fibrinolytic system is activated.

Fibrinolysis works at three possible sites: the hemostatic plug that seals a defect in a vessel wall, the pathologic intravascular thrombus, and circulating fibrinogen (where it is more accurately called *fibrinogenolysis*). Plasminogen is the precursor of the active fibrinolytic enzyme, plasmin. Plasminogen is converted to plasmin by "plasminogen activators." These include the naturally occurring substances, tissue plasminogen activator (t-PA) and urokinase, as well as the foreign compound, streptokinase.

Plasminogen is produced by the liver and is found in the circulation in a "free" state. When clot forms, this free plasminogen is incorporated into the thrombus and is bound to fibrin. The ideal thrombolytic agent would move into the thrombus and work only on fibrin-bound plasminogen, but most of the thrombolytic agents activate free, circulating plasminogen as well, producing plasmin and the so-called "lytic state" (Fig. 15-2). Free plasmin digests circulating fibrinogen and other clotting factors, producing an hypocoagulable state.

Thrombolytic Drug Preparations

Streptokinase (STK) works on both circulating and fibrin-bound plasminogen and thus produces a lytic state. Following streptokinase treatment, fibrinogen levels are markedly depleted. Because it is a foreign compound, it is antigenic, and allergic reactions occur in 1.7% of patients treated. It should not be used if STK was administered during the previous year. Transient hypotension develops in 10%, responding to recumbency or elevation of the legs. This vasodilator response is not an allergic reaction.

Anisoylated plasminogen streptokinase activator complex (APSAC) was designed to have greater tissue affinity and longer half-life than STK. The compound has greater tissue activity, but in clinical trials it proved equally anti-

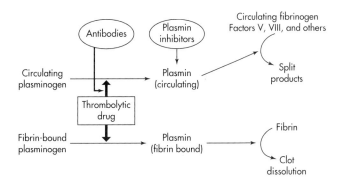

FIG. 15-2
Sites of action of thrombolytic drugs. Ideally, thrombolytics move into the thrombus and activate fibrinbound plasminogen, leading to prompt clot dissolution. In varying degrees, and depending on tissue affinity, thrombolytic drugs also work on circulating plasminogen, producing free plasmin. Free plasmin may also dissolve clot, but it also lyses circulating fibrinogen and other clotting factors. High levels of free plasmin and low levels of circulating fibrinogen constitute the "lytic state." Plasmin inhibitors may neutralize circulating plasmin, and antibodies may neutralize streptokinase.

From Taylor GJ: *Thrombolytic therapy for acute myocardial infarction*, Cambridge, Mass, 1992, Blackwell Science.

genic and no more efficacious than STK. Because of its expense it is rarely used.

Urokinase is an endogenous protein found in urine. It has less fibrin affinity than other agents, and uptake into thrombus is limited. It thus induces a systemic lytic state and relies on the free plasmin that is formed to digest thrombus. It is no more effective than STK in opening occluded coronary arteries, and no clinical trials have established a survival benefit. It is not approved for intravenous treatment of acute MI.

Tissue plasminogen activator, either native (t-PA) or recombinant (rt-PA), works primarily at the tissue level on fibrin-bound plasminogen, so there is less depletion of circulating fibrinogen. It relies on fibrin as a cofactor, and when bound to fibrin, its activity in cleaving (activating) plasminogen is increased 500-fold. That is why it is referred to as a "clot specific," or "tissue level" plasminogen activator. When not bound to fibrin and free in the circulation, it is not as potent. Fibrinogen is somewhat depleted during rt-PA treatment because of the huge dose of rt-PA that is given relative to physiologic, circulating levels of native t-PA. However, patients are not as hypocoagulable as they are after STK therapy, and anticoagulation is necessary after infusion of rt-PA.

There are two available forms of tissue plasminogen activator: recombinant t-PA (alteplase) and its mutant form, reteplase. The altered structure of reteplase results in slower clearance, so it can be given as a bolus rather than as a continuous intravenous infusion.

Choice of Agent

The GUSTO-1 study (the mother of all clinical trials, with 41,021 patients) showed that rt-PA (alteplase) is more effective than STK when front-loaded dosing is used[21] (Table 15-3). The 14.6% reduction in 30-day mortality with rt-PA is probably explained by more rapid and complete thrombolysis. Angiography 90 minutes after starting therapy showed a higher rate of TIMI grade 3 flow in the rt-PA group.[22] The newer t-PA preparation, reteplase, has efficacy and risks similar to alteplase.[23] It may be given as two intravenous bolus injections, and our nurses find this more convenient than the 90-minute infusion of alteplase. The cost of the two drugs is similar.

An often discussed drug selection issue is the increase in hemorrhagic stroke with rt-PA, raising the possibility that elderly patients who have a higher risk of stroke should be treated with STK (see the earlier discussion of older patients). A careful analysis of the data indicates that for patients less than 85 years old, rt-PA treatment is better than STK in lowering the combined rate of death and disabling stroke (there are a few more strokes, but many fewer deaths, for a net clinical benefit).[17] An elderly patient with a large anterior MI who can be treated early, especially within 1 to 2 hours from the onset of symptoms, would clearly benefit from more rapid thrombolysis with rt-PA. On the other hand, if therapy is begun more than 4 hours from the onset of MI, there is less muscle salvage, and the benefits of thrombolysis may be limited to other effects of an open infarct artery.[9] Speed of thrombolysis is less critical with late therapy, and STK would be a reasonable choice, especially when the risk of stroke is higher than usual.[28] Tailoring thrombolytic therapy to the risk of the MI (see Table 15-2), the risk of complications, and the timing of treatment applies to younger patients as well.[24]

A practical note: The nuances of drug selection may elude you in the middle of the night when dealing with an acutely ill patient. *When in doubt, you cannot go wrong using one of the t-PA preparations.* Dosing schedules for STK and the t-PAs are presented in Table 15-3.

Adjunctive Therapy and Hospital Management after Thrombolysis
Antiplatelet Therapy

The ISIS-2 trial established that chewed aspirin at the time of presentation increases survival for those treated with STK[25] (Fig. 15-3). Platelet inhibition has a number of beneficial effects. First, thrombolytic drugs work on fibrin, and there is little fibrin in the fresh clot. This platelet-rich thrombus is relatively resistant to fibrinolytic therapy, because aggregated platelets secrete plasminogen activator inhibitor-1 (PAI-1), which blocks fibrinolysis (Fig. 15-3). Second, when fibrin is lysed, there is exposure of thrombin. Thrombin is a potent activator

Table 15-3	*Intravenous Fibrinolytic Agents*			
Drug	**Cost***	**Dose**		**Adjunctive Therapy**
Streptokinase	$511	1.5 million IU in 45 ml, infused within 1 hour. Some recommend an initial loading bolus of 50,000-100,000 IU.		1. Aspirin 325 mg, chewed immediately 2. Intravenous or subcutaneous heparin of no proven benefit
rt-PA (alteplase)	$1925	15 mg bolus, then 0.75mg/kg for 30 min (to a maximum of 50 mg), then 0.5 mg/kg for the next 60 min (to a maximum of 30 mg).		1. Aspirin as above 2. Intravenous heparin 5000 U bolus, then 1000 U per hour (reduce to 800 U per hour for those who weigh <80 kg)
Mutant rt-PA (reteplase)	$1950	Two bolus doses of 30 MU given 30 minutes apart		1. Aspirin as above 2. Heparin as above

*Average cost to your hospital pharmacy. In most hospitals the cost is marked up. We are aware of some that charge twice this amount. That may not be a problem for a third-party payer, who negotiates the charge, but remember this when working on the behalf of the self-pay patient.

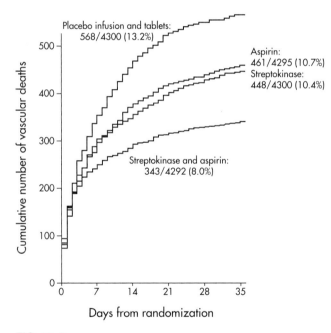

FIG. 15-3
The ISIS-2 trial consisted of four study groups: placebo, aspirin, streptokinase, and streptokinase plus aspirin. Chewed aspirin was as effective as streptokinase. The result secures the role of antiplatelet therapy as an important adjunct to coronary thrombolysis.

From ISIS-2 Collaborative Group: *Lancet* 2:349,1988.

of platelets, so fibrinolysis has the paradoxical, procoagulant effect of promoting platelet aggregation.[26]

Unlike thrombolytic therapy, the survival benefit with aspirin does not depend on early therapy. Those treated within 4 hours and other treated 12 to 24 hours after the onset of MI both had a 20% to 25% reduction in mortality. Because of its low risk, aspirin can be used in those with suspected MI or when the diagnosis is uncertain.

Low-dose aspirin effectively inhibits cyclooxygenase and reduces thromboxane A_2. However, this requires several days of therapy with a 75 mg dose. For this reason a loading dose, 160 to 325 mg, is given during acute MI. The aspirin is chewed, since buccal absorption produces a more rapid blood level. Prescribe an aspirin suppository (325 mg) if a patient is vomiting. After MI continue aspirin therapy indefinitely. The 75 mg dose is effective, and may cause fewer gastric side effects than 325 mg. Enteric-coated preparations also work.

In the early stage of acute MI, an antiplatelet strategy appears more important than a "red clot," antithrombotic strategy. However, aspirin has only a modest antiaggregatory effect on platelets during the acute phase of MI. The GUSTO-1 trial found that only 54% of patients had achieved TIMI grade 3 flow in the infarct artery after 90 minutes of rt-PA plus aspirin therapy. Pilot studies suggest that more effective antiplatelet agents produce more rapid and complete thrombolysis, with TIMI class 3 flow in >80% (Table 15-4). It is possible that lower dose t-PA (to minimize the procoagulant effect of fibrinolysis) plus aggressive platelet inhibition will emerge as the ideal thrombolytic regimen.[26]

Antithrombotic Therapy

Thrombolysis stimulates thrombin generation. (This is a general theme: clot dissolution and formation are simultaneous processes, and one provokes the other.) Clinical trials have documented no benefit when heparin is given after streptokinase. Of course, the patient is

Table 15-4	*Platelet Glycoprotein IIb/IIIa Inhibitors*

Agents	Mechanism
Abciximab (ReoPro)	An antibody fragment that directly blocks the receptor
Integrilin	A peptide that competes with the receptor's primary ligand, fibrinogen
Tirofiban, lamifiban, sibrafiban, lefradafiban, xemilofiban, orbofiban, and others	Small molecules that are also competitive inhibitors

*The glycoprotein (GP) receptor on the surface of the platelet is the final common pathway for platelet aggregation. Stimulation of platelets leads to activation of the receptor.

anticoagulated, as STK induces a lytic state, and there is marked depletion of fibrinogen and other clotting factors. Antiplatelet therapy is critical, but heparin is not.

On the other hand, those treated with t-PA preparations have less fibrinogen depletion and are not anticoagulated. Heparin therapy is essential after treatment with rt-PA (both alteplase and reteplase, Table 15-4), and the aPTT should be in the therapeutic range, 1.5 to 2 times control. It is common for the aPTT to be longer during the first 24 hours. *Do not interrupt heparin therapy or reduce the dose.* Instead, recheck the aPTT at 24 hours and adjust the dose.[21] It is noteworthy that earlier trials comparing STK and rt-PA showed similar effects of the two drugs. The difference that was shown by the GUSTO-1 trial may be explained by adequate heparin therapy for patients treated with rt-PA. (Note: when antithrombotic therapy is combined with STK, aPTT 100 seconds is a risk factor for hemorrhagic stroke.[20] Nevertheless, we agree with the GUSTO protocol, which continues heparin during the 24 hours after rt-PA therapy regardless of the aPTT.)

The more effective, direct antithrombotic agent, hirudin, has been studied and found no better than heparin as an adjunct to STK therapy for MI with ST segment elevation. Newer antithrombotics, both hirudin and hirulog, appear superior to heparin for treating other unstable coronary syndromes, including non–Q wave MI and unstable angina.[27] These were long-term studies of medical therapy that did not include angiography and revascularization, our usual approach with high-risk patients. They are mentioned because they indicate the utility of the "red-clot," antithrombotic strategy in addition to platelet inhibition for unstable coronary syndromes in which there is continued antegrade flow. For acute MI with a fresh, occlusive thrombus, fibrinolysis plus a "white-clot" strategy (platelet inhibition) appears more important.

Other Medical Therapy

Beta-adrenergic blockade during acute MI has been shown to reduce mortality in patients not receiving thrombolytic therapy (see Chapter 14). The TIMI-2 trial evaluated intravenous metoprolol as an adjunct to coronary thrombolysis and found no effect on survival or LV function.[28] Cases of recurrent ischemia and reinfarction were decreased. We use beta blockade for those with sinus tachycardia or hypertension if there is no evidence of heart failure (Table 14-4).

Calcium channel blockers, intravenous nitroglycerine, angiotensin-converting enzyme inhibitors, and intravenous magnesium have been proposed as treatment that may reduce infarct size. None has been shown to augment the benefits of reperfusion therapy.

Assessment of Reperfusion and Prognosis

Coronary angiography is the gold standard for identifying an open infarct artery after thrombolytic therapy. Relief of pain, when dramatic, is a fair marker of reperfusion. However, many with an open artery and myocardial salvage continue to have some discomfort, and there is often uncertainty based on symptoms. Reperfusion arrhythmias have not proved reliable markers, either. With reperfusion, there is rapid washout of CK-MB and other enzymes from the infarct zone, and this, combined with relief of chest discomfort and reduction in ST segment elevation, provides the best noninvasive index of reperfusion.

Improvement in ST segment elevation is an indicator of better prognosis after thrombolysis. Those with <50% reduction in ST elevation 1 hour from the start of therapy had worse LV function, increased morbidity, and higher short- and long-term mortality.[30] Another study found that <30% reduction in ST segment elevation at 3 or 4 hours indicated persistent coronary occlusion, lower LVEF, and higher mortality.[30] Yet another stratified resolution of ST elevation as complete

(<30% residual elevation), partial (30% to 70% residual elevation), or none (70% residual elevation). Patients with complete resolution at 3 hours had a 35-day mortality of just 2.5%. Mortality doubled in the group with partial resolution, and was ninefold higher in those with no resolution.[30] Thus repeating the ECG at 1 and 3 hours after starting thrombolytic therapy is useful for estimating prognosis. It is noteworthy that reteplase was more effective in achieving early and complete resolution of ST elevation than was streptokinase in one of these trials.[30]

Assessment of prognosis after MI is reviewed in Chapter 17. These principles generally apply to patients who have had thrombolytic therapy. Evidence for residual ischemia, based on exercise testing or ambulatory ECG monitoring, would be an indication for early angiography. Other important clinical indicators of poor prognosis have included advanced age, heart failure, and angina. When studied together with careful monitoring of ST segment resolution and either exercise ECG or ambulatory ECG, thallium 201 exercise testing did *not* provide additional prognostic information. In one study, those with high-risk scans fared no worse than the group with low-risk scans.[30] Perfusion imaging does not appear a necessary element of evaluation after thrombolysis.

Angiography and Revascularization

Ideally, angiography would be recommended for patients with successful thrombolysis and salvage of myocardium who are at high risk for reocclusion. Others could be treated medically. It may be possible to identify treatment failure: late application, no resolution of pain or ST elevation, and slow washout of CK-MB (or another of the cardiac enzymes). If this is clear cut, medical therapy to optimize LV function and reduce morbidity would be reasonable.

For many, perhaps a majority of patients, the status of the infarct artery is uncertain. Exercise testing may be misleading; one study reported that ST depression with exercise was more common with an occluded than an open infarct artery.[31] You not only want to identify the patient with an open infarct artery, but also the one at risk of reocclusion. Perfusion imaging does not reliably identify a patient with a poor prognosis.[31] Because of uncertainty, the trend in clinical practice has been angiography for a majority after coronary thrombolysis.

The TIMI-2 trial is the most influential study of revascularization, and it found no benefit with an invasive treatment strategy compared with a conservative approach that used medical therapy.[28] The invasive strategy included early angiography for all, and subsequent revascularization for the 66% considered to have critical stenosis of the infarct artery and viable muscle in the in-

farct zone. It might be assumed that TIMI-2 indicates that revascularization, and therefore angiography, are unnecessary after thrombolytic therapy.

There are a few problems with this interpretation. The first has to do with the management of patients in the conservative wing of the study. These patients were not sent home after the heart attack without evaluation. All of them had an exercise radionuclide angiogram before hospital discharge to look for residual ischemia. Those with a positive exercise ECG or scan had angiography.

If you elect to follow the conservative treatment model of TIMI-2, you must incorporate a similar exercise study pre-discharge as a screen for ischemia.

We see three possible explanations for similar outcomes in the conservative and aggressive treatment groups in TIMI-2. First, a large number of patients in the conservative wing crossed over; within a year of MI, 39% had revascularization, and twice that had angiography.

Second, TIMI-2 was not a trial of revascularization, but of culprit lesion angioplasty. Angioplasty was the technique used for 86%, and only 14% had bypass surgery. Patients with recent MI often have high-risk lesions, with ragged plaque surface and thrombus. Follow-up angiography was not a part of the study, and we wonder about reocclusion after angioplasty using what are now considered primitive techniques. Percutaneous coronary revascularization has undergone radical change at the end of the century. A trial from the 1980s makes no sense as a guide to treatment in a new era that includes stenting and more effective antiplatelet therapy.

Finally, because of recent MI and stunned nerves, reocclusion after angioplasty would have been clinically silent in 70% to 80% of patients.[13,14] We agree that TIMI-2 has shown that an initial strategy of balloon angioplasty after thrombolytic therapy is no better than medical treatment, but it has not excluded benefits of early coronary bypass surgery or newer catheter-based techniques.

A more recent Danish trial randomized patients with inducible ischemia after thrombolysis to invasive or conservative strategies.[32] There was less crossover from medical therapy to angiography and revascularization. The invasive strategy halved the rate of reinfarction, reduced unstable angina by 40%, and mortality by 18% (the mortality result was not significant in this small study).

Only a few U.S. centers follow the TIMI-2 conservative strategy for *all* patients. We, like others, recommend angiography for patients with moderate or large MI who appear to have reperfused.[33] Patients with small inferior MI, or those who do not seem to have opened the infarct artery, may have screening for residual ischemia (exercise testing with an imaging study, ambulatory ST segment monitoring where it is available), reserving angiography for patients with a positive study. Revascularization is recommended when there is evidence of an incomplete infarction, based on time to treatment, creatine kinase curve, response of ST segments, or persistence of contractility in the infarct zone.[33] This is the approach that made sense, clinically, a decade ago, and it has been widely adopted.[33,34]

PRIMARY ANGIOPLASTY

Angioplasty is an effective method for opening the infarct artery, and it works faster than thrombolytic therapy. Patients who come to our emergency department with acute MI have at least a 90% chance of having an open infarct artery within 60 minutes if they can be taken directly to catheterization. No study of thrombolytic drug therapy comes close to that result, and it is the approach that we take whenever possible. The problem, of course, is logistical. Accomplishing the goal—an open artery within 60 minutes—requires an open catheterization laboratory and a qualified team that is ready for the patient. Most programs are not organized to provide 24-hour or weekend service. Most important, only a minority of patients are initially treated in hospitals with angioplasty services. The time required to transfer the patient removes the major advantage of the procedure, speed.

The GUSTO-2b trial compared primary angioplasty with rt-PA therapy and found a lower 30-day risk of a composite end point including death, reinfarction, and nonfatal disabling stroke (9.6% vs. 13.7%). However, at 6 months no difference was demonstrated between the two treatments, and the report points to a "small-to-moderate, short-term clinical advantage" with angioplasty.[35] The study was conducted in 57 experienced international centers, and although not specifically reported, we expect that most of the patients presented initially to the hospital with the catheterization laboratory. Median time to angioplasty from onset of symptoms was 3.8 hours, about 2 hours after arrival at the hospital. (This means they frequently waited for a catheterization laboratory to become available.) On the plus side, more than 75% of those having angioplasty achieved TIMI grade 3 flow, and this subset of patients with excellent flow had a 30-day mortality of just 1.6%.

This result supports the use of angioplasty when it can be done quickly by an experienced team. On the other hand, we do not find the results compelling enough to either warrant delay of treatment or to justify cross-country transfer for a midnight balloon. Nor would it indicate a need to install catheterization laboratories at major crossroads. Despite enthusiasm for this technique (and interventional cardiologists love their work), we expect that most patients with acute MI in the United States will be properly treated in the emergency departments of community hospitals using thrombolytic therapy. The emphasis in your practice and in your hospital should be on rapid treatment.

REFERENCES

1. Fibrinolytic Therapy Trialists' (FTT) Collaborative Group: Indications for fibrinolytic therapy in suspected acute myocardial infarction: collaborative overview of early mortality and major morbidity results from all randomised trials of more than 1000 patients, *Lancet* 343:311, 1994.
2. White HD, Norris RM, Brown MA, et al: Effect of intravenous streptokinase on left ventricular function and early survival after acute myocardial infarction, *N Engl J Med* 317:850, 1987.
3. Bassand JP, Machecourt J, Cassagnes J, et al: Multicenter trial of intravenous APSAC in acute myocardial infarction: effects on infarct size and left ventricular function, *J Am Coll Cardiol* 13:988, 1989.
4. Guerci AD, Gerstenblith G, Brinker JA, et al: A randomized trial of intravenous tissue plasminogen activator for acute myocardial infarction with subsequent randomization to elective coronary angioplasty, *N Engl J Med* 317:1613, 1987.
5. Tiefenbrunn A, Sobel B: Timing of coronary recanalization: paradigms, paradoxes, and pertinence, *Circulation* 85:2311, 1992.
6. Califf RM, Newby LK: How much do we gain by reducing time to reperfusion therapy? *Am J Cardiol* 78 (suppl 12A):8, 1996.
7. Moses HW, Bartolozzi JJ, Koester DL, et al: Reducing delay in the emergency room in administration of thrombolytic therapy for myocardial infarction associated with ST elevation, *Am J Cardiol* 68:251, 1991.
8. The GUSTO Angiographic Investigators: The effects of tissue plasminogen activator, streptokinase, or both on coronary artery patency, ventricular function, and survival after acute myocardial infarction, *N Engl J Med* 329:1615, 1993.
9. Kim C, Braunwald E: Potential benefits of late reperfusion of infarcted myocardium: the open artery hypothesis, *Circulation* 88:2426, 1993.
10. Lamas GV, Flaker GC, Mitchell G, et al: Effects of infarct artery patency on prognosis after acute myocardial infarction, *Circulation* 92:1101, 1995.
11. Kloner RA: Does reperfusion injury exist in humans? *J Am Coll Cardiol* 21:537, 1993.
12. Solomon SD, Ridker PM, Antman EM: Ventricular arrhythmias in trials of thrombolytic therapy for acute myocardial infarction: a meta-analysis, *Circulation* 88:2575, 1993.
13. Meijer A, Verheugt FWA, Werter CJPJ, et al: Aspirin versus Coumadin in the prevention of reocclusion and recurrent ischemia after successful thrombolysis: a prospective placebo-controlled angiographic study: results of the APRICOT study, *Circulation* 68:251, 1993.

14. Taylor GJ, Katholi RE, Womack K, et al: Increased incidence of silent ischemia after acute myocardial infarction, *JAMA* 268:1448, 1992.
15. Lincoff AM, Topol EJ: Illusion of reperfusion: does anyone achieve optimal reperfusion during acute myocardial infarction? *Circulation* 87:1792, 1993.
16. Bates ER: Revisiting reperfusion therapy in inferior myocardial infarction, *J Am Coll Cardiol* 30:334, 1997.
17. White HD, Barbash GI, Califf RM, et al: Age and outcome with contemporary thrombolytic therapy: results from the GUSTO-1 trial, *Circulation* 94:1826, 1996.
18. Honan MB, Harrell FE Jr, Reimer KA, et al: Cardiac rupture, mortality, and the timing of thrombolytic therapy: a meta-analysis, *J Am Coll Cardiol* 16:359, 1990.
19. LATE Study Group: Late assessment of thrombolytic efficacy (LATE) study with alteplase 6-24 hours after onset of acute myocardial infarction, *Lancet* 342:759, 1993.
20. Simoons M, Maggioni A, Knatterud G, et al: Individual risk assessment for intracranial hemorrhage during thrombolytic therapy, *Lancet* 342:1523, 1993.
21. The GUSTO Investigators: An international randomized trial comparing four thrombolytic strategies for acute myocardial infarction, *N Engl J Med* 329:673, 1993.
22. The GUSTO Angiographic Investigators: The effects of tissue plasminogen activator, streptokinase, or both on coronary artery patency, ventricular function, and survival after acute myocardial infarction, *N Engl J Med* 329:1615, 1993.
23. The GUSTO-3 Investigators: A comparison of reteplase with alteplase for acute myocardial infarction, *N Engl J Med* 337:1118, 1997.
24. Simoons ML, Arnold AE: Tailored thrombolytic therapy: a perspective, *Circulation* 88:2556, 1993.
25. ISIS-2 Collaborative Group: Randomized trial of intravenous streptokinase, oral aspirin, both, or neither among 17,187 cases of suspected acute myocardial infarction: ISIS-2, *Lancet* 2:349, 1988.
26. Topol EJ: Toward a new frontier in myocardial reperfusion therapy: emerging platelet preeminence, *Circulation* 97:211, 1998.
27. Chesebro JH: Direct thrombin inhibition superior to heparin during and after thrombolysis: dose, duration, and drug, *Circulation* 96:2118, 1997.
28. The TIMI Study Group: Comparison of invasive and conservative strategies after treatment with intravenous tissue plasminogen activator in acute myocardial infarction: results of the Thrombolysis in Myocardial Infarction (TIMI) Phase II Trial, *N Engl J Med* 320:618, 1989.
29. Christenson RH, Ohman M, Topol EJ, et al: Assessment of coronary reperfusion after thrombolysis with a model combining myoglobin, creatine kinase-MB, and clinical variables, *Circulation* 96:1776, 1997.
30. Pepine CJ: Prognostic markers in thrombolytic therapy: looking beyond mortality, *Am J Cardiol* 78 (suppl 12A):24, 1996.
31. Stevenson R, Ranjadayalan K, Robert H, et al: Failure of post infarction exercise testing to predict coronary anatomy after thrombolysis: significance of reciprocal ST depression, *J Am Coll Cardiol* 21:87, 1993.
32. Madsen JK, Grande P, Saunamski K, et al: Danish multicenter randomized study of invasive versus conservative treatment in patients with inducible ischemia after thrombolysis in acute myocardial infarction (DANAMI), *Circulation* 96:748, 1997.
33. Guetta V, Topol EJ: Pacifying the infarct vessel, *Circulation* 96:713, 1997.
34. Taylor GJ, Mikell FL, Moses HW, et al: Intravenous versus intracoronary streptokinase therapy for acute myocardial infarction in community hospitals, *Am J Cardiol* 54:256, 1984.
35. The GUSTO IIb Angioplasty Substudy Investigators: A clinical trial comparing primary coronary angioplasty with tissue plasminogen activator for acute myocardial infarction, *N Engl J Med* 336:1621, 1997.

16 Complications of Myocardial Infarction

George J. Taylor
Sarah E. Stapleton

CARDIOGENIC SHOCK

Before the reperfusion era, cardiogenic shock developed in about 20% of patients with myocardial infarction (MI), and the mortality rate was as high as 80% (see Table 14-3, from the classic study of Killip and Kimble). With modern therapy, the incidence has fallen to 7%. Effective circulatory support and early revascularization have lowered the mortality rate to about 40%.[1] Still, left ventricular failure and cardiogenic shock remain the leading cause of in-hospital death from MI.

Pathophysiology

In 80% of cases, shock is caused by excessive damage to the left ventricle (LV). Autopsy studies have shown that the pump loses its ability to maintain blood pressure when 40% of the LV is infarcted. The remaining cases result from other mechanical complications of MI (Table 16-1). It is important to recognize these quickly, since the treatment approach may be different.

When LV injury, or pump failure, causes cardiogenic shock, it initiates a series of potentially harmful compensatory responses. An increase in sympathetic tone and activation of the renin-angiotensin system raise peripheral vascular resistance and ventricular afterload, further depressing LV function (see Chapter 2). The drop in arterial pressure lowers coronary perfusion pressure, aggravating ischemia; this further depresses LV contractility. Unfortunately, most patients with cardiogenic shock have multivessel disease. Collateral vessels thus are supplied by a stenosed artery, which magnifies the effect of lower perfusion pressure. A vicious cycle is set into motion, with decreasing coronary flow, further ischemic injury, and depression of LV function in a progressive, stuttering fashion.

Only 10% of those who develop shock have it at the time of admission. Loss of muscle at the edge of the infarct zone, often referred to as "infarct extension," may promote LV failure during the next few days. This rim of viable muscle dependent on collateral flow is salvageable in the early hours of infarction, but, with low perfusion pressure, becomes a late casualty.[1] Prolonged elevation of CK-MB may reflect the stuttering pattern of injury.

Clinical Presentation

The hemodynamic definition of cardiogenic shock includes (1) persistent hypotension with systolic arterial pressure <80 mm Hg, (2) low cardiac index (cardiac output corrected for body surface area <1.8 l/min/m²), and (3) elevated LV filling pressure (pulmonary wedge pressure >18 mm Hg). It is important to exclude other causes of low cardiac output and circulatory collapse (see Table 16-1). Acute mitral regurgitation, for example, may cause a tall V wave on the pulmonary wedge pressure tracing, causing elevation of the mean wedge pressure.

Most patients with shock and elevated LV filling pressure also have severe pulmonary congestion, and the clinical diagnosis is strongly suggested by low blood pressure, pulmonary edema, and clinical evidence of poor perfusion (including cool, clammy skin, low urine output, and altered sensorium).

Those with shock in a setting of a first MI usually have a large anterior MI. A small infarction may cause LV failure if a patient has had a previous infarction or heart failure; remember that LV injury is cumulative (see Chapter 14). Shock is more common in older patients and those with multivessel coronary artery disease (CAD). These features also indicate a worse prognosis.

Management

Laboratory Evaluation

The clinical findings suggest the diagnosis. Hemodynamic measurements confirm it, and monitoring helps with adjustment of inotropic support. An echocardiogram at the bedside shows severe LV dysfunction and excludes other conditions. If your hospital does not routinely use pulmonary artery catheterization in its intensive care unit, an echocardiogram would be the next best diagnostic study. The ECG usually shows a large MI.

Treatment

Supportive care of patients with shock is aimed at maintaining blood pressure and end-organ perfusion. The goal is to raise coronary perfusion pressure and stop the cycle of continued ischemia and LV injury. When there is hypotension but no pulmonary congestion, a fluid

Table 16-1	*Causes of Hypotension, Cardiogenic Shock, or Heart Failure after Acute Myocardial Infarction (MI)*	
	Clinical Findings, ECG, and Echocardiogram	**Hemodynamic Profile**
Cardiogenic shock (LV failure)	Large anterior MI; history or ECG evidence or prior MI; usually pulmonary congestion; echo = LV dysfunction and diffuse regional hypokinesis or akinesis	Elevated LV filling pressure (pulmonary wedge pressure), low or normal right atrial pressure, low cardiac output (CO), hypotension
RV infarction	Inferior MI, ST elevation in right precordial leads (V_{4R}), pulmonary congestion usually not present, jugular venous distention and later, edema; echo = RV dilation and hypokinesis, possibly normal LV function	Elevated right atrial and RV diastolic pressure, low or normal LV filling pressure (although it may be high with associated LV failure), low CO
Acute mitral regurgitation (MR)	Murmur of MR (but it may be soft), severe pulmonary congestion; echo = flail mitral leaflet and MR on the Doppler study; LV function may be only minimally depressed	Elevated LV filling pressure and tall V wave on the pulmonary wedge tracing, low CO
Ventricular septal defect (VSD)	Inferior or anterior MI, systolic murmur (may be soft or absent), often pulmonary congestion; echo = left-to-right shunt on the Doppler study, and no MR; LV function may not be depressed	Elevated LV filling pressure, but no V wave; "step-up" in oxygen saturation documents the shunt
Rupture of the ventricular free wall	Often a small, first MI (see text for clinical profile); usually sudden death, with no time for an echocardiogram; cardiac tamponade	Findings of cardiac tamponade, but rarely time for catheterization

challenge is a good initial maneuver (Table 16-2). Give 200 ml normal saline quickly, intravenously, and repeat it at 30-minute intervals. Carefully monitor the chest examination during fluid loading and stop if you find any evidence of congestion.

Catecholamine therapy is usually needed to treat hypotension due to LV failure, but it does not improve survival. Indeed, catechols increase myocardial oxygen demand and may aggravate ischemia. Consider pharmacologic support of blood pressure and cardiac output a short-term measure. The preferred agents are dobutamine, a pure inotropic agent with few noncardiac effects and low arrhythmogenic potential, and dopamine, which also is a renal vasodilator that promotes diuresis. At high doses, above 10 μg/kg/min, the selective actions of these drugs disappear; they work as pure vasoconstrictors, and LV filling pressure rises. Combining dopamine and dobutamine is useful. When each is given at rates as high as 7.5 μg/kg/min, cardiac output

and blood pressure rise without an increase in LV filling pressure.[2]

Intraaortic balloon pump (IABP) counterpulsation raises blood pressure, lowers afterload, and improves cardiac output and therefore coronary and coronary collateral perfusion pressure. At the same time, it reduces the work load of the heart (see Chapter 51). Of all possible supportive therapies, it is the most effective. However, without revascularization, the IABP does not improve survival. The classic study of IABP treatment from the early 1970s showed a short-term hemodynamic benefit, but 83% in-hospital and 91% 1-year mortality.[3] Many of these patients became "balloon dependent"; they were fine while the pump was working, but back in shock when it was turned off. That is a risk of using IABP support when there is no hope of reversing the shock syndrome with revascularization.

Reperfusion probably improves survival. The reason for hedging is that the placebo-controlled trials included few patients who were in shock at the time of thrombolytic therapy, and some of them received no benefit.[1] Once shock is established, there are significant obstacles facing thrombolytic therapy: reperfusion may be more difficult to achieve when pressure is low, and even with an open artery, low perfusion pressure may not allow excellent (TIMI grade 3) flow.[1] Nevertheless, early administration (within 3 to 4 hours of the onset of MI) of a fast-acting thrombolytic agent, one of the rt-PA preparations, may help patients in shock. Late therapy does not help once shock is established.

On the other hand, it is well established that reperfusion therapy prevents shock. The incidence of shock was reduced by about 50% in placebo-controlled studies. The GUSTO 1 trial found less shock and heart failure with rt-PA, which opens arteries faster than streptokinase[1] (see Chapter 15).

Revascularization appears to be the key to successful treatment. Although no randomized trials have been conducted, observational studies suggest that a mortality rate of about 40% may be achieved with primary angioplasty early in the course of cardiogenic shock. Survival is better with a successful procedure.[1] At this time, the multicenter SHOCK trial is in progress, testing urgent revascularization against medical therapy.

For revascularization to work, it must be accomplished early. The day after MI is no good. In fact, the odds are against angioplasty helping when a patient has been in shock for more than 10 to 12 hours. You want successful revascularization within 6 hours of the onset of MI and preferably within 4 hours.

Treatment Strategy

1. As soon as you make a clinical diagnosis of cardiogenic shock and agree with the patient and family that aggressive treatment is the correct approach, begin moving the patient to the catheterization laboratory (Table 16-2). Do this even if the patient has received thrombolytic therapy.
2. Initiate supportive measures to raise blood pressure to 80 to 90 mm Hg.
3. In the catheterization laboratory a few things are done: the diagnosis is confirmed, an IABP is inserted, and angiography and angioplasty are performed. The IABP is particularly helpful, because it raises coronary perfusion pressure and prevents reocclusion of the dilated artery. It usually can be removed within a couple of days.

If your hospital does not have revascularization capabilities, shock is an indication for emergency transfer (by helicopter if the distance is substantial). Do not take the patient to the coronary care unit with plans to try medical therapy, a Swan Ganz catheter, and so forth, unless you have made the decision to avoid revascularization. It is a waste of time.

Table 16-2	*Diagnosis and Treatment of Hypotension During Acute Myocardial Infarction (MI)*
Clinical Settings	**Response**
1. Small MI	1. Fluid challenge (200 ml normal saline, repeat in 1/2 hr); monitor for rales
2. Inferior MI	2. Rule out other causes of hypotension (RV infarct, VSD, or MR; see Table 16-1)
3. No prior MI	3. Catecholamines; consider pulmonary artery catheterization if no response to fluids
1. Anterior MI	1. If there is no pulmonary congestion, fluid challenge; monitor for rales
2. Large MI	2. Rule out other causes of hypotension (see Table 16-1)
3. History of prior MI or heart failure	3. Catecholamine therapy; consider pulmonary artery catheterization to monitor LV filling pressure a. Intraaortic balloon pump if no response to catechols b. With a clinical diagnosis of cardiogenic shock, emergency angiography and revascularization. *This should be accomplished within 6 hours of the onset of MI.* (Do not lose time doing other diagnostic studies if cardiogenic shock is the clinical diagnosis.)

RIGHT VENTRICULAR INFARCT SYNDROME [4,5]

The right ventricular (RV) infarct syndrome is a cause of shock that may complicate inferior MI. About one half of all patients with inferior infarction have demonstrable RV dysfunction, with hemodynamically significant RV failure in less than 10%.

Pathophysiology

Occlusion of the proximal right coronary artery interrupts flow in the branches to the free wall of the RV, as well as distal branches to the inferior wall of the LV. Ischemic injury and depression of the RV causes a reduction of the transpulmonic delivery of blood to the LV. Inadequate LV filling pressure leads to a drop in cardiac output and shock.[4]

LV filling pressure may be in the normal range, but this may be misleading, and LV preload may actually be low. Abrupt dilation of the ischemic RV is limited by the pericardium, and increased pressure in the pericardial space is transmitted to the LV.[5] This explains the presence of signs of tamponade during RV infarction (Box 16-1). With animal models of RV infarction, hemodynamics improve when the pericardium is opened and pericardial crowding is relieved. Excessive fluid loading may increase pericardial pressure, limiting diastolic return to the heart.

BOX 16-1

DIAGNOSIS OF RIGHT VENTRICULAR INFARCTION SYNDROME

CLINICAL FINDINGS
Inferior MI
Hypotension without pulmonary congestion
Jugular venous distention (and after fluid administration, peripheral edema and hepatic congestion)
Kussmaul's sign and pulsus paradoxus (see text)

CONFIRMATORY FINDINGS
ECG: ST segment elevation in right precordial leads (V_{4R}) (ST elevation in V_1 is suggestive)
Echo: right ventricular dilation and hypokinesis plus fair overall LV function
Hemodynamic study: elevated RA and RV diastolic pressure, normal or low LV filling pressure (may be elevated if there is concomitant LV failure)

Many with RV infarction also have coexisting LV dysfunction and require an elevated LV filling pressure (above 15 to 18 mmHg) to maintain stroke volume. LV dysfunction is severe enough in some patients that shock is the result of both RV and LV failure.

Clinical Presentation, Diagnosis, and Management

Consider RV infarction in a hypotensive patient with a large acute inferior MI (Box 16-1). Physical examination demonstrates right heart failure, with jugular venous distension and, with volume resuscitation, peripheral edema. There also may be pulsus paradoxus (>10 mm Hg drop in systolic blood pressure with inspiration) and Kussmaul's sign (a rise in jugular venous pressure with inspiration)—features that suggest pericardial tamponade, but instead reflect a crowded pericardial space following RV dilation. The clinical setting of acute inferior MI favors RV infarction, but when uncertain, an echocardiogram excludes tamponade.

ST segment elevation in lead V_{4R} (a right precordial lead in the V_4 position; see Chapter 5) is sensitive and specific for RV ischemia. It indicates a worse prognosis with inferior MI, but right precordial ST elevation does not indicate that shock is imminent. Shock does not develop in a majority with this finding. The echocardiogram shows dilation of the right atrium and RV, reduced contractility of the RV, and excludes pericardial effusion. Right heart catheterization documents elevation of right atrial pressure, with minimal or no elevation of pulmonary artery pressure, and low or normal LV filling pressure (see Table 16-1).

Treatment

RV infarction syndrome is prevented by early reperfusion. This is one more reason that large inferior MI is an indication for reperfusion therapy. Early right coronary artery reperfusion may hasten RV recovery, and even late reperfusion therapy with angioplasty has been recommended.[4]

The initial treatment for hypotension during inferior MI is volume expansion. As long the patient has no pulmonary congestion, a fluid challenge is safe, giving 300 ml normal saline per hour for a couple hours. If this does not correct hypotension, the patient needs hemodynamic monitoring with a pulmonary artery catheter. It is important to keep the pulmonary wedge pressure below 20 to 22 mm Hg to avoid pulmonary congestion. Above a certain level, the response of blood pressure and cardiac output flattens, indicating that increased pericardial pressure is limiting both RV and LV filling.

Intravenous nitroglycerine may aggravate hypotension because of reduced venous return to the heart. On the other hand, arterial vasodilator therapy may help, because lower left atrial and pulmonary artery pressures reduce RV afterload. If both LV and RV dysfunction are present, dobutamine is indicated for treatment of hypotension. Improved contractility of the interventricular septum boosts RV stroke volume.

Refractory hypotension often improves with the IABP, particularly for those with coexisting LV dysfunction. In addition, balloon pumping improves coronary perfusion pressure, augmenting ventricular septal performance. Spontaneous recovery of RV function is common, and there is less chance of "balloon dependence" than there is with cardiogenic shock caused only by LV injury.

Patients with RV infarction are heart rate sensitive. For this reason, the threshold for treating bradyarrhythmias with A-V sequential pacing is lower.

Clinical Course

Although many with RV dysfunction have spontaneous improvement within 2 to 3 days, it can be a more serious illness, and the mortality rate with RV infarction plus shock is 40%. Without shock it is <10%. Chronic right heart failure with peripheral edema and jugular venous distension is rare in survivors. This favorable long-term outlook is attributed to good collateral flow and the favorable oxygen supply-demand profile of the RV. Lower right heart pressure provides a favorable gradient for the transfer of coronary blood flow from the LV to the RV through collateral vessels.

CONGESTIVE HEART FAILURE

The risk of death from heart diseases that affect adults usually is linked to LV systolic function, and low LVEF predicts mortality after MI. About 20% of the survivors of MI are disabled by heart failure within 6 years.[6] Based on the Framingham studies, we used to teach that hypertension is the major cause of heart failure in the United States. However, a review of more recent, randomized trials of heart failure therapy indicates that CAD is now the most common cause.[7]

Pathophysiology

The most obvious cause of LV dysfunction after MI is loss of contractile units, translating to a loss of LVEF points. Occlusion of a large artery supplying a broad myocardial region has a greater effect on LVEF than occlusion of a small side branch. Ischemia also increases myocardial stiffness, and diastolic dysfunction contributes to an increase in pulmonary wedge pressure and congestion.

Remodeling

"Infarct expansion" and the associated change in LV geometry also have a role in the genesis of heart failure. During the week after infarction the necrotic muscle

softens and becomes "mushy." The LV wall thins, with bulging and expansion of the soft infarct zone. This is most common with anterior MI, and the result is a change in the shape of the LV apex (Fig. 16-1). Instead of the normal elliptical shape, the LV apex has a rounded, mushroom shape. The most extreme form of this is LV aneurysm (Fig. 16-1).

As subsequent healing takes place, scar is laid down in the "mold" provided by the altered infarct zone, resulting in a permanent alteration in shape. At that point the shape of the infarct zone is "cast in scar." The goal of afterload reduction therapy is prevention of early bulging, before scarring occurs.

Alteration in the shape of the apex has a negative effect on LV function. The radius of curvature of the LV is increased. Because of the Laplace relationship (Wall tension = Pressure × Radius), increased radius means an elevation of wall tension. LV wall tension is a determinant of myocardial oxygen demand, so overall MVO_2 is higher. In addition, the bulging segment of myocardium "absorbs" some of the contractile energy of the LV that would otherwise have gone toward ejection of blood.

Early reperfusion therapy preserves some muscle within the infarct zone and tends to prevent infarct expansion. The reperfused infarct zone has a marbled appearance, with patches of normal tissue mixed with injured muscle. This may explain improvement in clinical course despite depression of systolic function and only minimal improvement in LVEF. Even with little preservation of contractile function, when enough muscle is saved to prevent infarct expansion, there is clinical benefit.

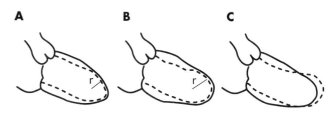

FIG. 16-1
Three patients who have had anterior MI. Solid line represents diastolic contour, and dashed line represents systolic contour. *Patient A,* The anterior wall is akinetic, but in diastole the LV still has its ellipsoidal shape (there has been no remodeling of LV shape). *Patient B,* In addition to anterior akinesis, the apex has changed to a rounded, more mushroom-like shape. This increases the radius *(r)* at the apex and thus increases wall tension (Tension = Radius × LV pressure). *Patient C,* There is an apical aneurysm. In addition to the rounded apex during diastole, there is aneurysmal bulging of the apex during systole. Not only is wall tension increased because of increased radius, but contractile energy also is "absorbed" by the bulging apex. This is the most extreme form of LV remodeling.

Reducing impedance to ejection with vasodilator therapy also has been shown to prevent LV remodeling after large MI. Afterload reduction using ACE inhibitors is now the standard of care for large MI and should be started during the first day for those with anterior infarction.

Treatment and Clinical Course

Congestive heart failure is a common illness, but one of the interesting differences between the practice of cardiovascular medicine at the end of the century and practice before 1985 is a noticeable decrease in the number of young patients with ischemic cardiomyopathy. We attribute this to reperfusion therapy, which has been shown to prevent heart failure, as well as boost survival. Other treatments that preserve muscle during acute infarction, such as beta-adrenergic blockade, also may be critical in preventing heart failure (see Chapter 14).

For those with large MI, including all patients with anterior MI, treatment with ACE inhibitors is the key to preventing infarct expansion, and treatment should be started within 24 hours of the onset of MI.[8] Trials testing ACE inhibition for smaller MIs also found a short-term survival benefit, and some advocate their use for all patients with MI who do not have a contraindication (e.g., bilateral renal-artery stenosis, renal failure, or history of adverse effects with prior treatment).[8,9] If there is LV dysfunction (usually defined as LVEF <40%), therapy should be continued long-term, at least 3 years. It is uncertain whether long-term treatment is of any benefit for those with smaller MI. Large, randomized trials of long-term ACE inhibition for all patients with MI are under way. (Table 14-7 provides a dosing schedule for captopril, but other ACE inhibitors have been found equally effective.[10])

As one in seven patients using ACE inhibitors stops the medicine because of cough, there is interest in angiotensin II (A-II) blockers as a substitute. ACE inhibitors also increase cardiac levels of bradykinin, as the enzyme that degrades kinins is similar to ACE. The kinins have been shown to reduce infarct size. A-II blockers do not have an effect on kinins. Nevertheless, early studies suggest that the A-II blocker, losartin, has a comparable, if not better effect on LV function and mortality after MI when compared with captopril, and large trials are underway.[11,12] We do not hesitate to prescribe losartin for the patient with ACE blocker intolerance. Whether to recommend it as initial treatment will depend on studies that should be completed by the end of the decade.

Treatment Tip: ACE Inhibitors and Renal Function

Some have expressed concern about using ACE inhibitors or angiotensin-II blockers in patients with mild renal dysfunction, with a creatinine level >1.5 mg/dL.

Perhaps there is underlying renal artery stenosis, and therapy will aggravate it. What do you look for? First, blood pressure; a precipitous drop in blood pressure might indicate especially high plasma renin activity and underlying renal artery stenosis. Second, creatinine; recheck it 24 to 48 hours after starting therapy. If the creatinine does not increase by more than 0.3 mg/dL, continue treatment. A small increase in creatinine necessitates repeat measurements. Be prepared to stop therapy if it continues to rise. A rise in creatinine with ACE inhibition is an indication to screen for renal artery stenosis.

Clinical Course

Patients with heart failure during the course of acute infarction have a higher mortality risk (see Table 14-3) and often develop chronic heart failure. They have complex ventricular arrhythmias, and sudden death is common. It is for this reason that careful monitoring of serum potassium and magnesium is critical for those requiring diuretics.

LV aneurysm is the most extreme case of infarct expansion (see Fig. 16-1). It is more common after anterior MI, usually involving the LV apex. Persistent ST segment elevation may be an indicator of aneurysm, but it may also occur with large infarction in the absence of aneurysm. This is a relatively uncommon condition with widespread use of reperfusion therapy. The diagnosis is easily made with an echocardiogram.

An aneurysm increases the mortality rate sixfold compared with those who have similar LVEF. Symptoms include the clinical triad of ventricular arrhythmias, heart failure, and angina. Rupture of a mature aneurysm is uncommon. Surgical repair is a good option if it can be delayed for 4 to 6 weeks after MI (allowing development of sufficiently strong scar tissue to hold sutures). The indication for aneurysmectomy is any one of the clinical triad plus a resectable aneurysm and a good opportunity for revascularization. Success depends on the contractility of the viable muscle, or the "residual ejection fraction" when the aneurysm is subtracted.

ARRHYTHMIAS

Complex Ventricular Arrhythmias Including Ventricular Fibrillation

It is important to distinguish between complex ventricular arrhythmias (VA) that develop during the early hours of MI and those occurring in the late hospital phase (after day 3 or 4).

Early Ventricular Tachycardia or Fibrillation

Ventricular tachycardia (VT) or ventricular fibrillation (VF) within the first day of MI appears to be an electrical phenomenon that is unrelated to infarct size. It may occur with small or large infarctions. Because the arrhythmia is not a marker of depressed LV function, it does not indicate poor long-term prognosis (providing, of course, that the patient survives the arrhythmia). We commonly teach students that sinus tachycardia at rest is a worse prognostic sign after MI than successfully treated VF during the first day of infarction.

Late Hospital-Phase VT/VF

The electrical storm that may complicate the early hours of infarction usually resolves in a day or two. The pathophysiology of complex VAs in the late hospital phase is different. They are limited to those with large MI. In fact, studies in the 1970s found that the best predictor of complex VAs was low LVEF, and the best predictor of low LVEF was complex VAs on a predischarge 24-hour monitor. After MI, documenting normal LV function indicates a low risk of complex VAs, and it is unnecessary to get a 24-hour monitor.

A patient with a depressed LV and complex VAs tends to have ectopy throughout the day. It is not intermittent or sporadic, as is commonly the case with supraventricular tachycardia, the spells of which may be separated by weeks. A 24-hour monitor done at random shows complex VAs (pairs of nonsustained VT). Conversely, a normal 24-hour monitor excludes them with fair certainty. There is no need to repeat monitoring for fear of having missed the arrhythmia.

Treatment

Control of ventricular arrhythmias during the first day of MI is discussed in Chapter 14. Lidocaine lowers the risk of VF and is given when there are frequent ectopic beats. It is no longer recommended as prophylactic therapy for all patients with acute MI. When lidocaine fails to prevent recurrence of VT or VF, intravenous amiodarone, bretylium, or procainamide may be effective. An occasional patient with refractory VT will respond to intravenous magnesium.

Late Hospital Phase and Postdischarge VAs

Those with sustained VT, VT causing syncope, or VF should have an electrophysiologic evaluation (see Chapter 26). Prophylactic antiarrhythmic therapy for patients with low LVEF and complex VAs is a controversial issue. This group has the highest mortality in the year after MI, and more than half of the deaths are sudden. The first step in treatment is to exclude conditions that may aggravate ventricular ectopy, including recurrent ischemia and electrolyte abnormalities. Look for low magnesium and low potassium.

The Cardiac Arrhythmia Suppression Trial (CAST) specifically studied the role of antiarrhythmic drug therapy after MI for patients with depressed LVEF and complex ectopy.[13] A pilot study screened a number of drugs

and identified those best at suppressing VAs on 24-hour monitors. Encainide, flecainide, and moricizine were the most effective, whereas quinidine and procainamide were less effective. The next, and largest, phase of the study compared the most effective drugs with placebo. The result was surprising: death or cardiac arrest was 2.64 times higher with drug treatment than with placebo (Box 16-2). The proarrhythmic effects of these drugs were more important than expected. Membrane-active agents suppress ectopy on the monitor, but they do not prevent sudden death.

BOX 16-2

LESSONS FROM THE CARDIAC ARRHYTHMIA SUPPRESSION TRIAL (CAST)[13]

1. Suppression of asymptomatic PVCs or non-sustained ventricular tachycardia (NSVT) after MI with class IC drugs increased the risk of sudden death. CAST demonstrated that proarrhythmia is more important than expected.
2. CAST did not study class IA drugs (quinidine or procainamide). They also have proarrhythmic effects, and the safety of long-term therapy is uncertain.
3. Suppression of PVCs on an ambulatory monitor did not predict improved survival with drug therapy. The mechanisms responsible for PVCs may differ from those causing sustained arryhthmias and sudden death.
4. The rate, length, and frequency of nonsustained VT had no influence on prognosis. A single 3-beat burst of VT at a rate of 120/min carried the same prognostic weight as multiple 8 to 10 beat runs at 150/min.
5. On the other hand, VT rates <100 beats/min indicated a mortality rate lower than VT rates above 100/min.
6. CAST did *not* include patients with normal LV function. With normal LVEF after MI, treatment of asymptomatic PVCs and NSVT with drugs other than beta-blockers is not indicated.
7. CAST did not study patients without CAD. The data may not apply to others with LV dysfunction (e.g., dilated cardiomyopathy).
8. CAST did not exclude possible efficacy of other drugs such as amiodarone.

Interestingly, beta-blockers have the opposite effect. As a rule, they do not suppress ectopy on the 24-hour monitor, but the incidence of sudden death is lower. There is an apparent difference between suppressing PVCs and preventing sustained VAs including VF. For asymptomatic VAs, beta blockade is the treatment of choice.

Studies of other antiarrhythmic agents including sotalol (with both class III antiarrhythmic and beta blocking activity), d-sotalol (a pure class III agent), and mexiletine and other class I drugs have shown no reduction in mortality when given as prophylaxis for patients with depressed LVEF and complex VAs after MI.[14] More recently, amiodarone has been studied in Canadian and European trials.[15] Neither study showed a decrease in cardiac death, but both found a decrease in arrhythmic death. The reason for this is uncertain, but the possibility that amiodarone increases nonarrhythmic cardiac death has not been excluded. In the Canadian trial, reduction in arrhythmic death was greatest among patients with congestive heart failure and those with a history of multiple MIs (those with the highest risk had the greatest benefit).

So where do we stand at this point? Table 17-2 provides a protocol for evaluation and treatment of ventricular arrhythmias after MI. Patients with long runs of VT or symptomatic VT should have electrophysiologic testing. Implantable defibrillator therapy may be life saving for this group. Those with brief spells of NSVT and those who do not have inducible VT in the EP laboratory should be treated with beta-blockers. We believe that amiodarone can be justified for those with heart failure and NSVT, especially when beta blockade is not feasible.

We emphasize that amiodarone is the only membrane-active agent that does not appear to *increase* the risk of sudden death in patients with previous MI and depressed LV function. It can be used with confidence in a few clinical settings. First, it may prevent symptomatic VT, and control of symptoms is one indication for its use. Second, those with an implantable defibrillator need to have VT suppressed to prevent the device firing. Finally, amiodarone is effective for treatment and prevention of atrial fibrillation; it can be used for this purpose in the post-MI patient with depressed LV function with less risk of sudden death than other drugs.

Atrial Tachyarrhythmias

Atrial fibrillation, supraventricular tachycardia, and sinus tachycardia tend to develop in patients with large MI. They are markers of low LVEF. Recognition and treatment are reviewed in Chapter 25. The prognosis is determined by the degree of LV dysfunction.

Bradyarrhythmias

Recognition and treatment of heart block after MI is reviewed at length in Chapter 27. As a rule, when conduction is blocked at the level of the AV node, the takeover pacemaker is reliable and has an intrinsic rate above 40 beats/min. The AV node usually recovers, and permanent pacing is seldom needed. Infranodal block is a much bigger problem, with a slow take-over pacer and little chance of recovery. It is an indication for a permanent pacemaker.

In general, a narrow QRS complex indicates nodal block, and a wide QRS means infranodal block.

RECURRENT MYOCARDIAL ISCHEMIA
Epidemiology and Pathophysiology

The incidence of postinfarction angina (PIA) is 20% to 30%. It is more common in patients with non–Q wave MI, since the infarct is incomplete and the infarct artery is tightly stenosed and unstable (see Chapter 14). Coronary occlusion and recurrent MI also are more common in this group. Other risk factors for recurrent ischemia are obesity, female sex, diabetes, and early peaking CK (an indicator of spontaneous thrombolysis).

Patients with MI and ST elevation treated with thrombolytic therapy also have "incomplete infarction" and are at risk for PIA and recurrence, or "completion" of the MI (see Chapter 15).

Primary angioplasty leaves the patient with a more stable artery, and there is less chance of reocclusion and reinfarction than there is after thrombolytic therapy. However, the risk of recurrent ischemia is still appreciable, and careful monitoring is necessary during the 2 to 3 days after the procedure.

Reocclusion of the infarct artery and "extension" of the infarct has a bad effect on prognosis. Mortality and heart failure are both increased. This holds true with clinically silent infarct artery reocclusion.

Remember that silent reocclusion of the infarct artery is common. In fact, it is probably more common than symptomatic reocclusion, as nociceptive dysfunction may occur after transient coronary artery occlusion (see Chapter 15). Think of recurrent ischemia if a patient has an unexplained increase in ventricular ectopy, has more elevation of ST segments on the telemetry ECG, or has unexpected or vague symptoms such as anxiety, restlessness, or dyspnea. Reocclusion of the infarct artery is promptly identified by reelevation of the ST segments on a 12-lead ECG.

Management

Prevention of recurrent ischemia is reviewed in Chapters 14 and 15. Aspirin and beta-blockers both lower the risk of recurrent angina and infarction. Diltiazem has that effect in patients with non–Q wave MI. Nitrates have not been shown to prevent ischemia after MI. After reperfusion therapy, most infarct artery reocclusion is missed. Prevention of this complication is the rationale for angiography and revascularization, which are aimed at "pacifying" the unstable vessel.[16]

If there is recurrence of angina at rest, get an ECG during pain to document new ST segment elevation. Standard medical therapy may be applied—even before the ECG—including nitrates, beta-blockers (intravenous or oral), aspirin, and heparin. Unless there is a dramatic response to nitroglycerin, urgent angiography and angioplasty is the best treatment for recurrent of ischemia. Thrombolytic therapy may be used for re-occlusion, but we consider it a second choice because of the higher risk of myocardial rupture with late thrombolysis.

PERICARDITIS

Fibrinous Pericarditis Early after Myocardial Infarction

Transient pericarditis is common during the week, and usually within 3 days, of transmural infarction. It is more common with large MI, occurring in 25% of those with Q wave infarction, and less than 10% with non-Q MI.[17] Limiting infarct size with early reperfusion therapy may prevent it.

Most patients have a transient friction rub without pain. A few have inflammation severe enough to cause pain that raises the possibility of postinfarction angina. The history and physical examination make the diagnosis straightforward in most cases: The pain is typical of pericarditis and different from the pain of the recent MI. It is "pleuritic" and improves with sitting and leaning forward. Radiation of the pain to the trapezius ridge indicates pericarditis. The ECG usually is unchanged, and it is uncommon to see diffuse ST segment elevation. Pneumonitis is uncommon.

The echocardiogram may confirm a small pericardial effusion. Tamponade is rare. When it occurs, it usually is caused by ventricular rupture or hemopericardium. As antiplatelet and anticoagulant therapy are commonly used after MI, there is concern about transforming fibrinous pericarditis to hemopericardium and tamponade. This is a rare complication, and mild pericarditis is not considered an indication for stopping anticoagulants when the patient is already taking them.[18] Careful monitoring of clotting function is indicated.

We would not hesitate to start anticoagulant therapy when the need is great. For example, recent angioplasty or stent placement, discovery of an LV thrombus, or development of unstable angina would weigh in favor of anticoagulation, despite the presence of a friction rub. Again, carefully monitor clotting parameters and watch for signs of tamponade.

The best treatment for early pericarditis is aspirin at doses that suppress inflammation (650 mg at 4 to 6 hour intervals). Both steroids and nonsteroidal inflammatory drugs may increase the risk of rupture when given early after MI. They also may aggravate infarct expansion.

The pericarditis is transient, generally has no direct clinical consequences, and does not recur. If a rub and fever redevelop more than 10 days after MI, it is Dressler's syndrome, a different illness. On the other hand, early pericarditis is a marker of larger infarction and thus a more complicated clinical course.

Late Pericarditis (Dressler's Syndrome)

Dressler's syndrome is a postmyocardial infarction syndrome characterized by fibrinous pericarditis that is localized to the region of infarction. It is much less common now than when it was first described in 1957, occurring in about 1% of patients with MI. Symptoms begin 10 days to 8 weeks after MI. In addition to typical pericarditis, there is evidence of generalized inflammation with fever, malaise, aching muscles (a flulike syndrome), elevation of the sedimentation rate, leukocytosis, and pericardial effusion. Pneumonitis is possible, with patchy infiltrates evident on chest x-ray. It is a rare cause of pericardial tamponade. Clinically, it is similar to the postpericardiotomy syndrome that occurs after heart surgery, an illness that you are more likely to encounter in a general medical practice (see Chapter 52).

No single test confirms the diagnosis. You are safe making the call based on the clinical picture and marked elevation of the sedimentation rate. A normal sedimentation rate makes it unlikely.

The best treatment for pericarditis occurring within 4 weeks of MI is high-dose aspirin. An occasional patient with severe inflammation requires steroids, which we try to avoid because of possible effects on scar formation. Treatment with steroids or nonsteroidal antiinflammatory agents within 2 weeks of MI increases the risk of rupture.[18] Their use 2 to 4 weeks after MI may be risky, although this is uncertain. After 4 weeks, steroids and nonsteroidal antiinflammatory agents are considered safe.

Clinical Course

With antiinflammatory therapy, symptoms resolve within a week. We usually stop therapy a week later or when inflammation has resolved. A falling sedimentation rate would favor stopping therapy. Continued treatment will not prevent recurrence. A minority of patients have recurrent symptoms, and treatment can be restarted. Later episodes are not as severe or as close together as earlier spells. In time the illness seems to burn itself out, and it is uncommon for flare-ups to develop more than 6 months after MI.

LEFT VENTRICULAR THROMBUS AND PERIPHERAL EMBOLIZATION

Without anticoagulation, mural thrombus develops in as many as 20% with Q wave MI, and the incidence rises to 40% with anterior MI. It is more common with large infarction. About 10% of those with LV thrombus have peripheral embolization. Thus the risk of embolization ranges from 1% to 4% with acute MI, depending on the size and location of infarction.

The pathogenesis of ventricular clot is uncertain. A loss of wall motion may lead to stagnation of blood in contact with the surface; normal contraction keeps blood moving along (that seems the case when comparing atrial fibrillation with flutter). It has also been suggested that inflammation of the endocardial surface of infarcted muscle may be thrombogenic. Embolization is more likely when a clot is mobile, protrudes more into the chamber, or is large (and is visible in multiple echo views).

Management

Heparin administered during acute MI lowers the chance of LV thrombus by 50%. No trials have been large enough to show a reduction of peripheral embolization. Thrombolytic therapy also reduces the chance of thrombus formation, but there has been a report of late thrombolytic therapy dislodging an LV thrombus, shaking an embolus loose.

The transthoracic echocardiogram is sensitive and specific for the diagnosis of LV thrombus; it is not necessary to do a transesophageal study. The current recommendations for prevention and therapy are outlined in Table 16-3.[19]

PULMONARY EMBOLUS

The best prevention for venous thrombus and pulmonary embolism is early ambulation. When MI was treated with prolonged bed rest, pulmonary embolus

Table 16-3 *Anticoagulation Therapy after Acute Myocardial Infarction: a Summary of Practice Guidelines*[19]

Short-term, treatment in hospital: heparin*	Prevention of arterial embolism	1. Heparin for large, Q wave anterior MI; continue until discharge 2. Heparin for those with acute MI, LV dilation, and low LVEF
Long-term treatment: warfarin†	Prevention of arterial embolism	1. Warfarin after heparin for those with mural thrombus or a dilated, akinetic LV apex. Continue for at least 3 months and stop only if the echo shows no thrombus. 2. Indefinite warfarin therapy with LV dilation and low LVEF or if there is persistent thrombus
Antiplatelet plus heparin therapy*	Short-term, immediately after thrombolytic therapy	Prevents recurrence or extension of MI for those managed medically. Long-term therapy with aspirin alone is adequate.
Aspirin plus warfarin†	Medical treatment, no thrombolytic therapy	Treatment with warfarin plus aspirin for at least 1 month *may* prevent extension of MI (evidence favors but does not prove efficacy).
Warfarin, no aspirin†	Secondary prevention of MI	Aspirin is the first choice, but warfarin may be used if there is intolerance to aspirin.
Subcutaneous heparin	Prevention of venous thrombosis and pulmonary embolism	Heparin 5000 U bid for 2 days. Continue heparin until fully ambulatory if the patient is high risk (age >70, heart failure, large MI, previous MI, obesity, previous PE or venous disease, prolonged bed rest).

*Intravenous heparin to prolong the activated partial thromboplastin time to 1.5 to 2.0 times control.
†Adjust warfarin so that INR = 2.0 to 3.0.

was responsible for 10% of deaths; currently it is a rare cause of death after MI. Patients at high risk should have prophylaxis with subcutaneous heparin (see Table 16-3). The Practice Guidelines call for routine treatment of all patients during the first 2 days in hospital. It is not a bad idea for the unusual patient not receiving full-dose heparin after MI.

NEW MURMUR AFTER MYOCARDIAL INFARCTION
Acute Ventricular Septal Defect

Acute mitral regurgitation and ventricular septal defect (VSD) are the causes of new systolic murmur after MI. The incidence of septal rupture with MI is about 2%. It is more common with advanced age, hypertension, and poorly developed collateral circulation; most have multivessel CAD. Like free wall rupture, thrombolytic therapy more than 12 hours from the onset of MI may predispose to rupture of the septum.

The interventricular septum is supplied by branches from both the anterior descending and posterior descending arteries, the two coronary branches that encircle the septum in the interventricular groove. Thus both anterior and inferior MI may cause septal rupture. The prognosis is worse with inferior infarction, possibly because of the basal location of the defect and difficulty with surgical repair. A VSD caused by anterior MI is positioned nearer the LV apex.

VSD develops during the first day of MI in 20%, and the majority occur within the first week. A loud, harsh, holosystolic murmur is the rule, and many have a thrill. Biventricular failure follows. With medical therapy, half die within a week, and 85% by 2 weeks.

Management

A new murmur is an indication for an urgent echocardiogram. The Doppler study demonstrates flow across the ventricular septum and excludes mitral regurgitation. *The next step is prompt transfer for angiography and surgical repair.* Do not delay, since a neglected, sicker patient has a much higher mortality risk with surgery.

While transfer is being arranged, blood pressure may be supported with catecholamines, and congestion treated with diuretics. Hypotension or a low cardiac output syndrome are indications for an IABP. Right heart catheterization confirms the diagnosis: the oxygen saturation in the pulmonary artery is higher than in the vena cavae and right atrium (there is a "step-up" in oxygen saturation at the level of the RV).

Immediate surgical repair is indicated for the usual patient with VSD who depends on catecholamine or IABP support. Surgical success is predicted by good ventricular function and brief duration of shock. A rare patient stabilizes without support. In such cases, surgery

may be delayed 3 to 4 weeks, with the hope that partially healed tissue will be easier to repair. During this time careful monitoring is necessary, because rapid deterioration is possible.

Acute Mitral Regurgitation

Papillary muscle rupture occurs in about 1% with MI. The posteromedial papillary muscle is supplied by the right coronary artery, and the anterolateral muscle by the circumflex. Inferior MI is a more common cause of mitral regurgitation (MR) than lateral infarction. Unlike VSD, a tiny MI may cause MR, as infarction of just the tip of a papillary muscle may lead to rupture. The patient may have single-vessel CAD.

Clinically, the patient has abrupt onset of heart failure, and pulmonary congestion predominates. Many have a loud holosystolic murmur, but no thrill. When cardiac output and blood pressure are low, the murmur may be soft. Unlike chronic MR, there is no S_3 gallop.

If heart failure unexpectedly develops in a patient with a small MI, obtain an echocardiogram to rule out MR, regardless of the presence or absence of a murmur.

The echocardiogram demonstrates MR and often a flail mitral leaflet. LV function often is near-normal. The pulmonary wedge pressure tracing typically shows a tall V wave, analagous to the V wave in the venous pulse in patients with tricuspid regurgitation.

If pulmonary congestion is severe and cardiac output is low, support with nitroprusside and use an IABP to provide a bridge to surgery. Immediate surgical repair is indicated. The biggest problem is the failure to recognize MR as the cause of heart failure.

RUPTURE OF THE VENTRICULAR FREE WALL

Rupture of the free wall of the LV is the second most common cause of death in patients hospitalized with MI (after LV failure) and is responsible for 10% of deaths. It occurs 3 to 7 days after MI, at about the same time as acute VSD or MR. It is at this time after MI that the necrotic zone is softest. It commonly happens after a first MI and may occur with small as well as large infarctions (usually anterior or lateral in location). Single-vessel CAD and poorly developed collaterals are common. Risk factors for rupture are late coronary thrombolysis (>12 hours from the onset of MI), hypertension, and advanced age. It is not uncommon in young patients. Steroids and nonsteroidal antiinflammatory agents probably increase the risk of rupture, but this is uncertain. As antiinflammatory therapy blunts healing and scar formation, they probably should be avoided for 1 month after MI.[20]

The clinical picture is one of acute tamponade and death. We have observed a number of ruptures in hospitalized patients. Mild agitation or other vague symptoms may be present just before rupture, but no chest pain. Telemetry shows no arrhythmia. Electromechanical dissociation occurs after the patient collapses. Resuscitation is unsuccessful, and there is not enough time for emergency surgery. It is a cause of sudden cardiac death for which there is no successful treatment. (We are familiar with case reports describing emergency surgical repair and survival, but we have never seen it.[21])

Pseudoaneurysm

In an occasional patient the rupture is contained by adherent pericardium, probably because of inflammation of the infarcted muscle and overlying pericardium. Clot usually is within the bulging aneurysmal sack that provides support, but which also may embolize. A pseudoaneurysm tends to have a narrow neck at the level of communication with the LV, distinguishing it from a true aneurysm. It may become quite large and may rupture. There are no clinical findings indicating its presence, and it usually is an unexpected finding on an echocardiogram after MI. Because of possible rupture, surgical repair is indicated.

If you hear of a rare case of free wall rupture that was successfully treated, it probably involved rupture with some degree of containment by the pericardium, which prevented tamponade, circulatory collapse, and immediate death.

REFERENCES

1. Barry WL, Sarembock IJ: Cardiogenic shock: therapy and prevention, *Clin Cardiol* 21:72, 1998.
2. Richard C, Ricome JL, Rimailho A, et al: Combined hemodynamic effects of dopamine and dobutamine in cardiogenic shock, *Circulation* 67:620, 1983.
3. Scheidt S, Wilner G, Mueller H, et al: Intraaortic balloon counterpulsation in cardiogenic shock: report of a cooperative clinical trial, *N Engl J Med* 288:979, 1973.
4. Goldstein JA: Right heart ischemia: pathophysiology, natural history, and clinical management, *Prog Cardiovasc Dis* 40:325, 1998.
5. Dell'Italia LJ: Reperfusion for right ventricular infarction, *N Engl J Med* 338:978, 1998.
6. American Heart Association: *Heart and stroke facts: 1998 statistical supplement,* Dallas, 1998, American Heart Association.
7. Gheorghiade M, Bonow RO: Chronic heart failure in the United States: a manifestation of coronary artery disease, *Circulation* 97:282, 1998.
8. Hennekens CH, Albert CM, Godfried SL, et al: Adjunctive drug therapy of acute myocardial infarction: evidence from clinical trials, *N Engl J Med* 335:1660, 1996.
9. ISIS-4 Collaborative Group: ISIS-4: a randomised factorial trial assessing early oral captopril, oral mononitrate, and intravenous magnesium sulphate in 58,050 patients with suspected acute myocardial infarction, *Lancet* 345:669, 1995.
10. Latini R, Maggioni AP, Flather M, et al: ACE-inhibitor use in patients with myocardial infarction: summary of evidence from clinical trials, *Circulation* 92:3132, 1995.
11. Higginbotham MB, Russell SD: Angiotensin II antagonists: present applications and future prospects in cardiovascular disease, *Contemp Int Med* 10:16, 1998.
12. Linz W, Wiemer G, Scholkens BA: Beneficial effects of bradykinin on myocardial energy metabolism and infarct size, *Am J Cardiol* 80:118, 1997.
13. The Cardiac Arrhythmia Suppression Trial (CAST) Investigators: Preliminary report: effect of encainide and flecainide on mortality in a randomized trial of arrhythmia suppression after myocardial infarction, *N Engl J Med* 321:406, 1989.
14. Underwood RD, Sra J, Akhtar M: Evaluation and treatment strategies in patients at high risk of sudden death postmyocardial infarction, *Clin Cardiol* 20:753, 1997.
15. Pratt CM, Waldo AL, Camm AJ: Can antiarrhythmic drugs survive the survival trials? *Am J Cardiol* 81:24, 1998. (Note: a good review of all clinical trails of antiarrhythmic agents after MI, including the beta-blocker trials.)
16. Guetta V, Topol EJ: Pacifying the infarct vessel, *Circulation* 96:713, 1997.
17. Tofler GH, Muller JA, Stone PH, et al: Pericarditis in acute myocardial infarction: characterization and clinical significance, *Am Heart J* 117:86, 1989.
18. Galve E, Garcia-del-Castillo H, Evangelista A, et al: Pericardial effusion in the course of myocardial infarction: incidence, natural history, and clinical relevance, *Circulation* 73:294, 1986.
19. Gunnar RM, Passamani ER, Bourdillon PD, et al: Guidelines for the early management of patients with acute myocardial infarction. A report of the American College of Cardiology/American Heart Association Task Force on Assessment of Diagnostic and Therapeutic Cardiovascular Procedures, *J Am Coll Cardiol* 16:249, 1990.
20. Silverman HW, Pfeifer MP: Relation between use of antiinflammatory agents and left ventricular free wall rupture during acute myocardial infarction, *Am J Cardiol* 59:363, 1987.
21. Reardon MJ, Carr CL, Diamond A, et al: Ischemic left ventricular free wall rupture: prediction, diagnosis, and treatment, *Ann Thorac Surg* 64:1509, 1997.

17

Long-Term Treatment after Myocardial Infarction

George J. Taylor
Mark Kohnle
Leslye C. Pennypacker

RISK STRATIFICATION

Patients who survive the acute phase of myocardial infarction (MI) and who are preparing to leave the hospital also face the possibility of sudden cardiac death (SCD), recurrent infarction, progression of ventricular dysfunction, or peripheral embolization during the next year (Table 17-1). The current standard of care includes laboratory studies to identify those at high risk for these late complications of MI and treatment to prevent them.

The recommendations for screening and treatment outlined in the tables are compatible with those of the American College of Cardiology/American Heart Association (ACC/AHA) Practice Guidelines.[1-5] Although they are supported by data from clinical studies, the weight of evidence varies. Recommendations based on randomized trials are identified as "strongly recommended" in the tables. For others, evidence is not from randomized trials, but available data are favorable, and they are considered within the standard of care.

Consider the tables a "standard of care menu." As you work with your patient just before hospital discharge, review the menu for appropriate and useful diagnostic and treatment possibilities. If you elect not to screen or treat, and that is often appropriate, it would be advisable to document the basis for your decision.

Sudden Cardiac Death after Myocardial Infarction (Table 17-2)

Complex ventricular arrhythmias (VAs) and SCD are more frequent among those with large MI and subsequent depression of left ventricular ejection fraction (LVEF <40%).[6] Studies using both Holter monitoring and measurement of LVEF have found that patients with low LVEF usually have complex VAs, and those with complex VAs usually have low LVEF. A normal LVEF (above 50% to 55% on an echocardiogram) almost excludes the possibility of sudden arrhythmic death. For this reason, measurement of LVEF is the first step in screening for possible SCD. Patients with small, uncomplicated MI do *not* need ambulatory ECG monitoring to screen for VAs (Table 17-2).

On the other hand, those with LVEF <40% after MI commonly have complex VAs and would benefit from monitoring (Table 17-2). Clinical indicators of low LVEF are moderate to large MI based on peak creatine kinase (CK), anterior MI, a history of MI before the present infarction, and clinical evidence for heart failure before or during the acute infarction. In such cases an echocardiogram to document LV function is indicated. If the LVEF is low, get a 24-hour ambulatory monitor. Low LVEF plus complex VAs, especially nonsustained ventricular tachycardia (NSVT), is the substrate for sudden, arrhythmic death.

A practical question is whether telemetry on the ward just before discharge may be substituted for tape recorder monitoring. If the telemetry system does not have memory that allows review of 24 hours of monitoring, or if monitoring depends on a nurse watching the screen, then it is not adequate. Newer telemetry systems with expanded memory and review capabilities are reasonable substitutes for tape recorder monitoring, if they are used properly.

Newer screening techniques include the signal-averaged electrocardiogram (SAECG) and low heart rate variability (Table 17-3). Abnormal studies correlate with low LVEF and an increased risk of complex VAs. While relatively inexpensive and easy to perform, they are not widely available, and their role in the screening process is not yet established.

Treatment

Table 17-2 provides a protocol for patient selection, evaluation, and treatment. Before the Cardiac Arrhythmia Suppression Trial (CAST), patients with NSVT, defined as three or more sequential ectopic beats, were automatically treated with membrane-active agents. CAST and subsequent studies showed us that the proarrhythmic effects of these drugs outweigh their antiarrhythmic actions; they actually increase the risk of SCD.[7] We no longer "chase VPBs" using antiarrhythmic drugs to make Holter monitors look better (see Chapter 16).

Beta blockade lowers the risk of sudden death and is indicated for all patients after MI, particularly those with NSVT. Amiodarone does not have as much proar-

Table 17-1 | *Predischarge Screening after Myocardial Infarction (MI)*

Complication the Year after MI That Warrants Screening	Screening Studies
Sudden cardiac death (SCD)	Measurement of LVEF, 24-hour Holter monitoring, electrophysiologic study
Residual or recurrent ischemia or MI	Stress ECG, exercises or pharmacologic perfusion imaging, RNA or echocardiogram, coronary angiogram
Progression of LV dysfunction, LV remodeling	Echocardiogram
LV thrombus and peripheral embolization	Echocardiogram
Progression of atherosclerosis	Lipid study, risk factor modification

LV, Left ventricle; *LVEF*, LV ejection fraction (the percentage of blood ejected with each heart beat, normal >50% to 55%); *ECG*, electrocardiogram; *RNA*, radionuclide angiogram.

Table 17-2 | *Sudden Cardiac Death (SCD) after Myocardial Infarction (MI): Screening and Treatment*

Study or Therapy	Indications and Comments
No screening for SCD needed	Small (nonanterior), uncomplicated, first MI; ECG does not show left bundle branch block or LVH (must screen for residual or recurrent ischemia; see Table 17-4)
Measure LVEF (echo or RNA)	*Probably indicated:* moderate or large MI, anterior MI, complicated MI, evidence for heart failure at any time before or after MI, history of previous or multiple MI
24-hour Holter monitoring	*Probably indicated:* LVEF <40%, heart failure, persistent VAs on telemetry, possibly symptomatic arrhythmias (telemetry a possible substitute; see text)
Electrophysiologic study	*Strongly indicated:* sustained VT or cardiac arrest >48 hours after acute MI, cardiac arrest without evidence of a completed Q wave MI *Probably indicated:* NSVT plus high risk for future arrhythmia (e.g., low LVEF), symptomatic VT *Not indicated:* VT or VF during the acute phase of MI (< 48 hours), asymptomatic NSVT plus normal LVEF
Screening for residual ischemia (see Table 17-4)	Indicated for all patients after MI, but especially for those with complex VAs, where ischemia may aggravate the arrhythmia
TREATMENT TO PREVENT SCD AFTER MI	
Beta-adrenergic blockade	*Strongly indicated:* most patients after acute MI unless there is a contraindication; best therapy for short runs of VT that are asymptomatic
Normalize electrolytes (K+ and Mg+2)	*Strongly indicated* for all patients, but especially those taking diuretics or with low LVEF and/or complex VAs
Amiodarone	Reasonable therapy for VT and NSVT after MI; less proarrhythmic effect than other membrane-active agents; therapy usually guided by results of EPS
Implantable cardioverter defibrillator (ICD)	*Strongly indicated:* inducible VT on the EPS, symptomatic VT despite optimal drug therapy

LV, Left ventricle; *LVEF*, LV ejection fraction (normal is >55%); *LVH*, LV hypertrophy; *RNA*, radionuclide angiogram; *VT*, ventricular tachycardia (three or more sequential ventricular ectopics); *NSVT*, nonsustained VT; *VF*, ventricular fibrillation; *VA*, ventricular arrhythmia.
"Strongly indicated," Always acceptable and considered useful (usually based on clinical trials data); "Probably indicated," acceptable but not as well established by evidence.

Table 17-3	*New Screening Studies for Ventricular Arrhythmias (VA)*

Test	How It Works
Signal-averaged ECG	Computer summation of a large number of QRS complexes allows measurement of the tiny "late-potential" at the tail-end of the QRS in patients with reentrant ventricular arrhythmias. This current may come from the reentrant circuit. Late potentials correlate with low LVEF and complex VAs after MI*.
Heart rate variability (HRV)	Large MI and low LVEF lead to decreased parasympathetic (vagal) tone. Vagal discharge is responsible for sinus arrhythmia, the normal respiratory variation in heart rate (or HRV). With loss of vagal tone, HRV decreases (the rhythm, and the R-R interval, become more regular). *Technique:* A large number of R-R intervals is collected by a computer on the ECG machine and averaged. The *standard deviation* of the mean R-R interval is a measure of variation, or HRV. Low HRV correlates with low LVEF and complex VAs.*

*Based on available studies, it does not appear that HRV or the SAEGG adds novel information about prognosis over and above that provided by LVEF and Holter monitoring. I think of these techniques as possible alternatives to ECG monitoring.

R-R interval, The distance (or time) between two R waves on the ECG.

rhythmic potential as other membrane active drugs and can be used to suppress NSVT (see Chapter 16). In practice, amiodarone is most commonly prescribed after electrophysiologic study and for special clinical indications. For example, a patient with symptomatic ventricular tachycardia (VT) who has declined interventional evaluation or treatment may have symptoms controlled by amiodarone. Amiodarone is not recommended as routine treatment for asymptomatic NSVT observed on a Holter monitor.

Another therapy that has prevented sudden death in clinical trials is angiotensin-converting enzyme (ACE) inhibition. It is doubtful that ACE inhibitors have a direct antiarrhythmic action. However, prevention of infarct expansion with its associated increase in wall tension and ischemia also may prevent serious arrhythmias (see Chapter 16).

Patients with depressed left ventricular (LV) function often are taking diuretics. Meticulous attention to serum potassium and magnesium (the overlooked electrolyte) levels are critical elements of arrhythmia prevention.

Highest risk patients, identified by symptoms or screening studies, should have an electrophysiologic study (EPS) (see Table 17-2). Those with inducible, sustained VT receive an implantable cardioverter defibrillator, which is known to increase survival. Those without inducible VT have a good prognosis with medical therapy, usually beta blockade. The results of EPS also are used to guide drug therapy.

Residual or Recurrent Myocardial Ischemia

All patients with MI should be screened for the possibility of a future ischemic event, regardless of how small or uncomplicated the MI. This is the standard of care. Noninvasive screening for ischemia is summarized in Table 17-4. A recent meta-analysis found that ST segment depression on a stress ECG was 44% sensitive in predicting cardiac death or reinfarction within the year after MI.[8] Sensitivity was improved by adding an imaging study: up to 80% with an exercise perfusion scan, 71% with a pharmacologic perfusion scan, 62% with an exercise echocardiogram, and 55% with a pharmacologic stress echocardiogram. Most of the studies of exercise testing after MI excluded patients with poor LV function. A large MI, particularly if complicated by heart failure, is a relative contraindication to early exercise testing, and angiography is safer. Angiography also is preferable for those with angina soon after MI.

Can the low-risk patient have an exercise ECG alone, or must you add an imaging study? The practice guidelines do not indicate a preference, despite recognition that imaging studies add sensitivity.[1,8] I do not think that you could be faulted for doing a symptom-limited exercise ECG in a setting of small, uncomplicated first MI and doing no further workup if the study is negative and exercise tolerance is good (>7 minutes on the treadmill using the Bruce protocol).

A Warning about Imaging Studies

You should be aware that imaging studies are operator dependent. The studies demonstrating their accuracy were performed in centers that have dedicated teams doing nuclear cardiology or echocardiography full time. Although not widely discussed, there is a problem when translating these results to some practice

Table 17-4	*Screening and Treatment for Residual or Recurrent Ischemia after Myocardial Infarction*

Study or Therapy	Indications and Comments
No screening study	Appropriate only when a decision is made to avoid interventional treatment (e.g., an elderly or disabled person who is not a candidate for revascularization, or when that is the patient's preference).
Exercise ECG	Uncomplicated, completed MI. If a low-level stress test is done in hospital, a symptom-limited study should be done 2 to 4 weeks later. *Contraindication:* LVEF <40%, complicated MI*
Symptom-limited exercise ECG plus an imaging study †	*Strongly indicated:* When ECG changes prevent interpretation of ST segment changes *Possibly indicated:* Uncomplicated, completed MI; more sensitive than a stress ECG alone.
Pharmacologic stress imaging	An alternative if patient is unable to exercise. Dipyridamole perfusion imaging is better than exercise scanning when there is left bundle branch block.
Coronary angiography	*Strongly indicated:* 1. Patients with a positive screening study. 2. As the initial test without a screening study: post-MI angina, heart failure after MI or LVEF <40%, late hospital phase VT or VF. *Possibly indicated:* 1. As the initial test after "incomplete" MI: thrombolytic therapy or non Q–wave infarction (while controversial, this has become the usual approach in the United States[9,10]). 2. A need to return to an unusually vigorous job or where public safety is an issue.
TREATMENT TO PREVENT ISCHEMIA	
Aspirin	All patients, barring contraindication
Beta-adrenergic blockade	*Strongly indicated:* All patients with these exceptions: 1. A contraindication to beta-blockers or side effects with beta blockade 2. A low risk of future ischemia based on known coronary anatomy and LVEF, and/or recent revascularization
ACE inhibition	*Strongly indicated:* LVEF <40%, prevention of remodeling also may prevent ischemia (see text)
Risk factor modification	This includes lowering LDL cholesterol below 100 mg/dL, usually with drug therapy, to prevent progression of atherosclerosis.

*Complicated MI: heart failure, persistent angina, uncontrolled arrhythmia.
†None of these studies used low-level exercise testing plus imaging studies.

settings, where scans may be read by a radiologist with little training or experience with nuclear cardiac imaging. Local experience often dictates the choice of imaging technique. If you have an experienced echocardiography team, use echocardiography. If there is more experience with nuclear studies, that is the choice. If your hospital has little or no experience with either, be aware that buying a nuclear camera does not mean that you will automatically achieve dependable results.

Timing

Timing of exercise testing is a fielder's choice. Testing while the patient is in the hospital, within 4 to 6 days of MI, rules out ischemia that may occur early after discharge. There is also the logistic advantage of getting it done while the patient is still in the hospital. However, the early exercise test should not push the patient hard (the target heart rate is usually 120 beats/min). Exercise tolerance is not tested with early study.

The advantage of later testing, more than 10 days after MI, is that exercise tolerance may be measured with a symptom-limited test. That is important because poor exercise tolerance is a sensitive indicator of poor prognosis, even more sensitive than ST segment depression on the stress ECG.[8] For a low-risk patient with a small, apparently completed MI, you may want the more complete study done 10 to 14 days after MI. If there is uncertainty about the patient's stability, a predischarge study would be preferred.

Incomplete Myocardial Infarction

Patients with non–Q wave infarction and patients with Q wave MI treated with thrombolytic therapy usually have unstable coronary plaque and tight stenosis. Viable muscle is present in the region supplied by the diseased artery, and the infarct is considered "incomplete." They are at high risk for occlusion of the infarct vessel and probably should have angiography.[9] Delaying transfer for angiography makes no sense; occlusion and reinfarction may occur while the patient languishes (usually in the middle of the night). The day after acute MI is a good time for transfer, when early VAs and chest pain have resolved. Early transfer also positions the patient in the catheterization laboratory queue, ensuring timely study (an important consideration when a weekend or holiday approaches).

Some advocate noninvasive screening of selected patients within this high-risk population with incomplete MI.[10] The selection of patients for noninvasive study rather than angiography is complicated, and recommendations seem to change with each new study. I would suggest sending a high-risk patient with incomplete MI to a cardiologist for that decision, and if the decision is to avoid angiography, fine.

Therapy To Prevent Recurrent Ischemia or Infarction

Those with high-risk coronary anatomy usually have revascularization. The purpose of the screening protocol is to identify them. Treatment of lower risk patients is summarized in Table 17-4. Even low-risk patients should be treated with daily *aspirin*, and 81 mg/day is adequate.

Beta-adrenergic blockade is recommended for all patients after MI, as long as it can be tolerated. It is not contraindicated for those with moderate depression of LVEF (30% to 40%) in the absence of symptomatic congestive heart failure. Some patients with heart failure also tolerate beta-blockers, but regulation of therapy is tricky. Obstructive lung disease with bronchospasm is a contraindication.

In a couple of situations, *not* prescribing beta blockade after MI is reasonable: (1) single-vessel coronary artery disease (CAD) and completed MI, where the risk of future ischemia is low, and (2) after revascularization, where the risk of future ischemia is low. Both are common clinical situations, and it is sensible to avoid the difficulties of beta blockade when it is safe to do so.

LV Dysfunction after MI
Remodeling

During the week after infarction the necrotic muscle softens and becomes "mushy." There is thinning, bulging, and expansion of the soft infarct zone. This is most common with anterior MI, and the result is a change in the shape of the LV apex. Instead of the normal elliptical shape, the LV apex has a rounded, mushroom shape. The most extreme form of this is LV aneurysm (see Fig. 16-1).

As subsequent healing takes place, scar is laid down in the "mold" provided by the altered infarct zone, resulting in a permanent alteration in shape. At that point the shape of the infarct zone is "cast in scar." The goal of afterload reduction therapy is prevention of early bulging, before scarring occurs.

Alteration in the shape of the apex has a negative effect on LV function. The radius of curvature of the LV is increased. Because of the Laplace relationship (Wall tension = Pressure × Radius), increased radius means an elevation of wall tension. LV wall tension is a determinant of myocardial oxygen demand (MVO_2), so overall MVO_2 is higher. Thus prevention of infarct expansion and this "stretch effect" also may be considered a treatment to prevent ischemia. Trials of ACE inhibitor therapy have shown less sudden cardiac death, possibly because of this antiischemic effect.

For those with large MI, including all patients with anterior MI, treatment with ACE inhibitors prevents infarct expansion, and treatment should be started within 24 hours of the onset of MI (Table 17-5). Contraindications include known bilateral renal artery stenosis, renal failure, or history of adverse effects with prior treatment. An angiotensin II blocker (e.g., losartan) is an alternative if the patient has a history of ACE inhibitor intolerance. Therapy for LV dysfunction should be continued long-term, at least 3 years.

It is uncertain whether treatment benefits those with smaller MI, and randomized trials of ACE inhibition for all patients with MI are in progress.

Screening for Peripheral Embolization after Myocardial Infarction

Without anticoagulation, mural thrombus develops in as many as 20% with Q wave MI, and the incidence rises to 40% with anterior MI. It is more common with large infarction. About 10% of those with LV thrombus have peripheral embolization. Thus the risk of embolization ranges from 1% to 4% with acute MI, depending on the size and location of infarction.

Table 17-5	Screening and Treatment for LV Dysfunction and Remodeling after Myocardial Infarction

Study or Therapy	Indications and Comments
No screening study	Small, uncomplicated, first, nonanterior MI
Echocardiogram	1. Anterior MI 2. Heart failure before, during, or after MI 3. History of prior MI 4. Large inferior or lateral MI (based on enzyme rise or a complicated clinical course)
TREATMENT TO PREVENT INFARCT EXPANSION ("REMODELING") AND DETERIORATION OF LV FUNCTION	

Angiotensin-converting enzyme inhibitor (ACEI)	*Strongly indicated:* 1. Anterior MI
	2. MI complicated by heart failure
	3. LVEF <40% after MI
	Uncertain indication: smaller infarction as short-term therapy[7]
	Contraindications: systolic blood pressure <100 mm Hg. Bilateral renal artery stenosis, adverse reaction to ACEI (e.g., cough, allergy)
	Drug and dose:*
	  Captopril (Capoten) 12.5 to 50 mg tid
	  Enalapril (Vasotec) 5 to 20 mg bid
	  Lisinopril (Prinivil, Zestril) 2.5 to 10 mg once daily
	  Ramipril (Altace) 2.5 to 5 mg bid

Angiotensin II blocker (losartan)	A subsitute for ACE inhibitors for those who are intolerant (e.g., ACE inhibitor–induced cough).

*Start at the low dose and advance to the maximal tolerable dose based on blood pressure and serum creatinine level. In some cases the doses are higher than usual for the treatment of hypertension. These doses are from trials of heart failure therapy and from studies of ACE inhibition after MI.[7]

The pathogenesis of ventricular clot is uncertain. A loss of wall motion may lead to stagnation of blood in contact with the surface; normal contraction keeps blood moving along. It also has been suggested that the inflamed endocardial surface of infarcted muscle may be thrombogenic. Embolization is more likely when a clot is mobile, protrudes well into the chamber, or is large (and is visible in multiple echocardiographic views).

The transthoracic echocardiogram is sensitive and specific for the diagnosis of apical LV thrombus; a transesophageal study is not necessary for routine screening. The current recommendations for prophylactic therapy are outlined in Table 17-6.

Summary: A Treatment Checklist after Myocardial Infarction

The treatments listed in Box 17-1 have been shown to prevent reinfarction or improve survival *for properly selected patients.* One way to approach your patient who has survived the acute event and is preparing for discharge would be to look at each item on the list and to decide why it has not been prescribed, if it has not. The preceding tables summarize screening studies and patient selection for these therapies.

Limitations of Screening Studies

Screening studies identify high- and low-risk patients. They do not identify patients with no risk for a complication. This is as true for coronary angiography as it is for noninvasive tests. I am careful to point this out to patients and their families.

Cardiac rupture is the one complication of MI that we are not able to predict with screening studies. Unfortunately, it is a common cause of death after MI, ranking behind arrhythmias and LV failure (see Chapter 16). It may occur during the 5 to 14 days after MI, soon after discharge. It is more common after a first MI and may occur with small, nonanterior infarction. The patient seems to be doing well clinically and has an apparently good prognosis based on a smooth clinical course and a small or moderately sized MI. Rupture catches everyone by surprise, especially the doctor. Death is sudden, with rupture into the pericardial space and tamponade. It is not treatable.

We mention rupture as one more reason for moderation when counseling your "low-risk" patient. It is important to emphasize an optimistic prognosis, but you cannot and therefore should not guarantee it.

Table 17-6	Screening and Treatment for LV Thrombus after Myocardial Infarction

Study	Indications and Comments
No screening	Small, uncomplicated, first MI (nonanterior)
Echocardiogram	1. Anterior MI
	2. Heart failure before, during, or after MI
TREATMENT TO PREVENT ARTERIAL EMBOLIZATION*	
	Indications:
Warfarin (INR = 2.0	1. Dilated, akinetic LV apex, or LV thrombus; continue warfarin for 3 months and stop
to 3.0)	only if a repeat echocardiogram shows no thrombus
	2. Persistent LV thrombus: indefinite therapy
	3. LV dilation and low LVEF: indefinite therapy

*The treatment that is outlined has not been the subject of randomized clinical trials but is consistent with Practice Guidelines.[1] Note that aspirin is not recommended as prophylaxis for peripheral arterial embolism.

BOX 17-1

THERAPIES THAT MAY PREVENT REINFARCTION OR DEATH AFTER MYOCARDIAL INFARCTION FOR *SELECTED* PATIENTS

Beta-adrenergic blockers
Aspirin
ACE inhibitors
Angiotensin II blockers
Warfarin
Implantable cardioverter defibrillator
Lipid-altering drugs (reductase inhibitors and niacin)
Risk factor modification, including exercise therapy

LONG-TERM TREATMENT AND FOLLOW-UP AFTER MYOCARDIAL INFARCTION

The long-term future of a low-risk patient is determined by the rate of progression of atherosclerosis. Risk factor modification is the cornerstone of secondary prevention, and management of smoking, diet, diabetes, and hypertension is the duty of the primary care physician (see Chapter 11).

Clinical trials have proven that progression of disease is blunted and survival improved when the low-density lipoprotein (LDL) cholesterol level is pushed below 100 mg/dL. That goal has become the standard of care for all who have documented CAD. Reaching it usually requires therapy with reductase inhibitors or niacin (see Chapter 12).

Exercise Therapy and Activity after Myocardial Infarction

Training Effects

The best measure of cardiovascular fitness is the maximum amount of oxygen the body is able to use during exercise (VO_2 max).[11] This can be measured during a "metabolic, or cardiopulmonary, exercise test" with a device that collects expired air and measures oxygen uptake (as well as minute ventilation and carbon dioxide production). VO_2 max is influenced by the oxygen-carrying capacity of blood (which declines with anemia), pulmonary function, and an ability to raise cardiac output. Notice that the curve flattens when VO_2 max is reached (Fig. 17-1). At this VO_2 plateau, continued exercise is accomplished with a disproportionate rise in minute ventilation and carbon dioxide production relative to oxygen uptake (VO_2). In fact, the anaerobic threshold is reached some time before the VO_2 and is identified as the point at which carbon dioxide production increases disproportionate to VO_2 (usually at about 40% to 70% of VO_2 max).

Trained distance athletes have especially high VO_2 max, largely the result of greater cardiac reserve. Measurable differences include increased blood volume, LV dilation, and therefore increased stroke volume (see Chapter 2). Athletes also have more efficient skeletal muscles, with an increased capacity for oxidative metabolism. At a given level of VO_2 (oxygen use by the body, in ml/kg/min), the trained individual is doing a similar amount of external work (Fig. 17-1). However, that level of work (and VO_2) is accom-

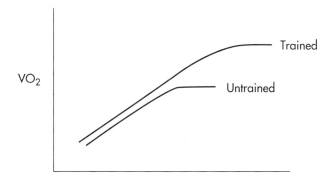

FIG. 17-1
Oxygen uptake by the body *(VO2)* increases during work. Cardiopulmonary reserve has a limit, and VO$_2$ reaches a plateau, referred to as *VO2 max,* which defines the level of fitness. Individuals who routinely engage in physical training have a much higher VO$_2$ max. Heart rate, blood pressure, and minute ventilation also increase with work. However, at any level of work (or level of VO$_2$), these are lower for trained individuals. Thus an individual who is physically trained has a more efficient body and a higher cardiopulmonary reserve.

plished with lower heart rate, blood pressure, and minute ventilation. That is a rough description of the "training effect."[11]

On the other hand, exercise training has little measurable effect on myocardial contractility. Small improvements in LVEF have been demonstrated with high-intensity exercise, but not at levels of exercise commonly used in cardiac rehabilitation programs.

The training effect is accomplished by patients with heart disease in aerobic exercise programs. VO$_2$ max is higher, and at any workload (with its associated VO$_2$), heart rate is lower. For a patient with severe exercise limitations, a small improvement in VO$_2$ max may be the difference between total disability and a return to simple activities outside the home.

Other benefits of exercise include weight loss, better control of diabetes, and increased high-density lipoprotein (HDL) cholesterol levels. The psychologic benefits cannot be overemphasized. Patients in formal exercise programs recover more quickly and are able to resume normal physical activity sooner.

Effect on Survival

Multiple studies have attempted to show a survival benefit of cardiac rehabilitation. Generally, they have not yielded statistical proof that exercise therapy reduces mortality.[13] These are tough studies to conduct. There is a lot of cross-over of control patients into exercise programs, and the studies have been small and have had short-term follow-up. They tend to show a benefit sim-

ilar to that reported for beta-blocker trials, but with too few patients to achieve statistical significance.

Patient Selection for Exercise Therapy

An important change in recent years is the discovery that patients with cardiac dysfunction benefit from exercise training.[13] In fact, those with lower VO$_2$ max tend to have a greater benefit in terms of percentage increase in exercise tolerance. We commonly send patients with low left ventricular ejection fraction (LVEF) and mildly symptomatic heart failure to cardiac rehabilitation. In such cases the exercise prescription and surveillance during training are critical.

A baseline exercise test is the basis for an exercise prescription. The major *contraindications* to training are exercise-induced ischemia, arrhythmias, and poorly controlled heart failure. When complications of exercise are identified on the baseline treadmill study, exercise training is avoided until they are corrected, which may not be possible. Those with persistent ischemia despite optimal therapy may proceed with exercise therapy but at levels well below the ischemic threshold. Similarly, a patient with heart failure may do well with shorter periods of exercise at a lower target heart rate.

Patients with the combination of *heart failure plus ischemia* are at higher risk for complications during exercise training. At the low level of exercise that is usually required, they seldom achieve a conditioning effect.

The Exercise Prescription

The baseline treadmill test is the key to designing a training program. It allows screening for exercise-induced ischemia or arrhythmias and definition of maximal heart rate and exercise tolerance. The symptom-limited exercise study performed a couple weeks after MI provides all the required data.

Conditioning depends on the frequency, intensity, and length of exercise sessions, and those are the elements of the "exercise prescription." The minimum *frequency* for cardiac fitness is three sessions per week. Once the patient is in shape, the target *intensity* is exercise to 75% to 85% of the maximal heart rate (based on the treadmill study). At the beginning the target rate should be lower, about 65% of the maximal rate, and this can be slowly advanced during the first 6 weeks of exercise. A fall in the perceived exertion with a given exercise is an indication that the intensity of exercise can be increased. The ideal *length* of exercise is 40 minutes of aerobic conditioning, preceded by a 10-minute warm-up and followed by a 10-minute cool-down.

The type of exercise is tailored to the patient. It should be aerobic. Strength training, especially isometric exercise, is avoided because it causes a disproportionate rise in blood pressure when compared with the increase in heart rate. Most patients are comfortable with dynamic leg training (walking or bicycling).

Supervised group exercise offers a number of benefits. An inexperienced patient learns how to exercise and often learns a bit about exercise physiology. Risk factors are addressed in the group setting. Unanticipated difficulties with exercise are detected. Many programs intermittently monitor even low-risk patients, screening for exercise-induced arrhythmias. Exercise groups tend to bond, and the community provides psychosocial support, as does the rehabilitation staff. Most insurance benefit programs provide 8 to 12 weeks of formal cardiac rehabilitation after MI.

Many patients exercise at home, outside the supervised setting. This is safe for those who do not have exercise-induced ischemia or arrhythmias. They should exercise to a prescribed target heart rate. It helps to suggest limits on perceived exertion as well. We tell patients that as long as they can talk, whistle, or sing, they probably are not pushing too hard.

Safety of Exercise Training

Aerobic exercise, as prescribed earlier, is safe for those without severe LV dysfunction or exercise-induced ischemia or arrhythmia. Risk stratification as outlined in this chapter is thus critical for a patient beginning exercise therapy.

High-risk patients are safest exercising in a supervised group with ECG monitoring. High risk is identified by symptoms or objective signs of any of the following: severe LV dysfunction, heart failure, exercise-induced ischemia, complex VAs, poor exercise tolerance, hypotension with exercise, or inability to self-monitor heart rate. Such patients may benefit from participation in a supervised group program for longer than the usual 8 to 12 weeks.

Supervised group exercise with either continuous or intermittent monitoring has a good safety record. The incidence of sudden death in a recent survey was 1.3 per 1 million patient hours of exercise and, of resuscitated cardiac arrest, 8.9 per million patient hours.[14]

Counsel Regarding Common Physical Activity

The exercise test conducted within 3 weeks of MI provides reassurance to you and your patient about the safety of exercise. The absence of exercise-induced ischemia or arrhythmias indicates that normal activities of daily living and a regular exercise program may be started safely.

Heart Rate 120 Beats/Min

This is a number worth remembering. Holter monitoring studies done early after uncomplicated MI have shown that normal activities such as walking up stairs and *light* housework may push the heart rate to 120 beats/min, but rarely higher. That is one reason why predischarge exercise testing is performed with a target heart rate of 120 beats/min. Tell the patient that it is a "safety test." Reaching 120 beats/min with no ECG abnormality or symptoms indicates that walking up stairs, carrying a bag of groceries, sweeping the kitchen floor, or making a bed also will be safe.

Sexual Activity[15]

The same Holter monitoring studies after MI found that sex with one's usual partner and in a familiar setting pushes the heart rate to 120 beats/min. On the other hand, sex in a novel setting or with an unfamiliar partner produces a much higher heart rate response. (There is good and bad news in those data.) If the patient can walk up two flights of stairs without symptoms, sexual intercourse is safe.

There are a few specific recommendations for your patient that make sex even safer:

1. Postpone sex for a couple hours after a large meal or immediately after drinking alcohol.
2. Use the sexual position that is most familiar and comfortable; adjustment may increase physical stress.
3. Have sex when relaxed and well rested.
4. When resuming sexual activity early after MI, consider a couple of warm-up sessions—intimacy without coitus for 1 or 2 days.

Symptoms, particularly new symptoms, indicate a need for prompt evaluation (starting with a stress test). These would include angina, unusual dyspnea or palpitations during sex, or excessive fatigue or prolonged tachycardia after sex. Checking the pulse rate after sex provides useful objective information.

Patients who are being treated medically for angina after MI may find that sublingual nitroglycerin just before sex prevents symptoms. There is no reason to recommend this for those who do not have angina.

A number of middle-aged men use fildenafil (Viagra). The drug blocks degradation of nitric oxide and thus has vasodilating properties. It is not contraindicated in patients with CAD or after MI. On the other hand, it is contraindicated for those taking nitrates because it enhances the hypotensive effects of nitroglycerin and may cause syncope. This may be a concern for the patient with angina who is not taking long-acting nitrates, but who uses intermittent sublingual nitroglycerin. If sexual activity provokes angina, nitroglycerin could be dangerous after taking fildenafil.

Sexual dysfunction after MI is common and usually results from transient situational depression. This improves with time and is helped by exercise therapy. There may be fear of precipitating another MI, and both the patient and spouse benefit from reassurance about safety, as well as specific recommendations about sexual activity.

A number of commonly prescribed drugs may cause impotence or depress the libido, including beta-blockers, diuretics, antiarrhythmic and lipid-lowering agents, major tranquilizers, and clonidine. Drug-induced impotence usually is an indication for changing medicines, and we are dismayed when we see a patient who does not mention his impotence.

Surveys have identified impotence as the most common problem for men after MI, and 10% of these patients become permanently impotent. Persistent sexual dysfunction necessitates further medical, urologic, and psychologic evaluation.

Follow-up after MI and Expected Clinical Course

Although infrequently described in texts, most patients are easily fatigued and have a general loss of energy after MI. Those who have had a moderate to large MI and who have depressed LV function are fatigued because of limits on cardiac performance, but patients with small infarction and normal LVEF also feel a loss of vigor. We tell them that this is the usual state during early healing after MI and that energy levels will return to normal a couple months after the infarction. (While you are reassuring the patient, also be sure that you have not missed unexpected LV dysfunction or aneurysm or silent ischemia.)

There is no protocol that prescribes frequency of clinic visits after hospital discharge. Those with complications such as heart failure or angina need more frequent evaluation. We usually see an uncomplicated, low-risk patient 1½ weeks, 6 weeks, 3 months, and 1 year after discharge. That schedule corresponds to the time of the initial symptom-limited exercise study, the time of return to work, and times for regulation of lipid-lowering therapy (see Chapter 12).

Return to Work and Disability Evaluation

Those in sedentary occupations are able to return to work 6 weeks after an uncomplicated MI. The average patient returns to work 2 to 3 months after MI. Those who do heavy physical work need a longer period of rehabilitation. Uncertainty about a patient's ability to handle heavy work is an indication for exercise testing before returning to work. In some cases, the occupation is a factor when recommending angiography.

Your attitude and approach have a major influence on the patient's decision to return to work. When the doctor outlines a timetable and exercise strategy

aimed at return to work, the time off work is shortened.[16] Earlier return has no adverse clinical effect, and there are financial and psychologic advantages for the patient.[16]

A number of patients seek medical disability after MI. The Social Security Administration (SSA) has specific criteria for awarding benefits, including depressed LVEF and heart failure, or objective evidence for ischemia (see Chapter 49). Although occupational stress is a real issue (see Chapter 46), it is not considered justification for disability benefits after uncomplicated MI. By establishing objective guidelines the SSA has at least lifted the burden of disability determination from the doctor, who remains the patient's friend and advocate. Patients who do physical labor, have less education, or are over 60 years of age are less likely to return to work after MI.[16]

Driving

A patient with a small, uncomplicated MI may safely drive within 3 weeks of MI. We advise against long trips that early, suggesting short drives in a nonstressful setting until later in recovery. A patient with large or complicated infarction is best advised to wait 6 weeks before starting to drive. It is wise to exclude arrhythmias and ischemia before agreeing to resumption of motor vehicle operation (using the risk stratification strategies described earlier).

Psychosocial Support and Canine Therapy

The CAST trial found that human social support was an independent predictor of survival after MI. It also found that dog, but not cat, owners lived longer (no surprise to those of us who are eccentric dog people).[17] We have all encountered an elderly patient who insists on early discharge from the hospital because of concern about the hound. Relationships give people a reason to live—however trivial the relationship appears to others.

REFERENCES

1. Ryan TJ, Anderson JL, Antman EM, et al: ACC/AHA Guidelines for the management of patients with acute myocardial infarction: executive summary. A report of the American College of Cardiology/American Heart Association Task Force on Practice Guidelines (Committee on Management of Acute Myocardial Infarction), *Circulation* 94:2341, 1996.
2. Ewy GA, Appleton CP, Demaria AN, et al: ACC/AHA guidelines for the clinical application of echocardiography. A report of the American College of Cardiology/American Heart Association Task Force on Assessment of Diagnostic and Therapeutic Cardiovascular Procedures, *J Am Coll Cardiol* 16:1505, 1990.

3. Knoebel SB, Crawford MH, Dunn MI, et al: Guidelines for ambulatory electrocardiography. A report of the American College of Cardiology/American Heart Association Task Force on Assessment of Diagnostic and Therapeutic Cardiovascular Procedures, *J Am Coll Cardiol* 13:249, 1989.

4. Ross J Jr, Brandenburg RO, Dinsmore RE, et al: Guidelines for coronary angiography. A report of the American College of Cardiology/American Heart Association Task Force on Assessment of Diagnostic and Therapeutic Cardiovascular Procedures, *J Am Coll Cardiol* 10:935, 1987.

5. Zipes DP, DiMarco JP, Gillette PC, et al: Guidelines for clinical intracardiac electrophysiological studies and catheter ablation procedures. A report of the American College of Cardiology/American Heart Association Task Force on Practice Guidelines (Subcommittee to Assess Clinical Intracardiac Electrophysiological and Catheter Ablation Procedures), *J Am Coll Cardiol* 26:555, 1995.

6. Underwood RD, Sra J, Akhtar M: Evaluation and treatment strategies in patients at high risk of sudden death post myocardial infarction, *Clin Cardiol* 20:753, 1997.

7. Pratt CM, Waldo AL, Camm, AJ: Can antiarrhythmic drugs survive survival trials? *Am J Cardiol* 81:24, 1998.

8. Peterson ED, Shaw LJ, Califf RM: Risk stratification after myocardial infarction, *Ann Intern Med* 126:561, 1997.

9. Guetta V, Topol EJ: Pacifying the infarct vessel, *Circulation* 96:713, 1997.

10. Quinones MA: Risk stratification after myocardial infarction: clinical science versus practice behavior, *Circulation* 95:1352, 1997.

11. Weber KT: What can we learn from exercise testing beyond the detection of myocardial ischemia? *Clin Cardiol* 20:684, 1997.

12. O'Connor GT, Buring JE, Yusuf S, et al: An overview of randomized trials of rehabilitation with exercise after myocardial infarction, *Circulation* 80:234, 1989.

13. Dafoe W, Huston P: Current trends in cardiac rehabilitation, *Can Med Assoc J* 156:527, 1997.

14. VanCamp SP, Peterson RA: Cardiovascular complications of outpatient cardiac rehabilitation programs, *JAMA* 256:1160, 1986.

15. Froelicher ES, Kee LL, Newton KM, et al: Return to work, sexual activity, and other activities after acute myocardial infarction, *Heart Lung* 23:423, 1994.

16. Dennis C, Houston-Miller N, Schwartz RG, et al: Early return to work after uncomplicated myocardial infarction: results of a randomized trial, *JAMA* 260:214, 1988.

17. Friedmann E, Thomas SA: Pet ownership, social support, and one-year survival after acute myocardial infarction in the Cardiac Arrhythmia Suppression Trial (CAST), *Am J Cardiol* 76:1213, 1995.

18 Mitral Valve Disease

Blase A. Carabello
Donald R. Graham

MITRAL STENOSIS
Etiology and Epidemiology

Almost all cases of adult mitral stenosis are caused by rheumatic heart disease. Rarely, calcium deposition in the mitral annulus can become severe enough to restrict mitral inflow, but rheumatic involvement of the mitral leaflets and chordae leads to valvular stenosis in most cases. Although the attack rate for rheumatic fever is similar between genders, the development of mitral stenosis after rheumatic fever is three to four times more common in women. Typically stenosis develops in the fifth and sixth decades of life in economically developed countries. In developing nations where the rheumatic process seems to be more aggressive, stenosis may occur much earlier. In some cases a woman with mitral stenosis is asymptomatic until pregnancy, when increased cardiac demand causes symptoms. Although the incidence of rheumatic fever is waning in the United States, mitral stenosis is still commonly seen in patients who emigrate from countries where rheumatic fever is prevalent.

Pathophysiology

In normal subjects, left atrial pressure changes little during ventricular systole. As ventricular relaxation occurs, pressure becomes higher in the left atrium than in the left ventricle, which in turn opens the mitral valve while producing rapid left ventricular filling. The gradient between the left atrium and left ventricle quickly dissipates, and pressures in the two chambers are equal for most of diastole because the wide open mitral valve forms a common chamber between the left atrium and the left ventricle (Fig. 18-1, *A*).

However, in mitral stenosis (Fig. 18-1, *B*), narrowing of the mitral orifice restricts emptying of the left atrium (and therefore filling of the left ventricle), and a persistent gradient develops between the left atrium and the left ventricle.[1] Thus mitral stenosis increases left atrial pressure while restricting left ventricular filling and therefore left ventricular output. Although in most cases left ventricular muscle function is normal, high left atrial pressure and decreased cardiac output

mimic the presence of congestive heart failure caused by left ventricular dysfunction.[2] The neurohumoral response to low cardiac output is the same (see Table 22-1).

Most of the propulsive force moving blood from the left atrium to the left ventricle is actually generated by the right ventricle. Thus the right ventricle sustains a pressure overload in mitral stenosis. It must generate the increased force needed to overcome the stenosis and fill the left ventricle. In addition, as mitral stenosis worsens, secondary pulmonary vasoconstriction may develop, further increasing pulmonary pressure and pressure overload on the right ventricle. Although the cause of this secondary pulmonary vasoconstriction is still unknown, some studies suggest that impaired nitric oxide release may be involved, as inhalation of nitric oxide may partially reverse pulmonary hypertension.[3]

Clinical Presentation

A patient with mitral stenosis complains of the symptoms of pulmonary congestion (Table 18-1). Dyspnea on exertion, orthopnea, and paroxysmal nocturnal dyspnea are common (one teacher was fond of stating that "mitral stenosis is a disease of the lungs"). As pulmonary hypertension develops, the symptoms of right-sided failure, ascites, edema, and fatigue also develop.

In addition to these symptoms common to any form of heart failure, hemoptysis is more specific for mitral stenosis. Hemoptysis occurs as left atrial hypertension leads to rupture of small bronchial veins. Enlargement of the left atrium may encroach on the left superior laryngeal nerve, causing hoarseness (Ortner's syndrome), or may encroach on the esophagus, causing dysphagia.

The history of rheumatic fever is often unreliable. Many patients previously diagnosed as having had rheumatic fever have no cardiac evidence that they ever sustained the illness, whereas other patients with clear rheumatic valvular deformity deny ever having had rheumatic fever.

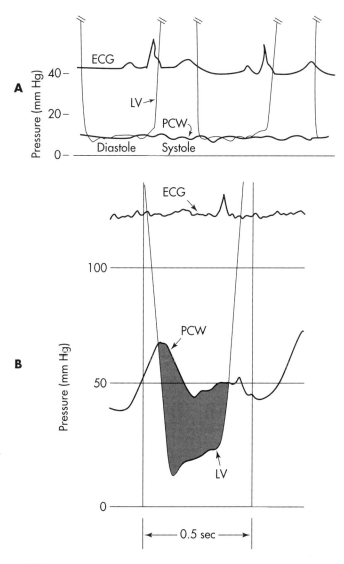

FIG. 18-1

Pressure tracings from the cardiac catheterization laboratory. **A,** A normal patient. During ventricular diastole, when the mitral valve is open, pressure in the left ventricle *(LV)* is no different from pressure in the left atrium (that pressure is identical to the pulmonary capillary wedge pressure, *PCW*). Both are about 10 mm Hg. During ventricular systole the mitral valve closes and LV pressure rises. **B,** A patient with mitral stenosis. Even when the mitral valve is open during diastole, a pressure "gradient" is present across the stenosed valve *(shaded area).*

From Carabello BA, Grossman W, editors: *Cardiac catheterization and angiography,* ed 3, Philadelphia, 1986, Lea & Febiger.

Physical Examination

Although the physical signs of mitral stenosis are easily recognized, the diagnosis is often missed because physical examination has been performed in a cursory manner. Palpation of the precordium finds a normal left ventricular apical impulse. A diastolic thrill may be noted especially when the patient is placed in the left lateral decubitus position. If pulmonary hypertension has developed, a parasternal lift may be noted.

Classically, S_1 is increased in intensity, and this may be the only clue to mitral stenosis in early cases. S_1 is loud because the transmitral gradient holds the mitral valve open throughout diastole, so ventricular systole closes the valve leaflets from a fully opened position. With more advanced disease, fusion of the commissures permits little mitral valve motion and S_1 becomes soft. S_2 is usually normal, although the pulmonic component may be increased in cases of pulmonary hypertension.

S_2 is followed by an opening snap (OS). The higher the left atrial pressure, the sooner the mitral valve opens. Thus with severe mitral stenosis the S_2-OS interval is shorter. An S_2-OS interval less than 0.10 second indicates severe mitral stenosis. A neat bedside trick helps with estimating the interval: the time between the "b" and the "t" in the word *butter* is about 0.14 second. The time between the "b" and the "l" in *blah* is about 0.11 second. Say those words to yourself while tapping the cadence with two fingers, then apply the "measurement" to the heart sounds. The OS is easily distinguished from an S_3 gallop, as it is higher pitched. Both the OS and S_3 tend to be localized at the apex.

After the OS a diastolic rumble is heard. If the patient remains in sinus rhythm, atrial contraction may cause presystolic accentuation of the murmur. Because the stenotic mitral valve restricts rapid left ventricular filling, third and fourth heart sounds are extremely rare in this condition.

Management

Laboratory Tests (Table 18-2)

Electrocardiogram. If the patient is in sinus rhythm, left atrial abnormality is usually demonstrated. However, atrial fibrillation is common in mitral stenosis. Right axis deviation and evidence of right ventricular hypertrophy are often seen.

Chest X-ray. Typical findings of the chest x-ray reflect the pathophysiology of the disease. Left atrial enlargement causes straightening of the left heart border and a double density at the right heart border where the left atrial shadow is found just inside the right atrial shadow. When pulmonary hypertension has developed, the pulmonary arteries may be enlarged. The lung fields may demonstrate Kerley B lines (thickened pulmonary lymphatics and septae).

Echocardiogram. The echo-Doppler study is the most important diagnostic test to be performed in patients with mitral stenosis[4] (Fig. 18-2). It demonstrates the rheumatic deformity of the valve and restricted leaflet motion. Calcification of the leaflets and disease in the subvalvular apparatus also can be assessed and are important guides to the suitability for balloon valvotomy (see below). Left atrial enlargement is almost

Table 18-1	*Clinical Synopsis of Severe Mitral Valve Disease*

	Etiology	Pathophysiology	Symptoms	Physical Findings
Mitral stenosis	Rheumatic fever	RV pressure overload	Dyspnea	RV lift
	Annular calcification (rare)	Reduced LV filling	Orthopnea	Diastolic rumble
		Increased left atrial pressure	PND	Loud S_1
			Hemoptysis	Opening snap
			Hoarseness	
			Edema	
Mitral regurgitation	Myxomatous valve degeneration	LV volume overload Enhanced LV filling	Dyspnea Orthopnea	Displaced apical impulse
	Endocarditis			Holosystolic murmur
	Myocardial ischemia	Increased LA pressure	PND	Soft S_1
	Chordal rupture			S_3 gallop
	Marfan syndrome			

RV, Right ventricle; *LV,* left ventricle; *PND,* paroxysmal nocturnal dyspnea.

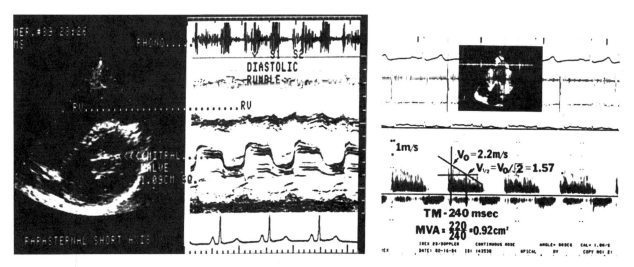

FIG. 18-2

Echocardiographic *(left panel)* and Doppler flow *(right panel)* patterns are shown for a patient with mitral stenosis. In the parasternal short axis view on the left, the narrowed mitral valve orifice is seen and planimetered to have a area of 1.09 cm². In the right panel the pressure half-time is calculated and used to derive the valve area, 0.92 cm². This figure provides an insight into the raw data used by an echocardiographer.

From Pepine CJ: *Diagnostic and therapeutic cardiac catheterization,* Baltimore, 1998, Williams & Wilkins.

Table 18-2	Diagnostic Studies in Mitral Valve Disease			
	Electrocardiogram	**Chest X-Ray**	**Echocardiogram**	**Indications for Surgical or Mechanical Intervention**
Mitral stenosis	Atrial fibrillation RVH	Double density at right heart border Kerley's lines RV enlargement	↑LA MVA <1.2 cm² RV enlargement Pulmonary hypertension	More than mild symptoms Pulmonary hypertension Atrial fibrillation
Mitral regurgitation	Atrial fibrillation LVH	Cardiomegaly Pulmonary congestion	↑LA ↑ LV Doppler color flow showing MR	More than mild symptoms EF ≤0.60 ESD ≥45 mm Atrial fibrillation

RV, Right ventricle; *RVH,* RV hypertrophy; *LA,* left atrium; *MVA,* mitral valve area; *LV,* left ventricle; *LVH,* LV hypertrophy; *EF,* LV ejection fraction; *ESD,* LV end-systolic dimension.

always present. If any tricuspid regurgitation is present, right ventricular and thus pulmonary artery pressure can be estimated using the Bernoulli principle to calculate the systolic pressure gradient between the right atrium and the right ventricle[5] (see Chapter 8).

The severity of mitral stenosis also can be adequately gauged using three different methods. In an en fosse view of the mitral valve the area of the open valve can be directly planimetered, giving an accurate measurement of the valve area, unless severe disease of the subvalvular apparatus causes the functional orifice to be less than the planimetered valve[6] (see Fig. 18-2). Alternatively, the gradient across the valve may be measured using the modified Bernoulli principle [Gradient = 4 × (Flow velocity)²]. Third, valve area can be estimated using an empiric device, the pressure half-time method[7] (see Chapter 8). With stenosis, mitral inflow velocity is increased and remains elevated throughout diastole, decaying slowly toward the end of diastole. The more severe the disease, the slower the decay. By dividing an empiric constant of 220 by the time it takes velocity to fall to its peak value divided by the square root of 2 (pressure half-time), valve area can be estimated (see Fig. 18-2). As pressure half-time (in the denominator) increases, valve area decreases.

Cardiac Catheterization. In most cases the combination of history, physical examination, chest x-ray, and echocardiography gives all the information needed to estimate the severity of the mitral stenosis. However, if severity degree is still unclear, cardiac catheterization can be used to measure the transvalvular gradient and cardiac output, data used to calculate valve area from the Gorlin formula:

$$\frac{CO/DFP \times HR}{38 \sqrt{gradient}}$$

where *CO* is cardiac output (ml/min), *DFP* is diastolic filling period (sec), and *HR* is heart rate (beats/min).[8]

In addition, since many patients with mitral stenosis are old enough to have coronary disease, coronary angiography is usually performed during catheterization if surgery is anticipated.

Treatment

Medical Therapy. Asymptomatic patients in sinus rhythm require no therapy other than antibiotic prophylaxis for bacterial endocarditis (see Chapter 21). If mild symptoms develop, diuretics lower left atrial pressure and relieve the symptoms of dyspnea and orthopnea. As cardiac output is limited by the stenotic valve, and not ventricular dysfunction, measures to improve ventricular function such as digoxin and afterload reduction therapy are ineffective.

Atrial fibrillation (AF) is a common development and carries the risk of systemic embolization and stroke. Reduced flow across the mitral valve and the enlarged left atrium make that risk much higher with mitral stenosis than it is with other causes of AF. Anticoagulation with warfarin is necessary, with the INR in the range of 2.5 to 4.0. Rate control with digoxin, beta-blockers, or calcium blockers is key in controlling symptoms.

Timing of Mechanical Relief of Stenosis of the Mitral Valve. Although medical therapy may be effective in mild disease, when more than mild symptoms develop or when pulmonary hypertension begins to develop, prognosis worsens[9,10] (Fig. 18-3). Then mechanical correction of mitral stenosis is advised. Many recommend surgery if AF cannot be reverted to sinus rhythm and maintained. In this case, relief of mitral stenosis may reduce left atrial size enough to allow restoration of normal rhythm.

Valvulotomy and Surgery. In many cases of mitral stenosis today, relief of the stenosis is achieved with percutaneous balloon valvotomy. Unlike aortic stenosis, mitral stenosis is caused by fusion of the mitral leaflets at their commissures. Inflation of a large balloon in the mitral orifice fractures these adhesions and restores both valve area and leaflet motion.[11] Echocardiography is performed to establish the suitability of the valve for this procedure.[12] Valves with only mild thickening of leaflets, little calcification, and scant involvement of the subvalvular apparatus are good candidates for balloon valvotomy. If more than mild mitral regurgitation is present, valvotomy is usually abandoned for surgical intervention because balloon dilation may significantly worsen mitral regurgitation.

Studies of balloon valvotomy demonstrate an excellent initial outcome, with an average doubling of mitral valve area and substantial improvement of cardiac symptoms.[13] Several years of follow-up are now available and indicate that most of the initial gains are maintained for more than 5 years after the procedure. In a controlled study of balloon versus surgical valvotomy, balloon valvotomy was superior when the initial anatomy was suitable for this procedure.[11] (Like all of medical therapeutics, correct patient selection is a key to success.)

If balloon valvotomy cannot be performed or if it is performed and fails to achieve a good result, surgery is warranted. In some cases, direct surgical repair of the valve is possible. Closed mitral commissurotomy is no longer performed. In other cases, severe rheumatic deformity prevents valve repair, so valve replacement is necessary.[14] Chapter 52 reviews the properties of artificial valve and model selection issues. After replacement, lifelong anticoagulation with warfarin is needed, with a target INR 3.0 to 4.0.

MITRAL REGURGITATION
Etiology

The mitral valve is composed of the mitral annulus, the mitral leaflets, the chordae tendineae, and the papillary muscles. Abnormalities of any of these components may lead to mitral regurgitation. The most common cause of mitral regurgitation in the United States today is myxomatous degeneration of the valve, its chordae tendineae, or both, leading to mitral valve prolapse.[15] Coronary artery disease, which causes papillary muscle ischemia, dysfunction, or necrosis, is the next most common cause. Endocarditis, the Marfan syndrome, and collagen vascular disease are other less common

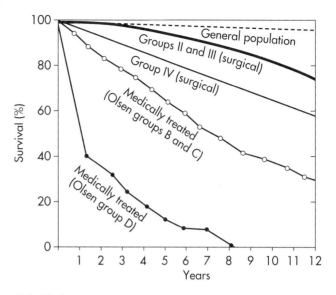

FIG. 18-3
Survivorship for medically and surgically treated patients with mitral stenosis. Olsen groups B, C, and D roughly correspond to New York Heart Association classes II, III, and IV, respectively. As symptoms worsen, the disparity between surgical and medical therapy becomes progressively greater.

From Roy SB, Gopinath N: *Circulation* 38(suppl 2):68, 1968.

causes of primary mitral regurgitation. The term *primary* implies that disease of the valve itself is responsible for the regurgitation. On the other hand, diseases of the left ventricle that cause it to dilate in turn produce papillary muscle malalignment and annular dilation, resulting in secondary mitral regurgitation. The regurgitation is caused by a ventricular rather than a valvular process.

Pathophysiology

The physiologic status of a patient with mitral regurgitation can be classified as acute, chronic compensated, or chronic decompensated.[16]

Acute Mitral Regurgitation. As shown in Figure 18-4, in acute mitral regurgitation there is a sudden emergence of a new pathway for ejection of blood from the left ventricle into the left atrium. The regurgitant volume and forward flow from the pulmonary veins combine to produce a volume overload on the left ventricle. It must pump these combined flows instead of just flow return from the lungs. This results in additional filling of the left ventricle, moving the left ventricle up and to the right on its pressure-volume curve, increasing both end-diastolic volume and end-diastolic pressure (see Chapter 2). The increase in end-diastolic volume is the Frank-Starling compensatory mechanism. Sarcomeres stretched toward their maximum length generate more work. The opening of the new pathway for ejection facilitates left ventricular emptying and

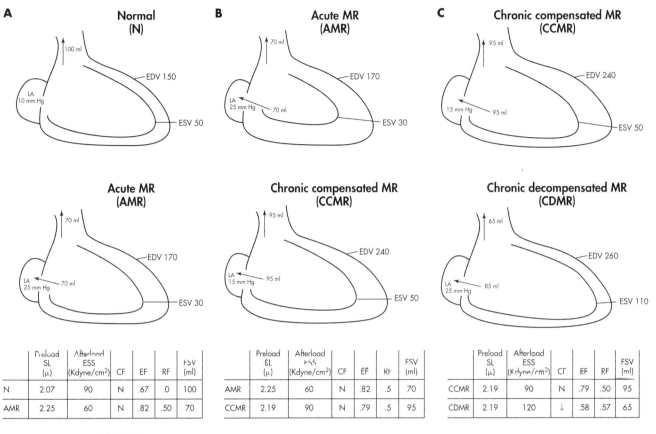

	Preload SL (μ)	Afterload ESS (Kdyne/cm²)	CF	EF	RF	FSV (ml)
N	2.07	90	N	.67	.0	100
AMR	2.25	60	N	.82	.50	70

	Preload SL (μ)	Afterload ESS (Kdyne/cm²)	CF	EF	RF	FSV (ml)
AMR	2.25	60	N	.82	.5	70
CCMR	2.19	90	N	.79	.5	95

	Preload SL (μ)	Afterload ESS (Kdyne/cm²)	CF	EF	RF	FSV (ml)
CCMR	2.19	90	N	.79	.50	95
CDMR	2.19	120	↓	.58	.57	65

FIG. 18-4

A, Acute mitral regurgitation is contrasted to normal physiology. Volume overload created by the acute mitral regurgitation increases sarcomere length *(SL)* and end-diastolic volume *(EDV)*—making use of the Frank Starling mechanism—allowing the left ventricle to increase stroke work. At the same time, the new pathway for ejection from the left ventricle into the left atrium *(LA)* decreases afterload (end-systolic stress, *ESS*), in turn reducing end-systolic volume *(ESV)*. Total stroke volume and ejection fraction *(EF)* increase. However, 50% of the total stroke volume is regurgitated into the left atrium (regurgitant fraction, *RF,* 0.50), in turn reducing forward stroke volume *(FSV)* and increasing left atrial pressure. At this time, contractile function *(CF)* is normal, yet the patient manifests the hemodynamics of congestive heart failure. **B,** Chronic compensated mitral regurgitation *(CCMR)* is compared to acute mitral regurgitation. In this stage eccentric hypertrophy has developed, allowing the ventricle to generate both increased total and forward stroke volumes. Forward stroke volume returns to normal, whereas left atrial enlargement permits lower left atrial pressure. **C,** Chronic decompensated mitral regurgitation *(CDMR)* is compared to CCMR. Reduced contractile function decreases ejection performance of the left ventricle, and end-systolic volume increases. Forward stroke volume decreases, and left atrial pressure becomes reelevated. It should be noted that at this time the still beneficial loading conditions permit a "normal" ejection fraction.

From Carabello BA: *Mod Concepts Cardiovasc Dis* 57:53, 1988.

decreases end-systolic volume. Together these changes increase total stroke volume and ejection fraction. However, because a large portion of this volume is regurgitated, or "wasted," forward stroke volume actually is diminished.

At the same time, ejection of blood into the small, unprepared, and relatively stiff left atrium increases left atrial and pulmonary venous pressures, resulting in pulmonary congestion. Although left ventricular muscle function is normal at this stage of the disease, the hemodynamics typical of left ventricular failure (reduced forward stroke volume and increased filling pressure) are present.

Chronic Compensated Mitral Regurgitation. In many cases, acute mitral regurgitation necessitates immediate corrective surgery. However, if the volume of regurgitation is not overwhelming, medical therapy allows for hemodynamic improvement, and the patient enters a chronic compensated phase. In this phase the development of eccentric cardiac hypertrophy greatly increases end-diastolic volume. Because left ventricular muscle function is normal, a large total stroke volume is ejected, in turn increasing forward stroke volume toward normal. At the same time, progressive left atrial enlargement and improved distensibility accommodate the regurgitant volume, absorbing the brunt of ventricular pressure, and the symptoms of pulmonary congestion abate. In this phase, relatively normal cardiac output and left ventricular filling pressure may allow the patient to be asymptomatic even during moderately strenuous physical activity.

Chronic Decompensated Mitral Regurgitation. The patient may remain in the chronic compensated phase for months or years, but eventually left ventricular contractile dysfunction develops. Ejection fraction falls, and end-systolic volume increases—the ventricle is unable to squeeze down to a normal volume. Total and forward stroke volumes decline, eliciting the neurohumoral responses to low cardiac output (see Table 22-1). The greater residual volume left in the ventricle at the end of diastole elevates left ventricular filling pressure. Additional dilation of the left ventricle may further distort the valve, worsening the mitral regurgitation.

In many cases the symptoms of left ventricular failure now develop. However, some patients enter the decompensated phase with deterioration of left ventricular function but remain asymptomatic. It should be noted that, although decompensation has occurred and left ventricular ejection is impaired with a fall in ejection fraction, the still favorable loading conditions permit an ejection fraction in the "normal" range. A left ventricular ejection fraction below the normal range is an ominous prognostic finding with mitral regurgitation.

Clinical Presentation

Mitral regurgitation causes the typical symptoms of left-sided heart failure, including dyspnea on exertion, orthopnea, and paroxysmal nocturnal dyspnea. In addition, there may be clues regarding the etiology of the mitral regurgitation, such as a history of endocarditis, myocardial infarction, or mitral valve prolapse syndrome.

The physical examination of a patient with *chronic* mitral regurgitation shows evidence of cardiac enlargement with displacement of the apical impulse downward and to the left (see Table 18-1). The apical impulse is typically hyperdynamic. S_1 may be reduced in intensity. In chronic disease the typical holosystolic apical murmur often radiates to the axilla. The murmur intensity does not vary with the R-R interval. It is usually accompanied by an S_3, which, in the presence of severe mitral regurgitation, does not necessarily indicate the presence of congestive heart failure. Instead, increased

left atrial volume causes an increase in rapid early filling of the left ventricle and generates the S_3 gallop.

Acute mitral regurgitation does not cause LV dilation, and the apex impulse is not displaced. Atrial contraction is usually maintained and forces a larger than normal volume into the relatively stiff (nondistended) ventricle, creating an S4 gallop. The murmur may be deceptively soft; the rapid rise in left atrial pressure (large V wave) leads to rapid equilibration between left ventricular and left atrial pressure during systole and a reduction in retrograde flow. These hemodynamics reduce both the length and the intensity of the murmur, potentially misleading the examiner into thinking that the mitral regurgitation is mild.

If pulmonary hypertension has developed, a loud pulmonic component of S_2 and parasternal lift will be found. If right ventricular failure has developed, neck vein elevation, ascites, and edema also will be present.

Management
Laboratory Studies

The echocardiogram in chronic mitral regurgitation typically shows left atrial abnormality. There may be left ventricular hypertrophy. Because volume overload and left ventricular dilation are responsible for increased left ventricular mass, high QRS voltage is the rule. Since there is no pressure overload of the left ventricle, there may not be T wave inversion in the lateral leads. If myocardial infarction is the cause of the mitral regurgitation, Q waves may be recognized. The chest x-ray should demonstrate cardiomegaly. A normal-sized cardiac silhouette indicates that either the mitral regurgitation is acute (without time for cardiac dilation) or is mild.

Echocardiography. Echocardiography is the most widely employed and important diagnostic study for the detection and quantification of mitral regurgitation. If the disease has been prolonged and severe, both the left atrium and left ventricle will be enlarged. Examination of the mitral valve in many cases demonstrates the valvular pathology responsible for regurgitation. Doppler interrogation of the mitral valve demonstrates systolic turbulence in the left atrium. Of the many schemes available to quantify the severity of mitral regurgitation, none is completely reliable.[17-19] Doppler flow interrogation of the mitral valve in mitral regurgitation can successfully determine whether regurgitation is absent, mild, or severe. However, intermediate grades of mitral regurgitation are more difficult to quantify (see Chapter 8).

Equally important is the measurement of left ventricular size and function. An enlarged left ventricular dimension at end-systole and reduced ejection fraction indicate advanced disease and a worse prognosis.

Cardiac Catheterization. While in some cases noninvasive studies are entirely adequate to demonstrate both the pathology responsible for mitral regurgitation and the severity of the lesion, in other cases additional information from cardiac catheterization is required to judge the severity of mitral regurgitation and therefore the timing of surgery. In symptomatic patients the left atrial pressure (pulmonary capillary wedge pressure) is increased, providing a hemodynamic explanation for the symptoms.

In many cases a large V wave is present in the pulmonary capillary wedge pressure tracing. As a rule, a tall V wave is more common with acute mitral regurgitation. On the other hand, large V waves may be present in the absence of mitral regurgitation. Thus V wave height in general is of only modest use in clinical decision making in mitral regurgitation.

Left ventriculography is used to further assess the severity of the lesion. Unlike color-flow Doppler interrogation of the valve, actual regurgitant flow rather than velocity is visualized, adding more information regarding regurgitant severity. Coronary arteriography is also performed, since ischemia is a potential cause for this lesion.

Medical Therapy

Acute Mitral Regurgitation. The goal of medical treatment of acute mitral regurgitation is to increase forward cardiac output while simultaneously decreasing regurgitant volume and left atrial pressure. Vasodilators form the cornerstone for meeting these objectives. Peripheral systemic vasodilation allows for a preferential increase in forward flow, simultaneously decreasing regurgitant flow and left atrial pressure. In addition, vasodilator therapy usually leads to a modest reduction in heart size, in turn reducing annular dilation, which may improve mitral valve function. Sodium nitroprusside has been the agent of choice for initiating vasodilator therapy because its short half-life allows easy titration to maximal vasodilation without hypotension.[20]

If the mitral regurgitation is so severe that compromised forward output leads to shock, vasodilators cannot be used because they will lower blood pressure further. In such cases, intraaortic counterpulsation lowers systolic afterload and increases forward flow while concomitantly augmenting diastolic systemic blood pressure.

Chronic Mitral Regurgitation. Because vasodilator therapy is used effectively in the treatment of acute mitral regurgitation and because vasodilators have been successful in treating the other left-sided regurgitant lesion, aortic regurgitation, it might seem intuitive that vasodilators would be successful in the treatment of chronic mitral regurgitation. However, this premise has not been proved. In asymptomatic patients with mitral regurgitation, vasodilators have done little to reduce cardiac size.[21] Unlike studies demonstrating that nifedipine can forestall the need for surgery in aortic regurgitation, no studies have been performed to demonstrate its efficacy in mitral regurgitation. Furthermore,

the two regurgitant lesions produce very different hemodynamic and loading conditions.[22] In aortic regurgitation, systolic hypertension leads to pressure overload and excess afterload. Thus afterload reduction with a vasodilator is logical and also has been shown effective. However, in mitral regurgitation, where afterload is normal, reduction in afterload to subnormal levels produces a physiologic state with which there is very little experience and for which the success cannot be judged without the experience from large controlled therapeutic trials.

Angiotensin-converting enzyme (ACE) inhibitors have been demonstrated to be effective in reducing left ventricular volumes in patients with symptomatic mitral regurgitation.[23] However, the standard therapy for such patients is surgical correction of the mitral regurgitation; there is no evidence that vasodilators are an adequate substitute for surgery. Thus vasodilators in mitral regurgitation should be reserved for acute symptomatic mitral regurgitation or for chronic symptomatic regurgitation in patients in whom surgery is not being contemplated because of the presence of comorbidity such as severe lung disease, neoplasia, and other conditions.

Surgical Therapy

Three operations are currently performed for the treatment of mitral regurgitation: (1) "standard" mitral valve replacement, in which the mitral valve and the subvalvular apparatus are removed and a prosthetic valve inserted; (2) mitral valve replacement with chordal preservation, in which a prosthesis is inserted but continuity between the papillary muscles, the subvalvular apparatus, and the mitral leaflets is maintained; and (3) mitral valve repair, in which no prosthesis is used but rather the native mitral valve is repaired to restore mitral valve competence.

It is now clear that the mitral valve apparatus has a far greater role than simply to prevent mitral regurgitation during systole. The mitral valve apparatus—including papillary muscles and chordae tendineae—is an integral part of the left ventricle that coordinates left ventricular contraction and maintains the efficient prolate ellipsoid shape of the ventricle.[24] Because damage to the apparatus by itself causes left ventricular dysfunction, the "standard" mitral valve replacement should be practiced only in those few situations in which the apparatus is so badly damaged (as in rheumatic fever) that it cannot be saved[25-27] (Fig. 18-5). Mitral valve replacement with chordal preservation ensures postoperative mitral valve competence while at the same time retaining the mitral valve apparatus and its important role in left ventricular function.[28] However, this operation carries all the postoperative risks of the presence of a valve prosthesis (potential for prosthetic valve degeneration,

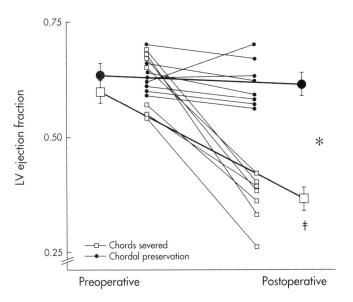

FIG. 18-5
Ejection fraction for patients with mitral regurgitation is demonstrated preoperatively and postoperatively in patients in whom the mitral valve apparatus was destroyed (chords severed) versus those in whom the mitral valve apparatus was entirely or partially preserved (chordal preservation). Ejection fraction fell substantially when the apparatus was destroyed, but it remained normal when the apparatus was preserved.

From Rozich JD, Carabello BA, Usher BW, et al: *Circulation* 86:1718, 1992.

relative valve stenosis, and thromboembolism). Pure mitral valve repair requires greater skill on the part of the surgeon but is the preferred operation when it can be performed, since it restores mitral valve competence, preserves left ventricular function, and does not require postoperative anticoagulation.

Timing of Surgery, Symptoms, and Left Ventricular Function

With the aid of transesophageal echocardiography, the valvular abnormality responsible for mitral regurgitation can be documented. This allows prediction of the kind of operation necessary to fix it and influences the timing of surgery. For instance, posterior chordal rupture can usually be repaired, and there is little point in delaying surgery. On the other hand, extensive rheumatic deformity may defy a successful repair. Currently, preoperative predictions are 80% accurate in predicting the operation ultimately performed. Although this percentage seems impressive, it still means that a number of patients predicted to have a mitral valve repair will leave the operating room with a valve prosthesis and its inherent risks.

Symptomatic Patients. Patients who become even mildly symptomatic with chronic mitral regurgitation probably should have surgical repair. A recent study of

patients with flail leaflets suggests that the presence of symptoms, even in the face of good left ventricular function, indicates a worse prognosis unless surgery is performed.[29] *Symptoms summarize the patient's overall pathophysiologic condition and indicate decompensation.* Surgery relieves the symptoms, improves the quality of life postoperatively, and almost certainly improves prognosis when compared with medical therapy. (Note that no randomized trials have compared surgery and medical therapy in mildly symptomatic patients. Although it might be possible to relieve symptoms medically, this strategy might mask left ventricular dysfunction and lead ultimately to a worsened prognosis.[29])

Asymptomatic Patients with Left Ventricular Dysfunction. It is clear that left ventricular dysfunction in mitral regurgitation can develop without causing symptoms. If this situation is unrecognized and is allowed to persist, dysfunction worsens and may become permanent. Thus, whether or not mitral valve repair or replacement is ultimately performed, asymptomatic patients with left ventricular dysfunction should have surgery. Implicit in this concept is the ability to determine when left ventricular dysfunction has developed using noninvasive preoperative surveillance of left ventricular function. Because several studies point to worsened prognosis if either ejection fraction falls below 60% (Fig. 18-6) or if the ventricle is unable to contract to an end-systolic dimension of 45 mm (Fig. 18-7), these two parameters, although not perfect, are good guidelines for when to perform surgery.[30,31] Thus, if follow-up of asymptomatic patients demonstrates a gradually falling ejection fraction toward 60% or a gradually increasing end-systolic dimension toward 45 mm, elective surgery should be performed. We usually recommend surgery at the earliest convenient date and would be uncomfortable waiting months.

Asymptomatic Patients with Normal Left Ventricular Function. This group currently is the most problematic in the timing of surgery. If mitral valve repair can be performed, a strategy similar to that of management of atrial septal defect could be followed. In atrial septal defect, asymptomatic patients routinely undergo operation because surgery does not involve a prosthesis or postoperative anticoagulation and can be performed with a low risk; the benefit of "prophylactic" surgery is prevention of persistent atrial arrhythmias or pulmonary hypertension.

If mitral valve repair can be performed, the situation is similar to atrial septal defect; the procedure is performed at low operative risk, does not use a prosthesis, and prevents the postoperative complication of eventual left ventricular dysfunction. However, to employ this strategy it is necessary to be able to predict with nearly 100% accuracy whether repair can be performed. If an unanticipated valve replacement is required for a

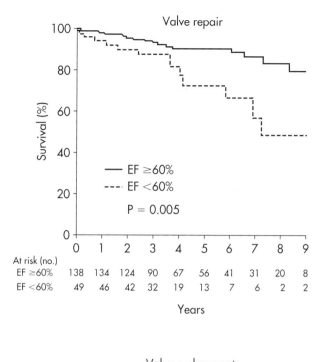

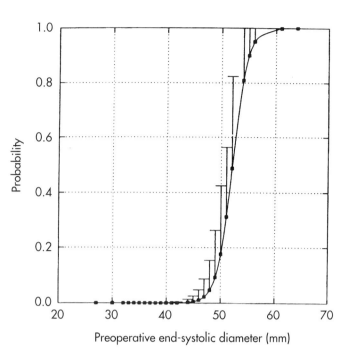

FIG. 18-7
The probability of a poor postoperative outcome is plotted against preoperative and systolic echocardiographic minor axis diameter. The probability of a poor outcome rose abruptly once preoperative and systolic dimension exceeded 45 mm.

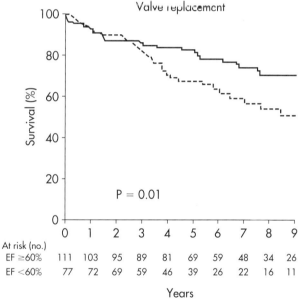

FIG. 18-6
Survivorship among patients with mitral regurgitation after surgery. Whether mitral valve repair or mitral valve replacement was performed, survival was excellent as long as preoperative ejection fraction (EF) was greater than 60%. However, when EF was below 60% preoperatively (dashed line) long-term survival was worse.

From Enriquez-Sarano M, Tajik AJ, Schaff HV, et al: *Circulation* 90:830, 1994.

young, otherwise asymptomatic healthy patient, that person is unnecessarily committed to the risks of a valve prosthesis. As already noted, in many centers preoperative prediction is not far enough advanced to allow this strategy at the present time.

Far-Advanced Left Ventricular Dysfunction. The question often arises of whether it is ever too late to perform surgery for mitral regurgitation. Mitral valve replacement with removal of the subvalvular apparatus usually leads to catastrophe in patients with ejection fraction of less than 40%. Thus it should not be performed in those patients. However, mitral valve annuloplasty has been performed successfully in patients with LV ejection fraction as low as 15%.[32] Again the type of operation performed to correct the mitral regurgitation is critical. In far-advanced disease it must be certain that either a mitral valve repair or replacement with chordal preservation can be performed; otherwise surgery should be avoided.

Surgery and the Etiology of Mitral Regurgitation

Ischemic Mitral Regurgitation. Coronary disease may cause mitral regurgitation by rupturing a papillary muscle or causing papillary muscle dysfunction. Regardless of the mechanism, the prognosis of mitral regurgitation with coronary disease is substantially worse than it is with other etiologies.[33] This probably is because of the coexistence of two potentially fatal cardiac diseases (mitral regurgitation and coronary artery disease). Coronary disease tends to progress even when mitral valve surgery is successful. Although some centers report a low operative mortality for mitral valve surgery in ischemic mitral regurgitation, the average operative risk is approximately 20%, and fewer than 50% of patients survive for 5 years.

Mitral Valve Prolapse (MVP). MVP is the most common cause of mitral regurgitation. The severity of MVP determines the prognosis. In some cases, mild prolapse is due to physiologic changes that cause a small left ventricle, does not represent true valve pathology, and does not increase the risk of valve complications. For example, atrial septal defect may lead to a small left ventricle and MVP, which are relieved once the defect is repaired. There is little risk to this type of prolapse.

At the other end of the spectrum, myxomatous degeneration of the valve leads to severe valve deformity, valve thickening, and valve redundancy, causing a billowing, or parachute, valve. Patients with this disease are most susceptible to the complications of MVP: endocarditis, stroke, and progression to severe mitral regurgitation.[34] Even in this group of patients prognosis varies. The condition is more likely to result in complications in men and older patients. Overall the risk of the complications of endocarditis, stroke, or progression to severe mitral regurgitation is less than 10%.

MITRAL VALVE PROLAPSE SYNDROME

MVP may be caused by other diseases. It is invariably present in Marfan's syndrome and is common in patients with Ehlers-Danlos syndrome, osteogenesis imperfecta, pseudoxanthoma elasticum, periarteritis nodosa, hyperthyroidism, Ebstein's anomaly of the tricuspid valve, the straight-back syndrome, coronary artery disease, and a number of other conditions. In such cases the clinical course and prognosis are usually governed by the underlying illness. MVP most commonly occurs in the absence of other illness and is referred to as *MVP syndrome.*

A majority of patients with MVP syndrome are asymptomatic. However, in some the prolapse is associated with palpitations, chest pain, or postural syncope. In such patients the presence of prolapse appears to coincide with autonomic dysfunction, although a definite link between the two conditions has yet to be defined.

Clinical Presentation and Physical Diagnosis

The diagnosis of MVP is made during physical examination by noting the characteristic midsystolic click followed by a late systolic murmur. These findings occur as the elongated chordae tendineae are stretched taut in midsystole, causing the click. At this point, one or both leaflets moves past the point of coaptation into the left atrium, resulting in mitral regurgitation and the late systolic murmur.

The Valsalva maneuver reduces left ventricular volume, causing the click to occur earlier in systole and the murmur to become louder and longer in duration. As the condition worsens, the mitral regurgitation and its attendant murmur become progressively more holosystolic. In most cases the diagnosis is made during physical examination.

Echocardiogram

Occasionally prolapse is seen on an echocardiogram when one or both of the classic physical findings (click or murmur) are absent. Even when the classic findings are present, at least one echocardiogram should be performed to establish whether the leaflets are thick and misshapen, thus adding prognostic information about the potential for later complications.

When it was first described, MVP was a common echocardiographic diagnosis. It was especially common in thin, asthenic young women, many of whom had vague symptoms. Stricter diagnostic criteria are now in favor and require marked prolapse with a myxomatous appearance of the valve.

Management
Endocarditis Prophylaxis

The failure to provide prophylactic therapy to patients with MVP constitutes one of the major preventable causes of endocarditis today. Patients with misshapen valves who have the murmur of mitral regurgitation require prophylaxis. Since turbulence is a key predisposing factor to the development of endocarditis, it may be unnecessary to administer prophylactic therapy to those patients who have prolapse but do not have a murmur.

Stroke Prophylaxis

Many recommend low-dose aspirin therapy to prevent stroke in patients with misshapen valves. However, no controlled studies are available to demonstrate the efficacy of this therapy. Patients with MVP and transient ischemic attack (TIA) are treated with aspirin. If TIA recurs, warfarin therapy is usually recommended.

Palpitations and Chest Pain

In patients with palpitations, beta-blockers may be effective. Clinical experience shows that they often are not. When that is the case, event monitoring often shows no arrhythmia while the patient has symptoms. As a general rule, documentation of an arrhythmia makes sense when considering antiarrhythmic therapy for any patient with palpitations.

Atypical, nonanginal chest discomfort also has been treated with beta blockade. The results are highly variable, particularly with mild MVP, where the symptoms may have nothing to do with the cardiac condition. More severe MVP, with definite physical findings and a parachute valve on the echocardiogram, may generate increased wall tension and ischemia in the region of the papillary muscle. The stress ECG may be abnormal, and an occasional patient has a small perfusion abnormality in the region of a papillary muscle. In such cases, beta-blockers may prove useful. (It is also important in such cases to be sure there is no coexisting coronary disease.)

Expected Clinical Course

The most frequent complication is progressive mitral regurgitation, which develops in about 10% of patients with MVP and a clearly myxomatous valve. The risk of serious mitral regurgitation is increased in men over 50 years old and in those with both a click and murmur. It is less common with an isolated click.

Endocarditis, stroke, and sudden death are much less common complications of MVP. The probability of having any one of them or of needing surgery for mitral regurgitation is about 1% per year. The risk of sudden death is higher when there is significant mitral regurgitation, a long QT interval, or a history of palpitations or syncope.

Follow-up and Referral. A patient with minimal or no symptoms, no murmur, and mild MVP on an echocardiogram needs reassurance and no specific therapy.

Endocarditis prophylaxis is indicated for those with a persistent or intermittent murmur and mitral regurgitation detected on Doppler study (see Chapter 21). A repeat echocardiogram at 2- to 3-year intervals may be considered.

Those with moderate mitral regurgitation should be followed with a cardiology consultant and have annual Doppler echocardiography in addition to endocarditis prophylaxis. The goal of monitoring is valve repair before left ventricular dysfunction develops.

REFERENCES

1. Carabello BA, Grossman W: Calculation of stenotic valve orifice area. In Grossman W, editor: *Cardiac catheterization and angiography,* ed 3, Philadelphia, 1986, Lea & Febiger.
2. Gash AK, Carabello BA, Cepin D, Spann JF: Left ventricular ejection performance and systolic muscle function in patients with mitral stenosis, *Circulation* 67:148, 1983.
3. Mahoney PD, Loh E, Blitz LR, et al: Effects of inhaled nitric oxide in patients with severe mitral stenosis and normal left ventricular function, *J Am Coll Cardiol* 31(suppl A):205, 1998.
4. Assey ME, Carabello BA, Usher BW: The patient with valvular heart disease. In Pepine CJ, Hill JA, Lambert CR, editors: *Diagnostic and therapeutic cardiac catheterization,* ed 3, Baltimore, 1998, Williams & Wilkins.
5. Currie PJ, Seward JB, Chan KL, et al: Continuous wave Doppler determination of right ventricular pressure: a simultaneous Doppler-catheterization study in 127 patients, *J Am Coll Cardiol* 6:750, 1985.
6. Martin RP, Rakowski H, Kleiman JH: Reliability and reproducibility of two-dimensional echocardiographic measurement of the stenotic mitral valve orifice area, *Am J Cardiol* 43:560, 1979.
7. Hatle L, Brubakk A, Tromsdal A, Angelsen B: Noninvasive assessment of pressure drop in mitral stenosis by Doppler ultrasound, *Br Heart J* 40:131, 1978.
8. Gorlin R, Gorlin SG: Hydraulic formula for calculation of the area of the stenotic mitral valve, other cardiac valves, and central circulatory shunts. I. *Am Heart J* 41:1, 1951.
9. Ward C, Hancock BW: Extreme pulmonary hypertension caused by mitral valve disease: natural history and results of surgery, *Br Heart J* 37:74, 1975.
10. Roy SB, Gopinath N: Mitral stenosis, *Circulation* 38(suppl 2):68, 1968.
11. Reyes VP, Raju BS, Wynne J, et al: Percutaneous balloon valvuloplasty compared with open surgical commissurotomy for mitral stenosis, *N Engl J Med* 331:961, 1994.
12. Wilkins GT, Weyman AE, Abascal VM, et al: Percutaneous balloon dilatation of the mitral valve: an analysis of echocardiographic variables related to outcome and the mechanism of dilatation, *Br Heart J* 60:299, 1988.
13. Bassand J, Schiele F, Bernard Y, et al: The double-balloon and Inoue techniques in percutaneous mitral valvuloplasty: comparative results in a series of 232 cases, *J Am Coll Cardiol* 18:982, 1991.
14. Cohn LH, Allred EN, Cohn LA, et al: Long-term results of open mitral valve reconstruction for mitral stenosis, *Am J Cardiol* 55:731, 1985.
15. Waller BF, Howard J, Fess S: Pathology of mitral valve stenosis and pure mitral regurgitation, II. *Clin Cardiol* 17:395, 1994.
16. Carabello BA: Mitral regurgitation. 1. Basic pathophysiologic principles, *Mod Concepts Cardiovasc Dis* 57:53, 1988.
17. Spain MG, Smith MD, Grayburn PA, et al: Quantitative assessment of mitral regurgitation by Doppler color flow imaging: angiographic and hemodynamic correlations, *J Am Coll Cardiol* 13:585, 1989.
18. Recusani F, Bargiggia GS, Yoganathan AP, et al: A new method for quantification of regurgitant flow rate using color Doppler flow imaging of the flow convergence region proximal to a discrete orifice: an in vitro study, *Circulation* 83:594, 1991.
19. Simpson IA, Shiota T, Gharib M, Sahn DJ: Current status of flow convergence for clinical applications: is it a leaning tower of "PISA"? *J Am Coll Cardiol* 27:504, 1996.
20. Horstkotte D, Schulte HD, Niehues R, et al: Diagnostic and therapeutic considerations in acute, severe mitral regurgitation: experience in 42 consecutive patients entering the intensive care unit with pulmonary edema, *J Heart Valve Dis* 2:512, 1993.
21. Wisenbaugh T, Sinovich V, Dullabh A, Sareli P: Six month pilot study of captopril for mildly symptomatic, severe isolated mitral and isolated aortic regurgitation, *J Heart Valve Dis* 3:197, 1994.
22. Wisenbaugh T, Spann JF, Carabello BA: Differences in myocardial performance and load between patients with similar amounts of chronic aortic versus chronic mitral regurgitation, *J Am Coll Cardiol* 3:916, 1984.
23. Schön JR: Hemodynamic and morphologic changes after long-term angiotensin-converting enzyme inhibition in patients with chronic valvular regurgitation, *J Hypertens* 12(suppl 4):95, 1994.

24. Rushmer RF: Initial phase of ventricular systole: asynchronous contraction, *Am J Physiol* 184:188, 1956.

25. Rozich JD, Carabello BA, Usher BW, et al: Mitral valve replacement with and without chordal preservation in patients with chronic mitral regurgitation: mechanism for differences in postoperative ejection performance, *Circulation* 86:1718, 1992.

26. Hansen DE, Sarris GE, Niczyporuk MA, et al: Physiologic role of the mitral apparatus in left ventricular regional mechanics, contraction synergy, and global systolic performance, *J Thorac Cardiovasc Surg* 97:521, 1989.

27. Goldman ME, Mora F, Guarino T, et al: Mitral valvuloplasty is superior to valve replacement for preservation of left ventricular function: an intraoperative two-dimensional echocardiographic study, *J Am Coll Cardiol* 10:568, 1987.

28. David TE, Burns RJ, Bacchus CM, Druck MN: Mitral valve replacement for mitral regurgitation with and without preservation of chordae tendineae, *J Thorac Cardiovasc Surg* 88:718, 1984.

29. Ling LH, Enriquez-Sarano M, Seward JB, et al: Clinical outcome of mitral regurgitation due to flail leaflet, *N Engl J Med* 335:1417, 1996.

30. Enriquez-Sarano M, Tajik AJ, Schaff HV, et al: Echocardiographic prediction of survival after surgical correction of organic mitral regurgitation, *Circulation* 90:830, 1994.

31. Wisenbaugh T, Skudicky D, Sareli P: Prediction of outcome after valve replacement for rheumatic mitral regurgitation in the era of chordal preservation, *Circulation* 89:191, 1994.

32. Bach DS, Bolling SF: Improvement following correction of secondary mitral regurgitation in end-stage cardiomyopathy with mitral annuloplasty, *Am J Cardiol* 78:966, 1996.

33. Cohn LH, Rizzo RJ, Adams DH, et al: The effect of pathophysiology on the surgical treatment of ischemic mitral regurgitation: operative and late risk of repair versus replacement, *Eur J Cardiothorac Surg* 9:568, 1995.

34. Mills P, Hollingsworth J, Amara I, Craige E: Long-term prognosis of mitral-valve prolapse, *N Engl J Med* 297:13, 1977.

BIBLIOGRAPHY

Nishimura RA, McGoon MD: Perspectives on mitral valve prolapse, *N Engl J Med* 341:48, 1999. An editorial that clears the air about diagnostic criteria for MVP syndrome. Only patients with billowing, thickened, myxomatous valves appear at risk for the late complications of MVP. Using stricter diagnostic criteria, two other articles in this issue of the *Journal* indicate a relatively low incidence (2.4%) of MVP in a community population (p. 1 of the July 1 issue) and an absence of any connection between MVP and stroke in young patients (p. 8).

Otto CM, Lind BK, Kitzman DW, et al: Association of aortic valve sclerosis with cardiovascular mortality and morbidity in the elderly, *N Engl J Med* 341:142, 1999. A thickened aortic valve with minimal outflow tract obstruction is a common finding among elderly patients, about 30% in this study. The risk of progression to significant stenosis is low, about 8% per year. However, this paper from the Cardiovascular Health Study group reported that there is an increased risk of myocardial infarction and cardiovascular death with aortic sclerosis, probably because it is a marker for underlying coronary artery disease (see the editorial by Carabello in the same issue).

19 Aortic Valve Disease

Blase A. Carabello

AORTIC STENOSIS
Epidemiology, Etiology, and Natural History

Aortic stenosis is the most common acquired valve disease. Approximately 1% of the American population is born with a bicuspid aortic valve. Aortic stenosis develops in approximately one third of these predominantly male patients between the ages of 40 and 60. Other patients, born with an apparently normal tricuspid aortic valve, may develop senile calcific degeneration of the valve leaflets leading to aortic stenosis in their sixth, seventh, and eighth decades. Why stenosis develops in some patients with a previously normal tricuspid aortic valve is unclear.

The initial lesion of aortic stenosis in such patients resembles the plaque of coronary disease.[1] Although rheumatic heart disease used to be a common cause of aortic stenosis, it now accounts for less than one fifth of all cases diagnosed in the United States. Since rheumatic heart disease nearly always involves the mitral valve, the diagnosis of rheumatic aortic stenosis should not be made if the mitral valve is entirely normal. In still other patients, congenital aortic stenosis that escaped detection in childhood has been noted for the first time in adults.

As shown in Figure 19-1, the natural history of aortic stenosis is crucial because it predicts outcome.[2] In asymptomatic patients, survival is nearly normal, and the risk of sudden death is less than 1% per year.[2-4] However, once the classic symptoms of angina, syncope, or heart failure develop, prognosis changes dramatically. Of the 35% of patients with aortic stenosis who have angina, 50% are dead within 5 years unless the aortic valve is replaced. With syncope, 50% survival is only 3 years, and for heart failure it is just 2 years if not surgically corrected. Thus management of patients with aortic stenosis should concentrate on carefully establishing the presence or absence of these symptoms.

Pathophysiology

As the aortic valve narrows to less than one third of its normal orifice area (normal, 3 to 4 cm²), the normal free flow of blood from the left ventricle (LV) into the aorta during systole is impeded. A pressure gradient develops at the aortic valve, causing a difference in pressure on either side of the open valve. The LV must pro-

duce higher pressure to maintain normal pressure and perfusion of the aorta and distal circulation[5] (Fig. 19-2). Pressure overload of the LV occurs, and it worsens as the aortic valve progressively narrows. Compensation for this pressure overload is afforded by the development of LV concentric hypertrophy.[6,7] The law of Laplace states that the stress on any portion of the ventricle is equal to pressure (p) times radius (r) divided by twice the thickness (th) of the LV:

$$\text{LV wall stress} = (p \times r) / 2 \text{ th}$$

As pressure in the numerator increases with tighter stenosis, it can be offset by an increase in wall thickness in the denominator. Stress is an expression of LV afterload. Hypertrophy helps to normalize afterload and maintain normal ejection performance despite the large increase in LV pressure.

Hypertrophy thus serves a compensatory role, but it also contributes to deterioration. Coronary blood flow to hypertrophied muscle is reduced, either because capillary density is reduced or because high ventricular diastolic filling pressure reduces the gradient driving blood flow across the coronary bed.[8] In either case, coronary blood flow and blood flow reserve are diminished, eventually leading to ischemia and angina. As noted, once symptomatic evidence of ischemia develops (onset of angina), mortality risk increases.

Syncope occurs when cerebral perfusion is inadequate. In aortic stenosis, syncope usually occurs with exertion. Its pathophysiology is still debated. In normal subjects, total peripheral resistance falls and cardiac output rises during exertion. The increase in cardiac output exceeds the fall in total peripheral resistance, causing blood pressure to increase. According to one theory of aortic stenosis, cardiac output during exercise is limited by obstruction at the aortic valve, and thus the fall in total peripheral resistance cannot be compensated. The result is hypotension and syncope. Another theory suggests that an abrupt increase in LV wall stress during exercise triggers a vasodepressor response. Alternatively, ischemia during exercise might induce cardiac arrhythmias, leading to a fall in cerebral perfusion.

Heart failure is classified as diastolic (impairment in LV relaxation and filling) or systolic (impairment in LV emptying). Both forms of heart failure may occur in aortic stenosis.[7, 9-11] Increased LV wall thickness causes an

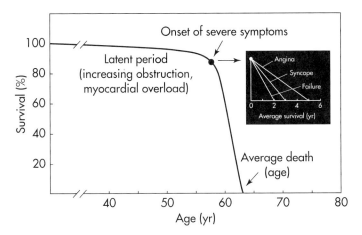

FIG. 19-1

The natural history of aortic stenosis. As long as patients have no symptoms, survival is nearly normal. However, once the symptoms of angina, syncope, or congestive heart failure develop, survival declines rapidly unless the aortic valve is replaced. As shown in the inset, average survival is 5 years after the development of angina, 3 years after the development of syncope, and just 2 years after the development of congestive heart failure.

From Ross J Jr, Braunwald E: Circulation 38(suppl 5):61, 1968.

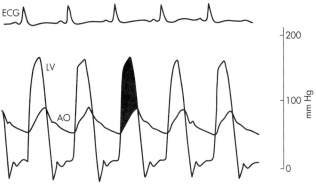

FIG. 19-2

Left ventricular pressure (LV) and simultaneously recorded aortic pressure (AO) in a patient with aortic stenosis. The blackened area represents the gradient across the aortic valve—the excess pressure that the left ventricle must generate in this disease.

From Grossman W, editor: Cardiac catheterization and angiography, ed 2, Philadelphia, 1980, Lea & Febiger.

obligate increase in wall stiffness. Thus a higher pressure is required to fill the concentrically hypertrophied ventricle to any given volume. Increased diastolic pressure in turn is transmitted back through the left atrium to the lungs, causing pulmonary congestion. Early relaxation may also be impaired in hypertrophic states, presumably as a result of abnormalities in diastolic calcium handling, delaying active relaxation.

LV emptying during systole depends on contractility (the innate ability of the myocardium to generate force) and afterload. Initially, hypertrophy normalizes afterload and allows normal systolic function. Eventually, hypertrophy is not adequate to normalize afterload; it increases, and ejection performance is impaired.[7] In addition to afterload excess, ventricular contractility may also be impaired with pressure overload. Impairment in contractility may result from abnormal calcium handling, ischemia, or cytoskeletal abnormalities of individual myocytes.

Clinical Presentation

History

The importance of obtaining an in-depth, probing history of a patient with aortic stenosis cannot be overemphasized. As noted earlier, the presence or absence of symptoms determines therapy. If there are no symptoms, the prognosis is excellent and surgery unnecessary. However, once symptoms develop the short-term prognosis is worse, and immediate aortic valve replacement is required. Not only should the physician care-

fully question for the presence of angina, syncope, or heart failure, but the asymptomatic patient should be given instructions in lay terms describing the key symptoms. Their appearance should prompt the patient to contact the physician immediately.

Physical Examination

Aortic stenosis is usually recognized during the physical examination by the presence of a systolic ejection murmur that radiates to the neck (Table 19-1). With mild to moderate disease the murmur typically peaks early in systole, may be quite loud, and is often associated with a systolic thrill. As the disease worsens and cardiac output decreases, the murmur peaks progressively later in systole and may actually become softer. Indeed, in patients with advanced disease who may still be candidates for surgery, the murmur may be nearly absent. After an extrasystolic beat, post-extrasystolic potentiation increases stroke volume, which greatly accentuates the loudness of the murmur.

Further clues to the presence of significant aortic stenosis are gleaned from simultaneous palpation of the carotid upstroke and LV apical impulse. The palpation of a forceful apex beat simultaneously with the classic weakened and delayed carotid upstrokes is highly suggestive of hemodynamically significant disease. However, in some patients, particularly older subjects, increased stiffness of the carotid arteries may pseudonormalize the carotid upstroke.

S_1 is usually normal. In young patients with congenital aortic stenosis the lack of calcification permits a systolic opening sound (click). S_2 often becomes single as the calcified, immobile aortic valve moves insufficiently to create A_2, leaving only the soft closing sound of the

Table 19-1 | *An Overview of Aortic Valve Disease*

	Symptoms (If Present)	Signs	ECG	Chest X-ray	Echocardiography	Timing of Surgery	Medical Therapy
Aortic stenosis	Angina common (35% to 50%)	Systolic ejection murmur	LV hypertrophy	Normal heart size	LV chamber normal in size	Predicated on symptomatic status	None
	Syncope uncommon (<20%)	Delayed carotid pulses			Concentric LV hypertrophy		
	Congestive heart failure (CHF) common (>50%)	Single S₂			Doppler showing gradient across the valve		
		Forceful nondisplaced apical impulse (PMI)			Need for periodic echo surveillance uncertain		
		Pulse pressure normal or reduced					
Aortic regurgitation	Angina (<20%)	Diastolic blowing murmur	LV hypertrophy	Enlarged heart	LV chamber enlarged	Predicated on objective evidence of LV dysfunction plus symptomatic status	Vasodilators for asymptomatic patients with normal LV function
	Syncope rare (<10%)	Diastolic rumble			Eccentric LV hypertrophy with modest concentric LV hypertrophy		
	CHF common (>60%)	Sharp carotid upstroke			Doppler showing regurgitation		
		Normal S₂			Periodic echo surveillance required to monitor LV size		
		Displaced hyperdynamic PMI					
		Widened pulse pressure causing a myriad of signs					

pulmonic valve. If S_2 is audible to the left of the sternum (the pulmonic area) but not to the right (the aortic area), then A_2 is absent. Occasionally the combination of LV dysfunction and outflow obstruction may delay the aortic component of S_2, causing paradoxical splitting (see Chapter 4).

Management

Laboratory Evaluation

Electrocardiogram (ECG) and Chest X-ray. The findings of these noninvasive studies are nonspecific in aortic stenosis. Typically the ECG demonstrates left atrial abnormality and LV hypertrophy (see Chapter 5). Radiographic examination of the chest shows normal heart size. However, the heart often assumes a boot-shaped configuration consistent with concentric LV hypertrophy. Occasionally, the densely calcified aortic valve can be seen in the lateral view.

Echocardiography. Echo-Doppler examination is indispensable in the assessment of aortic stenosis. The two-dimensional echocardiogram shows the degree of valve leaflet immobility, the amount of LV hypertrophy, and the state of LV ejection performance. Doppler interrogation of the valve provides an accurate estimation of the severity stenosis (see Chapter 8). As shown in Figure 19-3, because flow is the product of luminal area and velocity, when area decreases (as it does at a stenotic valve), velocity must increase for flow to remain constant.[12] This increase in velocity at the site of stenosis can be detected by Doppler interrogation. The acceleration of the red blood cells at the site of stenosis (Fig. 19-4, A) compresses the sound waves and causes the frequency of the return echo to be higher than the initial velocity of the transmitted signal. This Doppler "shift" is then used to calculate the velocity of the stream flow (Figure 19-4, B).[13] In turn, the area (A_2) at the site of stenosis can be calculated when the velocity on both sides of the stenosis and the area of the outflow tract are known. Alternatively, the gradient can be calculated using the modified Bernoulli equation, $G = 4V^2$. A peak velocity just distal to the aortic valve of greater than 4

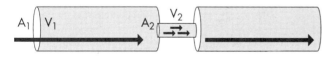

$$A_1 \cdot V_1 = A_2 \cdot V_2$$

FIG. 19-3
The characteristics of flow through a tube. When flow reaches a narrowing (reduced orifice area), velocity increases proportionally to the decrease in area so that flow remains constant ($A_1 \times V_1 = A_2 \times V_2$, the continuity equation). By knowing A_1, V_1, and V_2, A_2 can be calculated.
From Carabello BA: Cardiol Rev 1:59, 1993.

m/s indicates severe aortic stenosis, whereas peak velocities less than 3 m/s indicate milder disease. However, when cardiac output is severely reduced because of LV dysfunction, lower velocities may still be consistent with severe disease.

Cardiac Catheterization. Since most patients with aortic stenosis are of an age when coronary disease might be present, coronary arteriography is usually performed before surgery. In addition, the gradient may be confirmed at the time of cardiac catheterization by retrograde passage of a catheter across the stenotic valve.

Invasive hemodynamic studies have long been considered the gold standard for assessment of valvular heart disease. Unfortunately, with attention being given to therapeutic techniques in recent years, hemodynamic practices in some laboratories have been degraded. You may assume that data are reliable only if standard hemodynamic principles have been adhered to strictly.[14]

Exercise Testing. Exercise testing in patients with aortic stenosis previously had been contraindicated because of an increased risk of complications. Indeed, it is unwise to exercise a patient with clear-cut symptoms of aortic stenosis. However, occasionally patients complain of vague symptoms, making it difficult to determine their status. Since symptomatic status is the most crucial decision point in deciding whether to perform valve replacement, cautious exercise testing in these patients under the guidance of a trained physician may be revealing and safe.[15] If it is clear that exercise tolerance is limited by dyspnea or fatigue, then symptomatic status should be ascribed to the patient. On the other hand, excellent exercise tolerance with a normal rise in blood pressure indicates that the patient is well compensated. It should be noted that the ST segment response, so important in making the diagnosis of coronary disease, has no proven meaning in the presence of aortic stenosis and LV hypertrophy. Although exercise-induced ST segment depression in children with aortic stenosis is a bad prognostic sign, it has unknown significance in adults.

Therapy

Medical. In general, medical therapy is not indicated in patients with aortic stenosis. If the patient has no symptoms, no therapy is required. If symptoms have developed, prompt surgery is necessary to prevent sudden death. In patients with heart failure awaiting surgery, the judicious use of diuretics helps to relieve pulmonary congestion. However, angiotensin-converting enzyme inhibitors, useful in other types of heart failure, should be avoided, because vasodilator-induced reduction in peripheral vascular resistance may cause syncope. With aortic stenosis the afterload comes from the valve, and afterload reduction therapy with vasodilators does not address the problem.

Surgical. As already noted, surgery is usually not indicated in the absence of symptoms,. Even if a patient has a large transvalvular gradient, the risk of surgery, which is small (2% to 3% operative mortality), still outweighs the risk of sudden death, which is approximately 1% per year. This policy unfortunately overlooks a small percentage of patients who proceed from the asymptomatic phase, through symptoms, to sudden death within a very short period of time.[16] Currently, there is no satisfactory way to identify these patients. Until there is, it is not acceptable to expose all patients with asymptomatic aortic stenosis to unnecessary surgery to preserve the life of the 1% or 2% of patients who will have this tragic course. In general, aortic valve replacement is indicated promptly after symptoms develop provided that diagnostic studies indicate that critical aortic stenosis is causing the symptoms.

What is the critical valve area or pressure gradient at which symptoms occur? Unfortunately, the exact critical valve area is unknown.[17,18] Symptoms usually do not appear until valve area is less than 0.7 cm^2. However, if symptoms are present and the valve area is less than 0.9 cm^2, the symptoms can be attributed to aortic stenosis. Once surgery is performed, prognosis returns to that of the normal age-matched population[19] (Fig. 19-5).

Palliative. Aortic valve replacement is impossible in some patients because the patient either refuses to consent to surgery or co-morbidity deters operation. In such cases aortic balloon valvotomy may temporarily relieve symptoms. In this procedure a large balloon is passed across the aortic valve and inflated. Valvotomy helps to restore some leaflet mobility and leads to a modest reduction in stenosis severity. However, more than 50% of patients have complete loss of effect within 6 months, and the overall mortality for patients treated with balloon valvotomy is the same as that of untreated patients.[20]

In addition to balloon valvotomy, digoxin and diuretics may help to relieve symptoms but not improve longevity (see Chapter 53 for a discussion of palliative care).

Postoperative Follow-up. If a mechanical valve has been inserted, treatment with warfarin therapy is indicated. The INR should be regulated according to the type of prosthesis, other risks for embolization, and the risk of bleeding. For instance, in a young normotensive subject with a low-risk (St. Jude) valve, an INR of 2.0 probably represents adequate anticoagulation. On the other hand, for an older patient with a history of a previous neurologic event after valve implantation, an INR of 3.5 may be required. The correct level of anticoagula-

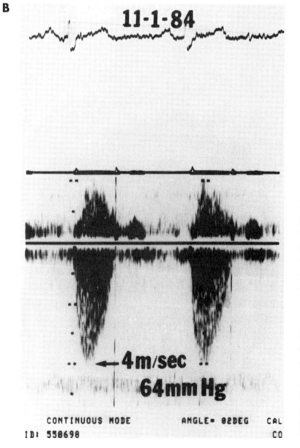

FIG. 19-4
A, In the upper panel a transducer emits sound waves toward a stationary truck. The frequency emitted is the same as the frequency received. In the lower panel the truck is moving toward the transducer. In this case the frequency received is higher than the frequency emitted because the sound waves are compressed by the movement of the truck toward the transducer. **B,** The Doppler signal acquired from a patient with aortic stenosis. Velocity across the aortic valve is 4 m/s, which, when applied to the Bernoulli equation, yields a peak gradient of 64 mm Hg.

A from Carabello BA: Cardiol Rev 1:59, 1993; **B** from Assey ME, Usher BW, Carabello BA: The patient with valvular heart disease. In Pepine CJ, Hill JA, Lambert CR, editors: Diagnostic and therapeutic cardiac catheterization, ed 2, Baltimore, 1994, Williams & Wilkins.

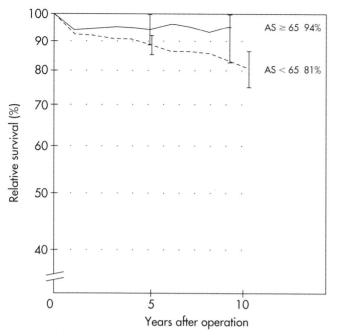

FIG. 19-5
Survival after surgery for aortic stenosis (AS). Survival for patients 65 years of age or older after surgery is not significantly different from normal survivorship. For younger patients, age-corrected survival was still excellent at 81%.

From Lindblom D, Lindblom U, Qvist J, Lundström H: J Am Coll Cardiol 15:566, 1990.

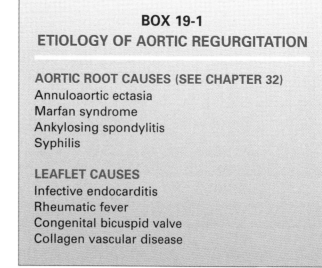

BOX 19-1
ETIOLOGY OF AORTIC REGURGITATION

AORTIC ROOT CAUSES (SEE CHAPTER 32)
Annuloaortic ectasia
Marfan syndrome
Ankylosing spondylitis
Syphilis

LEAFLET CAUSES
Infective endocarditis
Rheumatic fever
Congenital bicuspid valve
Collagen vascular disease

tion should be determined by a cardiac surgeon and cardiologist (see Chapter 52).

If a bioprosthesis is implanted, yearly physical examination for valve deterioration is warranted. The physician should listen carefully for a new murmur indicating aortic regurgitation.

AORTIC REGURGITATION
Etiology and Epidemiology

Aortic regurgitation is caused by disease either of the valve leaflets or of the aortic root (Box 19-1). Aortic root causes of aortic regurgitation include dilation (Marfan syndrome, or annuloaortic ectasia associated with aging and hypertension), aortic dissection, and syphilis. Diseases involving the leaflets leading to aortic regurgitation include endocarditis, bicuspid aortic valve, rheumatic valve disease, and collagen vascular disease.

Pathophysiology

Acute aortic insufficiency leads to rapid decompensation and is usually a surgical emergency (see later discussion). Diastolic aortic pressure drives blood across the incompetent aortic valve into a relatively small, unpre-

pared left ventricle.[21] LV volume overload increases LV preload and produces a modest increase in end-diastolic volume. Total stroke volume increases slightly, but this modest increase cannot compensate for the volume regurgitated (Fig.19-6).

End-diastolic pressure increases dramatically, leading to pulmonary congestion. In fact, LV diastolic pressure becomes higher than left atrial pressure, forcing the mitral valve to close before the onset of systole (mitral valve "preclosure").[22] These events combine to decrease forward cardiac output and at the same time decrease the gradient for coronary blood flow (aortic diastolic pressure minus LV diastolic pressure). This latter event may produce LV ischemia, resulting in a rapid downhill course of decompensated LV function. Severe acute aortic regurgitation resulting in even mild congestive heart failure or in mitral valve preclosure mandates urgent valve surgery.[2]

Chronic aortic regurgitation is rarely a medical emergency. Patients are managed medically into a chronic compensated phase. In this phase the development of eccentric cardiac hypertrophy causes LV enlargement and an increase in end-diastolic volume, in turn increasing both total and forward stroke volumes. The enlarged left ventricle can accommodate the regurgitant volume with little increase in diastolic pressure (and therefore no pulmonary congestion).

The increase in stroke volume increases systemic pulse pressure, resulting in systemic hypertension. Thus a simultaneous pressure and volume overload is placed on the LV in aortic regurgitation.[23] Compensation occurs by the development of both eccentric and concentric cardiac hypertrophy.[24] This is unlike mitral regurgitation, in which LV wall thickness is not increased and may even be decreased in the face of volume overload.

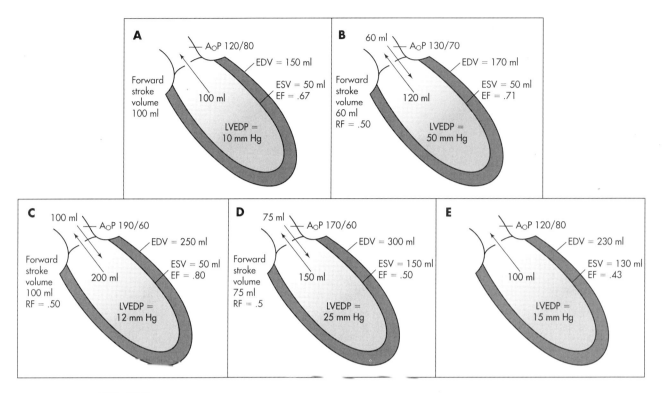

FIG. 19-6

A, Normal physiology. **B,** Pathophysiology of acute aortic regurgitation. **C,** Pathophysiology of chronic compensated aortic regurgitation. **D,** Pathophysiology of chronic decompensated aortic regurgitation. **E,** Physiology after aortic valve replacement for chronic aortic insufficiency. In acute aortic insufficiency, end-diastolic volume (EDV) increases slightly as existing sarcomeres are stretched toward their maximum. Afterload and contractility are unchanged, and therefore end-systolic volume (ESV) is unchanged. Ejection fraction (EF) increases slightly. Total stroke volume has increased to 120 ml, but because 50% of the total stroke volume (regurgitant fraction, RF, 0.50) is regurgitated back into the left ventricle, total stroke volume falls to 60 ml. At the same time the volume overload on the left ventricle increases left ventriclar end-diastolic pressure (LVEDP). If surgery can be avoided in this acute phase, or if the severity of aortic regurgitation increases gradually, the chronic compensated phase will be achieved. Now, eccentric cardiac hypertrophy has increased end-diastolic volume substantially, allowing a large total stroke volume to be ejected, causing a widened pulse pressure. It also compensates forward stroke volume back to normal. The now-enlarged left ventricle can receive the regurgitant volume of 100 ml at a much lower filling pressure. The chronic compensated phase may be maintained for years, but LV dysfunction eventually develops. The now-weakened left ventricle is unable to eject blood well, so end-systolic volume is greatly increased. This is represented echocardiographically as an increased end-systolic dimension. End-diastolic volume also may increase, in turn reelevating LV filling pressure. However, at this point in the progression of the disease the increase in end-diastolic volume is not enough to maintain forward stroke volume. If surgery is performed now, a fall in afterload after surgery causes a decrease in end-systolic volume and forward stroke volume returns to normal. However, ejection fraction is moderately depressed. With time, additional LV remodeling may allow ejection fraction to return to normal if LV dysfunction has been present for less than 18 months.

From Carabello BA: Aortic regurgitation: hemodynamic determinants of prognosis. In Cohn LH, editor: Aortic regurgitation, New York, 1986, Marcel Dekker.

A patient may remain in this compensated phase of aortic regurgitation for years, but the LV eventually fails. In this phase afterload increases, contractility decreases, and decompensation ensues. Reduced contractility and increased afterload result in a large increase in end-systolic volume, a further increase in end-diastolic volume, and no increase in stroke volume. The increase in end-diastolic volume increases LV end-diastolic pressure, and pulmonary congestion develops. In general, valve surgery may restore normal ventricular function if fewer than 18 months of decompensation have elapsed.

Clinical Presentation and Diagnosis
(Table 19-1)

Many patients with aortic regurgitation are asymptomatic. The most prominent symptoms are those of congestive heart failure. Thus the patient has dyspnea on exertion, fatigue, orthopnea, and occasionally paroxysmal nocturnal dyspnea. With physicians becoming aware of the need for early intervention, right heart failure in chronic aortic regurgitation has become uncommon

Patients with aortic regurgitation also may have angina pectoris, although this is a less frequent complaint than aortic stenosis (about 20% of patients).[24] Angina in patients with aortic insufficiency and normal coronary arteries is thought to result from reduced coronary blood flow reserve, possibly due to reduced aortic diastolic pressure, which reduces the driving pressure for coronary blood flow. Syncope occurs rarely, again presumably because of decreased diastolic pressure. Other symptoms include carotid artery pain and an unpleasant awareness of the heartbeat.

Physical Examination

The hyperdynamic circulation in aortic regurgitation produced by a large total stroke volume entering the circulation driven by high aortic systolic pressure causes distinctive findings during physical examination. The apical impulse is displaced downward and to the left and is hyperdynamic. S_1 and S_2 are typically normal, and gallop sounds are usually absent unless there is heart failure. The typical murmur is a diastolic blowing murmur heard best along the left sternal border when the patient is sitting up and leaning forward. An audible murmur to the right of the sternum may indicate a dilated aortic root, as with Marfan's syndrome.

With severe aortic regurgitation a diastolic rumble may be heard at the apex (the Austin Flint murmur). It originates from the mitral valve, probably from a combination of the aortic regurgitant jet impinging on the mitral valve, causing it to vibrate, and functional mitral stenosis caused by aortic valve back flow partially closing the mitral valve in diastole.

The wide pulse pressure produces a myriad of physical signs. These include Corrigan's pulse (sharp upstroke and rapid descent of the carotid pulse), DeMusset's sign (head bobbing), Quincke's pulse (systolic plethora and diastolic blanching of the nail bed when traction is placed on the nail), and Hill's sign (augmentation of systolic pressure in the leg by greater than 40 mm Hg compared with the arm).

Physical Diagnosis in Acute Aortic Regurgitation

Because cardiac dilation has not yet developed in acute cases, the physical examination usually does not uncover the characteristic findings of chronic disease. The examination may only demonstrate a short diastolic murmur and a soft S_1. This latter finding indicates mitral valve preclosure and is an ominous sign.

Management
Laboratory Examination

ECG and Chest X-ray. The ECG in chronic aortic regurgitation demonstrates LV hypertrophy and left atrial abnormality. Chest x-ray shows cardiac enlargement. A normal-sized heart indicates that either the aortic regurgitation is mild or that it is not chronic enough to permit cardiac dilation. Dilation of the aorta may be seen on the lateral view.

Echocardiogram. Echocardiography is indispensable in the diagnosis and management of a patient with aortic regurgitation. The echocardiogram gives clues to the severity of the aortic regurgitation and its physiologic consequences. Chamber dilation and LV function should be assessed carefully, because these are the keys to deciding when a patient should be referred for surgery (see later discussion). Doppler interrogation of the aortic valve is useful in quantifying the severity of the aortic regurgitation. Severity in part is gauged by color-flow Doppler examination using the depth and breadth to which the regurgitant jet penetrates the left ventricle.[25] The pressure half-time method is also used to gauge severity.[26] Using continuous wave Doppler the decay of the diastolic flow velocity across the aortic valve into the left ventricle is noted. In severe aortic insufficiency, rapid equilibration of pressure occurs between the aorta and left ventricle and the pressure half-time (the time it takes for the velocity to decay from its peak divided by the square root of 2) is brief (less than 400 msec). In milder aortic insufficiency the gradient between the aorta and left ventricle is maintained throughout diastole, the decay is slow, and the pressure half-time is long.

Cardiac Catheterization. Cardiac catheterization in patients with aortic insufficiency is performed when surgery is contemplated. In patients with risk factors for coronary artery disease, coronary arteriography is important. If the severity of aortic insufficiency is still in doubt after noninvasive testing, hemodynamic clues of severity (wide pulse pressure, rapid rise of LV diastolic pressure, and Hill's sign) are sought. In addition, aortography is performed to assess the flow of contrast from the aorta into the LV during diastole, helping to gauge the severity of the aortic regurgitation.

Treatment

Medical. In patients with more than mild symptoms, surgical therapy is preferred. However, medical therapy is appropriate for asymptomatic patients or patients with mild symptoms and preserved LV function. In such patients, vasodilators have been noted to improve hemodynamics, and, specifically, the vasodilator nifedipine (at a dose of 20 mg twice daily) can forestall the need for surgery.[27] Whether this is the ideal vasodilator is unknown, since no studies have compared vasodilators. It is usually impossible to return systolic pressure to normal. The degree to which systolic blood pressure must be reduced for optimal benefit of vasodilator therapy is currently unknown.

Surgical. Occasionally it is possible to repair the aortic valve in patients with aortic regurgitation, but aortic valve replacement is usually necessary. Therefore the risks of a valve prosthesis (thromboembolism, valve failure, and anticoagulation) must be weighed against the risks of delaying surgery. Over the last 2 decades useful guidelines have been developed to guide the timing of referral and of surgery[28,29] (Fig. 19-7). The onset of symptoms and the worsening of existing symptoms are important indicators of deterioration. Moderate symptoms alone may pose an increased risk and thus should be managed surgically rather than medically.

On the other hand, asymptomatic LV dysfunction develops in some patients with aortic insufficiency and substantially worsens the prognosis if left unattended.[28,29] Thus, unlike aortic stenosis, symptom assessment alone is not a satisfactory strategy for monitoring aortic regurgitation. Instead, periodic echocardiographic follow-up is necessary to monitor LV function. *If the LV ejection fraction falls below 55%, or if the end-systolic dimension exceeds 55 mm, prognosis worsens.*

If the end-systolic dimension is less than 40 mm, significant LV dysfunction likely will not develop within 2 years, and a follow-up echocardiogram can be performed at that time. For end-systolic dimensions between 40 and 50 mm, yearly echocardiographic surveillance is warranted; if end-systolic dimension exceeds 50 mm, there is little point in delaying surgery. Those who already have LV dysfunction may have surgery even though the risk is high and the long-term outcome may be suboptimal. After surgery these patients with "burned-out ventricles" are managed similarly to those with cardiomyopathy.

After surgery, guidelines for anticoagulation and for monitoring prosthetic valve function are like those used after correction of aortic stenosis.

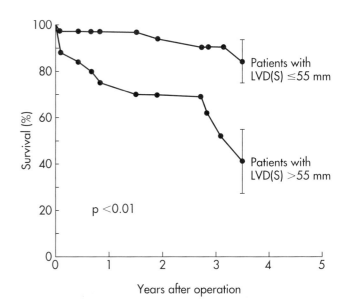

FIG. 19-7

Survival for patients with aortic regurgitation after aortic valve replacement is plotted for those patients with a preoperative LV end systolic dimension [LVD(S)] of less than 55 mm versus a dimension of greater than 55 mm. Survival was much better when surgery was performed before the left ventricle had decompensated to the point at which it could no longer contract to an end-systolic dimension of 55 mm.

From Bonow RO, Rosing DR, Kent KM, Epstein SE: Am J Cardiol 50:325, 1982.

REFERENCES

1. Otto CM, Kuusisto J, Reichenbach DD, et al: Characterization of the early lesion of "degenerative" valvular aortic stenosis: histological and immunohistochemical studies, *Circulation* 90:844, 1994.
2. Ross J Jr, Braunwald E: Aortic stenosis, *Circulation* 38(suppl 5):61, 1968.
3. Kelly TA, Rothbart RM, Cooper CM, et al: Comparison of outcome of asymptomatic to symptomatic patients older than 20 years of age with valvular aortic stenosis, *Am J Cardiol* 61:123, 1988.
4. Pellikka PA, Nishimura RA, Bailey KR, Tajik AJ: The natural history of adults with asymptomatic, hemodynamically significant aortic stenosis, *J Am Coll Cardiol* 15:1012, 1990.
5. Grossman W, editor: *Cardiac catheterization and angiography,* ed 2, Philadelphia, 1980, Lea & Febiger.
6. Grossman W, Jones D, McLaurin LP: Wall stress and patterns of hypertrophy in the human left ventricle, *J Clin Invest* 56:56, 1975.
7. Huber D, Grimm J, Koch R, Krayenbuehl HP: Determinants of ejection performance in aortic stenosis, *Circulation* 64:126, 1981.
8. Marcus ML, Doty DB, Hiratzka LF, et al: Decreased coronary reserve: a mechanism for angina pectoris in patients with aortic stenosis and normal coronary arteries, *N Engl J Med* 307:1362, 1982.

9. Peterson KL, Tsuji J, Johnson A, et al: Diastolic left ventricular pressure-volume and stress-strain relations in patients with valvular aortic stenosis and left ventricular hypertrophy, *Circulation* 58:77, 1978.

10. Carabello BA, Green LH, Grossman W, et al: Hemodynamic determinants of prognosis of aortic valve replacement in critical aortic stenosis and advanced congestive heart failure, *Circulation* 62:42, 1980.

11. Koide M, Nagatsu M, Zile MR, et al: Premorbid determinants of left ventricular dysfunction in a novel model of gradually induced pressure overload in the adult canine, *Circulation* 95:1601, 1997.

12. Carabello BA: Aortic stenosis: how to recognize and assess severity, *Cardiol Rev* 1:59, 1993.

13. Assey ME, Usher BW, Carabello BA: The patient with valvular heart disease. In Pepine CJ, Hill JA, Lambert CR, editors: *Diagnostic and therapeutic cardiac catheterization*, ed 2, Baltimore, 1994, Williams & Wilkins.

14. Carabello BA, Grossman W: Calculation of stenotic valve orifice area. In Grossman W, Baim DS, editors: *Cardiac catheterization, angiography and intervention*, ed 5, Baltimore, 1996, Williams & Wilkins.

15. Areskog NH: Exercise testing in the evaluation of patients with valvular aortic stenosis, *Clin Physiol* 4:201, 1984.

16. Carabello BA: Indications for valve surgery in asymptomatic patients with aortic and mitral stenosis, *Chest* 108:1678, 1995.

17. Otto CM, Burwash IG, Legget ME, et al: Prospective study of asymptomatic valvular aortic stenosis: clinical, echocardiographic, and exercise predictors of outcome, *Circulation* 95:2262, 1997.

18. Carabello BA: Timing of valve replacement in aortic stenosis, *Circulation* 95:2241, 1997.

19. Lindblom D, Lindblom U, Qvist J, Lundström H: Long-term relative survival rates after heart valve replacement, *J Am Coll Cardiol* 15:566, 1990.

20. Otto CM, Mickel MC, Kennedy JW, et al: Three-year outcome after balloon aortic valvuloplasty: insights into prognosis of valvular aortic stenosis, *Circulation* 89:642, 1994.

21. Carabello BA: Aortic regurgitation: hemodynamic determinants of prognosis. In Cohn LH, DiSesa VJ, editors: *Aortic regurgitation: medical and surgical management*, New York, 1986, Marcel Dekker.

22. Sareli P, Klein HO, Schamroth CL, et al: Contribution of echocardiography and immediate surgery to the management of severe aortic regurgitation from active infective endocarditis, *Am J Cardiol* 57:413, 1986.

23. Wisenbaugh T, Spann JF, Carabello BA: Differences in myocardial performance and load between patients with similar amounts of chronic aortic versus chronic mitral regurgitation, *J Am Coll Cardiol* 3:916, 1984.

24. Timmermans P, Willems JL, Piessens J, De Geest H: Angina pectoris and coronary artery disease in severe aortic regurgitation, *Am J Cardiol* 61:826, 1988.

25. Perry GJ, Helmcke F, Nanda NC, et al: Evaluation of aortic insufficiency by Doppler color flow mapping, *J Am Coll Cardiol* 9:952, 1987.

26. Teague SM, Heinsimer JA, Anderson JL, et al: Quantification of aortic regurgitation utilizing continuous wave Doppler ultrasound, *J Am Coll Cardiol* 8:592, 1986.

27. Scognamiglio R, Rahimtoola SH, Fasoli G, et al: Nifedipine in asymptomatic patients with severe aortic regurgitation and normal left ventricular function, *N Engl J Med* 331:689, 1994.

28. Henry WL, Bonow RO, Borer JS, et al: Observations on the optimum time for operative intervention for aortic regurgitation. I. Evaluation of the results of aortic valve replacement in symptomatic patients, *Circulation* 61:471, 1980.

29. Bonow RO, Lakatos E, Maron BJ, Epstein SE: Serial long-term assessment of the natural history of asymptomatic patients with chronic aortic regurgitation and normal left ventricular systolic function, *Circulation* 84:1625, 1991.

20 Tricuspid and Pulmonic Valve Disease

Blase A. Carabello

TRICUSPID VALVE DISEASE
Tricuspid Regurgitation
Epidemiology and Etiology

Most tricuspid regurgitation results from processes that raise pulmonary artery pressure and cause right ventricular dilation, rendering the tricuspid valve insufficient.[1,2] Left ventricular failure and mitral stenosis are common cardiac etiologies. Pulmonary hypertension may also develop in patients with chronic lung disease and may lead to mild tricuspid regurgitation (see Chapter 35).

Primary tricuspid regurgitation caused by structural damage to the valve is relatively uncommon. Rheumatic fever, carcinoid syndrome, infective endocarditis, and right ventricular infarction can injure the tricuspid valve. Of these, by far the most common is infective endocarditis, usually seen in drug abusers (Box 20-1).

Pathophysiology

The primary function of the right ventricle (RV) is to provide the hemodynamic impetus that fills the left ventricle (LV). Normally, the work requirements of the RV to fulfill this function are minimal. It must overcome the small resistance offered by the pulmonary vasculature. It also supplies some of the force needed to generate the initial gradient between left atrium and LV, which helps to open the mitral valve and initiate left ventricular filling. This work requirement is small enough that in patients with tricuspid atresia, the RV is bypassed and the LV fills passively from systemic venous pressure (see Chapter 30).

The work of the RV may be increased when either the LV requires a high filling pressure or pulmonary vascular resistance increases. When either the left atrial pressure (the equivalent of the LV filling pressure) or the pressure gradient across the pulmonary vascular bed is increased, there is pressure overload of the RV. Although modest concentric hypertrophy develops as it does in left ventricular pressure overload, right ventricular dilation also occurs and commonly leads to tricuspid regurgitation. Diseases that cause a primary right ventricular volume overload, such as atrial septal defect, also cause right ventricular dilation and tricuspid regurgitation.

The development of tricuspid regurgitation may substantially reduce forward output by giving the RV an alternative (but useless) pathway for ejection. Right atrial pressure is much lower than pulmonary artery pressure, favoring regurgitant flow across the tricuspid valve. Tricuspid regurgitation shifts the right ventricular pressure volume relationship rightward, further increasing right atrial pressure and producing systemic venous congestion.

Primary tricuspid regurgitation in the absence of pulmonary hypertension is tolerated remarkably well. For instance, in some patients with tricuspid endocarditis, the tricuspid valve is removed to effect a bacteriologic cure, leaving wide-open tricuspid regurgitation.[3] Although such patients may develop fatigue and a low output state several years later, initially they remain remarkably well compensated. Thus the RV appears to tolerate a volume overload quite well. In fact, a recent study demonstrated that even after years of torrential experimental tricuspid regurgitation, right ventricular muscle function remained nearly normal.[4]

Clinical Presentation

The typical symptoms of tricuspid regurgitation are those of right ventricular failure and include ascites, edema, and fatigue. Occasionally, tricuspid regurgitation may lead to rapid passive hepatic congestion, in turn causing right upper quadrant pain.

Palpation of the precordium demonstrates a sternal lift indicative of right ventricular enlargement. If pulmonary hypertension is present, the pulmonic component of S_2 may be increased. Right-sided gallop sounds may be heard over the sternum (see Chapter 4). The typical murmur of tricuspid regurgitation is audible along the right sternal border, is holosystolic, and increases with inspiration. The murmur does not always change with inspiration. Inspiration may increase the distance between the chest wall and the heart, obscuring the change in murmur intensity. Furthermore, with right ventricular failure, inspiration may fail to increase right ventricular output and thus fail to augment murmur intensity.

The neck veins are elevated and may demonstrate a large V wave (Chapter 4). However, if the tricuspid regurgitation is chronic or if the right atrium is large and compliant, the V wave may be absent. The liver is enlarged and pulsatile. There often is ascites and edema.

Management

Laboratory Evaluation. The electrocardiogram may show right atrial abnormality, evidence of right ventricular hypertrophy, and right axis deviation. The chest x-ray may demonstrate enlargement of the RV, indicated by loss of the retrosternal air space in the lateral view.

The most important study in assessing tricuspid regurgitation is the echocardiogram, which may be helpful in establishing the etiology. The central issue is the presence or absence of left heart disease. If left ventricular failure or mitral stenosis has led to pulmonary hypertension, the echocardiogram reveals these etiologies. Conversely, if lung disease is the cause of pulmonary hypertension, left-sided structures and function will be normal and right ventricular pressure elevated.

The right ventricular systolic pressure (which is the same as the pulmonary systolic pressure in the absence of pulmonic stenosis) is measured by the echo-Doppler study using the reverse gradient from the RV into the right atrium during systole.[5] The modified Bernoulli formula (gradient $= 4V^2$) gives the peak pressure gradient across the tricuspid valve. By adding right atrial pressure to this value, the peak right ventricular and peak pulmonary pressures can be obtained. Thus, if the peak velocity of the regurgitant jet from RV to right atrium is 3 m/s, a peak pressure gradient of 36 mm (4×3^2) is obtained. If the right atrial pressure is 15 mm Hg, a peak

right ventricular systolic pressure of 51 mm Hg (15 + 36) is estimated. On the other hand, if primary disease of the tricuspid valve (endocarditis, carcinoid, and so on) is the cause of the tricuspid regurgitation, a normal pulmonary pressure is found in conjunction with abnormalities of the valve itself.

Cardiac catheterization has little role to play in the diagnosis of tricuspid regurgitation. Although the height of the right atrial V wave may be of some use in judging severity, its correlation with the amount of tricuspid regurgitation is inconsistent. Left ventriculography is commonly used to demonstrate mitral regurgitation, but right ventriculography is not used in the assessment of tricuspid regurgitation because passage of a catheter across the tricuspid valve to perform right ventriculography may itself cause tricuspid regurgitation.

Treatment. Since most tricuspid regurgitation is secondary to either left ventricular failure, left-sided valvular heart disease, or pulmonary hypertension resulting from pulmonary disease, therapy for tricuspid regurgitation is usually centered on treating the primary problem. Effective treatment of left heart disease that lowers pulmonary artery pressure can be expected to improve the tricuspid regurgitation as well.[6] If lung disease has caused pulmonary hypertension, better oxygenation and ventilation may reduce pulmonary artery pressure, thereby helping to restore tricuspid valve competence (see Chapter 35).

For primary tricuspid regurgitation, as with infective endocarditis, therapy is aimed at relieving symptoms and consists primarily of diuretics. As noted earlier, severe isolated tricuspid regurgitation may be tolerated well for years.

When surgery is necessary, tricuspid valve repair using an annuloplasty ring leads to better results than tricuspid valve replacement.[7,8] Isolated tricuspid valve surgery is unusual. In practice, you will see it more commonly as an adjunct to mitral valve surgery. Often the surgeon evaluates the tricuspid valve after replacing the mitral valve. If there is still a lot of tricuspid regurgitation, the valve is repaired.

Tricuspid Stenosis

Tricuspid stenosis is a rare disease with two possible etiologies. It may occur with extensive rheumatic heart disease, in which other cardiac valves are always affected, or it may be seen in the presence of carcinoid syndrome. The exact cause of tricuspid stenosis in carcinoid heart disease is uncertain, but it appears to result from agents secreted by the carcinoid tumor. Levels of serotonin and its metabolites are higher in patients with carcinoid syndrome and tricuspid valve disease than in patients with carcinoid syndrome without tricuspid valve disease.

Clinical Presentation

Tricuspid stenosis causes the symptoms of systemic venous congestion, including edema and ascites. It has the clinical appearance of "right heart failure," although the stenotic valve protects the RV, and right ventricular size and function are normal. If rheumatic heart disease is the cause of the tricuspid stenosis, there are associated symptoms from rheumatic mitral valve disease. When carcinoid syndrome is the cause, other carcinoid symptoms will have been present for several years (diarrhea and flushing). It is likely that the diagnosis of carcinoid will be known. Rarely, carcinoid syndrome presents as primarily right-sided heart failure with ascites and edema.

On physical examination the precordium is quiet, the neck veins are elevated, and a diastolic rumble is heard at the right sternal border that increases with inspiration. Ascites, edema, and hepatic enlargement are evident.

Management

The diagnosis of tricuspid stenosis can be confirmed echocardiographically with demonstration of thickening and immobility of the tricuspid valve leaflets. The gradient across the valve can be calculated and a valve area obtained. If tricuspid stenosis is caused by rheumatic heart disease, the echocardiogram also demonstrates typical rheumatic mitral stenosis. If tricuspid stenosis results from carcinoid syndrome, the other heart valves look normal. Isolated tricuspid stenosis causes right atrial enlargement; right ventricular size is normal.

During cardiac catheterization the gradient across the tricuspid valve can be measured by placing one catheter in the right atrium and another in the RV. A small gradient is consistent with fairly severe disease.

Therapy. Diuretics are the cornerstone of therapy for tricuspid stenosis. If symptoms persist and valve surgery is contemplated to repair or replace other cardiac valves in the face of rheumatic heart disease, tricuspid commissurotomy can be performed at the time of surgery. For tricuspid stenosis in isolation that does not respond to diuretics alone, balloon tricuspid valvotomy is usually effective in relieving symptoms.

PULMONARY VALVE DISEASE
Pulmonic Stenosis
Epidemiology

Pulmonary stenosis is a congenital disease usually detected in childhood. Occasionally, however, it is noted for the first time in adulthood when a loud murmur is noted.[10]

Pathophysiology

Pulmonic stenosis produces pressure overload on the RV that is present from birth. This type of hypertrophy or hyperplasia differs from acquired valvular stenosis that occurs later in life, as ejection performance is almost always enhanced with congenital disease.[11,12] It appears that ventricular hypertrophy beginning early in life is associated with more effective contractility.

Clinical Presentation

Unless the pulmonic stenosis is extreme, right ventricular failure and its symptoms are usually absent. More common symptoms of pulmonary stenosis include angina, which is presumably caused by right ventricular hypertrophy, and syncope, which is caused by outflow obstruction from the RV (a pathophysiology similar to that of tetralogy of Fallot, see Chapter 30).

There is a harsh systolic ejection murmur heard best in the pulmonic area. Because the valve is not calcified with this congenital abnormality, the murmur is preceded by a systolic click that varies with respiration. During inspiration the valve is partially opened by passive flow, and the click may diminish or disappear. In expiration, the click is louder.

There usually is a right ventricular lift. In rare cases in the adult there may also be ascites and edema.

Management

The electrocardiogram shows right ventricular hypertrophy. If the transvalvular gradient is above 50 mm Hg, there may also be evidence of right ventricular strain in the right precordial leads. On chest x-ray there may be poststenotic dilation of the pulmonary arteries.

The echocardiogram is the key diagnostic test. It demonstrates doming of the pulmonic valve; Doppler interrogation demonstrates and quantifies the gradient across the valve.

Therapy. No treatment is required for asymptomatic patients with a gradient less than 50 mm Hg.[13] In symptomatic patients with a gradient of 50 mm Hg or more, or in asymptomatic patients with a gradient of 75 mm Hg or more, balloon valvotomy is performed and is usually successful.

REFERENCES

1. Waller BF, Howard J, Fess S: Pathology of tricuspid valve stenosis and pure tricuspid regurgitation. III. *Clin Cardiol* 18:225, 1995.
2. Waller BF, Moriarty AT, Eble JN, et al: Etiology of pure tricuspid regurgitation based on anular circumference and leaflet area: analysis of 45 necropsy patients with clinical and morphologic evidence of pure tricuspid regurgitation, *J Am Coll Cardiol* 7:1063, 1986.
3. Arbulu A, Asfaw I: Tricuspid valvectomy without prosthetic replacement: ten years of clinical experience, *J Thorac Cardiovasc Surg* 82:684, 1981.
4. Ishibashi Y, Nemoto S, Rembert JC, et al: Intrinsic myocardial function is normal in severe right ventricular volume overload, *Circulation* 98:1, 1998.

5. Skjaerpe T, Hatle L: Noninvasive estimation of systolic pressure in the right ventricle in patients with tricuspid regurgitation, *Eur Heart J* 7:704, 1986.

6. Skudicky D, Essop MR, Sareli P: Efficacy of mitral balloon valvotomy in reducing the severity of associated tricuspid valve regurgitation, *Am J Cardiol* 73:209, 1994.

7. Holper K, Haehnel JC, Augustin N, Sebening F: Surgery for tricuspid insufficiency: long-term follow-up after De Vega annuloplasty, *Thorac Cardiovasc Surg* 41:1, 1993.

8. Scully HE, Armstrong CS: Tricuspid valve replacement: fifteen years of experience with mechanical prostheses and bioprostheses, *J Thorac Cardiovasc Surg* 109:1035, 1995.

9. Lundin L, Norheim I, Landelius J, et al: Carcinoid heart disease: relationship of circulating vasoactive substances to ultrasound-detectable cardiac abnormalities, *Circulation* 77:264, 1988.

10. Johnson LW, Grossman W, Dalen JE, Dexter L: Pulmonic stenosis in the adult: long-term follow-up results, *N Engl J Med* 287:1159, 1972.

11. Leman RB, Spinale FG, Dorn GW II, et al: Supernormal ejection performance is isolated to the ipsilateral congenitally pressure-overloaded ventricle, *J Am Coll Cardiol* 13:1314, 1989.

12. Dorn GW II, Donner R, Assey ME, et al: Alterations in left ventricular geometry, wall stress, and ejection performance after correction of congenital aortic stenosis, *Circulation* 78:1358, 1988.

13. Sievert H, Kober G, Bussman WD, et al: Long-term results of percutaneous pulmonary valvuloplasty in adults, *Eur Heart J* 10:712, 1989.

21 Endocarditis

Donald R. Graham
Blase A. Carabello

Endocarditis mimics many diseases. Formerly a fatal illness in its classic subacute bacterial form (SBE),[1] it now is one of the few curable heart diseases. Its importance remains qualitative rather than quantitative, however. The average primary care clinician may encounter only one or two cases in a lifetime of practice. Even cardiologists see infective endocarditis (IE) infrequently, and most enlist the services of an infectious disease specialist to help with management of the infection. The symptoms are often subtle or obscured by other illnesses, and it is easy to miss the diagnosis. In general, however, the course of IE is relentless and will continue to haunt the patient and clinician until a diagnosis is made.

With the complexity of invasive procedures and the use of long-term indwelling vascular devices, the epidemiology of IE has evolved. Two forms of IE should be considered: acute and chronic (also known as "subacute"). The common acronym of medical school, SBE, is the less common of the two. The majority of patients now with infective valvular disease present with a history of some prior cardiac surgery or another form of invasive therapy before admission.

A recent controversy about the definition of IE has arisen. The term denotes infection of the endocardial surface of the heart and implies the physical presence of microorganisms in the valvular vegetation. However, diagnosis is generally made by indirect means. The leading schools of thought regarding diagnosis are led by von Reyn et al.,[2] who offer a definition that maximizes specificity, and Durack et al.[3] ("the Duke criteria"), who recommend a definition with optimal sensitivity. When blood cultures are repeatedly positive in the face of echocardiographic evidence of a valvular lesion, the diagnosis is simple. In a majority of cases it is not easy, since vague symptoms such as fatigue and fever, intermittently positive blood cultures, and previous antibiotic therapy make endocarditis difficult to diagnose on clinical grounds.

EPIDEMIOLOGY

The incidence of IE ranges from 0.16 to 5.4 cases per 1000 hospital admissions.[4,5] In Olmsted County, Minnesota, the incidence has been measured at 4.9 cases of IE per 100,000 person years, which of course reflects all persons in the community. This incidence ranks between rhinovirus infection (70,000 cases per 100,000 person years) and tetanus (0.03 cases per 100,000 person years).

In the days of Sir William Osler, acute endocarditis, a fulminant disease with high fever and severe toxicity marked by death in several days to weeks, was an unusual form of presentation. The vast majority of cases followed a slow course with fatigue, low-grade fever, malaise, weight loss, sweats, and myalgias. Now the tables have turned. With the rise of staphylococcal, fungal, and pyogenic streptococcal infections, classical SBE has been eclipsed. Moreover, the ready availability of antimicrobial therapy, although occasionally prescribed without clear-cut indications, has undoubtedly limited many incipient cases of IE before they could establish themselves, while delaying the diagnosis in other cases.

In recent years the mean age of patients with endocarditis has increased. Most patients are older than 50 years of age; the major exception is among young patients with congenital heart disease and others with structural valvular lesions. Men are slightly more likely than women to be infected.

Rheumatic heart disease used to be the leading risk factor for endocarditis (Box 21-1). As the incidence of rheumatic fever has diminished, so has the incidence of late complications. Congenital heart disease, acquired calcific aortic stenosis, other degenerative calcific valvular diseases, asymmetrical septal hypertrophy, mitral valve prolapse, and cardiac transplantation have assumed roles as important predisposing factors. Other forms of cardiac implantation such as stents, prosthetic valves, pacemakers, implantable defibrillators, patches, and aortic conduits can predispose to infection. Patients with acquired immunodeficiency syndrome (AIDS), regardless of the source of the infection, and all intravenous (IV) drug users are at special risk.

PATHOPHYSIOLOGY

As with all infections, IE requires a susceptible host to be exposed to an infecting organism. The primary component of susceptibility is a roughened valve or endovascular surface, generally caused by turbulent blood flow. Fibrin, platelets, and white blood cells combine to

BOX 21-1

POPULATIONS AT RISK FOR ENDOCARDITIS

Congenital heart disease
Valvular prosthesis
Patients with indwelling catheters and shunts
Degenerative valve disease
AIDS
Cardiac transplantation
Intravenous drug users
Rheumatic fever
Colon carcinoma
Marfan's syndrome
Post–myocardial infarction thrombi
Syphilis
Asymmetric septal hypertrophy
Mitral valve prolapse
Elderly

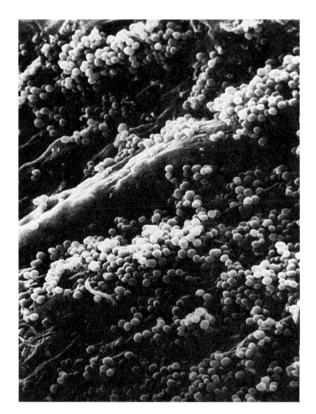

FIG. 21-1
Scanning electron micrograph of a pig valve 24 hours after infection by *Staphylococcus aureus*.

form thrombi. Eventually, circulating bacteria attach to the thrombi, multiply, invade locally, and spread systemically. Less important than the inciting episode of bacteremia, the bacteria attached to the roughened cardiac surface become an independent site of infection, able to seed the rest of the body. Although all bacteria can circulate through the bloodstream, it is primarily those that can adhere to valves and other endothelial surfaces that predispose to IE. Bacteria with the necessary adherence factors attach to valves during the first circulatory pass and within 24 hours can literally cover an area of the valve (Fig. 21-1). *Escherichia coli* and *Klebsiella pneumoniae* almost invariably pass a roughened valvular surface and do not cause IE, despite the relative frequency of bacteremia in such infections as ascending cholangitis and pyelonephritis. *Streptococcus mutans* is 450 times more likely than *S. pyogenes* to cause IE for any given episode of bacteremia.

Lesions with high degrees of turbulence promote bacterial colonization more than large defects or those with low flow. Thus patients with chronic atrial fibrillation and no valvular lesions rarely develop endocarditis, even though they often have a thrombus in the left atrium.

Many patients develop infections of more than one valve. Lepeschkin's autopsy series of 1024 cases of endocarditis through 1952 found that 86% involved the mitral valve, 55% the aortic valve, 20% the tricuspid valve, and 1% the pulmonic valve.[6]

Not only must the anatomy favor infection, but the cardiac lesion must be exposed to bacteremia. Not commonly appreciated is the high rate of bacteremia during our daily lives. Even chewing candy can cause a transient bacteremia in as many as one of five episodes.[7] Numerous other activities and minor surgical procedures can lead to bacteremia (Table 21-1).

Serologic factors may play a role in the development of endocarditis. Rheumatoid factor (the IgM antibody to IgG) develops in about half of the patients with IE lasting more than 6 weeks and one fourth of patients with staphylococcal endocarditis of short duration. It may block IgG opsonic activity and stimulate phagocytosis to accelerate microvascular damage. Antinuclear antibodies and circulating immune complexes occasionally develop. Patients with *Staphylococcus aureus* infections develop antibodies to lipoteichoic acid, a constituent of the cell wall of *S. aureus*. Another great mimic has been confused with endocarditis in recent years. Kaell[9] reported four cases of false-positive Lyme antibodies among patients with endocarditis. With treatment, most of the serologic changes revert to normal.

Pathology

IE can involve every organ in the body (Box 21-2). Depending on the time of presentation and chance, IE could conceivably be encountered by any physician. For example, a dermatologist may note splinter hemor-

Table 21-1 | *Incidence of Bacteremia after Procedures**

Procedure	Positive Blood Culture (%)
DENTAL	
Extraction	18-85
Periodontal surgery	32-88
Chewing candy or paraffin	17-51
Tooth brushing	0-26
Oral irrigation	27-57
UPPER AIRWAY	
Rigid bronchoscopy	15
Tonsillectomy	28-38
Nasotracheal intubation or suctioning	16
GASTROINTESTINAL	
Upper endoscopy	8-12
Sigmoidoscopy/colonoscopy	0-10
Barium enema	11
Porcutaneous liver biopsy	3-13
OBSTETRIC	
Normal vaginal delivery	0-11
Cervical punch biopsy	0
Placement and removal of IUD	0
UROLOGIC	
Urethral dilation	18-33
Urethral catheterization	8
Cystoscopy	0-17
Transurethral resection of prostate	12-46

*Data from Everett ED, Hirschmann JV: *Medicine* 56:61, 1977

rhages in the fingernails, tender subcutaneous peripheral nodules, or small peripheral pustules. A neurologist may encounter a person with a stroke. Nephrologists must consider IE as a cause of acute renal failure. Gastroenterologists may see acute bacterial hepatitis. Even ophthalmologists may be the first physicians to make the diagnosis when they see classic Roth spots with edema and hemorrhage in the retina.

CLINICAL PRESENTATION

The constitutional symptoms of IE include fever, weakness, sweats, fatigue, and weight loss. As noted, various clinical syndromes are possible, depending on the organ(s) affected (see Box 21-2). It is important to consider IE when dealing with potentially embolic conditions. In such cases, constitutional symptoms and a heart murmur would push IE to the top of the list.

The classic physical findings are fever and heart murmur. Although most of us learned about changing heart murmurs in medical school, the diagnosis of IE is rarely made by comparing a physical examination with one recorded earlier. Nevertheless, it is important to document the quality of the murmur during the first physical examination. Too often we find no description of the cardiac sounds and no comment about whether a murmur is present or absent at the time of the initial physical examination. Daily physical examinations may detect muffled prosthetic tones, a new pericardial or pleural friction rub, a new skin lesion, a subtle neurologic change, or a joint effusion.

Emboli are responsible for most other symptoms and signs. Although not all emboli are associated with infection, infections do represent some of the most treatable causes of emboli. Up to one third of patients with IE develop emboli, often to unusual areas. For

---

BOX 21-2

PATHOLOGIC CHANGES IN ENDOCARDITIS

HEART
Vegetation on valve
Perforation of valve leaflet
Rupture of chordae tendineae
Rupture of papillary muscle
Perivalvular abscess
Myocardial abscess
Purulent pericarditis
Myocardial infarction
Intracardiac embolus
Extracardiac embolus

SKIN
Janeway lesion
Osler node
Petechiae
Splinter hemorrhage

VASCULATURE
Mycotic aneurysm
Emboli
Rupture
Aortoenteric fistula

SPLEEN
Infarction
Abscess
Rupture

LUNG
Pneumonia
Septic embolus
Empyema
Abscess

LIVER
Abscess
Bacterial hepatitis
Hepatomegaly

CENTRAL NERVOUS SYSTEM
Embolus
Infarction
Cerebritis
Abscess
Hemorrhage
Meningitis
Delirium

EYE
Roth spot
Endophthalmitis
Retinal artery occlusion

KIDNEY
Abscess
Infarct
Glomerulonephritis
   Focal
   Diffuse
   Membranoproliferative
   Immune complex deposition
Renal failure
(Lesions are generally reversible with treatment of IE.)

ORTHOPEDIC
Septic arthritis
Osteomyelitis
Myositis

---

example, pulmonary emboli commonly arise from right-sided endocarditis infecting IV drug users (and patients who receive treatment through indwelling IV catheters). Stroke is a complication of IE in about one quarter of cases. Mycotic aneurysms of the cerebral circulation may develop, and diagnosis is important because of the greater tendency of such aneurysms to bleed during anticoagulation.

Classic skin lesions such as splinter hemorrhages, which are red or dark brown linear marks in the nails, are seen frequently in IE. Be mindful of the fact that carpenters and others who work with their hands often have benign splinters. Petechiae on the palate, conjunctiva, arms, and legs are common. They may be transient, even with untreated illness. However, fever and segmental skin lesions should lead you to consider the diagnosis of IE. Osler's nodes are uncommon but are often demonstrated first by the patient or family because they are painful nodules on the fingers, toes, and thumbs. They can also be localized distal to an infected renal arterial venous shunt or an infected graft. Disseminated gonococcal infections can cause similar lesions. Janeway lesions are hemorrhagic macules on the palms and soles, are generally painless, and are seen frequently with endocarditis caused by *S. aureus* (Fig. 21-2). Clubbing, common in chronic endocarditis, is not specific and always warrants a chest x-ray (lung cancer is another cause). The classic Roth spots are unusual, because of either the difficulties of funduscopy or the rarity of the lesions. They are present in only about 5% of cases of endocarditis and can also be seen in leukemia, systemic lupus erythematosus, and profound anemia. Suspected endocarditis is not a mandate for a dilated funduscopic examination. Splenomegaly and hepatomegaly occur in 25% to 60% of patients. Splenic infections can evolve into abscesses, which are extremely difficult to treat medically and often require splenectomy. Arthralgias and myalgias may be local or diffuse and may progress to frank intramuscular abscesses, septic joints, and osteomyelitis.

Right Heart Endocarditis

Intravenous drug use may inflame the tricuspid valve and rarely the pulmonary valve. Over half of addicts with IE have an infected tricuspid valve. The most common cause is *S. aureus* (especially methicillin-resistant strains [MRSA] in urban centers). Enterococci, viridans streptococci, and *Pseudomonas aeruginosa* are seen often.

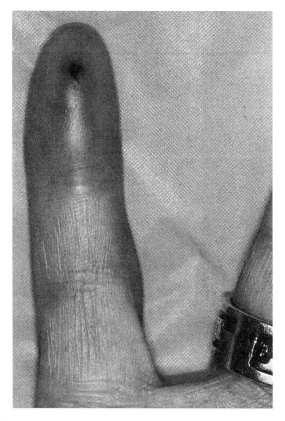

FIG. 21-2
Classic Janeway lesion on the palmar aspect of the fifth finger of a man with prosthetic valve endocarditis caused by *Acinetobacter* spp.

The source generally is the patient's skin; rarely is the apparatus or the drug itself contaminated. In this population, *Candida* spp. can cause culture-negative endocarditis, which may present with endophthalmitis or left-sided valvular disease. The illness may be hectic, but occasionally causes just nonspecific, flulike symptoms. Extracardiac manifestations are common and may direct the physician away from consideration of a valvular source.

Right-sided endocarditis is not limited to the drug-abusing population. With the frequent use of indwelling vascular catheters, it is possible to have bacteremia and subsequent valve infection. Particularly important is nosocomial bacteremia caused by *S. aureus*.

MANAGEMENT
Laboratory Studies

The hallmark of IE is the positive blood culture. Bacteremia in IE is continuous. Although not every culture is positive, especially after antibiotic treatment, as many as 95% of blood cultures are positive in established cases.[10] Most blood cultures yield so few organisms that quantitation may not differentiate a true positive blood culture from a contaminant. Samples that are repeatedly positive, those that yield "typical organisms," those that are positive without other explanation, and those that yield the same organism are all more likely to be true positives.

To make or exclude the diagnosis of IE, we recommend collection of three sets of blood cultures. The practice of collecting six blood cultures is not necessary. In the absence of antimicrobial therapy, the first blood culture is positive in 96% of cases of streptococcal endocarditis, and one of the first three cultures is positive in 98% of cases. However, if antimicrobial therapy has been given within the previous 2 weeks, the rate of positive blood cultures falls to about 65%.[11] The first blood culture is positive in 86% of IE caused by organisms other than streptococci, and one of the first three blood cultures is virtually always positive. Ideally three samples of blood (both aerobic and anaerobic) should be obtained in the first 24 hours. Common laboratory practice, which calls for two sets to be obtained at one time or even 30 minutes apart, does not distinguish transient bacteremia from persistent bacteremia because many organisms that cause IE can be inhibited by relatively trivial therapy.

The patient who has had antibiotics should have repeated cultures 2 to 10 days after antimicrobial therapy ends. This may be accomplished efficiently in the outpatient setting. In the managed care era the luxury of admitting a patient to the hospital and waiting for positive blood cultures may no longer be affordable.

Obtain at least 10 ml of blood for each blood culture. Special culture techniques may help with IE that is initially culture negative (e.g., addition of 0.05% to 0.1% L-cysteine or 0.001% pyridoxal phosphate to grow nutritionally deficient streptococci). Antimicrobial-removing resins generally do not improve the yield of true-positive blood cultures; in fact, the incidence of false-positive blood cultures rises.

Cultures of the bone marrow may help in mycobacterial infections, deep fungal infections, brucellosis, and typhoid fever. Antibody studies are necessary to diagnose Q fever *(Coxiella burnetii)* and psittacosis *(Chlamydia psittaci)*. Antibodies to *Brucella*, *Legionella*, and *Rochalimaea* spp. may be the only clues to IE caused by these organisms. Similarly, in cases of suspected culture-negative endocarditis, a second look at the fungi may be valuable. Tests to detect fungal, mycobacterial, and bacterial antigens are generally disappointing. Teichoic acid antibodies can be helpful; in titers greater than 1:4 they indicate disseminated staphylococcal disease.

Anemia is present in most cases, generally normochromic and normocytic and worse with time. Thrombocytopenia is infrequent. The white blood count is elevated occasionally in chronic cases and very commonly in acute endocarditis. About 25% of patients have large mononuclear cells; they correspond to the chronicity of the illness, but also may appear in tuberculosis, typhus, typhoid fever, and malaria.

Serologic studies are more commonly positive with chronic IE. Rheumatoid factor is found in nearly half of patients. Reduced levels of serum complement should be sought in patients with abnormal renal function to help determine the role of IE. Petersdorf found a mean Westergren sedimentation rate of 57 mm/hr.[2] The absence of an elevated sedimentation rate, however, does not exclude endocarditis. False-positive results of Venereal Disease Research Laboratory (VDRL) and Lyme antibody tests have been reported in fewer than 1% of cases. Circulating immune complexes may be measured by various techniques, but these measurements are not specific unless levels greater than 100 µg of aggregated gamma globulin equivalent per milliliter are found. Mixed cryoglobulins may be seen, and hypergammaglobulinemia occurs in about 20%.

Echocardiogram

Sonographic technology has greatly enhanced the definition of IE and is a standard component of the workup (see Chapter 8). A mass, or at least a dense cluster, of irregular echoes is found on the surface of one or more valve leaflets. Insufficiency of valves and perivalvular abscesses may be detected. In recent years transesophageal echocardiography (TEE) has enabled the detection of small vegetations. It is especially helpful in defining abscesses around sewing rings of prosthetic valves. However, even TEE is subject to false-positive and false-negative readings and must always

be interpreted in conjunction with clinical and laboratory information.

Valvular vegetations may persist for 2 or more years after infection has been eradicated. Thus a vegetation does not prove active infection. It is possible that a patient with a vegetation and no clinical evidence for IE had a prior infection that was successfully treated with antibiotics given for another illness.

A major difference between the Duke criteria and the von Reyn criteria for the definition of IE is Duke's use of echocardiography.[2,3] The Duke echocardiographic criteria include one of the following:

1. Oscillating intracardiac mass, on the valve or supporting structures, in the path of regurgitant jet, or on implanted material in the absence of an alternative anatomic explanation
2. Abscess
3. New partial dehiscence of a prosthetic valve

Unfortunately, small growths, irregularities, or thick valve surfaces are often seen and may be difficult to resolve, even with TEE. In such cases serial examinations may be helpful.

Other Imaging Studies

Gallium scans, indium scans, computed tomography (CT), and magnetic resonance imaging (MRI) seldom help. Cardiac catheterization simply to diagnose IE is not indicated. It has been suggested that collection of blood cultures from various cardiac locations would help pinpoint the site of infection, but this has limited clinical utility. Invasive techniques may be dangerous; angiography has caused acute decompensation in patients with aortic insufficiency caused by endocarditis.

Electrocardiogram and Chest X-ray

The ECG may be important, because a conduction defect develops in some patients. Likewise, the chest x-ray may show changes in cardiac size that can indicate congestive heart failure (CHF) and pericardial effusions. There may be pulmonary infiltrates and cavitary lesions consistent with IE. These are especially common in patients with right-sided endocarditis related to IV drug use and other vascular manipulations.

CAUSES

The most common causes of IE are listed in Table 21-2, but almost every bacterium, mycobacterium, and fungus has been reported to cause it. Often organisms thought to be contaminants or nonpathogens first enter the medical literature described in isolated case reports of IE. In time the organism may be found in other areas. For example, *Moraxella nonliquefaciens*, first identified as a cause of IE, has been found to cause septic arthritis and other invasive disease.[14]

Table 21-2	Causes of Endocarditis

Organism	Incidence* 1981	1994	Notes on Therapy†
Viridans streptococci	34%	23%	Highly susceptible to PCN; PCN + gentamicin for 2 weeks followed by PCN alone for 2 more weeks. Shorter course of therapy possible if there is no extracardiac infection.
Enterococcus	6%	7%	Harder to treat than streptococcus. Usually PCN or ampicillin + an aminoglycoside needed. Drug resistance common, and low MICs needed for drug synergy.
Streptococcus bovis	3%	6%	Therapy similar to viridans streptococci
Other streptococci	11%	8%	S. pneumoniae an especially devastating infection, requiring high-dose PCN.
Staphylococcus aureus, coagulase positive	25%	37%	No prosthetic material: start with nafcillin + gentamicin for 5 days, then nafcillin alone for 6 weeks; with PCN allergy, substitute cefazolin. For MRSA give vancomycin alone. Prosthetic material: often MRSA; therapy may be complex; vancomycin (6 weeks) + gentamicin (2 weeks). May need rifampin.
Coagulase-negative staphylococci	3%	7%	Same as for coagulase positive.
HACEK	7%	3%	Ampicillin + gentamicin (4 weeks). Drug resistance now common. Large vegetations and emboli common with Haemophilus. Mortality with actinobacillus IE 30%.
Candida albicans	2%	0	Surgery frequently needed.
Other species	7%	6%	Quinolones may be helpful.
Culture negative	5%	3%	Usually include vancomycin.

*The 1981 study included 104 cases diagnosed with the von Reyn criteria.[2] The 1994 series comprised 204 cases using the Duke criteria.[3]
†The drug choice assumes that the organism is susceptible to the drug(s); substitutions are commonly required for drug resistance or inadequate sensitivity.
PCN, Penicillin; MRSA, methicillin-resistant Staphylococcus aureus; MIC, minimal inhibitory concentration. HACEK, Haemophilus, Actinobacillus, Cardiobacterium, Eikenella, and Kingella.

Occasionally organisms are recognized for their unusual associations with other conditions. For example, more than half the patients with *Streptococcus bovis* endocarditis have serious lesions of the colon, including malignancies. Equally important, although not always indicative of IE, are bacteremias caused by *Clostridium septicum*, *Listeria monocytogenes*, group B beta-hemolytic streptococci, and *Capnocytophaga canimorsus* (formerly known as DF2), which may herald underlying malignancy.

Since the days of Osler, the incidence of viridans streptococcal endocarditis has diminished from virtually 100% of the cases to only 23% of the Duke cases[3] (Table 21-2). The change in etiology underscores the importance of applying stricter case definitions to IE. Because most organisms can cause IE, the diagnosis must be considered in all patients with positive blood cultures.

The enterococci deserve special attention. Formerly thought to represent transient bacteremia in most cases, they are now known to rival *S. aureus* in frequency as causes of IE. About one third of community-acquired enterococcal bacteremias represent endocarditis.[15] In addition to undergoing a full gastrointestinal evaluation, patients should have an echocardiogram, and strong consideration should be given to treatment for 2 to 6 weeks.

The HACEK group *(Haemophilus, Actinobacillus, Cardiobacterium, Eikenella, and Kingella)* and *Haemophilus* spp. including *H. aphrophilus, H. parainfluenzae,* and *H. paraphrophilus* can cause large vegetations and emboli.

Even though bacteremia is common, gram-negative aerobes are unusual causes of endocarditis because they are less adherent to roughened valve surfaces. When IE does occur there usually is an underlying disease such as cirrhosis, a prosthetic heart valve, or a history of narcotic use. Mortality is high, and bacteremia may persist despite apparently adequate therapy. The leading causes are *Salmonella* species, *E. coli, Serratia marcescens, Klebsiella* species, and *P. aeruginosa.*

Gram positive rods are increasingly recognized. In the past such organisms as *Corynebacterium* sp. have been dismissed as simple diphtheroids. However, not only Corynebacteria, but also *Listeria, Actinomyces, Oerskovia, Rhodococcus, Rothia, Erysipelothrix,* and a host of others can cause IE.

Anaerobes are unusual as the sole cause of IE. When anaerobic endocarditis is found a gastrointestinal or oral source should be sought. *Fusobacterium* is one of the leading anaerobic causes of IE.[16] Medical treatment alone may suffice.

The case of Q fever endocarditis is almost unique in medicine. Diagnosis is generally made serologically. Occupational exposure such as abattoir, shepherding, or laboratory work is common. Culture techniques are very difficult. Histologic evaluation of the valve aids the diagnosis, as does the presence of any antibody to the phase I antigen or a fourfold rise in titer to the phase II antigen. Therapy for several *years* is necessary.

Slowly and rapidly growing mycobacteria can cause IE, but the clinical importance of IE is overshadowed by the prolonged therapeutic courses for all mycobacterial infections. When therapy lasting 4 to 12 months is already required, the therapeutic implications of a 6-week course for IE are lessened.

Fungal infections caused by *Candida* sp. are increasingly common. Endophthalmitis and major emboli may occur. Cultures may be negative with conventional media or may require prolonged incubation to grow. The only manifestation may be elevated liver enzyme levels, which serve as a clue to presence of hepatosplenic candidiasis. Subtle presentations tend to be common. We treated a former drug addict who initially had weight loss, back pain, and low-grade fever. The presumptive diagnosis of Hodgkin's disease could not be confirmed. Aspirate of a lumbar disc yielded *Candida parapsilosis.*

Other *Candida* sp. may also cause IE. *Aspergillus* sp. and other fungi (histoplasmosis, blastomycosis, and coccidioidomycosis) are rare causes. As with mycobacteria, the therapeutic implications of fungal infections are minimized because all deep fungal infections require prolonged therapy. Serologic and echocardiographic diagnoses are often more useful than culture techniques, but in recent years radiometric techniques have increased the yield of organisms in blood cultures.[1]

Viruses do not cause endocarditis, although the theoretic possibility may exist, especially with chronic infections such as cytomegalovirus, which can cause a retinitis that mimics the retinitis seen in bacterial endocarditis. Given the high frequency of enteroviruses as causes of pericarditis, it is surprising that they do not cause endocarditis, but to date none have been implicated.

Parasites can cause chronic infections but generally lead to abscesses within organs rather than vegetations on heart valves.

Staphylococcal Bacteremia and the Risk of Endocarditis

Several early reports indicated that IE complicated *S. aureus* bacteremia in half or more of the cases. However, many patients treated briefly for staphylococcal bacteremia do not develop IE. The origin of the staphylococcal infection determines the risk of IE. Patients who have a defined source of infection generally manifest their *S. aureus* bacteremia as a secondary bacteremia and are less likely to develop IE. Those who have a primary bacteremia, with no recognizable source, have a better chance of having endocarditis. An intermediate-risk group includes patients with an infected IV site, a small boil, or a small foreign body that is easily removed, and these patients are defined as "those with a removable focus." Recommendations for treatment of such patients range from 2 weeks of IV therapy to a 4- to 6-week course, but the problem remains difficult to resolve.

Most authorities agree that a patient with nosocomial *S. aureus* bacteremia should be treated with high-dose therapy for at least 2 weeks. We often measure teichoic acid antibodies at that time. If the result is negative and the patient has no sign of deep infection and is doing well clinically, we usually discontinue parenteral therapy but may continue oral antibiotics for another 2 weeks. When in doubt, treat patients parenterally for 4 to 6 weeks simply because the consequences of valvular destruction are so great in comparison with the relative ease of administration of antistaphylococcal therapy.

Culture-Negative Endocarditis

Despite the best attempts at identifying an organism, some patients still have negative blood cultures in the face of a clinical syndrome consistent with endocarditis. One major cause is infection by nutritionally variant *Streptococcus*, which accounts for about 5% of all cases of IE and about 10% of cases of IE by viridans group streptococci. The culture media must be supplemented with pyridoxal phosphate. An alternative technique is streaking the media first with *S. aureus*, then by the sample in question. Nutritionally variant streptococci form satellites around *S. aureus*. The incubation period averaged 17 weeks among a group of patients referred to the Mayo Clinic.[18]

There are multiple causes of culture-negative IE, including the following:

- Right-sided endocarditis
- Cultures taken late in the course of an illness when the intensity of bacteremia is low
- Infection relating to mural thrombus or a ventricular septal defect
- Fastidious organisms
- Recent or current antimicrobial therapy either for other bacterial infections or for misdiagnosed cases of sinusitis or other upper respiratory tract infections (the practice of empiric antimicrobial therapy for flulike illnesses or fevers requires constant reexamination and should be discouraged)
- Fungal endocarditis, or IE caused by *Chlamydiae, Rickettsia,* or *Mycobacteria*
- Misinterpreted blood cultures (*Staphylococcus epidermidis* may be a contaminant or the real pathogen)
- Noninfective endocarditis (Box 21-3)

Before culture-negative IE is diagnosed, most patients have had a bone marrow biopsy, CT, or MRI scans of the abdomen and brain, spinal tap, and consultation with a rheumatologist.

Pseudoendocarditis

Although not traditionally described in journals and textbooks, pseudoendocarditis is most perplexing to the clinician. The myriad causes of false-positive blood cultures add to the complexity of diagnosis. Determining the importance of the blood culture is even more difficult if the blood culture does not come from the patient himself or herself. Such errors as incomplete cleaning of the skin by the phlebotomist, mix-up of samples, misreading of samples by radiometric systems, and use of topical thrombin to speed coagulation of blood[21] can all produce false-positive blood cultures. Interpretation is difficult enough with true-positive blood cultures. Laboratories should constantly strive to increase quality control to prevent false-positive results.

It is important to realize that the echocardiogram, while sensitive, is not that specific. Many conditions other than IE cause thickening of the valve leaflets. Even TEE has false-positive results. If the diagnosis is uncertain, it may help to repeat the echocardiogram several days after the initial study.

BOX 21-3

CAUSES OF NONINFECTIVE ENDOCARDITIS

NEOPLASM
Atrial myxoma
Marantic endocarditis (adenocarcinoma)[19]
Neoplastic disease (lymphoma, rhabdomyosarcoma)
Carcinoid

AUTOIMMUNE DISEASES
Rheumatic heart disease
Systemic lupus erythematosus (Libman-Sacks endocarditis)
Antiphospholipid antibody syndrome
Polyarteritis nodosa
Behcet's disease

POSTVALVULAR OPERATIONS
Thrombus
Sutures
Other postvalvular surgical changes

MISCELLANEOUS
Eosinophilic heart disease
Ruptured mitral chordae tendineae
Myxomatous degeneration
Atrial septal defect
Ventricular septal defect

Data from Berbari EF, Cockerill FR III, Steckelberg JM: *Mayo Clin Proc* 72:532, 1997.

Treatment of Infective Endocarditis

Although patients with bacterial infections need antimicrobial therapy as expeditiously as possible, full analysis of the case at the early stages can save trouble in the end. For example, early antimicrobial treatment for patients who have prosthetic valves may do them a disservice when they do not have a simple strep throat or a bacterial bronchitis, but instead have early IE. We have all seen nonspecific illnesses treated with one, two, or even three antimicrobial courses only to be ultimately diagnosed as IE.

Selection of therapy is difficult in cases of partially treated IE. Similarly, selection of the dose for IE requires a different approach from selection of therapy for mild infections. Therapy now has evolved to a consensus for treatment of the most common forms of IE, published in December 1995 by the American Heart Association (AHA).[22]

Microbiologic information is crucial in the selection of therapy for these patients. Whereas for many infections identification of an organism simply as an alpha streptococcus may enable the clinician to manage the condition, for IE that organism should be identified to the level of species. Moreover, antimicrobial susceptibility testing should determine the minimal inhibitory concentration (MIC) of the antimicrobial agents most likely to be used in the treatment. Simply determining whether the organism is susceptible (S), intermediate (I), or resistant (R) by standard Kirby-Bauer testing is insufficient for these complex infections. Similarly, epidemiologic information may be gleaned from full identification of the species. Extracardiac infections can be linked to the endocarditis. Blood cultures that turn positive after therapy can be identified more precisely. Whether a patient has a relapse (resurgence of the original infection) or a recurrence (a second infection) can guide whether antimicrobial therapy should be strengthened or whether surgery should be added to the therapeutic plan.[23]

Therapy is also dictated by location of the vegetation. Right-sided IE generally responds to antimicrobial therapy alone. Indeed, many patients who receive therapy of IE related to IV drug abuse stop therapy ahead of schedule yet still do well.

Patients with left-sided IE, especially cases caused by *Staphylococcus aureus*, *Streptococcus pyogenes*, and *S. pneumoniae* are more likely to require surgery. The aortic valve is more commonly injured than the mitral valve. Serial ECGs are necessary to detect conduction defects. In the early stages, continuous cardiac monitoring may be warranted.

Choice of Antibiotics and When To Refer

General cardiologists and primary care physicians see too few cases of IE to develop competence with the management of antibiotic therapy. An infectious disease specialist should be consulted during the evaluation and should direct antibiotic therapy. A detailed review of antimicrobial therapy is beyond the scope of this book. Drug regimens for the common infections are summarized in Table 21-2. For a large number of patients adjustment is necessary because of drug resistance or inadequate sensitivity.

Empiric Therapy

Some patients are so seriously ill that immediate therapy is necessary. Empiric selection of antimicrobial agents then is justified. When cultures return to document IE, therapy can be adjusted to suit the organism isolated. Initial empiric antimicrobial therapy could in-

clude vancomycin, gentamicin, and rifampin or a fluoroquinolone. Persons with the acute onset of native valvular IE should be given nafcillin or vancomycin plus an aminoglycoside. Some clinicians prefer ceftriaxone plus gentamicin.

The acute onset of prosthetic valvular IE could be treated with the same drug combination, with additional consideration of early valvular replacement. Subacute onset of IE on a native valve should be treated with ampicillin/sulbactam plus an aminoglycoside. This program would treat the HACEK group, *Enterococcus*, *Streptococcus*, and *Staphylococcus*. An alternative regimen would be vancomycin, ceftriaxone, and an aminoglycoside. For subacute onset of prosthetic valvular IE, a program of vancomycin plus an aminoglycoside and rifampin should be given. For intravenous drug users, nafcillin or vancomycin should be given with an aminoglycoside. Consideration might be given to the addition of an oral quinolone.

Monitoring Therapy

Blood cultures should be obtained within the first week after beginning therapy. Although *S. aureus* infections may produce bacteremia for several days after appropriate therapy begins, the blood is usually sterile by the end of the first week. Blood cultures should be obtained 1 and 4 weeks after therapy ends.

The Westergren sedimentation rate, often elevated in endocarditis, can be a useful guide to the course of therapy. However, neither it, the C-reactive protein, nor the rheumatoid factor may return to normal by the end of therapy, especially if a short course is chosen.

Aminoglycoside and vancomycin levels should be measured weekly during therapy. Mild acute renal insufficiency might be present early in the course. As the renal function improves, excretion of antimicrobial agents also improves, leading to subtherapeutic concentrations. Similarly, renal or drug toxicity may be present as rising drug levels in the later days of therapy as all of the renal excretion sites are saturated.

Weekly blood counts should be obtained because beta-lactam agents, especially oxacillin, can cause anemia, thrombocytopenia, and neutropenia. If oxacillin is used, liver enzyme levels should be measured weekly. The risk of oxacillin-induced hepatitis and neutropenia rises in the later weeks of therapy. Teichoic acid antibodies may be negative initially, but can become positive in the second and third weeks of infection. Such a development provides further justification for continuing a course of antistaphylococcal therapy in a patient with *S. aureus* bacteremia and no identified vegetations or other sources of infection.

Serum bactericidal testing, also known as Schlichter testing, may have methodologic inconsistencies. We measure a peak serum bactericidal level, obtained by collecting a sample of blood 30 to 60 minutes after infusion of the principal agent used to treat the infecting organism. The sample of blood is diluted serially by powers of two to a level of 1:512. The organism causing IE, previously saved by the laboratory for the purpose of testing, is inoculated into the diluted aliquot of serum. The greatest dilution (lowest concentration) of serum that still produces killing of the bacteria is known as the serum bactericidal concentration, level, or titer (SBC, SBL, SBT). Levels of 1:8 or greater usually predict cure. The test must be interpreted with caution because of potential variations. Not all authorities recommend its routine use.[22]

Clinical monitoring must continue to evaluate for fever, dyspnea, neurologic findings, and new skin lesions. Fever may indicate persistent infection, but late in the course it may simply reflect a reaction to therapy.

Surgical Therapy

The classic indications for surgery are persistent bacteremia, heart failure caused by valve dysfunction, and major embolic disease.[24] In recent years we have become persuaded of the value of earlier replacement of infected valves. Our extremely effective methods of treatment can mask advancing cases of congestive heart failure (CHF). If a patient with an apparently stable course requires new or additional diuretics, strong consideration should be given to valve replacement. This is especially true for aortic valvular disease. Mitral valvular infections can lead to the insidious development of myocardial or perivalvular abscess, complete heart block, fistulas, or mycotic aneurysms.

Other indications for surgery include infections caused by organisms known to be difficult to treat, such as fungi, *P. aeruginosa,* and certain unusual organisms for which fever resolves very slowly.

Patients who have prosthetic valvular IE often require surgery. One exception is the patient with a late-onset (more than 60 days after surgery) infection caused by a susceptible agent such as viridans streptococci.[16] Dysfunction of a valve, such as a perivalvular leak, usually requires surgery. It is important to listen carefully for the murmur of aortic regurgitation.

Continuation of or addition to antimicrobial therapy in the face of standard indications for surgery is generally a mistake. Patients who have indications for surgery fare as well or better when sent for surgery early. Delay of surgery portends a worse prognosis if the infection has been poorly controlled. The organism has a greater opportunity to burrow into the myocardium, cause abscesses, and generate more emboli. Even though the new valve is placed into an area that may not be completely sterile, rarely does it become infected by the original organism.

The replacement valve may not sit as securely into the valve ring because it has been sewn into weakened tissue. If the resulting valvular insufficiency is hemodynamically significant, the patient may require a second replacement, postponed, if possible, until the antimicrobial course is complete. Persistent valve dysfunction complicates about 15% of operations for active IE.

Some features of late prosthetic valve IE may warrant surgery. They include infection by a nonstreptococcal pathogen, development of a regurgitant murmur, fever lasting more than 10 days during therapy, and development of moderate to severe CHF.

Postoperative antimicrobial therapy may depend on the findings at surgery. Patients who undergo surgery early in the course of their planned antimicrobial therapy should finish the full 4 to 6 weeks of therapy postoperatively. Patients who completed therapy before surgery may be treated with only standard valve replacement prophylaxis. If surgery is performed in the final 2 weeks of a planned course of therapy, then another 2 weeks should be prescribed postoperatively. If inflammation is noted at the time of surgery, however, 4 extra weeks of therapy should be given. Patients with fungal endocarditis are treated with amphotericin. Rather than days of therapy, the total dose is the goal (1 to 3 g after surgery). After surgery for fungal endocarditis, long-term follow-up with blood culture is recommended (2, 6, and 12 months after therapy ends).[20]

PREVENTION OF ENDOCARDITIS

Despite our best efforts, IE cannot always be prevented. Furthermore, no randomized clinical trial has proved a benefit of antimicrobial prophylaxis (nor should there be one). Most cases of IE arise with no possible correlation to a procedure. Nevertheless, we know that certain localized infections and certain procedures lead to bacteremia, and patients with structural cardiac defects are at risk. If a simple measure can be offered with just the possibility of prevention, it should be considered. With that rationale, the American Heart Association and the American Dental Association have for several decades cooperated in their attempts to provide an efficient program of prevention.[25]

Risk Stratification (Box 21-4)

Patients at high risk of IE should always be considered for prophylaxis when invasive procedures are performed (Box 21-4). Moreover, they should be treated more aggressively than the general population when they have simple bacterial infections. Persons at high and moderate risk are treated similarly.

Patients with mitral valve prolapse but no murmur rarely develop IE. Those with murmurs or Doppler evidence of insufficiency should receive prophylaxis. When myxomatous valvular degeneration causes regurgitation, prophylaxis is indicated for invasive procedures. Men older than 45 years of age with mitral valve prolapse—even without a consistent systolic murmur—warrant prophylaxis. Children with mitral valve prolapse also may be at higher risk of IE. Patients with negligible risk do not require prophylaxis for IE per se but continue to require prophylaxis for other indications, such as prevention of local infection in contaminated surgery.

Procedures Causing Bacteremia *(Box 21-5)*
These procedures include such simple activities such as tooth brushing or chewing. Therefore not every episode of bacteremia can be treated. Prophylaxis is not necessary for routine cardiac catheterization and angioplasty. Currently, no data exist about placement of vascular prostheses and the risk of infection during the procedure itself. However, the vast experience of placement of intracoronary stents and the extreme rarity of subsequent infection suggests that prophylaxis is not necessary. Procedures that cause bacteremia for a discrete period warrant prophylaxis for the high- and moderate-risk groups (Box 21-5). Many common low-risk procedures do not warrant prophylaxis.

Antibiotic Recommendations *(Table 21-3)*
Prophylactic regimens are designed for the area of the body under treatment and have been simplified since the previous recommendations in 1990. For example, a single dose of 2 g of amoxicillin is given before most procedures. It is followed by 1.5 g orally afterward. Azithromycin, clarithromycin, clindamycin, and cephalexin are recommended instead of erythromycin, which causes dyspepsia.

Most dentists are aware of the requirements for antibiotic prophylaxis and prescribe the appropriate antibiotic when informed by the patient about the need for prophylaxis. Perhaps your most important job is to be sure that your high-risk patient understands his or her condition and the need for prophylaxis.

REFERENCES
1. Osler W: Chronic infectious endocarditis, *Q J Med* 2:219, 1908-09.
2. von Reyn CF, Levy BS, Arbeit RO, et al. Infective endocarditis, *Ann Intern Med* 94:505, 1981.
3. Durack DT, Lukes AS, Bright DK, and the Duke Endocarditis Service: New criteria for the diagnosis of infective endocarditis, *Am J Med* 96:200, 1994.
4. von Reyn CF, Levy BS, Arbeit RD, et al: Infective endocarditis: an analysis based on strict case definitions, *Ann Intern Med* 94:505, 1982.
5. Kaye D: Definitions and demographic characteristics. In Kaye D, editor: *Infective endocarditis*, Baltimore, 1976, University Park Press.
6. Lepeschkin E: On the relation between the site of valvular involvement in endocarditis and the blood pressure resting on the valve, *Am J Med Sci* 224:318,1952.
7. Everett ED, Hirschmann JV: Transient bacteremia and endocarditis prophylaxis: a review, *Medicine* 56:61,1977.
8. Parker MT, Ball LC: Streptococci and aerococci associated with systemic infection in man, *J Med Microbiol* 9:275,1976.
9. Kaell AT, Volkman DJ, Gorevic PD, Dattwyler RJ: Positive Lyme serology in subacute bacterial endocarditis: a study of four patients, *JAMA* 264:2916, 1990.

BOX 21-5
MEDICAL-SURGICAL PROCEDURES AND ENDOCARDITIS PROPHYLAXIS

HIGH-RISK PROCEDURES: ANTIBIOTIC PROPHYLAXIS RECOMMENDED

Dental

Extraction

Periodontal procedures (surgery, scaling, root planning, probing, and recall maintenance)

Dental implant placement

Reimplantation of avulsed teeth

Endodontic (root canal) instrumentation or surgery beyond the apex

Subgingival placement of antibiotic fibers or strips

Initial placement of orthodontic bands, but not brackets

Intraligamentary local anesthetic injections

Prophylactic cleaning of teeth or implants when bleeding is anticipated

Respiratory Tract

Tonsillectomy

Adenoidectomy

Surgical operations on respiratory mucosa

Rigid bronchoscopy

Gastrointestinal Tract

Esophageal variceal sclerotherapy

Esophageal stricture dilation

Endoscopic retrograde cholangiography with biliary obstruction

Biliary tract surgery

Surgical operations through intestinal mucosa

Genitourinary Tract

Prostatic surgery

Cystoscopy

Urethral dilation

LOW-RISK PROCEDURES: ENDOCARDITIS PROPHYLAXIS *NOT* RECOMMENDED

Dental

Restorative dentistry (filling cavities, replacement of missing teeth with or without retraction cord)*

Local anesthetic injection (nonintraligamentary)

Intracanal endodontic treatment; after placement and buildup

Placement of rubber bands

Postoperative suture removal

Placement of removable prosthodontic or orthodontic appliances

Taking of dental impressions

Fluoride treatments

Taking of oral radiographs

Orthodontic appliance adjustment

Shedding of primary teeth

Respiratory Tract

Endotracheal intubation

Flexible bronchoscopy with or without biopsy*

Tympanostomy tube insertion

Gastrointestinal Tract

Transesophageal echocardiography*

Endoscopy with or without biopsy*

Genitourinary Tract

Vaginal hysterectomy*

Vaginal delivery*

Cesarean section

In uninfected tissue:

    Urethral catheterization

    Uterine dilation and curettage

    Therapeutic abortion

    Sterilization procedures

    Insertion or removal of intrauterine devices

Other

Cardiac catheterization including balloon angioplasty

Implanted cardiac pacemakers, implanted defibrillators and coronary stents

Incisional biopsy of surgically scrubbed skin

Circumcision

*Prophylaxis is optional for high-risk patients.

Table 21-3	*Prophylactic Regimens for Endocarditis*

Situation	Agent	Regimen
DENTAL, ORAL, RESPIRATORY TRACT, OR ESOPHAGEAL PROCEDURES		
Standard general phylaxis	Amoxicillin	Adults: 2 g (children: 50 mg/kg) po 1 hour before the procedure
Nothing allowed orally (NPO)	Ampicillin	Adults: 2 g IM or IV (children: 50 mg/kg IM or IV) within 30 minutes before the procedure
Allergy to penicillin	Clindamycin	Adults: 600 mg (children: 20 mg/kg) po 1 hour before the procedure
	Cephalexin or cefadroxil	Adults: 2 g (children: 50 mg/kg) po 1 hour before the procedure
	Azithromycin or clarithromycin	Adults: 500 mg/kg (children: 5 mg/kg) po 1 hour before the procedure
Allergy to penicillin or NPO	Clindamycin	Adults: 600 mg (children: 20 mg/kg) IV within 30 minutes before the procedure
	Cefazolin	Adults: 1 g (children: 25 mg/kg) IM or IV within 30 minutes before the procedure
GENITOURINARY OR GASTROINTESTINAL (EXCLUDING ESOPHAGEAL) PROCEDURES		
High-risk patients	Ampicillin plus gentamicin	Adults: ampicillin 2 g IM/IV plus gentamicin 1.5 mg/kg (maximum 120 mg) within 30 minutes of starting the procedure; 6 hours later ampicillin 1 g IM/IV or amoxicillin 1 g po Children: ampicillin 50 mg/kg IM/IV (not to exceed 2 g) plus gentamicin 1.5 mg/kg within 30 minutes of a procedure; 6 hours later ampicillin 25 mg/kg IM/IV or amoxicillin 25 mg/kg po
High-risk patients allergic to ampicillin	Vancomycin plus gentamicin	Adults: vancomycin 1 gram IV over 1 to 2 hours plus gentamicin 1.5 mg/kg IM/IV not to exceed 120 mg; infusion should end within 30 minutes of starting the procedure Children: vancomycin 20 mg/kg IV over 1 to 2 hours plus gentamicin 1.5 mg/kg IM/IV; infusions must end within 30 minutes of starting the procedure
Moderate risk patients	Amoxicillin or ampicillin	Adults: amoxicillin 2 g po 1 hour before the procedure or ampicillin 2 g IM/IV within 30 minutes of starting the procedure Children: amoxicillin 50 mg/kg 1 hour before the procedure or ampicillin 50 mg/kg IM/IV within 30 minutes of starting the procedure
Moderate-risk patients allergic to ampicillin	Vancomycin	Adults: vancomycin 1 gr IV over 1 to 2 hours to complete infusion within 30 minutes of starting the procedure Children: vancomycin 20 mg/kg over 1 to 2 hours to complete infusion within 30 minutes of starting the procedure

10. Werner AS, Cobbs CG, Kaye D, Hooke EW: Studies on the bacteremia of bacterial endocarditis, *JAMA* 202:199, 1967.

11. Pazin GJ, Saul S, Thompson ME: Blood culture positivity: suppression by outpatient antibiotic therapy in patients with bacterial endocarditis, *Arch Intern Med* 142:263, 1982.

12. Pelletier LL Jr, Petersdorf RG: Infective endocarditis: a review of 125 cases from the University of Washington Hospitals, 1963-72, *Medicine* 56:287, 1977.

13. Sullivan D, Coleman D: *Candida dubliniensis:* characteristics and identification, *J Clin Microbiol* 36:329, 1998.

14. Graham DR, Band JD, Thornsberry C, et al: Infections caused by *Moraxella, Moraxella urethralis, Moraxella*-like groups M-5 and M-6 in the United States, 1953-1980, *Rev Infect Dis* 12:423, 1990.

15. Maki DG, Agger WA: Enterococcal bacteremia: clinical features, the risk of endocarditis, and management, *Medicine* 64:248, 1988.

16. Graham DR, Rodriguez-Larrain J, Woodruff RC III: *Fusobacterium* valve endocarditis 24 years after placement of a Starr-Edwards valve: successful treatment with penicillin, *J Long Term Effects Med Implants* 3:203, 1993.

17. Graham DR, Drake C, Barenfanger JE: Recovery of *Histoplasma* from BACTEC TB media, *J Clin Microbiol* 34:208, 1996.

18. Steckelberg JM, Melton LJ III, Ilstrup DM, et al: Influence of referral on the apparent clinical spectrum of infective endocarditis, *Am J Med* 88:582, 1990.

19. Cohen B, Taylor GJ, Graham DR, Myers RE: Unsuspected aortic valve vegetation in a patient with a heart murmur, *Ill Med J* 164:92, 1984.

20. Berbari EF, Cockerill FR III, Steckelberg JM: Infective endocarditis due to unusual or fastidious microorganisms, *Mayo Clin Proc* 72:532, 1997.

21. Graham DR, Wu E, Highsmith AK, Ginsburg ML: An outbreak of pseudobacteremia caused by *Enterobacter cloacae* from a phlebotomist's vial of thrombin, *Ann Intern Med* 95:585, 1981.

22. Wilson WR, Karchmer AW, Dajani AS, et al: Antibiotic treatment of adults with infective endocarditis due to streptococci, enterococci, staphylococci, and HACEK microorganisms, *JAMA* 274:1706, 1995.

23. Noreuil TO, Katholi RE, Graham DR: Recurrent bacterial endocarditis in a man with tetralogy of Fallot: earliest recurrence on record, *South Med J* 83:455, 1990.

24. Karchmer AW, Stinson EB: The role of surgery in infective endocarditis, *Infect Dis Clin North Am* 7:124, 1993.

25. Dajani AS, Taubert KA, Wilson W, et al: Prevention of bacterial endocarditis: recommendations by the American Heart Association, *JAMA* 277:1794, 1997.

22

Congestive Heart Failure: Systolic Dysfunction

Adrian B. Van Bakel
Reneé P. Meyer

The definition of congestive heart failure (CHF) is simple: a clinical syndrome resulting from the inability of the heart to pump a sufficient amount of blood to meet the metabolic demands of the body. Although the causes of CHF are many and the pathophysiology complex, left heart failure syndrome is usually characterized by exercise intolerance because of dyspnea. As the syndrome progresses, other symptoms of congestion such as orthopnea, paroxysmal nocturnal dyspnea, and peripheral edema occur. This disease carries a decreased life expectancy and, as with many other chronically debilitating diseases, accounts for an ever-increasing share of health care resources. This chapter discusses CHF primarily caused by systolic dysfunction. Other pathophysiologic mechanisms leading to the same clinical syndrome are discussed in Chapters 23 and 24.

EPIDEMIOLOGY, ETIOLOGY, AND NATURAL HISTORY

CHF is a disease that affects an aging population. Significant strides have decreased morbidity and mortality in the treatment of coronary artery disease and primary valvular disease. However, these improvements have left an older population with previous cardiac injury at risk for developing CHF. Between 2.3 and 3 million patients have been diagnosed with heart failure in the United States alone, with approximately 400,000 new cases diagnosed annually. The incidence of CHF more than doubles with each decade over age 45.[1] Including all patients with a diagnosis of CHF, the 1-year mortality is approximately 10% and the 10-year mortality approaches 50%. In its more advanced forms, even with current medical therapy, the 1-year mortality approaches 20%.[2]

The disease primarily responsible for the development of CHF caused by systolic dysfunction is coronary artery disease. The second most prevalent disease causing significant CHF is idiopathic dilated cardiomyopathy. Many of these cases may in fact be viral cardiomyopathies, but this remains unproven. Primary valvular disease and hypertension, once significant causes of CHF, have declined as a result of timely valve repair or replacement and aggressive treatment of asymptomatic hypertension. Incessant tachycardia is now a well-recognized, although infrequent, cause of cardiomyopathy and CHF, as are peripartum cardiomyopathy and various congenital cardiac defects. A myriad of other diseases also can cause systolic dysfunction and CHF, and these are reviewed in Chapter 24 and Box 22-1.

The natural history of CHF is somewhat difficult to define. Most papers published on the natural history of this disease have two weaknesses. First, many contain a referral bias, having been published by academic centers that were referral centers for patients with severe, advanced disease. Second, much of the information in the literature concerning mortality in CHF is derived from populations in the period before the use of angiotensin-converting enzyme (ACE) inhibitors. Nonetheless, some conclusions may be drawn.[3] The Framingham Study, conducted between 1949 and 1971, included all patients with the diagnosis of CHF and showed a 40% 3-year mortality. Patients followed by the Mayo Clinic from 1960 through 1978 had a similar mortality. In contrast, a trial conducted at the University of Minnesota between 1979 and 1984 found an approximately 75% 3-year mortality with severe CHF.[3]

These rather dismal survival statistics may be somewhat misleading because of referral bias. In a study subsequently published by the Mayo Clinic, patients referred with an initial diagnosis of idiopathic dilated cardiomyopathy had a 40% 4-year survival compared with a population-based group showing a 75% survival at 5 years.[4]

The natural history of CHF in the era of ACE inhibitors is even more difficult to define. Data derived from the many ACE inhibitor trials published since the mid-1980s are difficult to compare because of different inclusion and exclusion criteria as well as length of follow-up. A general sense of the natural history of CHF in the ACE inhibitor era can, however, be discerned from survival rates between placebo and treated groups. Table 22-1 summarizes the results of some of the more important early survival trials.

In the largest single center retrospective analysis to date, a total of 737 patients referred to the University of

BOX 22-1
ETIOLOGY OF CONGESTIVE HEART FAILURE (SYSTOLIC DYSFUNCTION)

CORONARY ARTERY DISEASE

IDIOPATHIC DILATED CARDIOMYOPATHY

VIRAL MYOCARDITIS

Coxsackie A and B	Arbovirus
Echovirus	Cytomegalovirus
Influenza A and B	Mumps
Polio virus	

OTHER BACTERIAL AND FUNGAL INFECTIONS

ACUTE RHEUMATIC FEVER

TOXINS

Alcohol	Ethylene glycol	Adriamycin
Cocaine	Cobalt	Cyclophosphamides
Heroin	Arsenic	Sulfonamides
Amphetamines	Lead	

NUTRITIONAL DEFICIENCIES

Protein	Selenium
Thiamine	L-carnitine

ELECTROLYTE DISORDERS

Hyponatremia	Hypocalcemia
Hypokalemia	Hypophosphatemia

COLLAGEN VASCULAR DISEASES

Systemic lupus erythematosus	Systemic sclerosis
Hypersensitivity vasculitis	Rheumatoid arthritis
Reiter's syndrome	Takayasu's syndrome
Periarteritis nodosa	

ENDOCRINE DISORDERS

Diabetes mellitus	Hypoparathyroidism
Hyperthyroidism	Hypothyroidism
Pheochromocytoma	

TACHYCARDIA-INDUCED CARDIOMYOPATHY

Atrial fibrillation
Incessant supraventricular tachycardia, ventricular tachycardia

MISCELLANEOUS

Peripartum cardiomyopathy	Sleep apnea
Hypereosinophilic syndrome	Sarcoidosis
Giant cell myocarditis	Hemochromatosis
Amyloidosis	

| Table 22-1 | *CHF Survival Trials* | | | | | | |

Trial	Patients	Inclusion Criteria	Therapy	Mean Follow-up(mo)	Treatment Mortality (%)	Placebo Mortality (%)
V-HeFT-I[5]	642	NYHA II-III EF <45% CTR >0.55	Hydralazine/ isosorbide vs prazosin vs placebo	0	325 (hydralazine/ isosorbide)	34
CONSENSUS[6]	253	NYHA IV	Enalapril vs placebo	6	25	44
V-HeFT-II[7]	804	NYHA II-III	Hydralazine/isosorbide vs enalapril	24	18 enalapril, 25 hydralazine/ isosorbide	NA
SOLVED[8]	2561	NYHA II-III EF <35%	Enalapril vs placebo	42	35.2	39.7

California at Los Angeles (UCLA) for transplant evaluation were followed longitudinally with total mortality broken down by era.[2] The 3-year mortality in this group of patients between 1986 and 1988 and between 1989 and 1990 was approximately 30%. The 3-year mortality in the years between 1991 and 1993 was approximately 16%. A dramatic decrease in total mortality was paralleled by a decrease in sudden death. The authors attributed this improvement to a combination of factors, including significantly increased use of ACE inhibitors and amiodarone, and a decreased use of type I antiarrhythmic agents.

Distilled results from these trials and the UCLA experience suggest that, in the ACE inhibitor era, more mild (New York Heart Association Functional Classes II and III) CHF continues to carry a 4-year mortality approaching 30%, with severe CHF continuing to have a significant mortality at 1 year.

PATHOPHYSIOLOGY

Our understanding of the pathophysiology of the CHF syndrome has improved dramatically over the past decade. Patients with similar systolic ejection performance may not have similar symptoms. There is a complex interplay of decreased mechanical performance with two (or perhaps more) interrelated compensatory neurohormonal/autocrine-paracrine systems that determines the severity of symptoms.

The adrenergic nervous system and the renin-angiotensin-aldosterone system are the two compensatory mechanisms that have been most thoroughly explored. These two systems are known to cross-regulate each other, with activation of one leading to activation of the other. Activation of the sympathetic nervous system leads to increased heart rate and contractility through beta-adrenergic receptors. Decreased renal blood flow leads to activation of the renin-angiotensin-aldosterone system. Angiotensin II is a major stimulator of aldosterone secretion, causing salt and water retention. Preload therefore increases, and cardiac output increases through the Frank-Starling mechanism (see Chapter 2). Beta-adrenergic and angiotensin II receptor mechanisms in the neurohypophysis cause the release of arginine vasopressin. Both norepinephrine and angiotensin II are powerful mediators of cardiac myocellular hypertrophy. Activation of both the adrenergic and renin-angiotensin-aldosterone systems cause vasoconstriction, which is beneficial in the short term but, in the long term, increases peripheral resistance and left ventricular wall stress, further reducing systolic performance.

The eccentric hypertrophy that occurs as a result of co-stimulation by both of these neuroendocrine systems eventually leads to ventricular remodeling, increasing the spherocity of the ventricle and further decreasing ejection performance. Changes already outlined that occur in both the myocardial cell and the ventricular chamber increase the metabolic demands of the cardiac myocyte when, due to increased diffusion distance, oxygen delivery to myocardial cells is limited. Direct myocellular toxicity appears to be mediated by beta-adrenergic mechanisms, leading to myocardial cell death and eventual fibrosis. The final pathway of contractility is calcium influx into the cell, which activates the contractile proteins. With increased beta-adrenergic tone, calcium overload occurs at the level of the contractile proteins. Additionally, myocytes may be lost as a result of apoptosis, or programmed cell death. This probably occurs as a result of prolonged growth stimulation by various cytokines.

The role of cytokines and other autocrine-paracrine mechanisms, including tumor necrosis factor (TNF) alpha, TGF-beta, endothelin, and cardiotrophin, is in the early stages of investigation. A simplified diagram of the better-studied neurohormonal pathways in CHF is depicted in Figure 22-1. The elucidation of these pathways has provided specific target areas for the development of medical therapy for CHF. Eichhorn and Bristow[9] have authored a concise review of the foregoing pathophysiology.

CLINICAL PRESENTATION

The clinical syndrome of CHF is characterized by symptoms that may be attributed to either inadequate arterial perfusion of various organs (brain, kidney, skeletal muscle), leading to what has been called "forward failure," and venous congestion of other organs such as lungs, liver, bowel, and lower extremities, or so-called "backward failure." The classically described symptoms of CHF include fatigue and dyspnea on exertion, which lead to progressively impaired exercise tolerance. Both of these manifestations of heart failure are caused by poor arterial perfusion of various organs. Pulmonary congestion from chronically elevated left atrial pres-

sures often worsens during exercise as well. Congestive symptoms may lead to any or all of the following: orthopnea, paroxysmal nocturnal dyspnea, abdominal fullness, pain and bloating, generally due to congestive hepatomegaly, nausea, vomiting, and diarrhea resulting from chronic bowel edema (with concomitant poor absorption of oral medications), and peripheral edema, which is generally dependent edema of the lower extremities but may worsen to the point of anasarca. Protein-losing enteropathy, which can result from chronic severe CHF, may also contribute to generalized peripheral edema. CHF is often the consequence of another cardiac disease. It might be diagnosed easily when the patient has an antecedent cardiac history. In younger people and in those without a previous cardiac history, CHF is often misdiagnosed. Common misdiagnoses include bronchitis, pneumonia, asthma or chronic obstructive pulmonary disease, cirrhosis with ascites, and chronic venous insufficiency. You can minimize delay in diagnosing CHF by maintaining a high index of suspicion, particularly if initial symptoms are slow to resolve. You suspect CHF as a possible etiology

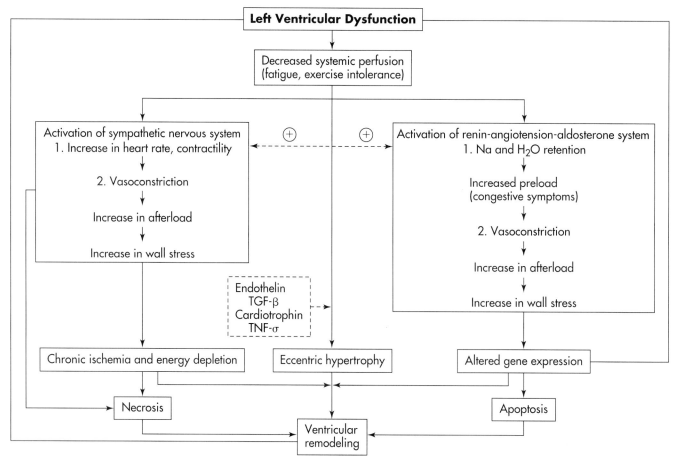

FIG. 22-1
The pathophysiology of congestive heart failure.

if (1) upper respiratory symptoms persist for more than 2 weeks on initial empiric therapy, (2) spirometry is unexpectedly better than suspected given the patient's symptoms, (3) ascites is present with an enlarged liver instead of the small, fibrotic liver expected with cirrhosis, (4) peripheral edema is noted in a younger patient, and (5) there is acute or subacute onset of peripheral edema in an older patient.

Physical examination findings in a patient with new-onset CHF may be subtle or dramatic. In a patient with severely decompensated CHF, there may be all of the signs listed in Box 22-2. With reasonably compensated CHF, many of these may be absent.

As with any disease process, a comprehensive history and physical examination are the essential first requirements in making a diagnosis and establishing a possible cause. The symptoms of CHF should be treated regardless of cause. However, certain diseases resulting in CHF

BOX 22-2

PHYSICAL FINDINGS WITH CONGESTIVE HEART FAILURE AND SYSTOLIC DYSFUNCTION

VITAL SIGNS
Resting tachycardia
Increased respiratory rate
Cheyne-Stokes respiration
Low pulse volume

NECK EXAMINATION
Elevated jugular venous pressure

PULMONARY SIGNS
Decreased breath sounds (pleural effusion)
Rales

CARDIAC SIGNS
Increased heart rate
S_3 gallop
Murmurs of mitral or tricuspid insufficiency
    with marked ventricular dilation

ABDOMINAL EXAMINATION
Hepatomegaly
Hepatojugular reflux
Diffuse abdominal tenderness
Ascites with associated right ventricular failure

EXTREMITIES
Peripheral edema

---

have specific treatment, and a rational search for etiologic factors in appropriate patients is necessary.

DIAGNOSTIC STUDIES
Routine

In addition to the comprehensive history and physical examination, all patients suspected of having CHF should routinely have the following studies: complete blood count (CBC) and urinalysis, serum chemistries including electrolytes, renal function tests, liver function tests, albumin and thyroid function studies (if more than 65 years old or in atrial fibrillation), chest x-ray, electrocardiogram (ECG), and echocardiogram with Doppler flow studies. These tests are used to do the following: (1) confirm the diagnosis of CHF, (2) search for any contributing causes of heart failure symptoms, and (3) attempt to elucidate a specific cause of CHF (Table 22-2).

Ancillary

Laboratory studies obtained under the category of ancillary diagnostic studies are generally tailored to investigate possible causes of CHF. These studies should be chosen when evidence in the history and physical examination makes one suspicious of a specific cause. Other tests include radionuclide ventriculography, stress perfusion testing, coronary angiography, hemodynamic monitoring, endomyocardial biopsy, cardiopulmonary stress testing, signal-averaged ECG, Holter monitor, and electrophysiologic study. Indications for these ancillary studies are listed in Table 22-3.

MANAGEMENT
Nonpharmacologic Therapy

All patients with moderate to severe CHF should restrict their dietary sodium intake. Generally, a 3 g sodium diet is palatable and can be made more so by using salt substitutes. Some patients find that hot pepper sauces help. Occasionally, it is necessary to restrict dietary sodium to 2 g or less, but the palatability of such a diet makes it difficult to maintain for most patients. Dietary counseling has now become an integral part of the treatment of any patient with CHF, and dietary compliance cannot be overemphasized.

Patients should be instructed to restrict their fluid intake as well. Those with mild congestive symptoms may be instructed to drink when thirsty, but no more. Those with more advanced disease should restrict their fluid intake to approximately 1500 to 2000 ml/day. Significant hyponatremia (serum sodium level ≤130) may require fluid restriction to 1 L/day or less.

Patients should be asked to maintain aerobic activity despite even severe symptoms of CHF. This has been

Table 22-2	*Routine Diagnostic Studies Useful in the Initial Evaluation of Patients with Suspected CHF*

Diagnostic Study	Clinical Issue(s)
CBC with differential	Anemia (may aggravate CHF; exclude high-output failure)
Serum chemistry profile	Electrolyte disturbances Diabetes mellitus Renal insufficiency Hypoproteinemia
Thyroid function tests	Hyperthyroidism/hypothyroidism
Urinalysis	Proteinuria (nephrotic syndrome, acute glomerulonephritis, both causes of edema)
Electrocardiogram	Myocardial infarction Ventricular hypertrophy Incessant tachycardia (arrhythmia)
Chest x-ray	Confirm congestion as the cause of dyspnea (especially important when there is obstructive lung disease) Pulmonary infiltrates/fibrosis Presence of pleural effusion Cardiomegaly
Echocardiogram	Differentiate systolic from diastolic dysfunction Document left ventricular dysfunction and chamber size Wall motion abnormalities (coronary artery disease as cause) Valvular abnormalities Pericardial effusion Intracardiac masses

shown to increase functional capacity by keeping skeletal muscles in better tone as well as maintaining better cardiovascular fitness. We generally ask that our patients build up to walking 45 to 60 minutes 3 to 4 days each week at whatever pace is sustainable for that period. Patients should avoid isometric activity because this abruptly increases systemic vascular resistance and afterload. Weight reduction is also advisable in patients who are significantly overweight.

Pharmacologic Therapy
Conventional

ACE inhibitors. The objectives of pharmacologic therapy are to improve functional capacity, improve signs and symptoms of CHF, improve survival, and minimize the use of health care resources for patients with CHF. Afterload reduction therapy with ACE inhibitors is the mainstay of treatment of CHF at all levels of severity.[10] It is the only treatment shown to improve survival with severe CHF, as well as to retard the progression of heart failure in patients with less severe disease. The ra-

tionale for the use of ACE inhibitors in CHF stems from the known activation of the renin-angiotensin-aldosterone system in patients with decreased left ventricular systolic function. ACE inhibitors inhibit the conversion of angiotensin I to angiotensin II, a potent vasoconstrictor. Through various mechanisms, including decreased aldosterone secretion and down-regulation of the sympathetic nervous system, ACE inhibitors decrease both afterload and preload, improving the symptoms of heart failure. The evidence for the clinical usefulness of ACE inhibitors in patients with CHF is based on multiple clinical trials that have shown improved survival as well as reduced hospitalization and other cardiac events. Some of these studies are summarized in Table 22-4.

These studies confirm that ACE inhibitors not only improve survival but retard the progression of CHF in asymptomatic and minimally symptomatic patients. ACE inhibitors are recommended as first-line therapy for any patient with decreased left ventricular systolic function, regardless of etiology, and are now being used

| Table 22-3 | *Ancillary Diagnostic Testing for Congestive Heart Failure* |

Diagnostic Study	Indication/Suspected Cause	Comment
Serum iron/ferritin	Hemochromatosis	
ACE level	Sarcoidosis	
Toxicology screening	Heavy metal toxicity, other environmental toxin	
Blood cultures	Bacterial and fungal infectious etiologies	
Viral titers	Viral myocarditis	
Sedimentation rate, ANA, rheumatoid factor	Collagen vascular disease	
Radionuclide angiogram (RNA)	Poor quality echocardiogram Prognostication for potential revascularization or cardiac transplantation	LVEF useful for prognosis throughout its range, although loses prognostic discrimination between 15% and 25%; RNA potentially inaccurate in patients with atrial fibrillation
Stress perfusion studies	Patients with CHF, without angina but with an intermediate risk of coronary artery disease as a possible etiology Determination of myocardial viability in patients who may be candidates for revascularization	Nonischemic cardiomyopathy may show patchy perfusion abnormalities
Coronary angiography*	All patients with CHF and a history consistent with angina or previous myocardial infarction (with or without recurrent angina) Patients with CHF and significant risk factors for coronary artery disease	
Hemodynamic monitoring ("tailored therapy")*	Patients who respond poorly to initial empiric therapy Patients being evaluated for cardiac transplantation to rule out fixed pulmonary hypertension	Tailoring therapy generally accomplished by optimizing filling pressures and cardiac output with a combination of intravenous inotropes and vasodilators, then substituting oral medicines
Endomyocardial biopsy*	Recent onset of CHF with rapid clinical deterioration Past or present use of specific chemotherapy Presence of systemic disease with possible cardiac involvement	Recent data do not support the use steroids or other immuno-suppressants in the long-term treatment of viral myocarditis[10]
Cardiopulmonary stress testing*	Objective measurement of functional capacity Useful for risk stratification (peak VO_2 <14 ml/kg/min indicates poor vascular prognosis); may be used to follow patients	Test is very effort dependent; other diseases such as chronic lung disease and peripheral disease may make interpretation difficult
Evaluation for cardiac arrhythmia (see Chapters 25 to 27)		

*Patients are referred to a cardiologist for this study. *LVEF,* Left ventricular ejection fraction.

Table 22-4 | *Trials of ACE Inhibitors for Congestive Heart Failure*

Trial	N	Inclusion Criteria	Therapy	Mean Dose	Mean Follow-up	Results
CONSENSUS[6]	253	NYHA IV	Enalapril vs placebo	18.4 mg/d	6 mo	31% reduction in mortality at 1 year; no difference in incidence of sudden cardiac death between groups
V-HeFT-II[7]	804	NYHA II-III	Hydralazine/ isosorbide vs enalapril	Hydralazine 199 mg/d Isosorbide 100 mg/d Enalapril 15 mg/d		28% reduction in mortality in enalapril vs hydralazine/ isosorbide attributed to a reduction in the incidence of sudden death
SOLVED[8] Treatment	2561	NYHA II-III EF <35%	Enalapril vs placebo	11.2 mg/d	42 mo	16% reduction in mortality in enalapril group
SOLVED[12] Prevention	4228		Enalapril vs placebo	12.7 mg/d	37 mo	8% mortality reduction in enalapril group, not statistically significant; 29% reduction in the combined end-point of death or progression to heart failure in enalapril group
SAVE[13]	2231	NYHA I-II EF ≤35%	Captopril vs placebo	Not reported, but 79% reached target dose of 150 mg/d	42 mo	20% reduction in mortality in captopril group; 21% reduction of combined fatal and nonfatal cardiovascular events in captopril group
AIRE[14]	2006	EF ≤40% after acute myocardial infarction with or without symptoms of CHF	Ramipril vs placebo	Mean dose not reported; target dose 5 mg bid	15 mo	27% reduction of all-cause mortality in treatment group
ATLAS[15]	3000	Acute myocardial infarction + clinical evidence of CHF NYHA II-IV LVEF <30%	High- vs low-dose lisinopril	2.5-5.0 mg/d vs 32.5 to 35 mg/d	46 mo	8% reduction in mortality in high-dose group (not significant); 24% reduction in CHF hospitalization in high-dose group (p = 0.003)

EF, Ejection fraction; *LVEF,* left ventricular ejection fraction.

routinely after myocardial infarctions in which there is demonstrated left ventricular systolic dysfunction.

Multiple ACE inhibitors are on the market for use in patients with CHF. Although most of the earlier studies were performed using enalapril or captopril, the benefits of ACE inhibition in CHF are believed to be a class effect. The doses of ACE inhibitors used in most clinical trials have been relatively high, usually higher than primary care physicians are accustomed to prescribing.

The ATLAS trial confirms the usefulness of higher dosing.[15] It randomized 3164 patients to receive lisinopril 2.5 to 5 mg qd versus 32.5 to 35 mg qd with a median follow-up of 46 months. The high-dose group had an 8% lower risk of death compared to the low-dose group, but this difference was not statistically significant. Hospitalization for CHF was 24% lower in the high-dose group (p = 0.003). Our current recommendation is to push the ACE inhibitor dose to tolerance, attempting to reach the doses used by the clinical trials (see Table 22-4). When postural hypotension develops, we back off. Although there is no clinical trial evidence that twice-daily dosing of long-acting ACE inhibitors is beneficial, in practice, more frequent dosing seems to cause less orthostatic hypotension.

The adverse effects of ACE inhibitors are well known and include cough, which occasionally responds to cough suppressants, but usually necessitates stopping the drug. In addition, symptomatic orthostatic hypotension with worsening renal function is possible. Check renal function 36 to 48 hours after starting the drug; if there is no change at that time the patient probably does not have renal artery stenosis. Follow-up electrolyte measurements are important, as hyperkalemia may occur (usually when there is renal dysfunction). Angioedema is an unusual complication and requires discontinuation of ACE inhibitors with no further rechallenge (even using a different preparation). ACE inhibitors are contraindicated in pregnancy because of the significant fetal and neonatal morbidity and mortality associated with their use.

Practical Tips for Starting ACE Inhibitors. Patients with CHF and depressed serum sodium levels have elevated plasma renin activity. They are particularly sensitive to ACE inhibitors. Begin treatment with a lower dose than is usual (e.g., captopril 12.5 mg bid, or even half that). Remember that volume depletion increases the chance of symptomatic hypotension when starting vasodilator therapy. A "diuretic holiday"—withholding furosemide for a couple days—before starting the ACE inhibitor may be considered for a patient with a borderline systolic pressure or when you believe that your patient is "dry." This is particularly useful when the serum sodium level is below 140.

Digoxin. Digitalis, derived from the foxglove plant, has been used to treat the symptoms of CHF for over 200 years. It is an inotropic agent that inhibits sodium potassium ATPase on the sarcolemmal membrane. This increases intracellular calcium levels, making more calcium available to the contractile elements. Digitalis has a narrow therapeutic window, and it is excreted by the kidneys. Toxicity may develop rapidly with an abrupt change in renal function (e.g., with decreased cardiac output or excessive diuresis). As is often the case with drugs that have been in use for a long time, the clinical

utility and risk-to-benefit status of digitalis has not been well studied until recently.

The RADIANCE trial stabilized patients on digitalis, diuretics, and ACE inhibitors, then randomly placed them on placebo or continued digoxin.[16] After 12 weeks the patients taking placebo had worsening heart failure. This study showed that digitalis controls symptoms but does not address survival. Detractors have for many years claimed that digitalis contributes to more frequent mortality. The results of the DIG trial were published in 1997.[17] In this trial 3397 patients were randomized to receive digoxin and compared with 3403 patients on placebo. After 4 years of therapy, there was no difference in mortality between the two groups. However, the risk of the combined end point of death or hospitalization due to worsening heart failure was significantly reduced in the group receiving digitalis. Based on these studies, we no longer hesitate to prescribe digoxin for patients with CHF whose symptoms are not controlled by ACE inhibitors and diuretics.

Diuretics. Diuretics are used for the treatment of congestive symptoms in chronic heart failure. They are classified by site of action within the nephron. Basically, all diuretics increase urinary sodium excretion with a resultant decrease in total body volume. On balance, these medications improve symptoms, although it must be remembered that intense diuresis may stimulate the renin-angiotensin-aldosterone system, which, if not adequately blocked, can lead to worsening of cardiac systolic performance. Diuretics may cause electrolyte abnormalities, including hypokalemia, hypomagnesemia, hyponatremia, or hypercalcemia as well as glucose intolerance, hyperlipidemia, hyperuricemia, and renal failure. Diuretics are not known to influence survival in severe CHF. Their use requires frequent monitoring of renal function and electrolyte levels, with appropriate adjustments of dose as well as potassium and magnesium supplementation.

Table 22-5 summarizes some of the more frequently used diuretics. Loop diuretics are often used initially because of their potency. Potassium-sparing diuretics such as spironolactone are, in general, weak diuretics that are primarily used for their potassium-sparing effects. It is currently unclear if specific aldosterone inhibition provides further benefit. Often, as CHF progresses and, in particular, if renal function deteriorates, higher doses of loop diuretics are required for adequate diuresis. Diuretic dosing must be individualized. Despite the low risk of ototoxicity with higher oral doses of the loop diuretics, metolazone is generally added as an adjunctive diuretic when loop diuretic doses exceed the equivalent of furosemide 200 mg/day. Torsemide (Demadex), a newer loop diuretic, has been found useful in some patients resistant to other loop diuretics such as furosemide and bumetanide (see Chapter 53).

Table 22-5	*Selected Diuretics Used in the Treatment of Congestive Heart Failure*

Site of Action	Diuretic	Dosage	Comments
Ascending loop of Henle	Furosemide Bumetanide	40-400 mg/d 1-5 mg/d	Higher doses required with progressive renal insufficiency Risk of ototoxicity related to peak plasma levels Risk is low with even high doses of these two medications due to prolonged absorption time and lower peak plasma levels Cannot be used with sulfa-allergic patients
	Torsemide	Half the furo-semide dose	May be useful when resistance develops to other loop diuretics
	Ethacrynic acid	50-100 mg/d	High ototoxicity risk but can use in sulfa-allergic patients
Distal tubule	Metolazone	2.5-20 mg/d	Promotes significant kaliuresis Most often used in combination with loop diuretic
	Thiazide diuretics Hydrochlorothiazide Chlorthalidone Chlorothiazide	25-100 mg/d 25-200 mg/d 500-1000 mg/d	Not as potent as loop diuretics Ineffective if GFR <30
Late distal tubule	Spironolactone	50-400 mg/d	Efficacy depends on level of aldosterone secretion Potassium sparing

GFR, Glomerular filtration rate.

Hydralazine/Isosorbide Dinitrate. The combination of hydralazine and isosorbide dinitrate was the first vasodilator regimen found to improve survival in CHF. Results of the V-HeFT-I trial published in 1986 compared placebo versus prazosin versus the combination of hydralazine and isosorbide dinitrate in the treatment of patients with CHF who were already taking digitalis and diuretics.[5] The combination of hydralazine and isosorbide dinitrate was the only non–ACE inhibitor vasodilator that showed improved survival. In the V-HeFT-II trial, enalapril had a greater effect on survival than hydralazine and isosorbide dinitrate, but exercise tolerance and left ventricular function were improved only by the hydralazine/isosorbide dinitrate combination.[7] Current recommendations for use of hydralazine/isosorbide dinitrate include patients who are intolerant to ACE inhibitors and patients with progressive symptoms of CHF and elevated systolic blood pressure despite full-dose ACE inhibition. Nitrates alone may be added for relief of concomitant angina and are occasionally used to prevent nocturnal dyspnea and orthopnea.

Beta-blockers. Activation of the sympathetic nervous system is an adaptive response that, in the short-term, supports cardiac output and perfusion of central organs. Chronically, however, this leads to increased afterload, further decreases systemic perfusion, and aggravates fatigue and exercise intolerance. Additionally, high levels of serum and myocardial norepinephrine produce chronic ischemia. The resultant calcium overload produces frank necrosis of cardiac myocytes. Chronic overstimulation by catecholamines leads to down-regulation and decoupling of beta$_1$ receptors. It has further been shown that this response is partially responsible for the reduced contractility of individual myocytes. Blunting these maladaptive responses with beta blockade may be beneficial in the long-term treatment of CHF. Initially, beta$_1$ selective antagonists were studied. Further research has found that the beta$_1$ receptors are down-regulated in CHF and that in this disease the cardiac beta$_2$ receptors have a much more important role.

A summary of beta-blocker trials in heart failure is presented in Table 22-6. The beta$_1$ selective blocking agents

Table 22-6	*Trials of Beta-Blockers in Congestive Heart Failure*				
Trial Criteria	**n**	**Inclusion**	**Therapy**	**Follow-up**	**Results**
MDC[18]	383	IDC EF <40%	Metoprolol vs placebo	12-18 mo	No reduction in all-cause mortality but 34% reduction in the metoprolol group for combined end-point of death or need for transplantation
CIBIS[19]	641	NYHA III-IV EF <40%	Bisoprolol vs placebo	1.9 yr	No reduction in mortality observed; however, patients taking bisoprolol required fewer hospitalizations for cardiac decompensation
ANZUS[20]	415	NYHA II-III EF <40%	Carvedilol vs placebo	18-24 mo	No effect on mortality or exercise tolerance; primary end-point was exercise tolerance.
US Trial[21]	1094	NYHA II-IV stratified by 6 min walk test EF <35%	Carvedilol vs placebo	6 mo	65% reduction in carvedilol mortality with carvedilol; significant reduction in hospitalizations for CHF in carvedilol group
BEST	2800 (projected)	NYHA III-IV EF <35%	Bucindolol vs placebo	≥18 mo	Ongoing

metoprolol and bisoprolol showed no survival advantage. However, the studies using these two drugs were underpowered for their stated end points. Based on data from the U.S. Carvedilol Trial Group, which included the PRECISE and MOCHA trials as well as the Australia–New Zealand Heart Failure Research Collaborative Group, carvedilol, a nonselective beta-blocker with vasodilating properties, improves survival in a dose-dependent manner in patients with New York Heart Association Functional Class II and III heart failure.

Carvedilol was approved by the Food and Drug Administration (FDA) for use in patients with mild to moderate heart failure in 1997. Starting carvedilol can be tricky, as it may initially exacerbate heart failure symptoms. The benefits both in symptom relief and in increased ejection performance are often not observed until 2 to 3 months of therapy. Patients are generally started at the lowest possible dose (3.125 mg bid), and the dose increased every 2 weeks to a maximum dose of 25 to 50 mg bid. Other medications may require adjustment in the initial titration phase (increasing diuretics, decreasing ACE inhibitors) to allow full titration. Another nonselective beta blocker with vasodilator properties, bucindolol, is currently under study in a long-term survival trial (BEST Trial). If the projected enrollment goals are met and the study is continued, the results should more fully elucidate the use of nonselective beta blockade in a wide spectrum of patients with CHF.

Promising New Therapies

Angiotensin II Blockers. The benefits of ACE inhibitors are well established. They reduce morbidity and mortality with chronic heart failure and retard the progression of heart failure, particularly after myocardial infarction. ACE inhibitors not only block the conversion of angiotensin I to angiotensin II but also inhibit the breakdown of bradykinin. Bradykinin has been associated with the release of nitric oxide and prostacyclin, which may contribute to the hemodynamic effects of ACE inhibition. Increased levels of bradykinin have also been implicated as the etiology of some of the more common adverse reactions such as chronic cough, angioedema, renal dysfunction with concomitant hyperkalemia, and hypotension.

Angiotensin II may be produced by alternate pathways (chymase), which may mitigate some of the beneficial effects of ACE inhibition. Several orally active, nonpeptide angiotensin II receptor antagonists have been developed that, in theory, more completely block the effects of angiotensin II. These drugs block angiotensin II receptors without increasing bradykinin levels and, in general, are somewhat better tolerated than ACE inhibitors (cough is not a side effect). Angiotensin II receptor antagonists currently available include losartan, valsartan, and irbesartan.

In one study, losartan was compared with captopril in 722 patients over age 65 who had never received ACE inhibitors.[22] The study group included patients with left ventricular ejection fraction less than 40% with NYHA Class II-IV CHF. Losartan was titrated to 50 mg qd and captopril to 50 mg tid for a follow-up period of 48 weeks. The primary end point was tolerability with regard to renal function, with secondary end points of death and/or hospital admissions for heart failure. Although there was no difference in renal dysfunction (creatinine increased 10.5% in both groups) or in hospital admission for heart failure, losartan was generally better tolerated, and fewer losartan patients discontinued therapy. The losartan group had an unexpected lower all-cause mortality, which will be evaluated in further trials.

The Val-HeFT trial is currently in progress and is testing the angiotensin II receptor blocker valsartan in combination with an ACE inhibitor therapy versus placebo. The primary end point is mortality.

Calcium Channel Blockers. The usefulness of calcium channel blockers in the treatment of chronic CHF due to systolic dysfunction is a subject of continued debate. First-generation calcium channel blockers such as verapamil, diltiazem, and nifedipine are contraindicated because of their negative inotropic effects. Second-generation dihydropyridine calcium channel blockers may be effective afterload reducers. The PRAISE study[23] randomly assigned 1153 patients with chronic heart failure of either ischemic or nonischemic etiology and an ejection fraction less than 30% to treatment with placebo or amlodipine in addition to standard triple therapy.[23] The primary end point for the study was death from any cause and hospitalization for major cardiovascular events. There was a 9% reduction in the combined risk of fatal and nonfatal events with amlodipine versus placebo. This did not reach statistical significance. Patients with nonischemic heart failure had a greater benefit, with a 31% reduction in the combined risk of fatal and nonfatal events and a 46% reduction in risk of death. There was no difference in these two end points in those with ischemic CHF. This study demonstrated the safety of amlodipine in patients with left ventricular systolic dysfunction of any etiology. A follow-up study (PRAISE-2) is ongoing, and is a mortality trial of amlodipine in nonischemic heart failure.

Another calcium channel blocker, felodipine, was tested in a much smaller population (n = 451) of patients with ejection fractions less than 45% and NYHA Classes II-III. This study compared felodipine versus placebo added to standard therapy with digoxin, diuretics, and ACE inhibitors. The mean follow-up period was 9.5 months with results showing no benefit or specific disadvantage to felodipine therapy on either mortality or exercise tolerance.[24]

Our current approach is to use amlodipine for patients with CHF and poorly controlled hypertension despite optimal doses of ACE inhibitors, angiotensin II blockers, or hydralazine/nitrate combinations. It may also be used cautiously in patients with CHF and angina that is unresponsive to the highest tolerable doses of nitrates.

Endothelin Blockers. Endothelin-1 (ET-1) is the most potent endogenous vasoconstrictor studied to date. Binding to two receptors (ET_A and ET_B), ET-1 produces long-lasting, intense vasoconstriction. ET-1 levels are elevated in CHF in proportion to the severity of disease. Plasma levels correlate with both exercise capacity and pulmonary artery pressure. Several ET_A and ET_B receptor antagonists are in clinical trials. There is hope that these potent receptor antagonists will provide additional survival benefit in patients with heart failure, particularly those with pulmonary hypertension.

Palliative Therapy for Refractory CHF

Intravenous Inotropes. Most treatment of CHF is directed toward interrupting the neurohormonal/autocrine-paracrine responses that exacerbate left ventricular pump dysfunction. Thus far no oral inotropic medication (a drug that increases contractility) has improved survival. With the exception of digitalis, all inotropic medications have had deleterious effects on survival. The adverse effects of chronic catecholamine stimulation of the myocardium have been reviewed.

Nevertheless, as a patient's clinical condition deteriorates, use of intravenous inotropes may become necessary for acute exacerbations of heart failure. It may be the only therapy that keeps the patient out of the hospital. It is now becoming common to use intravenous inotropes for the relief of symptoms, realizing that their chronic use will not enhance survival and, in fact, may hasten the patient's ultimate demise.

Of the group of beta-adrenergic agonists, dobutamine and dopamine are the most widely used. Both of these are now commonly given in the home setting with visiting nurse supervision. Other catecholamines such as epinephrine and norepinephrine may be used in the hospital when systemic hypotension is predominant.

Dobutamine is usually the first choice for outpatient treatment. It stimulates both $beta_1$ and $beta_2$ receptors and has a mild agonist effect on alpha receptors. It is superior to dopamine in heart failure because of its ability to increase cardiac output, decrease pulmonary capillary wedge pressure, and lower both systemic and pulmonary vascular resistance, without raising heart rate. The dose is 2 to 20 µg/kg/min as a continuous infusion in acute situations. Higher doses can exacerbate both atrial and ventricular arrhythmias, particularly if electrolyte levels are abnormal. The selective actions of this and other catecholamines are lost at higher doses, and the drug functions as a pressor agent; we try to keep the dose below 5 to 8 µg/kg/min. An occasional patient has an increased heart rate that may precipitate angina when there is coronary artery disease (CAD). The beneficial effects of dobutamine have been shown to persist for weeks after an infusion is terminated. Many patients are helped by a 6-hour infusion just once or twice a week. On the other hand, tachyphylaxis is possible.

Dopamine is seldom used for its inotropic properties but rather to enhance diuresis in patients with severe CHF. At doses of 1 to 3 μg/kg/min, it activates dopamine-specific receptors in the renal and splanchnic arterial beds, improving blood flow to these regions. It can be a useful adjunct when added to an intravenous inotrope in patients with difficulty maintaining their volume status.

Phosphodiesterase inhibitors (milrinone and amrinone) comprise a second class of intravenous inotropic agents. These agents inhibit intracellular phosphodiesterase III, leading to an increase in the cellular concentrations of cyclic adenosine monophosphate (AMP). Cyclic AMP is known to increase intracellular calcium influx via the slow channel, increasing contractility. It also sensitizes the contractile proteins to calcium, inhibits calcium uptake by the sarcoplasmic reticulum, and blocks adenosine receptors. Increased cyclic AMP levels also relax vascular smooth muscle, decreasing systemic vascular resistance.

Milrinone has supplanted amrinone as the phosphodiesterase inhibitor of choice when this class of medication is desired for intravenous inotropic support. This is largely due to amrinone's propensity to cause thrombocytopenia. Milrinone is generally given as a 50 μg/kg bolus over 10 minutes followed by continuous infusion at rates between 0.3 and 0.75 μg/kg/min. Studies have shown little or no increase in heart rate and myocardial oxygen consumption, which makes milrinone good for patients with ischemic cardiomyopathy. Its vasodilator effects are potent, and systemic hypotension can at times be severe. The dose of milrinone must be adjusted downward with concomitant renal dysfunction.

Toborinone (OPC-18790) is an intravenous positive inotropic agent that works in part by inhibiting phosphodiesterase III. This drug has some unique properties and has been shown to clearly improve clinical status in patients with heart failure. It is currently in clinical trials.

Home therapy with dobutamine or milrinone has gained favor over the past several years. Early studies with dobutamine showed increased mortality with higher doses. The decision to maintain a patient on chronic home inotropic infusion must take into consideration the expected beneficial effects as well as the potential risk. We often begin with a brief hospital stay, where hemodynamics are measured with a Swan-Ganz catheter before and after beginning the infusion. We thus identify the lowest effective dose. This minimal efficacious dose is used at home, with 6-hour infusions one to four times a week. In addition, patients are given intermittent rather than continuous infusion. Supervision by a visiting nurse and frequent follow-up are necessary. It is especially important to maintain electrolyte balance.

Ultrafiltration. As the severity of CHF progresses, patients often become resistant to increases in diuretic therapy. There is a lack of correlation of urinary sodium and water excretion with cardiac index. Instead, diuresis is related to a combination of hemodynamic and neuroendocrine variables (renin, aldosterone, and norepinephrine). Ultrafiltration has been used successfully to control volume and reestablish diuretic responsiveness.

Various methods of ultrafiltration have been tried for CHF, including peritoneal dialysis (PD), intermittent isolation ultrafiltration (IIUF), continuous arteriovenous hemofiltration (CAVH), and continuous venovenous hemofiltration (CVVH). Of these different techniques, CVVH has been used most successfully in severely decompensated CHF. The technique requires a double-lumen venous dialysis catheter, and it uses an external blood pump to generate adequate blood flow through the system. Net volume loss can be as high as 500 ml/hr and is generally hemodynamically well tolerated. CAVH uses the patient's systemic blood pressure to provide perfusion pressure through the membrane and is, in all other ways, similar to CVVH. The disadvantage of this technique is that an arterial catheter is required. Intermittent forms of ultrafiltration such as IIUF run a significant risk of systemic hypotension in patients with severe CHF. Anticoagulation, however, is only needed intermittently as opposed to continuously with the other techniques. Although peritoneal dialysis has been used, it often causes abdominal distention, which aggravates respiratory distress.

Adjunctive Medical Therapy

Antiarrhythmics. Patients with heart failure and concomitant atrial fibrillation require ventricular rate control. An attempt at cardioversion is appropriate for new-onset atrial fibrillation or atrial fibrillation of uncertain duration. Drugs such as digoxin, diltiazem, and beta-blockers may be used for rate control. However, with severe CHF, diltiazem and beta-blockers may exacerbate congestive symptoms. Amiodarone is the drug of choice in patients with heart failure both for rate control (if digoxin is unsuccessful) and for cardioversion. Occasionally, patients require atrioventricular nodal ablation with implantation of a permanent DDD pacemaker.

Ventricular arrhythmias are common in patients with CHF caused by systolic dysfunction. Most antiarrhythmic drugs have proarrhythmic effects or depress ventricular contractility, or both. Currently, no data support the use of antiarrhythmic therapy for asymptomatic ventricular arrhythmias, including nonsustained ventricular tachycardia. The evaluation and treatment of symptomatic or sustained ventricular arrhythmias is reviewed in Chapter 26.

If an antiarrhythmic drug is needed, class I agents should be avoided. Amiodarone has been shown to be reasonably safe and well-tolerated in patients with CHF. Results of the STAT-CHF trial found that amiodarone was effective in suppressing ventricular arrhythmias in asymptomatic patients.[25] An increase in LV ejection fraction was also noted in the treatment group. There was a trend toward improved survival in patients with non-ischemic cardiomyopathy (although statistically insignificant). The study showed no reduction in overall survival or in the rates of sudden death with amiodarone. The empiric use of amiodarone in asymptomatic patients with CHF remains controversial.

Indications for implantable cardioverter defibrillators (ICD) include survival after sudden cardiac death, inducible ventricular fibrillation, and inducible sustained ventricular tachycardia with or without hemodynamic compromise. The SCD-HeFT Trial is currently under way randomizing patients with asymptomatic nonsustained ventricular tachycardia to placebo, empiric amiodarone therapy, or ICD placement.

Anticoagulation. Routine anticoagulation with warfarin in patients with significant left ventricular systolic dysfunction and CHF is controversial. Retrospective analysis of several clinical trials reveal that the incidence of arterial thromboembolism ranges from 0.9% to 5.5% per 100 patient years, with the largest studies reporting an incidence of 2% and 2.4% per 100 patient years. Many physicians anticoagulate patients with left ventricular dysfunction, sinus rhythm, and a documented intracardiac thrombus. There are, however, no clinical trial data supporting this approach. Patients with atrial fibrillation should be fully anticoagulated with warfarin, with a target INR of 2.0 to 3.0 (see Chapter 25).

Surgical Therapy

High-Risk Coronary Revascularization

Although the operative mortality for coronary artery bypass grafting is higher in patients with poor left ventricular systolic function, it is this population that derives the most survival benefit from successful revascularization. Every patient with ischemic cardiomyopathy should be assessed for possible revascularization. If angiography reveals adequate distal vessels, a test of myocardial viability may be performed in an effort to identify "hibernating" myocardium. Thallium perfusion imaging and positron emission tomography (PET) scanning are the two most widely used methods. Although PET scanning appears to be a more sensitive method, it is not widely available.

The risk of revascularization must be weighed in each individual patient. If LV ejection fraction is more than 20%, the end-diastolic dimension is less than or equal to 7 cm, and "hibernating" myocardium is apparent, revascularization may be considered.

High-Risk Valve Repair or Replacement

Severe impairment of left ventricular systolic function may occur as a result of aortic stenosis, aortic regurgitation, or mitral regurgitation. Fortunately, patients who present in this manner are becoming rarer because of the effective noninvasive means of monitoring the progression of these lesions. The risk of performing valve surgery is higher with CHF, and it depends on the particular lesion and the degree of left ventricular dysfunction.

Aortic valve lesions, both stenosis and insufficiency, significantly increase afterload in the left ventricle. This afterload mismatch may be severe and can result in poor left ventricular systolic performance. Aortic valve replacement for both of these lesions may decrease afterload, possibly improving systolic function after surgery.

Valve replacement or repair for mitral insufficiency is, however, a different proposition. Numerous studies have documented poor survival for patients with ejection fractions less than 40% at the time of operation. The papillary muscles play an important role in maintaining ventricular geometry and systolic and diastolic function. Newer techniques of mitral valve surgery use chordal-sparing procedures, and mitral valve repair is considered better than replacement for those with marginal left ventricular function. Although a few published studies have specifically addressed the issue, mitral valve repair may be considered even with ejection fractions as low as 25% to 30%. When ejection fraction is lower, perioperative mortality is high, and left ventricular dysfunction progresses.

Dynamic Cardiomyoplasty

Dynamic cardiomyoplasty is still investigational. The latissimus dorsi muscle is harvested with its neurovascular pedicle intact, and it is relocated to the anterior chest cavity, where it is wrapped around the heart. It is "trained" over a period of approximately 8 weeks, then stimulated in gated fashion with a pacemaker to assist myocardial contraction. Most nonrandomized studies of this procedure have shown an improvement in symptoms and in the patient's perceived quality of life. However, no study has shown improvement in objective measures of cardiac function such as peak oxygen consumption or pulmonary capillary wedge pressure. The operative mortality in high-risk patients (NYHA Class IV, biventricular CHF, pulmonary hypertension, and elevated pulmonary vascular resistance) is quite high. The aggregate of studies suggests no survival benefit compared with medical therapy, and this procedure is clearly inferior to cardiac transplantation with regard to long-term survival. Progression of heart failure and ventricular arrhythmias are the major causes of late death after this procedure. A large, multicenter, prospective randomized trial comparing dynamic cardiomyoplasty and medical therapy is ongoing.

Surgical Left Ventricular Remodeling

Surgical left ventricular remodeling, or partial left ventricular resection with mitral valve repair, has been developed over the past decade by the Brazilian cardiac surgeon Randas V. Batista. The procedure is being performed in a few centers in the United States, and the Cleveland Clinic Foundation currently has the most extensive experience. A triangular section of the left ventricle between the anterolateral and posteromedial papillary muscles is resected, and the ventricle is sutured together. The procedure requires mitral valve repair. The goal of the surgery is to normalize the left ventricular diastolic dimension (dramatically decreasing left ventricular wall stress) and to eliminate mitral insufficiency.

Short-term studies have shown that this can be performed with an acceptable operative mortality even in very ill patients. There is a significant decrease in left ventricular end-diastolic dimension and near-doubling of the ejection fraction. Cardiac index rises as left ventricular filling pressure falls. Although the operative mortality is low, there have been a number of late deaths due to ventricular arrhythmias. Approximately 30% of patients have required the placement of ventricular assist devices and re-listing for cardiac transplantation.

This procedure is still undergoing refinement, and more data are needed to predict which patients will derive the most benefit.

Left Ventricular Assist Device

Left ventricular assist devices (LVADs) have been extensively refined over the past 20 years. Currently two different LVAD systems have been approved by the FDA for use in the United States. LVAD is currently restricted to use as a bridge to cardiac transplantation. Many of these patients have had prolonged waiting times, so much has been learned about the long-term safety and tolerability of these devices. Currently, a randomized study (Randomized Evaluation of Mechanical Assistance for the Treatment of Congestive Heart Failure—REMATCH) is ongoing comparing survival with a long-term LVAD and conventional medical therapy in patients who do not meet criteria for cardiac transplantation. This study should more clearly define the role of implantable LVADs in the long-term treatment of CHF.

Cardiac Transplantation

Currently, cardiac transplantation is the only surgical therapy that has been proven to significantly extend survival in patients with severe CHF. Although survival rates between 70% and 80% at 5 years have been achieved, cardiac transplant recipients continue to suffer significant morbidity over the years as a result of immunosuppressive therapy. The number of cardiac transplant operations is limited by the availability of suitable donor organs. Even with strict selection criteria, the number of patients who could potentially benefit from cardiac transplantation is estimated to be between three and five times the number of heart transplant procedures performed each year.

With ever-growing numbers of patients being added to transplant waiting lists and with over 50% of transplants each year being performed on hospitalized patients of high acuity, more emphasis has been placed on identifying and selecting patients who have a very poor 1-year survival. Current indications for cardiac transplantation are outlined in Box 22-3.

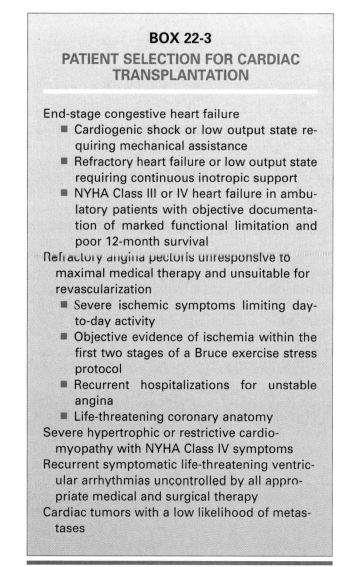

BOX 22-3
PATIENT SELECTION FOR CARDIAC TRANSPLANTATION

End-stage congestive heart failure
- Cardiogenic shock or low output state requiring mechanical assistance
- Refractory heart failure or low output state requiring continuous inotropic support
- NYHA Class III or IV heart failure in ambulatory patients with objective documentation of marked functional limitation and poor 12-month survival

Refractory angina pectoris unresponsive to maximal medical therapy and unsuitable for revascularization
- Severe ischemic symptoms limiting day-to-day activity
- Objective evidence of ischemia within the first two stages of a Bruce exercise stress protocol
- Recurrent hospitalizations for unstable angina
- Life-threatening coronary anatomy

Severe hypertrophic or restrictive cardiomyopathy with NYHA Class IV symptoms

Recurrent symptomatic life-threatening ventricular arrhythmias uncontrolled by all appropriate medical and surgical therapy

Cardiac tumors with a low likelihood of metastases

Once the need for cardiac transplantation is established using these criteria, a patient's suitability for the procedure must also be demonstrated. There are multiple potential contraindications to cardiac transplantation, including fixed pulmonary hypertension, concurrent infection, history of uncured malignancy, peripheral or cerebrovascular disease, active peptic ulcer, diverticular or gallbladder disease, psychiatric disease, substance abuse, and other systemic illnesses that would limit posttransplant survival or rehabilitation. Selection criteria and contraindications as well as the rigor with which these are sought out in any potential transplant recipient vary from program to program, but on the whole remain fairly consistent

WHEN TO REFER A PATIENT WITH CHF

Patients with CHF caused by systolic dysfunction should be referred to a general cardiologist for consultation whenever specific cardiologic diagnostic testing is deemed necessary. This would include testing required to establish a cause as well as any specialized or invasive testing required to define the prognosis. Patients with persistent NYHA Class III symptoms on standard conventional therapy and patients with other active primary or secondary cardiac problems, including angina pectoris, arrhythmias, and significant valvular problems, should also be followed intermittently by a general cardiologist.

The increase in the prevalence of CHF in the general population has prompted the establishment of specialized clinics for CHF. They are staffed by cardiologists and nurses who have special expertise in the management of CHF. Along with aggressive medical management, patient education, including diet, activity, and medication compliance, is repeatedly emphasized. In addition, many of these clinics have access to investigational medications and devices.

Multiple reports have been published on the positive effect of these specialized clinics with regard to reported patient compliance, functional status, quality of life, and number of hospitalizations for CHF. Consider referral to the Heart Failure Clinic for the following reasons:

1. The patient has a poor understanding of CHF or the necessary dietary, activity, and medication requirements.
2. There are persistent NYHA Functional Class III-B and IV symptoms despite optimal conventional therapy.
3. There have been frequent hospitalizations for CHF.

In our practice even general cardiologists have found the special services of the Heart Failure Clinic helpful for the management of patients with poorly controlled CHF.

REFERENCES

1. Ho KKL, Pinsky JL, Kennel WB, Levy D: The epidemiology of heart failure: the Framingham Study, *J Am Coll Cardiol* 22:6, 1993.
2. Stevenson WG, Stevenson LW, Middlekouff HR, et al: Improving survival for patients with advanced heart failure: a study of 737 consecutive patients, *J Am Coll Cardiol* 26:1417, 1995.
3. Costanzo MR: Current status of heart transplantation, *Curr Opin Cardiol* 11:161, 1996.
4. Sugrue DD, Rodeheffer RJ, Codd MD, et al: The clinical course of idiopathic dilated cardiomyopathy: a population-based study, *Ann Intern Med* 117:117, 1992.
5. Cohn JN, Archibald DG, Ziescte S, et al: Effect of vasodilator therapy on mortality in chronic congestive heart failure, *N Engl J Med* 314:1547, 1986.
6. The CONSENSUS Trial Study Group: Effects of enalapril on mortality in severe congestive heart failure: results of the Cooperative North Scandinavian Enalapril Survival Study (CONSENSUS), *N Engl J Med* 216:1409, 1987.
7. Cohn JN, Johnson G, Ziesche S, et al: A comparison of enalapril with hydralazine-isosorbide dinitrate in the treatment of chronic congestive heart failure, *N Engl J Med* 325:303, 1991.
8. The SOLVED investigators: Effect of enalapril on survival in patients with reduced left ventricular ejection fraction and congestive heart failure, *N Engl J Med* 325:293, 1991.
9. Eichhorn EJ, Bristow MR: Medical therapy can improve the biological properties of the chronically failing heart: a new era in the treatment of heart failure, *Circulation* 94:2285, 1996.
10. Brown NJ. Vaughan DE: Angiotensin converting enzyme inhibitors, *Circulation* 97:1411, 1998.
11. Mason JW, O'Connell JB, Herskowitz A, et al: A clinical trial of immunosuppressive therapy for myocarditis, *N Engl J Med* 333:269, 1995.
12. The SOLVED investigators: Effect of enalapril on mortality and the development of heart failure in asymptomatic patients with reduced left ventricular ejection fractions, *N Engl J Med* 307:685, 1992.
13. Pfeffer MA, Braunwald E, Moye LA, et al: Effect of captopril on mortality and morbidity in patients with left ventricular dysfunction after myocardial infarction: results of the survival and ventricular enlargement trial, *N Engl J Med* 327:669, 1992.
14. The Acute Infarction Ramipril Efficacy Study investigators: Effect of ramipril on mortality and morbidity of survivors of acute myocardial infarction with clinical evidence of heart failure, *Lancet* 342:821, 1993.
15. Packer M: *Assessment of treatment with lisinopril and survival (ATLAS).* Presented at the Annual Scientific Session of the American College of Cardiology, Atlanta, March 30, 1998.
16. Packer M, Gheorghiade M, Young JB, et al: Withdrawal of digoxin from patients with chronic heart failure treated with angiotensin-converting enzyme inhibitors, *N Engl J Med* 329:1, 1993.

17. The Digitalis Investigators Group: The effect of digoxin on mortality and morbidity in patients with heart failure, *N Engl J Med* 336:525, 1997.
18. Waagstein F, Bristow MR, Swedberg K, et al: Beneficial effects of metoprolol in idiopathic dilated cardiomyopathy, *Lancet* 342:141, 1993.
19. CIBIS Investigators and Committees: A randomized trial of beta blockade and heart failure: the cardiac insufficiency bisoprolol study (CIBIS), *Circulation* 90:1765, 1994.
20. Australia–New Zealand Heart Research Collaborative Group: Effects of carvedilol, a vasodilator-beta-blocker, in patients with congestive heart failure due to ischemic heart disease, *Circulation* 92:212, 1995.
21. Packer M, Bristow MR, Cohn JN, et al for the US Carvedilol Heart Failure Study Group: The effect of carvedilol on morbidity and mortality of patients with chronic heart failure, *N Engl J Med* 334:1349, 1996.
22. Segal B, Martinez R, Meures FA, et al: Randomized trial of losartan vs captopril in patients over 65 with heart failure (Evaluation of Losartan in the Elderly Study, ELITE), *Lancet* 349:747, 1997.
23. Packer M, O'Connor CM, Ghali JK et al: Effect of amlodipine on morbidity and mortality in severe chronic heart failure, *N Engl J Med* 335:1107, 1996.
24. Cohn JN, Ziesche S, Smith R, et al: The effect of the calcium antagonist felodipine as supplementary vasodilator therapy in patients with chronic heart failure treated with enalapril V-HeFT III, *Circulation* 96:856, 1997.
25. Singh SN, Fletcher RD, Fisher SH, et al: Amiodarone in patients with congestive heart failure and asymptomatic ventricular arrhythmia, *N Engl J Med* 333:77, 1995.

BIBLIOGRAPHY

ACC/AHA Task Force Report: Guidelines for the evaluation and management of heart failure, *J Am Coll Cardiol* 26:1376, 1995.

Blake P, Paganini EP: Refractory congestive heart failure: overview and application of extracorporeal ultrafiltration, *Adv Renal Replacement Ther* 3:166, 1996.

Bonow RO, Nikas D, Elefteriades JA: Valve replacement for regurgitant lesions of the aortic or mitral valve in advanced left ventricular dysfunction, *Cardiol Clin* 13:73, 1995.

Fonarow GC, Stephenson LW, Waldon JA, et al: Impact of a comprehensive heart failure management program on hospital re-admission and functional status of patients with advanced heart failure, *J Am Coll Cardiol* 30:725,1997.

Hozenpud JD, Greenberg BH, editors: *Congestive heart failure: pathophysiology, diagnosis, and comprehensive approach to management*, New York, 1994, Springer-Verlag.

Miller LW: Outpatient dobutamine for refractory congestive heart failure: advantages, techniques, and results, *J Heart Lung Transplant* 10:482, 1991.

Starling RC: Radical alternatives to transplantation, *Curr Opin Cardiol* 12:166, 1997.

Wenger NK, Goodman JF, Roberts WC: Cardiomyopathy and myocardial involvement in systemic disease. In Hurst JW, editor: *The heart*, New York, 1996, McGraw-Hill.

23 Diastolic Heart Failure

Kirk W. Walker
Douglas J. Thompson

Congestive heart failure (CHF) is responsible for more than 700,000 hospital admissions annually. Mortality is high. According to recent Framingham statistics, every other patient with the diagnosis of heart failure dies within 5 years.[1] Dyspnea, fatigue, and weakness handicap the survivors. Despite these grim statistics, many physicians are unaware that one third of their heart failure patients have normal systolic function—they have diastolic CHF.

The word *diastole* is Greek and means "to dilate or expand." Diastolic dysfunction is an inability to fill the ventricle to a normal end-diastolic volume without increasing end-diastolic pressure (EDP). A patient with diastolic CHF has normal left ventricular ejection fraction (LVEF) but high LVEDP and therefore elevated pulmonary venous pressure. The heart ejects blood easily but cannot fill because it is stiff and cannot relax.

Differentiating diastolic from systolic CHF is important. Each is treated differently, and the prognosis is better with diastolic disease.[2] We frequently see these patients because of recurrent hospital admission for CHF. Both the patient and physician are frustrated because standard triple therapy (digoxin, diuretics, and angiotensin-converting enzyme [ACE] inhibitors) is not working. Despite taking their medications, patients remain dyspneic, but also are hypotensive, dizzy, and weak.

Although digoxin and vasodilators help the heart eject blood, they do not help it fill. Using the same treatment strategy for both systolic and diastolic heart failure is like treating viral, bacterial, and fungal infections with one antibiotic.

PATHOPHYSIOLOGY

Systolic CHF and diastolic CHF involve different physiologic mechanisms. Simply stated, systolic CHF results from an inability of the myofibrils to shorten against a load. The ventricle weakens, becoming unable to eject blood into a high-pressure aorta, and the LVEF and cardiac output decline. This is represented graphically as a decline in the contractility curve and a stable diastolic filling curve (Fig. 23-1).

In contrast, diastolic CHF results from impaired filling. The heart is strong. The LVEF is normal or even high (the left ventricle is "hyperdynamic"). It ejects blood easily. However, myocardial relaxation is impaired or passive stiffness is increased. The heart is stiff, and the diastolic filling (compliance) curve is shifted up and to the left (Fig. 23-1). It cannot fill completely at normal filling pressures. Because of inadequate filling, the amount of blood ejected per beat falls and cardiac output drops. The underperfused kidneys produce less urine, fluid is retained, and intravascular filling pressures increase. These high pressures stretch out the stiffened heart, fill it with more blood, increase the stroke volume, and raise the cardiac output back toward normal. However, these high pressures push fluid from the pulmonary capillaries into the interstitial space, causing dyspnea and eventually pulmonary edema.

Like systolic dysfunction, the severity of diastolic dysfunction varies greatly from one patient to another. In its earliest stages diastolic dysfunction may be detected serendipitously in asymptomatic hypertensive patients with left ventricular hypertrophy. In these patients the echocardiogram may reveal abnormal filling caused by slowed relaxation, increased passive stiffness, or both. However, normal filling pressures and stroke volumes are maintained even with exertion.

As diastolic function deteriorates, symptoms are first noted with stress or exertion, when the cardiac output is elevated. In contrast to normal hearts, hearts with diastolic dysfunction cannot increase their relaxation rate in step with increased heart rate. Filling pressures may remain normal under resting conditions, but at higher cardiac output the pulmonary venous pressure increases, causing dyspnea.

At the extreme end of diastolic dysfunction, filling is impaired even at rest. Any additional problem such as increased sodium intake, ischemia, hypertension, or tachycardia may precipitate pulmonary edema.

Patients with *combined systolic and diastolic CHF* have the worst of both worlds. Their hearts can neither contract nor fill normally. For any given reduction in LVEF they are more symptomatic and their prognosis worsens. In general, these patients are best treated according to the guidelines outlined for systolic dysfunction. The rest of this chapter discusses patients with more "pure" diastolic heart failure, which can be defined as patients with heart failure and LVEF greater than 40%.[2]

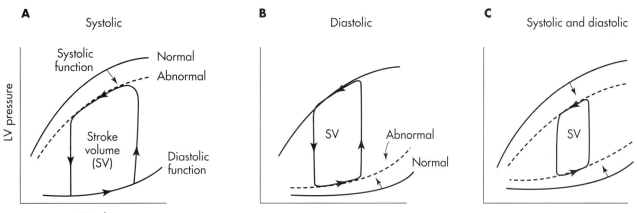

FIG. 23-1

Cardiac function in heart failure. The upper curves describe systolic performance of the ventricle. With increased left ventricular volume, the left ventricle develops greater pressure during systole (Starling's law, see Chapter 2). The lower curves describe left ventricular diastolic compliance or stiffness; with rising left ventricular volume, diastolic pressure rises. Stroke volume is proportional to the area under the box. **A,** Pure systolic heart failure. When contractility is impaired, the heart generates less pressure for any given end-diastolic volume (preload). The stroke volume is reduced. The body compensates by retaining salt and water, thus increasing left ventricular diastolic volume and stroke volume but at the expense of left ventricular diastolic pressure that causes pulmonary congestion. **B,** Pure diastolic heart failure. The left ventricle contractility curve is unchanged; however, the diastolic filling curve has been displaced upward. There is increased diastolic stiffness ("reduced compliance"), limiting the ability of the left ventricle to fill. For a given left ventricular filling pressure, the cardiac volume is smaller. To achieve adequate filling, left ventricular diastolic pressures must be increased (by retaining salt and water) into the range that produces pulmonary congestion. **C,** Both systolic and diastolic heart failure. Both the systolic and diastolic function curves have shifted, putting a big squeeze on stroke volume. The combination of these conditions produces marked elevation of filling pressures and low cardiac output.

Normal and Abnormal Diastolic Function

Diastole is a complex sequence of interrelated events.[3] The complexity is increased by our division of the cardiac cycle in different ways. When described hemodynamically, diastole is divided into four phases: isovolumic relaxation, early rapid filling, diastasis, and atrial systole. When describing muscle mechanics, there are only two important processes: active relaxation and passive stiffness. The hemodynamic description is more helpful for understanding how *to diagnose* diastolic dysfunction and the mechanical description is more helpful for understanding how *to treat* it.

The Four Hemodynamic Phases of Diastole: How Blood Flows into the Ventricle During Diastole

Diastole is divided into four hemodynamic phases: isovolumic relaxation, rapid filling, diastasis, and atrial systole. Doppler-echocardiography of mitral inflow velocities characterizes these phases quite well (Fig. 23-2).

The first phase is the isovolumic relaxation time (IVRT), which is the time between the closing of the aortic valve and the opening of the mitral valve. During this phase LV pressure falls rapidly, but no blood flows into the left ventricle, hence the term "isovolumic." The IVRT ends when LV pressure falls below left atrial pressure, the mitral valve flies open, and blood begins pouring into the left ventricle. This phase is very short, normally about 0.1 second. The IVRT is longer if relaxation is impaired. IVRT lasting more than 0.1 second suggests impaired relaxation caused by conditions such as hypertension or ischemia.

The second phase is early rapid filling. Doppler-echocardiography of LV inflow through the mitral valve measures this as an E wave. It begins the moment blood begins pouring from the left atrium into the left ventricle. Normally 80% of ventricular filling occurs at this time, but this may be reduced to 60% if relaxation is impaired.[4] This decreases the velocity of the E wave and

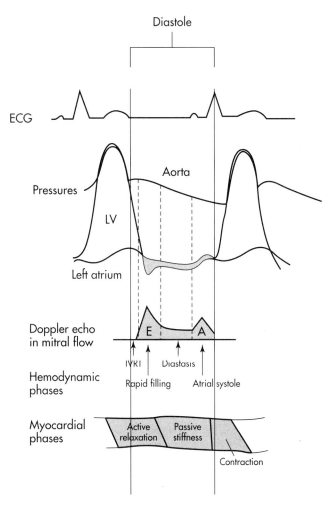

FIG. 23-2

Normal diastolic events. Flow across the mitral valve measured by Doppler- echocardiography defines the hemodynamic phases of diastole. The isovolumetric relaxation time *(IVRT)* begins with aortic valve closure and ends with mitral valve opening and the beginning of flow across the valve. Early rapid filling occurs as the left ventricular pressure falls below left atrial pressure; it is measured as the E wave on the Doppler tracing. Little flow occurs during diastasis, when the left atrial and left ventricular pressures equalize (note the pressure curve). Atrial systole pushes additional blood into the ventricle at the end of diastole (A wave). The myocardial phases illustrate the timing of active relaxation, passive stiffness, and contraction.

produces the characteristic E < A wave Doppler recordings of diastolic dysfunction caused by impaired relaxation (Fig. 23-3).

The third phase is diastasis and begins as left atrial and LV pressures equalize and rapid early filling ceases. During this phase little blood enters the ventricle and the ventricular volume increases only slightly. *The duration of diastasis is inversely related to heart rate.* As heart

rate increases, diastasis shortens and eventually disappears. The duration of the rest of the cardiac cycle changes little—it simply crowds out diastasis. This is not a problem in the normal heart. However, if filling is impaired, the loss of diastasis associated with tachycardia may lead to an insufficient time for filling. Slowing the heart rate in these patients is essential to improve filling and decrease dyspnea.

The final phase is atrial systole, generating the A wave on the Doppler tracing. The final pulse of blood acts to prime the LV pump. In the normal heart the left atrial kick is relatively unimportant, contributing less than 20% of total ventricular filling and raising stroke volume 10% to 15%. This is not essential for the performance of typical activities. However, that extra boost provided our ancestors with a distinct survival advantage when running to catch dinner or to avoid being dinner themselves. Those lacking this 20% atrial booster kick were severely penalized. With diastolic dysfunction the ventricle may depend on the atrial booster kick for as much as 40% of filling, raising stroke volume by 25% or more. The loss of the atrial booster kick, as with atrial fibrillation, can have devastating effects on cardiac function. To compensate for an abrupt drop in stroke volume and cardiac output, the kidneys retain salt and water, and pulmonary edema can rapidly ensue.

Active Relaxation and Passive Filling

Understanding the four hemodynamic phases of diastole is important for diagnosing diastolic dysfunction. However, the hemodynamic filling indices are only signs of the problem, like fever is a sign of infection. The problem is myocardial, either impaired relaxation, increased stiffness, or both.[3,5]

Ventricular Relaxation. Muscle relaxation begins long before diastole. It begins in mid systole, as the peak systolic pressure begins to fall, and it wanes about one third of the way through diastole. The process of relaxation is metabolically active. It "burns" adenosine triphosphate (ATP). Hydrolysis of ATP is necessary for pumping calcium from the cytosol back into storage in the sarcoplasmic reticulum. Without ATP the ventricle stays locked in a cramped, contracted state. If the cytosolic calcium concentration falls below a critical threshold, the calcium ions bound to the myofibrils are released from their binding sites, allowing the actin-myosin cross-bridges to release their hold on each other. This permits the myofibrils to slide back to their relaxed length.

The rate of relaxation depends on the rate at which calcium can be pumped into the sarcoplasmic reticulum. If ATP is scarce, as with ischemia, relaxation is slowed because calcium cannot be pumped out. If depolarization is delayed, by bundle branch block or ven-

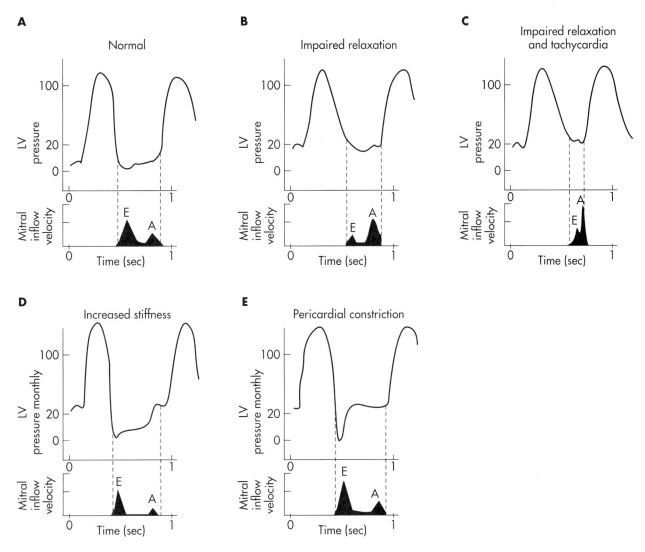

FIG. 23-3
The relationship between left ventricular pressure and mitral inflow velocity patterns.
A, Normal: rapid relaxation leads to a predominance of filling during early diastole
(E > A). Left ventricular end-diastolic pressure *(LVEDP)* is about 10 mm Hg. **B,** If relaxation is impaired, early filling is diminished and the E wave becomes smaller than
the A wave. LVEDP is elevated. A loss of atrial contraction (A wave) would substantially reduce ventricular filling. **C,** Tachycardia accentuates any problem with relaxation, the loss of diastasis leading to a summation of the E and A waves. The mitral
inflow velocities are even more elevated because the body must markedly elevate the
filling pressures (by retaining salt and water) to push enough blood into the ventricle
during the shortened diastole. LVEDP is elevated. **D,** "Pseudonormalization" of the
mitral flow pattern is possible when diastolic pressure is increased by elevated passive stiffness, as in a restrictive cardiomyopathy such as amyloidosis. The filling pressures are elevated, and the majority of the blood is pushed into the left ventricle during diastole. Although diastolic function is markedly abnormal, the E and A wave
ratios look deceptively normal; however, LVEDP is elevated. **E,** Pseudonormalization
of the E/A ratio when myocardial relaxation is normal, but filling is constrained by a
thickened, noncompliant pericardium. Again, the LVEDP is elevated.

tricular pacing, repolarization is delayed and relaxation is prolonged.

Passive Ventricular Stiffness. Active myocardial relaxation becomes less important and passive myocardial stiffness becomes more important as the early filling (E) wave finishes.[3] After the E wave, ventricular filling is determined primarily by the inherent stiffness of the myocardium and pericardial restraint.

The best way to describe the left ventricle's passive stiffness is to look at a diastolic pressure-volume curve (Fig. 23-4). This curve shows the two determinants of passive ventricular stiffness. The first determinant is volume—which moves you rightward and upward along the curve. It is analogous to stretching a rubber band. The more it is stretched, the stiffer it gets. The other determinant of the pressure-volume curve is the intrinsic stiffness of the ventricular muscle wall. Increased stiffness occurs when the ventricular wall becomes thickened with hypertrophy or when the elasticity of the wall is diminished by infiltration with collagen (from hypertrophy or infarction) or abnormal substances such as amyloid.

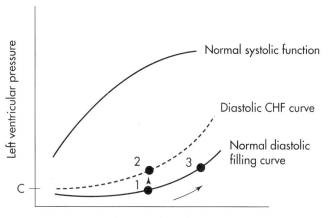

FIG. 23-4
Left ventricular end-diastolic pressure depends on two factors: left ventricular stiffness and ventricular volume. Increasing ventricular stiffness shifts the entire filling curve up (moving from position *1* to *2*). Increasing ventricular volume does not change the shape of the curve but does produce increased pressure (moving from position *1* to *3*). With enough volume overload, left ventricular diastolic pressure becomes high enough to force fluid from pulmonary capillaries into the interstitium *(C)*. At this point the patient has "congestive heart failure." Note that the diastolic function curve is curvilinear. When a volume-overloaded patient is at the far end of the curve, where it is steep, it is possible to greatly reduce filling pressure and therefore relieve congestion with just a small amount of diuresis or salt restriction or with venodilation (nitrates). Patients with diastolic dysfunction are thus "volume or preload sensitive."

MANAGEMENT
Steps in Making a Diagnosis
Step 1—Establish the Clinical Diagnosis of Congestive Heart Failure

Establishing the clinical diagnosis of CHF may not be as easy as it appears. Although the clinical diagnosis is straightforward in a patient who has dyspnea, rales, edema, and a chest x-ray showing cardiomegaly and pulmonary edema, most patients do not present like this. In actual practice up to 50% of heart failure diagnoses are incorrect.[6] Many misdiagnoses result from noncardiogenic causes of dyspnea that mimic CHF (Box 23-1). These alternative diagnoses must be ruled out. Given the morbidity and mortality associated with CHF, the initial clinical diagnosis should be confirmed with further testing.

Step 2—Measure the LVEF

Even if you are certain that a patient has heart failure by clinical examination, you cannot determine if it is systolic or diastolic CHF unless you measure the LVEF. This should be done at least once. No matter how good your history and physical examination, no matter how well you interpret the electrocardiogram (ECG) and chest x-ray, you cannot be certain[7] (Table 23-1). It does not matter how you measure the ejection fraction (Table 23-2), and precision is not critical. All you need to know is whether the LVEF is greater than or less than 40%. If your patient has CHF and an LVEF less than 40%, then your patient has systolic CHF and you need to treat it accordingly. On the other hand, if your patient has CHF and an LVEF greater than 40%, then you are dealing with diastolic CHF and you need to treat it differently.

BOX 23-1
NONCARDIAC CAUSES OF DYSPNEA AND EXERCISE INTOLERANCE

DISORDER	CAUSE OF DYSPNEA
Chest wall deformity	Inadequate ventilation
Obesity	Deconditioning/increased workload
Deconditioning	Poor muscle efficiency
Lung disease	Obstructive or restrictive lungs
Anemia	Low O_2-carrying capacity

The echocardiogram is the most useful noninvasive test for helping you assess both the LVEF and the cause of heart failure. In addition to obtaining the LVEF, a good echocardiogram can provide information on ventricular wall thickness, segmental wall motion, valvular function, and Doppler hemodynamics (see Chapter 8). These hemodynamic indices, discussed later, help establish the diagnosis of diastolic CHF. Unfortunately, the Achilles' heel of echocardiography is the poor image quality obtained in many patients, particularly those who are obese or emphysematous. If the echocardiogram is inadequate, obtain a radionuclide angiogram or go straight to cardiac catheterization.

Catheterization has both advantages and disadvantages. It allows a certain diagnosis of diastolic CHF. If the ventriculogram shows a normal LVEF and the LVEDP is elevated at rest or during exercise, this diagnosis is unquestionable. In addition, it can also demonstrate the presence of coronary artery disease (CAD) or valvular disease. We are especially inclined toward cardiac catheterization for patients with angina and heart failure (systolic or diastolic), which is an ominous combination, suggesting extensive CAD and a need for revascularization when feasible.

The principal disadvantage of cardiac catheterization is its invasiveness. The risk of a serious complication in a patient with compensated heart failure is about 0.1%. However, the risk of death from CHF within the next 12 months ranges from 10% to 50%, depending on the severity of the CHF. Keep these statistics in mind for patients with CHF who need catheterization. You may tell patients that there is a risk with cardiac catheterization, but that failing to make a correct diagnosis could be even riskier.

Step 3—Evaluate Noninvasive Indices of Filling: IVRT, E Wave, and A Wave

Left heart catheterization with direct measurement of the LVEDP may be the gold standard for diagnosing diastolic CHF, but it is impractical as a screening tool. Moreover, it may be unnecessary if your patient does not have angina and you can obtain a high-quality echocardiogram.

Doppler-echocardiography measures the velocity of blood flow in the heart. It is a routine part of a regular echocardiographic study and does not need to be ordered as a separate test (*although it helps to tell the echocardiographer that you are looking for diastolic dysfunction*). It can provide an excellent analysis of the four hemodynamic phases of diastole by measuring the inflow velocity pattern across the mitral valve during

Table 23-1 | *Clinical Similarity of Systolic and Diastolic Congestive Heart Failure*

	CHF Systolic	Diastolic
HISTORY		
Coronary artery disease	XX	X
Hypertension	X	XX
Diabetes	XX	X
Paroxysmal nocturnal dyspnea	X	XX
Acute decompensation	X	XX
PHYSICAL EXAMINATION		
Displaced PMI	XX	X
S₃ gallop	XX	X
S₄ gallop	X	XX
Mitral regurgitation	XX	X
Rales	XX	XX
Edema	XX	XX
Jugular venous distention	XX	XX
CHEST X-RAY		
Cardiomegaly	XX	X
Pulmonary congestion	XX	XX
ECG		
Left ventricular hypertrophy	X	XX
Q waves	XX	X

XX, Common; X, uncommon but still frequently present.

Table 23-2 | *Assessment of Left Ventricular Ejection Fraction*

	Advantages	Disadvantages
Echocardiography	Noninvasive Can evaluate wall thickness, left ventricular size, valves, wall motion, and diastolic function	Many patients cannot be imaged (poor windows)
Radionuclide angiography	Excellent LVEF measurement, noninvasive Virtually all patients can be imaged	Little information on cardiac structures or diastolic function
Cardiac catheterization	Excellent LVEF measurement and hemodynamic assessment	Invasive

diastole, especially the isovolumic relaxation time, the early rapid filling (E) wave, and the atrial filling (A) wave (see Fig. 23-3). Normally the isovolumic relaxation time is about 0.1 second, and the E wave is larger than the A wave. When relaxation is prolonged by ischemia or hypertension, the isovolumetric relaxation time is prolonged, early filling and the E wave are reduced, and the A wave is increased.

Regrettably, many factors affect these hemodynamic indices of filling. At times, patients with severe diastolic dysfunction can have a "pseudonormalized" pattern (E wave > A wave, see Fig. 23-3). A patient with diastolic dysfunction and the classic E < A pattern can have the filling pattern pseudonormalize if the preload becomes severely elevated by volume overload and congestion; blood is jammed into the ventricle during early diastole. Similarly, patients with increased passive stiffness may be unable to accept more blood at the end of diastole, making the E wave greater than the A wave. These "pseudonormalized" patterns can be difficult to distinguish from normal unless all the details of the case are properly integrated.[5] Other conditions that complicate the interpretation of the Doppler filling indices include aortic insufficiency, mitral regurgitation, and atrial fibrillation.

Radionuclide angiography has also been studied as a method to evaluate diastolic function by analyzing the time-activity curves of the radioactive counts in a cardiac chamber. These studies have shown that the diastolic phases of rapid filling, diastasis, and atrial filling can be identified and analyzed. However, this technique cannot reliably diagnose diastolic dysfunction in any individual patient, limiting its clinical usefulness to assessment of the LVEF.[8]

Step 4—If The Diagnosis Is Uncertain, Catheterize the Patient To Document an Elevated Left Ventricular End-Diastolic Pressure or Pulmonary Capillary Wedge Pressure

Nothing clinches a diagnosis like a gold standard test. If your patient has CHF symptoms and a normal LVEF and you cannot obtain a good echocardiogram, or if symptoms are not improving with appropriate therapy, do the catheterization.

Some patients with dyspnea and a normal LVEF may not have heart failure. Cardiac catheterization reveals normal filling pressures at rest and during exercise, ruling out diastolic dysfunction. Excluding disease is invaluable, since it properly redirects diagnostic efforts, redefines prognosis, and avoids the cost and adverse effects of unnecessary medications.

Cardiac catheterization can be helpful in patients who have recurrent diastolic heart failure but a relatively benign physical examination and few symptoms at the time of your evaluation. During cardiac catheterization their resting filling pressures may be relatively

normal. However, with exercise the filling pressures rise dramatically. This dramatic exertional rise in filling pressures may be the only evidence that diastolic CHF is the cause of symptoms.

An occasional patient with diastolic CHF has chronically elevated filling pressures at rest but no pulmonary rales and no congestion on chest x-ray. He or she may still have dyspnea with exertion and improve with diuresis. Right heart catheterization documents elevated LV filling pressures and confirms the diagnosis of diastolic heart failure.

Determining the Cause of Diastolic Congestive Heart Failure

In general, one third of patients with heart failure have diastolic CHF. However, the prevalence of diastolic heart failure is higher among elderly patients, especially women (Table 23-3). Ischemia, hypertrophy, and fibrosis are the usual underlying pathologic processes for ventricular diastolic dysfunction. The common diseases that produce these pathologic changes are CAD, systemic hypertension, diabetes mellitus, and aortic stenosis.

Age has important effects on diastolic function. Just like knees and backs, the normal ventricle stiffens with age, worsening diastolic function. This results in decreased early diastolic ventricular filling (E wave) and increased atrial systolic filling (A wave). Diastolic function in the elderly is also frequently impaired by hypertension or aortic stenosis, both causes of LV hypertrophy. Many elderly persons have subclinical impairment of ventricular diastolic function and are predisposed to developing overt diastolic CHF in the setting of ischemia, sustained tachycardia, atrial fibrillation, anemia, episodes of elevated blood pressure, or volume overload.

Table 23-3	Percentage of Congestive Heart Failure (CHF) due to Diastolic CHF According to Clinical Site, Patient Age, and Gender

Location	Age	Gender
Tertiary referral: 25%	60 years: 10%	Male: 25%
Community hospital: 33%	70 years: 30%	Female: 50%
Nursing home: 50%	80 years: 50%	

Prognosis

The annual mortality for patients with heart failure and preserved LVEF ranges from 1.3% to 17.5%, averaging about 5%.[7] Mortality is highest in the elderly and in those with concomitant CAD. These figures are better than those for patients with systolic CHF but not as good as for age-matched controls. To put these mortality figures into perspective, the 5-year mortality for systolic CHF is about 50%, for diastolic CHF about 25%, and for age-matched controls about 5%.

Treatment

Therapy for *systolic* CHF is based on multicenter, placebo-controlled trials, allowing well-substantiated evidence-based therapy. No analogous studies have been performed on patients with diastolic CHF. Hence management cannot be guided by evidence-based medicine but rather by information derived from small clinical trials, clinical experience, and knowledge of the pathophysiology of diastolic function.

The goal of treatment is to improve exercise tolerance by reducing pulmonary congestion and improving left ventricular filling. The following six strategies may accomplish this:

1. Reduce preload
2. Treat hypertension and left ventricular hypertrophy
3. Treat ischemia
4. Reduce heart rate
5. Maintain atrial booster function
6. Avoid digoxin and arterial vasodilators

Reduce Preload and Congestion

Dyspnea, orthopnea, and paroxysmal nocturnal dyspnea caused by pulmonary venous congestion usually can be effectively relieved with gentle diuresis. The importance of education about salt restriction cannot be overemphasized. Good dietary instructions about a salt-restricted diet given by a nurse or dietician can often reduce costly middle-of-the-night emergency room visits. It is often not enough to simply tell the patient to watch his or her salt intake; you have to inform both the patient and the cook which foods contain salt and explain why salt needs to be avoided.

A compliant patient doing everything right—takes medicine precisely as directed, records daily weight, and removes the salt shaker from the table—innocently eats pickles just before pulmonary edema "inexplicably" develops. It's not simply knowing that salt is bad; it's also knowing which foods contain salt.

Since hearts with diastolic dysfunction have a steep pressure-volume curve, small doses of diuretics often produce marked reductions in filling pressures (see Fig. 23-4). Although many patients require larger doses of diuretics, it is important to titrate the dose carefully, because too much diuresis may precipitate hypotension. A good starting dose in relatively stable patients is 12.5 to 25 mg/day of hydrochlorothiazide or 20 mg of furosemide once or twice daily.

Nitrates also can help by producing venodilation and reducing ischemia. Isosorbide dinitrate can be started at 5 to 10 mg tid in most patients. These doses may need to be titrated up relatively quickly in patients with marked hypertension or in those hospitalized for CHF.

Treat Hypertension and Reduce Hypertrophy

Lowering blood pressure has an immediate benefit. In a normal heart, an acute increase in afterload elicits a compensatory rise in contractility and accelerates relaxation, but this does not occur with diastolic CHF. Relaxation is slowed in diastolic CHF, and excessive afterload caused by hypertension slows relaxation even further. The reason for this may be that the function of the sarcoplasmic reticulum is impaired and cytosolic calcium resequestration is slowed. However, lowering blood pressure can rapidly improve left ventricular relaxation in patients with diastolic heart failure.

Over the longer run, reducing pressure leads to the regression of left ventricular hypertrophy. Myocardial hypertrophy can be adaptive, as thickening the wall normalizes wall stress according to the law of Laplace (see Chapter 2). However, this increases myocardial oxygen demand and can be associated with reduced myocardial blood flow reserve. Although a little hypertrophy may improve systolic function without adversely affecting function in well-trained athletes, pathologic myocardial hypertrophy impairs diastolic filling.

Several antihypertensive agents are known to reduce left ventricular mass, including ACE inhibitors, calcium channel blockers, centrally acting sympatholytic agents, and beta-blockers.

A growing body of evidence suggests that excessive deposition of collagen is important in the pathogenesis of diastolic CHF.[3] The recently introduced concept of remodeling has emphasized the potential use of so-called remodeling drugs to prevent or cause the regression of cardiac fibrosis. However, regression of myocardial collagen content seems to occur more slowly than regression of myocyte hypertrophy.

Various ACE inhibitors and aldosterone inhibitors appear to be the most efficient remodeling drugs currently available. Although no currently available drugs selectively inhibit collagen deposition or promote its reabsorption, several molecules designed to degrade or digest it are being studied. The theoretical goal is to optimize the ratio of the amount of collagen III to the amount of contractile protein. However, the clinical applicability and benefits of these experimental agents remain unproven.

Treat Ischemia

Chronic subendocardial ischemia at rest or with exertion impairs myocardial relaxation and may contribute to cell dropout and replacement fibrosis. Both improving myocardial blood flow and decreasing heart rate reduces ischemia (see Chapter 13). We favor drugs that lower the heart rate when treating angina pectoris in a patient with suspected diastolic dysfunction.

Revascularization therapy for CAD improves left ventricular diastolic relaxation and filling in patients with severe coronary stenosis. Because of the salutary effects of revascularization on symptoms and survival in selected patients, it is important to exclude CAD when there is unexplained diastolic dysfunction. This is especially true when there is angina, but remember that silent ischemia is common in elderly patients and those with diabetes.

Reduce Heart Rate to about 60 to 70 Beats/Minute

Since the duration of systole is relatively constant at all heart rates, tachycardia occurs at the expense of diastole. Tachycardia can have devastating effects on patients with prolonged filling caused by diastolic dysfunction. Slowing the heart rate can reduce pulmonary venous congestion by providing more time for relaxation and filling, allowing the heart to fill more completely at lower filling pressures. Because of these effects, beta-adrenergic blocking agents, calcium channel blocking agents, and (occasionally when the patient is in atrial fibrillation) digitalis have all successfully improved exercise tolerance in patients with diastolic heart failure and tachycardia.[3]

Maintain Atrial Booster Function (Sinus Rhythm)

Maintenance of a properly timed atrial contraction is important, so every effort must be made to preserve or restore normal sinus rhythm (for those with atrial fibrillation or flutter) and to maintain atrioventricular synchrony. Since loss of atrial contraction caused by atrial fibrillation can precipitate diastolic heart failure, cardioversion can produce rapid symptomatic improvement.

Avoid Inotropes and Pure Arterial Dilators

Digoxin acts as an inotropic agent by increasing intracellular calcium. Because excess intracellular calcium causes abnormal left ventricular relaxation, digoxin therapy may be counterproductive. The one instance in which it may be helpful is atrial fibrillation, where it may be needed to control the heart rate. However, heart rate can usually be controlled with a combination of beta-blockers and calcium channel blockers, and they are the first choice.

Potent vasodilators, such as hydralazine, may be detrimental. With diastolic dysfunction, these agents lower blood pressure without increasing cardiac output. This drug-induced hypotension is associated with reflex tachycardia and fluid retention caused by reflex sympathetic activation. These agents should be reserved for patients who remain markedly hypertensive despite treatment with beta-blockers, calcium channel blockers, diuretics, and nitrates.

No drugs safely and selectively enhance relaxation. Interestingly, catecholamines enhance the rate of left ventricular relaxation by increasing intracellular cyclic adenosine monophosphate (AMP). They also increase contractility, and it is hard to imagine using them when the left ventricle is hyperdynamic. There has been no study of the efficacy of these agents in diastolic CHF, and the tendency of these drugs to cause serious arrhythmias in heart failure patients may limit their long-term usefulness.

General Treatment Strategy

Specific treatment goals for diastolic CHF depend on how severely affected the patient is and which of the six problem areas (outlined earlier) need to be addressed. In general, five classes of medications are useful for the treatment of diastolic heart failure (Table 23-4).

Patients who have severe diastolic dysfunction or who come to the emergency department with florid pulmonary edema appreciate initial intravenous diuresis and venodilation with nitrates. Sublingual nitroglycerin may be given in the emergency department while waiting for intravenous access. This often provides some relief from congestive symptoms within minutes of administration, even when the patient does not have myocardial ischemia.

More stable patients, with only exertional dyspnea, likely benefit from therapy that controls blood pressure and exercise heart rate, either beta-blockers or rate-lowering calcium channel blockers. If heart rate and blood pressure have been controlled, the addition of nitrates and diuretics can help relieve congestion. Metoprolol is our initial choice of beta-blocker because it is relatively inexpensive. Start at 50 orally bid and increase to 200 orally bid. Carvedilol is a newer beta-blocking agent with alpha-blocking capability as well. It is also quite effective in decreasing blood pressure and heart rate, but it is expensive. The primary use for carvedilol is CHF caused by systolic dysfunction, not diastolic dysfunction. It has no specific advantage for diastolic heart failure.

The use of rate-lowering calcium channel blockers is also an excellent way to lower blood pressure and control the heart rate. Diltiazem is usually well tolerated. The starting dose is 30 mg qid of the generic or 60 mg bid of the extended-release form. It can be titrated up to 360 mg/day. Verapamil is also good and has an even greater rate-lowering effect. The starting dose of the generic form is 40 mg tid, titrated to 480 mg/day. Several extended-release forms are available.

Table 23-4	Drugs Used To Treat Diastolic Heart Failure			

	Positive Effects	Negative Effects	Indications	Contraindications
Beta-blockers Metoprolol 50-200 mg bid Atenolol 50-200 mg qd	Treat ischemia Slow heart rate Lower BP	Do not dilate coronaries	*After Q wave MI* Ischemia Hypertension HCM	Lung disease Brittle diabetes ?Depression Bradycardia
Rate-lowering calcium channel blockers Diltiazem 30-90 mg qid Verapamil 80-160 mg tid	Treat ischemia Slow heart rate	May theoretically slow relaxation	Ischemia Hypertension HCM	Bradycardia
Nitrate Isosorbide dinitrate 5-40 mg tid	Treats ischemia Venodilator (decreases congestion)	Headaches	Ischemia Congestion	Hypotension
Diuretics HCTZ 12.5-25 mg qd Furosemide 20-120 mg/day	Decrease congestion Lower BP	Hypotension Dehydration	Congestive symptoms Hypertension	Hypotension Dehydration
ACE inhibitors Captopril 6.25-100 mg tid Enalapril 2.5-20 mg bid	Lower BP Promote remodeling	Cough	Hypertension Hypertrophy	Renal artery stenosis Hyperkalemia Angioedema
Other antihypertensive agents	Lower BP	Hypotension	Continued hy- pertension after above agents maximized	Normotensive diastolic dysfunction

HCM, Hypertrophic cardiomyopathy; *HCTZ,* hydrochlorothiazide; *BP,* blood pressure.

In an asymptomatic patient with diastolic dysfunction and hypertension, the appropriate approach is control of hypertension (see Chapter 31).

SPECIFIC CLINICAL ISSUES
Restrictive Cardiomyopathy versus Constrictive Pericarditis

Restrictive cardiomyopathies and constrictive pericarditis can result in the clinical syndrome of diastolic CHF. Restrictive cardiomyopathy may result from endocardial abnormalities (e.g., pseudoxanthoma elasticum, Loeffler's endocarditis, or endomyocardial fibrosis) or myocardial infiltration (amyloid, sarcoid, hemochromatosis, connective tissue disease, cardiac transplant rejection, or diabetes mellitus).

Endomyocardial fibrosis is endemic in tropical countries and practically never seen in the United States. Idiopathic familial restrictive cardiomyopathy is suggested by a positive family history and the presence of associated skeletal myopathic characteristics. Amyloid infiltra-

tion should be considered in diastolic CHF patients with left ventricular hypertrophy demonstrated by echocardiogram and low voltages on ECG, especially if they also have peripheral neuropathy or digestive problems. Hemochromatosis is suggested by bronze skin and diabetes and can be detected by an elevated ferritin or iron/TIBC ratio.

Constrictive pericarditis must also be considered in patients with CHF and a normal LVEF, particularly if an echocardiogram shows no evidence of hypertrophy. Differentiating constrictive pericarditis from restrictive cardiomyopathy is challenging. It often requires an echocardiogram, left and right heart catheterization, computed tomography (CT) or magnetic resonance imaging (MRI) scan to evaluate pericardial thickness, and a room full of cardiologists and cardiothoracic surgeons studying the data.

In both conditions the ventricular cavity is normal or small, and biatrial enlargement may be present. Constrictive pericarditis is suggested by the presence of pericardial thickening (more than 4 mm on CT or MRI), pericardial calcium, normal ventricular wall thickness, a dilated inferior vena cava that remains unchanged with forceful inspiration, and pronounced respiratory variations of the transmitral inflow velocities. Although this condition is rare, it is important to diagnose because it is surgically curable.

Features that favor the possibility of a restrictive cardiomyopathy include thick ventricular walls, thickened cardiac valves, and interatrial septum. The echocardiographic myocardial texture may be abnormal. Doppler-echocardiography shows an absence of respiratory variation in transmitral flow velocities and the presence of atrioventricular valve regurgitation. Ventricular systolic function may be normal or mildly depressed.

If you suspect either a restrictive cardiomyopathy or constrictive pericarditis, refer your patient to a cardiologist for further evaluation. The diagnosis is challenging and the treatment options both risky and potentially curative. It is not unusual to send a patient to surgery for a pericardial stripping procedure and, with thoracotomy, find that the correct diagnosis is cardiomyopathy.

Hypertrophic Cardiomyopathy

Hypertrophic cardiomyopathy (HCM) is uncommon but important because of its hereditary transmission and association with sudden death in young athletic patients. The hallmark of HCM is an increase in left ventricle mass and wall thickness in the absence of an increase in external cardiac work (e.g., hypertension or aortic stenosis). The hypertrophy may be either concentric or asymmetric. Inheritance is autosomal dominant in half of these patients, with different families demonstrating different genetic defects of the contractile proteins. The identification of the particular genetic defect is potentially important for genetic counseling of family members at risk, since the prognosis appears to vary depending on the particular genetic defect. HCM is one of the few conditions associated with advanced paternal age. Because of its rarity and prognostic variability, patients with HCM should be referred to a cardiologist. In general, patients with nonobstructive HCM should be treated according to the same general guidelines already described.

Hypertrophic Obstructive Cardiomyopathy

Patients with HCM and outflow obstruction represent a special case. This condition is called by many names: hypertrophic obstructive cardiomyopathy (HOCM), asymmetric septal hypertrophy (ASH), or idiopathic hypertrophic subaortic stenosis (IHSS). Outflow tract obstruction is caused by a number of interacting mechanisms; hypertrophy of the proximal septum "crowds" the outflow tract, reducing its dimension. The size and length of the mitral leaflets are often increased, and the leaflet is often anteriorly displaced into the outflow tract. Hyperdynamic left ventricular ejection with a high-velocity jet pulls the mitral leaflets toward the ventricular septum (the Venturi effect), contributing to obstruction.

The clinical syndrome is more complicated than simple diastolic dysfunction. Outflow tract obstruction provokes ventricular hypertrophy, worsening diastolic CHF. Angina pectoris is common and is more likely if there is a large outflow tract gradient. Arrhythmias also may occur, and HOCM is one of the causes of sudden death in apparently healthy young people.

Echocardiography demonstrates septal hypertrophy and systolic anterior motion (SAM) of the anterior leaflet of the mitral valve. The Doppler study measures the outflow tract pressure gradient.

Medical therapy for patients with HOCM includes calcium channel blockers, beta-blockers, and disopyramide. All these agents depress contractility and therefore reduce outflow tract obstruction, and calcium channel and beta-blockers lower heart rate, improving diastolic function. Verapamil, nifedipine, and diltiazem improve both noninvasive and invasive indexes of diastolic dysfunction, but nifedipine is our last choice because it is a more potent vasodilator. Half of the asymptomatic patients with HOCM have thallium perfusion defects with exercise, and verapamil has been found to correct them. Verapamil also improves congestive symptoms. Beta-blockers are more likely to improve angina than exertional dyspnea. Many patients who obtain little improvement with beta-blockers are better while taking verapamil, and verapamil has become our first choice. All the medicines work by lowering heart rate and reducing contractility, thus improving myocardial oxygen supply-demand. No evidence has demonstrated a direct myocardial relaxing effect with drug therapy.[9] We believe that reducing the outflow tract gradient, improving diastolic function, and controlling symptoms with medical therapy also lower the risk of sudden death, but there are no data from clinical trials to support this approach.

The risk of sudden death is higher in younger patients (15 to 35 years old), in those with greater degrees of left ventricular hypertrophy, and when there is a family history of sudden death. Syncope or nonsustained ventricular tachycardia (NSVT) on an ambulatory monitor indicate a bad prognosis. For this reason, consider ambulatory monitoring for high-risk patients. Amiodarone may reduce the mortality risk for those with NSVT, but no randomized studies have been done.[10]

For patients refractory to medical therapy, some success has been achieved with myotomyectomy, wherein a large section of the enlarged septum is surgically resected. Unfortunately, it is technically difficult surgery. Results have been mixed, and the surgery is currently performed in relatively few centers.

Dual-chamber pacing appeared to help some patients with dynamic left ventricular obstruction. However, the only randomized trial of pacing failed to show a benefit. Another new technique is catheter ablation of the septum. An angioplasty-type catheter is advanced into the septal perforating arteries of the thickened septum, and a small dose of alcohol is injected, which causes myocardial necrosis and septal thinning.

Hypertrophic cardiomyopathy "burns out" in 10% to 15% of patients who develop left ventricular dilation, hypokinesis, and thinning of the ventricular wall. The outflow tract gradient may disappear. They have essentially developed dilated cardiomyopathy with systolic dysfunction and are treated accordingly (see Chapter 22).

AMERICAN HEART ASSOCIATION/ AMERICAN COLLEGE OF CARDIOLOGY PRACTICE GUIDELINES FOR EVALUATING DIASTOLIC DYSFUNCTION (A SUMMARY)

Doppler echocardiography or radionuclide imaging is of value in assessing systolic function and detecting diastolic dysfunction; the latter by measuring indexes of the rate of diastolic filling. Alternatively, cardiac catheterization may be used and may be of particular value when noninvasive studies are nondiagnostic. Unless another diagnosis has been established, most of these patients should be evaluated for underlying coronary artery disease and myocardial ischemia. Noninvasive testing to detect coronary artery disease may be used as in patients with systolic dysfunction. Alternatively, one could proceed directly to cardiac catheterization/coronary arteriography (1) when there is a high suspicion of occlusive coronary artery disease as the cause of the diastolic heart failure (e.g., presence of angina or previous myocardial infarction) and is potentially treatable by revascularization, (2) when the possibility of occlusive coronary artery disease cannot be reliably or safely assessed by other methods, and (3) when a patient with two or more risk factors for coronary atherosclerosis is slated to undergo cardiac surgery for what is believed to be the primary cause of the diastolic heart failure (e.g., aortic stenosis). Constrictive pericarditis, a surgically treatable condition, must be excluded in patients whose diastolic dysfunction appears to be secondary to a restrictive cardiomyopathy; in this setting, echocardiography, computerized tomography, or MRI or the finding of significant myocardial pathology by endomyocardial biopsy (e.g., myocardial amyloidosis, hemochromatosis) can be very helpful in guiding management.

REFERENCES

1. Ho KKL, Anderson KM, Kannel WB, et al: Survival after the onset of congestive heart failure in Framingham Heart Study subjects, *Circulation* 88:107, 1993.
2. Gaasch WH: Diagnosis and treatment of heart failure based on left ventricular systolic or diastolic dysfunction, *JAMA* 271:1276, 1994.
3. Brutsaert DL, Sys SU, Gillebert TC: Diastolic failure: pathophysiology and therapeutic implications, *J Am Coll Cardiol* 22:318, 1993.
4. Goldsmith SR, Dick C: Differentiating systolic from diastolic heart failure: pathophysiologic and therapeutic considerations, *Am J Med* 95:645, 1993.
5. Nishimura RA, Tajik AJ: Evaluation of diastolic filling of left ventricle in health and disease: Doppler echocardiography is the clinician's Rosetta stone, *J Am Coll Cardiol* 30:8, 1997.
6. Vasan RS, Benjamin EJ, Levy D: Congestive heart failure with normal left ventricular systolic function: clinical approaches to the diagnosis and treatment of diastolic heart failure, *Arch Intern Med* 156:146, 1996.
7. Vasan RS, Benjamin EJ, Levy D: Prevalence, clinical features, and prognosis of diastolic heart failure: an epidemiologic perspective, *J Am Coll Cardiol* 26:1565, 1995.
8. Spencer KT, Lange RM: Diastolic heart failure: what primary care physicians need to know, *Postgrad Med* 101:63, 1997.
9. Lenihan DJ, Gerson MD, Hoit BD, Walsh RA: Mechanisms, diagnosis and treatment of diastolic heart failure, *Am Heart J* 130:153, 1995.
10. McKenna WJ, Oakley CM, Krikler DM, et al: Improved survival with amiodarone in patients with hypertrophic cardiomyopathy and ventricular tachycardia, *Br Heart J* 53:412, 1985.

24

Cardiomyopathy and Cardiac Muscle Disease

Stephen H. Jennison
Barbara A. Mulch

DILATED CARDIOMYOPATHY

Epidemiology

Disease of the heart muscle, as distinct from valvular, coronary, pericardial, or congenital heart disease, was recognized as early as 1891. In the latter half of this century the term *primary myocardial disease* was introduced, with *primary* subsequently being designated to idiopathic afflictions of the heart muscle, as distinguished from diseases of other organ systems that affect the heart secondarily. According to the World Health Organization (WHO) definition, heart muscle disease secondary to specific causes or disease entities (e.g., thiamine deficiency, hemochromatoses, amyloidosis, or muscular dystrophy) are no longer included among the cardiomyopathies.[1] However, the similar clinical presentations and therapeutic problems have led to widespread continuation of the use of the term *cardiomyopathy* for such cases, especially the frequently encountered entity of congestive heart failure secondary to chronic ischemic heart disease, generally referred to as *ischemic cardiomyopathy.*

In developed countries the annual incidence of cardiomyopathy ranges from 0.7 to 7.5 cases per 100,000 population, and about 1% of cardiac deaths in the United States are attributed to cardiomyopathy. The mortality is twice as high for males and twice as high for blacks. It is generally believed that dilated cardiomyopathy constitutes greater than 90% of all cardiomyopathies encountered.

Pathophysiology

The original concept that most idiopathic cardiomyopathies are attributable to a single specific cause has been discarded. More than 75 specific heart muscle diseases may cause dilated cardiomyopathy, and it is now apparent that this is a multifactorial disease. Contributing pathogenetic mechanisms include genetic susceptibility, metabolic disturbances, hormonal imbalances, toxins, calcium overload, altered vascular reactivity, hypoxia, free radicals, infection, and immune and autoimmune processes.

Table 24-1 classifies the cardiomyopathies as dilated (congestive), nondilated (restrictive), or hypertrophic. This classification is based on simple clinicophysiologic principles, especially those related to the predominant mechanism by which each type produces heart failure.

The entity "dilated cardiomyopathy" is characterized by a reduction in left ventricular ejection fraction (LVEF). The diseases that cause cardiac impairment principally through the effect on systolic contractility do not cause heart failure unless LVEF falls below 40%. This specificity of the designation (dilated cardiomyopathy) is enhanced by insisting that LVEF be 40% before the designation is applied. Heart failure occurs because impairment of LVEF requires that the left ventricle dilate (Starling mechanism) to mitigate the fall in stroke volume that would otherwise occur. With increased diastolic volume, left atrial and left ventricular (LV) diastolic pressures rise. The degree to which the left atrial pressure is elevated depends on the degree of LV dilation (which is influenced by a number of factors, including dietary sodium intake, the effect of diuretic drugs, and the presence or absence of anemia, hypoxemia, or obesity) and on the passive pressure-volume relation of the left ventricle, or LV compliance (concepts that are explained more completely in Chapters 2, 22, and 23). LV dilation and a greatly reduced LVEF are more constant features of dilated cardiomyopathy than is decreased cardiac output or elevated left atrial pressure.

Right ventricular (RV) failure may follow LV failure. It is still not understood why biventricular heart failure develops in some patients and only left heart failure exists in others. Pulmonary vascular resistance is elevated in a few patients with dilated cardiomyopathy, but RV failure is not limited to patients whose pulmonary vascular resistance is elevated, as it is in patients with mitral or aortic stenosis.

Clinical Presentation and Course

The early symptoms of congestive heart failure (CHF) have been described (see Chapters 3 and 22). Dyspnea is the usual symptom of left atrial hypertension and pulmonary congestion. However, it may be overshadowed by fatigue or a nonspecific decline in exercise tolerance and vigor in the early stages of the illness.

A common physical finding is resting tachycardia. Mitral regurgitation is present in as many as two thirds of patients with dilated cardiomyopathy but is usually

Table 24-1	Classification of the Cardiomyopathies			
Classification	**LVDV**	**LVEF**	**Mechanism Of Heart Failure**	
Dilated (congestive)	Increased	<40%	Impaired systolic contractility	
Nondilated (restrictive)	Decreased or normal	30% to 70%	Compliance abnormality	
Hypertrophic	Decreased or normal	45% to 95%	Compliance abnormality	

LVDV, Left ventricular diastolic volume; *LVEF,* left ventricular ejection fraction.

mild or moderate. The most definitive auscultatory finding is a third heart sound or a summation gallop, one of which is virtually always present if heart failure exists.

The course and prognosis of dilated cardiomyopathy are a function of how early the diagnosis is made. Significant cardiomegaly, low cardiac output, and frank CHF are associated with a poor prognosis. The severity of histopathologic abnormalities correlates inversely with life expectancy, with cardiac hypertrophy having a favorable affect on prognosis, presumably by limiting systolic wall stress. (Increased LV thickness on an echocardiogram suggests a better prognosis than a thin-walled left ventricle despite equivalent LVEF values.) The presence of etiologic or contributory factors that can be eliminated, for example, ethanol, thiamine deficiency, hypertension, anemia, and thyrotoxicosis, also may affect the prognosis favorably.

Causes of Dilated Cardiomyopathy

Rare causes of dilated cardiomyopathy are outlined in Box 24-1. For the most part, they do not cause heart failure in the absence of other manifestations of the underlying disease. They account for a small percentage of patients with CHF, and more common illnesses that cause or aggravate heart failure are reviewed later.

Heredity

The familial occurrence of dilated cardiomyopathy is best known in the specific heart muscle diseases associated with hereditary disorders such as glycogen storage diseases, Fabry's disease, muscular dystrophy, and Friedreich's ataxia. Recently, X-linked autosomal dominant and autosomal recessive inheritance patterns of dilated cardiomyopathy have been reported. The use of echocardiography in systematic surveys of relatives of patients with dilated cardiomyopathy promises to reveal a familial prevalence much more frequently than suspected. Although not well documented in the literature, we have

observed familial clustering of alcoholic cardiomyopathy, suggesting a genetic susceptibility to cardiotoxins.

Thiamine Deficiency

Thiamine deficiency may cause "wet" beriberi. In this case "wet" refers to pulmonary congestion, and dry beriberi would be the deficiency syndrome without CHF (peripheral neuropathy or the Wernicke-Korsakoff syndrome). It is caused by dietary deficiency of thiamine or vitamin B1, a coenzyme essential to the decarboxylation of alpha ketoacids, a part of the hexose monophosphate shunt. In the absence of thiamine, oxidative phosphorylation, and hence myocardial energy production, is impaired.

Clinically, thiamine deficiency first manifests as a high output state, secondary to peripheral vasodilation, at least in part attributable to the accumulation of intermediate carbohydrate metabolites. With high output there is increased preload. The depressed myocardial function in the face of increased preload and wall stress leads to CHF, first in the presence of normal to high cardiac output and later in association with a low output state.[2] Undoubtedly, peripheral vasodilation delays the onset of LV failure. Indeed, the administration of thiamine reverses the peripheral vasodilation and has been reported to precipitate LV failure. A similar protective role of naturally occurring LV unloading by peripheral vasodilation is seen in hyperthyroidism and in cirrhosis of the liver.

Thiamine deficiency may aggravate cardiomyopathy caused by other illnesses. Be aware of this possibility in an elderly patient who has a poor diet.

Chronic diuretic therapy may cause thiamine deficiency. The mechanism of thiamine wasting is uncertain. We are reluctant to treat all patients taking diuretics with thiamine because there is no evidence-based support for it, and advanced CHF necessitates a large medicine load without adding more. But think of this

```
┌─────────────────────────────────────┐
│              BOX 24-1               │
│       RARE CAUSES OF DILATED        │
│            CARDIOMYOPATHY           │
├─────────────────────────────────────┤
```

Tuberculosis	Dermatomyositis
Endocardial	Selenium deficiency
fibroelastosis	Acromegaly
Cobalt poisoning	Glycogen storage
Lead poisoning	disease
Phosphorus	Fabry's disease
poisoning	Osteogenesis
High-dose	imperfecta
combination	Systemic carnitine
chemotherapy	deficiency
Combination	Acute leukemia
antituberculous	Duchenne's muscular
drugs	dystrophy
Sulfonamide	Myotonic dystrophy
Amphetamine	Fibrocystic disease
Heroin	Chronic tachycardia
Irradiation	Scleroderma
Systemic lupus	Dermatomyositis
erythematosus	Wegener's
Rheumatoid arthritis	granulomatosis
Acute rheumatic	Peripartum
fever	cardiomyopathy
Scleroderma	Hemochromatosis

possibility in a frail person who has been taking diuretics for some time, particularly if there is evidence for poor nutrition. Serum thiamine levels may be measured but do not reflect tissue levels. A therapeutic trial may be considered if symptoms of CHF are worsening. The maximum amount that may be absorbed is 2.5 to 5 mg thiamine per day. Many adult multivitamins contain 1.5 mg thiamine, which may or may not be enough to prevent deficiency.

Obesity-Induced Cardiomyopathy

It is now well established that morbidly obese individuals (i.e., body weight approximately 135 kg or more) may develop a syndrome of chronic circulatory congestion associated with diastolic and sometimes systolic LV dysfunction (see Chapter 43). Its pathologic, physiologic, and clinical features appear sufficiently distinctive to warrant classification as obesity heart muscle disease or cardiomyopathy. Regional blood flow with marked obesity is characterized by a significant increase to adipose tissue, a modest increase to the splanchnic vascular bed, and little change in flow to other organs. This results in high cardiac output at

rest in absolute terms and is directly related to the incremental increase in body oxygen consumption. Indices of LV systolic performance such as ejection fraction may be normal or depressed.

The prevalence of CHF in extremely obese subjects is about 10%. Body weight is usually twice the predicted norm, and rapid weight gain may precipitate or exacerbate congestive symptoms. Progressively increasing dyspnea and orthopnea are characteristic, whereas acute pulmonary edema is uncommon. Significant weight loss in subjects with marked obesity may result in favorable hemodynamic alterations and a reduction in chamber size and LV hypertrophy. The decrement in body oxygen consumption, blood volume, and cardiac output are proportional to the amount of weight loss. If previously impaired, ejection fraction may improve with weight loss.

Sleep Apnea and Obesity Hypoventilation Syndrome

Although sleep apnea occurs in various clinical settings, somewhat more than 50% of patients so afflicted are obese. They are usually men, 40 to 60 years of age, with degrees of obesity varying from moderate to extreme. Daytime hypersomnia is frequent. Significant increases in systemic and pulmonary artery pressures occur during apnea, and with a rapid succession of apneic spells there may be a progressive rise in both. Cardiac arrhythmias are frequent during apnea involving sinus arrest, asystole up to 6 seconds, heart block, and ventricular tachycardia. All of the hemodynamic and arrhythmic effects induced by sleep apnea may be reversed in some cases by tracheostomy, and when hypertension coexists, blood pressure may fall toward normal.

Chronic hypoxemia and hypercapnia stimulate pulmonary vasoconstriction, so the effects of augmented pulmonary vascular resistance are superimposed on the underlying hemodynamic derangements of severe obesity, specifically, increased circulating blood volume and flow with systemic hypertension. Hypoventilation is reversible with weight reduction, and the attendant improvement in arterial blood gas levels is accompanied by a fall in pulmonary artery pressure and a reduction or elimination of the transpulmonary diastolic pressure gradient.

When an obese patient develops cardiomyopathy, the potential reversibility of sleep apnea makes it important to consider. It is especially important for those with biventricular failure, who may have pulmonary hypertension. Pulmonary heart disease is reviewed in Chapter 35.

Toxins and Drugs
Alcoholic Cardiomyopathy

Depression of myocardial function by chronic intake of ethanol has been demonstrated in humans and in experimental animals. Considerable evidence favors a view that other factors may be required for full expression of the clinical syndrome of dilated cardiomyopathy associated with alcoholism, including genetic predisposition, malnutrition, infection, and other toxins. Clinically, the identification of a history of alcoholism in a patient with dilated cardiomyopathy is important, since the prognosis may improve with abstention.

Impaired diastolic relaxation of the left ventricle by echo-Doppler appears to be an early, preclinical manifestation of alcoholic cardiomyopathy. There may be LV hypertrophy with increased wall thickness and normal LV diameter. Finally, there is progression to LV dilation. The type of beverage consumed does not appear to be a determinant, since these abnormalities have been observed in individuals drinking predominantly wine, beer, or spirits.

Although CHF is common, many individuals have arrhythmias without heart failure as the first abnormality. Classic angina pectoris despite a normal coronary arteriogram may be the presenting symptom. The progression of the heart failure syndrome and complications are those of CHF due to any cause.

The course of alcoholic cardiomyopathy varies, depending to a large degree on the extent of cardiac involvement. The outlook is relatively poor for patients who continue to ingest ethanol in substantial amounts. The role of cardiac transplantation in the treatment of alcoholic cardiomyopathy must be judged case by case. Obviously the patient should have discontinued the use of alcohol (usually for a mandatory 6 months), and there should be no organic disease except the heart disease.

Chemotherapeutic Agents

Doxorubicin (Adriamycin) and daunorubicin, among the most effective agents in the chemotherapy of malignant neoplasms, are highly cardiotoxic. The overall incidence of clinically apparent heart failure is reported in up to 9% of patients, with subclinical LV dysfunction probably being more frequent. The chronic effects, which include dilated cardiomyopathy, have been studied extensively in humans and have led to the conclusion that we may be dealing with a multifactorial pathogenesis, including altered nucleic acid synthesis, altered mitochondrial respiration, release of vasoactive substances, formation of free radicals, and calcium overload.

With doxorubicin the incidence of CHF is 1.5% at a total cumulative dose of 300 mg/m², 4.9% at 400 mg/m², 7.7% at 450 mg/m², and 20.5% at 500 mg/m².[3] The risk of cardiomyopathy is markedly increased by mediastinal radiation therapy, preexisting heart disease, uncontrolled hypertension, or treatment with other chemotherapeutic agents (cyclophosphamide). A higher incidence is also reported in young children and older adults. Oncologists usually monitor LVEF with serial echocardiograms or radionuclide angiograms, especially as higher doses are reached. A fall in LVEF is an indication to discontinue doxorubicin therapy.

The clinical presentation of doxorubicin heart muscle disease is similar to that of idiopathic dilated cardiomyopathy. It may develop within days of treatment and usually within the first year. Later presentation is uncommon but possible. The clinical course varies from an acute fulminating heart failure and cardiogenic shock to a gradually progressive deterioration. A few patients improve and appear to regress with medical therapy for CHF, but the overall mortality has been reported to be as high as 61%. Those over 45 years old are more likely to have progression of CHF.

The cardiac toxicity of daunorubicin is similar to that of doxorubicin. Electrocardiographic (ECG) changes may be transient and do not predict subsequent cardiomyopathy. The incidence of CHF is 1.5% with a total dose less than 600 mg/m²; the incidence increases to 12% with a dose greater than or equal to 1000 mg/m². Children seem to be at greater risk. The onset of symptoms may be a little later than with doxorubicin. There are some instances of myocarditis-pericarditis during treatment. The literature also suggests that daunorubicin cardiomyopathy is less likely to respond to therapy.

Catecholamines

Studies of the cardiac effects of catecholamines have dealt primarily with acute effects, including myocardial necrotic foci resembling ischemic lesions that have been attributed to macrovascular spasm and hypoxia, altered membrane permeability, and calcium overload. Late effects of acute administration of isoproterenol to rats, however, include cardiomyopathy and CHF.

Catecholamine-induced dilated cardiomyopathy in humans may occur with pheochromocytoma. This form of cardiomyopathy is reversible by removing the tumor or by adrenergic blockade. Of wider interest is the evidence that catecholamines play a role in anthracycline cardiotoxicity and diabetic cardiomyopathy.

Tachyarrhythmia

Persistent supraventricular tachyarrhythmias, including rapid atrial fibrillation, may cause LV dysfunction and heart failure. There is usually no other evidence for heart disease. At times it is difficult to know whether LV depression is the cause of the arrhythmia or its consequence. A possible mechanism is myocardial calcium overload and decreased concentrations of cyclic adenosine monophosphate (AMP) at high frequencies of stimulation. The condition is usually reversible with restoration of a normal ventricular rate. Observing improved LVEF with control of the arrhythmia confirms the diagnosis of tachycardia-induced myopathy.

Peripartum Cardiomyopathy

Peripartum cardiomyopathy is a disease of unknown etiology with an incidence between 1 in 4000 and 1 in 15,000 gestations. Risk factors for its development include increased maternal age, black race, multiparity, twinning, malnutrition, toxemia, and hypertension. The mortality in the acute and subacute phases ranges from 30% to 60%. Markers of poor prognosis are cardiomegaly persisting more than 6 months and particularly low LVEF.[2]

Endomyocardial biopsies have been performed to elucidate the mechanism of disease, but the findings of myocyte hypertrophy, interstitial fibrosis, and alterations in nuclear chromatin are nonspecific and do not differentiate peripartum cardiomyopathy from idiopathic dilated cardiomyopathy.

The effects of subsequent pregnancy on LV contractility in this condition have never been systematically examined. Historically, pregnancy has been discouraged and sterilization advocated to avoid the risks of progressive deterioration in LV contractility as a result of the increased hemodynamic workload and the altered immunologic status of pregnancy.

Recent prospective studies have demonstrated that about half of the patients with postpartum cardiomyopathy have a return of LV size and function to normal within 6 months with conventional heart failure therapy. Some patients with recovery of cardiac function wish to become pregnant again, either because the illness occurred with the first pregnancy or because of intrauterine or perinatal deaths, which occur in almost one fifth of cases. Recent case reports, albeit few, have suggested that patients waiting at least 3 years after the initial episode of postpartum cardiomyopathy who have made a complete recovery may get through another pregnancy and delivery without symptoms or clinical signs of LV dysfunction. In such cases the patient should understand that she is taking a chance of developing recurrent heart failure.

Infection

All infectious organisms that can invade the bloodstream may reach the myocardium. Acute necrotic inflammatory lesions have been associated with many bacterial, spirochetal, rickettsial, viral, mycotic, protozoal, and helminthic infections. Some forms of acute myocarditis have long been recognized as precursors of chronic dilated cardiomyopathy. Increasing evidence also points to dilated cardiomyopathy as a late sequel to acute viral myocarditis.

Acute, as well as chronic, dilated cardiomyopathy is encountered with increasing frequency in patients with acquired immunodeficiency syndrome, often associated with evidence of myocarditis. It may be the result of opportunistic infections. It remains an open question whether the human immunodeficiency (HIV) virus itself is responsible for cardiomyopathy. Box 24-2 lists some of the infectious causes of acute dilated cardiomyopathy.

Diabetic Cardiomyopathy

Clinical and pathologic reports have documented the existence of a diabetic cardiomyopathy or heart muscle disease independent of coronary atherosclerosis. It is more common in women. Pathologic studies have shown myocardial hypertrophy and interstitial fibrosis.

Controversy exists regarding the presence and significance of small vessel disease, involving intramural coronary arteries, arterioles, and capillaries. Capillary microaneurysms have been demonstrated. Interestingly, experimental studies support the view that the diabetic state itself affects ventricular performance. Experimentally induced diabetes in dogs is associated with reduced LV compliance and increased interstitial connective tissue.

Hypertension combined with diabetes accelerates the myocardial complications of diabetes, and careful blood pressure control is essential.

Distinguishing Dilated Cardiomyopathy from Other Types of Cardiomyopathy

In both the nondilated and the hypertrophic cardiomyopathies the left ventricle is only slightly dilated, if at all, and the LVEF, although impaired in some instances, is seldom as reduced as it is in dilated cardiomyopathy. The distinction between dilated cardiomyopathy and other types of cardiomyopathy is not difficult if the physician understands that the classification of car-

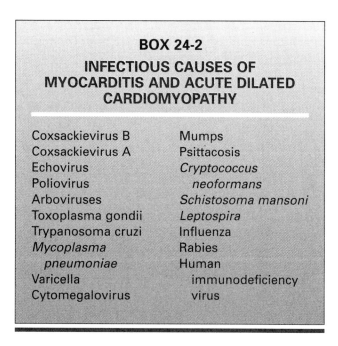

BOX 24-2

INFECTIOUS CAUSES OF MYOCARDITIS AND ACUTE DILATED CARDIOMYOPATHY

Coxsackievirus B	Mumps
Coxsackievirus A	Psittacosis
Echovirus	*Cryptococcus*
Poliovirus	*neoformans*
Arboviruses	*Schistosoma mansoni*
Toxoplasma gondii	*Leptospira*
Trypanosoma cruzi	Influenza
Mycoplasma	Rabies
pneumoniae	Human
Varicella	immunodeficiency
Cytomegalovirus	virus

diomyopathies is based on LV volume and LV ejection fraction, that is, on ventriculographic features (see Chapter 23).

The left ventricle may be dilated and the LVEF may be less than 40% in conditions of extreme afterload, such as aortic stenosis or uncontrolled hypertension. Such conditions can usually be distinguished easily from dilated cardiomyopathy during physical examination, but in a few patients with advanced aortic stenosis the typical murmur and abnormal carotid pulse are inconspicuous because of low cardiac output. Similarly, mitral stenosis may be a correctable cause of heart failure. An echocardiogram as a part of the initial evaluation of CHF excludes occult valvular disease.

Patients with LV aneurysm have left ventricle dilation and LVEF <40%. The ECG of almost all patients with a LV aneurysm shows Q waves, so confusion with idiopathic congestive cardiomyopathy is a problem only if left bundle branch block is present. Again, the echocardiogram documents a regional contractile abnormality and the aneurysm, rather than the global hypokinesis of dilated cardiomyopathy. Cardiac catheterization is often a part of this evaluation.

Table 24-2 suggests a screening process for distinguishing idiopathic cardiomyopathy from reversible causes of dilated cardiomyopathy. Although in some cases this is an oversimplification, it summarizes the laboratory studies we usually obtain as a part of our initial evaluation of cardiomyopathy (in addition to studies of cardiac function).

RESTRICTIVE CARDIOMYOPATHY

Restrictive cardiomyopathy is reviewed in Chapter 23. There is impaired diastolic filling of the heart caused by increased stiffness of the left ventricle. The most prevalent form of restrictive cardiomyopathy worldwide is endomyocardial fibrosis, which is not really a disease of muscle but primarily a disease of the endocardium, which becomes scarred and thickened, leading to diastolic dysfunction.

In the West, myocardial restriction is more common than endocardial restriction. The most frequent forms are idiopathic myocardial fibrosis and amyloid heart disease. Other infiltrative or fibrotic diseases include hemochromatosis, sarcoid heart disease, tumor infiltra-

Table 24-2	*Screening Procedure for Distinguishing Idiopathic Dilated Cardiomyopathy (CM) from Reversible Causes of Dilated CM*	
Possible Diagnosis	**Tests**	**Treatment**
Alcoholic CM	Repeated questioning of the patient and family members	Complete abstinence from alcohol
Uremic CM	BUN, serum creatinine	Renal dialysis
Hypophosphatemia	Serum phosphorus	Phosphate repletion
Hypocalcemia	Serum calcium	Calcium repletion
Iron overload	Serum iron studies: endomyocardial or liver biopsy in some cases	Treatment for hemochromatosis
Pheochromocytoma	Urinary screening tests	Operative removal of tumor
Sarcoid heart disease (if the chest x-ray suggests sarcoidosis)	Thallium scan, tissue biopsy, angiotensin I-converting enzyme (serum)	Corticosteroids
Acute inflammatory myopericarditis	Serum antibody titers for enteroviruses, toxoplasma, cold agglutinins, ANA, rheumatoid factor, ASLO, endomyocardial biopsy	Immunosuppressive treatment for postviral or noninfectious cases

ANA, antinuclear antibody; *ASLO,* antistreptolysin O.

tion, Fabry's disease, and radiation fibrosis. All can present as restrictive cardiomyopathy.

The diagnosis of restrictive cardiomyopathy, the rarest form of cardiomyopathy, should be entertained in patients with CHF in the presence of slight or no cardiomegaly. Elevation of jugular venous pressures is usually quite prominent. Patients with restrictive physiology may need endomyocardial biopsy to rule out specific heart diseases such as amyloidoses.

Amyloid Heart Disease

Cardiac dysfunction due to amyloid infiltration has been reported in the systemic amyloidoses, familial amyloidotic polyneuropathy, familial amyloidotic cardiomyopathy, and senile cardiac amyloidoses. Manifestations in the cardiovascular system may be diverse, and CHF is common. The features may also simulate, both on clinical observation and at cardiac catheterization, constrictive pericarditis or restrictive cardiomyopathy. Abnormal impulse formation and conduction disturbances are common in cardiac amyloidoses. Uncommon features include rupture of the heart, myocardial infarction, pericardial tamponade, and valvular dysfunction.

The laboratory findings are nonspecific. Low voltage on ECG can also be found in pericardial disease, in obesity, and in emphysema, but it is the ECG finding seen most frequently in patients with amyloidosis. An echocardiographically increased LV mass can also be found in other infiltrative cardiomyopathies, in hypertrophic cardiomyopathy, and with left ventricular pressure overload. However, the *combination* of an increased echocardiographic cardiac mass and a low voltage ECG point to amyloidosis.

Amyloidosis is characterized by organ function loss due to extracellular deposition of a fibrillar protein with a beta-pleated sheet confirmation. In clinical medicine, amyloidoses associated with inflammatory conditions (AA amyloid) and amyloidoses associated with plasma cell dyscrasia (AL amyloid) are of major importance. AA amyloid is derived from the immunochemically related acute phase serum reactant SAA, whereas AL amyloid is derived from the immunoglobulin light change. Heart failure is rarely ever found in AA amyloidoses but is not uncommon in the AL type.

Echocardiography appears to be the best method of predicting the degree of cardiac involvement in amyloidoses, since the degree of echocardiographic change parallels the reduction in myocardial function and the clinical condition. Unlike many forms of hypertrophic cardiomyopathy, amyloid infiltration may lead to RV and LV thickening.

The diagnosis of cardiac amyloidosis requires myocardial biopsy, but the first step in diagnosis is a search for systemic amyloidosis (orthostatic hypotension, neuropathy, weight loss, malabsorption, macroglossia, purpura, hepatomegaly, hypothenar wasting, and so on).

Serum and urine protein electrophoresis shows a monoclonal protein in more than 75% of cases.[4] The best noncardiac site for biopsy confirmation may be the abdominal fat pad, which is 88% sensitive.[4] The next step would be endomyocardial biopsy.

Amyloid heart disease has been considered a contraindication for cardiac transplantation based on the hypothesis that it is a systemic disease and that amyloid deposition would occur in the cardiac allograft. Recent surveys from international heart transplant centers have continued to demonstrate that patients undergoing cardiac transplantation for systemic amyloidoses have ongoing progression of the systemic disease in other organs despite the fact that the allograft is infrequently affected. Furthermore, the data suggest that current immunosuppressive protocols do not appear to alter the progression of systemic amyloid deposition.[3,4]

Hemochromatoses

Heredity hemochromatosis is the most common autosomal recessive disorder affecting Caucasians. It is a disease of iron overload that is HLA linked and genetically determined by an inappropriate increase in intestinal iron absorption. Individuals who are homozygous for the abnormal iron-loading gene developed significant amounts of excess iron deposition.[5] Older studies demonstrated a male:female ratio of as high as 10:1 for individuals with significant amounts of iron overload, but more recent studies have shown ratios of 2:1 or 3:1. The decreased frequency of significant iron overload in women probably results from physiologic losses of iron from menstruation and pregnancy.

The full clinical expression of hereditary hemochromatoses is influenced by age, gender, dietary habits, and other known factors. Although some patients in their twenties present with symptoms of organ damage, it is more usual for men in their forties to fifties to have hereditary hemochromatosis and women about 10 years later. Patients generally have at least 10 to 20 g of excess storage iron at the time of diagnosis. Because the liver is the primary organ for storage of iron, it is invariably affected and often damaged early in the course of the disease. The pancreas and heart are other organs that accumulate excess amounts of iron and are susceptible to tissue damage, although to a lesser degree than the liver.

Symptoms of CHF are seen in 0 to 40% of patients with hereditary hemochromatosis. Blood studies used to confirm the diagnosis of hereditary hemochromatoses include tests for serum iron, transferrin, and ferritin concentration. Since serum iron concentration and the transferrin saturation can be falsely elevated in nonfasting individuals, blood should be obtained in a fasting state. A transferrin saturation greater than 60% is seen in 90% of homozygous patients and should be considered abnormally elevated when it is greater than 55%.

The treatment of hereditary hemochromatoses is relatively straightforward and simple, since the vast majority of patients can be treated with regular phlebotomy. As with other diseases, the goals of treatment are to initiate therapy before the development of end-stage complications.

Hypertrophic Cardiomyopathy

Despite its rarity, hypertrophic cardiomyopathy has held the fascination of cardiologists because of its dramatic aberrations of geometry and function and its importance as a cause of disability and death in young, otherwise healthy adults. Hypertrophic cardiomyopathy, conceptually, is a disorder characterized by asymmetric septal hypertrophy and dynamic outflow tract obstruction. Interventions aimed at reducing the dynamic outflow gradient, including the use of negative inotropic agents such as propranolol and surgical ablation of the gradient using the myotomy-myectomy procedure, have been developed.

Necropsy studies in these patients demonstrated the consistent finding of disorganization and malalignment of the myofibrils (myofibrillar disarray), findings that are not unique to hypertrophic cardiomyopathy but that are more extensive in this disorder than in secondary hypertrophy from pressure overload or congenital heart disorders.

Not all patients have severe outflow tract pressure gradients. Most have an abnormality of diastolic performance. A systolic murmur indicative of a LV outflow gradient is not an invariable feature of the disease, or in the natural history of an individual followed from adolescence through adulthood. In individuals with dramatic signs of outflow obstruction in young adulthood, clinical deterioration in middle age is frequently associated with disappearance of the dynamic systolic murmur and the development of physiologic features resembling those of restrictive cardiomyopathy. The extent of septal hypertrophy and duration of mitral leaflet–septal apposition correlate well with the magnitude of the systolic gradient. However, the cardiac morphology does not correlate well with either symptoms or natural history. Severe symptoms of angina, pulmonary congestion, and syncope occur in patients with either the obstructive or the nonobstructive forms of the disease, and many but not all investigators believe that little relation exists between the magnitude of the systolic gradient and the severity of symptoms or improvement in functional status with pharmacologic agents.

Two morphologic forms of hypertrophic cardiomyopathy merit particular attention: apical hypertrophy and midventricular hypertrophy. These atypical forms are of interest not because of their prevalence but because they underscore the fact that our perception of hypertrophic cardiomyopathy has been significantly shaped by the capabilities and limitations of the tools available for the study of patients. Both of these forms of hypertrophic cardiomyopathy are associated with nonspecific physical findings, escape detection by M-mode echocardiography, and have come to attention with two-dimensional imaging using either contrast ventriculography or two-dimensional echocardiography.

Since the initial case reports, sudden cardiac death has been an ominous feature of hypertrophic cardiomyopathy distinct from its hemodynamic abnormalities. Similar to dilated cardiomyopathy, major obstacles include the ability to identify individual patients at high risk of sudden death and to find treatment strategies that reduce risk. Although the overall annual mortality for patients studied at referral centers is estimated to be 2% to 3%, the risk of premature death is skewed by a high incidence of sudden cardiac death in children and young adults. In about 50% of patients, death occurs suddenly, is unexpected, and can be the index presentation of hypertrophic cardiomyopathy. Risk factors for sudden death include young age (first 3 decades of life), prior syncope, and a family history of sudden death. It is still controversial whether the extent of hypertrophy is an independent predictor of sudden death. Otherwise, sudden death is not predicted by symptoms, functional limitations, hemodynamic abnormalities (including the presence or absence of LV outflow obstruction), or rest ECG abnormalities.

The true prevalence of familial versus sporadic forms of hypertrophic cardiomyopathy is still somewhat uncertain, partly because of the techniques used to detect occult disease and also because morphologic expression of the disease may not be apparent until young adulthood. Hypertrophic cardiomyopathy appears to be familial in nearly 60% of cases and sporadic in the remainder. A single pattern of inheritance is not characteristic, an observation that suggests that several genetic defects may contribute to the pool of patients now diagnosed as having hypertrophic cardiomyopathy.

REFERENCES

1. Abelmann WH, Lorel BH: The challenge of cardiomyopathy, *J Am Coll Cardiol* 13:1219, 1989.
2. Carvalho A, Brandao A, Martinez EE, et al: Prognosis in peripartum cardiomyopathy, *Am J Cardiol* 64:540, 1989.
3. *Physicians' Desk Reference*, ed 52, Montvale, NJ, 1998, Medical Economics.
4. Hosenpud JD, Uretsky BF, Griffith BP, et al: Successful intermediate term outcome for patients with cardiac amyloidoses undergoing heart transplantation: results of a multi-center survey, *J Heart Transplant* 9:346, 1990.
5. McCarthy RE III, Kasper EK: A review of the amyloidoses that infiltrate the heart, *Clin Cardiol* 21:547, 1998.
6. Barton JC, McDonnell SM, Adams PC, et al: Management of hemochromatosis. Hemochromatosis Management Working Group, *Ann Intern Med* 129:932, 1998.

25 Atrial Arrhythmias

Walter A. Brzezinski
Robert B. Leman

ATRIAL ARRHYTHMIAS
Pathophysiology

Atrial arrhythmias are the result of reentry or increased automaticity. Unlike ventricular arrhythmias, triggered events from after-depolarizations do not seem to cause atrial arrhythmias. Box 25-1 is a classification of arrhythmias and indicates the presumed pathophysiology of each.

Reentry occurs when two pathways exist with differing conduction velocities and refractory periods (Fig. 25-1). A premature beat usually finds the fast pathway refractory, as it usually has a longer refractory period. It thus proceeds down the slow pathway. Current exits this protected focus when the fast pathway has recovered and is excitable. Normal tissue is depolarized, and a retrograde circuit is established. Retrograde conduction through the rapid pathway depolarizes the atria, and slow conduction through the abnormal pathway completes the circuit.

Automaticity occurs when an area of tissue has a change in its action potential so that there is spontaneous depolarization and repetitive firing. In essence, the focus becomes more like nodal tissue. It functions like a fixed-rate pacemaker.

Clinical Presentation

Atrial arrhythmias cause a wide range of clinical symptoms. Palpitations direct attention to the heart. Other, more vague symptoms like dizziness, fatigue, lethargy, shortness of breath, and weight loss also may be caused by atrial arrhythmias and must be considered in the diagnostic workup. Recent reports show that some panic attacks are in fact paroxysmal atrial arrhythmias. Transient ischemic attacks (TIAs) and stroke may be provoked by arrhythmias.

ATRIAL FIBRILLATION AND FLUTTER
Epidemiology, Etiology, and Natural History

Atrial fibrillation (AF) is the most frequent cardiac rhythm disturbance requiring treatment in hospitalized patients. It is rare in infancy and childhood, increasing in frequency with advanced age. It commonly becomes a chronic rhythm. Atrial flutter tends to be short lived, with spontaneous conversion back to either normal sinus rhythm or AF.

Both AF and atrial flutter can occur intermittently or in chronic form. Paroxysmal AF in normal people may follow periods of extreme emotional or physical stress. Electrolyte abnormalities, drugs, and acute alcohol toxicity can lead to paroxysms of these arrhythmias. Chronic AF more commonly develops in patients with underlying heart or lung disease. Most heart diseases can be associated with these arrhythmias, including coronary and valvular heart disease (especially mitral valve disease), and cardiomyopathy. Hypertensive heart disease is the most commonly identified cause in older patients. Lung disease with associated hypoxia may cause AF, and it may complicate pulmonary embolism. AF may be the presenting complaint in elderly patients with hyperthyroidism who may not have other signs or symptoms of thyroid dysfunction.

Atrial flutter is often provoked by conditions that elevate right heart pressure. Consider pulmonary embolus when flutter develops in a bedridden elderly patient. It is common in those with advanced lung disease as well. Transient flutter may complicate other acute illnesses and is a common postoperative arrhythmia. Chronic flutter is more common in those with advanced pulmonary disease.

Pathophysiology
Mechanism of Atrial Flutter

The reentrant circuit causing flutter is at the base of the right atrium (isthmus between tricuspid valve and inferior vena cava). The atrial rate is close to 300 beats/min. Fortunately, the atrioventricular (AV) node does not allow conduction of a rate this fast, and typically every other beat reaches the ventricles (2:1 conduction), and the ventricular rate is about 150 beats/min (Fig. 25-2). A rare patient has 1:1 conduction and a ventricular rate of 300 beats/min. This does not allow adequate time between contractions for ventricular filling, and stroke volume, cardiac output, and blood pressure fall.

The electrocardiogram (ECG) shows a typical "saw-toothed" atrial activity, usually best seen in the inferior

BOX 25-1

ATRIAL ARRHYTHMIAS

Sinus tachycardia (automatic focus)
Atrial fibrillation/flutter (reentry)
Paroxysmal supraventricular tachycardia
(reentry)
   AV nodal reentry
   Atrial reentry
   Sinus node reentry
   Accessory pathways
      Wolff-Parkinson-White (WPW) syndrome
      Lown-Ganong-Levine (LGL) syndrome
      Mahaim fibers
Automatic ectopic tachycardia (automatic
focus)
   Atrial ectopic tachycardia
   Junctional tachycardia
   Multifocal atrial tachycardia

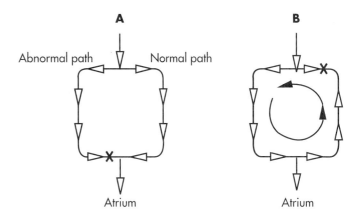

FIG. 25-1
Schematic representation of reentry. There are two pathways: conduction through the normal pathway is rapid, and conduction through the "reentrant focus" is slow. **A,** A normal sinus beat conducts antegrade, discharging tissue that surrounds the protected, reentrant focus. Current exiting the reentrant focus finds the surrounding tissue refractory and thus is blocked. **B,** A premature atrial contraction finds the normal pathway refractory (from the preceding sinus beat) and does not conduct antegrade. However, the abnormal, reentrant pathway is not refractory and allows antegrade conduction. Current exits the protected focus, finds the atrium excitable, and generates an ectopic atrial beat (an atrial "echo"). If the timing is right, this ectopic beat reenters the protected focus, and a circuit is established, with antegrade conduction through the abnormal pathway and retrograde conduction through the normal pathway, leading to sustained supraventricular tachycardia. Most commonly the reentrant focus is within the body of the AV node (leading to AV node reentrant tachycardia), but it also may be located in the SA node or the body of the atria.

leads. In the absence of aberrant conduction the QRS complex looks normal.

Mechanism of Atrial Fibrillation

AF comes from a more diffuse reentrant circuit within the atria, and electrical activity seen on the ECG is totally chaotic. The rate of atrial depolarization can be as high as 600 beats/min. The pattern of conduction through the AV node is irregular. Even though the atrial rate is faster than with atrial flutter, the ventricular rate is usually slower because of decremental conduction within the AV node. In the absence of aberrant conduction, the QRS complex is narrow.

Clinical Presentation

Most patients with AF have palpitations and are aware of an irregular heartbeat. Some are asymptomatic. If conduction through the AV node is slow enough that the ventricular response to the atrial arrhythmia is not excessive, the patient may not sense palpitations. An occasional elderly patient with a rapid ventricular response is also unaware of a rhythm change.

Other cardiac symptoms are common. If the ventricular rate is too high or too low, cardiac output falls, and a variety of "low output" symptoms may result: syncope, postural dizziness, fatigue, weakness, shortness of breath, and so forth. A rapid ventricular rate may provoke angina in those with coronary artery disease (CAD), or TIAs or stroke in those with cerebrovascular disease. With AF the loss of atrial contraction leads to a

decline in stroke volume, even when the ventricular rate is in a physiologic range (see Chapter 2). This is a greater problem for those with left ventricular diastolic dysfunction (see Chapter 23), who may have a 25% drop in cardiac output when going from sinus rhythm into AF. There may be a worsening of congestive heart failure or other low output symptoms.

Laboratory Studies

Electrocardiogram

In addition to identifying the arrhythmia, an ECG may help identify underlying heart disease (e.g., prior myocardial infarction [MI] or ventricular hypertrophy). AF is recognized by the irregularly irregular pattern of QRS complexes, the absence of P waves, and baseline undulation, or fibrillatory waves. Should the ventricular response be rapid with aberrant conduction and wide QRS complexes, AF can be confused with ventricular tachycardia. *Even when the rhythm is rapid, irregularity identifies it as AF.* Close scrutiny for the presence or ab-

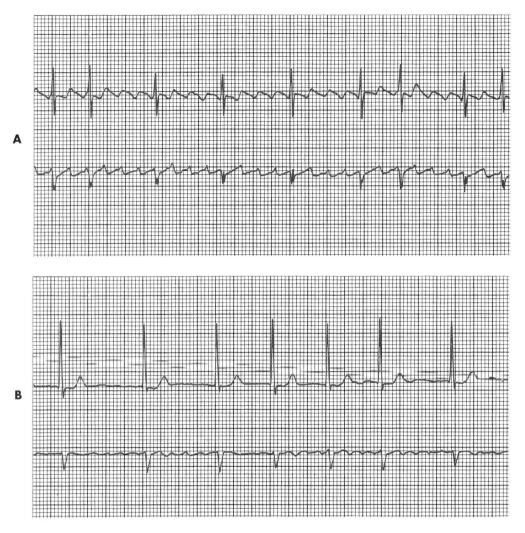

FIG. 25-2
A, Atrial flutter with saw-toothed flutter waves and a regular ventricular rate. **B,** Atrial fibrillation *(AF).* The rhythm is grossly irregular. Fibrillatory waves may or may not distort the baseline.

sence of P waves may help with the diagnosis. This may require either carotid massage or pharmacologic slowing (adenosine) of conduction through the AV node to prove the absence of the P waves. Generally, atrial flutter is easier to identify because of the obvious saw-toothed appearance of flutter waves in the inferior leads and the *regular* ventricular response at 150 beats/min. Atrial flutter on occasion can have an irregular pattern because of variable block. Shifting from 2:1 (150 beats/min) to 3:1 (100 beats/min) block may be confusing, but flutter waves identify the rhythm.

Ambulatory Monitoring

Episodic or paroxysmal atrial flutter or AF can be missed by a resting ECG. Twenty-four-hour Holter monitoring is useful when the arrhythmia occurs daily. Unfortunately, most do not occur daily.

The *loop monitor* (also called the *event monitor*) is a recording device that constantly monitors and records the ECG. At the end of 5 minutes, it "loops" and records over the beginning of the 5-minute tape. There is a button that the patient pushes when there is a symptom. This freezes the loop, preserving the last 5 minutes of rhythm data. The monitor is then removed and attached to the telephone to transmit the rhythm strip. Loop monitors can be worn for long periods; we typically send them home with the patient for 3 weeks. The device is useful for identifying the cardiac rhythm during intermittent symptoms, including palpitations. It works well regardless of the nature of the arrhythmia.

Table 25-1	*Drugs That Slow AV Node Conduction and Control the Ventricular Rate in Atrial Fibrillation and Flutter*	

Drug	Dose	Comments
Digoxin	1.0 to 1.125 mg loading dose; may start with 0.5 mg IV, then 0.25 mg PO at 2-hour intervals	Does not convert to sinus rhythm; a good choice when there is heart failure
Diltiazem	20 mg IV bolus, then continuous infusion at 5 to 15 mg/hr	Rapidly establishes rate control; safe when there is mild heart failure; now considered drug of choice
Metoprolol	5 mg IV bolus, repeat in 10 min	Poorly tolerated with heart failure or bronchospasm
Esmolol	0.5 mg/kg iv loading dose, then 0.05 mg/kg/min IV infusion	Beta blocker with short half-life
Amiodarone	15 mg/min IV for 10 min, then 0.5 to 1.0 mg/min maintenance infusion	Only used in refractory cases

Although event monitoring has been useful for evaluating palpitations and presyncope, it has been less effective for syncope. An unconscious patient is unable to press the button and activate the monitor.

General Medical and Cardiac Evaluation

In addition to ECG techniques, evaluation of atrial arrhythmias requires the measurement of electrolytes, including calcium and magnesium. Thyroid function studies are routine. Possible hypoxemia is evaluated with oximetry or arterial blood gases. A thorough review of all drugs—both legal and illegal—is important, and measurement of levels is occasionally appropriate (e.g., when binge drinking causes AF). An echocardiogram is useful for diagnosing valvular heart disease, cardiomyopathy, and prior ischemic injury. In many situations a transesophageal echocardiogram can better delineate valvular abnormalities. It is also more helpful in evaluating the patient for atrial thrombus.

Management
Rate Control

Control of the ventricular rate is the first priority in a stable patient. Table 25-1 lists the drugs that slow the ventricular response by blocking the AV node. Digoxin is our first choice and is given when the ventricular rate is above 110 to 120 beats/min. Controlling the rate quickly with intravenous drug therapy is important if tachycardia is responsible for symptoms.

You may not have time to control the rate when a patient is unstable. *Life-threatening symptoms, such as unsta-ble angina or marked hypotension, are indications for immediate DC cardioversion.*

An occasional older patient has a ventricular rate less than 100 beats/min because of conduction disease within the AV node. Further rate-lowering therapy is not indicated. Rarely, AV nodal block is severe enough to require pacemaker therapy.

In a stable, asymptomatic patient, oral digoxin is suitable for controlling the rate both soon after the onset of AF and chronically. Some active patients have better control of tachycardia and fewer side effects with calcium channel or beta-adrenergic blockers. Chronically, most with AF have adequate rate control with a single agent. An exception is the patient with hyperthyroidism, who may not have adequate rate control until thyroid dysfunction is corrected. Atrial flutter may be more difficult to control, and two-drug therapy is commonly required.

Rate control cannot be achieved for an occasional patient with chronic AF. In such cases the treatment of choice is radiofrequency catheter ablation of the AV node in the electrophysiology laboratory plus a permanent ventricular pacemaker.

Anticoagulation

AF is a rare cause of death, and we often encounter patients who have been in AF for more than 5 years. Morbidity and mortality are more commonly the result of peripheral embolization, a common complication of AF. The risk of embolic stroke is increased 17-fold with AF and rheumatic heart disease (as high as 8% per year) and 6-fold without rheumatic mitral valve disease (about 3% per year).[1,2] Stroke is more common when the patient converts from AF to sinus rhythm, and the risk remains high for the following 6 weeks. Patients with paroxysmal AF have a 2% to 6% per year risk of stroke.[3,4]

In the absence of valvular heart disease, risk factors for stroke with AF include advanced age, hypertension, diabetes, and a history or prior stroke or TIA. With any of these risk factors the annual risk of stroke is above 4%, and warfarin reduces the risk by 68%.[2] Left atrial enlargement, left ventricular dysfunction, and congestive heart failure also may increase the risk of embolization.

On the other hand, patients with AF younger than age 60 who have a normal echocardiogram have a low risk of stroke (about 1% per year).[2] These younger patients with "lone atrial fibrillation" do not require anticoagulation with warfarin. No clear benefit has been shown with aspirin in this group, but it is commonly prescribed because of the low risk (the effective dose for AF is 325 mg/day).[5]

Anticoagulation with warfarin is thus indicated for all patients in AF except those with lone atrial fibrillation under the age of 60 or those with a contraindication to anticoagulation (e.g., gastrointestinal bleeding, severe uncontrolled hypertension, or recent surgery). If a patient with new AF can be converted to sinus rhythm within 48 hours of the onset of AF, anticoagulation is not required. Beyond 48 hours, the present recommendation is anticoagulation with warfarin and achievement of a prothrombin time (PT) in the therapeutic range for 3 weeks before cardioversion. After cardioversion, warfarin is continued for 6 weeks.

Some patients with AF are unable to take warfarin because of medical contraindications. Another common problem is the noncompliant patient who does not report for monitoring of PT or who takes the medicine improperly despite the best efforts of caregivers. After frank discussion, we tell such patients that we are unable to prescribe warfarin. Aspirin 325 mg/day is an alternative. While not as effective as warfarin, it has been shown to reduce the incidence of embolization by 44%.[2]

Atrial flutter is different from AF, as there is recognizable contraction of the atria. With AF the atrial wall just quivers. The risk of stroke with flutter is lower than it is with AF, but there is still a risk. Warfarin therapy is currently recommended for atrial flutter.

Monitoring Warfarin Therapy Using the International Normalized Ratio (INR)

We use the PT to adjust the warfarin dose, but there are problems with accuracy because of variation in the potency of thromboplastin used by different laboratories to measure PT. In fact, the thromboplastin you are using this month may be different from what you were using 3 months ago. The result is variability in PT results. The INR method of PT reporting relates a laboratory's thromboplastin activity to that of a preparation standardized by the World Health Organization, thus eliminating any variability.[6,7]

Multicenter trials have shown a substantial reduction in risk of stroke and peripheral embolization with warfarin therapy. Fortunately, low-dose warfarin is effective, and the current recommendation is adjustment of the dose so that the INR is between 2.0 and 3.0 (a PT of 14 to 17 seconds).[5,6] By comparison, for patients with a mechanical heart valve or recent pulmonary embolus, the INR should be 3 to 3.5, corresponding to a PT around 20 seconds.

Cardioversion

There are a couple of predictors of an *inability* to convert to and maintain sinus rhythm: prolonged AF and marked left atrial enlargement. A patient with recent-onset AF and a near-normal or normal left atrium should have cardioversion. On the other hand, it is not worth trying when AF has been present for years or when the left atrium is huge. An attempt to cardiovert is worthwhile for the intermediate patient who has been in AF for a few months and has a near-normal left atrium.

Cardioversion with Drugs. Table 25-2 lists drugs that have been used to chemically convert atrial fibrillation to sinus rhythm. Contrary to popular belief, digoxin is no more effective than placebo and is used only for rate control. Most of the class IA (quinidine, procainamide), IC (flecainide, propafenone), and III (ibutilide, amiodarone, sotalol) agents are effective, and the choice is based on side effects and risk of proarrhythmia. In addition to cardioversion, these drugs help the patient stay in sinus rhythm. That is the rationale for a few days of drug therapy before DC cardioversion: some patients will convert with drug therapy, and all will have a better chance of remaining in sinus rhythm after cardioversion.

Quinidine or procainamide used to be our first choice. Because these class IA agents may have a proarrhythmic effect in patients with normal LV function, we use them less frequently.[8] If left ventricular function is normal, our initial choice for oral therapy is flecainide or propafenone. With left ventricular dysfunction the proarrhythmic effect of the IC agents increases. For such patients we prefer amiodarone (or quinidine, whose proarrhythmic action is less influenced by left ventricular dysfunction than IC agents).

Hospital Admission and Telemetry During Cardioversion. The risk of provoking ventricular tachycardia is low for those with normal left ventricular ejection fraction who are given class IC agents, but the risk is not zero. About half the proarrhythmia occurs within a couple days of starting IA or IC antiarrhythmics. Our current

Table 25-2	*Drugs Used To Convert Atrial Fibrillation or Flutter to Sinus Rhythm*	
Drug	**Dose**	**Comments**
Ibutilide	1 mg infusion over 10 minutes; may repeat once after 10 min pause	Class III antiarrhythmic; half convert with drug alone, and most with DC cardioversion after ibutilide.[10]
Amiodarone	15 mg/min for 10 min load; 0.5 to 1.0 mg/min maintenance	Only in refractory cases in critically ill patients
Propafenone	High-dose oral loading (450 to 600 mg single dose)	Proarrhythmic effect more common in congestive heart failure (CHF)
Flecainide	High-dose oral loading (200 mg single dose)	Proarrhythmia common with CHF

practice is to have patients in the hospital and on telemetry for 3 days during chemical cardioversion. If AF persists, DC cardioversion is done on the third day. We often do not hospitalize a patient treated with amiodarone; with a 50-day half-life, it may be weeks before a therapeutic level is reached.

New-onset AF is common in hospitalized patients, especially after surgery. It often converts spontaneously or with correction of electrolyte levels. Pushing the serum Mg^{+2} level to above 2.0 mg/dL is especially effective, and correcting serum potassium concentration is also a critical element of treatment. *Ibutilide* is particularly effective for new-onset AF and is our usual therapy (Table 25-2). One advantage of intravenous ibutilide is that you know immediately whether or not it works. If it does not, DC cardioversion may be done later in the day. Large single doses of flecainide or propafenone have also been used for acute chemical cardioversion.[9] As noted, anticoagulation is unnecessary when cardioversion is accomplished less than 48 hours from the onset of AF.

Ibutilide may also be used for cardioversion of established AF. A logistically neat approach is admission to hospital and ibutilide cardioversion the same day. If it does not work, DC cardioversion is done a half hour later.[10] Regardless of which of these techniques works, a IC or IA agent is started after cardioversion to maintain sinus rhythm.

Electrical Cardioversion. Hemodynamic compromise or unstable angina provoked by rapid AF or atrial flutter is a medical emergency. DC cardioversion is usually successful and should be used without hesitation. In the nonacute situation, cardioversion may be considered when drug therapy does not work.

Our DC cardioversion protocol for AF starts at 100 joules, followed by 200 joules, then 360 joules applied twice. If that does not work, we stop. Remember that when a patient has been in AF for more than 48 hours,

anticoagulation is needed for at least 3 weeks before elective cardioversion.

Atrial flutter converts more easily than AF. Cardioversion using 10 to 15 joules may work, and we usually begin with 25 joules. It is common for a patient with flutter to go into AF with the initial shock. When that happens, proceed immediately with the AF cardioversion protocol.

Maintenance of Sinus Rhythm

After cardioversion, antiarrhythmic therapy must often be used to maintain normal sinus rhythm. All the drugs used for cardioversion work. Drugs that slow AV conduction and control rate (digoxin, calcium channel blockers, and beta-blockers) are not effective for this purpose. We often use sotalol 120 to 160 mg bid. Propafenone, flecainide, disopyramide, quinidine, and procainamide are reasonable choices. For a patient with heart failure, amiodarone is especially effective; after a loading period of 2 to 4 weeks (600 to 1000 mg/day), we prescribe 200 mg/day as long-term therapy.

Invasive and Possibly Curative Therapy for AF and Flutter

Catheter ablation for recurrent atrial flutter has become possible. A line of scar generated by a radiofrequency ablation catheter is formed from the tricuspid annulus to the inferior vena cava, which interrupts the reentrant circuit and maintains sinus rhythm.

Similar catheter techniques are being developed for AF, but the success rate is low. A surgical procedure called the Maze procedure has been shown to be effective in restoring sinus rhythm in those with chronic atrial fibrillation. It is a major operation that requires extensive surgical incisions in both atria, and the mortality and morbidity have been high.

AV nodal (His) ablation plus permanent pacing has been effective in those with refractory AF and poor rate control. This causes complete heart block, and the patient is pacemaker dependent. However, it does restore rate control and regularity. In addition, the new variable-rate pacemakers allow a physiologic increase in heart rate with exercise.

SINUS TACHYCARDIA

Sinus tachycardia is not considered an arrhythmia if it is an appropriate response to a stress, exercise, or depressed cardiac function. If the cause is not obvious, screen for congestive heart failure, anemia, volume depletion, thyroid disease, or infection (usually with fever). Typically sinus tachycardia comes on gradually and resolves gradually, and carotid massage will simply cause a very gradual slowing of the overall rate. This distinguishes it from many of the other supraventricular tachycardias, which may change abruptly with carotid massage. An additional clinical clue to the presence of sinus tachycardia comes from careful analysis of the overall rate. Maximal predicted heart rate can be grossly predicted as 220 minus the patient's age. Should the rate go beyond this value, sinus tachycardia is unlikely.

In general, sinus tachycardia should not be treated because it is a normal physiologic response to a stress. Instead, treat the underlying disorder. For example, a patient who is dehydrated with fever and sinus tachycardia might respond to beta blockade with lowering of the heart rate. A much more appropriate treatment would be volume replacement with intravenous fluids and aspirin for fever.

A rare patient has an increased sinus rate without a specific cause, called "inappropriate sinus tachycardia." It may be a persistent arrhythmia and usually is an abnormality of automaticity. Radiofrequency ablation therapy has been used when drug therapy is not tolerated (beta-blockers or calcium channel blockers).

PAROXYSMAL SUPRAVENTRICULAR TACHYCARDIA

Reentry is the usual mechanism of paroxysmal supraventricular tachycardia (PSVT). This reentrant circuit may be in normal cardiac structure such as the sinus node, AV node, or tissue in the body of the atria. It may involve an accessory pathway, as is commonly seen in Wolff-Parkinson-White syndrome.

Electrophysiologic Studies

Electrophysiologic study (EPS) is often the most definitive test for the evaluation of arrhythmia. It is similar to a heart catheterization. A sheath introducer is placed in the femoral vein, and recording electrodes are advanced to atrial and ventricular sites. One of them is positioned across the tricuspid valve to record

bundle of His activity (see Chapter 27). An arterial line is inserted for pressure monitoring when the arrhythmia is induced. EPS is thus invasive, but it poses less risk than left heart catheterization and angiography. The mortality with EPS is 1 in 10,000. Other complications include bruising or hematoma at the catheter insertion site and induction of an arrhythmia that requires cardioversion.

The EPS protocol for supraventricular arrhythmias involves provoking the reentrant arrhythmia by stimulating the atrium with an atrial electrode. Once the arrhythmia is initiated, the recording electrodes are used to "map" the location of the reentrant circuit. Observation of the arrhythmia in the laboratory allows measurement of the ventricular response rate; this determines the risk of hemodynamic compromise. EPS is diagnostic for evaluating reentry involving the sinoatrial (SA) node, intraatrial pathways, the AV node, and accessory pathways. If an automatic focus is responsible for the arrhythmia, it can be mapped and evaluated with this technique.

AV Nodal Reentrant Tachycardia

AV nodal reentrant tachycardia (AVNRT) is the most common form of PSVT in adults. It causes the abrupt onset of a supraventricular tachycardia, with heart rates ranging from 140 to 220 beats/min. The arrhythmia is usually initiated by a premature atrial contraction. The pathophysiology is best explained by the presence of dual AV nodal pathways. With typical AVNRT (Fig. 25-3), conduction is down the slow pathway and up the fast pathway, producing a narrow QRS complex with retrograde P waves that most often are buried in the next QRS. In atypical AVNRT the reverse happens and leads to a tachycardia that has a long R-P interval. The P wave is closer to the next QRS, and it looks like sinus tachycardia except that the P wave axis is abnormal (the P waves are inverted in inferior leads, Fig. 25-4).

Treatment is aimed at slowing conduction in the slow pathway. This may be accomplished by carotid sinus massage or the Valsalva maneuver. The drug of choice for acute conversion is intravenous adenosine. It produces a profound, transient conduction block in the sinus and AV nodes and terminates the arrhythmia 90% of the time.[11] Its short half-life of 1.5 seconds requires it to be given as a 6 to 12 mg rapid IV bolus. Alternative treatments are digoxin, beta-blockers, and verapamil or diltiazem. Beta blockade and calcium blockers are first choices for prophylaxis to prevent a recurrence. Quinidine, flecainide, and amiodarone can be used but may have significant long-term side effects; we do not like committing an otherwise healthy young patient to prolonged therapy with such agents. A better approach for a patient with recurrent symptoms is an electrophysiologic study and ablation therapy. The success rate is

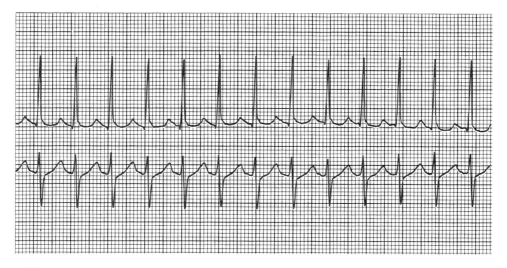

FIG. 25-3
Supraventricular tachycardia *(SVT),* most commonly AV node reentrant tachycardia *(AVNRT).* The P waves are buried within the T waves.

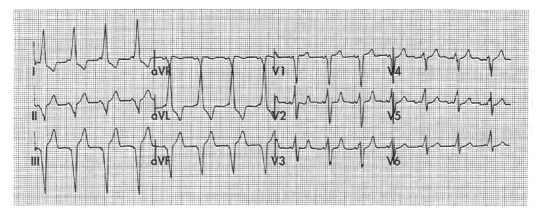

FIG. 25-4
Preexcitation, Wolff-Parkinson-White (WPW) syndrome. The PR interval is short. The upstroke of the QRS complex is slurred, creating a "delta wave" that is most noticeable in the limb leads. The QRS complexes have the general configuration of left bundle branch block, and it is easy to mistake the broad delta wave caused by WPW syndrome with a ventricular conduction abnormality. The short PR interval helps establish a diagnosis. In addition, in this tracing the initial part of the QRS is slurred, typical of preexcitation (see V₅). With bundle branch block it is the terminal portion of the QRS that is slurred.

above 90%, the risk is low, and subsequent drug therapy is unnecessary.[12]

Atrial Reentrant Tachycardia

There is a two-track reentrant circuit within the body of the atrium. It usually has a different P wave configuration than the sinus node P wave because it comes from a different location. Pharmacologic treatment of atrial reentrant tachycardia is similar to therapy of AVNRT,

but it may be more difficult to control. Radiofrequency ablation of the pathway is often curative.

Sinus Node Reentry

Because the reentrant circuit is within the SA node, the P wave configuration is normal. There is an abrupt change in sinus rate, with a normal-looking P wave initiating the arrhythmia (Fig. 25-5). It is an uncommon arrhythmia. Typically during sinus tachycardia the PR

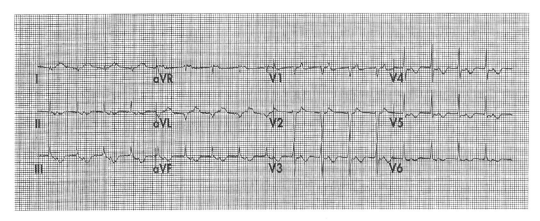

FIG. 25-5
Nodal tachycardia, just above 100 beats/min and with retrograde P wave distorting the T waves. It is common for there to be no apparent P waves.

interval gets shorter. That is not the case with SA node reentry, and a long PR interval associated with what looks like sinus tachycardia suggests this arrhythmia. The treatment outlined for AVNRT is generally useful. Ablative therapy can be done but carries a risk of SA node injury, requiring a pacemaker.

Accessory Pathway Arrhythmias and "Preexcitation"

Normally the atria are insulated from the ventricles, the only point of electrical contact being the AV node. Think of accessory pathways as defects in this insulation, small bundles of atrial-like muscle that cross the AV groove between the atria and the ventricles. The wave of atrial depolarization is normally funneled through the AV node. An accessory tract transmits current to the ventricles, "bypassing" the AV node.

It is possible for a reentrant circuit to be established, with the AV node its slow path and the accessory tract the fast conducting path. When a circus rhythm develops, the current usually travels antegrade through the AV node and retrograde through the accessory pathway. As current enters the ventricles from the AV node and bundle of His, the ventricles are depolarized simultaneously, and the QRS complex is narrow. The arrhythmia looks like PSVT (a narrow QRS complex tachycardia).

The reverse may occur, with retrograde conduction in the AV node and antegrade conduction in the accessory path. Ventricular depolarization begins in either the left or the right ventricle, the contralateral ventricle depolarizing late. The QRS complex is wide, and the SVT is a wide QRS complex tachycardia.

In the absence of arrhythmia there are two common ECG findings (see Fig. 25-4). Current traveling antegrade through both the AV node and accessory pathway activates the ventricles. As accessory pathway conduction is more rapid, it reaches the ventricle first, "preexciting" it and generating a delta wave. The second finding is a short PR interval. AV node conduction time is not shorter, but the early-appearing delta wave occupies part of the PR on the surface ECG.

Atrial fibrillation or atrial flutter is particularly dangerous in the presence of an accessory pathway. Rather than current passing through the AV node, which conducts slowly and allows just a fraction of the impulses to pass, it may travel antegrade through the bypass tract. This conducts much more rapidly and may allow a ventricular rate as high as 200 to 250 beats/min. The result may be circulatory collapse.

About 10% to 15% of patients with preexcitation have multiple pathways. It is possible to have reentrant circuits with antegrade conduction through one and retrograde conduction through another of them.

Syndromes

The Wolff-Parkinson-White (WPW) syndrome is caused by the Kent bundle, which connects the atrium to the ventricle. Typically the ECG shows a very short PR interval with slurring of the upstroke of the QRS complex (delta wave). There are latent cases of WPW syndrome, with occasional conduction through the bypass tract and, therefore, intermittent appearance of the delta wave. Concealed WPW syndrome only conducts retrograde over the Kent bundle and thus never causes a delta wave. The concealed form is occasionally discovered during an electrophysiologic study of a patient with presumed AVNRT.

WPW syndrome may be asymptomatic, and no therapy is indicated. It commonly causes PSVT and requires treatment. If the patient is hemodynamically compromised, DC cardioversion is the treatment of choice. Drugs that may be given intravenously to interrupt PSVT include adenosine, procainamide, beta-blockers, ibutilide, and verapamil or diltiazem. Drugs given long-term to prevent recurrent PSVT include beta-blockers, IA and IC agents, sotalol, and amiodarone. Two-drug therapy often is required. *Digoxin as single-drug therapy is not recommended;* it may slow conduction in the AV node and promote more rapid conduction through the accessory pathway in the event of AF. In practice, drug therapy to prevent PSVT is tricky. Long-term control is unusual, and patients tend to spend a lot of time and money on the process.

Radiofrequency ablation of the bypass tract has become the therapy of choice for patients with WPW syndrome and recurrent PSVT. The success rate is 90% to 95%, and continued drug therapy is unnecessary (i.e., it is a "cure").

Lown-Ganong-Levine (LGL) syndrome is caused by "James fibers" that connect the atrium directly to the bundle of His. Since ventricular activation originates from the bundle of His, there is no delta wave, but there is a shorter PR interval. LGL syndrome may cause PSVT. More worrisome are AF or atrial flutter because of the rapid transmission of impulses from the atrium to the ventricle. The treatment approach is similar to that with WPW syndrome; ablation therapy is possible if PSVT is not easily controlled.

Less common than the WPW or LGL syndrome is PSVT caused by the Mahaim pathway, fibers connecting the AV node to the ventricular fascicle. This may cause narrow QRS complex PSVT or PSVT with left bundle branch block that is difficult to distinguish from ventricular tachycardia. The diagnosis is made with EPS, and ablation therapy is possible.

AUTOMATIC ECTOPIC TACHYCARDIA

In addition to reentry, it is possible to have enhanced automaticity of pacemaker fibers as a cause of supraventricular tachycardia. Cells with spontaneous depolarization and pacemaker potential are found in the atria, the AV node, and the bundle of His, and any of them can be involved in the development of an automatic ectopic tachycardia.

Atrial ectopic tachycardia is a rare cause of sustained supraventricular tachycardia. The 12-lead ECG shows a rapid rate, occasionally higher than 200 beats/min, but usually 140 to 160 beats/min. At this rate it may be difficult to distinguish from atrial flutter with 2-1 block (150 beats/min). This tachycardia may occur in patients with no underlying heart disease, and it tends to be sustained rather than paroxysmal. It often is refractory to medical therapy. When terminated, it may recur without an antecedent premature atrial contraction. Confirmation of the diagnosis usually requires EPS. Ablation of the ectopic focus is the most effective therapy.

Junctional tachycardia is another rare cause of supraventricular tachycardia. The usual mechanism is enhanced automaticity of AV nodal tissue. Inflammation after heart surgery, infection, electrolyte abnormalities, and drug toxicity may cause it. Most cases result from digitalis toxicity. The 12-lead ECG shows a regular, narrow QRS complex tachycardia, often with AV dissociation (P waves that do not appear to be related to any of the QRS complexes). Others have retrograde conduction to the atria and retrograde P waves (see Fig. 25-5). Proper therapy is correction of the underlying disorder. If the arrhythmia persists, drugs to reduce automaticity are indicated. Most effective are beta-blockers, calcium channel blockers, and amiodarone. EPS is infrequently needed for refractory cases, and radiofrequency ablation is possible.

Multifocal atrial tachycardia (MAT) is also caused by enhanced automaticity. The most common clinical setting is severe pulmonary disease, but it may also occur in acutely ill elderly patients. The diagnosis is made when there are at least three different P wave patterns, variation in PR intervals, and an irregular atrial rate averaging more than 100 beats/min (Fig. 25-6). It occasionally is mistaken for AF because of the irregularity, but a P wave before each QRS excludes that diagnosis. Treatment is aimed at correcting the underlying disease. MAT indicates a bad prognosis in patients with lung disease, not because of the arrhythmia, but because it is a marker of end-stage lung disease. Beta-blockers are the best medical therapy, but they cannot be used when there is severe bronchospasm. Verapamil or diltiazem may slow the rate, but digoxin does not work well. Correcting electrolyte abnormalities, especially hypomagnesemia, may help. The heart rate is rarely fast enough to compromise cardiac function. In the absence of severe tachycardia, no specific antiarrhythmic therapy is indicated.

TACHYCARDIA-INDUCED CARDIOMYOPATHY

An uncommon and curious side effect of sustained atrial tachyarrhythmias is cardiomyopathy. We have seen a number of cases with atrial fibrillation.[13] Typically, a patient with nonspecific complaints (fatigue, weakness, decreased exercise tolerance) is found to have rapid AF, and an echocardiogram shows reduced left ventricular ejection fraction and mild dilation. In such cases, it may be that cardiomyopathy is the cause of the arrhythmia, but the reverse is also possible. The correct approach is treatment of the depressed left ventricular fraction with afterload reduction therapy. Congestive symptoms may necessitate diuretic therapy as well, but it may be unnecessary to continue treatment for heart failure long term. With restoration of sinus rhythm and a heart rate below 100 beats/min, it is common for left ventricular size and function to normalize. Repeat the echocardiogram 2 to 3 months after cardioversion.

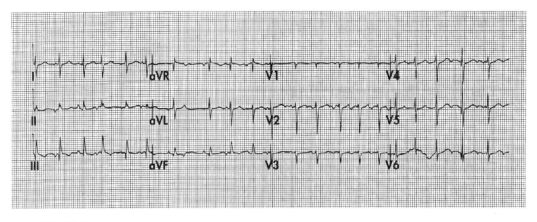

FIG. 25-6
Multifocal atrial tachycardia (MAT). The rhythm is grossly irregular, but there are P waves before each QRS. P wave morphology varies, as does the PR interval.

REFERENCES

1. Golari H, Cebul R, Bahler R: Restoration and maintenance of sinus rhythm and indications for anticoagulation therapy, *Ann Intern Med* 125:311, 1996.
2. Wolf PA, Dawber TR, Thoma HE Jr, Kannel WB: Epidemiologic assessment of chronic atrial fibrillation and risk of stroke: the Framingham study, *Neurology* 28:973, 1978.
3. Atrial Fibrillation Investigators: Risk factors for stroke and efficacy of antithrombotic therapy in atrial fibrillation: analysis of pooled data from five randomized controlled trials, *Arch Intern Med* 154:1449, 1994.
4. Peterson P, Godtfredsen J: Embolic complications in paroxysmal atrial fibrillation, *Stroke* 17:622, 1986.
5. Stroke Prevention in Atrial Fibrillation Investigators: Patients with nonvalvular atrial fibrillation at low risk of stroke during treatment with aspirin, *JAMA* 279:1237, 1998.
6. Hirsh J, Dalen JE, Deykin D, Poller L: Oral anticoagulants: mechanism of action, clinical effectiveness, and optimal therapeutic range, *Chest* 102(suppl 4):312, 1992.
7. Kirkwood TBL: Calibration of reference thromboplastin and standardization of the prothrombin time ratio, *Thromb Haemost* 49:238, 1983.
8. Fenster PE, Comess KA, Marsh R, et al: Conversion of atrial fibrillation to sinus rhythm by acute intravenous procainamide infusion, *Am Heart J* 106:501, 1983.
9. Boriani G, Cappuci A, Lenzit T, et al: Propafenone for conversion of recent onset atrial fibrillation, *Chest* 1008:355, 1995.
10. Oral H, Souza JJ, Michaud GF, et al: Facilitating transthoracic cardioversion of atrial fibrillation with ibutilide pretreatment, *N Engl J Med* 340:1849, 1999.
11. DiMarco JP, Miles W, Akhtar M, et al: Adenosine for paroxysmal SVT, *Ann Intern Med* 113:104, 1990.
12. Kay GN, Epstein AE, Dailey SM, Plumb VJ: Role of radiofrequency ablation in the management of supraventricular arrhythmias, *J Cardiovasc Electrophysiol* 4:371, 1993.
13. Fenelon G, Wijns W, Andries E, Brugada P: Tachycardiomyopathy: mechanisms and clinical implications, *Pacing Clin Electrophysiol* 19:95, 1996.

BIBLIOGRAPHY

Ganz L, Friedman P: Supraventricular tachycardia, *N Engl J Med* 332:162, 1995.

Golari H, Cebul R, Bahler R: Atrial fibrillation: restoration and maintenance of sinus rhythm and indications for anticoagulation therapy, *Ann Intern Med* 125:311, 1996.

Seidl K, Hauer B, Schwick NG, et al: Risk of thromboembolic events in patients with atrial flutter, *Am J Cardiol* 82:580, 1998. Documented embolism in 11 of 191 consecutive patients referred for flutter during 26 months' follow-up. We now recommend anticoagulation, although evidence for this is not as clear as it is for AF.

Ventricular Arrhythmias

Elisha L. Brownfield
Robert B. Leman

PREMATURE VENTRICULAR CONTRACTIONS

Premature ventricular contractions (PVCs) are common and may be symptomatic or asymptomatic. The major goal of management is identification and treatment of patients at high risk for sustained ventricular arrhythmia and sudden cardiac death.

Epidemiology, Etiology, and Natural History

PVCs, especially asymptomatic ones, are the most commonly encountered ventricular arrhythmia and may occur in both healthy and ailing hearts. They are seen on 1% of resting electrocardiograms (ECGs), and 40% to 75% of 24- to 48-hour ambulatory ECGs in clinically normal people.[1] Patients without heart disease have an excellent prognosis. Conversely, patients who have had a myocardial infarction and have frequent or complex PVCs have a twofold to threefold increased risk of sudden cardiac death compared with similar patients without ventricular arrhythmias.[2] Patients with reduced systolic function—with and without coronary heart disease—are also at increased risk for sudden arrhythmic death. The prevalence of PVCs increases with several factors, which should be considered when evaluating patients (Box 26-1).

Pathology, Pathophysiology, and Definition

Arrhythmias are generated in the ventricles by one of three mechanisms: spontaneous firing of ventricular cells (automaticity), the slow trip of an electrical impulse through a reentrant pathway that emerges and reexcites surrounding tissue (reentry), or the triggering of a cardiac cell by the preceding impulse (triggered). The most common mechanism for isolated PVCs is automaticity, whereas reentry is usually responsible for ventricular tachycardia. Regardless of the mechanism, PVCs appear roughly the same on ECG as wide QRS complexes with no preceding P wave, and they are typically followed by a compensatory pause. Therefore you can plot the normal R-R interval through the PVC and following pause, and the subsequent beat will arrive on time (Fig. 26-1). Two PVCs in a row are a couplet, and three or more together are termed *ventricular tachycardia* (Fig. 26-1). The interval between the normal QRS complex and the PVC can be variable or fixed to create bigeminy (every other beat), trigeminy (every third beat), quadrigeminy, and so on. Evaluation and treatment are the same regardless of the pattern.

Clinical Presentation

PVCs may be symptomatic and are described most frequently as skipped beats or palpitations. Many are asymptomatic and are incidental findings on the ECG. Because the prognosis depends on the underlying condition of the heart (Box 26-2), a careful review of car-

---

BOX 26-1

FACTORS THAT INCREASE FREQUENCY OF PREMATURE VENTRICULAR CONTRACTIONS

Increasing age
Male sex
Caffeine
Alcohol
Sympathomimetic drugs
    Cocaine
    Amphetamines
    Amphetamine-like compounds
Phenothiazines
Tricyclic antidepressants
Thyroid disease
Hypokalemia
Hypoxia
Exercise
Systemic infection
Myocardial irritation
    Ischemia
    Inflammation
Anesthesia
Surgery
Emotional excitement
Left ventricular dysfunction

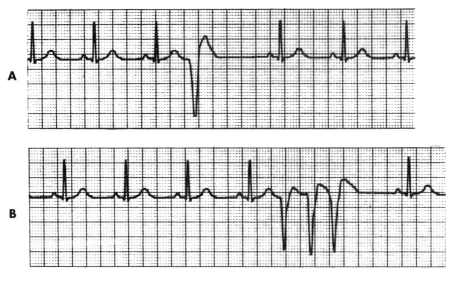

FIG. 26-1

A, Premature ventricular contraction. The QRS complex is greater than 0.14 ms, and there is no preceding P wave. Using calipers, one can mark out the normal R-R interval through the PVC. The ventricular depolarization does not depolarize the atrium and thus does not "reset" the atrial rhythm. P waves march through the ectopic beat. A failure to reset the atrium results in a "compensatory pause" after the PVC. **B,** A triplet of PVCs; three or more PVCs constitute ventricular tachycardia *(VT).*

From Taylor GJ: *150 practice ECGs: interpretation and board review,* Cambridge, Mass, 1997, Blackwell Science.

BOX 26-2

RISK OF CARDIAC MORTALITY IN PATIENTS WITH PREMATURE VENTRICULAR CONTRACTIONS

LOW RISK
Normal heart
Mitral valve prolapse

HIGHER RISK
Cardiac ischemia
Angina
Myocardial infarction
Cardiomyopathy
Ischemic
Dilated
Hypertrophic
Family history of sudden death

---

diac systems is important. Specifically ask about caffeine, alcohol, and illicit drug use. The physical examination should focus on the cardiac evaluation, as well as peripheral signs of cardiac dysfunction.

Laboratory Studies

Studies used in the evaluation of PVCs are summarized in Table 26-1. A resting ECG may identify PVCs as the cause of palpitations. In a patient with symptoms, 24-hour ambulatory ECG (Holter) monitoring, particularly with a symptom calendar, is useful for identifying the cause of the subjective complaint. An event monitor can be used when the symptoms are infrequent. This ECG device contains a tape that records for 5 minutes and then loops so that the sixth minute of recording overrides the first minute. A patient-operated button starts and stops the machine, and the 5-minute ECG strip can then be sent over the telephone for evaluation. The machine can be worn for months.

Serum potassium and magnesium levels should be measured whenever an arrhythmia is suspected, especially in a patient taking diuretics. Eating disorders may also cause electrolyte abnormalities.

A key element of the evaluation is definition of left ventricular (LV) function. Echocardiography (see Chapter 8) identifies dilated or hypertrophic cardiomyopathies and mitral valve prolapse. Exercise stress testing (see Chapter 6) or other cardiac stress testing should be considered in a patient with symptoms or a history suggesting coronary disease, with coronary angiography generally reserved for a subgroup of those patients with positive noninvasive tests.

Table 26-1	*Studies for Evaluation of Premature Ventricular Contractions*

Clinical Status	Asymptomatic	Symptomatic
Low risk—young patient with no clinical evidence of heart disease	K^+, Mg^{2+} Echocardiogram* Stress ECG* Ambulatory ECG (Holter monitor)*	K^+, Mg^{2+} Echocardiogram* Stress ECG* Ambulatory ECG
High risk—any clinical evidence for poor LV function, cardiomyopathy, or active myocardial ischemia	K^+, Mg^{2+} Echocardiogram to measure LV function Screen for coronary disease Ambulatory ECG (and signal-averaged ECG if available) Consider EPS if the above screening studies are positive	K^+, Mg^{2+} Echocardiogram to measure LV function Screen for coronary disease Ambulatory ECG (and signal averaged ECG if available) EPS if the above screening studies are positive

*Optional; may be performed for patients with frequent or multifocal PVCs or couplets, if underlying disease is suspected, or if there are special concerns such as excessive patient or family anxiety despite reassurance.

Table 26-2	*Management of Premature Ventricular Contractions**

Clinical Status	Asymptomatic	Symptomatic
Normal heart or mitral valve prolapse	No treatment	Trial of beta blockade
Ischemic heart disease or cardiomyopathy	Optimal therapy for underlying condition; possible cardiology referral	Cardiology referral to consider EPS or arrhythmia suppression therapy

*All patients should have K^+ and Mg^{2+} normalized.

Management

Management of PVCs is summarized in Table 26-2. All patients should have electrolyte levels normalized. Patients with normal LV function have an excellent prognosis despite PVCs. For them, the risks of arrhythmia suppression therapy outweigh any benefits. They should be reassured and left untreated. If the patient has symptoms impairing quality of life, beta-blocker therapy may be started to reduce PVCs. These should be given at the lowest effective dose, and an attempt to discontinue therapy should be made after an agreed-on interval. Avoidance of triggering factors such as caffeine and alcohol is also warranted.

A patient with PVCs and an abnormal heart presents a more challenging management problem. PVCs in ischemic heart disease and cardiomyopathies are associated with increased risk of sudden death, but treatment has not been shown to significantly alter that risk. In fact, the Cardiac Arrhythmia Suppression Trial (CAST) tested the effect of three different antiarrhythmic agents in asymptomatic or symptomatic patients with PVCs after myocardial infarction (MI) and showed an increase in the mortality of the treated group when compared to placebo[3] (see Chapter 17).

Presently, there is no indication to treat asymptomatic simple or complex PVCs in a patient with ischemia or cardiomyopathy. For a symptomatic patient, beta-blocker therapy should be used. Antiarrhythmic drugs, amiodarone in particular, can also be helpful, with the caveat that all such agents can provoke arrhythmia—the so-called proarrhythmic effect. Consultation with a cardiologist is in order before initiating any treatment in this subset of patients.

Follow-up

Patients with normal LV function and a negative screen for ischemia, whether asymptomatic or symptomatic, can be followed by their primary care practitioner. Consider cardiology consultation if the diagnosis is uncertain or if a patient has symptoms despite beta-blocker therapy. A patient with asymptomatic complex PVCs and cardiac ischemia or cardiomyopathy may warrant a visit with a cardiology consultant, particularly in view of the rapid changes in medical knowledge regarding the treatment of these patients. Symptomatic patients with abnormal hearts should also be referred, because specialized studies may be indicated and drug treatment can be proarrhythmic.

VENTRICULAR TACHYCARDIA

Ventricular tachycardia (VT) can be a life-threatening arrhythmia and usually signifies underlying heart disease. It is the most common cause of wide QRS complex tachycardia, and a patient may appear clinically stable despite the arrhythmia. There are several underlying causes, and management frequently is dictated by the inciting factors.

Epidemiology, Etiology, and Natural History (Box 26-3)

Ischemic Heart Disease

About half the cases of VT and sudden cardiac death occur during the early stage of acute MI (see Chapter 16). Even a small MI may be complicated by ventricular tachycardia or ventricular fibrillation (VF) during the acute phase of infarction. After the acute phase, beyond 36 to 48 hours from the onset of MI, complex ventricular arrhythmias are limited to those with large MI. Predictors of late hospital phase VT include reduced LV ejection fraction, ventricular aneurysm, congestive heart failure, new bundle branch block, and hypotension during MI. Early reperfusion therapy reduces infarct size and therefore lowers the risk of ventricular arrhythmias. Patients with incomplete infarction and open arteries may have VT with recurrent ischemia (see Chapter 16).

Left Ventricular Dysfunction

Both dilated and hypertrophic cardiomyopathies carry a risk of VT. Patients with *dilated* cardiomyopathy have a 15% to 30% risk of sudden death per year, and complex ventricular arrhythmia on an ambulatory ECG is an independent risk factor for mortality.[4] Syncope, nonsustained VT on ambulatory monitoring, and family history of sudden death all increase the risk of sudden cardiac death in patients with *hypertrophic* cardiomyopathies.

Prolonged QT Syndromes

Prolonged QT syndromes may be familial or acquired, usually as a result of prescription drugs (Table 26-3). The incidence of familial long QT is unknown, but it has been found on every continent and in every race. Long QT syndrome can be associated with congenital deafness, and 1 to 2 per 1000 congenitally deaf patients have this on ECG. About 25% of congenital long QT cases are sporadic. The mortality without treatment in the congenital form is estimated at 1.3% per year, and risk factors for cardiac events include associated congenital deafness, history of syncope, female sex, and documented malignant tachyarrhythmias. As with other long QT syndromes, torsades de pointes is the usual pattern of VT.

Right Ventricular Dysplasia

Right ventricular dysplasia is an uncommon disorder characterized by irregular fatty infiltration and fibrosis within the right ventricle. Patients more often are male, and the ECG in sinus rhythm tends to show T wave inversion in the right precordial leads with occasional atrioventricular (AV) node conduction abnormalities. The echocardiogram may show right ventricular enlargement. Angiography may also reveal localized sacculations in the right ventricle.

Normal Heart VT

Normal heart VT is a rare cause of sustained VT, and patients tend to be young. The arrhythmia may or may not be symptomatic. Patients with structurally normal hearts, normal LV function, and VT have an excellent prognosis.[5]

Mitral Valve Prolapse

Although PVCs are common and nonsustained VT has been reported, sustained VT is rarely associated with mitral valve prolapse. Fewer than 100 cases of sudden death with mitral valve prolapse have been reported.

BOX 26-3

UNDERLYING CARDIAC PATHOLOGY IN VENTRICULAR TACHYCARDIA

Ischemic heart disease (usually with LV dysfunction)	40% to 67%
LV dysfunction	4% to 22%
Dilated cardiomyopathy	20%
Hypertrophic cardiomyopathy	2%
Prolonged QT syndromes	4% to 8%
Right ventricular dysplasia	Rare
Normal heart	17% to 28%
Valvular disease	8% to 10%
Mitral valve prolapse	Rare

Table 26-3	*Causes of Prolonged QT syndrome*

FAMILIAL
Jervell and Lange-Nielsen syndrome
(congenital deafness, autosomal recessive)
Romano-Ward syndrome (normal hearing, autosomal dominant)
Sporadic

ACQUIRED

Drugs
Quinidine
Procainamide and metabolites
Sotalol
Amiodarone
Disopyramide
Phenothiazines
Tricyclic antidepressants
Astemizole with or without ketoconazoles
Terfenadine with or without ketoconazoles
Erythromycin
Pentamidine
Some antimalarial agents
Cisapride (Propulsid)

Electrolytes
Hypokalemia
Hypomagnesemia
(Both are common with
diuretic therapy, but may be
seen with lipid protein diets
or starvation)

Others
CNS lesions
Bradycardia

Pathology and Pathophysiology

Three major mechanisms are behind VT, and different treatments have been advocated for each. For all practical purposes, the mechanism responsible for a particular case cannot be ascertained without electrophysiologic studies (EPS), which is discussed later.

Automaticity, which causes most PVCs, comes in two varieties—enhanced and abnormal. Enhanced automaticity is seen with adrenergic stimulation, common in the post-MI period. Abnormal automaticity may occur as a result of myocardial ischemia, electrolyte abnormalities, and hypoxia.

Reentry occurs when conduction through a protected region of the ventricle is unidirectional and slow. Current exiting the protected focus reexcites surrounding tissue, establishing a "circuit." This is the usual mechanism of VT with cardiomyopathy and coronary artery disease.

Triggered automaticity occurs when there are oscillations in cell membrane potentials, also called *after-depolarizations* (early and delayed). This mechanism is the driving force behind torsade de pointes and digitalis toxicity.

Clinical Presentation

Three or more sequential ventricular beats at 120 beats/min or faster is termed *VT.* Nonsustained VT is 3 or more such beats lasting less than 30 seconds; sustained VT lasts more than 30 seconds or is associated with hemodynamic compromise. It is important to remember that VT is uncommon, and a minority of the patients in your practice with syncope or palpitations will turn out to have VT as the etiology. On the other hand, sorting out and managing wide QRS complex tachycardia can be a daunting task (Fig. 26-2).

A patient with VT can present in many different ways. Despite the gravity we often assign to this rhythm, it may be found incidentally in an asymptomatic patient. It is often seen on the Holter monitors of patients with nonischemic cardiomyopathy. Symptoms influence management, so any history of syncope, presyncope, heart failure, dizziness, palpitations, or hypotension is important. Associated cardiac conditions also dictate prognosis and management, and the general cardiac evaluation is an important element of the arrhythmia workup.

A patient with familial long QT syndrome often presents at a young age with syncope when confronted by intense emotion, such as fright or anger, physical activity, or sudden awakening. There is often a higher incidence of symptoms at the time of menses. There may be a family history of syncope or early death.

If a patient is having the arrhythmia in your presence, remember to treat the patient and not just the ECG. Check the airway, breathing, and blood pressure before reaching for the defibrillator. A stable patient often responds to antiarrhythmic medications such as lidocaine

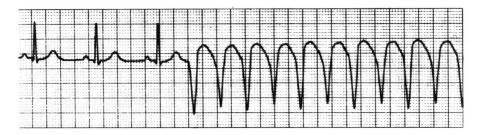

FIG. 26-2

Ventricular tachycardia. A VT episode that exceeds 30 seconds is called *sustained VT.* The QRS complexes are wide (greater than 0.14 ms) and the rate is over 120 beats/min with no apparent P waves. This is monomorphic VT, since all the ventricular beats have the same appearance (morphology).

From Taylor GJ: *150 practice ECGs: interpretation and board review,* Cambridge, Mass, 1997, Blackwell Science.

FIG. 26-3

A-V dissociation in ventricular tachycardia. Note the P waves that occur intermittently between QRS complexes. P waves are difficult or impossible to see on most surface ECGs because of the magnitude and rate of the VT complexes. In the electrophysiology laboratory, a recording can be taken from an electrode in the right atrium, resulting in giant, obvious P waves, and making it possible to document A-V dissociation. This is how EPS determines whether wide complex tachycardia is ventricular or supraventricular. With supraventricular rhythms, there is a regular relationship between P waves and QRS complexes.

From Taylor GJ: *150 practice ECGs: interpretation and board review,* Cambridge, Mass, 1997, Blackwell Science.

(see Chapter 50). *Any instability, including decreased blood pressure, shortness of breath, or chest pain, requires immediate, synchronized cardioversion, even if the wide complex tachycardia is an aberrantly conducted atrial rhythm.*

You may be asked to determine the cause of a wide complex tachycardia. If you guess VT on all, you will be wrong only 20% of the time, but some guidelines help to determine its cause. Basically, a wide complex tachycardia could be VT, a supraventricular tachycardia with a bundle branch block, or a supraventricular tachycardia that preexcites the ventricles through an accessory tract. A history of previous cardiac ischemia or congestive heart failure would be a good indication that the rhythm is ventricular.

There are several methods for determining the cause of a VT from the resting ECG, but Andries, Brugada, and Brugada[6] have developed a four-step approach that had a 96% specificity and a 98.6% sensitivity for detecting VT. This involves inspecting the precordial

leads for an RS complex, measuring the interval between the onset of the R wave and the deepest part of the S, looking for dissociation between atrial and ventricular firing (Fig. 26-3), and looking at the morphology of the QRS in leads V_1 and V_6 (Box 26-4). This rather complex exercise is interesting and useful once the patient's condition has been stabilized. However, when treating an acutely ill patient, particularly if there is hypotension, rapid treatment of wide QRS tachycardia is critical. Assume that it is VT and apply DC countershock.

Laboratory Studies

Initial diagnostic tests for ventricular arrhythmias include the ECG and Holter monitor. If the arrhythmia is prevalent, these studies easily make the diagnosis. However, the arrhythmias often are not prevalent, decreasing the sensitivity. A loop monitor can be used for a clinically stable patient without syncope or near-syncope.

BOX 26-4

FOUR-STEP METHOD FOR DIAGNOSING WIDE QRS COMPLEX TACHYCARDIA

1. Evaluate all precordial leads for RS complex
   None found → VT
   Found → Go to 2
2. Measure interval between onset of R wave and deepest part of S in multiple leads
   Interval >100 ms in lead with longest RS → VT
   Interval <100 ms → Go to 3
3. Look for dissociation of the atrial and ventricular depolarizations.
   Found → VT
   Not found → Go to 4
4. Inspect morphology of V_1 and V_6
   If V_1 is a positive deflection (right bundle branch block pattern)
     Look for monomorphic or QR pattern in V_1
       Found → VT
     R:S ratio → 1 in V_6
       Found → VT
   If V_1 is a negative deflection (left bundle branch block pattern)
     r >30 ms in V_1 or V_2
       Found → VT
     Slurred or notched downstroke of S in V_1 or V_2
       Found → VT
     Interval from onset of QRS to nadir of QS or S >70 ms
       Found → VT
     Any Q wave in V_6
       Found → VT
     All negative → not VT
     Present in both V_1 and V_6 → VT

Adapted from Andries EW, Brugada J, Brugada P: *Primary Cardiol* 18:29, 1992.

Additional noninvasive tests that indicate an increased probability of VT are heart rate variability and the signal-averaged ECG (see Table 17-3).

It is interesting that a critical initial study for patients with suspected VT is a measure of LV function, usually with an echocardiogram. Normal LV function, normal serum electrolyte levels (including Mg^{+2}), and a normal QT interval exclude VT in most cases.

EPS is often used in patients with syncope and possible ventricular arrhythmias. The goal is to induce VT in the electrophysiology laboratory using paced PVCs. EPS is always done before the implantation of a cardiac defibrillator, not only to diagnose the arrhythmia, but also to determine the best VT-terminating pacing protocol for the specific arrhythmia. EPS may identify an arrhythmia that can be ablated (e.g., bundle branch reentry).

Coronary angiography is often a part of the VT workup. Correction of ischemia with revascularization may prevent VT. Even more reliable is resection of a ventricular aneurysm.

Management

Treatment of VT depends on cardiac function, the presence of ischemia, and symptoms related to the arrhythmia. Acutely, the clinician should treat any electrolyte disturbances and follow the advanced cardiac life support (ACLS) protocol (see Chapter 50), always remembering to evaluate the patient before treating the ECG. Long-term management varies depending on the cause. (Table 26-4).

Ischemia

As has been demonstrated in the CAST study and subsequent follow-up, medical treatment of asymptomatic or mildly symptomatic ventricular arrhythmias does not always prolong life[3] (see Chapter 17). There is no consensus regarding the treatment of VT in patients after MI, but everyone would agree that treating any correctable ischemia is a good place to start. Moss and colleagues[7] found that implantable cardiac defibrillators (ICD) were better than medical therapy for patients with asymptomatic, nonsustained VT that was inducible during EPS. These results have been criticized because some patients in the defibrillator group received antiarrhythmic medications and some patients in the drug treatment group were not taking antiarrhythmic agents at the time of death. The AVID study, however, also showed a benefit of ICDs over medical treatment.[8]

In our institution, we evaluate post-MI patients based on symptoms and other tests before starting therapy. Patients with *asymptomatic* nonsustained VT have an evaluation of LV function and a signal-averaged ECG. If these are normal, no therapy is prescribed. If either is abnormal, EPS is done, and an ICD is implanted if the study indicates a high risk of sudden death. Patients with *symptomatic* complex PVCs receive beta-blockers, LV function testing, and signal-averaged ECG. If the tests are abnormal, EPS is done. Symptomatic VT is an indication for EPS, and therapy is guided by the results.

Drug Therapy

It has long been known that VT is a marker for sudden death. However, little conclusive evidence shows that the eradication of ventricular arrhythmias by anti-

Table 26-4	*Management of Nonsustained Ventricular Tachycardia**	
Clinical Status	**Asymptomatic (Brief Run of VT)**	**Symptomatic (More Prolonged VT)**
Ischemic heart disease	Echocardiogram normal—no therapy	EPS-guided therapy (drugs versus ICD)
Dilated cardiomyopathy	Possibly no therapy, possibly a candidate for clinical trials	Probably EPS, then ICD versus drugs versus transplant
Hypertrophic cardiomyopathy	Beta blockade—no further therapy versus EPS, depending on the length of VT	EPS, then a choice of beta blockade, calcium blocker, amiodarone, or ICD
Long QT syndrome	Stop inciting factors (see Table 26-3); high-risk familial—beta-blockers	Familial—beta-blocker, pacemaker, surgery (sympathectomy), or ICD
Right ventricular dysplasia	No therapy	EPS-guided therapy
Mitral valve prolapse	No therapy	If hemodynamically significant, EPS; if not, beta blockade
Normal heart VT	No therapy	Beta blocker, calcium blocker, EPS, radiofrequency ablation

*The first principle of management is optimal treatment of the underlying condition.

arrhythmic agents prolongs life. All antiarrhythmics (Box 26-5) can cause arrhythmias, and many have significant side effects and need drug monitoring with levels and other laboratory work. It has been clearly shown that sodium channel blocking antiarrhythmics do not promote survival (class I). Class II agents (beta-blockers) have a beneficial effect on survival, but this may not be because of their antiarrhythmic properties. Beta-blockers also prevent ischemia, and larger trials have shown a reduction in recurrent MI, which also has a favorable effect on survival.

Amiodarone (class III) has been shown to control VT, but it does not prolong survival (see Chapter 17).

Implantable Cardioverter-Defibrillator

The ICD is the most effective therapy for preventing sudden cardiac death, according to two recent studies, the MADIT and AVID.[7,8] With ICD therapy for VT or VF, survival is 99% at 1 year and 96% at 5 years. The third-generation ICDs have greatly improved in correcting and controlling ventricular arrhythmias. The ICD can act as a pacemaker and can pace the heart from the ventricular position or AV sequentially (both atria and ventricles). It is able to sense VT and then pace-terminate it using a preprogrammed pacing protocol. If pacing is unsuccessful, various energy levels of cardioversion can be used. The device also identifies fast VT or VF and proceeds immediately to cardioversion.

The ICD is inserted transvenously and does not require a thoracotomy. The battery pack is placed in the left pectoral region, with wire electrodes going to the right atrium and right ventricular apex. The electrodes are two coils—one in the right ventricle and the other in the superior vena cava region. With discharge, current travels from the two coils to the battery pack in the left pectoral region. The mortality from implantation of an ICD is usually less than 1%. At the time of implantation, VT or VF is provoked. The device is programmed to convert this arrhythmia. Most ICDs can deliver between 29 to 37 joules, and the defibrillator's threshold is set about 10 joules less than maximum output (19 to 27 joules). However, if ventricular thresholds are not adequate for the transvenous system, then surgery may be performed to place a patch on the left ventricle.

The third-generation ICDs have a tremendous selection of programming features that can be adjusted during the follow-up visits of the patient. Patients with ICDs are seen every 3 to 6 months. During follow-up the device is evaluated for its effectiveness in pacing and the lead's integrity. The newer ICDs can record up to 15 minutes of Holter data from the events that are activated by the machine. These machines indicate if the electrogram (intracardiac ECG) is normal or abnormal (wide).

The ICD also records its activity, providing ongoing quality control. It records the electrogram at the time of

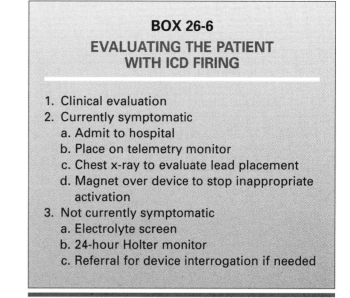

BOX 26-5

ANTIARRHYTHMICS

Class I	Sodium channel blockers
	A Moderate kinetics (quinidine)
	B Fast kinetics (lidocaine)
	C Slow kinetics (propafenone)
Class II	Antiadrenergics (beta-blockers)
Class III	Potassium channel blockers
	(amiodarone)
Class IV	Calcium channel blockers
	(verapamil)

BOX 26-6

EVALUATING THE PATIENT WITH ICD FIRING

1. Clinical evaluation
2. Currently symptomatic
   a. Admit to hospital
   b. Place on telemetry monitor
   c. Chest x-ray to evaluate lead placement
   d. Magnet over device to stop inappropriate activation
3. Not currently symptomatic
   a. Electrolyte screen
   b. 24-hour Holter monitor
   c. Referral for device interrogation if needed

discharge, documenting the arrhythmia. If it shocked the wrong rhythm, it can be reprogrammed. The longevity of these devices ranges from 4 to 8 years and hopefully will be increased further. Battery life is determined by the number of shocks delivered, because this is the highest energy drainage.

ICDs are followed in our "device clinic" by a cardiologist expert in their management. Interrogation of ICD function and ICD programming are technical exercises unfamiliar to most cardiologists. The generalist, including the primary care physician, should understand several things about the machine. It gives you recorded data indicating why the machine was activated. If a patient has syncope after the machine is implanted and the machine is not activated, then tachyarrhythmia is an unlikely cause. A bradyarrhythmia is a possible cause, since the ICD does not record or treat slow rhythms.

If a patient has a shock and is asymptomatic afterward, he or she should see a primary care physician for a measurement of electrolyte levels and a Holter monitor. Patients who have multiple shocks (two or three in a row) should be transported to the emergency department immediately and hospitalized. Again, electrolyte levels should be measured and the patient placed on telemetry. A chest x-ray should be obtained, since the leads can be misplaced (Box 26-6). The most common causes of multiple shocks are development of atrial fibrillation, increasing ventricular arrhythmias, and lead displacement. Atrial fibrillation must be corrected and the ventricular rate slowed so that the machine does not sense the fast heart rate as VT. If a patient has increasing ventricular arrhythmias, antiarrhythmic agents should be started to suppress them. These drugs may affect the defibrillation threshold of the device. Lead misplacement must be corrected.

Occasionally in the emergency department a patient is shocked inappropriately for atrial fibrillation, often frightening both the patient and medical personnel. Placing a magnet over the battery pack eliminates this because sensing is turned off, disabling the machine. With the magnet in place the ICD will not sense VT either, and the patient should be on telemetry. If VT is noted on telemetry, the magnet can be removed, and the ICD will sense and terminate the arrhythmia.

Left Ventricular Dysfunction

Patients with idiopathic dilated cardiomyopathy and normal coronary arteries have a 40% incidence of nonsustained VT and a 17% incidence of sudden cardiac death. Unfortunately no evidence has shown that eradicating nonsustained VT reduces mortality risk. Those with syncope tend to do poorly. Cardiologists may use ambulatory monitoring, the signal-averaged ECG, or EPS to identify patients at highest risk of sudden cardiac death, but there is no standard workup. Unfortunately EPS is helpful only if it induces VT. A negative EPS does not exclude VT as the cause of symptoms. A patient with symptomatic ventricular arrhythmias or documented sustained VT may be treated with an ICD. Cardiac transplantation may be the best treatment for those with end-stage cardiomyopathy and recurrent VT.

Patients with *hypertrophic cardiomyopathy* have a 19% incidence of nonsustained VT and an 8% incidence of sudden cardiac death. Those who are asymptomatic or mildly symptomatic with brief and infrequent nonsustained VT are thought to have a low mortality risk. Treatment is controversial and usually reserved for symptomatic patients. EPS may help to separate high-risk from low-risk patients. Treatment may consist of antiarrhythmic agents, calcium channel blockers, beta-blockers, or the ICD.

Long QT Syndromes

Acquired long QT syndrome should be treated by correcting the inciting factors. Correction of torsade de pointes includes intravenous magnesium, isoproterenol, and temporary pacing to increase the heart rate, in addition to DC cardioversion.

When an index case of long QT syndrome is found, all family members should have screening ECGs, and ambulatory monitoring should be used for those with a long QT interval. An asymptomatic patient usually does well, but occasionally a patient may die as a result of the first symptomatic cardiac episode. High-risk groups include those with congenital deafness, neonates through age 1 year, and siblings of children who have died suddenly. Generally speaking, no patients with familial long QT should engage in competitive sports.

Beta-blockers should be used in symptomatic patients with a history of syncope or aborted cardiac arrest and some asymptomatic patients from high-risk families. The dose should be maximized so that the heart rate is less than 130 beats/min with exercise testing. A pacemaker can be added for patients who have bradycardia on beta blockade. Patients who continue to have recurrent syncope or aborted cardiac arrest may be treated with a surgical procedure in which the sympathetic nervous system is disconnected from the heart (left cervicothoracic sympathetic ganglionectomy) or with an automatic implantable cardiac defibrillator.

Many gene mutations are associated with this condition, and drug therapy specific to the mutation is now being used. For example, mexiletine has been found to be effective in patients with a mutation of SCN5A sodium channels. Potassium and spironolactone have been used with good results in patients with mutations of the delayed rectifier potassium channels.[7,9]

Here again, treatment decisions should be made in conjunction with a cardiologist. The family pediatrician should be involved as well if the children see a separate practitioner. Because these patients are often young and female, pregnancies may occur and neonates should be screened.

RV Dysplasia

Patients with this condition are rare and should be followed by a cardiologist. Patients usually have a left bundle branch block, and the VT also has a left bundle pattern. It may respond to antiarrhythmic treatment, which should be guided by Holter monitor or EPS.

Normal Heart VT

The patient should be evaluated to ensure the heart is normal, with an assessment of LV function and a screen for coronary artery disease. Because this group has an excellent prognosis with an extremely low incidence of sudden cardiac death, treatment should be reserved for symptomatic patients. Symptom relief can often be achieved with beta-blockers or calcium antagonists. EPS-guided radiofrequency ablation should also be considered, especially if drug treatment fails to control symptoms. The ablation also has the advantage of freeing the relatively young patient from lifelong medication.

Mitral Valve Prolapse

The prognosis is good in the mitral valve prolapse group. Beta-blockers or calcium channel blockers can be used in symptomatic patients. If the arrhythmia is hemodynamically significant, EPS should be considered. The signal-averaged ECG is not helpful in this group because it is often falsely positive.

Follow-up

Patients with VT should be followed by their primary care practitioner and a cardiologist. Those taking antiarrhythmic drugs may need to have drug levels checked and electrolyte levels monitored regularly. If a patient with an implantable defibrillator suspects the device is firing, he or she should come in for an electrolyte screen and 24-hour Holter monitor. The device can be turned off by placing a magnet over it (see Box 26-6).

The psychologic aspects of care for these patients should not be overlooked. They are frequently anxious about performing usual activities and may be especially fearful of defibrillation if they have an ICD. This is not a comfortable experience, and many of our patients have described a sensation of "being kicked in the chest." Antianxiety drug therapy may help in these cases. Often our patients report avoiding sex for fear of starting an arrhythmia. In such cases a low-level exercise test to exclude exercise-induced VT is reassuring. Open discussions can be very helpful.

TORSADES DE POINTES
Epidemiology, Etiology, and Natural History

Torsades de pointes originates in the setting of a long QT. It can be inherited or acquired through drug therapy or electrolyte abnormalities. Lesions of the brain can rarely cause this arrhythmia. The various underlying causes are outlined in Table 26-3. There tends to be a twofold to threefold higher incidence of this arrhythmia in women. A long QT interval may happen with normal doses of antiarrhythmic agents and therapeutic drug levels, while noncardiac drugs generally must reach high plasma concentrations before causing the derangement. The prognosis is good because most causative agents can be corrected, and familial long QT syndrome can be treated.

Pathology and Pathophysiology

Torsades de pointes is a triggered arrhythmia that occurs when an after-depolarization of the action potential reaches a threshold to allow for repetitive firing. This can occur more easily with a long QT interval. There are two varieties: pause dependent and adrenergic dependent. The pause-dependent type is acquired and is the underlying mechanism for torsades de pointes with bradycardia, electrolyte imbalances, and drug therapy. A PVC occurs and is followed by a sinus beat with a long QT. A second PVC then falls during the long QT, and tachycardia is initiated. Torsadse with familial long QT and neurologic lesions is adrenergic dependent. Excess adrenergic tone is thought to contribute to triggered automaticity.

Clinical Presentation

Torsades de pointes may manifest as any other ventricular tachycardia—symptomatically or asymptomatically. Patients taking drugs known to cause torsades de pointes may be at higher risk of developing the arrhythmia when the QT interval is greater than 500 ms. There may be frequent nonsustained episodes or sustained tachycardia at a rate of 160 to 250 beats/min. Occasionally this rhythm degenerates into VF.

The ECG has a distinctive appearance. Wide QRS complexes are polymorphic when viewed over several leads and seem to become gradually larger, then smaller (Fig. 26-4). The QRS axis appears to be "turning around a point." Recognizing the ECG image of torsades de pointes is especially crucial because acute and chronic therapy for this VT differ from those for all the others.

The drug history is important, including any over-the-counter agents. Antihistamines and other phenothiazine derivatives may be responsible. A celebrated epidemic of torsade resulted from combined treatment with erythromycin and the popular antihistamine, terfenadine (Seldane). Erythromycin competes for cytochrome P450 sites, and terfenadine levels rise. Azithromycin (Zithromax), another macrolide antibiotic with similar spec-

trum, does not have this interaction with antihistamines. We have seen torsades and syncope in some patients who were taking other antihistamines in addition to quinidine (initially prescribed for atrial fibrillation).

Family history of syncope or early death is important if no causative agents can be found. All family members should be screened if familial long QT syndrome is suspected. Ischemia can also cause a long QT, so cardiac history and symptoms of ischemia should be determined.

Management

Laboratory studies include Mg^{+2} concentration, electrolyte levels, and measurement of drug levels when appropriate.

The acute treatment of torsades de pointes is aimed at shortening the action potential and eliminating triggered activity. Intravenous magnesium can be given to the patient at the time of the arrhythmia to decrease triggering (see Chapter 50). Over the long term, beta-blockers help to prevent triggered activity in many patients with long QT syndrome. Full recommendations for the treatment of familial long QT can be found in Table 26-4. In the acute setting, temporary cardiac pacing at a rate of 90 to 100 beats/min or isoproterenol infusion to increase heart rate also shortens the action potential. Electrolyte levels should be corrected immediately and offending drugs discontinued.

Follow-up

Patients with acquired long QT do quite well over the long term. After correction of the underlying cause, ECGs should be repeated to measure the QT_c interval. This should ideally remain below 500 ms to prevent recurrence. Amiodarone rarely causes torsades de pointes and should be considered as an optional antiarrhythmic agent in patients who continue to have a long QT. Electrolyte levels should be monitored as well to ensure adequate and sustained correction. Persistent bradycardia may require permanent pacing. Cardiology consultation would be recommended, at least until any inciting factors are gone.

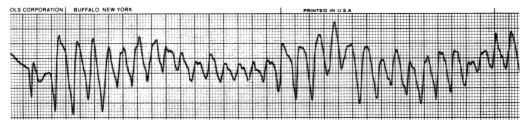

FIG. 26-4
Torsades de pointes. QRS complexes are wide and polymorphic and become gradually larger and then smaller over several seconds. The axis of the QRS is shifting, "around a point."

From Taylor GJ: *150 practice ECGs: interpretation and board review,* Cambridge, Mass, 1997, Blackwell Science.

Familial long QT syndrome deserves special follow-up with the patient's primary care provider and a cardiologist. Patients who are not adequately treated with beta-blockers may need pacemakers, surgery, or automatic implantable defibrillators. Recently therapy targeted to the specific gene mutation has been suggested, and the patient may need gene testing to determine which portion of the depolarization process is being affected. These patients need life-long management by the primary care practitioner in conjunction with a cardiologist.

VENTRICULAR FIBRILLATION AND SUDDEN CARDIAC DEATH

Prognosis for ventricular fibrillation and sudden cardiac death depends on the speed of defibrillation. The overall prognosis is poor, with the exception of patients who experience this in the setting of an acute MI.

Epidemiology, Etiology, and Natural History

Approximately 300,000 cases of sudden cardiac death occur annually, accounting for more than 50% of all cardiovascular deaths in the United States. Patients at high risk for sudden cardiac death include those with coronary artery disease, cardiomyopathies, and documented ventricular arrhythmias. Other, less common etiologies include hypoxia, atrial fibrillation with very rapid ventricular responses, electrical cardioversion or accidental electrical shock, and competitive ventricular pacing used to terminate VT. Valvular, inflammatory, and infiltrative heart disease have also been associated with this lethal arrhythmia.

Resuscitation is effective in the short term for many patients found immediately after cardiac collapse. The rapidity of correction is directly proportional to survival. The automatic external defibrillator (AED) is becoming more widely used and should improve prognosis. Unfortunately, 40% to 60% of patients resuscitated out of the hospital die during that initial hospitalization. Only 10% of these deaths are caused by arrhyth-

mias. Most of these deaths are from central nervous system injury and the remainder are from a low cardiac output state in the patient with advanced structural heart disease. Predictors of mortality in survivors of VF include low left ventricular ejection fraction, cardiac wall motion abnormalities, history of congestive heart failure, history of MI, and the presence of known ventricular arrhythmias.

If VF occurs early after the onset of acute MI, a patient's prognosis is no worse than that for others with similar infarction and no VF. In fact, acute MI as the cause of out-of-hospital VF is a good prognostic indicator. Those with VF and no acute MI have a poor prognosis because recurrence of VF is more likely.

Clinical Appearance and Evaluation

The ECG in VF reveals a disordered rhythm (Fig. 26-5). The patient is in a state of cardiovascular collapse without blood pressure or pulse. There is no such thing as stable VF.

Survivors should have serial cardiac enzyme measurements and serial ECGs to determine the presence of an acute MI. Resuscitation may cause a short-term elevation in cardiac enzyme levels. An echocardiogram (see Chapter 8) may be used to show acute wall motion abnormalities and to evaluate LV function. Coronary angiography and EPS are indicated for all patients who have unexpected, sudden cardiac death.

Management

Acutely, the ACLS protocol should be applied with cardiopulmonary resuscitation and immediate defibrillation (see Chapter 50). Intravenous lidocaine, amiodarone, bretylium, or procainamide can be administered once a stable rhythm is achieved to prevent recurrences. A determination of cause is made after the patient is stable. If the patient has had an acute MI, conventional therapy for the treatment of MIs should be used. Arrhythmogenic agents should be withdrawn. Further treatment is determined by the results of EPS and coronary angiography.

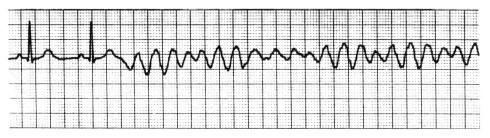

FIG. 26-5
Ventricular fibrillation. The rhythm is apparent over baseline, but disordered.

From Taylor GJ: *150 practice ECGs: interpretation and board review,* Cambridge, Mass, 1997, Blackwell Science.

REFERENCES

1. Kennedy HL, Whitlock JA, Sprague MK, et al: Long-term follow-up of asymptomatic healthy subjects with frequent and complex ventricular ectopy, *N Engl J Med* 312:193, 1985.
2. Braunwald E: *Heart disease,* ed 5, Philadelphia, 1997, WB Saunders.
3. Cardiac Arrhythmia Suppression Trial (CAST) investigators: Preliminary report: effect of encainide and flecainide on mortality in a randomized trial of arrhythmia suppression after myocardial infarction, *N Engl J Med* 321:406, 1989.
4. Holmes J, Kubo SH, Cody RJ, Kligfield P: Arrhythmias in ischemic and nonischemic dilated cardiomyopathy: prediction of mortality by ambulatory electrocardiography, *Am J Cardiol* 55:146, 1985.
5. Lemery R, Brugada P, Bella PD, et al: Nonischemic ventricular tachycardia: clinical course and long-term follow-up in patients without clinically overt heart disease, *Circulation* 79:990, 1989.
6. Andries EW, Brugada J, Brugada P: An algorithm for diagnosing wide QRS complex tachycardia, *Primary Cardiol* 18:29, 1992.
7. Multicenter Automatic Defibrillator Implantation Trial investigators: Improved survival with an implanted defibrillator in patients with coronary disease at high risk for ventricular arrhythmia, *N Engl J Med* 335:1933, 1996.
8. Hallstrom AP, AVID Investigators: Antiarrhythmics versus implantable defibrillators (AVID): rationale, design and methods, *Am J Cardiol* 75:470, 1995.
9. Schwartz PJ: Long QT syndrome patients with mutations of the SCN5A and HERG genes have differential responses to Na+ channel blockade and to increases in heart rate, *Circulation* 92:3383, 1995.

BIBLIOGRAPHY

Fu EY, Clemo HF, Ellenbogen KA: Acquired QT prolongation: mechanisms and implications, *Cardiol Rev* 6:319, 1998. A good review of torsades de pointes.

Roden DM: A practical approach to torsade de pointes, *Clin Cardiol* 20:285, 1997.

Wolfe DA, Kosinski D, Grubb BP: Update on implantable cardioverter-defibrillators, *Postgrad Med* 103:115, 1998.

Zimetbaum P, Josephson ME: Evaluation of patients with palpitations, *N Engl J Med* 338:1369, 1998.

27

Bradyarrhythmias and Evaluation of Syncope

Leonard S. Lichtenstein
Robert B. Leman

BRADYARRHYTHMIAS

Bradyarrhythmias have been defined in the past as heart rate lower than 60 beats/min. However, this definition may be spurious because some young, healthy, athletic people have rates even lower. Therefore the cutoff for bradycardia may actually be lower in certain groups, even as low as 45 beats/min.

Clinical Patterns

The cardiac conduction system has been described in Chapter 2 (see Fig. 2-11). Conduction delay or block may occur at any level of the system, beginning with the sinoatrial node.

Sinoatrial (SA) Node Syndromes

Probably the most common type of arrhythmia seen by the general internist occurs in asymptomatic patients with sinus bradycardia. Again, this is relatively common in trained, athletic individuals. However, in patients with heart disease or in the elderly, bradycardia may be an ominous sign and must be evaluated further, especially if symptoms are present.

Sinus node dysfunction presents as sinus bradycardia and is the most common bradyarrhythmia. SA node conduction problems are classified in the same way as atrioventricular (AV) node block—first, second, and third degree. Except for second-degree block, which has a Wenckebach periodicity (group beating and a progressive shortening of the P-P interval before a pause), the degree of sinus node dysfunction cannot be distinguished by surface electrocardiogram (ECG). First- and third-degree sinus node dysfunctions are indistinguishable on surface ECG from sinus bradycardia. An electrophysiologic study (EPS), which provides direct sinus node recording or indirect sinoatrial conduction times must be done to establish the degree of dysfunction.[1]

Another type of sinus node dysfunction is chronotropic incompetence, which is the inability of the sinus node to respond to normal physiologic needs. The heart rate does not increase appropriately with exercise.

Sick Sinus Syndrome

Sinus node dysfunction can present as a combination of both tachycardia and bradycardia, the so-called tachy-brady, or sick sinus, syndrome. There may be rapid tachycardia (often atrial fibrillation) followed by an abrupt pause. At other times a patient has marked and inappropriate sinus bradycardia. When documented, this combination of arrhythmias establishes the diagnosis. Sick sinus syndrome is common in the elderly and is a frequent cause of palpitations followed by dizziness, near-syncope, or syncope.

Vasovagal Fainting Spells

Another type of bradyarrhythmia occurs as a result of vagal discharge, without abnormality of the SA node or cardiac conduction. Pain or stress causes vagal discharge and leads to sinus node arrest, severe sinus bradycardia, or even AV nodal block. This is the usual mechanism of fainting in an otherwise healthy person (the "common faint").

AV Node Syndromes and Heart Block

AV nodal conduction disease is classified as first-degree, second-degree, and third-degree block (Table 27-1).[1] First-degree AV block is a decrease in conduction velocity through the AV node and is recognized on the surface ECG as prolongation of the PR interval (>220 ms). It does not cause symptoms, and it usually does not progress to higher-degree AV block.

Second-degree AV nodal block is subdivided into two types—Mobitz type I, also called Wenckebach, and Mobitz type II (Table 27-1). The Wenckebach pattern shows (1) a progressive prolongation of PR intervals, with the initial progression being the longest and subsequent progressions being less; (2) shortening of the R-R intervals; and (3) a dropped beat (Fig. 27-1). The level of block is within the AV node. Because infranodal conduction is normal and the ventricles are activated simultaneously, the QRS duration is normal. Mobitz type I block may occur in healthy young people, particularly athletes. It commonly develops during sleep. In the absence of other heart disease, it is a benign condition. However, Mobitz type I heart block may be the first indication of conduction problems in an elderly patient with symptoms.

Second-degree Mobitz type II block is commonly associated with a wide QRS complex because the conduction defect is within or below the His bundle. The pause following the blocked P wave equals that of the

| Table 27-1 | *Atrioventricular (AV) Nodal Block* | | |

Clinical Pattern	Level of Block	ECG Identification	Possible (Reversible) Causes
First-degree block	AV node	Long PR interval (>0.22 sec)	Digoxin, beta blockade, calcium blockers, elevated K^+, Mg^{+2}, inferior myocardial infarction
Second-degree block, Mobitz type I	AV node	The Wenckebach pattern: progressively longer PR, decreasing RR interval, dropped beat; narrow QRS complex	All of the above. The ventricular rate may increase, or heart block resolve with atropine or isoproterenol treatment.
Second-degree block, Mobitz type II	Below the AV node	Fixed PR and RR intervals, dropped beats; wide QRS complex	None. Usually caused by irreversible conduction system disease. Infranodal block does not respond to atropine or isoproterenol.
Third-degree block	1. Within the AV node	1. AV dissociation, ventricular rate >40 beats/min, narrow QRS complex	1. Digoxin, beta blockade, calcium blockers, elevated K^+, Mg^{+2}, inferior myocardial infarction. Block may improve with atropine.
	2. Below the AV node	2. AV dissociation, slower ventricular rate, wide QRS complex	2. None. Usually caused by irreversible conduction system disease.

preceding P to P wave interval. The PR interval of this type of block does not prolong and is steady, as are the PP and RR intervals (Figure 27-1). Mobitz type II may progress to complete heart block and is an indication for treatment when there are symptoms.

Second-degree AV block can present with a 2:1 pattern. Because there is no opportunity to observe PR interval prolongation, it is difficult to determine whether it is Mobitz type I or II. As a rule, a narrow QRS complex indicates Mobitz type I block (block within the AV node), and a wide QRS complex indicates Mobitz type II (infranodal) block.

Third-degree, or "complete," AV block has no conduction of P waves to the QRS (Fig. 27-2). Block may occur within the AV node or below it. When it is infranodal, the ventricular escape rhythm is slow (fewer than 30 beats/min) and the QRS complex is wide. Because it originates from a ventricular pacer, the QRS complex looks like an ectopic ventricular beat. (Do not give lidocaine, because you do not want to suppress it.) Patients with infranodal block usually have evidence of ventricular conduction disease (a wide QRS complex) on ECGs done before the development of complete heart block.

If the level of complete heart block is the AV node, the take-over pacemaker is high in the bundle of His, before the division of the bundle branches. For this reason, the QRS is narrow and the intrinsic rate is faster, usually above 40 beats/min. This pacer may respond to atropine or isoproterenol with an increase in rate.

Another form of third-degree block is paroxysmal. Multiple, nonconducted P waves are interspersed with periods of sinus rhythm without heart block. In the absence of reversible causes of heart block (Table 27-1), both paroxysmal and fixed third-degree AV block require pacemaker implantation.

Pathophysiology

Bradyarrhythmias are caused by abnormal automaticity (abnormal impulse generation) in the SA node or by delayed or blocked conduction in neural structures below it. The most common causes of abnormal automaticity are electrolyte disturbances, cardioactive drugs, or other metabolic disturbances. Conduction system problems may occur as part the normal process of aging—a degenerative, fibrotic process in the conduction system (Lev's or Lenegre's disease). Other disease processes that may influence conduction are ischemia,

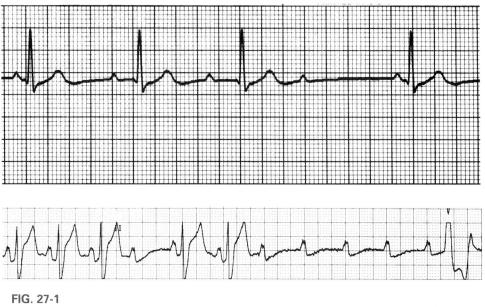

FIG. 27-1

Two patients with second-degree AV block. *Top:* Mobitz type I (Wenckebach). There is progressive lengthening of the PR interval, and the fourth P wave is not conducted. Following the dropped beat, the PR interval is short. The R-R interval decreases before the blocked beat. The QRS complex is narrow, and the level of block is the AV node. *Bottom:* Mobitz type II block. The fourth P wave is not conducted. There is no progressive lengthening of the PR interval before the blocked beat. Later in the tracing there are four blocked P waves, a short spell of complete heart block. The QRS complex is wide (the 12-lead ECG showed bifascicular block), further evidence that the level of block is below the AV node.

From Taylor GJ: *150 practice ECGs: interpretation and board review,* London, 1997, Blackwell Science.

thyroid disease, infiltrative diseases, neuromyopathic disorders, surgical trauma, or infectious diseases (Lyme disease or myocarditis).[1]

Clinical Presentation

The usual symptoms are syncope or near-syncope, but you should be aware of unusual presentations. Fatigue and lack of energy are common with sinus node abnormalities and bradycardia. There may be an inability to exercise because of chronotropic incompetence. In the elderly, mental lapses may result from brady-arrhythmias. Shortness of breath and other symptoms of heart failure may worsen with bradycardia. Stroke or transient ischemic attacks may be precipitated by a drop in cardiac output caused by bradycardia. A patient with the tachybrady syndrome may have a drop in cardiac output with associated symptoms during periods of tachycardia.

The physical examination provides little diagnostic information. The pulse is slow. S_1 often is soft with first-degree AV block (during the long PR interval the AV valves drift toward the closed position, reducing excursion during closure). S_1 may vary with variable con-

duction problems. Cannon A waves are seen in the jugular venous pulse in patients with third-degree AV block.

Laboratory Evaluation

The general laboratory evaluation should include measurement of electrolytes, thyroid function (particularly if the tachybrady syndrome is considered), and digoxin level when appropriate.

The surface ECG can easily diagnose most brady-arrhythmias. It is critical to document the arrhythmia while symptoms are present, because some symptoms, such as dizziness, may have another cause. Unfortunately the symptoms and the arrhythmia are often transient. A Holter monitor is helpful if symptoms occur daily. For less frequent symptoms the 24-hour monitor is usually unrewarding.

The loop monitor is an event monitor that can be used to correlate intermittent symptoms with the cardiac rhythm. The patient can wear it for weeks and activates it when a symptom occurs. Unfortunately with syncope, the loop may not be activated in sufficient time to make the diagnosis. Also elderly patients tend

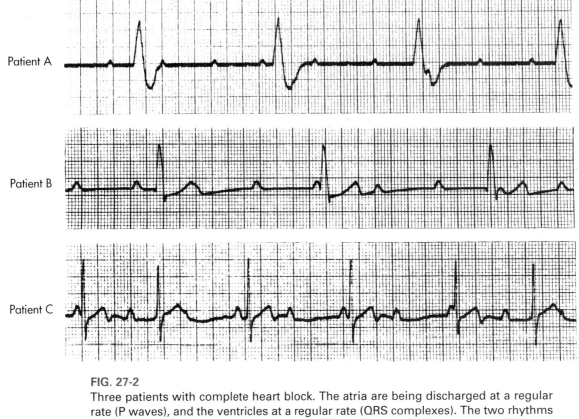

FIG. 27-2

Three patients with complete heart block. The atria are being discharged at a regular rate (P waves), and the ventricles at a regular rate (QRS complexes). The two rhythms appear unrelated; there is *AV dissociation.* There is a temptation to say that P waves positioned before QRS complexes could be conducted, but these do not alter the regularity of the ventricular rhythm. Patients *A* and *B* have wide QRS complexes and slow ventricular rates; they probably have block below the AV node, and the takeover pacemakers are ventricular in origin. Patient *C* has a more rapid escape rate (55 beats/min), and the QRS complex is narrow; the level of block is the AV node, and the takeover pacer is high in the His-Purkinje system, before the division of the bundle branches.

From Taylor GJ: *150 practice ECGs: interpretation and board review,* London, 1997, Blackwell Science.

not to like using these devices and may not be wearing them when the arrhythmia occurs.

EPS can be used to define conduction system physiology and thus identify bradyarrhythmias when the diagnosis is uncertain. It is possible to test both sinus node and conduction system function. If abnormal, the EPS result usually defines the bradyarrhythmia as the cause of symptoms. However, a normal EPS does not eliminate the possibility of a bradyarrhythmia as the cause of intermittent symptoms, so it is not as sensitive as one would prefer. Our usual approach is to do an EPS if the patient has severe symptoms (such as syncope) and there is suspicion of bradyarrhythmia. In this case an EPS may prove expeditious in making a diagnosis.

A new diagnostic tool is an implantable monitor that works for 2 years. It can store 45 minutes of ECG data that can be downloaded using a radiotelemetry device. The implantable monitor has been effective in determining the cause of syncope in difficult cases. However, it is expensive and requires minor surgery. It may take a significant period of time before defining the cause of syncope (or at least ruling out an arrhythmia).

Management

The first step is to eliminate possible extrinsic causes (Table 27-1). Antihypertensive agents are the usual culprits; nodal blocking agents such as beta-blockers, calcium channel blockers, and reserpine should be stopped and vasodilators substituted for control of blood pressure. When checking for drugs as the cause of bradycardia, ophthalmic solutions are often overlooked. These often contain beta-blocking agents, and a systemic effect is possible. Electrolyte disturbances

should be corrected. Treatment of hypothyroidism may eliminate the need for pacing.

Pacemaker therapy is the usual treatment. There are no drugs that enhance conduction or increase heart rate. Pacemaker therapy has become more physiologic with the development of dual-chamber pacemakers (see Chapter 28). They are now able to improve chronotropic capabilities with the use of sensors that increase heart rate with exercise.

Specific Syndromes
Sick Sinus Syndrome

Sick sinus syndrome usually occurs in the elderly and is uncommon in those under 50 years of age. (A rare familial variant affects young adults.) It is the major indication for pacing in the United States, leading to more than 50% of the new pacemaker implants.[2]

Sick sinus syndrome is defined as abnormal sinus node function that correlates with symptoms. It includes tachybrady syndrome, with the patient intermittently having either tachycardia or bradycardia. The initial treatment goal is control of tachyarrhythmia, often atrial fibrillation. Unfortunately, the drugs needed to control rapid rates aggravate bradyarrhythmia. The pacemaker provides the patient rate support so that the medication needed to control the tachycardia can be tolerated.

Initially sick sinus syndrome was treated with just ventricular pacemakers, and mortality was unchanged by pacing. Dual-chamber pacing appears to improve survival, possibly by decreasing the incidence of atrial fibrillation, thus lowering the risk of stroke.

Carotid Sinus Syncope

Carotid sinus massage causes a fall in heart rate and blood pressure. A hyperactive carotid baroreceptor reflex may cause syncope. A tight collar, turning or tilting the head, or other maneuvers that place pressure on the carotid sinus may provoke it. Most patients (80%) have syncope because of a fall in heart rate, but 20% of the time symptoms are the result of decreasing both heart rate and blood pressure (the vasodepressor response).[3]

Carotid sinus syncope is caused by an overly sensitive carotid baroreceptor reflex and is diagnosed when carotid sinus stimulation for 5 seconds leads to a 3-second or greater pause. Treatment of this syndrome is with a physiologic dual-chamber pacemaker, which is effective in the 80% of patients whose syncope results from bradycardia.

Heart Block
Congenital

Heart block commonly accompanies congenital heart diseases, including transposition of the great vessels, fibroelastic disease, and ventricular septal defect. It com-

monly occurs in the absence of other structural cardiac problems.[1] Because the level of block is the AV node, the take-over pacemaker has a rate above 50 beats/min, which may increase slightly with exercise. For these reasons, congenital heart block may be asymptomatic, and no intervention is needed. However, if a patient has a wide QRS complex, or the average heart rate is less than 50 beats/min, he or she may not be truly asymptomatic and pacing should be instituted.

Acquired (Stokes-Adams Attack)

Complete, or third-degree, heart block is a common illness of advanced age. Contrary to popular belief, it is rarely caused by coronary artery disease. Instead, a fibrotic, degenerative process affecting the infranodal conduction system is usually responsible (Lev's disease). Because the level of block is usually below the AV node, the take-over pacemaker is from the ventricular level and is slow (usually less than 30 beats/min). Without pacemaker therapy, there is a risk of sudden death. Complete heart block in an elderly person is a definite indication for pacing.

The classic Adams-Stokes attack causes severe dizziness or syncope from third-degree AV block. Since it is intermittent, it may not be seen with a routine ECG. However, the ECG may provide clues, including conduction disturbance (first-degree block, hemi-block, bundle branch block, or a combination). Holter monitoring is occasionally helpful. EPS documents prolongation of the HV interval (the conduction time from the His deflection, next to the AV node, to the beginning of the QRS; Fig. 27-3). Pacing is indicated if the duration of the HV interval is more than 70 ms.

Myocardial Infarction. Heart block is often seen with inferior myocardial infarction. A combination of increased vagal tone and ischemia of the AV node is responsible. Because it is AV nodal block, there may be a progression from first-degree to Mobitz type I second-degree block (Wenckebach, Table 27-1). Occasionally it progresses to third-degree heart block. With inferior myocardial infarction, even complete heart block resolves over time, and permanent pacing is not necessary. As with other forms of nodal block, heart rate increases with either atropine or isoproterenol therapy. Occasionally temporary pacing is needed because of hypotension, bradycardia that aggravates heart failure, or other problems. Heart block usually resolves within a couple of weeks.

Heart block with anterior myocardial infarction tends to be infranodal, usually because of ischemic injury of the conducting tissue in the interventricular septum. It is an ominous development, primarily because it occurs with unusually large infarctions. Even when the bradyarrhythmia is easily controlled, a number of patients succumb to left ventricular failure. Transient

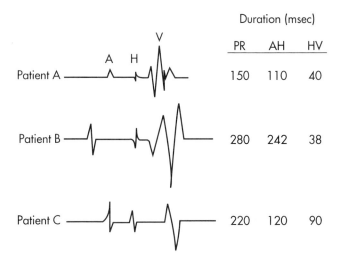

	Duration (msec)		
	PR	AH	HV
Patient A	150	110	40
Patient B	280	242	38
Patient C	220	120	90

FIG. 27-3
Bundle of His recordings from three patients. In evaluating heart block with electrophysiologic study (EPS), the goal is to determine the anatomic level of conduction delay, whether block is within the AV node or below it. A bipolar recording catheter is positioned next to the AV node and is used to record the electrical discharge of the bundle of His (the H spike), as well as atrial (A) and ventricular (V) activation. The bundle of His spike originates from tissue immediately below and adjacent to the AV node. Patient A: The PR interval is normal as is the H-V interval (<55 ms) Patient B: There is PR interval prolongation. Marked prolongation of the A-H interval identifies a delay in conduction above the bundle of His, within the AV node. Infranodal conduction, the H-V interval, is normal. Patient C: There is PR interval prolongation. The A-H interval is normal, so there is no delay in conduction through the AV node. There is prolongation of the H-V interval, indicating infranodal conduction delay. With infranodal conduction disease this patient has a higher risk of developing symptomatic heart block.

third-degree heart block with an anterior myocardial infarction is an indication for permanent pacing because sudden death is common in this group.

Another indication for permanent pacing after myocardial infarction is new bifascicular block (right bundle plus left anterior fascicular block); progression to complete heart block and sudden death are common. Left bundle branch block, if new, is an indicator for temporary pacing during acute myocardial infarction, especially if the patient's condition is unstable. However, complete heart block is not as common as it is with bifascicular block.

SYNCOPE

Syncope is a sudden loss of consciousness associated with loss of cerebral blood flow.[4] It usually occurs when systolic pressure falls below 70 mm Hg.

Epidemiology

Syncope is common, accounting for 6% of emergency department visits. The condition occurs in people of all ages. In fact, the classic faint is very common in youth. In the elderly there is a 6% annual occurrence rate with a very high (approximately 30%) recurrence rate. Specific causes vary with age.

Pathophysiology

The brainstem is the origin of the syncopal symptom complex. The reticular activating system located in the midbrain and pons is responsible for maintenance of the conscious state. Alteration of supply of oxygen through decreased blood flow in the vertebral artery is the cause of altered function. The time of diminished blood flow determines the symptoms. After 5 to 15 seconds the patient develops pallor, loss of consciousness, and then decreased muscle tone. If flow is interrupted longer than 15 seconds, myoclonus develops.

Etiology

Specific causes of syncope are summarized in Box 27 1. Diminished cardiac output is the most common final pathway (in at least 50% of cases). This may result from cardiac arrhythmias, valvular disease, cardiomyopathies, acute ischemic events, or a sudden loss of vascular tone (neurocardiogenic syncope).

Neurocardiogenic syncope, a variant of orthostatic hypotension, is the most common cause of syncope in this group, occurring in approximately 30%.[4,5] The initiating event is relative hypovolemia caused by venous pooling, usually after a shift to upright posture. This causes decreased left ventricular volume and cardiac output. Baroreceptors are stimulated, causing increased adrenergic tone. The inotropic state of the heart and the heart rate both increase. At this point the response—diminished venous return—is normal. However, for unknown reasons these patients overshoot, with an excessive increase in the inotropic state. The marked increase in contractility activates mechanical receptors in the heart, provoking vagal discharge. This decreases the heart rate. The reflex also includes increased central sympathetic tone, which causes vasodilation in the periphery. The result is bradycardia and hypotension with dizziness, near-syncope, or syncope. Of note, this complex reaction to upright posture takes some time. Patients usually are upright for 2 to 5 minutes before dizziness begins. A typical history: "I got up, walked to the kitchen, and fell while standing at the sink."

Orthostatic hypotension may occur without activation of the neurocardiogenic syncope reflex. It is common in elderly patients treated with antihypertensive drugs. In this form, dizziness tends to occur immediately on rising, and syncope is less common.

BOX 27-1

CAUSES OF SYNCOPE

DIMINISHED CARDIAC OUTPUT
Alteration in Vascular Tone
Neurocardiogenic syncope
Orthostatic hypotension
Vasodepressor (vasovagal) syncope
Situational, reflex-mediated syncope (micturition, cough, defecation, swallowing)
Carotid sinus syncope
Glossopharyngeal neuralgia
Autonomic neuropathy
Tachyarrhythmias
Ventricular tachycardia
Supraventricular tachycardia
Bradyarrhythmias
Sick sinus (tachybrady) syndrome
Atrioventricular block (Stokes-Adams)
Valvular Heart Disease and Outflow Obstruction
Aortic stenosis
Hypertrophic subaortic stenosis
Mitral stenosis
Aortic regurgitation (rare)
Atrial myxoma (with valve obstruction)
Right ventricular outflow obstruction (pulmonic stenosis, pulmonary hypertension, pulmonary embolus)
Cardiomyopathy (Increased Risk of Ventricular Arrhythmia)
Congestive cardiomyopathy
Restrictive cardiomyopathy

Ischemic Heart Disease
Ventricular arrhythmias with acute ischemia
Ventricular arrhythmia with ischemic cardiomyopathy

OCCLUSIVE VASCULAR DISEASE
Vertebrobasilar ischemia
Arterial embolization
Pulmonary embolism with or without paradoxical embolism
Bilateral carotid artery stenosis (rare)
Subclavian steal syndrome

VASCULAR VOLUME LOSS (may act in concert with other etiologies)
Acute hemorrhage
High volume paracentesis, urinary bladder drainage, thoracentesis, or dehydration
Severe anemia

OTHER ETIOLOGIES IN THE NEUROAXIS
Seizures (partial complex)
Hysteria
Migraines (rare)
Intoxicants
Hypoxia, hypoglycemia (not truly syncope)
Head trauma

Vasovagal syncope, or the common faint, is characterized by marked sinus bradycardia in most patients. Another less common form is pure vasodepressor syncope with a loss of arterial pressure and minimal change in heart rate.

Syncope caused by other forms of dysautonomia occurs. Diabetes mellitus may be complicated by orthostatic hypotension as part of the autonomic neuropathy of that disorder. A loss of efferent adrenergic discharge has been demonstrated. Glossopharyngeal or trigeminal neuralgia may initiate vasodepressor neural reflexes.

Cardiac arrhythmia is the second most common cause of transient loss of cardiac output. The arrhythmia tends to occur just before the clinical event, frequently is transient, and thus is not observed by the clinician. Ventricular tachycardia (see Chapter 26) is the most common arrhythmia causing syncope, ahead of brady-

arrhythmias. Among the bradycardias, sick sinus syndrome accounts for the largest proportion of patients, followed by Stokes-Adams attack (AV block).

Structural heart disease, either valvular or myocardial, may present as syncope. The echocardiogram is an important tool in the syncope workup. A history of *effort* syncope should raise suspicion of the presence of left ventricular outflow tract obstruction, either valvular or subvalvular. Hypertrophic subaortic stenosis is one of the causes of syncope or sudden death in young athletes (see Chapter 23). Arrhythmias—atrial fibrillation or ventricular arrhythmias—may occur with this as well as other cardiomyopathies.

Coronary artery disease does not directly cause syncope as an "anginal equivalent." On the other hand, acute ischemia may provoke ventricular tachyarrhythmias, and left ventricular dysfunction after myocardial

infarction is the most common substrate for ventricular tachycardia.

Cerebrovascular disease is an unusual cause of syncope. About 5% of transient ischemic attacks or strokes cause syncope, and these are usually due to vertebrobasilar ischemia. Most of these patients also have other neurologic symptoms, including vertigo, ataxia, and paresthesia. Carotid artery disease causes hemiparesis, not syncope. (A rare exception is severe bilateral carotid stenosis.) With a thorough and normal neurologic examination and no other neurologic symptoms, cerebrovascular disease is excluded as a cause of syncope, for all practical purposes. Carotid Doppler studies, although commonly ordered, contribute little to the syncope workup because they do not evaluate the vertebral circulation.

The subclavian steal syndrome is a more common vascular cause of syncope (see Fig. 34-1). The vertebral artery serves as the source of collateral blood flow when the subclavian artery is stenosed at its origin. With arm exercise, there is increased flow from the carotids, through the circle of Willis, and retrograde through the vertebral artery to the subclavian artery. In effect, blood is "stolen" from the vertebrobasilar circulation, causing syncope. Stenosis of the subclavian artery may be acquired (atherosclerosis or arteritis) or caused by a congenital abnormality of the thyrocervical trunk. Consider it when syncope occurs with arm exercise, and listen for a subclavian bruit.

Vertebrobasilar insufficiency may also occur with compression or occlusion of the spinal portions of the vertebral arteries. Cervical spondylosis may be responsible, and this may be a complication of rheumatoid arthritis. Atherosclerosis or vasculitis may affect the vertebral arteries, but both are rare.

Some neuropsychiatric conditions can mimic syncope, but seizures (major motor) usually do not. Partial complex seizures may confuse physicians. Recurrent and unexplained syncope warrants electroencephalographic (EEG) evaluation in selected cases. Hysteria and related hyperventilation may cause syncope through the alteration of $PaCO_2$. Emotional trauma usually causes syncope through vasovagal mechanisms.

Unexplained Syncope. It is important to make a diagnosis because the prognosis of syncope is variable.[6] Patients with noncardiac syncope have a lower mortality risk than some with cardiac syncope. For this reason, a principal aim is the exclusion of serious heart disease.

Evaluation

The history and physical examination are diagnostic in as many as 50% of cases. Important historical data include premonitory symptoms, frequency and severity of episodes, posture and activity during episodes, medication history, and use of alcohol or other toxins. Associated medical illnesses often point to a diagnosis. For example, a history of myocardial infarction and heart failure increases the chance of ventricular arrhythmia. An elderly person with no history of heart disease but with known bundle branch block is at risk for Stokes-Adams attacks.

Important elements of the physical examination are vital signs with special attention to orthostatic changes in blood pressure and pulse. You should measure the blood pressure intermittently for 5 minutes after standing. Auscultation excludes the murmurs of aortic stenosis or hypertrophic subaortic stenosis. A thorough and normal neurologic examination may eliminate the need for extensive neurologic diagnostic testing (including imaging studies and EEG). General laboratory evaluations include measurements of serum electrolytes, glucose, hemoglobin, and hematocrit, and, in selected cases, thyroid-stimulating hormone (TSH), thyroid function tests, and cortisol.

Cardiovascular Studies

The cardiovascular evaluation of syncope includes a number of possible studies (Table 27-2). It begins with the ECG (Fig. 27-4). Early detection of third-degree AV block can be made at that time. A normal ECG does not exclude intermittent arrhythmia as a cause of the event. The next step in the evaluation of the syncopal patient depends on whether there is underlying cardiac disease.[7,8] If the patient is young and has no cardiac symptoms, a normal physical examination, and a normal echocardiogram, the most productive assessment is the tilt-table test[5,9] (Fig. 27-5). In patients with normal ventricular function the diagnostic yield of the tilt-table test varies from 70% to 80% (sensitivity, 0.61; specificity, 0.93). However, the yield of this test is low with abnormal left ventricular function, since these patients are more likely to have an arrhythmia. The next test for an otherwise healthy person with a normal tilt-table test is the loop monitor. Again, patient selection is the key to yield; event monitoring is sensitive in patients with palpitations or dizziness (Table 27-3).[10] It is less useful for the evaluation of syncope because the patient has no antecedent warning and cannot activate the monitor. It still is worth obtaining when other studies have not helped, especially when there are other, possibly presyncopal, symptoms.

Poor left ventricular function on the echocardiogram redirects the evaluation toward detection of ventricular tachycardia. Most electrophysiologists believe that EPS is the next step. Holter monitoring is commonly performed, but the yield is low. Even with a normal 24-hour monitor, EPS would be justified for a patient with syncope and depressed left ventricular ejection fraction. Our diagnostic yield with EPS in patients with abnormal cardiac function is above 70% (Table 27-4).

Table 27-2	*Diagnostic Studies Used in the Evaluation of Syncope*

Study	Findings and Commens
ECG	Heart block often present in symptomatic patients. Ventricular conduction abnormality common in elderly patients with intermittent heart block (normal QRS duration makes infranodal block less likely). Q waves indicate prior left ventricular injury (raising the possibility of left ventricular dysfunction).
Echocardiogram	Valvular disease, myxoma Left ventricular outflow tract obstruction Low left ventricular ejection fraction or left ventricular aneurysm (Ventricular tachycardia is rare when left ventricular ejection fraction is normal.) Hypertrophic cardiomyopathy (or severe left ventricular hypertrophy)
Tilt table	Postural hypotension (the key to making the diagnosis of neurocardiogenic syncope)
Holter monitor	Ventricular tachycardia is usually detected by a single, 24-hour monitor. Bradyarrhythmias and supraventricular arrhythmias may be intermittent (and can be missed by a 24-hour study).
Loop recorder	Patient-activated ("event monitor"), it records the cardiac rhythm during symptoms.
EPS	Normal study excludes ventricular tachycardia as a cause of syncope but is not as accurate in ruling out bradyarrhythmia.
Angiography	Detection of vertebrobasilar disease, subclavian steal syndrome

ECG may identify patients at high risk for intermittent heart block. An elderly patient with syncope and a wide QRS complex, including bundle branch block with or without fascicular block, may have intermittent complete heart block. This is an indication for EPS with a bundle of His electrogram.

Management
Neurocardiogenic Syncope

Treatment goals are augmentation of vascular volume and blocking the inappropriate increase in left ventricular contractility. Low-dose beta blockade and salt tablets control symptoms for most patients. Disopyramide, fludrocortisone (Florinef), clonidine, scopolamine, fluoxetine, ephedrine, and phenylephrine are other agents that may be used.

A variant of neurocardiogenic syncope is malignant bradycardia, with prolonged asystole after vagal discharge.[11,12] Treatment of this unusual group has been slightly controversial; some believe that conservative treatment with beta blockade and volume augmentation is adequate. Others believe that pacemaker implantation is indicated for prolonged pauses.

The treatment of ventricular arrhythmias is discussed in Chapter 26, and indications for pacemaker therapy are reviewed in Chapter 28.

Cardiology Consultation

Referral is unnecessary for healthy individuals who have a fainting episode. The common faint is usually obvious from the history and physical examination.

If the workup for syncope identifies left ventricular dysfunction (echocardiogram), cardiology evaluation may prove useful. This is especially true of patients with nonischemic cardiomyopathy (no Q waves, no history of myocardial infarction, but poor left ventricular function).[13] The combination of left ventricular ejection fraction <35%, no coronary artery disease, and syncope indicates a high mortality risk. EPS is indicated.

A cardiologist may help with screening for active ischemia, although stress testing may be done by any qualified physician. Most tilt-table testing is done by cardiologists. An electrophysiology consultation is indicated for a survivor of cardiac arrest and may prove useful for a patient with recurrent, elusive, or complex symptoms.

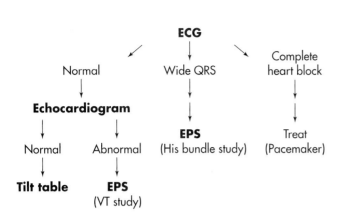

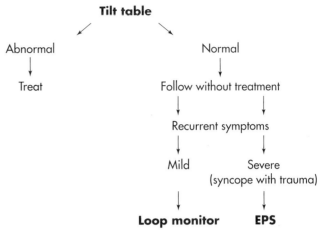

FIG. 27-4

An approach to a patient with no clinically apparent heart disease and unexplained syncope. If third-degree heart block and a slow ventricular rate are identified by the ECG, there is no need for further testing (proceed with pacemaker therapy). If the ECG is normal, an echocardiogram to exclude left ventricular dysfunction and other cardiac abnormalities is the next step. An abnormal study is an indication for cardiology consultation and possibly EPS. Holter monitoring is often done, but is a low-yield technique. An elderly patient with conduction disease apparent on the ECG (a wide QRS complex, or AV nodal block) may benefit from EPS. On the other hand, a narrow QRS and normal ECG indicate a low risk of heart block.

FIG. 27-5

Management of the patient with syncope, normal left ventricular function, and no structural heart disease. An abnormal tilt-table test indicates neurocardiogenic syncope (the most common cause of syncope). If the test is normal, loop monitoring may be used to diagnose intermittent arrhythmia.

Table 27-3	*The Chance of a Positive (Diagnostic) Loop Monitor**	
Symptoms	**Cardiac Status†**	**Positive(%)**
Palpitations	Heart disease	62
	Normal	68
Presyncope	Heart disease	17
	Normal	62
Syncope	Heart disease	8
	Normal	10

*The loop monitor is also known as an *event monitor.*
†*Heart disease,* The echocardiogram identifies an abnormality of left ventricular function (depressed left ventricular ejection fraction) or structure (including hypertrophic cardiomyopathy or severe left ventricular hypertrophy); *Normal,* normal echocardiogram.

Table 27-4	*The Chance of a Positive Test in a Patient with Syncope*	
Symptoms	**Cardiac Status***	**Positive(%)**
Tilt table	Normal	63
	Heart disease	19
Electrophysiologic study	Normal	29
	Heart disease	72

Data from the Medical University of South Carolina, 1994.
**Normal,* normal echocardiogram; *Heart disease,* echocardiogram identified an abnormality of left ventricular function (depressed left ventricular ejection fraction) or structure (including hypertrophic cardiomyopathy or severe left ventricular hypertrophy).

REFERENCES

1. Zipes D, Jalife J: *Cardiac electrophysiology: from cell to bedside,* Philadelphia, 1995, WB Saunders.
2. Bernstein AD, Parsonnet V: Survey of cardiac pacing and defibrillation in the United States in 1993, *Am J Cardiol* 78:187, 1996.
3. Madigan NP, Flaker GC, Curtis JJ, et al: Carotid sinus hypersensitivity: beneficial effects of dual-chamber pacing, *Am J Cardiol* 53:1034, 1984.
4. Kosinski D, Grugg BP, Temesy-Armos P: Pathophysiological aspects of neurocardiogenic syncope; current concepts and new perspectives, *Pacing Clin Electrophysiol* 18:716, 1995.
5. Bass EB, Elson JJ, Fogoros RN, et al: Long-term prognosis of patients undergoing electrophysiologic studies for syncope of unknown origin, *Am J Cardiol* 62:1186, 1988.
6. Kapoor WN: Work up and management of patients with syncope, *Med Clin North Am* 79(5):1153-1170, 1995.
7. Kapoor WN, Hammill SC, Gersh BJ: Diagnosis and natural history of syncope and the role of invasive electrophysiologic testing, *Am J Cardiol* 63:730, 1989.
8. Benditt DG, Remole S, Bailin S, et al: Tilt-table testing for evaluation of neurally mediated (cardioneurogenic) syncope: rationale and proposed protocols, *Pacing Clin Electrophysiol* 14:1528, 1991.
9. Fogel RI, Gest CR, Evans JJ, Prystowsky EM: Are event recorders useful and cost effective in the diagnosis of palpitations, presyncope and syncope? *J Am Coll Cardiol* 21(suppl):358, 1993.
10. Grugg BP, Ternesy-Armos P, Moore J, et al: Head-upright tilt-table testing in evaluation and management of the malignant vasovagal syndrome, *Am J Cardiol* 69:904, 1992.
11. Sra JS, Jazayeri MR, Avitall B, et al: Comparison of cardiac pacing with drug therapy in the treatment of neurocardiogenic (vasovagal) syncope with bradycardia or asystole, *N Engl J Med* 328:1085, 1993.

28 Pacemaker Therapy

H. Weston Moses
Roger L. Fulton

INDICATIONS FOR CARDIAC PACEMAKERS

The most important indication for cardiac pacing is a symptomatic bradyarrhythmia. Documenting this would appear to be straightforward but often is not (see Chapter 27). The obvious indications for pacing are complete heart block and sick sinus syndrome with symptomatic bradycardia. Table 28-1 reproduces the American Heart Association/American College of Cardiology practice guidelines for pacemaker therapy.[1] It ranks indications as definite and intermediate, and it also lists conditions that are not considered indications for pacing.

In the initial evaluation of patients with lightheadedness or syncope with bradyarrhythmias, one of the most important issues is a survey for medications that may cause or aggravate bradycardia. These include betablockers or calcium channel blockers (diltiazem or verapamil), which can slow the heart rate. Other drugs to investigate are disopyramide (Norpace) and other antiarrhythmic drugs, although most of these do not cause bradyarrhythmias and may instead provoke syncope through their proarrhythmic effects with ventricular tachycardia or torsades de pointes.

Sick Sinus Syndrome

The "bradycardia-tachycardia" syndrome is part of the sick sinus syndrome in which there are periods of inappropriate pauses associated with various types of supraventricular tachyarrhythmias. Drug therapy is essential to suppress the fast rhythm, but it aggravates bradyarrhythmias. Pacing is required to protect the patient from worsening bradyarrhythmias. On the other hand, neither asymptomatic transient bradycardia at the termination of a supraventricular tachycardia nor an asymptomatic pause of even a few seconds during atrial fibrillation is an indication for pacing.

Heart Block

Heart block can be a complex problem (for a thorough review see Chapter 27). It is useful to think of heart block as occurring either in the atrioventricular (AV) node or below the AV node (Fig. 28-1; see Fig. 27-3 and Table 27-1). First-degree AV block occurs at the level of the AV node. Second-degree AV block may be in the AV node or below it. This leads to the often confusing designations, Mobitz type I and Mobitz type II seconddegree AV block. Mobitz type I block (Wenckebach phenomenon) is caused by delayed conduction in the AV node. The duration of the QRS complex is *usually* short (rarely it is wide because of coincidental bundle branch block). This type of block is often seen in normal healthy individuals, and it is common in patients with athletic hearts resulting from high vagal tone. It tends to be more benign with a junctional escape rhythm as a backup. Infrequently, in elderly patients it becomes more severe and symptomatic and requires pacing. Drugs that slow AV node conduction may cause it, and Wenckebach phenomenon is an early sign of digitalis toxicity. It is characterized by a lengthening PR interval before the dropped beats. The PR interval may lengthen over several beats, and this may be a subtle change. In that case a useful approach is to look at the PR interval *after* the dropped beat. The PR interval will always be shorter after the dropped beat than before.

Mobitz type II block is caused by blocked conduction in the His-Purkinje system *below* the AV node. For practical purposes it is *always* associated with a wide QRS complex. A reasonable way to think about this is to consider the three fascicles below the AV node (right bundle, left anterior fascicle, and left posterior fascicle)—two are completely blocked and the third is conducting only intermittently. With two of the three fascicles gone, there must be a bundle branch block pattern and a wide QRS complex. The pattern of block is regular, with every other (2:1 block) or two of three (3:1) beats blocked. When third-degree, or complete, heart block develops in a patient with previous infranodal, Mobitz type II block, the escape rhythm is ventricular. The intrinsic rate of ventricular escape rhythms is slow and may lead not only to syncope but also to cardiac arrest and sudden cardiac death (see Fig. 28-1).

One concern prevalent a few years ago is chronic bifascicular block (left bundle branch block or right bundle branch block with left anterior hemiblock or left posterior fascicular block). When it is chronic, this is not a particularly ominous finding. There is no indication to push these patients to electrophysiologic testing unless they have symptoms. A patient with chronic stable bifascicular block who is scheduled for surgery does

| Table 28-1 | *Indications for Permanent Pacemaker Therapy: Practice Guidelines from the American College of Cardiology/American Heart Association*[1] |

Pacing Definitely Indicated*	Probably Indicated (Intermediate Indication)	Not Indicated
ACQUIRED ATRIOVENTRICULAR BLOCK IN ADULTS		

1. Third-degree AV block with any one of the following:
  a. Symptomatic bradycardia
  b. Drug therapy aggravating bradycardia is essential
  c. Asystole, ≥3.0 sec or an escape rate <40 beats/min
  d. After-catheter ablation of the AV node
  e. Postoperative AV block not expected to improve
  f. Neuromuscular disease with AV block (myotonic dystrophy, limb-girdle disease, peroneal muscular atrophy)
2. Second-degree AV block (regardless of the level of block) with symptomatic bradycardia
	1. Asymptomatic third-degree AV block with average awake ventricular rate ≥40 beats/min
	2. Asymptomatic Mobitz type II (second-degree AV) block
	3. Asymptomatic Mobitz type I block with EPS showing block below the AVN (rare)
	4. First-degree AV block and symptoms due to inadequate atrial contraction, plus proven improvement with temporary AV pacing
		1. Asymptomatic first-degree AV block
		2. Asymptomatic Mobitz type I (second-degree AV block)
		3. AV block expected to resolve (drug toxicity, Lyme disease)

CHRONIC BIFASCICULAR AND TRIFASCICULAR BLOCK		
1. Intermittent third-degree block 2. Mobitz type II block	1. Syncope not proven due to AV block, but other causes (VT) have been excluded 2. Marked prolongation of the HV interval (≥100 msec) when asymptomatic 3. Pacing-induced infra-His block at EPS	1. Fascicular block without symptoms or AV block 2. Fascicular block plus first-degree AV block without symptoms
AFTER THE ACUTE PHASE OF MYOCARDIAL INFARCTION		
1. Persistent second- or third-degree infranodal AV block 2. Transient advanced second- or third-degree infranodal AV block and associated bundle branch block (EPS may be needed to ascertain the level of block) 3. Persistent, symptomatic second- or third-degree AV block	Persistent second- or third-degree block at the level of the AV node†	1. Transient AV block with a narrow QRS complex (AV block is probably nodal) 2. Transient AV block with LAFB 3. New LAFB 4. Persistent first-degree AV block with chronic bundle branch block
SINUS NODE DYSFUNCTION, INCLUDING THE SICK SINUS SYNDROME		
1. Symptomatic bradycardia, including frequent sinus pauses; possibly the result of essential drug therapy for which there is no substitute 2. Symptomatic chronotropic incompetence	SA node dysfunction with necessary drug therapy and heart rate <40 beats/min but no documented symptoms	1. Sinus bradycardia (rate <40 beats/min) but no symptoms 2. Symptomatic sinus bradycardia with nonessential drug therapy

*Although not included in this table, the Practice Guidelines also review the nature of the data supporting these recommendations (large randomized clinical trials versus smaller or nonrandomized studies versus consensus among experts).

AV, Atrioventricular; *SA,* sinoatrial; *VT,* ventricualr tachycardia; *EPS,* electrophysiology study; *LAFB,* left anterior fascicular block.

Table 28-1	*Indications for Permanent Pacemaker Therapy: Practice Guidelines from the American College of Cardiology/American Heart Association—cont'd*		
Pacing Definitely Indicated*	**Probably Indicated (Intermediate Indication)**		**Not Indicated**

PACING TO PREVENT TACHYARRHYTHMIA

Sustained, pause-dependent ventricular tachycardia, with or without prolonged QT interval, with EPS documentation of the efficacy of pacing	High-risk patients with congenital long QT syndrome	1. Long QT syndrome due to reversible causes (drugs) 2. Frequent, complex ventricular ectopic activity without sustained VT and with a normal QT interval

NEURALLY MEDIATED SYNCOPE OR HYPERSENSITIVE CAROTID SINUS SYNDROME

Recurrent syncope due to carotid sinus hypersensitivity; minimal carotid pressure causes asystole of >3 sec duration, in the absence of medicines that depress the SA node	1. Recurrent syncope without provocation and a hypersensitive cardioinhibitory response 2. Syncope of unproven origin, but EPS documents major abnormalities of SA or AV node function 3. Syncope with a positive head-up tilt and significant bradycardia (many of thse patients also have vasodepression)†	1. Cardioinhibitory response to carotid sinus stimulation in the absence of syncope, or with vague symptoms (e.g., dizziness) 2. Situational vasovagal syncope where avoidance behavior is effective 3. Syncope of unproven cause

HYPERTROPHIC CARDIOMYOPATHY (HCM)

Arrhythmias, as described above	Medically refractory, symptomatic HCM with outflow tract obstruction†	1. Asymptomatic, medically controlled 2. No outflow tract gradient

DILATED CARDIOMYOPATHY (CM)

Arrhythmias, as described above	PR interval prolongation (and ineffective atrial contraction) when acute pacing studies document hemodynamic benefits of pacing†	1. Asymptomatic CM with or without drug therapy 2. Symptomatic ischemic CM

†An intermediate indication where usefulness/efficacy is less well established by evidence/opinion.

not need electrophysiologic preoperative evaluation other than the routine history and physical and general cardiac evaluation. Years ago there was concern that such patients may need a temporary pacemaker for surgery; this is not the case.

Heart Block after Myocardial Infarction

It is unusual for pacemakers to be required for heart block after myocardial infarction (MI). It is interesting how seldom we see heart block in the setting of an acute MI in this era of aggressive reperfusion therapy (see Chapter 15). Heart block still occurs because, of course, these therapies are not completely effective. An inferior wall MI usually leads to block at the level of the AV node, and this usually recovers with time (see Fig. 28-1). It is extremely rare to need a pacemaker for chronic AV nodal block after an inferior wall MI.

Heart block with anterior MI is infranodal. There is destruction of the His-Purkinje fibers within the interventricular septum, so heart block has a Mobitz type II pattern. Progression to complete heart block is common. Even the new onset of bifascicular block or bundle branch block alone would be an indication for establishing temporary backup pacing. When uncertain about the indication, we at least have the temporary transcutaneous pacemaker in place and ready to turn on. A patient with persistent, severe His-Purkinje system disease after an anterior wall MI is a candidate for a permanent pacemaker. With reperfusion therapy this is an unusual situation, and consultation with a cardiologist or electrophysiologist may be appropriate. Most patients who develop advanced heart block with anterior MI die, not because of the arrhythmia, but because heart attacks this size usually cause cardiogenic shock.

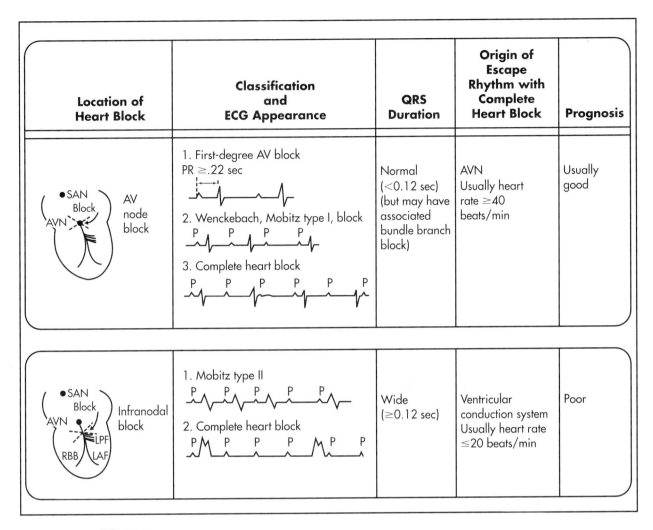

Location of Heart Block	Classification and ECG Appearance	QRS Duration	Origin of Escape Rhythm with Complete Heart Block	Prognosis
AV node block	1. First-degree AV block PR ≥.22 sec 2. Wenckebach, Mobitz type I, block 3. Complete heart block	Normal (<0.12 sec) (but may have associated bundle branch block)	AVN Usually heart rate ≥40 beats/min	Usually good
Infranodal block	1. Mobitz type II 2. Complete heart block	Wide (≥0.12 sec)	Ventricular conduction system Usually heart rate ≤20 beats/min	Poor

FIG. 28-1

Nodal versus infranodal heart block. A statistically and clinically significant association between ECG pattern and the anatomic location of block is shown. In general, block within the AV node has a good prognosis (with some exceptions), and block of second- or third-degree below the AV node has a poor prognosis. The unusual situation of Mobitz type I second-degree AV block in association with a wide QRS complex is not depicted here. This type of block can be caused by nodal or infranodal block and may require investigation with electrophysiologic studies. *SAN,* Sinoatrial node; *AVN,* atrioventricular node; *RBB,* right bundle branch; *LPF,* left posterior fascicle; *LAF,* left anterior fascicle.

From Moses HW, Moulton KP, Miller BA, Schneider JA: *A practical guide to cardiac pacing,* ed 3, Boston, 1991, Little, Brown.

Syncope

Most cases of syncope are unrelated to bradyarrhythmias. Vasodepressor syncope is the most common cause (see Chapter 27). Even with a bradyarrhythmic response with neurogenic syncope, pacing is usually *not* indicated because the mechanism of syncope is vasodilation and a sudden drop in blood pressure. A pacemaker cannot overcome that. When such patients are evaluated by an arrhythmia specialist, a pacemaker rarely is inserted for neurogenic syncope. On the other hand, in a primary care or general cardiology setting where there is less experience (and greater anxiety), pacemakers are used more commonly. Unfortunately, symptoms often continue afterward. You may want to refer these patients to an electrophysiologist before rushing in with the pacemaker. Often an electrophysiologist can make the correct decision on the basis of the clinical history alone, without needing a tilt-table study.

Most tilt-table studies rule out the need for a pacemaker rather than indicating need.

Hypersensitive carotid sinus syndrome is controversial. In the past pacemakers were recommended more commonly than they are now. The indication for pacing is excessive, prolonged, symptomatic bradycardia after gentle carotid sinus massage. Even when this is the case, about 25% of those given pacemakers continue to have symptoms.

This has been a simplified review of current pacemaker indications. We want to do the best for our patients. At the same time, decision making is influenced by medical-legal concerns on the one hand and by cost of care issues on the other. The complexity of pacemakers and their indications has led to the suggestion that pacemaker cardiology become a specialty in itself. In fact, most large cardiology group practices delegate decisions about pacemaker therapy to their electrophysiology sub-subspecialists. If, as a primary care physician, you are going to send patients directly for pacemaker implantation, it is important to be certain of the indications (Table 28-1). It is equally important to have a cardiology/electrophysiology consultation available for cases with equivocal indications.

PACEMAKER TECHNOLOGY[2]
Battery

Older physicians will recall the days of the mercury zinc battery, which had an average life span of $1\frac{1}{2}$ years. When I was in training one of the most common procedures done in our catheterization laboratory was replacement of the pacemaker generator (some centers do that in the operating room and others in the catheterization laboratory). Now pacemaker generator replacement is much less common because they are more reliable and because the lithium iodine batteries have such a long life.

One of the common questions your patients will ask how long their pacemaker is good for. There is no clear-cut answer to this, although I usually say "about 5 to 15 years." The life span depends on the pattern of use. If the pacer is sensing all the time and not pacing, little energy is drained. If the patient is completely pacemaker dependent, especially if it is a dual-chamber pacer with stimulation of the atrium and the ventricle with every heart beat, the battery life drains more quickly. We have seen battery depletion in just 3 years with dual-chamber pacing.

Other factors influence battery life, including the size of the battery and total resistance in the system. Here is a trivia question: would you prefer a high-resistance or a low-resistance system in your patient? Most answer that low resistance is good, but in fact the highest resistance that still allows capture of the myocardium is bet-

ter because it means there is less current drain, amperes, per pacing spike (in Ohm's equation, resistance is inversely proportional to amperage).

Pacemaker Leads

The terms *unipolar* and *bipolar* can be confusing. For a circuit to be completed there must be two poles (positive and negative). Bipolar leads are almost universally used in the United States. They have two wires, or poles, in the pacemaker lead. One goes to the exposed metal electrode at the tip of the pacing lead. The second wire goes to an exposed metal band about 1 to 2 cm back from the tip. Electrons travel from the tip electrode back to this second pole through the surrounding myocardium. It is the flow of electricity, or circuit, between these two electrodes that stimulates the heart.

A unipolar lead is less commonly used now. It is simply a single wire down to the tip of the lead. Electricity travels from the tip electrode through the heart and the surrounding tissue back to the pacemaker generator pack, completing the circuit. One part of the generator has exposed metal attached internally to the second pole of the battery. With this system, electricity may travel 12 to 18 inches through the chest wall. The current is so small that the patient does not feel it. This type of pacemaker may be more prone to interference from outside electromagnetic activity. A unipolar system may be recognized on the surface electrocardiogram (ECG) because of unusually tall pacing spikes.

ELECTROPHYSIOLOGY OF PACING

The pacing "threshold" is the minimum current needed to stimulate the myocardium. When the pacemaker lead is first implanted, it has its lowest threshold. For that reason the physician inserting the unit must find a lead position that is stable and has an excellent threshold. As scar tissue forms around the tip of the electrode, the threshold rises. Peak threshold usually occurs about 1 month after placement and results from inflammatory tissue around the tip of the pacing wire. An academic note: the increase in threshold is probably not caused by increased "resistance" of scar or inflamed tissue, but instead is caused by that tissue physically moving the electrode further from the excitable myocardium. The electricity that finally reaches the myocardium has a lower "charge density" and therefore the threshold rises.

After about 3 months, inflammation diminishes, chronic scar tissue stabilizes, and the pacing threshold becomes stable. The long-term threshold is higher than the threshold immediately after placement, but it is lower than the threshold at 1 month. Some pacing leads have a steroid-eluting electrode to reduce inflammation and scar tissue.

Your patients should always *see the electrophysiologist or implanting physician about 3 months after implantation and have the pacing threshold checked* to ensure the threshold has not risen dramatically. Although the threshold is elevated above the postinsertion level, it usually is relatively low. At this time the backup voltage can usually be reduced. For instance, if the pacer was initially programmed at 5 volts for long-term use and the threshold is still quite good, then it may be reprogrammed down to 2.5 volts. This adjustment may extend the battery life by years. Another common adjustment is narrowing the pulse width, which also reduces the energy per pacemaker spike and lengthens battery life. These changes are made using a radiofrequency, noninvasive programmer.

Occasionally a patient has such a high threshold at the time of implantation that the pacemaker voltage, pacemaker spike width, or both must be increased during the acute inflammatory phase, 3 to 6 weeks after insertion. Even more careful follow-up is needed, and the voltage and pulse width adjusted with resolution of inflammation to conserve battery life.

These manipulations are usually done by a cardiologist or electrophysiologist, but as the primary care physician, you need to be aware that they *should be done*. Furthermore, you must be sure that the doctor who inserts pacemakers for your patients is sophisticated enough to evaluate pacemaker function and make appropriate adjustments. You and your patient cannot be satisfied with a surgeon who has learned to insert pacemakers but cannot provide the necessary follow-up care.

TYPES OF PACEMAKERS AND HEMODYNAMICS OF PACING

The primary care physician will be following patients with various types of pacemakers. Table 28-2 outlines pacemaker nomenclature. The two most common pacemaker types are VVI and DDD. The first letter refers to the chamber paced; the next, to the chamber sensed; and the third to the "mode of response" (inhibited or triggered). For example, a VVI is a lead placed to the ventricle that paces in the ventricle, senses ventricular discharge, and, when it senses a ventricular beat, "inhibits" itself for a preset period of time. If it senses no ventricular beat (there is a pause), it paces the ventricle. It sets a fixed paced rate, and if the patient's heart rate rises above that, the pacemaker turns itself off. An AAI would be the same type of pacemaker in the atrium (SSI is a manufacturers' term for a single chamber, implying that it could be used either in the atrium or in the ventricle).

Dual-Chamber Pacing

The DDD pacemaker is used for dual-chamber pacing. There are pacing leads in both the right atrium and the

Table 28-2	Generic Pacemaker Nomenclature (usually a three-letter code)*

First Letter: Chamber(s) Paced	Second Letter: Chamber(s) Sensed	Third Letter: Response to Sensing
O = none	O = none	O = none
A = atrium	A = atrium	T = triggered
V = ventricle	V = ventricle	I = inhibited
D = dual	D = dual	D = dual
(A + V)	(A + V)	(T + I)

*A fourth letter added to the code indicates programming functions, and a fifth indicates anti-tachyarrhythmia functions. Occasionally a manufacturer will use "S" (single) in the first two positions, indicating that the single lead or pacemaker can be used in either the atrium or ventricle. Once the unit is implanted, it becomes A or V. This nomenclature has been adopted by the North American Society for Pacing and Electrophysiology and the British Pacing and Electrophysiology Group.

right ventricle. The first *D* refers to dual pacing (it can pace in the atrium or the ventricle). The second *D* refers to dual sensing (it can sense in the atrium or the ventricle). The third *D* refers to a dual mode of response (it can be inhibited or triggered).

The "triggered" term may be confusing to someone not involved in pacing and is best explained by understanding the historical predecessor of dual-chamber pacing. It became apparent early in pacing that it would be helpful to keep the P wave in front of the QRS complex. This does two things. First, it maintains AV synchrony so that the heart is more efficient (there is normal atrial contraction that augments ventricular filling). Second, it preserves the normal physiologic response of the sinoatrial (SA) node to exercise so that heart rate increases with exercise. Both of these components generally make a patient feel better. This was first accomplished with a two-lead pacemaker, one lead going to the ventricle and one to the atrium. With the simpler circuitry available, this original dual-chamber pacemaker was not sophisticated and could pace only the ventricle. The atrial electrode was for sensing. It sensed the P wave, and after an appropriate delay or PR interval, the generator delivered a ventricular stimulus. This came close to establishing physiologic electrical activity in the heart. This "VAT" pacemaker paced the ventricle, sensed the atrium, and *triggered* a spike in the ventricle. Multiple problems associated with this approach became apparent over the years. For instance, it would be better if the lead in the ventricle could sense ventricular beats as well as pace in the ventricle. VAT technology has been replaced by the more sophisticated DDD pacemakers.

Pacemaker-Mediated Tachycardia

With the onset of dual-chamber pacing, pacemaker management became more complicated. For instance, the pacemaker must be designed so that the ventricular lead does not sense the atrial lead and vice versa, avoiding "cross talk." There are built-in "blanking periods" that can be programmed to various intervals to prevent this problem.

An occasional patient has retrograde conduction from the ventricular beat backward through the His-Purkinje system and AV node to the atrium, causing atrial contraction. This paced premature atrial beat may be sensed, leading to another paced beat. This can lead to reentrant tachycardia with the pacemaker as a part of the reentrant circuit, referred to as *pacemaker-mediated tachycardia* (Fig. 28-2). This problem has been overcome by ingenious programming parameters and options in the pacemaker. Advanced programming of this type requires special skills in pacemaker management.

Rate Limits

A dual-chamber pacemaker does not automatically fire at a set rate. It has an upper and a lower rate limit. The lower rate limit would be set in case the patient's sinus node slows down dramatically (for instance, a patient with both sick sinus syndrome and heart block). There would be a lower limit below which the pacemaker would pace either or both chambers to avoid marked bradycardia. Conversely, an upper limit is placed so that the patient does not follow an atrial tachyarrhythmia with a very rapid ventricular response. For instance, atrial flutter at 300 beats/min would be disastrous if the flutter waves were followed one-to-one with ventricular beats.

Atrial Arrhythmia

The dual-chamber pacemakers also have to manage the problem of patients who intermittently or persistently have a supraventricular arrhythmia such as atrial fibrillation. This may require additional reprogramming and can cause confusion.

Programming

Modern pacemakers all contain at least simple and usually multiple programmable functions. For example, it became apparent early in the days of pacing that it would be beneficial to change a pacemaker's rate. These early devices included a screw on the pacemaker that could be turned to change the rate, but this adjustment required a surgical procedure. Current pacemakers are programmed noninvasively by "talking" to them through the skin using a radiofrequency transmitter. The pacemakers have built-in complex codes before they respond. This reduces the chance of external, inappropriate programming by radiofrequency waves that all of us are exposed to in the today's world. The sim-

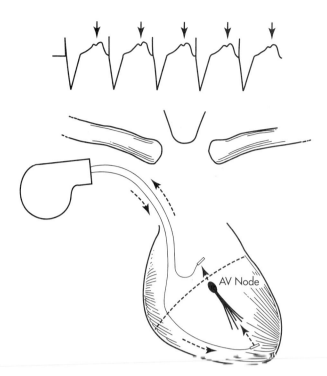

FIG. 28-2
Endless loop, or circus tachycardia. In this dual-chamber pacemaker, sensing occurs in the atrium that triggers a ventricular spike after an appropriate delay. Ventricular depolarization is followed by a retrograde P wave owing to ventricular-atrial conduction (demonstrated as an exaggerated inverted P wave marked by an arrow). The retrograde P wave sensed in the atrium causes the ventricle to fire again, and this creates a pacemaker-mediated tachycardia. It can be treated by mechanisms that cause a block of the retrograde ventricular-atrial conduction or by causing the atrium to stop sensing the retrograde P wave.

From Moses HW, Moulton KP, Miller BA, Schneider JA: *A practical guide to cardiac pacing,* ed 3, Boston, 1991, Little, Brown.

plest programmable function is changing the upper and lower rate limits. Other programmable features involve the sensing ability of the pacemaker. Sensitivity can be increased to better sense intrinsic beats or decreased if the pacer is sensing skeletal muscle or T-wave electrical activity.

More complex programmable features are also fairly routine, including adjustment of the refractory period, voltage, and mode (e.g., a DDD pacemaker should be switched to the VVI mode if the patient goes into chronic atrial fibrillation).

Physiologic Pacemakers

Newer pacemakers often have "rate modulation." This is a technologic effort to make the pacemaker more physiologic. A totally pacemaker-dependent patient with a VVI device will pace at a set rate, commonly 72

beats/min, with no change regardless of activity. With rate modulation, a sensor in the pacemaker increases the rate in response to activity. A common sensor is a piezoelectrode that detects motion and increases heart rate. This is a useful method but not perfect. For instance, a patient on a stationary bicycle moving only his or her legs may transmit little or no motion to the pacemaker. Conversely, a patient on a bumpy bus ride may have his or her heart rate go up simply because of the motion unrelated to physical activity.

Other sensing devices commercially available in pacemakers include sophisticated devices that measure relative minute ventilation, temperature change related to physical activity, and QT interval (the QT interval tends to shorten with increased catecholamine stimulation). The primary care physician is not normally involved with programming but may find it useful to monitor the function of these devices. You might see if the patient's heart rate does in fact increase with activity, or even measure the heart rate with a low-level treadmill test. This information could be used by the programmer to adjust the rate modulation.

TRANSCUTANEOUS TEMPORARY PACEMAKER DEVICE

The transcutaneous temporary pacemaker device may be one of the most important issues for the primary care physician. Before the development of this device by Dr. Zoll, temporary pacing was done through a venous stick with a pacemaker lead guided to the right ventricular apex. This required a fairly high level of sophistication and fluoroscopy guidance. Devices were

developed for insertion without fluoroscopy, but they were often unsuccessful.

Figure 28-3 demonstrates the concept of transcutaneous pacing. Large pads are placed on the anterior and posterior chest so that electricity, as it travels between these two pads, can stimulate the myocardium. The pads must be large to disperse the electrical charge over a fairly large area to minimize pain. Current transcutaneous pacemakers are often combined with defibrillators.

Figure 28-4 demonstrates one area of potential confusion with the use of this device. The pacing spikes generated are huge, and if the patient is on telemetry, nurses must turn the gain down much farther than usual. There will still be large spikes, but the QRS complexes essentially disappear from the screen. It may seem that the pacemaker is not capturing. One way to avoid confusion in this setting is to monitor arterial pressure (or to feel the pulse) when a patient is being paced with a transcutaneous pacemaker.

After the patient's condition is stable, we often switch either to a transvenous temporary pacemaker or to a permanent pacemaker, depending on the clinical situa-

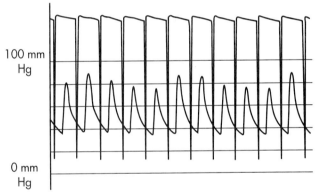

FIG. 28-4
This tracing came from a patient with an arterial line who is being paced with a transcutaneous pacemaker. The patient had dramatic, severe asystole and responded to transcutaneous pacemaking emergently. The patient's blood pressure is 85/40 and is stabilized with the transcutaneous pacemaker. Note the size of the transcutaneous pacemaker spikes, which were over 11 cm in height with routine standardization. The QRS complex is not easily noted, but one-to-one pacing is documented with the arterial line. If the massive transcutaneous pacing spikes were shrunk for a routine bedside monitor, the QRS complexes would be essentially invisible and monitoring would be difficult. The value of arterial monitoring is obvious. We have encountered a situation in which the transcutaneous pacemaker was felt not to be working because of the virtually invisible QRS complex after the massive spike.

From Moses HW, Moulton KP, Miller BA, Schneider JA: *A practical guide to cardiac pacing,* ed 3, Boston, 1991, Little, Brown.

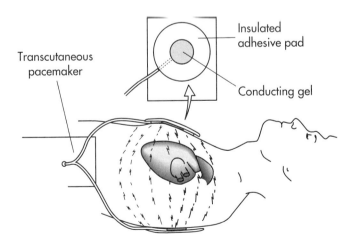

FIG. 28-3
Transcutaneous temporary pacing. Current is passed through the thorax of a patient attached to a transcutaneous pacemaker. From Moses HW, Moulton KP, Miller BA, Schneider JA: *A practical guide to cardiac pacing,* ed 3, Boston, 1991, Little, Brown.

tion. But the transcutaneous pacer is the emergency device that often saves the patient's life. It is effective for cardiac arrest caused by bradyarrhythmia. Other causes of cardiac arrest, such as pump failure, may include profound bradycardia. This is one characteristic of the "dying heart," and it will not respond to pacing. Sometimes the situation is uncertain, and a trial of transcutaneous pacing is warranted. If it does not work, there is nothing to be gained by a desperate attempt at transvenous or transthoracic (direct cardiac puncture) pacing.

PACEMAKER FOLLOW-UP

Another critical aspect of pacemaker therapy involving primary care physicians is follow-up. The most important point to emphasize is that *the patient must be enrolled in a pacemaker telephone follow-up clinic.* Among the services of the telephone clinics are monitoring the patient as the battery nears end-of-life, determining the appropriate time for elective generator replacement, and troubleshooting. The development of a new arrhythmia, such as atrial fibrillation, is often diagnosed by the clinic. It is common for patients to call in a rhythm strip when they notice a change in condition. The clinic thus serves as a source of reassurance and information for the patient.

An especially important reason for the clinic is that pacemaker leads and generators can fail unexpectedly. A manufacturer cannot guarantee perfection. Occasionally new models with excellent early performance show unexpected defects. You can imagine how confusing it would be if you received a letter from a pacemaker manufacturer indicating that a pacemaker your patient received 6 years ago is now displaying random, abrupt failure and that you need to reassess the patient. After 6 years you may have lost contact with the patient. The best way to find the patient is through the pacemaker follow-up clinic, and it can usually be done with remarkable simplicity.

Often physicians are surprised at the quality of recording obtained by the transtelephonic monitor. Figure 28-5 is an example of the monitoring system. A perfectly good rhythm strip is transmitted over the telephone from anywhere in the world to the receiving center.

Once the patient is enrolled in the pacemaker clinic, the primary care physician's follow-up is fairly simple. You would check for any recurrence of symptoms, such as dizziness or syncope, that may need evaluation. The pacemaker site itself should be checked as part of the routine physical examination. Occasionally (fortunately rarely) the pacemaker generator erodes through the skin. Even more peculiar is the "twiddler's syndrome," wherein the patient, usually unaware that he or she is doing it, turns the pacemaker generator under the skin,

leading to dislodgement of the pacemaker lead. At routine follow-up visits an ECG can be done, but it is not necessary annually.

Often patients and physicians are confused about the use of the magnet. In its simplest description, the magnet converts a VVI or a DDD pacemaker to a VOO or DOO pacemaker. In other words, the magnet disables the sensing function and the pacemaker discharges at a fixed rate. The most common use of this is simply to check capture. For instance, if a patient with a VVI pacemaker calls in with an intrinsic rate of 80 beats/min, appropriately has no pacing spikes because the pacemaker is set below 80 beats/min, it means one of two things: (1) that the pacemaker is working fine and is turned off because it is sensing the patient's intrinsic beats, or (2) the pacemaker is malfunctioning but you do not know it. By placing the magnet the spikes "march through" the patient's intrinsic rhythm and eventually fall into a "vulnerable" period, and appropriate capture is documented. When the magnet is removed, the pacemaker reverts to its original mode.

There is often concern expressed about the danger of a pacemaker spike falling on the T wave, leading to capture and precipitating ventricular tachycardia. For the average patient this is almost unheard of. Virtually all patients can have their pacemakers checked with and without the magnet over the telephone. The one clinical setting in which this may not be safe is acute MI. The heart is much more vulnerable to ventricular tachycardia during the early phase of MI, and this is the one time that the magnet should not be used for fear of precipitating ventricular tachycardia or fibrillation.

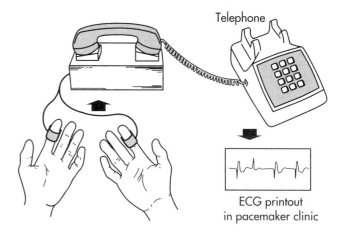

FIG. 28-5

Fingertip electrode transmitter. Electrodes are placed on two fingers and connected to the rhythm strip transmitter. *ECG,* Electrocardiogram.

From Moses HW, Moulton KP, Miller BA, Schneider JA: *A practical guide to cardiac pacing,* ed 3, Boston, 1991, Little, Brown.

SPECIAL CONCERNS AND MANAGEMENT OF CLINICAL PROBLEMS IN THE PACEMAKER PATIENT

Role of Pacemaker Manufacturer

When faced with special issues, it is often important to contact the pacemaker company through a local representative. These individuals are in sales (so they are readily available), but they also have special training and a large experience with the technology of pacing and with the particular features of their equipment. They are in direct contact with their engineering departments. Shielding technology has improved, so problems with external energy sources are rare, but in some situations there is uncertainty and the company should be contacted.

Household Appliances

A commonly asked question by patients with pacemakers concerns exposure to microwave ovens and simple electrical devices, such as a heating blanket or electric razor. It would be rare today for any of these devices to be a threat to the patient, and reassurance is all that is required. On the other hand, the shielding in pacemakers is not perfect, and exposure to very powerful electromagnetic sources such as a ham radio or an arc welder may in fact be dangerous. Consultation with the pacemaker company may be required.

Cellular Telephones

Considerable recent publicity has focused on cellular telephones. Again, this is a somewhat complicated issue, but basically patients can use cellular telephones *if they keep them away from the pacemaker generator.* If the patient believes that his or her pacemaker is interacting with a cellular phone, you should contact the pacemaker representative. It is not a simple issue because cellular telephone technology is different in the United States and Europe, and pacemaker manufacturing standards vary.

Electrocautery

A patient with a permanent pacemaker can undergo surgery, but special attention must be paid if electrocautery is used. The basic principle is that electrocautery can be used if it is not too close to the pacemaker generator and there is careful monitoring. There is a difference between bipolar and unipolar electrocautery. Bipolar may be preferable. If unipolar electrocautery is used, the "indifferent electrode" must be placed so that no current comes near the permanent pacemaker. If electrocautery is used near the pacemaker generator, it would probably be best to check with the pacemaker manufacturer regarding management.

Cardioversion or Defibrillation

Elective cardioversion is usually best carried out with anteroposterior placement of the paddles, avoiding a shock directly across the pacemaker lead, which may traverse from the right subclavian vein to the apex of the right ventricle. We routinely cardiovert atrial fibrillation/atrial flutter without difficulty in patients with permanent pacemakers, but it should be done cautiously. Telemetry for a few hours after cardioversion is useful to check pacemaker function.

With ventricular fibrillation (an immediately life-threatening emergency) the patient should be shocked immediately. The pacemaker can always be fixed later. Never be timid about shocking or cardioverting a patient who is clinically unstable. The same is true for atrial tachyarrhythmias causing hemodynamic instability or unstable angina.

Electroconvulsive Therapy

A psychiatric patient receiving electroconvulsive therapy needs ECG monitoring, but the shock tends to be away from the pacemaker. It is worth consulting the pacemaker company, but it is usually a safe procedure.

Hospital Telemetry

If a patient with a pacemaker is monitored, one potential problem is the development of ventricular fibrillation with pacemaker spikes still appearing. The telemetry warning system may interpret the pacer spikes as continued sinus rhythm and not alert the staff to cardiac arrest. Some sophisticated telemetry systems may recognize this situation, but this is not guaranteed and a patient at high risk for ventricular fibrillation needs to be more carefully monitored.

Magnetic Resonance Imaging

Magnetic resonance imaging (MRI) subjects the patient and the pacemaker to intense magnetic fields and is generally contraindicated. If absolutely necessary, then consultation with the pacemaker company is advised.

There had been some theoretical concern about patients who have an inactive pacemaker lead in the heart subjected to MRI. Theoretically the powerful magnetic fields could establish an electric circuit in the heart, leading to ventricular arrhythmias.

Radiation Therapy

Diagnostic radiation is not dangerous. However, radiation therapy for cancer may damage the delicate electronics in a pacemaker if the generator is directly in the beam.

Diagnosis of Acute Myocardial Infarction

When there is 100% capture, the QRS complex is wide, and it is like trying to diagnose myocardial infarction (MI) in a patient with bundle branch block. Some patients have striking ST segment changes in the paced complexes, and MI can be diagnosed from the ECG. However, if ST segment changes are not pronounced, it

may be difficult to diagnose infarction. It may be possible to reprogram the pacemaker to a slower rate, allowing the patient's intrinsic rhythm to take over and thus making an ECG diagnosis possible.

Lithotripsy

In general, lithotripsy is not dangerous if the pacemaker is located in the pectoral region. However, if the pacemaker generator is placed in the abdomen, interference from the powerful lithotripsy waves is possible, especially with a DDD pacemaker that senses lower voltage P waves. Consultation with the pacemaker company is recommended.

Pediatric Patients

Pediatric patients are generally followed by a pediatric cardiologist. They have the same potential for complications as adults, with the additional problem of lead displacement due to their growth.

Broken, Unused Pacing Leads

Failed pacing leads are seldom removed because scar tissue at the tip firmly anchors the lead to the right ventricular endocardium. The old leads have no adverse effect on cardiac function, although they make for a strange-looking chest x-ray. Removal is necessary when the lead is infected. The lead also must be removed is when it becomes displaced, with the proximal end floating freely in the right ventricle or into the pulmonary artery. A transvenous catheter snare can be used for extraction. As catheterization laboratory cases go, this is technically advanced work and should be referred to an experienced operator.

REFERENCES

1. Gregoratos G, Cheitlin MD, Conill A, et al: ACC/AHA guidelines for implantation of cardiac pacemakers and antiarrhythmia devices: a report of the ACC/AHA Task Force on Practice Guidelines (Committee on Pacemaker Implantation), *J Am Coll Cardiol* 31:1175, 1998. (A copy of the executive summary of this document is available from the American Heart Association by calling 800-242-8721; ask for reprint number 71-0136.)
2. Moses HW, Moulton KP, Miller BD, Schneider JA: *A practical guide to cardiac pacing*, ed 4, Boston, 1995, Little, Brown.

29 Pericardial Diseases

Mary B. Frankis
Kimberly D. Rakes

The pericardium is a sack-shaped fibrous structure that encloses the heart and the proximal portion of the great vessels and anchors the inferior surface of the heart to the diaphragm. It is a two-layered structure, composed of a fibrous outer layer and an inner serous membrane. The inner membrane lines the surface of the heart, the epicardium and epicardial fat, and is known as the visceral pericardium. The serous membrane reflects back on itself and, along with the fibrous outer layer, forms the parietal pericardium. Superiorly the great vessels pass through the pericardium, and the outer layer of the great blood vessels blends with the fibrous coat of the pericardium to form a firm attachment.[1]

The two layers of the pericardium, the visceral and the parietal, are usually separated by a thin layer of pericardial fluid. The composition of normal pericardial fluid suggests that it is an ultrafiltrate of plasma.[2] There is 15 to 50 ml of clear fluid present in the healthy state.

Although the pericardium fixes the heart anatomically in position and prevents excessive motion, the complete physiologic significance and role of the pericardium remain controversial. It is interesting to note that congenital absence of the pericardium is not associated with cardiac dysfunction or increased morbidity or mortality. In the healthy state the normal pressure within the pericardial sack is believed to be zero or slightly negative.

EPIDEMIOLOGY, ETIOLOGY, AND NATURAL HISTORY

Diseases of the pericardium generally become clinically apparent secondary to pain from inflammation or hemodynamic stress caused by the accumulation of fluid. Processes affecting the pericardium can be acute or chronic and include acute pericarditis, recurring pericarditis, chronic constrictive pericarditis, and cardiac tamponade.

Many systemic illness may involve the pericardium and lead to inflammation or the accumulation of pericardial fluid (Box 29-1). The etiologies most frequently identified in studies of acute pericarditis vary with the patient population evaluated. In referral centers, neoplastic disease is often the cause. In an unselected population of patients with primary acute pericarditis, Zayas et al.[3] reported that the most common cause was idiopathic, followed less frequently by neoplastic processes, tuberculosis, thyroid disorders, and collagen vascular disease. The category of idiopathic pericarditis likely includes many cases caused by viral infections. Although the incidence of pericardial inflammation on autopsy examination has been reported to be as high as 6%, clinically apparent pericarditis is much less infrequent and may account for approximately 1 of every 1000 hospital admissions.[2]

Viral/idiopathic pericarditis, postpericardectomy pericarditis, and post–myocardial infarction pericarditis are syndromes that are usually self-limited, with symptoms generally resolving after 2 to 4 weeks (see Chapters 16 and 52). The signs and symptoms of pericarditis associated with systemic illness can generally be expected to parallel the course of the systemic illness. Pericardial involvement after acute myocardial infarction appears to be related to the size of the infarction, and as such is a clinical marker for worsened prognosis. In patients who have received thrombolytic therapy, the reported incidence of post–myocardial infarction pericarditis is reduced.[4]

Up to 25% of patients with an episode of acute idiopathic pericarditis have at least one recurrent episode. Effective therapy for this disorder can be difficult and is discussed later. During the course of acute or chronic/relapsing pericarditis, the accumulation of significant amounts of pericardial fluid may lead to cardiac tamponade. A more insidious potential complication of an acute episode of pericarditis is the progression to constrictive pericarditis. It is not clear how frequently this occurs. Most with constriction have no history of acute pericarditis, suggesting subclinical inflammation. Signs of mild constriction that disappear within 3 months of the initial episode develop in as many as 9% of patients with acute idiopathic pericarditis with pericardial effusion.

BOX 29-1

POSSIBLE ETIOLOGIES OF PERICARDITIS

1. Idiopathic
2. Viral
   a. Coxsackie
   b. Adenovirus
   c. Human immunodeficiency virus
   d. Mononucleosis
3. Bacterial
   a. Tuberculosis
   b. *Staphylococcus*
   c. *Pneumococcus*
   d. *Brucella*
   e. *Salmonella*
   f. *Mycoplasma*
4. Neoplastic
   a. Breast carcinoma
   b. Lung carcinoma
5. Collagen vascular diseases
   a. Lupus erythematosus
   b. Rheumatoid arthritis
6. Drugs
   a. Procainamide
   b. Hydralazine
7. Thyroid disease
8. Uremia
9. After myocardial infarction (Dressler's syndrome)
10. After cardiac surgery (postcardiotomy syndrome)
11. After radiation exposure
12. Aortic dissection

PATHOPHYSIOLOGY

Acute Pericarditis

Regardless of cause, inflammation of the pericardial membranes can result in chest pain and accumulation of pericardial fluid. The pathologic changes are characteristic of acute inflammation, including the influx of inflammatory cells. If inflammation is severe, the adjacent epicardial myocardium can be involved. Normally a balance exists between production of pericardial fluid and drainage through the thoracic duct and the right lymphatic duct. Acute pericarditis may cause fluid accumulation if the balance between production and drainage is disturbed. The physiologic consequence of fluid accumulation in the pericardial sac depends on the rate of accumulation and the total volume of fluid.

Normal   Tamponade

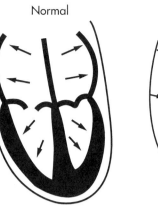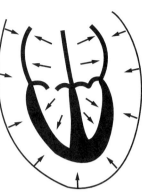

FIG. 29-1
The physiology of cardiac tamponade. In the normal state, pericardial pressure is near zero and intracardiac pressures in effect "inflate" the cardiac chambers. With tamponade, pericardial pressure increases and tends to compress the heart. Intracardiac pressure is the sum of pericardial pressure plus that pressure generated by volume within the cardiac chambers. During diastole the pericardial pressure is sufficiently high to be the major determinant of intracardiac pressure, and pressures in the four chambers tend to equalize. External compression of the atria also retards venous return to the heart, lowering cardiac output and blood pressure.

A small pericardial effusion may have more hemodynamic consequences than a large one if the small effusion accumulates rapidly. If pericardial fluid accumulates slowly, the pericardium can stretch and accommodate the fluid without an increase in intrapericardial pressure. For example, a huge effusion may be seen with severe hypothyroidism; tamponade is rare because the effusion develops slowly. On the other hand, the pericardium's ability to stretch may be hampered by fibrosis or tumor infiltration.

Cardiac Tamponade

Cardiac tamponade and a rise in intrapericardial pressure occur when fluid accumulates quickly and the pericardium has no time to stretch. Most causes of pericarditis can lead to tamponade (see Box 29-1). The most common causes are malignancy (more than half the cases), idiopathic/viral pericarditis, uremia, and bacterial infection. Anticoagulant therapy increases the risk.

The physiology of tamponade is illustrated in Figure 29-1. Inflation of any plastic structure is determined by *transmural* pressure, or the difference between internal (inflating) pressure and external (deflating) pressure. Normally, the pericardial pressure is zero, and the inflating pressure within the cardiac chambers is unopposed. With effusion and increased pericardial pressure, the transmural pressure declines, limiting diastolic filling. Pericardial pressure is high enough during tam-

ponade to govern intracardiac diastolic pressure, and diastolic pressure in the four chambers equalizes. That is the hemodynamic basis of the diagnosis: equalization of diastolic pressures. Pressures also are higher than usual, but they are higher because of *external pressure,* not because of increased filling of the chambers. Filling is lower, and the echocardiogram documents "collapse" of the atria.

The external pressure blocks blood return to the heart. With reduced cardiac filling during diastole, stroke volume and cardiac output fall. There is hypotension and reflex tachycardia.

Pulsus Paradoxus

There is nothing paradoxical about pulsus paradoxus. Normally the systolic blood pressure falls 10 mm Hg during inspiration. With pulsus paradox, it falls more. In extreme cases the peripheral pulse volume is appreciably lower. The technique for measuring the amount of pulsus is reviewed in Chapter 4.

The physiology of pulsus paradoxus is complex. Normally the intrathoracic and intrapericardial pressures become negative during inspiration, sucking blood into the chest and increasing venous return to the right heart. Right ventricular volume (preload) increases. The expanded right ventricle pushes the interventricular septum toward the left ventricle, reducing left ventricular volume. In addition, pulmonary venous return to the left atrium is decreased during inspiration. Physiologists talk of "respiratory preload variation" (right ventricular preload rises and left ventricular preload falls). The net effect of a smaller left ventricle during inspiration is a reduction in stroke volume and therefore systolic blood pressure.

Cardiac tamponade causes an exaggeration of these changes. Both ventricles are smaller than usual because of elevated pericardial pressure. With inspiration there is still a drop in intrapericardial pressure and flow to the right ventricle is increased. Bowing of the septum toward the left ventricle has an even greater effect because the left ventricle is already small.

Constrictive Pericarditis

If the inflammatory process of pericarditis results in thickening or fibrosis of the pericardium, chronic constrictive physiology may result. The adherent pericardium limits diastolic filling of the heart without a significant accumulation of fluid in the pericardial space. Unlike tamponade, early diastolic filling is normal, but it is limited in later diastole because further increases in volume are hampered by the encasement of the ventricles within the pericardium. Ventricular pressure tracings have a characteristic "dip-and-plateau" waveform. Although central venous pressures are also elevated in constrictive pericarditis, in contrast to the situation in car-

diac tamponade, systemic venous pressures do not fall during inspiration. In fact, jugular venous pressure, as reflected by the height of jugular venous distension, may increase during inspiration (Kussmaul's sign).

Clinical Presentation and Laboratory Evaluation

The most frequent chief complaint in acute pericarditis is chest pain, which varies in location but is often located substernally. For this reason it can be confused with the pain of myocardial infarction. The pain often has a positional component, with patients describing relief with sitting forward and increased intensity of pain while lying supine or with deep breathing, coughing, or swallowing. Subjective dyspnea can occur.

On physical examination the pathognomonic feature is the three-component friction rub, with components during atrial systole, ventricular systole, and early diastole. However, the rub often comprises one or two components instead of the classic three, and is frequently evanescent. The 12-lead electrocardiogram classically demonstrates diffuse ST segment elevation and can have accompanying PR segment depression. The electrocardiogram of pericarditis is described as progressing through several stages, but these are not always seen clinically. An echocardiogram is the most sensitive tool for the detection of accompanying pericardial fluid and may demonstrate other features reflecting the abnormal filling of the heart chambers.

If pericarditis is accompanied by a significant accumulation of pericardial fluid, heart sounds may become diminished on auscultation. If the fluid accumulation results in increased intrapericardial pressure, cardiac tamponade may result. The patient may become dyspneic and, as cardiac output falls, may have cool, clammy extremities. On physical examination there is elevation of the neck veins, reflecting high filling pressures, as described earlier. Often noted is a reduction in arterial pulse during inspiration—pulsus paradoxus. It is important to carefully measure the amount of paradox (see Chapter 4).

In chronic constrictive pericarditis there are several unique physical examination findings. A diastolic pericardial knock is heard along the left sternal border that corresponds to the time of rapid ventricular filling (soon after S_2). As in tamponade, jugular venous pressure is elevated. Unlike tamponade, an inspiratory increase occurs in jugular venous pressures (Kussmaul's sign), and severe pulsus paradoxus is uncommon. Hepatomegaly, ascites, and other signs of chronic liver dysfunction as a result of passive liver congestion may be noted on physical examination. (Constriction is one cause of "cryptogenic cirrhosis.")

The electrocardiogram of chronic constrictive pericarditis may feature low QRS voltage. Atrial fibrillation

is common. On chest x-ray, extensive calcification may be seen in the pericardium. Echocardiographic interrogation may reveal the characteristics of abnormal chamber filling.

In the setting of acute pericarditis, blood tests reflect the inflammatory process. Leukocytosis may be present, and elevation of the erythrocyte sedimentation rate is usual. Cardiac enzyme levels are usually normal but may be elevated if inflammation extends into the epicardium. Diagnostic testing should be tailored toward the individual patient and guided by clinical features and suspicion (Box 29-2). Blood cultures may be indicated if infective endocarditis is suspected. The tests that may be indicated on an individual basis include human immunodeficiency virus (HIV) testing, thyroid function analysis, and blood urea nitrogen (BUN) and creatinine to exclude uremia. It is seldom necessary to check viral titers because identifying the viral agent does not affect treatment and has not been shown to alter prognosis.

BOX 29-2

DIAGNOSTIC PROTOCOL FOR ACUTE PERICARDITIS

GENERAL LABORATORY EVALUATION
Complete blood count, erythrocyte sedimentation rate
Serum urea and creatinine
Blood cultures
Tuberculin skin test
ANA/RF
Serologic tests for *Toxoplasma, Mycoplasma, Salmonella, Brucella,* HIV
Thyroid hormones
Other tests as suggested by initial examination
  Suspicion for neoplasms
  Aortic dissection

PERICARDIAL FLUID
Red cell count
Total protein
Lactic acid dehydrogenase
Adenosine deaminase activity (high levels suggest tuberculosis)
Culture
Direct stain for tuberculosis bacilli
Cytologic study

PERICARDIAL TISSUE
Histologic and bacteriologic examinations

Several studies have attempted to define the diagnostic yield and clinical usefulness of performing pericardiocentesis with or without pericardial biopsy in the presence of a pericardial effusion. In one large series the highest diagnostic yield for invasive diagnostic strategy was found in the population in which pericardiocentesis and pericardectomy with biopsy was performed to relieve cardiac tamponade. The conclusion reached by the investigators was that the diagnostic yield of pericardiocentesis and biopsy in young patients with uncomplicated acute pericarditis was low and perhaps did not justify the risk of the procedures.[3]

Pericardiocentesis may prove diagnostic in a patient with suspected malignancy. The clinical setting involves a middle-aged or older patient with no history of pericarditis (e.g., pain and fever). The effusion may be an incidental finding on chest x-ray or echocardiogram. There may be no other evidence of cancer, and a laboratory screen for collagen vascular disease and hypothyroidism is normal. A bloody pericardial effusion in the absence of anticoagulant therapy points to tumor, and cytologies are usually positive (see Chapter 38).

MANAGEMENT

If a specific cause for pericarditis is identified, treatment is directed toward the underlying condition. The treatment of idiopathic and other inflammatory causes of pericarditis includes nonsteroidal antiinflammatory agents such as aspirin or indomethacin. It is reasonable to hospitalize patients with acute pericarditis and effusion, because tamponade can develop in up to 15% of patients.[6] If the pain and inflammation of pericarditis are not responding to nonsteroidal therapy after several days, corticosteroids may be administered. When symptoms have been controlled for several days to a week, doses of antiinflammatory agents may be tapered. Inflammation may recur with tapering of the antiinflammatory medications or may recur up to several months after the initial course of therapy. Such patients may respond to another course of nonsteroidal agents, but some patients have required long-term treatment with corticosteroids. Since long-term use of corticosteroids is associated with many adverse side effects, other therapies have been pursued. Pericardectomy has been proposed for relief of relapsing pericarditis, and colchicine has been reported to be effective in patients with recurrent pericarditis.[7] Box 29-3 reviews commonly used methods for the treatment of acute pericarditis.

Tamponade

Without prompt intervention, a patient may die if fluid accumulation causes hemodynamic compromise. The increased intrapericardial pressure can be relieved by evacuation of fluid with percutaneous pericardiocente-

---

BOX 29-3

TREATMENT MODALITIES FOR ACUTE PERICARDITIS

GENERAL
Bed rest
Aspirin, 3 to 4 grains/day
Indomethacin, 75 to 150 mg/day

REFRACTORY OR RELAPSING CASES
Prednisone, 20 to 60 mg/day
Colchicine, 0.5 to 1.5 mg/day

---

sis or by surgical procedures such as limited pericardectomy under local anesthesia or extensive surgical pericardectomy. Percutaneous pericardiocentesis is usually guided by fluoroscopic examination in the cardiac catheterization laboratory or, more recently, by echocardiographic imaging. This lessens the risk of the procedure, which, when done blindly at the bedside without imaging, has a complication rate as high as 20%.[2] With echocardiographic guidance the complication rate is generally less than 5%.

A patient with hypotension, neck vein distention, a small quiet heart, and a clinical setting that suggests pericarditis should have an echocardiogram as an emergency procedure. It is best to have an experienced person drain the effusion and to do so in the optimal setting (the cardiac catheterization laboratory with echocardiographic guidance). On the other hand, severe hypotension and shock may necessitate emergency needle pericardiocentesis based on a clinical diagnosis. In many cases this is life-saving. The procedure is described in Chapter 50. When done properly, it is relatively safe, even when the diagnosis is incorrect and there is no effusion.

REFERENCES

1. Snell RS: *Clinical anatomy for medical students,* ed 2, Boston, 1981, Little, Brown.
2. Lorell BH: Pericardial diseases. In Braunwald E, editor: *Heart disease: a textbook of cardiovascular medicine,* ed 5, Philadelphia, 1997, WB Saunders.
3. Zayas R, Anguita M, Torres F, et al: Incidence of specific etiology and role of methods for specific etiologic diagnosis of primary acute pericarditis, *Am J Cardiol* 75:378, 1995.
4. Correale E, Maggioni AP, Romano S, et al: Pericardial involvement in acute myocardial infarction in the post-thrombolytic era: clinical meaning and value, *Clin Cardiol* 20:327, 1997.
5. Sagrista-Sauleda J, Permanyer-Miralda G, Candell-Riera J, et al: Transient cardiac constriction: an unrecognized pattern of evolution in effusive acute idiopathic pericarditis, *Am J Cardiol* 59:961, 1987.
6. Permanyer-Miralda G, Sagrista-Sauleda J, Soler-Soler J: Primary acute pericardial disease: a prospective series of 231 consecutive patients, *Am J Cardiol* 56:623, 1985.
7. Adler Y, Zandman-Goddard G, Ravid M, et al: Usefulness of colchicine in preventing recurrences of pericarditis, *Am J Cardiol* 73:916, 1994.

BIBLIOGRAPHY

Mehta A, Mehta M, Jain AC: Constrictive pericarditis, *Clin Cardiol* 22:334, 1999. A thorough review of newer diagnostic methods, with great pictures of abnormal scans.

30

Congenital Heart Disease in Adults

George J. Taylor
Chad Alford

About 1 infant in 100 has congenital heart disease, and you may consider this group of illnesses the business of pediatricians. However, some of these conditions are not discovered until adulthood. Others are treated with success, and survival into adult life has become common for patients with complex congenital disease. The primary care physician and cardiologist must deal with the sequelae of both the illness and its surgical repair, including arrhythmias, heart failure, and pulmonary hypertension.

COMMON CONGENITAL HEART DEFECTS

The most common lesions, accounting for more than 90% of cases, are atrial septal defect (ASD), ventricular septal defect (VSD), patent ductus arteriosus (PDA), tetralogy of Fallot, coarctation of the aorta, Ebstein's disease, aortic stenosis (bicuspid aortic valve), and pulmonic stenosis. Other complex lesions such as transposition of the great vessels, truncus arteriosus, and tricuspid atresia make up just 5% of the cases in our pediatric cardiology registry (the Medical University of South Carolina).[1]

Atrial Septal Defect
Anatomy and Pathophysiology

ASD is a common cause of left-to-right ("left-right") shunt, or movement of blood from the left side of the heart to the right through an anatomic defect (Fig. 30-1). There are three possible sites of communication between the right and left atria. The most common (more than 80% of cases) is the *ostium secundum* defect , which is located in the mid-septum, well above the atrioventricular (AV) valves. The *ostium primum* defect (15% of cases) is a defect originating in the endocardial cushion, a structure in the center of the fetal heart that also contributes to the formation of the mitral and tricuspid valves and the upper part of the ventricular septum. The most extreme form of endocardial cushion defect is the absence of these structures, resulting in a single-chambered heart. With primum ASD, there may be cleft mitral or tricuspid leaflets and regurgitation. The interventricular conduction system also is affected, and left axis deviation (usually left anterior fascicular block) is a marker of primum rather than secundum defect. The *sinus venosus* defect is

the least common ASD, occurring at the entrance of either the superior or the inferior vena cava.

The usual ASD is large, often 2 cm in diameter. Because of its size, there is no jet effect and little turbulence. Thus the ASD itself does not generate a murmur. The large defect also means that pressures in the two atria are equal. Blood flows toward the right atrium because the right ventricle is more compliant than the left ventricle during diastole.

The major hemodynamic effects are right atrial (RA) and right ventricular (RV) volume overload (Fig. 30-1). When the catheterization report indicates a 2:1 shunt, it means that pulmonary blood flow is twice the systemic blood flow and that the right ventricle is handling twice as much volume as the left ventricle (Box 30-1).

Increased pulmonary blood flow may provoke a rise in pulmonary artery (PA) pressure, and a form of Eisenmenger's syndrome occurs in at least 10% of patients. This is lower than the incidence of Eisenmenger's syndrome with communication at the level of the ventricles (VSD) or arteries (PDA). With those conditions flow is increased to the PA, but, in addition, systemic pressure—either left ventricular (LV) or aortic pressure—is transmitted to the PA (Fig. 30-1). The combination of high pressure and high flow is a stronger stimulus of pulmonary vascular reactivity.

Clinical Presentation and Laboratory Evaluation

ASD is commonly diagnosed in adult life. Young adults are usually asymptomatic, and the diagnosis may be made during routine physical examination or chest x-ray. Middle-aged patients often have atrial arrhythmias. Heart failure may develop in patients 50 to 70 years old. It would seem that the left ventricle should be protected, but a common pattern is biventricular failure and not isolated RV failure.

Think how the interventricular septum works. It has to "choose sides," to work as a part of the left or right ventricle. It chooses the side with the greater workload, normally the left ventricle. With chronic RV overload, it works instead with the right ventricle, moving away from the lateral wall of the left ventricle rather than toward it during systole (Fig. 30-2). Loss of septal function may contribute to the eventual failure of the left ventricle when there is chronic RV volume overload.

347

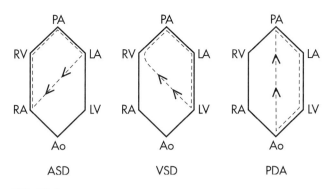

FIG. 30-1

Left-right shunting. Atrial septal defect (ASD). The right atrium *(RA)*, right ventricle *(RV)*, and pulmonary artery *(PA)* receive extra volume (blood that is "recycled" through the shunt). Notice that the extra volume misses the left ventricle *(LV)*. There is RV volume overload and increased PA flow. Ventricular septal defect (VSD). The RV receives the shunt volume, which must be handled by the left atrium *(LA)* and LV. The RV and PA are exposed to systemic pressure and increased flow. Patent ductus arteriosus (PDA). The PA is exposed to systemic pressure and increased flow. *Ao,* Aorta.

From Chizner MA: *Classic teaching in clinical cardiology,* Cedar Grove, NJ, 1996, Laennec.

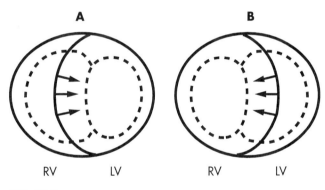

FIG. 30-2

Patterns of RV and LV contractility. *Solid line,* Diastolic contour; *dashed line,* systolic contour. **A,** Normal. The interventricular septum functions as a part of the left ventricle, moving toward the lateral wall during systole. **B,** RV volume overload. The septum functions as a part of the right ventricle, moving toward the right ventricle free wall and away from the lateral wall of the left ventricle during systole. This is identified by the echocardiogram as "paradoxical septal motion."

BOX 30-1

CALCULATING THE MAGNITUDE OF LEFT-RIGHT SHUNTING

The measurements obtained in the catheterization laboratory are O_2 saturation (sat) from the pulmonary artery (PA), aorta (Ao), and superior and inferior venae cavae (the average is the "mixed venous" sat).

Pulmonary blood flow/Systemic blood flow =
      Ao sat − Mixed venous sat/Ao sat − PA sat

Example: Ao sat = 95%, mixed venous sat = 65%, PA sat = 85% (a "step-up" in oxygen sat from the right atrium to the PA):

Pulmonary blood flow/Systemic blood flow =
      95 − 65/95 − 85 = 3/1

That is, the RV output and PA flow are three times the LV output and Ao flow.

BOX 30-2

CLINICAL FINDINGS IN ATRIAL SEPTAL DEFECT

PHYSICAL EXAMINATION
Fixed and widely split S2
Systolic flow murmur across the pulmonic valve
Possible RV lift with volume overload
Mitral or tricuspid regurgitation (primum defect)
Diastolic rumble at the left sternal border (increased tricuspid flow)

ECG
Incomplete right bundle branch block (rSR' in V1, caused by RV volume overload)
Left axis deviation or left anterior fascicular block (primum defect)

CHEST X-RAY
Increased pulmonary vascular markings ("pulmonary plethora," a sign of increased pulmonary blood flow)

ECHO-DOPPLER STUDY
Large right ventricle and right atrium
Paradoxical septal motion (Fig. 30-2)
Flow across the ASD (seen with echocardiographic contrast and Doppler)

The physical findings of ASD are not subtle (Box 30-2). S_2 is widely split, with no respiratory variation. Because of volume overload, emptying of the right ventricle is delayed, and P2 is late. The large ASD distributes the increased venous return to the heart during inspiration equally to both atria. *When you hear normal inspiratory splitting of S2, you have excluded ASD.* There is usually a short systolic murmur at the left base, the pulmonic area. This is not caused by flow across the ASD, but instead is generated by high flow across the normal pulmonic valve (when the shunt is 2:1, an average-sized ASD, flow across the pulmonic valve is twice normal). With a primum defect a cleft mitral or tricuspid leaflet causes the typical regurgitant murmur.

Because of RV volume overload, the electrocardiogram (ECG) invariably demonstrates incomplete right bundle branch block with an rSr' pattern in lead V_1 (see Chapter 5). The primum defect usually causes left anterior fascicular block, and checking the axis in a patient with ASD is a mark of clinical sophistication. Pulmonary plethora on the chest x-ray is an invariable finding, and experienced radiologists claim that it is not subtle (I have a hard time seeing it). A normal ECG and chest x-ray exclude significant left-right shunting and ASD.

The echocardiogram confirms RV enlargement and "paradoxical septal motion" (see Fig. 30-2). The ASD is easily visualized, and flow across the defect may be documented with echocardiographic contrast agents (agitated saline solution); Doppler study shows the flow as well. In addition, the echo-Doppler study allows estimation of PA pressure. In the cardiac catheterization laboratory the magnitude of the shunt is calculated (see Box 30-1) and PA pressure is measured. Angiography may be performed in older adults to exclude coronary artery disease before surgery.

Associated conditions include mitral or tricuspid regurgitation (with primum ASD), mitral valve prolapse (about 25% of cases), and, rarely, mitral stenosis (Lutembacher's syndrome, probably caused by associated rheumatic disease). A diastolic rumble may be caused by increased tricuspid valve flow, and the echocardiogram excludes mitral valve disease.

Management

Surgical repair of ASD is recommended when the pulmonary-to-systemic blood flow is above 1.5:1, especially when RV size is increased. Pulmonary hypertension, a rare complication, develops before age 30. In middle age, repair is done to prevent heart failure and atrial arrhythmias. There is a survival benefit with surgery even for patients older than 50 years, most of whom are symptomatic.[2] Because there is little turbulence and no jet effect, isolated ASD is not an indication for antibiotic prophylaxis for endocarditis.

Surgery is a cure, with no late complications for patients who were asymptomatic preoperatively. Older patients with atrial arrhythmias or heart failure may expect improvement but often need to continue medical therapy for those conditions.

Ventricular Septal Defect[3]
Anatomy and Pathophysiology

The clinical picture is determined by the size and position of the VSD. A small VSD causes no volume or pressure overload of the right ventricle and no increase in PA pressure or flow, but its jet produces a loud, pansystolic murmur (*maladie de Roger*). The high-velocity jet may injure the RV endocardial surface or a leaflet of the tricuspid valve and poses an endocarditis risk. Small VSDs often close spontaneously and thus are uncommonly seen in adults. The perimembranous types may form a septal aneurysm with closure, which is rarely of clinical consequence but is a curious finding on an echocardiogram.

The major hemodynamic effects of moderate and large VSDs are increased pressure and flow in the right ventricle and PA. Both LV and RV hypertrophy develop (both ventricles have increased loads, Fig. 30-1). As pulmonary vascular resistance increases, the left-right shunt decreases and, with this, the intensity of the systolic murmur decreases. Eisenmenger's syndrome develops in childhood in most patients with large VSDs. LV hypertrophy regresses with this development.

Clinical Presentation and Laboratory Evaluation

A moderate to large VSD without fixed pulmonary hypertension is rare in adult patients. Children with this syndrome have a loud, pansystolic murmur, a loud P_2 (usually without splitting of S_2), and biventricular hypertrophy on the ECG. There may be a diastolic rumble resulting from increased flow across the mitral valve. The echo-Doppler study confirms the diagnosis. A rare patient develops hypertrophy of the crista supraventricularis and RV outflow tract (infundibular) stenosis. This reduces flow into the PA, protecting the pulmonary vasculature, and may lead to right-left shunting across the VSD. The clinical course then mimics tetralogy of Fallot.

The diagnosis of VSD is easy when compared with ASD, since the pansystolic murmur is impossible to miss. With significant left-right shunting, chest x-ray shows biventricular enlargement and increased pulmonary vascular markings. Biventricular hypertrophy is evident on the ECG, and the echo-Doppler study images the defect in the septum and documents flow across it. Remember that with pulmonary hypertension, the pressure gradient between the left and right ventricles decreases, reducing the velocity of the jet and the intensity of the murmur. With high PA pressure a murmur of pulmonic regurgitation may develop (Graham Steell murmur). Significant aortic regurgitation develops in about 5% to 8% of patients because of lack of support of the aortic root.

Management

The only therapy needed for small VSDs is endocarditis prophylaxis. Surgery should be considered if endocarditis recurs despite antibiotic prophylaxis. Children with moderate to large VSDs (left-right shunt at least 2:1) should have surgical repair. This condition is uncommon in adults; surgery is indicated if it occurs and the shunt is at least 1.5:1. Pulmonary hypertension contraindicates surgery if the ratio of pulmonary to systemic vascular resistance is greater than 0.9, and surgery is considered safe if the ratio is less than 0.75. Some institutions will operate if shunting is bidirectional and the ratio is between 0.75 and 0.9. Management of adults with large VSDs and Eisenmenger's syndrome is reviewed later in this chapter.

Patent Ductus Arteriosus

Anatomy and Pathophysiology

Failure of the ductus arteriosus to close is another of the "big three" left-right shunts. The connection extends from the origin of the left PA to the aorta, just distal to the left subclavian artery. PDA may be a complication of maternal rubella, and it may coexist with other congenital defects (VSD, pulmonic stenosis, or coarctation or transposition of the great vessels). In older patients the ductus becomes atherosclerotic and calcified.

Small PDAs have high-velocity flow with low volume and have little effect on PA pressure. The degree of shunting across larger defects is determined by pulmonary vascular resistance. With equalization of resistance in the PA and aorta, shunt flow stops. When PA pressure exceeds aortic pressure, there is right-left shunting (Eisenmenger's syndrome). This results in the curious finding of "differential cyanosis." Oxygenation proximal to the shunt is normal (head and upper extremities), whereas that below the shunt is reduced. Thus clubbing and cyanosis are limited to the lower body and toes, with the head, arms, and fingers spared.

Clinical Presentation and Laboratory Evaluation

PDA is the most common cause of continuous (systolic plus diastolic) murmur. Causes of similar murmur include other connections between the central arterial and venous circulations: aortic-PA window, sinus of Valsalva aneurysm rupturing into the right atrium or ventricle, and coronary artery–PA fistula. VSD plus aortic regurgitation may mimic PDA. There are other causes of continuous murmur, but the murmur usually is not as loud. (Examples include venous hum, venous souffle in a lactating woman, and arteriovenous fistula involving coronary, pulmonary, or systemic vessels.)

The murmur of PDA often is louder in systole than in diastole and is best heard in the second left interspace. An associated thrill in the suprasternal notch is common. There is a wide pulse pressure, with bounding peripheral pulses, and a prominent LV lift. Large PDAs

cause pulmonary hypertension. With high pulmonary resistance and PA pressure, flow across the defect is reduced and the murmur is softer.

While there is left-right shunting, the ECG shows biventricular hypertrophy. The echo shows left atrial (LA) enlargement, and LA size is proportional to the magnitude of left-right shunt. The echo-Doppler study may image the shunt, and catheterization confirms a step-up in oxygen saturation at the level of the PA.

Management

Surgery is curative, and even small PDAs should be repaired in children and young adults to remove the risk of endarteritis. Transcatheter repair often is possible. Surgery may be more complicated for older patients, in whom the ductus may be calcified and brittle. For patients over age 60, the risk of surgery may exceed the risk of endocarditis.

Tetralogy of Fallot

Anatomy and Pathophysiology

The critical lesions of tetralogy of Fallot are VSD and RV outflow tract (infundibular) stenosis. The two other components are RV hypertrophy and an aortic root that overrides the VSD. The severity of infundibular stenosis determines the clinical picture. In most cases, severe stenosis protects the pulmonary vasculature, causes RV hypertrophy, and prevents left-right shunting. In fact, severe stenosis causes right-left shunting, and tetralogy is the most common lesion that causes cyanotic heart disease beyond infancy. More than half of the adults with cyanotic congenital heart disease have tetralogy of Fallot.

Much less common is the patient with minimal infundibular stenosis, and the effect of the VSD predominates (the so-called pink tetralogy). There is left-right shunting and eventually the development of pulmonary hypertension and Eisenmenger's syndrome.

Clinical Presentation and Laboratory Evaluation

A child with infundibular stenosis and right-left shunt is subject to hypoxic spells (more severe cyanosis, hyperpnea, and syncope). These may result from catecholamine release, which increases the contractility of muscle in the RV outflow tract, and worsened stenosis. The spells may be prevented with beta blockade. (It is a situation analogous to hypertrophic subaortic stenosis, in which blunting contractility also reduces outflow tract obstruction.) There often is a history of squatting after exercise. Squatting increases systemic vascular resistance, raises the common ventricular pressure, and forces more blood across the RV outflow tract.

Other complications of tetralogy include endocarditis, paradoxical cerebral embolism, brain abscess, and, uncommonly, RV failure.

Physical examination demonstrates a loud systolic murmur that originates from the RV outflow tract

(rather than the VSD). It has an ejection quality but no ejection click (distinguishing it from pulmonic valve stenosis). Radiographically, lung fields appear clear and the pulmonary arteries look small, as pulmonic blood flow is limited by infundibular stenosis. In one quarter of cases there is a right-sided aortic arch. The ECG shows RV hypertrophy.

Management

Because pulmonary vascular resistance is normal, surgical repair is possible and is recommended even for adult patients. Surgery includes patching the VSD and enlarging the RV outflow tract (Fig. 30-3). In earlier times, infants had palliative procedures, with a shunt constructed between the systemic and pulmonary circulations to increase pulmonary blood flow (the "blue baby operation"). Surgical correction is indicated even for patients who appear stable with a *Blalock-Taussig* or *Potts shunt.* Some patients have severe pulmonary atresia plus tetralogy, and it is not possible to achieve repair of the RV outflow tract. The *Rastelli operation* places a Dacron conduit from the right ventricle to the PA, usually with a prosthetic valve in the conduit.

Late complications of surgical repair include pulmonic regurgitation, ventricular arrhythmias originating from the RV outflow tract, right bundle branch block,

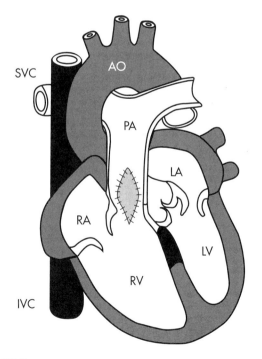

FIG. 30-3
Repair of tetralogy of Fallot. The pulmonary outflow tract is enlarged with a patch, and there is patch repair of the VSD.

From Alpert JS: *Cardiology for the primary care physician,* St Louis, 1996, Mosby.

leak from the VSD patch, and aortic regurgitation. Conduit obstruction is a risk with the Rastelli operation.

Valvular Heart Disease

Bicuspid aortic valve is the usual cause of aortic stenosis (AS) in young and middle-aged patients. In addition to the typical murmur, an ejection click is common and strongly suggests the diagnosis (see Chapter 19). A bicuspid valve is common in patients with Turner's syndrome. Subvalvular AS may be caused by a fibrous ring in the outflow tract and does not produce an ejection click. Supravalvular stenosis most commonly is a constriction of the aorta just above the coronary ostia (it may be a feature of Williams' syndrome with mental retardation and elfin facies).

Pulmonary stenosis may be valvular, infundibular, or peripheral in the pulmonary artery. Valvular stenosis is associated with an ejection click (see Chapter 20). A dysplastic pulmonic valve is a feature of Noonan's syndrome (along with short stature, low-set ears, ptosis, and mental retardation).

Coarctation of the Aorta
Anatomy and Pathophysiology

Most coarctations are short constrictions of the aorta just beyond the left subclavian artery, at the ligamentum arteriosum (in fetal life, the ductus arteriosus). In a minority of cases the narrowing extends proximally. A bicuspid aortic valve is present in 80% of cases, and congenital aneurysms may exist near the coarctation. Occasionally there is associated subvalvular aortic stenosis, aneurysms of the circle of Willis (berry aneurysm), PDA, or mitral valve abnormalities.

Arterial pressure is higher proximal to the constriction, and coarctation is considered one of the curable causes of hypertension. With severe obstruction, collateral circulation develops with marked dilation of branches of the subclavian, cervical, intercostal, internal mammary, and parascapular arteries. If collateral vessels are somewhat effective, distal pressure is only mildly depressed. If distal flow is inadequate, the renin-aldosterone system is activated, raising proximal pressure. (The effect is identical to that of bilateral renal artery stenosis.) End-organ complications of hypertension are limited to those proximal to the stenosis and include LV hypertrophy and failure, as well as stroke. Hypertensive renal disease does not occur.

Clinical Presentation, Laboratory Evaluation, and Management

Hypertension is the usual presentation of coarctation of the aorta in adults. Femoral pulses are faint, and blood pressure in the legs measured with a cuff below the knee is lower than arm pressure (normally it is at least 10 mm Hg higher). A systolic or late-systolic bruit is audible over the left anterior chest or posteriorly between the

scapulae, to the left of midline. The findings of a bicuspid aortic valve (ejection click plus murmur) supports the diagnosis of coarctation, as the two often coexist.

The ECG may show LV hypertrophy. Chest x-ray may demonstrate indentation of the aortic shadow at the level of obstruction, with poststenotic dilation (the "figure-3 sign"). Dilated intercostal arteries may cause rib notching (the third rib and lower). The transthoracic echocardiogram may not visualize the stenosed section of the aorta, but a transesophageal echocardiogram does.

Late complications of coarctation are those of poorly controlled hypertension (stroke and hypertensive heart disease). Dissection or rupture of the aorta is possible, as is bleeding from a berry aneurysm. Infective endarteritis may occur distal to the coarctation, and a murmur is an indication for antibiotic prophylaxis. Surgical repair is indicated when there is hypertension and collateral formation. Balloon dilation has been used in children, but aneurysm formation near the site of dilation is a possible complication. Interestingly, some patients have persistent hypertension after surgery.

LESS COMMON LESIONS IN ADULTS
Cyanotic Lesions

Tetralogy of Fallot accounts for almost 10% of all congenital heart disease and is the most common cause of cyanosis after infancy. However, most adult patients with cyanosis and clubbing have Eisenmenger's syndrome (usually from VSD and PDA and, less commonly, ASD).

Tricuspid Atresia

The tricuspid valve is virtually absent, with perhaps a dimple in the tissue connecting the right atrium and right ventricle (Fig. 30-4) . Both an ASD and VSD are necessary for survival. Blood return to the heart crosses from the right atrium, through an ASD, to the left atrium. The VSD allows blood to pass from the left ventricle to the pulmonary artery. A small VSD and the small right ventricle limit flow, protecting the pulmonary circulation. Oxygenated blood returning from the lungs to the left atrium mixes with blood coming from the right atrium, and cyanosis is present from birth. If the VSD is large and does not limit flow (essentially a single ventricle), the lungs are flooded and the infant dies early. Some infants with a single ventricle are saved by a pulmonary artery banding procedure.

Repair is possible in older children who do not have pulmonary hypertension using the Fontan procedure. A conduit is placed from the right atrium to the PA, and the ASD and VSD are closed. A modification of the Fontan connection places the conduit from the venae cavae to PA. Late complications of surgery include obstruction of the conduit and right heart failure, leak of the ASD patch (consider this if there is persistent cyanosis), atrial arrhythmias, mitral regurgitation, and LV failure.

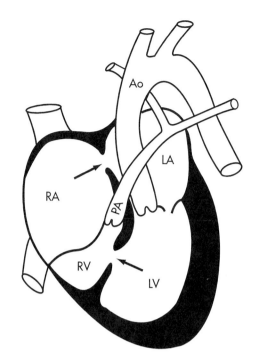

FIG. 30-4
Tricuspid atresia. Flow between the right atrium and right ventricle is blocked. ASD and VSD allow adequate mixing for the patient to live. Most patients have a small VSD and limited flow in the PA (the pulmonary circulation is "protected").

Ebstein's Anomaly

The tricuspid valve is displaced downward, into the body of the right ventricle, which is small and poorly contracting (Fig. 30-5). The unusually large right atrium has either an ASD or a patent foramen ovale, and this is the level of right-left shunt. Shunting occurs when RA pressure is raised by either tricuspid regurgitation or RV failure. Cyanosis may be mild or absent, and tricuspid regurgitation, atrial arrhythmias, and right heart failure are the clinical issues. Cyanosis may first appear in adolescence with the onset of RV failure and elevated RA pressure. Others do not have cyanosis, and Ebstein's disease may be discovered when evaluating an adult patient with unexplained right heart failure or atrial arrhythmias.

The anterior tricuspid valve leaflet is unusually large. Its increased excursion and late closure lead to a widely split S_1 (the "sail sound," like the resonant snap that occurs with the sudden filling of a sail). This second, tricuspid component of S_1 is louder than the mitral component. S_2 has fixed splitting (the effect of the ASD),

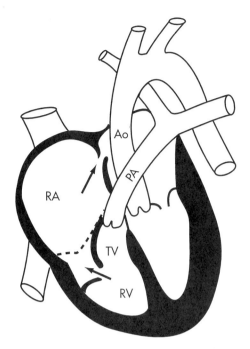

FIG. 30-5

Ebstein's anomaly. *Dashed line,* Normal position of the tricuspid valve. The tricuspid valve is set low within the body of the right ventricle (a portion of the right ventricle is "atrialized"). The septal leaflet is large and floppy, and tricuspid regurgitation usually is present. A patent foramen ovale (or an ASD) is commonly present. With tricuspid regurgitation and increased RA pressure, right-left shunting and cyanosis occur.

and there is a murmur of tricuspid regurgitation (that clearly increases with inspiration).

The ECG shows RA enlargement with unusually tall P waves, and most have right bundle branch block. The Wolff-Parkinson-White syndrome is present in 25% of patients. The chest x-ray shows cardiomegaly (RA enlargement) and clear lung fields. The echocardiogram easily identifies the abnormal tricuspid valve. Surgical repair of the tricuspid valve and closure of the ASD are considered for those with heart failure and severe disability. Since the results of surgery are unpredictable, medical therapy is the best option for mildly symptomatic patients with small shunts.

Cardiac Malpositions

Complete Transposition of the Great Vessels

Complete transposition of the great vessels is the most common of the transpositions. The aorta arises from the right ventricle, and the PA from the left ventricle (Fig. 30-6). For the infant to survive, there is an associated communication between the right and left heart (an ASD, VSD, or PDA). Cyanosis is usually present at birth and is soon followed by heart failure. Palliation of in-

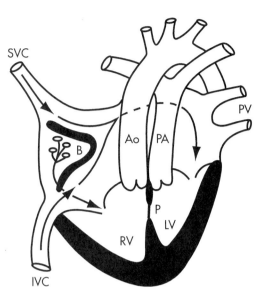

FIG. 30-6

Transposition of the great vessels, the aorta coming from the right ventricle and the PA from the left ventricle. The Mustard repair is an intraatrial "switch," with a baffle *(B)* in the atrium directing caval (superior vena cava and inferior vena cava) flow across an ASD to the left atrium and left ventricle, and pulmonary venous *(PV)* blood to the right atrium and right ventricle. The VSD is patched *(P).* One problem with this approach is that the anatomic right ventricle remains exposed to systemic arterial pressure (an unusually high afterload for the right ventricle), and RV failure may be a late complication of surgery.

fants is achieved with the *Rashkind procedure,* the creation of a large ASD using a balloon catheter.

There are two surgical approaches. It is common to encounter adults who had an atrial switch operation. The *Mustard procedure* constructs a baffle within the atria that directs flow from the vena cava toward the mitral valve and routes blood from the pulmonary veins to the right ventricle[4] (Fig. 30-6). About 80% of the patients having intraatrial switch surgery have survived to adulthood. There are a number of late complications. Atrial and ventricular tachyarrhythmias are common. Bradyarrhythmias may necessitate pacemaker therapy. Many patients develop cardiomyopathy, as the anatomic right ventricle cannot handle systemic loads.

The second approach to transposition, and the one currently in use, is an arterial switch. Both the aorta and the PA are relocated to their correct ventricles, and the coronary arteries are reimplanted. This allows the anatomic left ventricle to function as the systemic ventricle, decreasing the chance of heart failure.

Corrected Transposition

In corrected transposition, the ventricles and the great vessels are reversed. The defect itself usually causes no symptoms. However, most patients have an associated abnormality, most commonly VSD, mitral or tricuspid regurgitation, pulmonic stenosis, or heart block. Surgery may be required for the associated defect(s).

Double-Outlet Right Ventricle

Both the aorta and the PA come from the right ventricle, and oxygenated blood from the lungs reaches the aorta through a VSD. There may be associated pulmonary stenosis, PDA, coarctation of the aorta, or mitral valve obstruction. When the VSD is close to the aortic valve, flow from the left ventricle moves easily into the aorta and the clinical picture is similar to isolated VSD with pulmonary hypertension. When pulmonic stenosis is significant, the illness resembles tetralogy of Fallot. Surgical correction is done in early childhood.

Truncus Arteriosus

In truncus arteriosus a single large vessel comes from the two ventricles. PA branches originate from this vessel. Survival is possible because of a VSD. Most patients have some cyanosis, which is more severe if pulmonary blood flow is reduced by stenosis of large PA branches or by obliterative pulmonary vascular disease. Surgical correction involves a conduit from the right ventricle to the PA branches.

TREATMENT OF CONGENITAL HEART DISEASE

Surgical Correction

The surgical approach for specific conditions has been described. Table 30-1 summarizes the more commonly used operations. Many of these patients survive to adult life and are at risk for late complications, including atrial and ventricular arrhythmias, heart block, recurrent or residual VSD or ASD (patch leak), malfunction of prosthetic valves, and heart failure. Many are at risk for endocarditis and require appropriate antibiotic prophylaxis (see Chapter 21). The treatment of heart failure involves standard therapy: diuretics, afterload reduction, and digoxin (see Chapter 22). High pulmonary vascular resistance does not respond to vasodilator therapy.

Eisenmenger's Syndrome[5]

Most adults who are cyanotic and have a history of congenital heart disease have Eisenmenger's syndrome. The syndrome develops in about 8% of patients with congenital disease and 11% of those with left-right shunts. The most common causes are VSD, PDA, transposition of the great vessels, surgically created connection between the PA and aorta (e.g., Blalock-Taussig or Potts shunts), and ASD. The size of the shunt is the key factor in the development of pulmonary hypertension; Eisenmenger's syndrome develops in about half of the patients with large PDA or VSD.

Pathophysiology

High pulmonary blood flow is the cause. Lesions that also transmit systemic pressure to the PA more commonly provoke pulmonary hypertension (VSD and PDA, Fig. 30-1), and it develops during infancy. By contrast, the incidence of Eisenmenger's syndrome is less than 10% with large ASDs, which have high RV and PA flow, but less increase in pressure. Furthermore, pulmonary hypertension appears later in life with ASD, between puberty and age 30.

High pulmonary blood flow leads to irreversible microvascular changes. Why some patients have vascular injury while others do not is uncertain. Endothelial dysfunction, growth factors, and platelet aggregation appear to contribute to intimal proliferation and progressive occlusion of small arterioles. With these anatomic changes, high pulmonary vascular resistance is irreversible.

There tends to be overshoot, with pulmonary resistance exceeding systemic resistance. The direction of shunting reverses, becoming right to left. Desaturated blood reaches the left heart, and the resulting arterial hypoxemia stimulates erythrocytosis.

Clinical Presentation and Management

There may be a history of pulmonary congestion during infancy, when left-right shunting is dominant. As pulmonary resistance increases, congestion resolves. Cyanosis, erythrocytosis, and clubbing develop with shunt reversal later in infancy or soon after. It is uncommon for an adult patient to develop Eisenmenger's syndrome, although it is possible in young adults with ASD.

The symptoms and complications of Eisenmenger's syndrome are summarized in Table 30-2. Most patients have symptoms of low cardiac output, the result of pulmonary hypertension with elevated RV afterload, as well as the underlying congenital defect. Symptoms of right and left heart failure are possible. Fatigue is a common symptom.

Erythrocytosis with hyperviscosity is a day-to-day management issue. Formerly we used frequent phlebotomy to keep the hematocrit under 65%. That is not the current practice, and the indication for phlebotomy is clinical symptoms (Table 30-3). Most patients with hematocrits approaching 70% are symptomatic, with headache, fatigue, dizziness, visual disturbances, anorexia, or lethargy. Any of these is an indication for reducing the hematocrit to below 65% with isovolumic phlebotomy. Phlebotomy without volume replacement

Table 30-1 | *Surgery for Congenital Heart Disease and Late Complications*

Lesion	Operation	Residual Problems and Late Complications
Atrial septal defect (ASD)	Patch repair	Atrial arrhythmias Right atrium (RA) and right ventricle (RV) enlargement, possible RV failure Pulmonary hypertension (<10%)
Primum ASD	Patch repair; repair of cleft AV valve leaflet	As above, plus residual mitral or tricuspid regurgitation
Ventricular septal defect (VSD)	Patch repair	Leak of the VSD patch Left ventricle (LV) failure
Patent ductus arteriosus (PDA)	Ligation of the PDA; surgery is low risk	A cure for young patients; PDA is brittle in older patients, increasing the risk of surgery
Coarctation of the aorta	Resection and anastomosis, or Dacron graft	Recurrent coarctation Persistent hypertension (with its complications) Intracranial aneurysm, possible rupture Bicuspid aortic valve, aortic stenosis
Tetralogy of Fallot	Repair of VSD and patch repair of infundibular stenosis	(15% require reoperation) Persistent RV outflow tract obstruction Branch pulmonary stenosis Pulmonic regurgitation and RV failure Aortic regurgitation (common, due to dilation) Right bundle branch block Ventricular arrhythmia (originating from the RV outflow tract)
Tetralogy of Fallot	Rastelli procedure: VSD repair plus conduit from RV to pulmonary artery (PA) (when the infundibular-pulmonary stenosis cannot be repaired)	As above, plus conduit obstruction (there is a prosthetic valve in the conduit)
Tricuspid atresia	Fontan connection: RA to PA (or caval to PA) conduit, plus repair of associated lesions (ASD and VSD)	Conduit obstruction Atrial arrhythmias LV dysfunction Mitral regurgitation ASD patch leak (causing cyanosis) VSD patch leak
Transposition of the great vessels	Mustard procedure (mid-atrial baffle that "switches" the atria, directing venous return to the LV and PA, and pulmonary venous flow to the RV and aorta)	Vena cava obstruction (superior or inferior) Sinus node injury and bradyarrhythmia Atrial tacharrhythmia Midatrial baffle obstruction Residual subpulmonic obstruction Pulmonary venous obstruction Tricuspid regurgitation RV failure (inability to handle systemic loads)
Transposition of the great vessels	Arterial switch procedure, with reimplantation of the coronary arteries	*Comment:* Now more common than intraatrial surgery, with fewer late sequelae; with this operation, the anatomic LV is the pump for the systemic circulation

may worsen symptoms. Usually 500 ml of blood is removed and 500 ml of saline solution infused. Other volume expanders have no advantage over saline solution. Isovolumic phlebotomy relieves symptoms in about 24 hours. If symptoms are not relieved, a second unit of blood may be taken, but this is rarely needed.

Note: All intravenous lines should be equipped with a device to filter air bubbles to prevent paradoxical air embolism to the brain.

Phlebotomy leads to improved hemostasis (see Table 30-2), possibly because of increased blood flow and oxygen delivery to bone marrow and liver. Thus phlebotomy is recommended for those with a hematocrit of at least 65% who are to have surgery to decrease postoperative bleeding complications.

Iron deficiency and microcytosis are common, especially for patients who have had phlebotomy. The small red blood cells deform less than normal, do not pass through capillaries as easily, and thus aggravate sludging. When red blood cell indices indicate microcytosis, iron replacement therapy is indicated. Low serum iron, low ferritin, and decreased transferrin saturation are also indications for iron therapy.

Stroke may be caused by hyperviscosity, and that has been the rationale for aggressive phlebotomy in the past. More recently, phlebotomy has been identified as a risk factor for stroke in patients with Eisenmenger's syndrome.[6] This study also identified atrial fibrillation and hypertension as risk factors, but the most powerful predictor was microcytosis. It is important to look for other

---

Table 30-2	*Symptoms and Complications of Eisenmenger's Syndrome*

Clinical Problem	Comment
Low cardiac output Dyspnea on exertion, fatigue, syncope	High pulmonary resistance (increased afterload) leads to RV failure. An uncorrected congenital defect may also cause ventricular failure.
Erythrocytosis and hyperviscosity Headache, dizziness, visual disturbance, anorexia, fatigue, lethargy	Microcytosis increases viscosity (the small, stiff red blood cells are less deformable and promote sludging). If the MCV is low, treat with iron. Indications for phlebotomy: Table 30-3.
Hemostatic abnormalities Thrombocytopenia, prolonged bleeding, prothrombin and partial thromboplastin times	Deficiency of vitamin K–dependent clotting factors, abnormal fibrinolysis, and a von Willebrand factor abnormality have been described.
Stroke	Pathogenesis may include hyperviscosity (ischemic stroke), paradoxical emboli, and bleeding (berry aneurysm or impaired hemostasis).
Cerebral abscess	Paradoxical embolus or endocarditis.
Hemoptysis	Cause may be rupture of pulmonary arterioles or of an aortopulmonary collateral, pulmonary embolism, bronchitis, or bleeding diathesis.
Gout or hyperuricemia	Hyperuricemia with increased production and decreased renal clearance of uric acid. Clinical gout is uncommon (colchicine is the treatment of choice; avoid nonsteroidal antiinflammatory agents).
Cholelithiasis	Bilirubin stones result from erythrocytosis.
Hypertrophic osteoarthropathy Clubbing of fingers and toes, arthralgia	Arthritis is uncommon. There is also periostitis in long bones, metatarsals, and metacarpals. Synovial effusions are common. (Treat severe arthralgia with salsalate.)
Renal dysfunction	Glomerulopathy in one third of patients: proteinuria, urinary casts or red blood cells, reduced glomerular filtration rate, rarely the nephrotic syndrome. *Warning: try to avoid drugs that impair renal function (nonsteroidal antiinflammatory agents, contrast agents).*

etiologies of stroke, including paradoxical embolization and bleeding. Blood cultures should be drawn when cerebral embolism is suspected because the risk of *brain abscess* is increased by right-left shunting. This is critical when there has been a recent procedure that may have caused bacteremia, or when there is localized infection. Some have recommended treatment with antibiotics as soon as cultures are drawn, until negative culture results and imaging studies exclude abscess.

Special Clinical Issues

Pregnancy. Eisenmenger's syndrome is a strong indication for elective abortion because of the high risk for both mother and child. Maternal mortality is about 45%.[5] Most women die during delivery or during the week postpartum of thromboembolism, complications of hypovolemia, or preeclampsia. The mortality risk is no lower with cesarean section. Spontaneous abortion occurs in as many as 40%, and only 25% of pregnancies go to term. Intrauterine growth retardation is high, as is perinatal infant mortality (8% to 28%).[5] When abortion is declined, the patient usually is hospitalized during the third trimester of pregnancy and managed by an experienced team.

The safest method of contraception is tubal ligation. Oral contraceptives are contraindicated because of the higher risk of thromboembolism. Intramuscular medroxyprogesterone (at 3-month intervals) or a subcutaneous levonorgestrel implant are safe alternatives.

Noncardiac Surgery. With noncardiac surgery, perioperative mortality may be as high as 19%. As with pregnancy, an experienced team should be involved. In particular, the patient needs a cardiac anesthesiologist with experience managing patients with Eisenmenger's syndrome. Normalization of red blood cell indices well before surgery may lower the risk, and phlebotomy 2 weeks before surgery may be considered (Table 30-3). Excessive lowering of hematocrit must be avoided, as a normal hematocrit may not provide adequate oxygenation. Pulmonary artery catheters are often used to monitor cardiac function during surgery for patients with heart disease. This is not feasible for a patient with complex congenital disease or Eisenmenger's syndrome, and the risks of an indwelling catheter are excessive.

High Altitude and Airplane Travel. Lower oxygen tension at high altitude may provoke further pulmonary vasoconstriction and worsening of right-left shunting. Higher PA pressures may precipitate right heart failure. For these reasons we advise against travel to regions of high altitude, especially if a patient is marginally compensated.

Commercial air transportation in a pressurized cabin is usually tolerated if the patient receives supplemental oxygen, and that is considered necessary treatment. Regulation of oxygen flow is best accomplished by monitoring oxygen saturation with a portable oximetry device. The goal is to keep oxygen saturation at or above the patient's usual resting level.

Expected Clinical Course

The prognosis with Eisenmenger's syndrome is better than it is for other causes of pulmonary hypertension,

Table 30-3	*Management of Erythrocytosis in Patients with Eisenmenger's Syndrome*
Clinical Issue	**Treatment**
Dehydration (fever, burns, poor oral intake, renal or gastrointestinal loss, and so forth)	Rehydration
Hyperviscosity symptoms, normocytic indices	Isovolumic phlebotomy (500 ml)
Hyperviscosity symptoms, microcytic indices	Iron therapy, and monitor symptoms; phlebotomy if symptoms do not resolve
Hematocrit ≥65%, no symptoms, normocytic indices	Monitor symptoms
Hematocrit ≥65%, no symptoms, microcytic indices	Iron therapy, monitor symptoms, hematocrit and red blood cell indices
Surgery (cardiac or noncardiac) planned	Isovolumic phlebotomy to hematocrit <65%; iron therapy if microcytic (this must be done weeks before surgery to be effective)

including primary pulmonary hypertension. Survival is 80% at 10 years, 77% at 15 years, and 42% at 25 years.[5] Predictors of early mortality include syncope, elevated RV filling pressure and right heart failure, and more severe hypoxemia (oxygen saturation less than 85% at rest). The location of the shunt does not influence survival. Sudden cardiac death is common and is attributed to ventricular arrhythmias. Other causes of death are heart failure, hemoptysis, stroke, brain abscess, thromboembolism, and complications of surgery or pregnancy.

Because patients with Eisenmenger's syndrome constitute a small percentage of general medical practice, most patients are seen regularly in a specialty clinic. In fact, many who practice adult cardiology have little experience with complex congenital disease, and management of these adult patients has evolved as a subspecialty within cardiology. Since most patients do not have immediate access to the specialty clinic, the primary physician is an important member of the team and properly has a role in day-to-day care, including the treatment of erythrocytosis (Table 30-3).

Transplantation. Elevated pulmonary vascular resistance is fixed, with irreversible anatomic changes in small pulmonary arterioles. A transplanted heart with normal RV function would not be able to push blood through the lungs and would immediately fail. Thus heart transplantation can be done only with associated lung transplant.

Single lung transplantation and repair of the cardiac defect are possible for patients with Eisenmenger's syndrome who have correctable cardiac defects. Recovery of RV function and regression of hypertrophy have been the usual results. Survival after lung transplantation is 70% to 80% at 1 year and below 50% at 4 years.[5] Heart-lung transplant recipients have survival rates of 60% to 80% at 1 year and 30% at 10 years.

Poor short-term prognostic indicators are the usual indications for transplantation: syncope, refractory right heart failure, severe hypoxemia, and declining exercise tolerance (advanced New York Heart Association functional class).

REFERENCES

1. Gazes P: *Clinical cardiology, a cost effective approach*, ed 4, New York, 1997, Chapman & Hall.
2. Cowen ME, Jeffery RR, Drakeley MJ, et al: The results of surgery for atrial septal defect in patients aged fifty years and over, *Eur Heart J* 11:29, 1990.
3. Perloff JK, Child JS: *Congenital heart disease in adults*, Philadelphia, 1998, WB Saunders.
4. Vanden Belt RJ, Ronan JA Jr, Bedynek JL Jr: *Cardiology, a clinical approach*, Chicago, 1979, Mosby.
5. Vongpatanasin W, Brickner ME, Hillis LD, Lange RA: The Eisenmenger syndrome in adults, *Ann Intern Med* 128:745, 1998.
6. Ammash N, Warnes CA: Cerebrovascular events in adult patients with cyanotic congenital heart disease, *J Am Coll Cardiol* 28:768, 1996.

31 Hypertension

Richard E. Katholi
George J. Taylor
Marcey R. Ervin

EPIDEMIOLOGY

Since 50% of people over age 65 have hypertension, all physicians regularly treat this common illness. The recently released Sixth Report of the Joint National Committee on Prevention, Detection, Evaluation, and Treatment of High Blood Pressure (JNC-VI) provides a comprehensive guide for therapy.[1] The National High Blood Pressure Education Program has been issuing these reports since 1972, revising them periodically as new information has become available from clinical trials. These new guidelines still recommend diuretics and beta-blockers as initial drug choices in uncomplicated hypertension. However, other drug classes are also recommended when hypertensive patients have diabetes with proteinuria, heart failure, or isolated systolic hypertension.

This Sixth Report calls on physicians and public health officials to intensify their efforts to detect and treat high blood pressure because the incidence of hypertension-related morbidity and mortality has *stopped* declining, and fewer than 30% of hypertensive patients have their blood pressure under control. An important point in this Sixth Report is that the upper limit of normal blood pressure is no longer necessarily 140/90 mm Hg. Physicians must treat hypertension more aggressively, intervene with lifestyle modification and medication earlier, and, for some patients, pursue lower target blood pressures than in the past. These strategies are especially important for patients with risk factors for cardiovascular disease or those who already have target organ damage. Thus persons with the highest cardiovascular risk—those with diabetes, heart failure, or renal failure—should begin treatment with both lifestyle modifications and antihypertensive drugs, even if their blood pressure is in this high-normal range of 130 to 139/85 to 89 mm Hg. In these patients the goal blood pressure is 130/85 mm Hg or lower, whereas the goal for patients without these risk factors is 140/90 mm Hg or lower.

During the past two decades, mortality from coronary heart disease has fallen 50%, and mortality from stroke has fallen 75%.[2] Treatment of hypertension played a role in this decline. However, these trends have not continued to decrease, and in the past few years it appears that fewer patients are meeting recommended guidelines for proper control of blood pressure. Thus the Sixth Report should be studied carefully at this time.

In the United States and Western Europe approximately half of the hypertensive population is undetected, half of those detected are untreated, and half of those treated are not satisfactorily controlled. Another reason why the new recommendations are more aggressive is because age adjusted stroke rates have risen slightly since 1993, whereas the age-adjusted rate of coronary heart disease has remained stable.[1] Furthermore, the incidence of end-stage renal disease is increasing (hypertension is the second most common cause of renal failure, after diabetes), and the incidence of heart failure has been increasing, especially in elderly patients (the majority of heart failure patients have antecedent hypertension).

ETIOLOGY AND PATHOPHYSIOLOGY
Defining Hypertension

Blood pressure should be measured in a patient seated after 5 minutes of rest and at least 30 minutes after exposure to caffeine or tobacco. An elevated blood pressure should be reconfirmed in 5 to 10 minutes. If it is still elevated, hypertension should not be diagnosed until an elevated pressure has been confirmed on two or more subsequent measurements. Averaging the blood pressure readings indicates whether a patient has hypertension or not.

On initial evaluation, it is worthwhile measuring blood pressure in both arms. Slightly higher pressure may be noted in the right arm than in the left under normal conditions. Blood pressures in both arms are useful, particularly in older patients, to screen for subclavian stenosis and as a future reference if the patient ever has chest or back discomfort that might represent an ongoing aortic dissection. Systolic blood pressures in the arm and leg should be compared by palpation to rule out coarctation as a secondary cause of hypertension or in older patients as a screening tool for periph-

eral vascular disease. Normally the arterial pressure in the leg is about 10 mm Hg higher than in the arm. A normal cuff can be used to measure blood pressure in the leg by placing it below the calf and palpating the systolic pressure in the posterior tibial or dorsalis pedis pulses. The systolic blood pressure in the lower leg is then compared with a palpated systolic blood pressure in the radial pulse.

With increasing public awareness of the insidious nature of hypertension (patients can have high blood pressure with no symptoms) and the availability of blood pressure monitors that can be purchased or used in pharmacies and other public places, we hope to see a decrease in the number of undetected patients with high blood pressure before they have a cardiovascular event.

Systolic blood pressure is defined as the first appearance of sound after the cuff has been inflated to above the blood pressure, and the disappearance of sound has been used to define diastolic blood pressure. The JNC-VI report provides a new classification of elevated blood pressure based on the risk of target organ damage (Table 31-1). Increasing levels of hypertension justify increasingly aggressive treatment. Importantly, in recent years, epidemiologic and other studies indicate that systolic blood pressure is a more important predictor of future coronary heart disease events than is diastolic blood pressure.

Even borderline elevation of blood pressure mandates intervention because borderline high blood pressure often progresses and is linked to obesity and insulin resistance. Optimal blood pressure in respect to cardiovascular risk is less than 120/80 mm Hg.

Since blood pressure is often measured by paramedical personnel or by patients themselves, recognizing a change in the heart rhythm should be emphasized so that it can be brought to the physician's attention.

Premorbid States

Long-term population studies, including the Tecumseh and Framingham trials, have identified a number of risk factors for development of hypertension. Modification of these risk factors may lead to the "primary prevention" of hypertension.

Borderline Hypertension or High-Normal Blood Pressure

Finding borderline hypertension or high-normal blood pressure warrants careful education and follow-up; the Tecumseh study demonstrated that a previous history of elevated blood pressure in childhood or adolescence correlated with the development of hypertension in middle age.[3-4] The Framingham study demonstrated that hypertension developed at twice the normal rate in people with high-normal blood pressure (diastolic pressure of 85 to 89 mm Hg).[5] A subgroup with "labile"

Table 31-1	*Using Risk Factors in Deciding When to Initiate Drug Treatment for Hypertension*		
Blood Pressure	**Risk Group A** No risk factors* No target organ damage† No clinical cardiovascular disease	**Risk Group B** At least one risk factor, not including diabetes No target organ damage No clinical cardiovascular disease	**Risk Group C** Target organ damage Clinical cardiovascular disease, or diabetes, with or without other risk factors
High-normal 130/85 to 139/89 mm Hg	Lifestyle modification only	Lifestyle modification only	Drug therapy‡ (for those with heart failure, renal insufficiency, or diabetes)
Stage 1 140/90 to 159/99 mm Hg	Lifestyle modification trial (up to 12 months)	Lifestyle modification trial (up to 6 months) Or drug therapy (patients with multiple risk factors)‡	Drug therapy‡
Stages 2 and 3 ≥160/100 mm Hg	Drug therapy ‡	Drug therapy‡	Drug therapy‡

Modified from the Joint National Committee on Detection, Evaluation, and Treatment of High Blood Pressure: *Arch Intern Med* 157:2413, 1997.
*Smoking, dyslipidemia, diabetes mellitus, age >60 years, gender (men and postmenopausal women), family history of cardiovascular disease in women younger than 65 or men younger than age 55.
†Heart diseases (left ventricular hypertrophy, angina, previous myocardial infarction, previous coronary revascularization, heart failure), nephropathy, peripheral arterial disease, retinopathy, stroke, transient ischemic attack.
‡Lifestyle modification should be adjunctive therapy for all patients recommended for drug therapy.

hypertension have normal blood pressures at rest but inappropriately elevated blood pressures for the degree of exercise. Over time, end-organ changes, such as left ventricular hypertrophy, often develop in these patients. The diagnosis of hypertension should be suspected if these patients occasionally have an elevated blood pressure when seen in the office or an inappropriate elevation of blood pressure is observed during a graded exercise test.

Obesity

The Tecumseh study also demonstrated that increased skinfold thickness is a predictor of hypertension and is independent of past history of elevated blood pressure. An overweight child with an elevated blood pressure had a 90% probability of being hypertensive in middle age. Upper body obesity is worse, and those with increased hip ratio have the highest risk of developing hypertension. Commonly, the onset of hypertension is associated with weight gain, whether it be from a patient who suddenly becomes less active or one who gains weight after stopping smoking.

Insulin Resistance

Elevated insulin levels in euglycemic patients are often found in patients with hypertension. This is a more common finding in overweight patients, but there remains a positive correlation of hypertension and insulin resistance even when corrected for body weight.[6] Insulin has a number of potential deleterious effects that relate to control of blood pressure and to development of atherosclerosis. The mechanisms by which insulin may facilitate a hypertensive process include the fact that insulin causes increased renal absorption of sodium and stimulates the release of catecholamines with a resultant increase in arterial pressure. Insulin resistance in these patients is localized to skeletal muscle. Adipose tissue and other organ systems have normal insulin sensitivity. Hyperinsulinemia has been associated with altered microvascular architecture. Muscle biopsy in patients with insulin resistance has revealed an abnormality of the microcirculation with an apparent reduction in the number of arterioles surrounding muscle bundles. A lower total cross-sectional area of the microvascular bed may cause an increase in peripheral vascular resistance and, therefore, higher blood pressure. Insulin may also function as a "growth factor" in the arterial wall, promoting thickening of the arterial smooth muscles.

Exercise Patterns

Isometric (weight lifting) exercise causes an abrupt and profound rise in systolic and diastolic blood pressure. Low-level aerobic, isotonic exercise produces a fall in peripheral vascular resistance, an increase in heart rate and cardiac output, and little rise in arterial blood pressure. If pushed to extremes, even aerobic exercise is accompanied by a rise in blood pressure. These hemodynamic changes are accentuated in exercise that involves antigravity work, such as running uphill or running rather than walking. When running, you lift your body off the ground (antigravity work). Studies of young athletes have found that hypertension may be a complication of isometric training using heavy resistance, such as weight lifting.

These studies may fit the vascular architectural theory; that is, with isotonic training, such as low-level jogging or swimming, the number of "slow twitch" fibers increases, and these have a high number of arterioles per cross-sectional area around muscle bundles. High-resistance weight training causes an increase in the number of "fast twitch" fibers, which have a smaller number of arterioles per cross-sectional area around muscle bundles.

Family History of Hypertension

Subjects with a family history of hypertension should have more frequent blood pressure checks, since their tendency to develop high blood pressure is increased. Essential hypertension has a mosaic of causative factors, and studies have shown subtle renal abnormalities that predispose these patients to the subsequent development of hypertension. One European study found that normotensive young men with a positive family history of hypertension had delayed natriuresis and an exaggerated blood pressure response to an acute intravenous saline load.[7] Another study of similar patients described renal vasoconstriction and abnormally low renin and aldosterone secretion after a sodium load.[8] Both results suggest that some families have an inability to handle the large sodium load that characterizes the diet of the industrialized world. However, it is unlikely that a single, heritable mechanism is responsible for essential hypertension. It should also be noted that insulin resistance and obesity run in families.

Stress

Job stress can be influential on resting arterial blood pressure. The Framingham study reported that increased anxiety predicted the future development of hypertension in middle-aged men, but not in women. Members of the Luo tribe in Western Kenya who migrated to the city developed higher systolic blood pressure compared to their rural counterparts.[9] This study attributed much of the rise in blood pressure to increased sodium intake and body weight. However, an increase in the resting heart rate in this group suggests increased sympathetic nervous system activity, indicating some contribution of increased stress to hypertension. The Tecumseh study reported that 37 of 99 young patients with borderline hypertension

had evidence of a "hyperdynamic circulation," with increased heart rate and cardiac output and elevated plasma norepinephrine level suggesting excessive sympathetic activity as the mechanism. Although most of these patients had a positive family history for hypertension, psychologic stress was suggested as a contributor.

The Framingham investigators offered a thoughtful interpretation of their findings, suggesting that stress be considered as one of the many interacting risk factors for the development of hypertension. Future epidemiologic studies therefore should include analysis of psychosocial and biological factors (insulin levels, sodium and potassium intake, and so forth).

Smoking

Studies using ambulatory blood pressure monitoring have documented a direct pressor effect from cigarette smoking. Chronic smokers have a persistent 6 mm Hg rise in mean arterial blood pressure and an increase in heart rate while smoking two cigarettes per hour.[10] Tolerance does not appear to develop, since these findings are reproducible in chronic smokers. In addition, beta-adrenergic blockade does not blunt the rise in peripheral resistance caused by smoking, confirming a direct action rather than nicotine stimulation of the sympathetic nervous system.

Premorbid States and Other Cardiovascular Risk Factors

With an understanding of these premorbid conditions, patients at risk of developing hypertension may be identified. Many of the premorbid conditions for hypertension are also risk factors for coronary heart disease. The interactions of hypertension with coronary risk factors continue to be studied. Patients with borderline hypertension and hyperinsulinemia may have more rapid catabolism of high-density lipoprotein (HDL) and thus a lower HDL cholesterol level. Hypertension and lipid abnormalities coexist more frequently than can be explained by chance, and insulin resistance is the probable mechanism. Insulin itself has been implicated as a "trophic" factor that may promote the development of arterial plaque independent of its effect on plasma lipid levels. The obvious implication of this growing awareness is the importance of identifying and treating borderline hypertension as well as the premorbid states. In the medical literature this is referred to as the "primary prevention" of hypertension.

MANAGEMENT
Evaluation

The goals of evaluation of patients with confirmed hypertension are to search for correctable causes of the high blood pressure, to assess the presence or absence of target organ damage, and to identify other cardiovascular diseases that would guide therapy. Evaluation includes medical history, physical examination, and laboratory testing.

History

The medical history should include the duration of elevated blood pressure, family history of high blood pressure, history of recent changes in weight, exercise history, smoking history, sodium intake history, alcohol and caffeinated beverage intake history, use of illicit drugs, and a history of all prescribed or over-the-counter medications and herbal remedies. A history focused on the presence or absence of coronary heart disease, heart failure, cerebrovascular disease, peripheral vascular disease, renal disease, diabetes, dyslipidemia, gout, and sexual dysfunction should also be elicited. The results or adverse effects of previous antihypertensive therapy should be reviewed, as well as psychosocial environmental factors that may influence hypertension control.

As an example of how a medical history provides important cardiovascular implications, women 35 to 45 years of age who are smokers and use oral contraceptives have a risk of myocardial infarction 30 times the normal rate and an increased risk of subarachnoid hemorrhage 20 times normal. Compared with nonsmokers, smokers tend to drink more ethanol and caffeinated beverages and also tend to ingest more analgesics, laxatives, and hypnotics.

Physical Examination

The physical examination should include measurement of blood pressure in both arms and legs, funduscopic examination for hypertensive retinopathy, and examination of the neck for bruits, elevated venous pressure, or an enlarged thyroid gland. Physical examination should also include assessing the heart for abnormalities in rate or rhythm, increased size, precordial heave, murmurs, or gallops. (The S_4 is an early sign of increased LV stiffness.) When examining the abdomen, check for bruit, enlarged kidneys, masses, or abnormal aortic pulsation and examine the extremities for diminished or absent peripheral pulsations, bruits, or edema. Neurologic status should be assessed, including documentation of right- or left-handedness.

Laboratory Studies

Laboratory studies are recommended before initiating therapy to determine the presence of end-organ damage, screen for secondary causes, and identify other cardiovascular risk factors. Routine tests should include urinalysis, complete blood cell count, blood chemistries (potassium, sodium, magnesium, creatinine, calcium, phosphate, uric acid, fasting glucose, total cholesterol, low-density lipoprotein [LDL] and HDL cholesterol, and triglycerides), and 12-lead electrocardiogram (ECG).

The benefits of these recommended laboratory tests are as follows:

1. *Urinalysis.* Urine glucose testing is a screen for diabetes. Proteinuria, hematuria, or bacteriuria may indicate underlying renal disease that could contribute to the hypertensive process. A patient with borderline hypertension and diabetes who has proteinuria should be considered at high risk for nephropathy and needs aggressive therapy with an angiotensin-converting enzyme (ACE) inhibitor.

2. *Complete blood count.* Hemoglobin, white blood cell count, and platelet count provide a screen for underlying diseases but provide no specific information regarding the cause or management of hypertension.

3. *Blood chemistry.* Hypokalemia in an untreated patient may indicate primary aldosteronism as the cause of the hypertension. It may also reflect laxative abuse. Once the patient has been begun diuretic therapy, a low potassium level is less helpful as far as diagnosing underlying causes, but it is still an important finding, since hypokalemia is potentially a life-threatening complication of diuretic therapy, especially if there is heart disease. Thus if a patient's baseline potassium level is normal and diuretics are started, the potassium level should periodically be measured and kept between 4.0 and 5.0 mEq/L to decrease the chance of ventricular arrhythmias. *Potassium replacement also has blood pressure–lowering benefits.*

   Hypomagnesemia may be caused by chronic diuretic usage or by chronic diarrheal illnesses or diabetes. Hypomagnesemia exacerbates hypertension and also may provoke cardiac arrhythmias. Serum sodium measurement is less useful in patients with mild hypertension who are otherwise healthy. However, in patients with coexisting heart failure, hyponatremia indicates poor prognosis and serves as a marker of increased plasma renin activity and increased sensitivity to ACE inhibitors. Creatinine measurement is an important screen for underlying renal disease. Any evidence of early nephropathy justifies aggressive management. Fasting glucose level is a screen for diabetes. Hyperglycemia also may be associated with secondary causes of hypertension, including Cushing's syndrome, pheochromocytoma, and primary aldosteronism. Since diuretics can provoke or aggravate hyperglycemia, a baseline value is necessary. Measurements of total cholesterol, LDL and HDL cholesterol, and triglycerides are recommended for screening patients with cardiovascular disease. These are also important when deciding on therapy, because a number of antihypertensive medications may aggravate hyperlipidemia.

   Calcium and phosphate are screens for hyperparathyroidism. Half of all patients with hyperparathyroidism develop hypertension. Uric acid levels may increase during treatment with diuretics. Hyperuricemia has increasingly been found to be an independent risk factor for cardiovascular disease, particularly in women.

4. An *ECG* is recommended as a baseline measure of target organ damage, but also as a screen for unexpected coronary artery disease and unexpected conduction system disease, which could be influenced by nonhydropyridine calcium channel antagonists or beta-blockers. Sensitivity in detecting left ventricular hypertrophy by ECG is less than 50%. The early sign of hypertensive heart disease by ECG may be a left atrial abnormality, with a biphasic P wave in lead V_1 (see Chapter 5). If left ventricular hypertrophy is suspected, measurement of left ventricular wall thickness with the echocardiogram is the gold standard.

When their use is warranted, other specific tests are discussed under secondary causes of hypertension.

Ambulatory blood pressure monitoring is not required in the initial evaluation and management of patients with hypertension.[1] Ambulatory blood pressure monitoring is helpful in patients with suspected "white coat" hypertension. It is also helpful in patients with apparent antihypertensive medication resistance, in those with suspected hypotensive symptoms from antihypertensive medications, and in patients with autonomic dysfunctional states.

Although ambulatory blood pressure monitoring is not recommended for routine evaluation, much has been learned from clinical trials using this technique. The average daytime pressure recorded by monitors is about 5 mm Hg lower than office readings. The average daily blood pressure from ambulatory monitoring is superior to isolated cuff pressures in predicting future cardiovascular events. Pressure rises soon after awakening and rising from bed. This rise appears to be caused by increased sympathetic nervous system activity, which may contribute to the observed increase in the incidence of myocardial infarction and sudden death in the early morning hours.

A failure of the blood pressure to fall while the patient is asleep increases the risk of the patient developing left ventricular hypertrophy. Black patients, both with and without hypertension, are less likely to have this nocturnal decline in arterial blood pressure, possibly explaining their earlier onset of hypertension and worse prognosis.[11] Ambulatory blood pressure monitoring also is effective in detecting episodes of hypotension. Elderly patients in nursing homes who had fallen were found to have substantial decreases in arterial blood pressure when standing, after using nitroglycerin, or after taking blood pressure medications.

Secondary Hypertension

Essential hypertension accounts for approximately 90% of patients with elevated arterial pressure. Most of those with secondary hypertension have chronic renal disease, and these patients are identified by measuring serum creatinine. Of the remaining patients who have "curable hypertension," most have renovascular disease, which in some series represents 5% of the hypertensive population. The remainder of the curable hypertension cases include those with primary aldosteronism (0.5%), coarctation of the aorta (0.5%), Cushing's syndrome (0.1%), or pheochromocytoma (0.2%).

In the initial evaluation of a patient with hypertension, the history, physical examination, and routine laboratory work usually suggest whether further search for secondary causes of hypertension is necessary. An unexplained low potassium level may suggest primary aldosteronism. A lower systolic blood pressure in the leg compared with the arm suggests coarctation of the aorta. Cushing's syndrome causes cushingoid facies, skin changes, and hyperglycemia. Factors that would lead one to consider renovascular hypertension or pheochromocytoma are discussed later.

Renal Artery Stenosis

In view of the important role the kidney plays in the control of arterial blood pressure and the maintenance of fluid balance, physicians should maintain a high index of suspicion for renal artery stenosis when evaluating patients who have hypertension and renal dysfunction. Renovascular hypertension is suggested by the development of hypertension in patients under age 25, *especially if there is no family history of elevated blood pressure.*

In younger patients fibromuscular dysplasia is the usual cause of renal artery stenosis. Fibromuscular dysplasia is more common in women than in men. In older patients the sudden appearance of hypertension or the sudden worsening of controlled hypertension should raise the possibility of atherosclerotic stenosis of the renal artery. In patients having both renal dysfunction and hypertension, about one fourth have renal artery stenosis. Atherosclerotic disease in other vascular beds increases the likelihood of a patient having renal artery stenosis.[12] Severe multivessel coronary artery disease is associated with a higher incidence of renal artery stenosis. Forty-five percent of people with peripheral vascular disease have renovascular disease. There is a twofold higher prevalence of renovascular disease in diabetic persons.

An elderly patient should be evaluated for renal artery stenosis if there is worsening of previously stable hypertension, new-onset hypertension, or progressive renal impairment while taking ACE inhibitors. Bilateral renal artery stenosis should be suspected when acute renal failure develops after starting an ACE inhibitor, sug-gesting that intrarenal angiotensin II is required to maintain glomerular perfusion pressure. In these patients the acute worsening of glomerular filtration rate is usually reversible by stopping the ACE inhibitor. Bilateral renal artery stenosis should also be suspected in patients with unexplained recurrent pulmonary edema.

It is important to diagnose renal artery stenosis due to atherosclerotic disease, not only to improve arterial blood pressure control, but also to protect renal function. The natural history of atherosclerotic renal artery stenosis is one of progression toward renal insufficiency and end-stage renal disease despite good blood pressure control with medications. In patients with atherosclerotic renal artery disease having greater than 60% stenosis, there was a 4% per year rate of renal artery silent occlusion.

In laboratories with an experienced technician the renal artery duplex scan is an excellent method of screening for renal artery stenosis. In other laboratories pretreatment with captopril followed by isotope renography has been received enthusiastically. The gold standard for diagnosing renal artery stenosis is renal angiography, a relatively benign procedure. If a patient requires some other form of angiography, such as cardiac catheterization, and if there is an index of suspicion about associated renal artery stenosis, an abdominal aortogram can be performed to evaluate renal arterial circulation ("while in the neighborhood"). This is cost effective, adds only a minute to the procedure, and requires only an additional 20 to 40 mL of contrast medium.

If renal artery stenosis is caused by fibromuscular dysplasia, renal angioplasty effects an excellent long-term result. If renal artery stenosis results from atherosclerosis, angioplasty with stent placement is technically and clinically effective treatment. Prospective follow-up studies using renal artery duplex scan indicate improved arterial blood pressure control, stable serum creatinine levels, and no occluded renal arteries 1 year after angioplasty with stenting, suggesting that this approach beneficially alters the natural history of atherosclerotic renal artery stenosis.

Pheochromocytoma

Pheochromocytoma is a rare cause of hypertension and is suggested by the sudden development of hypertension in a young person with no family history. Associated symptoms are palpitations, headache, episodic sweating, anxiety attacks, flushing, weight loss, and hyperglycemia. Over half the patients have fixed elevated blood pressure, and others have paroxysmal elevations in blood pressure. Aggravation of hypertension by stress, including surgery, anesthesia, endotracheal intubation, and pregnancy, may occur. Ten percent of pheochromocytomas are malignant, 10% are bilateral, and 10% are extraadrenal. A 24-hour urine test for catecholamines

and metanephrine collected while the patient is hypertensive establishes the diagnosis in 95% of these patients. Patients with pheochromocytoma have markedly elevated catecholamine levels, not borderline elevated levels. Provocative testing is no longer necessary. If a hypertensive patient has mildly elevated urinary catecholamine levels and you need to differentiate whether this results from increased central sympathetic nervous system activity or a pheochromocytoma, the patient can be given oral clonidine, adjusting the dosage until the patient is normotensive. Repeating the 24-hour urine collection after the patient is normotensive reveals normal urinary catecholamine levels if the problem is essential hypertension. Patients with pheochromocytoma maintain elevated urinary catecholamine and metanephrine levels. If a patient appears to have a pheochromocytoma, computed tomography (CT) or magnetic resonance imaging (MRI) study of the adrenal glands would be the next step to identify the location of the tumor. Surgical removal of the tumor cures hypertension in 98% of patients who have a benign adenoma.

Other Causes of Hypertension

Baroreflex failure is a recently described, uncommon mechanism of hypertension that can mimic pheochromocytoma.[13] Hypertension may be labile and severe, and urinary catecholamine levels are extremely high. High norepinephrine levels are caused by unrestrained activation of the central sympathetic nervous system. Most cases are cause by injury of the glossopharyngeal or vagal afferent nerves that carry inhibitory messages from the baroreceptors to the brainstem centers controlling central sympathetic outflow. In almost all cases described, there is a history of neck surgery or irradiation. Blood pressure can be controlled with a central sympatholytic agent, such as clonidine, and very low doses should be initiated, since the patient can be quite sensitive to its effect. This clonidine suppression allows the exclusion of pheochromocytoma. The clinical setting should suggest the diagnosis, such as prior neck surgery or trauma.

Increasingly it appears that *sleep apnea* may contribute to the development and maintenance of hypertension. Although the mechanism is not well understood, it may occur through an enhancement of sympathetic nervous system activity. This is another reason for screening for sleep apnea during annual examinations and for increasing the public's awareness of sleep apnea. Most of these patients are also obese, and many have essential hypertension. Nevertheless, successful treatment of sleep apnea may dramatically improve blood pressure control.

Ethanol consumption and high blood pressure are directly related, and excessive ethanol use should be considered as a cause of secondary hypertension accounting for as many as 10% to 12% of cases of hypertension. Arterial blood pressure has been found to be consistently higher in those who chronically consume excessive amounts of ethanol. The mechanism is enhanced central sympathetic nervous system activity. The diagnosis may require interview of family members, and an ethanol history is an important part of the hypertension workup.

Treatment of Hypertension

The JNC-VI report provides helpful guidelines concerning when to initiate therapy for hypertension based on the patient's risk group and offers an algorithm for treating patients.[1] Like the previous report issued in 1993, the JNC-VI recommends diuretics or beta-blockers as initial drug choices for hypertension not complicated by other diseases. These are still the only classes of drugs proven in large-scale clinical trials to decrease morbidity and mortality. This recommendation, however, may change when the Antihypertensive and Lipid-Lowering Treatment to Prevent Heart Attack Trial (ALLHAT) concludes in 2002.[14]

Although it is well known that the risk of cardiovascular disease increases with high blood pressure (recent evidence shows that systolic blood pressure is more important than diastolic blood pressure), hypertension is only one of many risk factors. The JNC-VI revised a three-tiered risk classification (see Table 31-1). The urgency of starting antihypertensive drug therapy depends not only on the patient's blood pressure, but also on the other cardiovascular risk factors. As recommended, everyone with a blood pressure of 130/85 mm Hg or higher should modify their lifestyle to lower blood pressure, including weight reduction, increased low-resistance exercise, moderation of alcohol intake, and decreased salt intake while maintaining an adequate intake of potassium, magnesium, and calcium. While avoiding tobacco and eating less fat do not affect blood pressure per se, these modifications are recommended to decrease cardiovascular risk. As shown in Table 31-1, Risk Group A has the lowest risk (no cardiovascular risk factors other than hypertension, no target organ damage, and no clinical cardiovascular disease). Patients in this group with stage I hypertension (blood pressure 140/90 to 159/99 mm Hg) can then undergo a trial of lifestyle modification alone for up to 12 months. Those with higher blood pressures should start lifestyle modification and drug therapy immediately.

Risk Group B is defined as patients with at least one additional cardiovascular risk factor, not including diabetes, but no target organ damage or clinical cardiovascular disease. Patients in this group of stage 1 hypertension can try lifestyle modification alone for up to 6 months if they have only one risk factor. Patients with

higher blood pressure or with more than one risk factor should start lifestyle modification and drug therapy immediately.

Risk Group C has the highest risk: target organ damage and clinical cardiovascular disease or diabetes with or without other risk factors. As stated earlier, patients with heart failure, diabetes, or kidney failure should begin lifestyle modification and drug therapy immediately even if their blood pressure is in the high-normal range of 130/85 to 139/89 mm Hg. In these patients, the goal blood pressure is 130/85 mm Hg or lower.

Nonpharmacologic Therapy

All patients with high blood pressure benefit from lifestyle modifications that favorably influence hypertension as well as risk of future cardiovascular events. Nonpharmacologic interventions may normalize mild hypertension as well as facilitate antihypertensive drug therapy in patients with moderate or severe hypertension. Box 31-1 lists lifestyle modifications for hypertension prevention and management from the JNC-VI report. Weight loss is best accomplished by a combination of caloric restriction and increased low-resistance exercise. If a patient adds walking 1 mile daily to his or her regimen, this individual would lose 10

pounds over the course of 1 year. Even a 10-pound weight loss enhances the effects from antihypertensive drug therapy. Weight loss and exercise are the only effective treatments for insulin resistance. Weight gain and being overweight increase the risk of hypertension, whereas weight loss reduces the risk.

Box 31-1 summarizes the recommended limit for daily intake of beer, wine, and 100-proof whiskey.

Sodium restriction and adequate intake of potassium, magnesium, and calcium in combination with weight reduction also achieve some lowering of arterial blood pressure. Morton's Lite Salt is half potassium chloride and half sodium chloride and is a useful substitute for anyone without renal insufficiency because it increases the potassium intake and decreases the sodium intake. The taste of Morton's Lite Salt cannot be differentiated from normal table salt.

Discontinuing smoking and decreasing dietary saturated fat and cholesterol are recommended for overall cardiovascular health. In addition, there is a direct pressor effect of cigarette smoking. Patients do not appear to develop tolerance to this and will have a pressor response with each cigarette. Caffeine causes an acute rise in arterial pressure by triggering the release of catecholamines from nerve endings. Under stressful conditions the addition of caffeine leads to excessive norepinephrine release.

Drug Therapy

Figure 31-1 is an algorithm for treating hypertension from the JNC-VI report. Table 31-2 reviews indications and relative contraindications for using individualized antihypertensive drug therapy.

In a departure from the previous report the JNC-VI report emphasizes four indications for using classes of drugs other than diuretics and beta-blockers as first-line agents, as follows:

1. With type I diabetes mellitus with proteinuria, ACE inhibitors are indicated.
2. With heart failure due to systolic hypertension, ACE inhibitors and diuretics are indicated.
3. With isolated systolic hypertension in elderly patients, diuretics are preferred, but long-acting dihydropyridine calcium channel antagonists may also be indicated.
4. After myocardial infarction, beta-blockers without intrinsic sympathomimetic activity are indicated; ACE inhibitors are indicated for patients with systolic dysfunction (left ventricular ejection fraction of at least 40%).

The report also identifies several less compelling indications and some relative contraindications for specific classes of drugs (see Table 31-2).

If the initial drug at full dosage has no effect on blood pressure or causes troublesome side effects, JNC-VI recommends substituting a drug from a differ-

---

BOX 31-1

LIFESTYLE MODIFICATIONS FOR HYPERTENSION PREVENTION AND MANAGEMENT

Lose weight if overweight

Limit alcohol intake to no more than 1 oz (30 mL) of ethanol (e.g., 24 oz [720 mL] of beer, 10 oz [300 mL] of wine, or 2 oz [60 mL] of 100-proof whiskey) per day or 0.5 oz (15 mL) of ethanol per day for women and lighter-weight people.

Increase aerobic physical activity (30 to 45 minutes most days of the week)

Reduce sodium intake to no more than 100 mmol/day (2.4 g of sodium or 6 g of sodium chloride)

Maintain adequate intake of dietary potassium (approximately 90 mmol/day)

Maintain adequate intake of dietary calcium and magnesium for general health

Stop smoking and reduce intake of dietary saturated fat and cholesterol for overall cardiovascular health

ent class. However, if the initial drug produces a partial response and is well tolerated, JNC-VI recommends adding another drug from a different class, preferably a diuretic, if not already used (see Fig. 31-1). The JNC-VI report, more than earlier reports, references the published studies from which each prevention or treatment

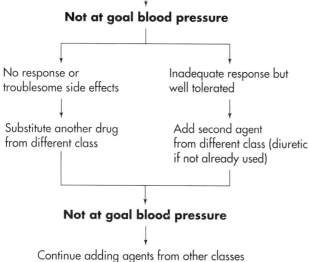

Begin or continue lifestyle modifications

↓

Not at goal blood pressure
<140/90 mm Hg, or lower for patients with diabetes or renal disease

↓

Initial drug choices
Use unless contraindicated; start with a low dose of a long-acting once-daily drug and titrate dose; low-dose combinations may be appropriate
    Uncomplicated hypertension
        Diuretics
        Beta-blockers
    Diabetes mellitus (type 1) with proteinuria
        Angiotensin-converting enzyme inhibitors
    Heart failure
        Angiotensin-converting enzyme inhibitors
        Diuretics
    Isolated systolic hypertension (older persons)
        Diuretics preferred
        Long-acting dihydropyridine calcium antagonists
    Myocardial infarction
        Beta-blockers without intrinsic sympathomimetic activity
        Angiotensin-converting enzyme inhibitors (patients with systolic dysfunction)

↓

Not at goal blood pressure

No response or troublesome side effects → Substitute another drug from different class

Inadequate response but well tolerated → Add second agent from different class (diuretic if not already used)

↓

Not at goal blood pressure

↓

Continue adding agents from other classes
Consider referral to a hypertension specialist

FIG. 31-1
Algorithm for treating hypertension.
Modified from the Joint National Committee on Detection, Evaluation, and Treatment of High Blood Pressure, *Arch Intern Med* 157:2413, 1997.

recommendation originated. Wherever possible the committee tried to base its recommendations on randomized, controlled trials.

The goal of pharmacologic therapy should be to control blood pressure with a convenient dosing schedule and minimal side effects. With the many classes of antihypertensive medications available, this should be possible in most patients. Table 31-3 demonstrates the oral antihypertensive medications with trade name, usual dosage range, and selected side effects. Table 31-4 contains the combination drugs for hypertension. Low doses of two agents may minimize the adverse effects of the individual agents. For example, a low-dose combination of an ACE inhibitor with a nonhydropyridine calcium channel antagonist may reduce proteinuria more than either drug used alone. The combination of a dihydropyridine calcium channel antagonist and an ACE inhibitor induces less pedal edema than does the calcium antagonist alone.

Immediate-release nifedipine may precipitate myocardial ischemia when given in doses above 60 mg/day, and an increase in mortality has been described for patients who have underlying coronary artery disease. Since long-acting calcium channel antagonists are available, immediate-release nifedipine usage should be avoided. Clinical trials are in progress with long-acting calcium channel antagonists that are currently approved for the treatment of hypertension, so the final answer about the safety of calcium channel antagonists compared with other agents will be determined.

Nondihydropyridines, specifically, diltiazem and verapamil, can cause slowing of the heart rate and even heart block in patients with underlying conduction system disease. The dihydropyridines cause more ankle edema than the nondihydropyridine calcium channel antagonists. One side effect that warrants greater publicity is that hypertensive patients with poor dental hygiene may develop gum hypertrophy when treated with calcium channel antagonists. If the patient is edentulous, this is of no concern. If a patient flosses once daily, he or she greatly decreases the chance of developing gum hypertrophy. A drug-food interaction has been reported, with hypotension occurring in patients given felodipine (Plendil) who drink significant amounts of grapefruit juice. Grapefruit juice inhibits the hepatic metabolism of felodipine, resulting in increased plasma levels with resultant hypotension.

Demographics and co-existing conditions may dictate drug choice for a specific patient. The following section emphasizes issues to consider when prescribing treatment for hypertension.

Atherosclerosis

Epidemiologic studies have shown decreases in stroke, renal failure, and heart failure with the treatment of hy-

Text continued on p. 372

Table 31-2	Indications and Contraindications for Using Particular Classes of Drugs To Individualize Antihypertensive Drug Therapy

Compelling Indications*	Less-Compelling Indications†	Relative Contraindications‡
Diabetes mellitus (type 1 with proteinuria) Angiotensin-converting enzyme (ACE) inhibitors	**Angina** Beta-blockers Calcium antagonists	**Bronchospastic disease** Beta-blockers (contraindicated)
Heart failure due to systolic dysfunction ACE inhibitors Diuretics	**Atrial tachycardia and fibrillation** Beta-blockers Calcium channel antagonists (nondihydropyridine)	**Depression** Beta-blockers Centrally acting alpha-agonists Reserpine (contraindicated)
	Cyclosporine-induced hypertension Calcium antagonists (caution with the dose of cyclosporine)	**Diabetes (type 1 and 2)** Beta-blockers Diuretics (in high doses)
Isolated systolic hypertension (older patients) Diuretics (preferred) Calcium channel antagonists (long-acting dihydropyridines)	**Diabetes mellitus with proteinuria** ACE inhibitors (preferred) Calcium channel antagonists	**Dyslipidemia** Beta-blockers without intrinsic sympathomimetic activity Diuretics (high doses)
	Diabetes mellitus (type 2) Low-dose diuretics	**Gout** Diuretics
	Dyslipidemia Peripheral alpha-blockers	
Myocardial infarction Beta-blockers without intrinsic sympathomimetic activity (e.g., atenolol, betaxolol, bisoprolol, metoprolol, nadolol, propranolol, timolol) ACE inhibitors (patients with systolic dysfunction)	**Essential tremor** Beta-blockers (noncardioselective)	**Heart block (second- or third-degree)** Beta-blockers (contraindicated) Nondihydropyridine calcium antagonists (contraindicated)
	Heart failure Carvedilol Losartan	**Heart failure** Beta-blockers (except carvedilol) Calcium antagonists (except amlodipine, felodipine)
	Hyperthyroidism Beta-blockers	
	Migraine Beta-blockers (noncardioselective) Calcium antagonists (nonhydropyridine)	**Liver disease** Labetalol Methyldopa (contraindicated)
	Myocardial infarction Diltiazem	**Peripheral vascular disease** Beta-blockers
	Osteoporosis Thiazides	**Pregnancy** ACE inhibitors (contraindicated) Angiotensin II receptor blocker (contraindicated)
	Preoperative hypertension Beta-blockers	
	Prostatic hypertrophy Peripheral alpha-blockers	**Renal insufficiency** Potassium-sparing agents
	Renal insufficiency ACE inhibitors (caution in renovascular hypertension and creatinine ≥3 mg/dL)	**Renovascular disease** ACE inhibitors Angiotensin II receptor blockers

Modified from the Joint National Committee on Detection, Evaluation, and Treatment of High Blood Pressure, *Arch Intern Med* 157:2413, 1997.
*Proved to have beneficial effects on comorbid conditions in randomized trials.
†*May* have favorable effects on comorbid conditions.
‡*May* have unfavorable effects on comorbid conditions; may be used with special monitoring unless contraindicated.

Table 31-3	*Oral Antihypertensive Drugs*

Drug	Trade Name	Usual Dose Range, Total mg/d* (Frequency per Day)	Selected Side Effects and Comments*
DIURETICS (PARTIAL LIST) Chlorthalidone (G)† Hydrochlorothiazide (G)	Hygroton HydroDIURIL, Microzide, Esidrix	12.5-50 (1) 12.5-50 (1)	*Short term:* increases cholesterol, triglyceride, and glucose levels; *biochemical abnormalities:* decreases potassium, sodium, and magnesium levels; increases uric acid and calcium levels; *rare:* blood dyscrasias, photosensitivity, pancreatitis
Indapamide Metolazone	Lozol Mykrox Zaroxolyn	1.25-5 (1) 0.5-1.0 (1) 2.5-10 (1)	(Less or no hypercholesterolemia)
Loop Diuretics Bumetanide (G)	Bumex	0.5-4 (2-3)	(Short duration of action, no hypercalcemia)
Ethacrynic acid Furosemide (G)	Edecrin Lasix	25-100 (2-3) 40-240 (2-3)	(Only nonsulfonamide diuretic, ototoxicity) (Short duration of action, no hypercalcemia)
Torsemide	Demadex	5-100 (1-2)	
Potassium-Sparing Agents Amiloride hydrochloride (G) Spironolactone (G)	Midamor Aldactone	5-10 (1) 25-100 (1)	Hyperkalemia Breast tenderness and/or gynecomastia, gastritis
Triamterene (G)	Dyrenium	25-100 (1)	
ADRENERGIC INHIBITORS ***Peripheral Agents*** Guanadrel sulfate Guanethidine monosulfate Reserpine (G)‡	Hylorel Ismelin Serpasil	10-75 (2) 10-150 (1) 0.05-0.25 (1)	(Postural hypotension, diarrhea) (Postural hypotension, diarrhea) (Nasal congestion, sedation, depression, activation of peptic ulcer)
CENTRAL SYMPATHOLYTIC AGENTS Clonidine hydrochloride (G)	Catapres/ Catapres-TTS	0.2-1.2 (2-3) 0.1-0.3 weekly	Sedation, dry mouth, bradycardia, withdrawal hypertension (More withdrawal)
Guanabenz acetate (G) Guanfacine hydrochloride (G) Methyldopa (G)	Wytensin Tenex Aldomet	8-32 (2) 1-3 (1) 500-3000 (2)	(Less withdrawal) (Hepatitis, lupus syndrome, and Coombs' positive hemolytic anemia; safest to use in pregnancy)

Modified from the Joint National Committee on Detection, Evaluation, and Treatment of High Blood Pressure, *Arch Intern Med* 157:2413, 1997.
*These dosages may vary from those listed in the *Physicians' Desk Reference,* ed 51, which may be consulted for additional information. The listing of the effects is not all-inclusive, and side effects are for the class of drugs except where noted for individual drug (in parentheses); clinicians are urged to refer to the package insert for a more detailed listing. Note the review of drugs in Part Three: Cardiology Drug Reference.
†Generic available.
‡Also acts centrally.

Continued

Table 31-3	*Oral Antihypertensive Drugs—cont'd*

Drug	Trade Name	Usual Dose Range, Total mg/d* (Frequency per Day)	Selected Side Effects and Comments*
PERIPHERAL ALPHA-BLOCKERS			Postural hypotension, increases HDL, decreases total cholesterol and triglycerides, stress incontinence in women, decreased prostatic obstruction in men
Doxazosin mesylate	Cardura	1-16 (1)	
Prazosin hydrochloride (G)	Minipress	2-30 (2-3)	
Terazosin hydrochloride	Hytrin	1-20 (1)	
BETA-BLOCKERS			Bronchospasm, bradycardia, AV block, heart failure, withdrawal may lead to exacerbation, to angina, and myocardial infarction, may mask insulin-induced hypoglycemia; less serious: impaired peripheral circulation, Raynaud's phenomenon, vivid dreams, insomnia, fatigue, decreased exercise tolerance, hypertriglyceridemia, decreased HDL cholesterol (except agents with intrinsic sympathomimetic activity, early in pregnancy may result in lower birth weight)
Acebutolol §‖	Sectral	200-800 (1)	
Atenolol (G)§	Tenormin	25-100 (1-2)	
Betaxolol hydrochloride§	Kerlone	5-20 (1)	
Bisoprolol fumarate §	Zebeta	2.5-10 (1)	
Carteolol hydrochloride ‖	Cartrol	2.5-10 (1)	
Metoprolol tartrate (G)§	Lopressor	50-300 (2)	
Metoprolol succinate§	Toprol XL	50-300 (1)	
Nadolol (G)	Corgard	20-320 (1)	
Penbutolol sulfate ‖	Levatol	10-20 (1)	
Pindolol (G)	Visken	10-60 (2)	
Propranolol hydrochloride (G)	Inderal	40-480 (2)	
	Inderal LA	40-480 (1)	
Timolol maleate (G)	Blocadren	20-60 (2)	
COMBINED ALPHA- AND BETA-BLOCKERS			Postural hypotension, bronchospasm, bradycardia, AV block
Carvedilol	Coreg	12.5-50 (2)	
Labetalol hydrochloride (G)	Normodyne, Trandate	200-1200 (2)	
DIRECT VASODILATORS			Headaches, fluid retention, tachycardia
Hydralazine hydrochloride (G)	Apresoline	50-300 (2)	(Lupus-like syndrome)
Minoxidil (G)	Loniten	5-100 (1)	(Hirsutism)

Modified from the Joint National Committee on Detection, Evaluation, and Treatment of High Blood Pressure, *Arch Intern Med* 157:2413, 1997.
§Cardioselective.
‖Has intrinsic sympathomimetic activity.
¶Approved in the United States for angina.

Table 31-3 | *Oral Antihypertensive Drugs—cont'd*

Drug	Trade Name	Usual Dose Range, Total mg/d* (Frequency per Day)	Selected Side Effects and Comments*
CALCIUM CHANNEL ANTAGONISTS *Nondihydropyridines*			Conduction defects, bradycardia, worsening of systolic dysfunction, gingival hyperplasia, mild ankle edema (Nausea, headache)
Diltiazem hydrochloride¶	Cardizem SR	120-360 (2)	
	Cardizem CD, Dilacor XR, Tiazac	120-360 (1)	
Mibefradil dihydrochloride¶ (T-channel calcium antagonist)	Posicor	50-100 (1)	(No worsening of systolic dysfunction; contraindicated with terfenadine [Seldane], astemizole [Hismanal], and cisapride [Propulsid]); see text regarding concomitant use with statins
Verapamil hydrochloride¶	Isoptin SR, Calan SR, Verelan, Covera-HS	90-480 (2) 120-480 (1)	(Constipation)
Dihydropyridines			Ankle edema, flushing, headache, gingival hyperplasia
Amlodipine besylate¶	Norvasc	2.5-10 (1)	
Felodipine	Plendil	2.5-20 (1)	(Hypotension when combined with grapefruit juice)
Isradipine	DynaCirc	5-20 (2)	
	DynaCirc CR	5-20 (1)	
Nicardipine hydrochloride	Cardene SR	60-90 (2)	
Nifedipine¶	Procardia XL, Adalat CC	30-120 (1)	
Nisoldipine	Sular	20-60 (1)	
ANGIOTENSIN-CONVERTING ENZYME INHIBITORS			Common: cough; rare: angioedema, hyperkalemia, rash, loss of taste, leukopenia, acute renal failure with bilateral renal artery stenosis or stenosis of the artery to a solitary kidney, increased fetal mortality
Benazepril hydrochloride	Lotensin	5-40 (1-2)	
Captopril (G)	Capoten	25-150 (2-3)	
Enalapril maleate	Vasotec	5-40 (1-2)	
Fosinopril sodium	Monopril	10-40 (1-2)	
Lisinopril	Prinivil, Zestril	5-40 (1)	
Moexipril	Univasc	7.5-15 (2)	
Quinapril hydrochloride	Accupril	5-80 (1-2)	
Ramipril	Altace	1.25-20 (1-2)	
Trandolapril	Mavik	1-4 (1)	
ANGIOTENSIN II RECEPTOR BLOCKERS			Angioedema (very rare), hyperkalemia, acute renal failure with bilateral renal artery stenosis or stenosis of the artery to a solitary kidney, increased fetal mortality
Losartan potassium	Cozaar	25-100 (1-2)	
Valsartan	Diovan	80-320 (1)	
Irbesartan	Avapro	150-300 (1)	(Also has a uricosuric effect)

¶Approved in the United States for angina.

Table 31-4 | *Common Combination Drugs for Hypertension*

Drug Name	Trade Name
BETA-ADRENERGIC BLOCKERS AND DIURETICS	
Atenolol, 50 or 100 mg/chlorthalidone, 25 mg	Tenoretic
Bisoprolol fumarate, 2.5, 5, or 10 mg/hydrochlorothiazide, 6.25 mg	Ziac*
Metoprolol tartrate, 50 or 100 mg/hydrochlorothiazide, 25 or 50 mg	Lopressor HCT
Nadolol, 40 or 80 mg/bendroflumethiazide, 5 mg	Corzide
Propranolol hydrochloride, 40 or 80 mg/hydrochlorothiazide, 25 mg	Inderide
Propranolol hydrochloride (extended release), 80, 120, or 160 mg/hydrochlorothiazide, 50 mg	Inderide LA
Timolol maleate, 10 mg/hydrochlorothiazide, 25 mg	Timolide
ANGIOTENSIN-CONVERTING ENZYME (ACE) INHIBITORS AND DIURETICS	
Benzapril hydrochloride, 5, 10, or 20 mg/hydrochlorothiazide, 6.25, 12.5, or 25 mg	Lotensin HCT
Captopril, 25 or 50 mg/hydrochlorothiazide, 15 or 25 mg	Capozide*
Enalapril maleate, 5 or 10 mg/hydrochlorothiazide, 12.5 or 25 mg	Vaseretic
Lisinopril, 10 or 20 mg/hydrochlorothiazide, 12.5 or 25 mg	Prinzide, Zestoretic
ANGIOTENSIN II RECEPTOR ANTAGONISTS AND DIURETICS	
Losartan potassium, 50 mg/hydrochlorothiazide, 12.5 mg	Hyzaar
CALCIUM ANTAGONISTS AND ACE INHIBITORS	
Amlodipine besylate, 2.5 or 5 mg/benazepril hydrochloride, 10 or 20 mg	Lotrel
Diltiazem hydrochloride, 180 mg/enalapril maleate, 5 mg	Teczem
Verapamil hydrochloride (extended release), 180 or 240 mg/trandolapril, 1, 2, or 4 mg	Tarka
Felodipine, 5 mg/enalapril maleate, 5 mg	Lexxel
OTHER COMBINATIONS	
Triamterene, 37.5, 50, or 75 mg/hydrochlorothiazide 25 or 50 mg	Dyazide, Maxzide
Spironolactone, 25 or 50 mg/hydrochlorothiazide, 25 or 50 mg	Aldactazide
Amiloride hydrochloride, 5 mg/hydrochlorothiazide, 50 mg	Moduretic
Clonidine hydrochloride, 0.1, 0.2, or 0.3 mg/chlorthalidone, 15 mg	Combipres
Prazosin hydrochloride, 1, 2, or 5 mg/polythiazide, 0.5 mg	Minizide

Modified from the Joint National Committee on Detection, Evaluation, and Treatment of High Blood Pressure, *Arch Intern Med* 157:2413, 1997.
*Approved for initial therapy.

pertension. They have shown less effect in preventing myocardial infarction. This is explained by the fact that high blood pressure is just one of the risk factors for coronary atherosclerosis. Furthermore, successful treatment of hypertension may, in part, have been counterbalanced by adverse effects on blood sugar and lipid levels. Table 31-5 shows the effect of the commonly recommended antihypertensive agents on total cholesterol, HDL cholesterol, LDL cholesterol, and triglycerides. The angiotensin II receptor antagonists, ACE inhibitors, calcium channel antagonists, and vasodilators are lipid-neutral. Diuretics can cause a rise in total and LDL cholesterol and in triglycerides, as well as aggravate insulin resistance. Beta-blockers without intrinsic sympathomimetic activity (ISA) tend to raise serum triglyceride levels and lower HDL cholesterol levels. Beta-blockers also provoke insulin resistance. These effects are less pronounced with cardioselective beta-blockers, such as metoprolol and atenolol, and are virtually nonexistent in beta-blockers having ISA, including pindolol and alprenolol. In contrast, peripheral alpha-blockers improve lipid profiles, lowering LDL cholesterol and triglyceride levels, and raise HDL cholesterol levels, possibly by as much as 25%.

Recommendation. When there is known coronary artery disease, dyslipidemia, glucose intolerance, or multiple other coronary risk factors, consider using ACE inhibitors, calcium channel antagonists, or peripheral alpha-blockers instead of diuretics or beta-blockers. If a diuretic is required, note that indapamide (Lozol) has minimal effect on lipids (see Table 31-5).

Left Ventricular Hypertrophy (LVH) and Heart Failure

LVH is associated with a number of detrimental effects on the myocardium, including prolongation of the QT

Table 31-5	*Lipid Effects of Antihypertensive Agents*

Drug	TC	HDL-C	TG	LDL-C
ACE inhibitors	NC to ↓	NC to ↑	NC to ↓	NC to ↓
Angiotensin II receptor blockers	NC	NC	NC	NC
Peripheral alpha-blockers	↓	↑	↓	NC to ↓
Beta-blockers				
Without ISA	NC to ↑	↓	↑	NC to ↑
With ISA	NC	NC to ↑	Variable	NC
Calcium channel antagonists	NC	NC to ↑	NC	NC
Central sympatholytic	NC to ↓	NC to ↑	NC to ↓	NC to ↓
Diuretics				
Thiazide	↑	↓	↑	↑
Loop	↑	↓	↑	↑
Indapamide	NC	NC to ↑	NC	NC
Vasodilators	NC	NC	NC	NC

TC, Total cholesterol; *TG,* triglyceride; *NC,* no change; *ISA,* intrinsic sympathomimetic activity.

interval, an increased proportion of collagen with resultant diastolic dysfunction, and abnormalities of perfusion of cardiac muscle.[15] In LVH secondary to essential hypertension, coronary perfusion is below that expected for the degree of hypertrophy. Clinical studies have supported the notion that cardiac hypertrophy is associated with a significant decrease in coronary flow reserve, a mechanism for angina and abnormal ECG changes in such patients during exercise. Others have documented LVH as a risk factor for cardiovascular mortality and morbidity, including congestive heart failure and sudden cardiac death. LVH in women is now considered to be a strong blood pressure–independent cardiovascular risk factor, and there is an increase in atrial fibrillation and sudden death. Concentric LVH may be disproportionate to the arterial pressure in obesity, suggesting a genetic basis for this problem. This occurs most often in women. Another factor contributing to LVH is sustained elevation of blood pressure through the night and the absence of the normal nocturnal fall of pressure. This may explain the higher incidence of LVH in hypertensive black patients, who often have persistent nocturnal hypertension.

Effective long-term antihypertensive therapy focused on regression of LVH is important. LVH regression necessitates effective arterial blood pressure lowering 24 hours a day. In patients who fail to regress, 24-hour ambulatory monitoring may help to determine whether arterial pressure is effectively controlled. In addition to controlling arterial pressure, weight loss facilitates regression of LVH.

Classes of antihypertensive medications that most rapidly induce the regression of LVH are ACE inhibitors, followed by calcium channel antagonists. ACE inhibitors may be so effective because angiotensin II is a growth factor promoting cardiac hypertrophy. Accordingly, the angiotensin II receptor blockers are probably also effective in facilitating the regression of LVH, but these newer agents are still being investigated.

ACE inhibitors also appear to be beneficial because they improve coronary endothelial cell function by bradykinin-mediated release of nitric oxide and decreased myocardial oxygen consumption by nitric oxide inhibition of mitochondrial respiration. Besides facilitating regression of LVH, calcium channel antagonists improve coronary blood flow. Several lines of evidence suggest that combining an ACE inhibitor with a calcium channel antagonist may have additive effects, not only for blood pressure reduction but also for regression of hypertrophy. Peripheral alpha-adrenergic blocking agents, central sympatholytic agents, thiazide diuretics, and even beta-adrenergic receptor blocking agents also promote the regression of LVH over time. Direct vasodilators, such as minoxidil and hydralazine, although effective in controlling blood pressure, do not induce the regression of LVH.

For patients with LVH, it is important to keep the potassium level at or above 4.0 mEq/L and magnesium level at or above 2.0 mEq/L to decrease the chance of ventricular arrhythmias. Recent evidence indicates that the aldosterone receptor blocker spironolactone effectively facilitates the regression of LVH. Thus if a diuretic is required, concomitant use of spironolactone is useful in conserving potassium and magnesium concentrations, as well as facilitating regression of LVH.

If a patient has a hyperadrenergic response to exercise, verapamil and diltiazem are appropriate choices for symptomatic relief, since these calcium channel antagonists attenuate both the heart rate and the blood pressure response to exercise, whereas beta-adrenergic receptor blocking agents may block only the heart rate response to exercise.

Ongoing studies may provide additional pharmacologic approaches to the treatment of patients with LVH. Because thyroxine stimulates hypertrophy of the left ventricular muscle, it appears that under-replacement therapy for hypothyroid patients facilitates regression of LVH. In postmenopausal women with normal epicardial coronary vessels and exertional angina, estrogen replacement appears to decrease the angina, perhaps by raising the patient's pain perception threshold or by improving coronary endothelial function.

With regard to patients with LVH and left ventricular systolic dysfunction, ACE inhibitors delay the development of congestive heart failure. In addition, antioxidant therapy with 400 IU of vitamin E daily may attenuate or prevent the lethal transition from LVH to congestive cardiomyopathy. These innovative approaches may prove to be adjunctive therapy in the treatment of patients with LVH.

Elderly Patients

Hypertension is common in patients over 65 years of age. Recently, it has become evident that an elevated pulse pressure, which indicates reduced vascular compliance in large vessels, may be an even better marker of increased cardiovascular risk than either systolic blood pressure or diastolic blood pressure. This is particularly relevant in older patients who frequently have an isolated elevation of systolic blood pressure. Essential hypertension is by far the most common form of hypertension in these patients, but, as mentioned previously, atherosclerotic renovascular hypertension should be considered if there is a sudden change in the patient's blood pressure level. If there is no target organ damage, clinicians should consider "white coat" hypertension or pseudohypertension resulting from increased vascular wall stiffness. Obtaining further readings outside of the office or a 24-hour ambulatory blood pressure monitor will help in the diagnosis of "white coat" hypertension. If systolic blood pressure by palpation is lower than systolic blood pressure by auscultation, pseudohypertension should be considered and *blood pressure managed according to the palpated blood pressure*. If a patient's blood pressure is much higher in one arm than the other, the higher blood pressure should be used in managing antihypertensive therapy.

Older patients are more likely than younger patients to exhibit an orthostatic fall in blood pressure; thus blood pressure should be measured with the patient in the standing as well as the seated or supine positions.

Hypertension in older patients is often volume sensitive. Modest salt reduction and weight loss may work without pharmacologic therapy. *Low-dose* diuretic therapy should be started because these agents have been effective in reducing mortality and morbidity in older patients with hypertension, especially isolated sys-

tolic hypertension. If diuretic therapy is not satisfactory, long-acting dihydropyridine calcium channel antagonists are considered appropriate alternatives in these patients. If these patients have associated angina, it should be noted that, of the dihydropyridines, only amlodipine and nifedipine have been approved for the treatment of angina. Of the nondihydropyridines, diltiazem and verapamil have been approved for the treatment of angina. Because of the effect on the conduction system and heart rate, nondihydropyridines should be used with caution. We have also noted the warning regarding concomitant drinking of grapefruit juice with felodipine, which results in increased levels of felodipine and a greater blood pressure–lowering effect than would be expected.

The goal of antihypertensive treatment in older patients should be the same as in younger patients with a target blood pressure less than 140/90, if at all possible. However, an intermediate goal of a systolic blood pressure below 160 mm Hg may be necessary for those with marked systolic hypertension. Any reduction in blood pressure appears to have benefit. Drugs that tend to exaggerate postural changes in blood pressure, such as peripheral alpha-blockers and high-dose diuretics, or drugs that can cause cognitive dysfunction, such as central sympatholytics, should be used with caution.

If an elderly patient is on diuretic therapy and has a poor diet, chronic diuretic therapy can result not only in potassium and magnesium depletion but also in *thiamine and zinc depletion*. Chronic thiamine depletion can result in a diuretic-induced beriberi heart disease with a decrease in contractility that is reversed on replacing the thiamine. Zinc depletion results in a metallic taste to the patient's food that may decrease a limited diet further; this can be corrected by replacement with zinc sulfate 220 mg daily over a few weeks.

Black Patients

Hypertension in black patients, particularly men, is more difficult to control and has a worse prognosis. Renovascular hypertension is less common in blacks. These patients are more sensitive to salt restriction and diuretics than whites. They are responsive to calcium channel antagonists and peripheral alpha-blockers. Beta-blockers and ACE inhibitors are less effective. Because of the severity of hypertension in this group of patients, multidrug therapy is frequently required. The absence of a nocturnal decline in blood pressure may explain why black patients have increased cardiovascular morbidity and mortality, including LVH and heart failure (which appears unrelated to the level of blood pressure). In addition, blacks with hypertension have more insulin resistance and non-insulin-dependent diabetes than whites. Weight loss may be particularly important in this racial group. Observational studies have

also suggested a greater increase in blood pressure response to alcohol in blacks than in whites.

Seven-year follow-up studies in patients in the MRFIT trial found that renal function worsened in blacks but actually improved in whites despite similar control of blood pressure in the two groups.[16] Even black patients with the best control of blood pressure (diastolic <95 mm Hg) had a rise in creatinine levels. It is possible that black patients require more aggressive control of blood pressure to prevent nephropathy. It has also been suggested that there is less renal bradykinin formation in black patients, and bradykinin may attenuate the effects of high blood pressure in other racial groups.

Latino Patients

Studies of Latinos indicate no increase in the incidence of hypertension despite an increase in the prevalence of obesity and non-insulin-dependent diabetes. Insulin resistance may be an especially important etiologic factor in this group of patients, and this should influence the choice of therapy. Accordingly, agents that aggravate hyperglycemia should be avoided.

Women

Young women are more commonly affected by fibromuscular dysplasia and renovascular hypertension. Oral contraceptives may raise blood pressure, although contraceptive-induced hypertension is less common owing to the reduction in hormone doses in current preparations. Studies of patients receiving combination estrogen and progesterone replacement after ovariectomy found that blood pressure actually fell. Thus long-term estrogen replacement has no adverse effect on arterial blood pressure. LVH may occur more readily in women in association with obesity, and LVH in women is now considered a blood pressure–independent cardiovascular risk factor. High blood pressure as the cause of heart failure is more common in women than in men, probably because men develop other illnesses (myocardial infarction) at a younger age, causing heart failure.

Pregnancy

Hypertension is more common in women with a past history of preeclampsia who are multiparous, obese, and have a family history of hypertension. The mechanism of hypertension in pregnancy is complex, but the effectiveness of aspirin in decreasing preeclampsia in some studies suggests an imbalance between the vasodilator, prostacycline, and the vasoconstrictor, thromboxane. Some studies have suggested that aspirin decreases the risk of preeclampsia, but others have not confirmed this, so this therapy is still under investigation. Since aspirin is a thromboxane inhibitor, it could be considered for high-risk patients. In low-risk populations, the risk of prophylactic aspirin therapy during pregnancy may exceed the benefits. Alpha methyldopa has been the most extensively used medication for treating hypertension during pregnancy and is recommended for those with a diastolic blood pressure over 100 mm Hg. Beta-blockers may retard fetal growth earlier in pregnancy but are considered safe during the later stages of pregnancy. Angiotensin II receptor blockers and ACE inhibitors may adversely affect the fetus and are contraindicated during pregnancy.

Diabetes

None of the antihypertensive classes are contraindicated in patients with diabetes. However, both beta-blockers and diuretics increase insulin resistance, and beta-blockers can mask signs of hypoglycemia. Peripheral alpha-blockers and ACE inhibitors tend to increase insulin sensitivity, while calcium channel antagonists do not influence glucose metabolism. Patients with diabetes often have exogenous obesity and dyslipidemia, so the choice of therapy should also be based on lipid profile. Weight loss and exercise can improve insulin sensitivity significantly. ACE inhibitors are also beneficial in attenuating the development of nephropathy in diabetic patients. Prospective studies with ACE inhibitors found that urinary albumin excretion decreased and glomerular filtration rate was maintained in even normotensive patients with diabetes and microalbuminuria. In patients with diabetes, hypertension is an additional risk factor for a patient developing chronic renal failure. ACE inhibition should be initial therapy in hypertensive diabetic patients. The benefit of using angiotensin II receptor antagonists in patients with diabetes and hypertension is under investigation.

Renal Insufficiency

Hypertension may be a complication of any form of chronic renal failure. Ruling out correctable factors, such as nephrolithiasis, renal artery stenosis, and hydronephrosis, is important. Calcium channel antagonists are safe in patients with renal dysfunction because glomerular perfusion pressure is maintained. However, with careful monitoring, any of the commonly used antihypertensive drug classes can be successfully used in patients with renal insufficiency. A target blood pressure of 130/85 mm Hg or less is recommended. In the advanced stages of renal failure, hypertension often is volume dependent and diuretics are critical. Once serum creatinine level exceeds 1.5 mg/dL, thiazides are less effective and loop diuretics are required.

As noted earlier, ACE inhibitors reduce proteinuria and retard the progression of diabetic nephropathy. However, when initiating ACE inhibitor therapy, renal function should be monitored carefully for a sudden decrease in glomerular perfusion pressure as a result of

---

BOX 31-2
CAUSES OF INADEQUATE RESPONSIVENESS TO ANTIHYPERTENSIVE THERAPY

PSEUDORESISTANCE
"White coat" hypertension
Pseudohypertension in older patients
Use of regular cuff on very obese arm

NONCOMPLIANCE TO THERAPY

VOLUME OVERLOAD
Excess salt intake
Progressive renal insufficiency (nephrosclerosis or silent occlusion of a renal artery)
Fluid retention from reduction of blood pressure
Fluid retention from vasodilator therapy
Inadequate diuretic therapy

DRUG-RELATED CAUSES
Doses too low or incorrect dosing schedule
Wrong type of diuretic
Drug actions and interactions
    Sympathomimetics
    Nasal decongestants
    Appetite suppressants
    Cocaine and other illicit drugs
    Caffeine
    Oral contraceptives
    Adrenal steroids
    Licorice (as may be found in chewing tobacco)
    Cyclosporine, tacrolimus
    Erythropoietin
    Antidepressants
    Nonsteroidal antiinflammatory drugs

ASSOCIATED CONDITIONS
Smoking
Increasing obesity
Sleep apnea
Insulin resistance/hyperinsulinemia
Ethanol intake of more than 1 oz (30 mL) per day
Anxiety-induced hyperventilation or panic attacks
Chronic pain
Intense vasoconstriction (arteritis)
Organic brain syndrome (e.g., memory deficit)

UNRECOGNIZED SECONDARY CAUSES OF HYPERTENSION

Modified from the Joint National Committee on Detection, Evaluation, and Treatment of High Blood Pressure, *Arch Intern Med* 157:2413, 1997

---

occult renal artery stenosis. We measure baseline serum creatinine levels before initiating ACE inhibitor therapy and then measure it again within the first week. If the serum creatinine level has increased more than 0.3 mg/dL, we consider either volume depletion or renal artery stenosis. ACE inhibitors may also precipitate hyperkalemia.

In advanced cases of renal failure the inability to excrete salt and water may lead to an acceleration of hypertension, rendering medical therapy ineffective and necessitating dialysis.

Patients with Bronchospastic Lung Disease or Chronic Airway Disease

Beta-blockers or combined alpha- and beta-blockers may exacerbate asthma. These agents should not be used in patients with asthma except under careful supervision. In addition, the topical ophthalmologic application of a beta-blocker, such as timolol maleate, used in the treatment of glaucoma, may exacerbate asthma. ACE inhibitors appear to be safe in most patients with asthma. If an ACE inhibitor–induced cough develops, angiotensin II receptor blockers are an alternative.

Patients with Gout

Hyperuricemia is a frequent finding in patients with untreated hypertension and may reflect a decrease in renal blood flow. Hyperuricemia may be a cardiovascular risk factor, particularly in women. All diuretics can increase serum uric acid levels, but rarely induce acute gout. In patients with gout, diuretics should be avoided if possible. Diuretic-induced hyperuricemia does not require treatment in the absence of gout or urate stones.

Quality of Life

In most large clinical trials, 20% to 40% of patients drop out because of side effects. It is important to distinguish between side effects from the drug and those from lower blood pressure. The newer antihypertensive drug classes, including ACE inhibitors, angiotensin II re-

ceptor blockers, calcium channel antagonists, and peripheral alpha-blockers, are better tolerated than diuretics and beta-blockers. This directly affects compliance.

Causes of Inadequate Responsiveness to Antihypertensive Therapy

About 60% of patients with moderate hypertension can be controlled with single-drug therapy. JNC-VI defines resistant hypertension as blood pressure that cannot be reduced below 140/90 mm Hg in patients who are adhering to an adequate and appropriate triple-drug regimen that includes a diuretic, with all drugs prescribed at near-maximal doses. For older patients with isolated systolic hypertension, resistance is defined as failure of an adequate triple-drug regimen to reduce systolic blood pressure to less than 160 mm Hg. Box 31-2 lists various causes of true resistance. The most common is volume overload due to inadequate diuretic therapy. Thiazide diuretics are more effective antihypertensive agents (because of their longer duration of action), but loop diuretics may be required if the patient's creatinine clearance is less than 50 mL/min or if the serum creatinine level is above 1.5 mg/dL. It should be emphasized that use of nonsteroidal antiinflammatory medications blocks intrarenal prostaglandin synthesis, causes renal vasoconstriction, and increases sodium retention. It is necessary to screen for their use because nonsteroidal, nonaspirin antiinflammatory medications can now be bought over the counter and patients often do not include them on their medication list. In evaluating a patient you believe has resistant hypertension, you should review again the possibility that the patient may have a secondary cause of hypertension and screen for common problems, such as excessive alcohol intake or sleep apnea. However, if the goal blood pressure cannot be achieved without intolerable adverse effects, even submaximal reduction of blood pressure contributes to decreased morbidity and mortality.

REFERENCES

1. JNC: The Sixth Report of the Joint National Committee on Detection, Evaluation, and Treatment of High Blood Pressure, *Arch Intern Med* 157:2413, 1997.
2. JNC: The Fifth Report of the Joint National Committee on Detection, Evaluation, and Treatment of High Blood Pressure, *Arch Intern Med* 153:143, 1993.
3. Julius S, Jamerson K, Mejia A, et al: The association of borderline hypertension with target organ changes and higher coronary risk: Tecumseh Blood Pressure study, *JAMA* 264:354, 1990.
4. Julius S, Krause L, Schork NJ, et al: Hyperkinetic borderline hypertension in Tecumseh, Michigan, *J Hypertens* 9:77, 1991.
5. Leitschuh M, Cupples LA, Kannel W, et al: High-normal blood pressure progression to hypertension in the Framingham Heart Study, *Hypertension* 17:22, 1991.
6. Skarfors ET, Lithell HO, Selinus I: Risk factors for the development of hypertension: a 10-year longitudinal study in middle-aged men, *J Hypertens* 9:217, 1991.
7. Widgren BR, Herlitz H, Hedner T, et al: Blunted renal sodium excretion during acute saline loading in normotensive men with positive family histories of hypertension, *Am J Hypertens* 4:570, 1991.
8. van Hooft IM, Grobbee DE, Derkx FH, et al: Renal hemodynamics and the renin-angiotensin-aldosterone system in normotensive subjects with hypertensive and normotensive parents, *N Engl J Med* 324:1305, 1991.
9. Poulter NR, Khaw KT, Hopwood BE, et al: The Kenyan Luo migration study: observations on the initiation of a rise in blood pressure, *Br Med J* 300:967, 1990.
10. Groppelli A, Giorgi DM, Omboni S, et al: Persistent blood pressure increase induced by heavy smoking, *J Hypertens* 10:495, 1992.
11. Harshfield GA, Hwang C, Grim CE, et al: Circadian variation of blood pressure in blacks: influence of age, gender, and activity, *J Hypertens* 4:43, 1990.
12. Katholi R, Lucore C: Cardiology of iodinated contrast. In *Iodinated contrast: past, present and future*, Philadelphia, Lippincott-Raven (in press).
13. Robertson D, Hollister AS, Biaggioni I, et al: The diagnosis and treatment of baroreflex failure, *N Engl J Med* 329:1449, 1993.
14. Davis BR, Cutler JA, Gordon DJ, et al: Rationale and design for the Antihypertensive and Lipid Lowering Treatment to Prevent Heart Attack Trial (ALLHAT). ALLHAT Research Group, *Am J Hypertens* 9:342, 1996.
15. Katholi RE, Ervin MR, Ginsburg G: Hypertensive heart disease syndrome in women in a cardiology practice, *Compr Ther* 23:508, 1997.
16. Neaton JD, Grimm RH Jr, Prineas RJ, et al: Treatment of Mild Hypertension Study. Final results. Treatment of Mild Hypertension Study Research Group, *JAMA* 270:713, 1993.

32 Diseases of the Aorta

Kimberly D. Rakes
George J. Taylor

Although many disease processes affect the aorta, all result from one of two general mechanisms: (1) weakness in the wall of the aorta (dissection, aneurysm, or rupture) or (2) obstruction of the aorta or its branches. They may be either congenital or acquired. In acquired disease, predisposing factors include aging, atherosclerosis, and hypertension and infectious, inflammatory, and autoimmune diseases.

ABDOMINAL AORTIC ANEURYSM
Epidemiology, Etiology, and Natural History

Three fourths of aortic aneurysms are confined to the abdomen, and all result from atherosclerotic vascular disease. Usually fusiform in shape, almost all originate below the renal arteries and extend to the aortic bifurcation or iliac arteries; the visceral circulation is usually spared.[1,2] Untreated, the chance of death is about 1 in 3. About half of those aneurysms with a diameter greater than 6 cm rupture within the year, compared with 15% to 20% when the aneurysm is 5 to 6 cm. Chance of rupture of aneurysms <4 cm is less than a 2%.

Aneurysms are rarely static, with 80% expanding over time. For this reason, time is another risk factor for rupture. Aneurysm in most patients gradually expand, but 20% expand rapidly (greater than 0.5 cm within a year).

Risk factors for developing abdominal aneurysm include advanced age (over 55 years for men, 70 years for women), male sex (the disease is five times as common in men), and a positive family history.[1] Cigarette smoking is the largest contributor to risk. It is estimated that 3% of people older than 50 years in the United States have abdominal aneurysms.

Pathophysiology

Aneurysms develop in areas of atherosclerosis. The aortic wall is eroded, and the elastic elements are destroyed, eventually leading to dilation of the aorta and aneurysm formation. Expansion is influenced by Laplace's law (see Table 2-5):

Wall tension = Intraluminal pressure ×
Radius of the aneurysm

As the aneurysm enlarges, wall tension increases, which promotes further expansion and increases the chance of rupture. High luminal pressure (hypertension) aggravates this situation.

The common location of abdominal aneurysm may result from the absence of vasa vasorum in the infrarenal aorta. Oxygen and nutrients must diffuse from the lumen to the inner part of the media. Atherosclerosis thickens this portion of the vessel wall, increasing the distance that the nutrient supply must traverse. Anything that increases wall tension further compromises diffusion.

Clinical Presentation

Most abdominal aneurysms are asymptomatic. They are typically detected on routine physical examination or abdominal x-ray. When symptoms develop, the pain is usually described as steady or gnawing and is located in the midabdominal, lumbar, or pelvic area. The pain is not affected by movement, is typically constant, and becomes more severe with a boring quality as the aneurysm expands. Unless the patient is obese, you can usually palpate a periumbilical abdominal mass that is pulsatile. If rapidly expanding, the aneurysm may be tender to palpation. There may or may not be bruits or diminished femoral pulses.

More than half of those patients with rupture die before reaching the hospital. Survivors appear critically ill and may have hemorrhagic shock. Most frequently, rupture occurs into the retroperitoneal space and is locally confined. There may be a hematoma in the flank area or a second area of rupture. Some bleed into the peritoneal space. Additionally, the rupture may occur into adjacent structures, presenting as a gastrointestinal hemorrhage or an arteriovenous fistula.

Diagnostic Studies

Although an abdominal x-ray may be helpful (and inexpensive), if eggshell calcification of the aorta is seen, at least one fourth of abdominal aneurysms are not seen on radiographs. Ultrasound (cross sectional) is currently the simplest way to detect and measure aneurysms and is the screening technique of choice. Computed tomographic (CT) scans have proven to be as sensitive as ultrasound and frequently give more definition; however, CT has some disadvantages (Table 32-1). Both ultrasound and CT are particularly useful

| Table 32-1 | *Diagnostic Procedures for Abdominal Aortic Aneurysm* |

	Ultrasound	CT	MRI	Angiography
Availability, convenience	+++	+	±	±
Inexpensive	+++	+	+	+
Safe (noninvasive)	+++	+	+	−
Sensitivity	++	++	++	+
Specificity	++	++	++	+

when following an abdominal aneurysm over time. Angiography may be helpful but is frequently misleading if a clot is present within the aneurysm. Remember that the angiogram paints only the lumen of the vessel (it is a "lumenogram"). The lumen may look normal despite the presence of a large aneurysm if there is a thick clot layered on the wall of the aneurysm. Magnetic resonance imaging (MRI) is also used and correlates closely with CT and ultrasound. It often is more difficult to obtain because of limited access to equipment. The increased length of testing adds to patient discomfort.

Management

Medical Therapy

Medical management consists of decreasing risk factors, including controlling hypertension and effectively treating hypercholesterolemia.

Surgical Therapy

Surgical repair is recommended for asymptomatic patients who have abdominal aneurysms with a diameter greater than 5 or 6 cm. A patient who is an excellent surgical candidate may have surgery for a 5 cm aneurysm. On the other hand, a patient with multiple medical problems who is considered a poor surgical risk may have surgery delayed until the aneurysm approaches 6 cm.

Surgery is also indicated if the aneurysm is actively expanding. Most would recommend surgery for an aneurysm that enlarges to more than 5 cm while it is being observed. Patients with symptoms require urgent repair, and rupture and acute expansion are true surgical emergencies.

The procedure consists of resecting the aneurysm and replacing it with a Dacron graft. In low-risk patients the

surgical mortality is less than 5%. Expanding aneurysms carry a surgical mortality between 5% and 15%, while surgery in a setting of acute rupture has a mortality risk closer to 50%.

The risk of elective surgery is higher in patients with coronary artery disease (CAD), so preoperative screening for CAD is indicated (see Chapter 48).

Follow-Up and Expected Clinical Course

The current recommendation for repeat imaging of a stable, small aneurysm is every 6 months.[3] If there is a higher risk, particularly if the aneurysm is expanding or is quite large, repeat imaging at 3-month intervals is sensible.

Patients who have had surgical repair of an abdominal aneurysm have a 5- to 10-year survival rate that parallels that of an age-matched population. Without surgical intervention for an aneurysm larger than 6 cm, the 5-year survival rate is only 5% to 10%, compared to 50% for those with aneurysms less than 6 cm.[4]

THORACIC AORTIC ANEURYSM

Epidemiology, Etiology, and Natural History

Approximately one fourth of aortic aneurysms are thoracic. These are either fusiform or saccular in shape and atherosclerotic in origin but also may result from infectious or inflammatory processes. Although aneurysms can occur anywhere along the thoracic aorta, the more common locations are the arch and descending portions, with frequent extension into the abdomen. The exception is syphilitic aortitis with aneurysm, which usually is saccular and located in the ascending aorta.

Survival is related to the size of the aneurysm. Aneurysms with a diameter greater than 7 cm are more prone to rupture.[5] Since expanding thoracic aneurysms tend to cause symptoms related to compression, asymptomatic rupture is less common. Studies have shown the 5-year survival of symptomatic thoracic aneurysms to be 25% to 30%, compared with greater than 50% if the patient is asymptomatic.[5] Since the illness is frequently associated with diffuse atherosclerosis, it is not surprising that only one third of the deaths are attributable to actual rupture, whereas over half are caused by other complications of atherosclerosis.

Pathophysiology

The pathogenesis of thoracic aneurysms is identical to that of abdominal aneurysms, that is, arteriosclerosis leading to weakening of the aortic wall, medial degeneration, and ultimately localized dilation. Once again, hypertension appears to play a major role. It is more common for cystic medial necrosis to cause a thoracic rather than abdominal aneurysm. In young patients thoracic aneurysm is usually caused by Marfan's or

Ehlers-Danlos syndromes (see Chapters 37 and 45). In these cases the aneurysm originates at the level of the aortic valve and involves the sinuses of Valsalva ("annuloaortic ectasia"), and the ascending aorta nearer the arch may look normal. With atherosclerosis the aneurysm usually spares the sinuses of Valsalva and is located in the distal portion of the ascending aorta and the arch.

Clinical Presentation

Since most thoracic aneurysms are also asymptomatic, they are frequently detected on chest x-ray or are suspected in a patient with aortic regurgitation. In symptomatic patients the most common complaint is chest pain, which is usually described as deep and aching or throbbing. Pain, which often radiates to the back, results from compression or erosion of adjacent musculoskeletal structures. Be aware that the onset of excruciating pain may signal acute expansion and threatened rupture or dissection. Aneurysms in the arch and proximal descending aorta may present with symptoms of compression of surrounding structures (Table 32-2). Rupture may present as exsanguination, hemoptysis, hemopericardium, or pericardial tamponade, depending on the rupture's location. Most commonly the aneurysm ruptures into the left intrapleural space or the pericardium. Less common sites of rupture are into the esophagus or right ventricle.

With most aneurysms the physical examination is normal. An occasional patient with a dilated aortic root has aortic valve regurgitation (AR). A useful physical sign that the AR is caused by a dilated root is an audible murmur to the right of the sternum (soft AR murmurs caused by valvular disease are usually heard only to the left of the sternum).

Diagnostic Studies

The chest x-ray may be used for screening, but it may not reveal a small, saccular thoracic aneurysm. Echocardiography, particularly transesophageal echocardiography (TEE), is especially good at visualizing the aortic root. TEE is widely used for the detection of aortic dissection. Aortography may help make the diagnosis and outline the anatomy of the aneurysm and should be performed on all patients considered for elective surgical repair. CT scanning and MRI have similar profiles for both thoracic and abdominal aneurysms (see Table 32-1).

Management
Medical Therapy

Two principles of medical therapy are followed for acute situations (i.e., rapid expansion or dissection). The first is to reduce blood pressure using parenteral therapy, commonly with nitroprusside. The second is to reduce the velocity of ventricular ejection with beta-blockers.

Table 32-2 *Symptoms Caused by Aortic Arch Aneurysms*

Compressed Structure	Symptom(s)
Recurrent laryngeal nerve	Hoarseness (vocal cord paralysis)
Trachea or mainstem bronchus	Airway obstruction, wheezing, cough, dyspnea, recurrent pneumonia, loss of lung volume
Esophagus	Dysphagia
Vena cava	Superior vena cava syndrome (edema of the head and neck)

Chronic beta blockade is recommended for patients with Marfan's syndrome and aortic dilation.

Surgical Therapy

Surgical excision currently is the treatment of choice for aneurysms of the ascending aorta that are 6 cm or larger. If the operative risk is high because of coexisting illness, surgery is often delayed until the aneurysm is 7 cm. Surgery is the treatment of choice for smaller aneurysms that produce symptoms, the urgency depending on the patient's condition. The survival rate for elective resection of thoracic aneurysms is currently reported as 90% to 94%.[5]

The most frequent perioperative complications are those related to the associated arteriosclerosis, including myocardial infarction, stroke, and renal failure. In addition, inadvertent interruption of blood flow to the spinal cord during surgery can cause spinal cord injury, with paralysis complicating 5% of operations.

Follow-up and Expected Clinical Course

The rate of expansion is between 4 and 5.5 mm/year. Current recommendations are to reimage thoracic aneurysms annually until they reach 5 cm. At that time the expansion rate increases fourfold, and biannual follow-up imaging is recommended.

THORACIC AORTIC DISSECTION
Epidemiology, Etiology, and Natural History

At least 2000 new cases of acute aortic dissection are reported annually, and an estimated 600 to 700 are never diagnosed. The true incidence is not known but is related to the prevalence of the risk factors for dissection,

which include untreated or poorly controlled hypertension, increased age, and disease of the aortic wall. Degeneration of the aortic media (loss of collagen and elastic tissue) occurs as a result of chronic stress, such as longstanding hypertension. There may be underlying defects in the connective tissue, as in Marfan's and Ehlers-Danlos syndromes, that predispose to dissection, particularly proximally.

Dissection consists of a longitudinal tear in the media by a dissecting hematoma. It is usually not circumferential but may involve the entire length of the aorta. The ascending portion is involved in about two thirds of all dissections, with the entry tear occurring just above the aortic valve. Isolated dissections of the descending aorta are less common, occurring in about one fourth of all cases. The DeBakey classification is used to describe the location and extent of dissection (Fig. 32-1). About half of all proximal dissections involve the aortic valve, causing AR.

External rupture is the most common cause of death. Proximal rupture can cause pericardial tamponade or hemothorax, usually on the left. Branch vessel obstruction is seen in about half of all proximal dissections and can be catastrophic, particularly if the brain or coronary circulations are compromised. Involvement of the iliac arteries is common but is not life-threatening.

Clinical Presentation

Aortic dissection is seen most frequently in men (at a ratio of 2:1) in the fifth to seventh decades of life. The most common presenting symptom is severe pain. The pain is severe at its onset and does not have a crescendo quality. Tearing, ripping, and stabbing qualities are frequently described, and some patients find the pain to be unbearable. The location may be anterior if the dissection is proximal and is intrascapular if it is distal. In addition, there may be vasovagal manifestations, such as vomiting, diaphoresis, and faintness. These manifestations are sometimes difficult to differentiate from those of myocardial infarction, pancreatitis, cholecystitis, perforated peptic ulcer, or severe back strain. If the femoral or subclavian arteries are occluded, aortic dissection may appear clinically identical to embolization.

Physical examination may reveal altered or asymmetrical pulses or a murmur of AR; these are most commonly seen with proximal dissections. Hypertension is common with distal dissections and may be severe, with diastolic pressures greater than 160 mm Hg. Conversely, hypotension is seen in about 20% of patients with proximal disease and usually indicates aortic rupture or tamponade.

Diagnostic Studies

On chest x-ray the aortic shadow is abnormal in 80% to 90% of patients, making it fairly sensitive but not specific. A finding that is more specific, but less common, is a progressively widening aorta with a "double-lumen" effect—intimal calcification greater than 6 mm inside the aortic margin.

The current recommendation is to start the evaluation with a transthoracic echocardiogram; if a dissection is still suspected and the patient is unstable, an emergency transesophageal echocardiogram should be obtained. TEE has been reported to have a sensitivity of up to 99% and a specificity as high as 98% in detecting descending dissection. If the patient's condition is stable, CT imaging with contrast medium or MRI would be the next step, depending on availability, since they are less invasive. Although angiography is a useful diagnostic tool, it is usually reserved for stable patients who have suspected compromise of an aortic branch.

High-resolution techniques (including echocardiography, CT, and MRI) are now able to detect intramural hematoma, which indicates rupture of the vasa vasorum, within a few hours of the onset of pain. This is frequently a precursor to the actual dissection.

Management

Management consists primarily of stopping the progression of the dissection. Emergency observation of blood

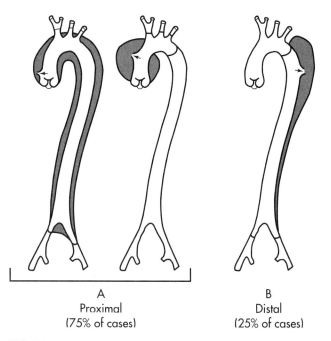

A
Proximal
(75% of cases)

B
Distal
(25% of cases)

FIG. 32-1
The standard classification of aortic dissection. The original, proposed by DeBakey, suggested three classes: I, dissection beginning proximally and going to the distal aorta; II, dissection limited to the proximal aorta; and III, dissection beginning distal to the left subclavian artery. Because all proximal dissections are treated surgically, the more current classification system combines types I and II lesions as class A. Distal dissection, which may be treated medically, is class B.

pressure, cardiac rhythm, central venous pressure, and urine output is critical. The goals of medical therapy at this point are control of systolic blood pressure, reduction of the velocity of left ventricular ejection, and pain control. Ideally the systolic pressure should be between 100 and 120 mm Hg, but should be dropped only to the level that the vital organs can tolerate. This is usually accomplished by using two drugs, nitroprusside and beta-blockers. Nitroprusside is used as a vasodilator but must be monitored very closely after 48 hours of use, since it can cause cyanide toxicity. Simultaneous use of a beta-blocker is necessary to counter the increase in ventricular ejection velocity caused by nitroprusside. Hydralazine, minoxidil, and diazoxide are all contraindicated at this point because they produce reflex inotropic stimulation.

Indications for emergency surgery are severe AR, threatened rupture, and an occluded branch artery. In addition, surgery improves survival with proximal dissection after the patient is hemodynamically stable. Surgery is no better than medical management for treating stable distal dissection. With type B, distal dissection, a patient who has survived the acute phase and has no indication for emergency surgery has a 1-year survival rate with both medical and surgical therapy that is approximately 90%. Surgery may be contraindicated with advanced age, severe comorbid diseases, and severe neurologic damage.

Follow-Up and Clinical Course

Residual aortic disease requires surgery within 10 years in 20% to 30% of the patients who survive aortic dissection, with or without initial surgical therapy. These patients should be followed by serial CT or MRI every 3 months for 1 year, depending on the size of the aorta and the rate of expansion.

AORTITIS

The three main types of aortitis are syphilitic, infectious, and inflammatory. Syphilitic aortitis involves the proximal aorta and is usually the result of occlusion of the vasa vasorum (endarteritis obliterans). The primary complications are aneurysm, aortic regurgitation, and coronary ostial stenosis. The aneurysm usually involves the sinuses of Valsalva. Symptoms are caused by pressure on adjacent structures, but rupture occasionally occurs. AR may range from mild to severe. Coronary stenosis is suspected when angina is out of proportion to the aortic regurgitation. Treatment includes antibiotics for persistent infection, usual therapy for congestive heart failure (if present), possible valve replacement for severe AR, aneurysm repair if indicated, or even coronary artery bypass grafting for coronary ostial stenosis.

Bacterial infectious aortitis usually results from either hematogenous spread or infection in contiguous tissue.

If it is caused by hematogenous spread, it usually results from endocarditis but can result from septicemia alone. The infection usually affects the aorta at a site that had been previously damaged. Tuberculosis in an adjacent node may cause caseous necrosis of the aortic wall. Treatment is decided on the basis of the underlying infection.

Takayasu's disease ("pulseless disease") is the classic example of noninfectious or inflammatory aortitis. It may present as stenosis or obstruction of the aorta and its branches, dilation or aneurysm, or aortic regurgitation. It is an autoimmune phenomenon with an unknown cause. Women 20 to 30 years of age are most commonly affected. Treatment consists of steroid administration in the active phase, possibly anticoagulation, and occasionally surgery for symptoms of arterial obstruction. Other causes of inflammatory aortitis are giant cell arteritis in older adults and aortitis associated with ankylosing spondylitis or Reiter's syndrome.

OCCLUSIVE DISEASE OF THE AORTA
Chronic Occlusive Disease

Chronic occlusive disease is usually atherosclerotic in origin but can result from an inflammatory, neoplastic, or infectious process. Vascular bifurcations are the areas most frequently involved, especially the proximal left subclavian artery. Chronic disease often has no symptoms because of collateral circulation that has developed over time. One exception to this, however, is the subclavian steal syndrome, which may cause cerebral ischemia with increased use of the upper extremities (see Chapter 34).

Other clinical syndromes include abdominal angina or renovascular hypertension. With aortoiliac disease the patient may have Leriche's syndrome, with impotence and diminished femoral pulses. Surgery is sometimes helpful if the distal vessels are patent. Angioplasty is only a temporizing measure.

Acute Occlusive Disease of the Aorta

Acute occlusion can be embolic, which is usually from the heart, or thrombotic, which is seen if preexisting atherosclerosis is accompanied by shock or severe heart failure. The presenting symptoms are limb ischemia or acute renal failure. Since collateral circulation has not had time to develop, immediate surgery is necessary, as is treatment of underlying causes. Embolectomy may fail, because smaller, distal emboli frequently are present.

AORTIC TRAUMA

The most common cause of aortic trauma is sudden high-speed deceleration from a motor vehicle accident. This creates shearing forces that are greatest at areas where mobile and fixed portions of the aorta meet, the

most common site being the aortic isthmus where the ligamentum arteriosum inserts. Another cause of rupture from trauma occurs with blast or crush injuries, which cause an acute increase in intraaortic pressure. The diagnosis is often hidden by the other serious injuries that almost always occur in these patients. A few symptoms arise from the rupture itself, but symptoms caused by localized hematoma, including dyspnea, stridor, dysphagia, or superior vena cava syndrome, may be present (see Table 32-2). An interscapular systolic bruit may be detected during physical examination, with no other findings except evidence of trauma.

The chest x-ray is abnormal in greater than 90% of patients with traumatic aortic rupture, with opacification between the aortic and pulmonary arteries and mediastinal widening being the most sensitive findings. A contrast CT scan should be obtained as soon as possible to confirm the diagnosis. If the situation is still unclear after CT, angiography should be performed. Eighty percent of victims die instantly; 70% of those who make it to the hospital survive after surgical intervention, which is the only treatment.

With penetrating injuries such as those caused by a bullet or knife, massive hemorrhage may rapidly ensue. If the aorta is penetrated within the pericardial sac, the patient may have cardiac tamponade. Immediate surgical repair is usually necessary, often with only a chest x-ray done beforehand, as the patient is hemodynamically unstable or becomes so very quickly.

REFERENCES

1. Davies MJ: Aortic aneurysm formation; lessons from human studies and experimental models, *Circulation* 98:193, 1998.
2. Van der Vliet JA, Boll APM: Abdominal aortic aneurysm, *Lancet* 349:863, 1997.
3. Brown PM, Pattenden R, Vernooy C, et al: Selective management of abdominal aortic aneurysms in a prospective measurement program, *J Vasc Surg* 23:213, 1996.
4. Coselli JS, de Figueiredo LFP: Natural history of descending and thoracoabdominal aortic aneurysms, *J Card Surg* 12:285, 1997.
5. Pitt MPI, Bonser RS: The natural history of thoracic aortic aneurysm disease: an overview, *J Card Surg* 12:270, 1997.

33 Peripheral Arterial Disease

Joseph R. Hartmann
Howard Roth

EPIDEMIOLOGY

Unlike other ischemic syndromes—coronary, carotid, or renal—patients with disabling claudication often are told to live with it. This recommendation must be tempered by the recognition that the 5-year mortality of patients with symptomatic peripheral arterial disease (PAD) is 30%.

PAD affects 12% to 14% of the general population; 3% to 7% have intermittent claudication.[1,2] In men over 40 years old, claudication develops at an annual rate of 8.6/1000 patients.[3] (Fig. 33-1) Approximately 25% to 33% of patients with claudication have deterioration of their symptoms after initial diagnosis; 1% to 5% eventually require amputation.[2] The prevalence of coronary artery disease (CAD) in patients with PAD ranges from 37% to 78% and accounts for the major morbidity and mortality associated with this disease (Fig. 33-1).

Criqui et al.[4] showed that the risk of dying within 10 years among subjects with large-vessel PAD increases sixfold even in the absence of symptoms. Cardiovascular mortality increases 15-fold in patients with severe, symptomatic PAD.

Unfortunately, claudication is frequently an excuse to avoid screening for CAD because of the patient's inability to walk on a treadmill. An inability to exercise contributes to the progression of CAD. There may be no warning of CAD because inactivity keeps patients from having angina. As a result, the initial symptom may be myocardial infarction or sudden death. This accounts for the increased mortality with PAD as compared with other forms of atherosclerotic disease.

In 1990 the National Hospital Discharge Survey documented that 50,000 to 60,000 peripheral angioplasties and 110,000 bypass operations were performed.[5,6] During the same year 100,000 amputations were reported. This is an amputation/revascularization ratio of 38%. With claudication reported in about 1.8% of patients under 60 years old, 3.7% of those 60 to 70 years of age, and 5.2% of patients over age 70, we suggest the following:

1. Too few patients with PAD are admitted to the hospital each year.
2. Too few have an angiogram or revascularization.
3. With an amputation/revascularization ratio of 38%, the medical community is not serving patients well with the current, conservative approach to this disease.
4. With a 5-year mortality of 30% (mostly due to CAD) in patients with lower limb ischemia, a more general evaluation for vascular disease is justified.

RISK FACTORS

Peripheral arterial disease shares the same risk factors as other atherosclerotic diseases (see Chapters 11 and 12).

Lipids

As with CAD, the presence of low-density lipoprotein (LDL) cholesterol increases the risk of developing PAD. The contribution of low high-density lipoprotein (HDL) and high triglyceride levels to PAD may be somewhat greater than with CAD.[9-12] Nevertheless, the goal of therapy with established PAD is the reduction of LDL levels to less than 100 mg/dL and the cholesterol:HDL ratio to less than 4:5, since this has been shown to block progression of disease.

Smoking

Smoking causes vasoconstriction of small arteries and arterioles, in addition to its atherogenic actions (see Chapter 11). Cessation of smoking may not immediately improve symptoms, but it lowers mortality, helps prevent the progression of disease, and reduces the need for amputation.[13] Review the (nonrandomized) data in Table 33-1 with your patient. The effect of continued smoking should impress any reasonable person.

Hypertension

Patients with hypertension have twice the incidence of PAD as coronary disease.[14] There is no evidence that medical therapy for hypertension changes the course of PAD. Beta-blockers have been known to aggravate symptoms of intermittent claudication, possibly because of vasospasm. The mechanism is uncertain but is probably related to loss of the vasodilating action of beta-adrenergic stimulation and leaving the vasoconstrictor alpha influence unopposed.[15] Beta-blockers should not be used as primary treatment for hypertension when there is PAD but should be reserved for

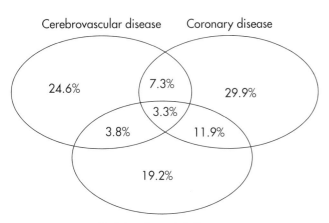

FIG. 33-1
The distribution of symptomatic atherosclerosis.

Table 33-1	*Effects of Smoking Cessation on Morbidity and Mortality in Patients with Peripheral Artery Disease (5-year follow-up)[13]*

	Continued Smoking (%)	Stopped Smoking (%)
Worsening claudication	60	44
Amputation	11	0
Mortality	27	12

patients with aortic aneurysms, coronary disease, or both.

Diabetes

Diabetes mellitus occurs in up to 30% of patients with intermittent claudication. Diabetes has a significant affect on morbidity and mortality. The amputation rate over 5 years is four times higher with diabetes.[15] There is no evidence that improved control of diabetes alters the progression of the disease. Diabetic foot care, on the other hand, is crucial in avoiding amputation. Diabetic patients should be educated about avoidance of injury and infections in the feet. Foot care should be managed by a professional with knowledge and experience with PAD. The occurrence of infection in the feet should be treated aggressively, including attempts to improve blood supply by interventional means when indicated.

EVALUATION OF PATIENTS WITH CLAUDICATION

Symptoms

Claudication is a reproducible discomfort in the calves, thighs, or buttocks. It may be described as pain, tightness, ache, or fatigue brought on by a particular exercise, usually walking a well-defined distance. Increasing the speed or adding elevation shortens the distance that provokes symptoms.

A detailed history is essential in separating true claudication from pseudoclaudication, which is not reproducible and may occur while walking or standing. Pseudoclaudication is relieved by sitting or lying down, which is not the case with true claudication.

Pain at rest occurs with critical ischemia and may be confused with neuropathy. Patients with resting ischemia frequently obtain relief by hanging their feet over the bed, particularly at night. Relief with the feet in a dependent position is a key feature of PAD.

Physical Examination

Examination usually confirms the diagnosis of PAD. Radial, ulnar, brachial, carotid, aortic, femoral, popliteal, dorsalis pedis, and posterior tibial pulses should be palpated in every patient. Auscultation of carotid, aortic, and femoral arteries for bruits is an important part of the examination. If foot pulses are normal (easily palpated and not delayed) in an asymptomatic person, it is unlikely that the ankle-brachial index (ABI) will be depressed. Suggestive symptoms indicate a need for noninvasive testing, even when pulses are present. Secondary signs of pallor, dependent rubor, delayed capillary and venous fill time, and loss of hair are all important clues to the presence of vascular disease and should not be overlooked. The high mortality of patients with even asymptomatic large-vessel PAD is an indication to look for these findings in all of our patients.

Noninvasive Testing

Noninvasive vascular testing is used to identify PAD and to determine its location and severity. It can also be used to differentiate PAD from pseudoclaudication. Finally, noninvasive testing is used to follow patients after surgical or percutaneous revascularization.

Ankle-Brachial Pressure Index

The resting ankle-brachial pressure index (ABI) is the most common noninvasive test. Brachial blood pressure and ankle pressure are measured using a Doppler device to sensitively identify systolic pressure as the arm or calf blood pressure cuff is slowly deflated. ABI is the ratio of the arm and ankle systolic pressures. Its measurement is easy and inexpensive, and some believe it should be performed for all patients in whom cardiovascular disease is suspected as a part of screening for

atherosclerosis. For example, the ABI has been shown to be an independent predictor of CAD and carotid artery disease. It also provides prognostic information. The relative risk for total deaths with an ABI of less than 0.9 is almost four times normal[17] (Table 33-2).

Patients with an ABI greater than 0.9 probably do not have obstructive PAD. Important exceptions to this are patients with heavily calcified arterial walls, including those with diabetes, renal failure, and idiopathic Mönckeberg's medial sclerosis. In these cases palpable foot pulses might also be misleading.

Doppler Examination

As simple and informative as resting ABI is, the information it can provide is limited. For example, it cannot localize the stenotic lesion or indicate the extent of disease. The peripheral vascular arterial Doppler (PVAD) examination is performed in conjunction with segmental pressures. This test can identify the location and severity of stenosis by detecting changes in blood flow velocity. It is frequently used to follow patients after interventional procedures.

Pulse Volume Recording

The pulse volume recording (PVR) test uses changes in the volume of blood between systole and diastole to detect obstruction at a given level of the lower extremity. It is more qualitative than PVAD and more subject to interpretive errors. In addition, obesity, edema, and muscular tremors can reduce its accuracy.

Exercise Doppler Testing

Some patients with symptoms of claudication have a normal resting ABI and equivocal PVAD. Stress testing allows confirmation of the diagnosis. The patient walks on a treadmill until symptoms prevent further exercise. The ABI is measured before and immediately after exercise. If the results are abnormal, the pressure is measured repeatedly until recovery occurs. If symptoms are caused by arterial disease, foot pressure drops and recovery is delayed. Normally, foot pressures rise with exercise. This useful test may uncover iliac disease but is limited by poor exercise tolerance. (Unlike the evaluation of CAD, there is no way to do a pharmacologic stress test of the lower extremity.)

Duplex Ultrasonography

Duplex ultrasonography images the atherosclerotic plaque. This sounds useful, but the technique has little role in screening for PAD. It is more expensive and time intensive than the other tests discussed. It provides anatomic information but little physiologic data. Duplex imaging is most useful when following patients after either surgical or endovascular intervention. In par-

	Table 33-2	Ankle-Brachial Index (ABI) As a Risk Factor for Cardiovascular Mortality (16-month follow-up)[17]

	ABI <0.9	ABI ≥0.9	Relative Risk*
Total deaths	6.9%	1.7%	3.8
CHD deaths	3.3%	0.9%	3.2
CVD deaths	4.6%	1.2%	3.7

Adapted from Newman AB, Sutton-Tyrell K, Vogt MT, Kuller LH: *JAMA* 270:487, 1993.
*A relative risk of 3.8 means that the risk is 3.8 times higher with the lower ABI.
CHD, Coronary heart disease; *CVD*, cardiovascular disease (including stroke, myocardial infarction, and other complications of CVD).

ticular, it is good for screening femoral-popliteal bypass grafts for new plaque.

Transcutaneous Oxygen Tension

In patients with gangrene or nonhealing ulcerations caused by vascular compromise, transcutaneous oxygen measurements ($TcPO_2$) can help predict healing both before and after vascular intervention. These patients typically have multisegmental lesions and extensive calcification, making other tests less reliable. $TcPO_2$ measurements may help determine whether revascularization should be done. In general, a $TcPO_2$ of 30 mm Hg or greater indicates a fair chance of an ulcer healing without revascularization.

Newer Technologies

Newer imaging techniques may someday replace or at least supplement angiography. These include CT angiography and MR angiography. Their advantages include three-dimensional reconstruction and rapid, noninvasive data acquisition. They have already proven beneficial in preoperative planning of surgical or endovascular aortic aneurysm repair. Neither is widely available, and they are not considered routine. They are expensive and thus may not be useful as screening tools.

Angiography As a Screening Tool ("While in the Neighborhood")

With the advent of digital catheterization laboratories, combined coronary, renal, and peripheral angiography can be performed in less than 30 minutes with less than 150 ml of contrast medium. Angiography of an additional vascular bed adds little to the risk of a procedure.

We do not hesitate to study the coronary arteries of patients having peripheral angiography, and we routinely study the renal or peripheral arteries in patients with difficult to control hypertension or intermittent claudication who are having coronary angiography. We believe that this "while-in-the-neighborhood" approach is safer for the patient than missing disease. It is also more cost effective than additional noninvasive studies, possibly followed by another angiogram. It is especially useful for avoiding multiple arterial procedures in a patient with PAD and difficult arterial access.

Angiography

Patients with a positive screening study for PAD should have angiography when they cannot do aerobic exercise because of their vascular disease. As a rough guide, a person unable to walk for 30 minutes at a pace brisk enough to produce mild breathlessness warrants an angiogram. Patients often wish to try medical therapy, and this is no situation for arm-twisting. However, it is our experience that the best medical therapy infrequently leads to normal exercise tolerance (an ability to walk briskly for 30 minutes).

Screening Patients for Vascular Surgery

Physicians are frequently asked to clear their patients with PAD for vascular surgery. Both the American Heart Association and the American College of Physicians practice guidelines identify vascular procedures as high risk and an indication for screening for CAD (see Chapter 48). Stress testing and perfusion imaging have been identified as suitable studies (see Chapter 48).

Another valid approach is coronary angiography at the time of peripheral angiography. The Cleveland Clinic studied 1000 patients admitted for elective peripheral vascular operations from 1978 to 1982 with coronary angiography before the vascular procedure.[18] In a subgroup of 381 patients with claudication and no cardiac history, CAD was found in 28%. The 5-year survival of patients in this group who were subsequently treated with bypass surgery was 72%, compared with 43% in those who did not have coronary revascularization (this was not a randomized clinical trial).

MEDICAL THERAPY FOR PERIPHERAL ARTERY DISEASE

PAD is a strong marker for future arterial thrombotic events, including myocardial infarction and cerebral vascular accidents. Detecting disease should be one goal of the physical examination in every adult patient. Once identified, aggressive modification of risk factors and appropriate treatment can significantly reduce morbidity and mortality (see Chapters 11 and 12).

Antiplatelet Agents

Platelet activation plays a pivotal role in acute thrombotic events complicating atherosclerosis, contributing to stroke, myocardial infarction, and vascular death.[20]

No randomized trials have compared aspirin to placebo in patients with PAD. One trial of 90 patients compared pentoxifylline (Trental, 400 mg tid) with aspirin (325 mg daily). No difference was reported at 6 weeks in ABI, pain, or activity. Absolute walking distance was improved in patients receiving pentoxifylline (2 miles versus 1.2 miles, p <0.05).[21] Neither low (110 mg) nor high (1000 mg/day) doses of aspirin had an effect on vessel patency after peripheral angioplasty or cumulative survival in a 216-patient randomized trial.[22] Aspirin has not been shown to have a beneficial effect in patients with PAD. However, aspirin may be used for other reasons in these patients, particularly if they have concomitant coronary or cerebrovascular disease.

There have been two clinical trials of ticlopidine (Ticlid) in patients with intermittent claudication. Ticlopidine significantly improved pain-free and total walking distance in both studies.[23,24] Another study tested whether ticlopidine prevents myocardial infarction, stroke, and transient ischemic attacks in patients with intermittent claudication.[25] A statistically significant benefit was found in reduction of the combined endpoints in favor of ticlopidine (relative risk reduction of 38%, p = 0.017). The difference disappeared, however, when an intention-to-treat analysis was performed (p = 0.24). Overall mortality was lower in the treatment group (18.5% versus 26.1%, p = 0.015).

Ticlopidine was more effective than aspirin in reducing the endpoints of stroke, myocardial infarction, and vascular death in a large group of patients with atherosclerosis in the Antiplatelet Trialists's Collaboration. However, the side effects of ticlopidine have limited its appeal as long-term therapy.

Clopidogrel (Plavix) is a newer thienopyridine derivative, chemically related to ticlopidine. It prevents arterial and venous thrombosis and reduces atherogenesis in animal models.[26,27] CAPRIE was a randomized clinical trial designed to assess the relative efficacy of clopidogrel (75 mg/day) versus aspirin (325 mg/day). It enrolled 19,185 patients with either recent stroke, myocardial infarction, or symptomatic peripheral arterial disease and followed them for an average of 1.9 years. Clopidogrel significantly reduced the combined endpoints of ischemic stroke, myocardial infarction, or vascular death when compared with aspirin in all entry groups (relative risk reduction of 8.7%, p = 0.043). Those with PAD had a relative risk reduction of 23.8% in combined endpoints. The side effect profile of clopidogrel is similar to aspirin. It does not cause the neutropenia seen with ticlopidine and thus is suitable for long-term therapy.

Our Recommendation. At the present time (fall 1999), clopidogrel has been found superior to aspirin for patients with symptomatic PAD. If its safety profile holds up with wider use, lifelong therapy with clopidogrel 75 mg/day should be prescribed for patients with intermittent claudication.

Pentoxifylline

Pentoxifylline (Trental) is a hemorheologically active compound that improves capillary blood flow. It decreases platelet aggregation and blood viscosity, and some studies report improvement in claudication in about half their patients.[29,30] However, controversy surrounds its efficacy, as other studies have not demonstrated benefit.[31,32]

If it is to be prescribed, the dose is 400 mg tid with meals to avoid nausea. Aplastic anemia has been reported rarely, so periodic blood counts are recommended. Objective determination of efficacy should be documented after 3 months of treatment. If there is no improvement, the drug should be stopped. Our own experience suggests that this drug has little effect on intermittent claudication.

Exercise

Exercise is an important part of the treatment of intermittent claudication. A structured walking program improves peak walking time and pain-free walking time by 100% to 150%. Treadmill exercise appears to be more effective than strength training. It may be difficult to get patients to exercise through pain. A structured hospital-based program usually is more successful, with greater sustained benefit than a home program.[33] Walking programs for patients with claudication can easily be incorporated into hospital-based cardiac rehabilitation programs.

Each patient should be given an individual exercise prescription based on the distance to pain threshold. Repeated walking until there is pain, separated by rest until pain disappears, should be continued for a total of 30 minutes of actual walking time at least five times a week. A written prescription reviewed with the patient along with an exercise form for documenting performance will help ensure compliance. Follow-up visits with a review of walking times and distance encourage continuation of the program.

REVASCULARIZATION THERAPY

Indications for revascularization include limb-threatening ischemia and intolerable symptoms. As already described, most patients consider an inability to walk briskly for 30 minutes as intolerable. This may not be the case with elderly or frail patients with many medical problems.

For a patient who has angiography soon after symptoms develop, we are more likely to find stenoses that can be easily treated with angioplasty or stenting. Angioplasty is the treatment of choice in stenotic peripheral arteries. The more difficult problems occur with either acute or chronic total occlusion. A treatment approach is outlined in Fig. 33-2.

When there is thrombosis in addition to atherosclerotic plaque, thrombolytic therapy is usually applied before balloon dilation or stenting. The usual approach is infusion of urokinase through an arterial catheter positioned next to the lesion.

Totally Occluded Arteries

The treatment of chronically occluded peripheral arteries remains a challenge for the interventional angiographer. Success rates are lower than for stenosed but nonoccluded vessels, complications rates are higher, and the time and expense to achieve patency are considerable. Thrombolysis has improved our ability to recanalize total occlusions and may improve long-term patency.

There are three mechanisms of arterial occlusion: (1) arterial emboli, (2) arterial thrombosis, and (3) arterial thrombosis superimposed on atheroma. The degree of thrombosis associated with total occlusion is not appreciated by most clinicians. This results in a conservative or surgical approach to total occlusion.

Embolization is suggested by an acute onset of pain. The patient seeks immediate help. In addition to pain there is numbness, coolness, and, later, paralysis. The pain is severe initially and tends to improve a little in the next hour. A cardiac source of embolus may be apparent (atrial fibrillation, mitral stenosis, or prior myocardial infarction with a regional wall motion abnormality). It is important to look for an embolic source with an echocardiogram in all patients, but particularly in patients with no previous history of claudication.

Thrombosis is suggested by a sudden worsening of stable claudication. Patients who could walk six blocks and now cannot walk one block have usually had a thrombosis on top of an atherosclerotic lesion. A change in the location of the claudication may indicate new thrombosis. A patient with stenosis of the iliac artery may complain of claudication in the calf. When thrombosis of the iliac occurs, the location may change to the buttock.

These changes in symptoms do not always bring patients to their physicians. Some of their reluctance may be based on the conservative approach physicians have taken to the original complaint of claudication.

Specific Lesions
Iliac Artery Occlusion

Catheter-based repair of the iliac artery is especially desirable because it allows the patient to avoid abdominal surgery. Clinically, a patient usually notices a significant

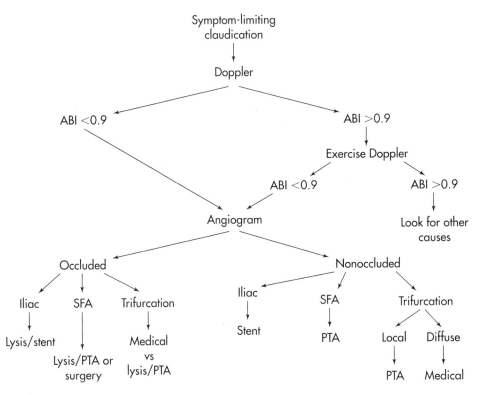

FIG. 33-2

Evaluation of peripheral artery disease. *ABI,* Ankle brachial index; *SFA,* superficial femoral artery; trifurcation = vessels below the knee; lysis = thrombolytic therapy (usually with urokinase infused locally); PTA = angioplasty (often with stent placement).

shortening of walking distance. If collateral vessels are not well developed, acute ischemia may develop. There is usually clot in the vessel. Thrombolysis followed by angioplasty is successful in total iliac occlusions in over 90% of cases. Stenting is especially effective in this vessel. It is rare for us to refer patients for surgery with iliac occlusion.

Superficial Femoral Artery Occlusion

Occlusion of the superficial femoral artery (SFA) requires careful assessment of collateral vessels and distal anatomy. Thrombolysis followed by angioplasty may be considered, but long-term patency is inconsistent. It is important to assess the lesion (and patient) together with a surgical colleague.

For a localized occlusion at the adductor canal less than 5 cm long, balloon angioplasty is almost always successful, and thrombolysis is unnecessary.

Occlusion of the lower two thirds of the SFA from the adductor canal and distally usually includes a large thrombus. The best approach is thrombolysis followed by angioplasty of the culprit atherosclerotic lesion at the adductor canal.

Occlusion from the origin of the SFA down to the adductor canal is the most difficult to treat. The vessel is usually filled with thrombus, extending from the adductor canal back to the next collateral vessel (in this case the profunda). This occlusion frequently requires surgical bypass. However, we have been surprised at how much thrombus is involved in these lesions. A 24-hour infusion of urokinase may result in marked resolution of clot with a short segment of residual occlusion or stenosis at the adductor canal that is easily treated with angioplasty. Our current approach is to attempt thrombolysis first and refer to surgery only if this fails.

Popliteal Occlusion

Popliteal occlusions usually have a large thrombus load. The initial approach is thrombolysis to visualize the culprit lesion. These cases are treacherous, requiring a significant amount of time in the catheterization laboratory for adjustment of catheter position before the lesion is cleared of thrombus and identified for angioplasty. Popliteal occlusion has the lowest success rate with angioplasty and the highest complication rate. Surgery is also more difficult with these lesions. We usually begin with thrombolysis of the occluded artery, which may uncover a popliteal artery aneurysm and better define the patient's anatomy. When surgery is needed, this improves the chance for success.

Occlusion of Trifurcation Vessels (Below the Knee)

Occlusion of vessels below the knee may cause limb-threatening ischemia. It is common in diabetics who have nonhealing ulcers. The small size of these vessels and the diffuse nature of the disease limit the success of revascularization. Surgical options are limited. Long-term patency is poor with either surgery or catheter-based procedures. However, opening an artery for just weeks to months may permit the ulcer to heal. Once healed, the area frequently remains healed even though the artery reoccludes (it takes less oxygen to maintain normal skin than it does to heal an ulcer). We always use thrombolysis before angioplasty with these lesions. Percutaneous techniques occasionally can be used to clean up the vessel, enabling a poor candidate for surgery to have a successful operation.

ACUTE LOWER LIMB ISCHEMIA

Patients with acute thrombotic or embolic occlusion of the lower extremities have life-threatening disease. Despite a century of surgical experience, mortality may be as high as 25% acutely and 42% at 1 year. Amputation rates average 40%.[34-38] The severity of concomitant disease in these patients accounts for the high mortality.

Two randomized trials have compared intraarterial thrombolysis and surgery versus surgery alone.[39,40] Both showed similar limb salvage rates and similar initial mortality. Unexpectedly, 1-year mortality was significantly reduced when thrombolytic therapy was used. This suggests that an initial lytic approach to acute occlusion is less traumatic and leads to fewer long-term complications. Event-free survival at 1 year was 75% versus 52% in the surgical group in one of the studies.[37] Our current approach is local infusion of urokinase with subsequent treatment (angioplasty or surgery) determined by the location and character of the lesion.

OTHER SYNDROMES
Buerger's Disease

Also called *thromboangiitis obliterans,* Buerger's disease is uncommon in the United States and more common in Asia. The diffuse vasculopathy is usually seen in young male smokers. The pathophysiology is uncertain, and it may represent hypersensitivity to some component of cigarette smoke. Pathologically, there is panarteritis of both small arteries and veins, with giant cells, lymphocytes, and thrombus. The inflammatory process is usually segmental.

The disease affects the small vessels of the feet and hands, resulting in digital ischemia. It may affect the arteries of the calves. Thrombophlebitis is common. Pain at rest caused by arterial insufficiency is an early symptom. When claudication occurs, it tends to involve the foot. Calf claudication is more consistent with atherosclerotic disease. Painful, tender ulcers on the tips of the digits lead to guarding. These lesions plus a history of migratory phlebitis and diminished distal pulses strongly suggest the diagnosis. Proximal pulses are usually normal. The diagnosis is confirmed by angiography showing segmental occlusion of small vessels in the feet and hands.

The only effective therapy is cessation of smoking, but the addiction is unusually strong in those with Buerger's disease. Vasodilators such as nifedipine may be beneficial but only if smoking is discontinued. These patients commonly require amputation.

Trash Foot

Trash foot (blue toe syndrome) is not a refined term, but we like it. Nothing better describes the lesions (and prognosis) of patients with this devastating problem. Although it can occur spontaneously as a complication of abdominal aortic aneurysm or a ragged plaque in the iliac or superficial femoral artery, it is most frequently seen after a vascular intervention such as cardiac catheterization or abdominal angiography. It is caused by a shower of small cholesterol emboli. The multiple small and painful gangrenous changes in the distal foot and the bilateral occurrence are pathognomonic.

Trash foot may be fatal, not because of limb ischemia, but because of emboli to the splanchnic and renal circulations. Progressive renal failure or intestinal ischemia in frail, elderly patients with vascular disease often leads to progressive deterioration and death. Anorexia, nausea, and abdominal pain suggest emboli to the bowel.

When trash foot occurs spontaneously and is bilateral, the patient should be screened for an abdominal aortic aneurysm with ultrasound. Repair of the aneurysm is necessary regardless of the size. If trash foot is unilateral, angiography is indicated to look for the offending lesion. Atherectomy is successful when the lesion is in the superficial femoral artery. Iliac stenting is the treatment of choice if the lesion is in the iliac artery.

If this condition results from an arterial procedure, warfarin anticoagulation may be helpful (although there is no evidence-based support and some controversy regarding its use). Close follow-up for renal failure is necessary.

REFERENCES

1. Criqui MH et al: The prevalence of peripheral arterial disease in a defined population, *Circulation* 71:510, 1985.
2. Kannel WB, McGee DL: Update on some epidemiologic features of intermittent claudication: the Framingham Study, *J Am Geriatr Soc* 33:13, 1985.

3. Bowlin SJ et al: Epidemiology of intermittent claudication in middle-aged men, *Am J Epidemiol* 140:418, 1994.

4. Criqui MH et al: Mortality over a period of 10 years in patients with peripheral arterial disease, *N Engl J Med* 326:381, 1992.

5. Gillum RF: Peripheral arterial occlusive disease of the extremities in the United States: hospitalization and mortality, *Am Heart J* 120:141, 1990.

6. McDaniel MD, Cronenwett JL: Basic data related to the natural history of intermittent claudication, *Ann Vasc Surg* 3:273, 1989.

7. Juergens JL, Barker NW, Hines EA Jr: Arteriosclerosis obliterans: review of 520 cases with special reference to pathogenic and prognostic factors, *Circulation* 21:118, 1960.

8. Humphries AW et al: Evaluation of the natural history and the results of treatment in occlusive arteriosclerosis involving the lower extremities in 1850 patients. In Wesolowski SA, Dennis C, editors: *Fundamentals of vascular grafting*, New York, 1963, McGraw-Hill.

9. Pomrehn P: The association of dyslipoproteinemia with symptoms and signs of peripheral arterial disease: The Lipids Research Clinics Program Prevalence Study, *Circulation* 73(suppl I):1, 1986.

10. Montanan G et al: Metabolic approach to the diagnosis and treatment of atherosclerotic peripheral vascular disease, *Int Angiol* 6:339, 1987.

11. Blankenhorn DH et al: The rate of atherosclerosis change during treatment of hyperlipoproteinemia, *Circulation* 57:355, 1978.

12. Blankenhorn DH et al: Effects of colestipol-niacin therapy on human femoral atherosclerosis, *Circulation* 83:438, 1991.

13. McDaniel MD, Cronenwett JL: Basic data related to the natural history of intermittent claudication, *Ann Vasc Surg* 3:273, 1989.

14. Davignon J et al: Plasma lipids and lipoprotein patterns in angiographically graded atherosclerosis of the legs and in coronary heart disease, *Can Med Assoc J* 116:1245, 1977.

15. Rodger JC et al: Intermittent claudication complicating beta blockade, *BMJ* 1:1125, 1976.

16. Schadt DC et al: Chronic atherosclerotic occlusion of the femoral artery, *JAMA* 175:937, 1961.

17. Newman AB et al: Morbidity and mortality in hypertensive adults with a low ankle/arm blood pressure index, *JAMA* 270:487, 1993.

18. Hertzer NR et al: Coronary artery disease in peripheral vascular patients: a classification of 1000 coronary angiograms and results of surgical management, *Ann Surg* 199:223, 1984.

19. Hertzer NR, Young JR, Beven EG, et al: Late results of coronary bypass in patients with peripheral vascular disease. I. Five-year survival according to age and clinical cardiac status, *Cleve Clin Q* 53:133, 1986.

20. Collaborative overview of randomised trials of antiplatelet therapy. I. Prevention of death, myocardial infarction, and stroke by prolonged antiplatelet therapy in various categories of patients, Antiplatelet Trialists' Collaboration, *BMJ* 308:81, 1994.

21. Ciocon JO, Galindo-Ciocon D, Galindo DJ: A comparison between aspirin and pentoxifylline in relieving claudication due to peripheral vascular disease in the elderly, *Angiology* 48:237, 1997

22. Minaret AL: Comparison of effects of high-dose and low-dose aspirin on restenosis after femoropopliteal percutaneous transluminal angioplasty, *Circulation* 91:2167, 1995.

23. Arcan JC et al: Multicenter double-blind study of ticlopidine in the treatment of intermittent claudication and the prevention of its complications, *Angiology* 39:802, 1988.

24. Balsano F, Coccheri S, Libretti A, et al: Ticlopidine in the treatment of intermittent claudication: a 21-month double-blind trial, *J Lab Clin Med* 114:84, 1989.

25. Janzon L et al: Prevention of myocardial infarction and stroke in patients with intermittent claudication: effects of ticlopidine. Results from STIMS, the Swedish Ticlopidine Multicentre Study, *J Intern Med* 227:301, 1990.

26. Herbert JM et al: Clopidogrel, a novel antiplatelet and antithrombotic agent, *Cardiovasc Drug Rev* 11:180, 1993.

27. Herbert JM et al: Inhibitory effect of clopidogrel on platelet adhesion and intimal proliferation following arterial injury in rabbits, *Arterioscler Thromb* 13:1171, 1993.

28. A randomized, blinded, trial of clopidogrel versus aspirin in patients at risk of ischemic events (CAPRIE), *Lancet* 348:1329, 1996.

29. Porter JM et al: Pentoxifylline efficacy in the treatment of intermittent claudication: multi-center controlled double-blind trial with objective assessment of chronic occlusive arterial disease patients, *Am Heart J* 113:864, 1982.

30. Johnson AK et al: Treatment of claudication with pentoxifylline: are benefits related to improvement viscosity? *J Vasc Surg* 6:211, 1987.

31. Donaldson DR et al: Does oxpentifylline have a place in treatment of intermittent claudication? *Curr Med Res Opin* 9:35, 1984.

32. Gallus AS et al: Intermittent claudication: a double blind crossover trial of pentoxifylline, *Aust N Z J Med* 15:402, 1985.

33. Regensteiner JG et al: Hospital vs home-based exercise rehabilitation for patients with peripheral arterial occlusive disease, *Angiology* 48:29, 1997.

34. Jivegard L et al: Acute limb ischemia due to arterial embolism or thrombosis: influence of limb ischemia vs pre-existing cardiac disease on postoperative mortality rate, *J Cardiovasc Surg* 29:32, 1988.

35. Blaisdell FE, Steele M, Allen RE: Management of acute lower extremity ischemia due to embolus and thrombosis, *Surgery* 84:822, 1978.

36. Lusby RJ, Wylie E: Acute lower limb ischaemia: pathogenesis and management, *World J Surg* 7:340, 1983.

37. Ouriel K et al: A comparison of thrombolytic therapy with operative revascularization in the initial treatment of acute peripheral arterial ischemia, *J Vasc Surg* 19:1021, 1994.

38. Comerota AJ et al: A prospective, randomized, blinded, and placebo-controlled trial of intraoperative intraarterial urokinase infusion during lower extremity revascularization: regional and systemic effects, *Ann Surg* 218:534, 1993.

34 Cerebrovascular Disease

Timothy D. Carter
Adrian B. Van Bakel

STROKE AND RELATED SYNDROMES

Epidemiology

In the United States, as in most developed countries, stroke is the third leading cause of death and a leading cause of adult disability. About 600,000 strokes occur annually in the United States, with 157,991 deaths from stroke in 1995.[1] Currently the number of stroke survivors in the United States is estimated at 4 million.[1] The economic burden is staggering, with an estimated cost of nearly $20 billion in 1994.[2]

Pathophysiology

The term *stroke* has varying degrees of specificity. Most neurologists use the term to apply to cerebrovascular disease and usually mean ischemic stroke. Broadly, cerebrovascular problems fall into two categories: hemorrhagic and ischemic. The most common bleeding problems are intracerebral and subarachnoid hemorrhage. Ischemic stroke includes both thrombotic and embolic stroke. Ischemic stroke is much more common than hemorrhagic events in the United States, with 70% to 80% of strokes being ischemic, about 10% to 15% secondary to intracerebral hemorrhage (ICH), and 5% to 10% secondary to subarachnoid hemorrhage (SAH).[3]

Thrombotic stroke is the most common and perhaps the most treatable type of stroke. Generally, this type of stroke is caused by atherosclerosis of the large intracranial arteries or the carotid and vertebral arteries in the neck.

Small vessel disease, usually the result of hypertension, can also lead to stroke. The small, penetrating arteries that branch directly from larger intracranial arteries seem to tolerate higher perfusion pressures poorly. The walls of these vessels break down, a process called *lipohyalinosis*.[4] As the walls of the vessel widen as a result of this process, the lumen becomes progressively smaller until it becomes occluded. Thrombosis may also occur within microaneurysms, which may develop as the vessel walls become progressively disorganized, or these vessels may be occluded by small embolic particles.[4] This results in a small area of infarction in the territory of the affected vessel, commonly referred to as a *lacune* or *lacunar infarct*. Although the area of infarction may be small, the resulting neurologic deficit can be great. For example, a well-placed lacune in the posterior limb of the internal capsule may cause a marked hemiparesis that affects the entire contralateral body. Alternatively, the weakened vessels may rupture, leading to intracerebral hemorrhage, which is frequently devastating because of destruction of the surrounding brain tissue from the mass effect of the hematoma. Thus lacunar infarcts and ICH tend to occur in the same areas in the brain, namely, where there are small, penetrating blood vessels (subcortical and cerebellar hemispheric white matter, basal ganglia, thalamus, and pons).

When large vessel intracranial disease leads to stroke, the cause is often intracranial atherosclerosis. However, extracranial carotid disease is also a common cause of stroke. The mechanisms by which extracranial disease may lead to stroke are likely multiple. Certainly, carotid stenosis may lead to hypoperfusion and result in infarction, but carotid to intracranial arterial embolization also seems to occur.

Embolism, usually from a cardiac source (cardioembolism), is an important cause of stroke, primarily because it may be one of the most preventable. Atrial fibrillation is the most prevalent risk factor for cardioembolic stroke, but numerous other cardiac sources of embolization are often identified (Box 34-1).

A small percentage of patients with ischemic stroke have less common causes for their stroke. Coagulopathies, vasculitis, antiphospholipid antibody syndrome, hemoglobinopathies, polycythemia, leukemia, thrombocythemia, arterial dissection, and cerebral venous occlusion can all cause stroke.

As noted earlier, ICH is most commonly seen with hypertension (frequently poorly controlled hypertension). Other causes include coagulopathies (including therapeutic anticoagulation), cerebral amyloid angiopathy, tumors, drugs (cocaine, amphetamines, and other sympathomimetics), and vascular anomalies.[5]

Nontraumatic SAH is most commonly the result of a ruptured berry aneurysm. These aneurysms tend to occur most frequently at branch points around the circle of Willis and may occasionally cause symptoms from their mass effect before rupture.

Prevention of Cerebrovascular Disease

Generally, strategies for stroke prevention are similar to those for the prevention of any type of vascular disease. Optimal management of vascular risk factors can greatly decrease stroke risk in most individuals (see Chapters 11

and 12). Specific medical and surgical options for stroke prevention are outlined in Table 34-1. Obviously, preventive strategies and management must be tailored to the clinical situation. For example, antibiotics would be the most appropriate therapy for a patient with infective endocarditis, whereas steroids might be the best choice for a patient with cerebral vasculitis.

Natural History

Survival after a stroke varies depending on the stroke subtype, with early mortality from ICH ranging from 30% to 80%, SAH from 20% to 50%, and ischemic stroke 8% to 20%.[6] Most early deaths (within 30 days) from ischemic stroke are the result of cardiopulmonary problems rather than cerebral edema, and neurologic deterioration in these patients is more likely to lead to increased disability rather than death.[6]

Recurrent stroke occurs commonly, with the immediate poststroke period carrying the highest risk. Since recurrent stroke results in the most stroke morbidity and mortality, appropriate evaluation and risk factor management are especially important in stroke survivors.[6]

Clinical Presentation

The sudden onset of a neurologic deficit should be considered to have a vascular cause until proved otherwise. The tempo of vascular events, either ischemic or hemorrhagic, is uniformly brisk. Stroke symptoms develop

---

BOX 34-1

POTENTIAL CARDIAC SOURCES OF EMBOLISM[7,38]

Atrial fibrillation
Spontaneous echocardiographic contrast
Mitral stenosis
Mitral valve prolapse
Sick sinus syndrome
Atrial myxoma
Prosthetic cardiac valves
Infective endocarditis
Recent myocardial infarction
Intracardiac shunt*
Left ventricular (LV) thrombus
Atrial septal aneurysm
LV aneurysm
Mitral annular calcification
Dilated cardiomyopathies
Calcific aortic stenosis
Rheumatic heart disease
LV wall motion abnormalities
Aortic arch atheromatous plaque

*Commonly atrial septal defect or patent foramen ovale.

Table 34-1	Specific Medical and Surgical Options for Stroke Prevention*

Therapy	Potential Clinical Applications
Aspirin (85 to 1300 mg qd)†	General stroke prevention (primary and secondary)
Ticlopidine (250 mg bid)	General stroke prevention for aspirin-intolerant patients TIA or stroke in patient taking aspirin
Clopidogrel (75 mg qd)	Same as ticlopidine
Warfarin (generally INR 2-3)‡	Patients with major cardiac source of embolism Possibly in patients on antiplatelet therapy who have a stroke or TIA Possibly in patients with a prothrombotic state
Carotid endarterectomy	Symptomatic carotid stenosis ≥ 70% Possibly symptomatic stenosis ≥ 50%, especially in men§ Asymptomatic stenosis ≥ 60%

*Adapted from references 7, 31, 32, and 39. Therapy should include vascular risk factor management and should be individualized to the patient. Referral to the referenced practice guidelines is encouraged.
†The appropriate dose of aspirin for stroke prevention remains controversial.
‡The intensity of anticoagulation depends on the indication being treated.
§Based on as yet unpublished data from the NASCET trial presented by Barnett HJM for the NASCET collaborators at the Twenty-third International Joint Conference on Stroke and Cerebral Circulation, Feb, 1998.

Table 34-2	*Some Common Patterns of Neurologic Deficits in Stroke Patients*

Signs and Symptoms	Localization/Cause
Amaurosis fugax	Ipsilateral ophthalmic artery occlusion causing retinal ischemia
Right hemiparesis (face, arm > leg) Right hemisensory deficit Aphasia Right hemianopsia	Dominant (left) hemisphere in middle cerebral artery territory
Left hemiparesis (face, arm > leg) Left hemisensory deficit Left-sided neglect/visuospatial disturbances Left hemianopsia	Nondominant (right) hemisphere in middle cerebral artery territory
Pure motor hemiparesis	Small vessel, subcortical, or brainstem
Pure hemisensory deficit	Small vessel, subcortical, or brainstem
Cross findings (cranial nerve deficits on one side, body deficits on the other) Ataxia Possibly quadriparesis or diffuse sensory loss Visual field defects	Brainstem/cerebellum, posterior circulation

Data from Fisher CM: *Neurology* 32:871, 1982; and Carter TD et al: *J SC Med Assoc* 90:310, 1994.

suddenly, over a period of minutes, hours, or perhaps a few days—not weeks, months, or years.

Clinical Syndromes That Mimic Stroke

Transient Ischemic Attack (TIA). Much has been made over the difference between stroke and TIA. The "official" definition of TIA is a neurologic deficit of vascular cause that totally resolves within 24 hours. Since most TIAs resolve in less than an hour, many stroke experts have suggested that this time frame should be shortened.[7] For example, in the NINDS tPA Stroke Study, only 2.7% of patients in the placebo group totally recovered by 24 hours.[8] Thus, if a patient has relatively unchanged, substantial neurologic deficits of 90 to 180 minutes' duration, then the likelihood of that event being a TIA is small. Since about one third of the 50,000 TIA patients seen annually in the United States subsequently have a stroke, prompt evaluation of TIAs is critical.[7] We almost always hospitalize patients who present emergently with TIAs, since the risk of stroke is greatest immediately after a TIA.[7] TIAs present an important opportunity to prevent a stroke, just as intervention in unstable angina may prevent a myocardial infarction (MI). Published practice guidelines recommend that the workup of patients seen within 1 week of a TIA be completed in, at most, a week and that hospi-

talization is frequently justified.[7] The diagnostic evaluation of a TIA is basically the same as that for a stroke patient (see Table 34-3 and subsequent text).

Syncope and Dizziness. A key component in our definition of an acute cerebrovascular problem such as a stroke or TIA is the presence of a focal neurologic deficit (Table 34-2). Thus an episode of fainting, passing out, syncope, the vapors, or whatever type of episodic loss of consciousness, when unaccompanied by a focal neurologic deficit, is unlikely to have a focal vascular cause (as would be seen with a stroke or TIA). A neurologist is often consulted when referring physicians are concerned about the possibility of TIA in syncopal patients. Much more common causes of syncope relate to cardiac output problems than to focal neurovascular difficulties (see Chapter 27). Dizziness is another common symptom for which I am asked to evaluate patients. Unless it is accompanied by other findings such as diplopia or other cranial nerve deficits, cerebellar signs, visual disturbances, or focal weakness, dizziness is unlikely to result from cerebral ischemia or hemorrhage. True vertigo (dizziness accompanied by a sense of movement on the part of the patient or the environment) is usually an inner ear problem. On rare occasions it may have a vascular cause, and it is more likely to have a cerebrovascular cause than nonspecific dizziness or lightheadedness. It

is important to have patients describe exactly what they mean by dizziness, since some may actually be describing gait or truncal ataxia, which would represent a focal neurologic problem.

Subclavian Steal Syndrome. One cause of episodic dizziness is the subclavian steal syndrome, in which stenosis affects the subclavian or brachiocephalic artery proximal to the origin of the vertebral artery, usually on the left side. With arm exercise there is lower vascular resistance. This promotes flow from the relatively high-pressure contralateral vertebral artery, across the circle of Willis, and retrograde through the ipsilateral vertebral artery back to the subclavian artery distal to the site of obstruction (Fig. 34-1). This can produce bouts of posterior circulation ischemia with vertigo and, less commonly, syncope. Usually symptoms of ipsilateral upper extremity ischemia (arm pain, weakness, coolness) predominate, and it is uncommon to have syncope or dizziness as the only symptom or sign of subclavian steal.

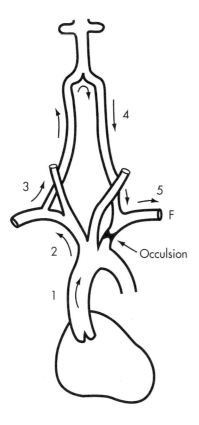

FIG. 34-1
A schematic of the subclavian steal syndrome. There is occlusion or stenosis of the left subclavian artery. Arterial blood supply to the left arm comes from the brachiocephalic artery *(2)*, through the right vertebral artery *(3)*, around the circle of Willis, through the left vertebral artery *(4)*, and to the left subclavian artery *(5)*. Left arm exercise increases the demand for arterial blood, "stealing" it from the vertebral circulation and causing syncope.

The physical examination commonly reveals relatively diminished and delayed upper extremity pulses and decreased blood pressure on the affected side. While patients may describe dizziness when using the affected limb, exercise of the arm does not provoke symptoms in most patients.[9] Many of these patients also have carotid disease and should be evaluated for it. Right subclavian steal is less common than left, but it can lead to carotid territory infarction from propagation of thrombus into the brachiocephalic and carotid arteries, thus warranting more aggressive management.[9]

History and Physical Examination

An important historical point is the time of onset of symptoms, especially if acute intervention is being considered. Probably the best way to get at this issue is not to ask when the problem started, but to ask when the patient was last normal. This time should be used as the time of onset of symptoms. It is also important to inquire about a history of similar problems, which could be suggestive of TIAs, seizures, hypoglycemia, structural lesions, or other causes of neurologic deficits that might require different management than stroke.

Physical examination should, of course, concentrate on first ensuring hemodynamic and respiratory stability. Next, a careful neurologic examination should be performed, searching for objective documentation of neurologic deficits. Patterns of deficits that correspond to particular vascular territories are especially helpful in confirming the clinical suspicion of stroke (see Table 34-2). Other physical findings such as evidence of meningeal irritation should be noted. Many physicians treating stroke patients are routinely beginning to use the NIH Stroke Scale, which is a scored neurologic examination that emphasizes deficits commonly seen in stroke patients and that was used by the NINDS tPA study group.[10]

Management of Stroke
Laboratory Evaluation

While the history and physical examination are being conducted in the emergency room, initial laboratory studies are obtained (Table 34-3). These typically include complete blood count, coagulation parameters, serum chemistry panel, and finger stick blood glucose measurement. An electrocardiogram (ECG) is also useful, since stroke may occur in conjunction with MI and an associated arrhythmia. This is particularly true for elderly patients who may have MI without chest pain.

The most important emergency test is a computed tomogram (CT) of the head. A noncontrast-enhanced scan is adequate because the main purpose of the CT is to evaluate for hemorrhage. Hemorrhagic events are managed differently than nonhemorrhagic events, and the CT determines the management path. Certainly, a CT is

Table 34-3 | *Diagnostic Tests in the Evaluation of TIA/Stroke Patient*

Test	Diagnostic Wave	Diagnostic Rationale	Management Rationale
Complete blood count with platelets	First (include this in the workup of all patients)	Screen for polycythemia, severe anemia, infection, leukemia, thrombocytosis, or thrombocytopenia	Correction of hematologic/hemorheologic problem may prevent recurrent stroke or improve current ischemic/hemorrhagic problem. Identification and treatment of infection may improve outcome or prevent further complications. Screen for contraindications to thrombolysis or other treatment
Prothrombin time (PT), partial thromboplastin time (PTT)	First	Screen for coagulopathy	Correction may improve hemorrhage/bleeding. Therapeutic levels in patients already taking anticoagulants. Screen for contraindications to thrombolysis or other treatments. Is further evaluation for a prothrombotic state or hemostatic problem needed?
Chemistry profile: electrolytes, renal, hepatic screen (including glucose, fasting lipid levels)	First	Screen for metabolic abnormalities	May influence a decision about thrombolysis (especially hypoglycemia/hyperglycemia. Correction of abnormalities may improve outcome, prevent complications, or prevent future problems
ECG	First	Screen for arrhythmias, cardiac ischemia	Help determine need for further cardiac evaluation. Atrial fibrillation indicates need for anticoagulation
Westegren sedimentation rate, syphilis serology	First	Screen for syphilis or evidence of other infection and vasculitis	Determine the need for further diagnostic evaluation for these conditions (which have management methods that would not otherwise be employed for stroke/TIA)
CT scan	First	Hemorrhage (ICH, SAH, SDH). Nonvascular cause for signs (tumor, etc). Vascular lesions (aneurysm, AVM, hyperdense MCA sign in acute stroke)	Determine specific management path (hemorrhage vs ischemia). Appropriate management of relatively unsuspected problems, such as tumor
Noninvasive carotid arterial imaging	First	Define presence and severity of carotid stenosis	Determine possible need for surgical treatment of carotid disease or need for further evaluation of this possibility

ICH, Intracranial hemorrhage; *SAH*, subarachnoid hemorrhage; *AVM*, arteriovenous malformation; *Abs*, antibodies; *SPEP*, serum protein electrophoresis; *MCA*, middle cerebral artery.

Table 34-3 | *Diagnostic Tests in the Evaluation of TIA/Stroke Patient—cont'd*

Test	Diagnostic Wave	Diagnostic Rationale	Management Rationale
Chest x-ray	First—stroke patients	Exclude pneumonia or other occult process Examine cardiac silhouette	Detects pulmonary complications that may need to be addressed
Echocardiography (transthoracic or transesophageal)	First/second	Determine cardiac source of embolus (See Box 34-1)	Useful in any patient in whom finding a cardiac source of embolus would alter management (such as a patient with no contraindication to anticoagulation) Situation-specific use, such as suspected endocarditis
Transcranial Doppler Cerebral angiography	Second (not performed in all patients and not a part of initial evaluation)	Answers more specific questions about cerebral and extracranial vasculature Degree of carotid or intracranial disease Vascular anomalies such as aneurysms, AVM May diagnose vasculitis	Useful in resolving issues of diagnostic uncertainty that would alter management, such as • Surgery for carotid disease or aneurysm • Anticoagulation for dissection or severe intracranial vascular disease • Steroids for vasculitis
Prothrombotic studies • Antiphospholipid Abs • Protein C & S • Antithrombin III • Thrombin time • Factor V lever mutation • Hemoglobin electrophoresis • SPEP	Second (for most patients) May be first for patients with suggestive clinical features, such as young (<50 yrs) patients or personal or family history of thrombotic events	Determine specific cause for hypercoaguability	Determine need for anticoagulation or other disease-specific treatment
MRI	First/second	Uncertain nature of cerebral pathology Useful for suspected small lesion or posterior circulation events	Need for disease-specific treatment
Ambulatory ECG monitoring	Second	Arrhythmias	Need for disease-specific treatment
Cerebrospinal fluid examination	Second (or first with suspected SAH and a negative CT)	Exclude infection (meningitis) SAH with negative CT	Need for disease-specific treatment

mandatory if thrombolytic therapy or anticoagulation are being contemplated.

General Management Principles

Prevent Hypotension. There are themes in the management of stroke that apply in all cases. Probably the most important is to prevent even relative hypotension. Lowering the blood pressure of an acute stroke patient is rarely helpful and often is the wrong thing to do. Recall that cerebral blood flow is autoregulated over a wide range of systemic blood pressure, but in acute stroke this autoregulatory system often malfunctions, so cerebral blood flow is more directly related to blood pressure. Furthermore, patients with chronic hypertension tend to shift their zone of cerebral autoregulation higher to correspond to their chronically higher blood pressures. *Even modestly lowering the blood pressure may substantially decrease cerebral blood flow and decrease perfusion to already ischemic areas of brain.*

If blood pressure must be lowered, avoid precipitous drops. Thus agents such as sublingual nifedipine should not be used. Many stroke neurologists use small intravenous doses of labetalol or perhaps captopril or nicardipine to lower blood pressure in small increments. Alternatively, a constant intravenous infusion of nitroprusside or a short-acting, easily titrated agent may be used.[2,12]

Metabolic Issues, Concurrent Illnesses, and Early Mobilization. Hypoxemia and hypoglycemia are neurologically detrimental under any circumstance and should be avoided in an acute stroke patient. There is also evidence that hyperglycemia can promote a worse outcome in stroke, and euglycemia should be maintained.[2,11] Infection and fever may result in neurologic worsening and thus should be prevented if possible and treated aggressively if they occur.[2,11] Cerebral edema may be promoted or worsened if there is volume overload, but dehydration should also be prevented. Because dysphagia may prevent oral intake in many cases, the early institution of nutritional support is important. In bed-bound patients, prevention of deep venous thrombosis may be accomplished with subcutaneous heparin or serial compression stockings. Early mobilization and rehabilitation in an organized stroke unit may stave off many complications before they occur and also improve outcome.[13]

Urinary tract infection is a complication that can be minimized by avoiding indwelling urinary catheters as much as possible. Deep venous thrombosis prophylaxis is important in all bed-bound patients. Early disposition planning involving the patient's family is useful in helping to reduce the length of the acute hospitalization.

Treatment of Specific Stroke Syndromes

Subarachnoid Hemorrhage. One of the major battles in the management of subarachnoid hemorrhage (SAH) is making the diagnosis. The acute onset of "the worst headache of my life" should always suggest the diagnosis. Although many of these patients present moribund with or without focal neurologic deficits, some may have only headache and neck stiffness. Diagnostically, CT scanning to evaluate for the presence of subarachnoid blood is the first step. If the CT is negative and diagnostic suspicion or uncertainty remains, then cerebrospinal fluid (CSF) examination should follow. Once the diagnosis is made, a neurosurgeon should be promptly involved, since the ultimate goal is to surgically repair the aneurysm that has bled. Cerebral angiography is necessary to determine the location of the suspected aneurysm(s).

Most patients should be given nimodipine, a cerebroselective calcium channel blocker that has been shown to help prevent cerebral vasospasm, a common, dangerous complication of SAH. Care is otherwise largely supportive and preventing complications is important. Again, the definitive therapy is neurosurgical.[14]

Intracerebral Hemorrhage. Unfortunately the care of a patient who has suffered an ICH is largely supportive (see general measures discussed earlier). Treatment of increased intracranial pressure may be beneficial. The best specific therapy remains undetermined, and surgical treatments seem to come in and out of vogue. One clear surgical indication is cerebellar hemorrhage, for which evacuation of the clot and decompression of the brainstem may be lifesaving and produce a good functional outcome. This may also be applicable in certain cases of cerebellar infarction.

Acute Ischemic Stroke. This is an exciting time in the management of patients with ischemic stroke because effective treatments are evolving. Intravenous thrombolytic therapy with recombinant tissue plasminogen activator (rt-PA) has been approved for the treatment of acute ischemic stroke. However, this therapy should be administered only to carefully selected patients according to a specific protocol. When patient selection is done properly, the treatment effect is remarkable. In the landmark NINDS rt-PA stroke trial, treated patients were 30% more likely to recover completely or with minimal neurologic deficits than patients receiving placebo.[15] Although rt-PA does increase the risk of intracerebral hemorrhage, the benefit to patients does not come at the expense of higher mortality. Overall, the level of benefit is comparable to the use of thrombolysis for MI.[16]

Therapy with rt-PA also compares favorably with other interventions for stroke when examined using number-needed-to-treat (NNT) analysis, which determines the number of patients needed to treat to obtain one additional favorable outcome. For example, the NNT with warfarin for chronic atrial fibrillation is 33, carotid endarterectomy for symptomatic carotid stenosis has a NNT of 11, and the treatment of acute ischemic stroke with t-PA has a NNT of 8.[17]

Intravenous rt-PA must be administered within 3 hours of the onset of symptoms to be safe and effective. Thus an organized, preplanned approach to the evaluation and treatment of these patients is mandatory.[18] Many hospitals use acute stroke teams to quickly and efficiently evaluate patients.[18,19]

The inclusion/exclusion criteria and protocol for using rt-PA[11,12,15,20] are listed in Box 34-2. A few points deserve special emphasis. One is treating within the 3-hour time window. The ECASS study, which had a 6-hour time to treatment, found no benefit from t-PA and increased mortality with later treatment (although this was not statistically significant).[21]

We cannot overemphasize the importance of determining the exact time of symptom onset. Again, it is helpful to ask when the last time the patient was known to be normal rather than when symptoms were first noticed. Thus a patient found to have symptoms on first awakening must be assumed to have the onset of stroke just after retiring, the time the patient was last observed to be normal. Thus 11 PM would be the symptom-onset time for someone who goes to bed at 11 PM and awakes at 7 AM with hemiparesis.

The major complication of rt-PA treatment is ICH. In the NINDS trial, treated patients had a tenfold increase (6.4% versus 0.6%) in ICH.[5] However, careful patient selection can help to minimize this risk. Elevated blood pressure is an important factor in selecting patients for thrombolysis. The NINDS study investigators did not use t-PA in patients with sustained pressure greater than 185/110 mm Hg or in patients who required "aggressive" therapy (more than nitropaste or a single dose of labetalol) to bring the blood pressure below that cut-off value. The ECASS trial, which showed no benefit with rt-PA treatment, did not exclude patients with uncontrolled hypertension.[21]

The CT is also important. No evidence of hemorrhage should be seen. It has also been found that patients with mass effect or hypodensity have an increased risk of hemorrhage.[22] Furthermore, patients with more subtle changes, seen early in the course of infarction, such as sulcal effacement affecting more than one third of the middle cerebral artery territory, have higher rates of hemorrhage.[21] However, such patients tend to do poorly in any event and have a better chance of a good outcome (little or no disability) with t-PA treatment despite an increased risk of hemorrhage.[22] Thus it may be reasonable to treat these patients after discussing these issues with the patient and family.

Another factor associated with an increased risk of hemorrhage is the size of the area of injury. Large infarcts are more likely to have hemorrhagic transformation than smaller ones. Analysis of the NINDS data showed an increased risk of hemorrhage in patients with large clinical deficits.[22] That study used the NIH Stroke Scale to clinically grade deficits. The NIH Stroke Scale is simply a standardized, scored neurologic examination with higher scores representing larger clinical deficits. Patients with NIH Stroke Scale scores of 20 or greater were at increased risk for hemorrhage when treated with t-PA.[22] An NIH Stroke Scale score of at least 20 may describe, for example, a lethargic patient with dense right hemiplegia affecting the face, arm, and leg, diminished sensation on the right, and global aphasia. A patient this sick tends to do poorly without intervention; thrombolytic therapy, although risky, may still be reasonable.

After administration of rt-PA the patient still requires close monitoring. The protocol prohibits the administration of any anticoagulants or antiplatelet agents in the 24 hours following rt-PA administration. Close attention also must be paid to blood pressure control after rt-PA. Blood pressure should be kept at or below 185/110 for the first 24 hours after rt-PA administration, and the recommended method for accomplishing this is described in Box 34-2.

Close attention to neurologic status is also important, and frequent neurologic checks may help to detect complications early, especially ICH. Clinical indicators of ICH include depressed level of consciousness, new headache or vomiting, increased weakness, and increasing blood pressure or pulse pressure.[22] Follow-up CT scanning to exclude ICH should be considered for patients who develop these findings. Such a high level of monitoring generally requires that patients be maintained in an intensive care unit or similar close observation unit for at least the first 24 hours after rt-PA administration.

What about the treatment of patients with ischemic stroke who are not candidates for intravenous rt-PA? Intraarterial thrombolytic therapy is being used at an increasing number of centers and appears promising, although a definitive trial has yet to be completed. The use of intravenous thrombolytic agents other than rt-PA cannot currently be recommended.[12,23-25] Three separate trials of intravenous streptokinase were stopped prematurely by their safety monitoring committees because of excess hemorrhage and mortality in treated patients.[12,20]

Heparin has been used in the acute treatment of stroke for years, but it has never been shown to be of benefit in a randomized, controlled clinical trial. The recently completed International Stroke Trial (IST) found an increased rate of hemorrhagic complications and no clinical improvement in outcome in patients treated with either high (12,500 U bid) or low (5000 U bid) doses of subcutaneous heparin.[26] Despite this lack of evidence, many neurologists use heparin in patients with *embolic infarcts* to prevent early recurrence of embolism. If heparin is used in such situations, we frequently delay its use, since hemorrhagic transformation (which occurs frequently in cardioembolic stroke) usually occurs within the first 48 hours.[27,28] We then obtain a follow-up

---

BOX 34-2

rt-PA PROTOCOL

INCLUSION CRITERIA
1. Clearly defined onset of symptoms ≤3 hours before treatment (see text)
2. CT scan without hemorrhage, early signs of infarction, or nonstroke cause of symptoms
3. Consent from patient, or family, or both

EXCLUSION CRITERIA
1. Previous stroke or serious head injury within the preceding 3 months
2. Major surgery within the last 14 days
3. History of intracerebral hemorrhage
4. Systemic blood pressure (BP) ≥185 or diastolic BP ≥110, or if aggressive treatment is required to reduce BP to those levels
5. Rapidly improving symptoms
6. Minor symptoms
7. Symptoms suggestive of subarachnoid hemorrhage
8. Gastrointestinal or urinary tract hemorrhage within the previous 21 days
9. Arterial puncture at a noncompressible site within the previous 7 days
10. Seizures at onset of stroke
11. Taking anticoagulants or received heparin within the preceding 48 hours and/or has:
    a. Elevated partial thromboplastin time (PTT)
    b. Prothrombin time ≥15 sec
    c. Platelets ≤100,000
12. Glucose ≤50 or ≥400
13. Any other complicating problems that might be thought to increase risk of this treatment
14. Possibly NIH stroke scale score ≥20 (see text)

DOSE
rt-PA 0.9 mg/kg to maximum dose of 90 mg, administered intravenously with 10% given rapidly and the remaining 90% infused over 60 min

FOLLOW-UP
1. Intensive care unit for 24 hours after rt-PA administered
2. Keep BP ≤185/110, monitor BP every 15 min for 2 hours, then every 30 min for 6 hr, then every 1 hr for 16 hr, then routine (see Box 34-3 for suggested BP management)
3. No anticoagulants or antiplatelet agents for 24 hours after treatment

---

CT to exclude hemorrhage before starting heparin. If heparin is used, we often start it without an initial bolus or with a smaller bolus (e.g., 2000 to 5000 U) than is typically used for other indications. We aim for prolongation of the activated partial thromboplastin time (aPTT) no longer than 1.5 times normal. Weight-based protocols may be helpful in this regard. Recall that patients with large clinical deficits have large areas of infarction and a higher risk of bleeding into the infarct; we usually do not use heparin in these patients.

Other than cardioembolic stroke, many believe that heparin may be useful in various other situations, in-cluding progressing stroke and crescendo TIA, possibly arterial dissection, and posterior circulation thrombosis. Again, realize that heparin has not been *proved* to be beneficial in any of these situations. Results of trials using low-molecular-weight heparins have shown mixed results, and the role of these agents remains unclear.[29,30]

Although the IST showed no benefit from heparin, it did show a small, but worthwhile, improvement in patients given aspirin within 48 hours after the onset of symptoms.[26] No significant complications were seen, so this may become one of the most frequently used specific therapies for stroke. The acute role of other agents

---

BOX 34-3

BLOOD PRESSURE (BP) MANAGEMENT FOR PATIENTS GIVEN INTRAVENOUS rt-PA[20]

---

1. Monitor BP as recommended in Box 34-2; for elevated BP ≥180/110, recheck at least twice, 5 to 10 min apart
2. For systolic BP = 180-230 or diastolic BP = 105-120:
   - Labetalol 10 mg IV over 1-2 min
     - May repeat or double dose every 10-20 min to max dose of 150 mg
     - Monitor BP every 15 min during labetalol treatment
3. For systolic BP ≥230 or diastolic BP = 120 to 140:
   - Labetalol as above
   - If response is not satisfactory, IV sodium nitroprusside 6.5-10 μg/kg/min
     - Consider continous arterial monitoring if nitroprusside used
4. For diastolic BP ≥140:
   - Nitroprusside as above

---

that affect platelet function, including ticlopidine, clopidogrel, and abciximab, has yet to be determined.

Various neuroprotective agents and strategies that interfere with the biochemical and molecular cascade of events initiated by cerebral ischemia have been proposed and tested in clinical trials. Unfortunately, so far, none of these agents have proved beneficial, although many still appear promising.

Secondary Prevention

Preventing recurrent stroke is important, and the cause of stroke defines the most appropriate secondary prevention strategy. The usual vascular risk factors should be addressed. In addition to neuroimaging (to evaluate for hemorrhage, tumor, and so forth), we obtain carotid duplex ultrasound studies, since the treatment of significant carotid stenosis involves surgical, in addition to medical, management.[31,32]

Echocardiography to evaluate for a cardiac source of embolization is also important. Recent studies suggest that transesophageal echocardiography (TEE) may be warranted and cost effective in all ischemic stroke patients.[33,34] For example, lacunar strokes were not considered cardioembolic, but a recent study with TEE found intracardiac thrombus in 28% of patients. As patent foramen ovale (PFO) has been more clearly defined as

cause of embolic stroke, screening for right-to-left shunting at the time of echocardiography may be useful. A recent study found that notching of the QRS in inferior leads may suggest an underlying PFO in stroke patients (the "crochetage" pattern).[35]

The intracranial circulation can be examined noninvasively with transcranial Doppler, magnetic resonance angiography (MRA), and CT angiography (possible with the advent of helical or spiral CT scanners), but angiography remains the gold standard. Recall that angiography is not without risk, with a 1.2% stroke rate in patients having arteriograms to evaluate asymptomatic carotid stenosis.[36]

Overall, the workup for each patient should be individualized (see Table 34-3). The outcome of the etiologic evaluation will determine the best options to prevent recurrent stroke. Early and aggressive rehabilitation will help patients recover as much functional ability as quickly as possible.

ASYMPTOMATIC CAROTID ARTERY DISEASE

The question of how to manage a patient with an asymptomatic carotid bruit arises not infrequently. Unfortunately, the presence of a bruit does not always herald critical carotid stenosis, and severe stenosis is not always associated with a bruit.[31] Thus further diagnostic testing is needed to define the underlying vascular lesion, since carotid endarterectomy has been shown to be beneficial in asymptomatic patients with low surgical risk who have at least 60% stenosis[32,36] (Table 34-4).

Although conventional angiography remains the gold standard, we usually start with carotid duplex ultrasound because it can be obtained quickly, is relatively inexpensive, and entails no risk to the patient. The quality of duplex ultrasonography is laboratory dependent, and there is a documented risk of misinterpreting high-grade stenosis (for which endarterectomy may be highly beneficial) as total occlusion (for which endarterectomy is not indicated).

MRA is another noninvasive technique for examining the carotid vessels, but it also may incorrectly define the degree of stenosis (usually overestimating the extent of stenosis in my experience). Despite these limitations, some centers consider endarterectomy on the basis of duplex studies or the combination of duplex and MRA results without always proceeding to angiography. It is also important to remember that the major published clinical guidelines regarding carotid endarterectomy[31,32] (also see Table 34-1) are based on studies that used angiography as the ultimate method for determining the degree of stenosis; generalizing these guidelines to duplex or MRA results, without the results of further studies, may not be valid. However, we still begin the evalu-

Table 34-4	*Diagnostic Studies for Evaluating Carotid Disease*

Test	Pros	Cons
Duplex ultrasound	Noninvasive, little risk Inexpensive	Quality results are laboratory dependent False positive rate (misidentification of high grade stenosis as occlusion) reported between 1% and 14%[31]
Magnetic resonance angiography	Noninvasive, little risk	May overestimate or underestimate the degree of stenosis More costly
Conventional catheter angiography	The gold standard Published surgical guidelines are based on angiographic results	Invasive, with an attendant risk of stroke (1.2% in asymptomatic patients in the ACAS trial [36]) More costly

ation with duplex ultrasonography and decide on the need for further testing based on those results.

REFERENCES

1. *1998 Cardiovascular statistics,* Dallas, 1998, American Heart Association.
2. Adams HP et al: Guidelines for the management of patients with acute ischemic stroke, *Stroke* 25:1901, 1994.
3. Sacco RL: Classification of stroke. In Fisher M, editor: *Clinical atlas of cerebrovascular disorders,* London, 1994, Mosby.
4. Fisher CM: Lacunar strokes and infarcts: a review, *Neurology* 32:871, 1982.
5. Feldmann E: Intracerebral hemorrhage. In Fisher M, editor: *Clinical atlas of cerebrovascular disorders,* London, 1994, Mosby.
6. Sacco RL: Frequency and determinants of stroke. In Fisher M, editor: *Clinical atlas of cerebrovascular disorders,* London, 1994, Mosby.
7. Feinberg WM et al: Guidelines for the management of transient attacks, *Stroke* 25:1320, 1994.
8. Grotta J: t-PA: the best current option for most patients, *N Engl J Med* 337:1310, 1997.
9. Caplan LR: *Stroke—a clinical approach,* ed 2, Boston, 1993, Butterworth-Heinemann.
10. Brott T et al: Measurements of acute cerebral infarction: a clinical examination scale, *Stroke* 20:864, 1989.
11. Schneck MJ: Acute stroke: an aggressive approach to intervention and prevention, *Hosp Med* Jan 1998, p 11.
12. Adams HP et al: Guidelines for thrombolytic therapy for acute stroke: a supplement to the guidelines for the management of patients with acute ischemic stroke, *Circulation* 94:1167, 1996.
13. Stroke Unit Trialist Collaboration: How do stroke units improve patient outcomes? A collaborative systematic review of the randomized trials, *Stroke* 28:2 139, 1997.
14. Mayberg MR et al: Guidelines for the management of aneurysmal subarachnoid hemorrhage, *Stroke* 25:2315, 1994.
15. NINDS rt-PA Stroke Study Group: Tissue plasminogen activator for acute ischemic stroke, *N Engl J Med* 333:1581, 1995.
16. Wilcox RG et al: Trial of tissue plasminogen activator for mortality reduction in acute myocardial infarction: AS-SET, *Lancet* 2:525, 1988.
17. Haley EC et al: Myths regarding the NINDS rt-PA Stroke Trial: setting the record straight, *Ann Emerg Med* 330:676, 1997.
18. *Proceedings of a National Symposium on Rapid Identification and Treatment of Acute Stroke,* Bethesda, Md, Aug 1997, The National Institute of Neurologic Disorders and Stroke, National Institutes of Health.
19. National Acute Stroke Team Group: Survey of acute stroke teams in the U.S., *Stroke* 29:314, 1998.
20. Practice Advisory: Thrombolytic therapy for acute ischemic stroke: summary statement. Report of the Quality Standards Subcommittee of the American Academy of Neurology, *Neurology* 47:835, 1996.
21. Hacke W et al: Intravenous thrombolysis with recombinant tissue plasminogen activator for acute hemispheric stroke, The European Cooperative Acute Stroke Study (ECASS), *JAMA* 274:1017, 1995.
22. The NINDS t-PA Stroke Study Group: Intracerebral hemorrhage after intravenous t-PA therapy for ischemic stroke, *Stroke* 28:2109, 1997.
23. Caplan LR et al: Thrombolysis (not a panacea for ischemic stroke, *N Engl J Med* 337:1309, 1997.
24. Wijdicks EFM et al: Intra-arterial thrombolysis in acute basilar artery thromboembolism: the initial Mayo Clinic experience, *Mayo Clin Proc* 72:1005, 1997.
25. Davis SM, Donnan GA, Grotta JC, Hacke W: *Interventional therapy in acute stroke,* Malden, Mass., 1998, Blackwell Science.
26. International Stroke Trial Collaborative Group: The International Stroke Trial (1ST): a randomized trial of aspirin, subcutaneous heparin, both, or neither among 19,435 patients with acute ischemic stroke, *Lancet* 349:1569, 1997.
27. Cerebral Embolism Task Force: Cardiogenic brain embolism, *Arch Neurol* 43:71, 1986.

28. Hart RG: Cardiogenic embolism to the brain, *Lancet* 339:589, 1992.
29. Kay R et al: Low-molecular weight heparin for the treatment of acute ischemic stroke, *N Engl J Med* 333:1588, 1995.
30. The Publications Committee for the Trial of ORG 10172 in Acute Stroke Treatment (TOAST) Investigators: Low molecular weight heparinoid, ORG 10172 (Danaparoid), and outcome after acute ischemic stroke: a randomized controlled trial, *JAMA* 279:1265, 1998.
31. Moore WS et al: Guidelines for carotid endarterectomy, *Stroke* 26:188, 1995.
32. Biller J et al: Guidelines for carotid endarterectomy, *Stroke* 29:554, 1998.
33. McNamara RL et al: Echocardiographic identification of cardiovascular sources of emboli to guide clinical management of stroke: a cost-effectiveness analysis, *Ann Intern Med* 127:775, 1997.
34. Lavados PM et al: Unsuspected intracardiac thrombus in patients with lacunar strokes, *Stroke* 29:284, 1998.
35. Ay H et al: An electrocardiographic criterion for diagnosis of patent foramen ovale associated with ischemic stroke, *Stroke* 29:1393, 1998.
36. Executive Committee for the Asymptomatic Carotid Atherosclerosis Study: Endarterectomy for asymptomatic carotid artery stenosis, *JAMA* 273:1421, 1995.
37. Lyden PD: Magnitude of the problem of stroke and the significance of acute intervention. In *Proceedings of a National Symposium on Rapid Identification and Treatment of Acute Stroke*, Bethesda, Md., Aug 1997, The National Institute of Neurologic Disorders and Stroke, National Institutes of Health.
38. Minematsu K: Cardioembolic stroke. In Fisher M, editor: *Clinical atlas of cerebrovascular disorders*, London, 1994, Mosby.
39. CAPRIE Steering Committee: A randomised, blinded, trial of clopidogrel versus aspirin in patients at risk of ischaemic events (CAPRIE), *Lancet* 348:1329, 1996.
40. Carter TD et al: Clinical syndromes of cerebral ischemia, *J SC Med Assoc* 90:310, 1994.
41. McDowell FH et al: Stroke: the first six hours: emergency evaluation and treatment, *Stroke Clin Updates* 4:1, 1993.

35 Pulmonary Heart Disease

Christopher D. Nielsen
David P. Malone

Pulmonary disease affects the right side of the heart, since the right atrium and ventricle are immediately upstream from the pulmonary circulation. The link between lung disease and the heart is invariably pulmonary hypertension. High pulmonary artery pressure functionally obstructs right heart outflow, eventually causing right heart failure. The combination of lung disease and right heart failure is called *cor pulmonale.* Primary cardiac conditions that affect the left side of the heart may also cause pulmonary hypertension. Since the pulmonary hypertension is not caused by lung disease, it is not considered cor pulmonale, even though the heart failure syndrome is similar.

The pulmonary circulation is a low-pressure, low-resistance circuit with a high capacitance. Normal pulmonary artery peak systolic pressure at sea level is 18 to 25 mm Hg. By definition, pulmonary hypertension is present if peak pulmonary artery systolic pressure exceeds 30 mm Hg or the mean pulmonary artery pressure exceeds 20 mm Hg. At higher altitudes, normal pulmonary artery pressures are higher. At 15,000 feet above sea level, normal peak pulmonary artery pressure may be up to 38 mm Hg, with a mean pressure of 25 mm Hg.

CHRONIC COR PULMONALE[1-5]
Epidemiology

Cor pulmonale may be defined as hypertrophy and dilation of the right ventricle with or without right ventricular failure. There are many causes of chronic cor pulmonale (Box 35-1). Because of its association with chronic lung disease, this is a common heart condition. About 50 million people in the United States have chronic obstructive pulmonary disease (COPD), with more than 80,000 deaths occurring annually. All cases of COPD do not lead to cor pulmonale. The prevalence of cor pulmonale is difficult to estimate because the diagnosis is often overlooked. Physical examination may be unimpressive in patients with pulmonary hypertension without right ventricular failure, or lung disease may be so severe that the cor pulmonale is masked or overlooked, leading to underdiagnosis.

Most patients with cor pulmonale are over 50 years old, and the majority are men. COPD is the most common cause, accounting for over 50% of cases. Any disease that affects ventilation, gas exchange, or the pulmonary vascular bed can potentially cause cor pulmonale.

Pathophysiology

There are three basic mechanisms by which chronic lung disease can lead to pulmonary hypertension and then right heart failure (Box 35-1): (1) hypoxic vasoconstriction, (2) obstruction of the pulmonary vascular bed, (3) obliteration of lung parenchyma with resulting loss of pulmonary vascular bed. Most disease processes lead to cor pulmonale by a combination of these mechanisms.

Hypoxia is a potent pulmonary vasoconstrictor. After prolonged hypoxia, there is intimal thickening and medial hypertrophy of the pulmonary vessels. This may eventually progress to irreversible fibrosis of the vessels. Hypercarbia and acidosis can also contribute to vasoconstriction in a hypoxic patient. Patients with COPD and hypoxia, most commonly those with chronic bronchitis (the "blue bloater"), are thus more prone to cor pulmonale than others with emphysema and equally severe airway obstruction but with normal arterial oxygen saturation (the "pink puffer").

Obstruction of the pulmonary vascular bed results in decreased effective vascular surface area and an increase in pulmonary vascular resistance. This may occur in several ways. Pulmonary emboli may obstruct flow. In situ thrombus formation, which is evident in primary pulmonary hypertension and sickle cell disease, can obstruct flow. Unusual causes include invasive tumors that compress pulmonary vessels, inflammation, arteritis, and parasite infestation.

Obliteration of a part of the pulmonary vascular bed occurs when a disease process destroys lung parenchyma, which reduces the pulmonary vascular surface area. Emphysema, bronchiectasis, cystic fibrosis, and many inflammatory disorders may cause cor pulmonale by this mechanism.

Clinical Presentation

Symptoms vary depending on the underlying lung disease and the degree of cor pulmonale. Most early complaints are nonspecific and could be caused by the

---

BOX 35-1

CAUSES OF CHRONIC COR PULMONALE GROUPED BY MECHANISM OF PULMONARY HYPERTENSION

HYPOXIC VASOCONSTRICTION
Chronic Obstructive Pulmonary Disease (COPD)
Chronic bronchitis
Emphysema
Idiopathic pulmonary fibrosis

Cystic Fibrosis

Chronic Hypoventilation
Obesity hypoventilation syndrome
Sleep apnea
Neuromuscular weakness
Dysfunction of chest wall (kyphoscoliosis, thoracoplasty)
Pleural fibrosis
Idiopathic hypoventilation

Chronic High-Altitude Dwelling

OBSTRUCTION OF THE PULMONARY VASCULAR BED
Pulmonary Embolism
Thromboembolism
Tumor
Air
Bone marrow
Amniotic fluid
Fat

Primary Pulmonary Hypertension
Parasites (Schistosomiasis and Others)
Sickle Cell Disease
Fibrosing Mediastinitis, Mediastinal Tumors
Pulmonary Venoocclusive Disease
Inflammatory Disorders of the Pulmonary Vessels
Collagen vascular diseases
Drug-induced lung disease

OBLITERATION OF LUNG PARENCHYMA WITH LOSS OF VASCULAR SURFACE AREA
Emphysema
Alpha-1-Antitrypsin Deficiency
Diffuse Bronchiectasis/Cystic Fibrosis
Diffuse Interstitial Diseases
Autoimmune disease (systemic lupus, rheumatoid arthritis, polymyositis, mixed connective tissue disease)
Tuberculosis
Chronic fungal infection
Sarcoidosis
Idiopathic pulmonary fibrosis
Histiocytosis X
Pneumoconiosis
Adult respiratory distress syndrome (ARDS)
Hypersensitivity pneumonitis

---

lung disease. Dyspnea is almost always present, a consequence of underlying lung disease. Fatigue is another common nonspecific complaint. Cough and atypical chest pain may be noted. Lower extremity edema is a usual finding with right-sided heart failure. Palpitations are common and are often caused by atrial arrhythmias.

Examination of the heart usually reveals an accentuated pulmonic component of the second heart sound indicating pulmonary hypertension. A right-sided S_3 gallop may be heard. A systolic murmur of tricuspid regurgitation or a diastolic murmur of pulmonic regurgitation may be present. Palpation may reveal a right ventricular lift and possibly a palpable pulmonary artery pulsation. Examination of the neck veins reveals an elevated jugular venous pressure. A prominent venous A wave can be seen with right heart failure, and a large V wave would indicate tricuspid regurgitation (see Chap-

ter 4). If right-sided failure is present, an inspiratory rise in the jugular venous pressure (Kussmaul's sign) is possible. Owing to the increased right-sided venous pressures, there may be enlargement of the liver and lower extremity edema. The pulmonary examination varies depending on the underlying disease. A near-normal examination does not exclude cor pulmonale. Abnormal lung sounds, hyperinflated lungs, and change in heart position can make the cardiac examination challenging.

Management
Laboratory Studies

Lung disease that progresses to the point of causing cor pulmonale usually is evident as an abnormal finding on chest x-ray. The x-ray findings of pulmonary hypertension and cor pulmonale are enlargement of the right ventricle and the central pulmonary arteries. The lack of vessel markings at the periphery of the lung fields in

contrast to the large central vessels produces the classic "pruned tree" appearance.

The electrocardiogram (ECG) is a nonspecific test for cor pulmonale. The classic findings of right ventricular hypertrophy and P-pulmonale are reviewed in Chapter 5. Remember that the absence of right ventricular hypertrophy on ECG does not rule out cor pulmonale. Atrial arrhythmias including atrial flutter, fibrillation, and multifocal atrial tachycardia are common. These arrhythmias are at times aggravated by treatment of chronic lung disease with beta-agonists and theophylline. On the other hand, successful treatment of the lung disease tends to improve arrhythmia control, and improving oxygenation and pulmonary mechanics is the most important antiarrhythmic strategy.

The echocardiogram is an invaluable tool for assessing right ventricular and atrial size and function. Right side chamber enlargement is the usual finding in cor pulmonale. RV wall thickness is difficult to assess, and the echocardiogram is not reliable for diagnosing or excluding RV hypertrophy. Mild tricuspid regurgitation is common when there is pulmonary hypertension. Doppler techniques allow estimation of pulmonary artery pressure. The echocardiogram is equally important in screening for nonpulmonary causes of pulmonary hypertension and right ventricular failure (e.g., occult mitral stenosis). In many patients with advanced lung disease, especially emphysema, cardiac structures may be difficult to visualize. The transesophageal echocardiogram may improve visualization but is potentially risky in patients with compromised lung function.

Radionuclide angiography using the first-pass technique can give an accurate right ventricular ejection fraction. Radiotracers can also be used to measure right ventricular wall thickness and volume.

Right heart catheterization is the only direct way to measure pulmonary artery pressure, cardiac output, and pulmonary capillary wedge pressure. This also allows the calculation of pulmonary vascular resistance. The information obtained is useful diagnostically and also can help in assessing the response to treatment acutely or chronically. The gradient between pulmonary artery diastolic pressure and pulmonary capillary wedge pressure (transpulmonary gradient) is elevated if lung disease is the cause of pulmonary hypertension. The pulmonary wedge pressure (equivalent to the left atrial pressure, see Chapter 2) is elevated, and the transpulmonary gradient is near normal if the cause of pulmonary hypertension is left heart disease (e.g., left ventricular failure or valvular disease).

Lung biopsy is occasionally needed to make a diagnosis of the underlying cause of cor pulmonale using transbronchial or open techniques.[1] Biopsy is most helpful in cases of pulmonary fibrosis, some connective tissue disorders, and in primary pulmonary hypertension.

Approach to the Workup. It is difficult to devise a single strategy for the workup of cor pulmonale because of the variety of lung diseases that can cause it. In addition to the above studies, many other tests can be helpful. In patients with airway or parenchymal disease, arterial blood gases, spirometry, lung volumes, and diffusing capacity can show the degree of impairment and possibly the cause of the impairment. Serologic testing for inflammatory or autoimmune disorders may be considered. Perfusion lung scanning or other tests for pulmonary emboli can be useful if no other obvious cause is suspected. If a patient has symptoms of sleep apnea, then a sleep study may be diagnostic. Obviously, a good history and physical examination are needed to focus the laboratory examination.

Treatment

The initial treatment of cor pulmonale is always aimed at reducing pulmonary hypertension. This strategy is also important in preventing the development of cor pulmonale in patients who have lung disease and early pulmonary hypertension but do not yet have right heart failure. Treatment of the underlying lung disease is important if a specific treatment is available. Many of these diseases unfortunately have no effective specific treatment, so the general approach described below applies. Improvement in oxygenation is of paramount importance, since most of these patients have some degree of hypoxia, and this must be the initial treatment. Secondary treatment is aimed at right-sided heart failure.

Improving Oxygenation. Patients with hypoxia should be treated with supplemental inhaled oxygen, with the goal of restoring the PaO_2 to ≥ 60 mm Hg. This must be done judiciously if there is concomitant hypercarbia and acidosis. Since chronic hypercarbia and acidosis depress the CO_2 respiratory drive, the main stimulus to respiration in these patients may be hypoxia. By improving the hypoxia too quickly, one can precipitate a worsening of respiratory depression, which may progress to apnea and death.

In addition to supplemental oxygen, it is important to make sure the oxygen can get to the alveoli and be absorbed into the blood. Inhaled bronchodilators are helpful in patients with a bronchospastic component to their disease. Theophylline can also relieve bronchospasm, as well as acting as a pulmonary vasodilator and as a direct stimulant to right ventricular function. Corticosteroids are useful in relieving bronchospasm and may also help treat some inflammatory lung conditions. Antibiotics treat infection and decrease secretions. Clearance of secretions is important and may be accomplished by endotracheal suctioning or by postural drainage. Avoidance of tobacco smoke and other inhaled irritants is imperative. Medications such as ben-

zodiazepines that depress respirations should be avoided if possible.

Treatment of Right Heart Failure

Diuretics decrease the volume of blood that passes through the pulmonary vasculature. This may lower pulmonary arterial pressure. Diuretics also relieve lower extremity edema and passive congestion of the liver. Isovolumic phlebotomy may be considered if the hematocrit is above 60%. This lowers viscosity and consequently improves flow through the pulmonary vasculature. This must be done cautiously and in small volumes of only 200 to 300 ml at a time. Microcytosis must be avoided (see Chapter 30).

Vasodilator therapy is of uncertain benefit in most patients with cor pulmonale but may be effective in a subset of patients with primary pulmonary hypertension. If the underlying disease cannot be improved, and if improved oxygenation does not relieve pulmonary hypertension, then vasodilators probably will not work. Nifedipine and diltiazem have been tried, but they must be given at much higher doses than are used for systemic hypertension. Hypotension may develop before adequate pulmonary vasodilation is achieved.

Digoxin is another medication of uncertain benefit. It is known to improve right ventricular function, but without improvement in pulmonary hypertension, it is unlikely to offer clinical benefit. For unclear reasons, patients with cor pulmonale seem to be more susceptible to digoxin toxicity.

The tachyarrhythmias of cor pulmonale, particularly atrial flutter and multifocal atrial tachycardia, are generally resistant to membrane-active antiarrhythmic agents. Rate control may be achieved with digoxin and verapamil (beta blockade is usually contraindicated by the lung disease). Cardioversion of atrial flutter may be considered if rate control is not possible, but maintenance of sinus rhythm is unlikely unless pulmonary function is improved. You must treat the lung disease to treat the arrhythmia.

Surgery

Surgical intervention should be considered for many situations. Patients with obstructive sleep apnea can benefit from removal of excess posterior pharyngeal tissue. Pulmonary embolectomy for acute, large emboli and pulmonary thromboendarterectomy for chronic pulmonary emboli are occasionally attempted. Single lung, double lung, and heart-lung transplantation is a consideration in selected patients with cor pulmonale. The most common diseases treated with transplantation are primary pulmonary hypertension, emphysema, idiopathic pulmonary fibrosis, and cystic fibrosis. The 5-year survival rate for lung transplantation is around 60%.[3]

ACUTE COR PULMONALE: PULMONARY EMBOLISM[6-15]

Pulmonary embolism (PE) is the most common cause of acute core pulmonale. Approximately 600,000 cases of PE are reported annually in the United States, and 150,000 are fatal.[1] PE is responsible for 5% of deaths in men 50 to 80 years old.[4] There is a slightly increased incidence of PE in men, especially in older age groups. The cumulative risk of having a pulmonary embolus is almost 11% in men by age 80.

Pulmonary embolism is a thromboembolic event, with the clot originating in the deep veins of the lower extremity. It is rarely caused by superficial thrombophlebitis or by thrombosis in the pelvic veins or upper extremities. Most who have phlebitis do not have embolism, as the inflamed vessel seems to hold the clot tightly. It is more common for asymptomatic phlebothrombosis to serve up the clot.

Thromboembolism originating from the heart is possible, especially in cases of atrial fibrillation or congestive heart failure. Other embolic sources such as air, bone marrow, fat, tumors, and amniotic fluid are rare causes of pulmonary emboli.

Pathophysiology

An embolus that travels into and obstructs a portion of the pulmonary circulation has several clinical consequences. Hemodynamically, there is a loss of vascular cross-sectional area and an increase in vascular resistance. As stated earlier, the pulmonary circulation is a circuit with low resistance and high capacitance. Small individual emboli may not cause an appreciable hemodynamic effect. However, multiple emboli or large emboli can increase resistance enough to cause right heart strain or even failure. Usually over 50% of the pulmonary circulation must be obstructed before there is a rise in pulmonary arterial pressure.[2]

From a respiratory standpoint, there is ventilation of nonperfused alveoli. The effect is an increase in dead space, causing hypoxemia. Unless the embolus is very large, patients generally do not have hypercarbia. In fact, many patients hyperventilate in response to hypoxemia and develop hypocarbia. Hypoxemia can further aggravate the situation by causing pulmonary vasoconstriction and worsening pulmonary hypertension.

Pulmonary infarction occurs in only half of those with pulmonary emboli. This is because there are several sources of oxygenation for lung tissue, and alternative sources can come into play when the pulmonary artery is obstructed. The bronchial artery circulation supplies collaterals to the obstructed area. There is some diffusion of oxygen from the airways. There can also be back diffusion of oxygen through the pulmonary veins. These mechanisms may not be effective in patients with other types of

lung or cardiac disease, who will be more likely to infarct lung tissue. Even small pulmonary emboli can be devastating in patients with already marginal lung function.

Deep Venous Thrombosis

Pulmonary emboli and deep venous thrombosis of the lower extremity can be considered elements of a single disease state. The risk factors that predispose to deep venous thrombosis are the same as those for pulmonary embolus. The primary risk factor is limb immobility in bedridden or wheelchair-bound patients and even in persons who sit for long periods (e.g., cross-country drivers.) A pulmonary embolus often occurs as a result of an illness or operation that necessitates being in bed for a long period. Trauma to a limb not only requires bed rest, but also may stimulate thrombosis. Old age, tobacco, and oral contraceptives also increase the risk of deep venous thrombosis and therefore pulmonary embolus.

Clinical Presentation

The clinical diagnosis of pulmonary embolism can be difficult to make (Box 35-2). Small pulmonary emboli produce few symptoms or vague and nonspecific symptoms. The diagnosis should be considered in a patient with unexplained dyspnea, tachycardia, atrial arrhythmia, or fever. PE (or another cause of hypoxia) should be considered in an elderly, bedridden person with a change in mental status. New atrial flutter may be the only sign of PE.

Larger pulmonary emboli that cause a pulmonary infarction often cause pleuritic chest pain, dyspnea, or hemoptysis. If the embolus occludes more than 50% of the pulmonary circulation, the patient may present with shock.

BOX 35-2

CONDITIONS THAT MAY BE CONFUSED WITH PULMONARY EMBOLISM

Myocardial infarction
Pneumonia
Exacerbation of lung disease
Congestive heart failure
Aortic dissection
Pericarditis/tamponade
Tumors of the lung and mediastinum
Musculoskeletal pain
Pneumothorax
Anxiety
Acute dementia (a reflection of hypoxia)

Although rarely diagnostic, the physical examination may provide supporting evidence or prognostic information. There may be a pleural rub or decreased breath sounds over a periinfarct pleural effusion. Examination of the neck may reveal elevated jugular venous pressure with a large venous A wave if the patient is in normal sinus rhythm. If there is tricuspid regurgitation, large V waves may be present as well. Rarely, Kussmaul's sign can be seen. Cardiac examination may reveal a right ventricular lift, a right-sided S_3 and S_4, and a loud pulmonic second sound indicative of pulmonary hypertension. Occasionally a systolic flow murmur is produced by turbulent flow around an embolus in the proximal pulmonary circulation. The systolic murmur of tricuspid regurgitation may also be heard.

Management
Laboratory Studies (Table 35-1)

The chest x-ray is frequently normal. The classic appearance of a pulmonary infarct is a wedge-shaped infiltrate, but this is infrequently seen. There may be atelectasis or a small pleural effusion. The pulmonary artery and the right ventricle may appear enlarged. Comparison with a prior x-ray is usually necessary to detect such subtle findings.

Acute PE can cause a variety of ECG changes. These changes are usually transient, and the transient nature is the most important diagnostic feature. The most common ECG patterns are a large S wave in lead I with a large Q wave in lead III (S_1-Q3 pattern), rightward axis deviation, transient complete or incomplete right bundle branch block (a sign of RV overload), and T wave inversion in the right precordial leads. Other findings include clockwise rotation, left axis deviation, QR pattern in lead V_1, R wave > S wave in V_1, R/S in V_1 >1, staircase ascent of the ST segment in lead I or II, isolated ST elevation in lead III, ST elevation or depression in the right precordial leads, P pulmonale pattern (right atrial enlargement), sinus tachycardia, atrial arrhythmia, first-degree atrioventricular block, and nonspecific ST and T wave changes in the left precordial leads.

Blood Gases. Arterial blood gases may be normal with small pulmonary emboli, but with larger emboli or multiple small emboli PaO_2 is decreased. As a screening test, a normal PaO_2 makes a moderate to large PE unlikely. On the other hand, a low value does not make the diagnosis (it is a nonspecific finding). One must keep in mind the age of the patient and other lung problems when interpreting the PaO_2.

Lung mechanics are usually not affected by PE, and pulmonary function testing is not a part of the early workup.

D-dimer. This is a by-product of endogenous fibrinolysis, and its can be useful in the diagnosis of pulmonary embolus. Any condition that involves thrombosis and lysis may cause an elevation of D-dimer, and pulmonary embolus is one of these conditions. Since

many clinical conditions may cause elevation of D-dimer, the test lacks specificity for PE. However, it is a highly sensitive test; if it is negative (<500 ng/ml), the chance of PE is low. There are several assays for measuring D-dimer. The enzyme-linked immunoabsorbent assay (ELISA) is the most accurate, and currently is the only method that should be relied on for this purpose. Many hospitals do not use this method, so it is useful to check with the hospital laboratory before ordering and relying on the results of this test.

Ventilation-Perfusion Scan. The V/Q nuclear scan is a useful diagnostic test for pulmonary embolus. Often times, only the perfusion portion of the test is performed. Unless there is significant air space disease, the ventilation portion of the scan is unnecessary. These scans are usually interpreted in four possible ways: normal, low probability, intermediate (or indeterminate) probability, or high probability. A normal scan means that a pulmonary embolus is extremely unlikely. A high probability scan means there is a 95% chance of having a pulmonary embolus. A low probability scan indicates the patient has a 20% chance of having had a pulmonary embolus. Do not interpret a low probability scan as normal. Instead, the result should be interpreted in the context of the clinical presentation and other laboratory values. For example, a bedridden patient with suggestive symptoms, low Pa_{O_2} and a low or intermediate probability scan may be treated with heparin until other studies exclude the diagnosis (D-dimer or angiography).

Venous Studies. Lower extremity venous studies such as ultrasound or contrast venography can be a useful tool in the diagnosis of pulmonary embolus. Contrast venography is the gold standard for diagnosis of thrombi in the deep veins, but the test is seldom needed. Ultrasound is now the screening study of choice because it is noninvasive, does not involve contrast administration, and may be performed at the bedside if necessary. Used alone, a positive or negative study for venous thrombosis does not automatically establish or rule out PE, but it can be useful when considered with other study results. For example, a patient with a low-probability perfusion scan and a normal

| Table 35-1 | *Diagnostic Tests for Pulmonary Embolus (PE)* |

Test	Comments
Chest x-ray	Lacks sensitivity and specificity. Findings may include wedge-shaped infarct, lack of vessels in area of embolus, and enlarged pulmonary arteries and right ventricle. Most useful in ruling out other conditions.
Electrocardiography	Multiple potential findings, but all nondiagnostic. Transient nature of changes is an important feature and may help in diagnosis.
Arterial blood gases	Not very useful by itself, but hypoxemia is usual with a moderate PE.
D-dimer	Very sensitive, not specific (if it is negative, then chance of pulmonary embolus is low). Must use ELISA method.
Ventilation-perfusion lung scan	Normal scan means that PE is unlikely. High probability scan means pulmonary embolus is likely. Low or intermediate probability scans must be interpreted along with clinical suspicion and other tests.
Venous ultrasound	Highly sensitive for deep venous thrombosis. Remember that deep venous thrombosis and PE are part of the same disease process.
Pulmonary arteriogram	Gold standard for diagnosis of pulmonary embolus.
Spiral CT scan	Noninvasive, but requires contrast. Useful for larger emboli in the proximal pulmonary circulation.
Magnetic resonance imaging	Can be used to look for thromboemboli in the pulmonary circulation or for lower extremity clots. Cine-MRI can also assess right ventricular function.
Echocardiography	Rapid bedside test. May be the only test possible in critically ill patients. Presence of RV dilation portends poorer prognosis. This finding may indicate a need for thrombolytic therapy.

ultrasound study probably does not have PE. It should be noted that all of the lower extremity studies may miss pelvic vein thrombus; if you suspect it, let the radiologist know before the venogram so that extra views are obtained.

Pulmonary Angiography. Contrast pulmonary angiography remains the gold standard in the diagnosis of pulmonary embolus. The test is invasive and requires contrast administration. With the other diagnostic studies available, it is rarely needed. It is used when other tests are inconclusive or even negative in the face of a high clinical suspicion of pulmonary embolus. It is especially useful for identifying small peripheral emboli. Although invasive, it can be performed in acutely ill patients. Those with chronic pulmonary hypertension, and particularly Eisenmenger's syndrome, have a higher risk of complications with pulmonary angiography. There is a definite learning curve for both the performance and reading of pulmonary angiograms, and it should be done in centers with experience.

Other Diagnostic Studies. Spiral or high-resolution CT scanning with contrast is another relatively new test for pulmonary embolus. It is best suited for identifying emboli in the large proximal pulmonary arteries; it may miss smaller, more peripheral emboli.

Magnetic resonance imaging (MRI) can identify emboli within the pulmonary vascular tree and can also assess right ventricular function, which may be important in deciding proper treatment. MRI has also been used to identify thrombus in the deep veins. These methods are currently not in wide clinical use.

Echocardiography. The echocardiogram may help with diagnosis, prognosis, and therapeutic choices. Those with cardiogenic shock due to pulmonary embolus usually have evidence of acute right ventricular pressure overload with a dilated and hypocontractile right ventricle. Because it can be done quickly and safely at the bedside, an echocardiogram may be the only test available for a hemodynamically unstable patient who is suspected of having PE. Those with PE who are in shock have a high mortality. Even in patients with stable hemodynamics, right ventricular dysfunction is a negative prognostic factor. Echocardiography is also useful in ruling out other causes of hemodynamic collapse such as myocardial infarction, aortic dissection, pericarditis, and tamponade.

Approach to the Workup. All these diagnostic studies need not be performed in each patient. Because each case is different, there are no set guidelines for which tests and how many tests are necessary to make or refute the diagnosis. For a bedridden patient with a change in condition but little else to suggest PE, you might be satisfied after a single test such as a normal ventilation-perfusion scan or perhaps even a normal Pao$_2$. However, if the clinical suspicion of PE is high and screening diagnostic studies are indeterminate, then you may pursue other tests, even pulmonary arteriography.

One useful initial strategy is to obtain a ventilation-perfusion study along with a D-dimer (ELISA). If these are both normal, then pulmonary embolism is unlikely. If these are indeterminate, then adding lower extremity venous ultrasound can be helpful. Patients who have a clinical history suspicious for pulmonary embolism with a documented deep venous thrombosis should be treated for pulmonary embolism. Other supporting studies may not be necessary, since both conditions require the same type of anticoagulation therapy.

Therapy

Anticoagulation. Anticoagulation is the mainstay of therapy for thromboembolic disease. The risks of bleeding and the usual contraindications for anticoagulation must be considered before proceeding with anticoagulation. Anticoagulation is accomplished acutely with intravenous heparin followed by several months of oral warfarin.

The usual dosing regimen for heparin is a bolus dose of 5000 to 10,000 U followed by a continuous infusion, which is adjusted at 4- to 6-hour intervals to maintain a partial thromboplastin time (PTT) of 60 to 80 seconds. Patients with large PE often are resistant to heparin, and this resistance diminishes over 2 to 4 days. Remember that the effects of heparin can be immediately reversed with protamine sulfate if life-threatening hemorrhage develops. The usual dose of protamine is 50 mg given slowly over 10 to 30 minutes (to reverse a bolus dose of heparin, give 1 mg protamine for each 100 mg heparin). Life-threatening allergic reactions are possible with protamine and are more common in diabetic patients who have been treated with NPH insulin.

Once anticoagulation with heparin is achieved, warfarin is begun. Warfarin may take 5 days to reach optimal anticoagulant activity, and overlap may shorten length of stay. Another reason to overlap heparin and warfarin therapy is a transient procoagulant effect of warfarin, which is blocked by heparin.

It may take several days or even weeks after that to adjust the dose of warfarin. The usual goal is an international normalized ratio (INR) of 2.0-3.0. Remember that heparin can prolong the INR slightly (by about 0.5), so this must be taken into account when stopping heparin therapy.

The optimal duration of anticoagulation is unknown, but most experts recommend at least 3 months and possibly 6 months of therapy. Patients with recurrent pulmonary emboli probably require lifelong anticoagulation.

Low-molecular-weight heparin has been shown in several studies to be just as safe and effective as unfrac-

tionated heparin in the treatment of venous thromboembolic disease. Low-molecular-weight heparin offers the advantages of being administered subcutaneously, not requiring frequent PTT checks, and causing less heparin-induced thrombocytopenia. This may offer cost advantages and may enable patients to leave the hospital sooner. It is now accepted therapy for venous thrombosis, and we anticipate that studies in progress will prove its utility for PE as well.

Thrombolytic Therapy. For patients who present in cardiogenic shock or with hemodynamic instability, thrombolysis can be life saving. These patients have a mortality rate greater than 30% if treated with anticoagulation alone. One must always keep in mind the risks of bleeding and the contraindications to thrombolysis when deciding on this therapy. Duration of symptoms should not necessarily be a deterrent to the use of thrombolysis, since it has been shown to be effective even 2 weeks after onset of symptoms.

The best choice of a thrombolytic agent remains uncertain. Various studies have used each of the available agents and have shown some benefit. The only currently approved regimen is recombinant tissue plasminogen activator (rt-PA) 100 mg administered as a continuous drip over 2 hours. Heparin is used as an adjunct to thrombolysis, and this must be followed by long-term oral anticoagulation. Patients with very small pulmonary emboli are unlikely to benefit from thrombolytic therapy.

An intermediate group with normal hemodynamics but an embolus large enough to cause right ventricular overload as seen on the echocardiogram may benefit from thrombolysis. There are no data from clinical trials to support the use of rt-PA in such patients. If future studies prove a benefit with thrombolysis, the echocardiogram will become an important part of the workup of seriously ill patients with PE.

Inferior Vena Cava (IVC) Filters. IVC filters are used to prevent large emboli from passing up through the inferior vena cava and into the lungs. They have been used for both primary and secondary prevention of PE in patients with documented lower extremity deep venous thrombosis. The usual indications are multiple emboli despite anticoagulation, critically ill patients for whom a PE would be deadly, or in patients with PE and a contraindication to anticoagulation.

Filters decrease the risk of PE but may provoke recurrent deep venous thrombosis. Placement of a filter does not obviate the need for anticoagulation. As a rule, a patient who receives a filter because of a contraindication for anticoagulation should be periodically reassessed to decide if the contraindication has resolved. Often, a contraindication such as a gastrointestinal hemorrhage or recent surgery may be temporary. Filters should not be thought of as an alternative to anticoagulation, but

as an adjunct to anticoagulation, and in some cases, a temporizing measure.

Embolectomy. Thrombolysis or anticoagulation is at times contraindicated or ineffective. Interventional radiologists are exploring techniques to break up or remove a clot through a pulmonary artery catheter. The pulmonary artery catheter can also be used to deliver thrombolytic drugs locally and at a lower than systemic dose. Surgical embolectomy is also used in rare circumstances to remove the thrombus.

Prevention

Patients at risk for PE should be identified, and measures must be taken to decrease the chances of a pulmonary embolus. Clinical trials have shown that prophylactic administration of either unfractionated or low-molecular-weight heparin lowers the risk of PE in patients having hip or knee replacement and for those having high-risk abdominal or pelvic surgery. There is consensus agreement that most patients having surgery should receive prophylaxis while bedridden. Those with obesity or cancer are at higher risk.

Patients with specific medical conditions are at higher risk for venous thrombosis. Although no data from clinical trials have proved a need for heparin prophylaxis, observational data support its use for patients on extended bed rest who are elderly, who are in the intensive care unit, who have congestive heart failure, who are obese, or who have a history of venous disease.

In addition to anticoagulation, sequential compression stockings are helpful in bedridden patients. If the immobility is expected to be prolonged, then long-term oral anticoagulation with warfarin can be considered. Early mobilization of patients is an important part of prevention.

An IVC filter may be considered as prophylaxis for a patient with recent PE or venous thrombus who must have a surgical procedure that would increase the risk of perioperative PE.

PRIMARY PULMONARY HYPERTENSION[16-18]

Primary pulmonary hypertension (PPH) is a sustained elevation of pulmonary arterial pressure without an identifiable cause. It is a diagnosis of exclusion, made after other causes of pulmonary hypertension have been ruled out. The National Institutes of Health diagnostic criteria include a mean pulmonary artery pressure greater than 25 mm Hg at rest (30 mm Hg with exertion), with exclusion of valvular heart disease, myocardial diseases, congenital heart disease, pulmonary parenchymal disease, connective tissue diseases, and thromboembolic disease. Other conditions such as portal hypertension, HIV disease, cocaine use, and weight-loss drugs (fenfluramine, dexfenfluramine, and amphet-

amines) have been implicated as causes of some cases of PPH.

There appears to be a genetic predisposition, since conditions reported to cause PPH do so in only a small percentage of the population. In addition, the disease has a familial form that is inherited as an autosomal dominant trait with incomplete penetrance.

The estimated incidence of PPH is 1 or 2 cases per million people. Most patients are 10 to 40 years old, and women predominate. The disease can progress to death within 2 to 3 years of diagnosis. However, patients often have had symptoms for several years before a diagnosis is made. Deaths may result from cor pulmonale and right heart failure, pneumonia, or pulmonary embolus. Sudden death is common.

Pathophysiology

PPH is a disease of the small pulmonary arteries and arterioles. Several pathologic changes have been noted in biopsy specimens or at autopsy, including medial hypertrophy, intimal proliferation and fibrosis, necrotizing arteritis, formation of plexiform lesions, and in situ thrombosis. These lesions may be adjacent to normal or near-normal vessels. The diagnosis is certain if all these features are present; however, often there are only one or a few of these findings.

In addition to structural changes, functional changes may occur in the pulmonary vascular bed, such as altered production of or response to endogenous vasoconstrictors and vasodilators. The net effect is vasoconstriction, loss of vascular surface area, and thrombosis in situ.

Clinical Presentation

As with other causes of cor pulmonale, the initial symptoms are relatively nonspecific. Dyspnea, fatigue, dizziness, syncope, chest pain, palpitations, orthopnea, cough, and hoarseness have all been described. Syncope and dizziness are usually exertional and are often the first symptoms that bring patients to medical attention. Keep a high index of suspicion for this disease in young female patients with these symptoms. Reynaud's phenomenon is present in 10% of cases.

The physical findings are those of cor pulmonale and right heart failure (described above). The major difference is that the physical examination is usually unobscured by changes related to other cardiac or pulmonary conditions.

Management
Laboratory Findings

PPH is a diagnosis of exclusion. It is important to exclude lung or heart disease as causes of right heart failure. Chest x-ray shows the typical changes described for pulmonary hypertension but without evidence of parenchymal disease. The ECG shows right ventricular hypertrophy. Pulmonary function testing is used to rule out lung disease. Echocardiography is useful in ruling out other causes and defining the extent of right heart failure. Perfusion lung scanning, as well as the other diagnostic tests for pulmonary embolism, can be used to rule out recurrent PE as a cause of pulmonary hypertension. Right heart catheterization is useful to accurately assess not only pulmonary artery pressures, but also response to treatment. Biopsy of the lung is diagnostic when the classic features described previously are seen.

Treatment

PPH has no known cure. Therapy is aimed at improving symptoms and functional capacity and at prolonging survival.

Vasodilators. Because vasoconstriction is such a prominent component of the disease, vasodilation is the key to treatment. Among the conventional systemic vasodilators, the calcium channel blocking agents, nifedipine and diltiazem, have been shown to be the most effective in pulmonary hypertension. The doses of these medicines necessary to relieve pulmonary hypertension are much higher than conventional doses used for systemic hypertension.

Not all patients respond favorably to vasodilator therapy. Before committing a patient to long-term vasodilators, a favorable response should be established, which can be achieved with use of right heart catheterization. Initial hemodynamics are measured, then the patient is challenged with a short-acting, potent vasodilator such as inhaled nitrous oxide, intravenous adenosine, or intravenous epoprostenol (prostacyclin). If pulmonary artery pressure decreases and cardiac output increases, and no significant change occurs in the systemic pressure or oxygenation, then a favorable response to oral vasodilators is expected. However, if pulmonary artery pressure increases or remains the same, systemic pressure falls dangerously, cardiac output decreases, or oxygenation worsens, then vasodilator therapy will not help. Vasodilation may aggravate hypoxemia if the vessels that dilate supply poorly functioning areas of lung, thus shunting blood supply from more normal regions.

Oral vasodilator therapy is adjusted to symptoms and clinical status. Often, a repeat right heart catheterization is useful to confirm clinical findings and assess whether medications are maximized.

Epoprostenol (prostacyclin) is useful not only as a diagnostic vasodilator, but also as an agent for chronic use. It must be administered by continuous intravenous infusion because of its short half-life. Epoprostenol is a potent pulmonary vasodilator, and it inhibits both platelet aggregation and the proliferation of vascular smooth muscle. Even patients who do not respond fa-

vorably to the short-term vasodilator challenge may have a good long-term result with epoprostenol as a result of its other actions. Tolerance to epoprostenol can be overridden by increasing doses. Although it improves symptoms (and possibly survival), epoprostenol has the disadvantage of requiring a constant infusion pump. One of its uses has been as a bridge to lung transplantation. Analogues of epoprostenol that can be given orally are being sought.

Since one of the prominent pathologic features of PPH is thrombosis in situ, anticoagulation with warfarin is recommended as part of the therapy. This has been shown to improve survival. The dose of warfarin is adjusted to achieve an INR of approximately 2.0.

Transplantation. Lung transplantation and heart-lung transplantation are therapeutic options for patients with end-stage primary pulmonary hypertension. This is generally a last resort and is used only if other treatments are failing. For unclear reasons, the mortality rate of lung transplant is higher with PPH than with other illnesses. The 1-year survival rate is approximately 65% to 70%, and the 5-year survival rate is below 60%. It is a therapy of last resort. After transplantation, right ventricular hypertrophy usually regresses, and heart failure improves. Although rejection of the transplanted lung is possible (bronchiolitis obliterans), a recurrence of PPH in the transplanted lung has not been reported.

REFERENCES

1. Fishman AP, Palevsky HI: Pulmonary hypertension and chronic cor pulmonale, *Heart Dis Stroke* 2:335, 1993.
2. Wiedemann HP, Matthay RA: Cor pulmonale in chronic obstructive pulmonary disease: circulatory pathophysiology and management, *Clin Chest Med* 11:523, 1990.
3. White J, Bullock RE, Hudgson P, Gibson FJ: Neuromuscular disease, respiratory failure, and cor pulmonale, *Postgrad Med J* 68:820, 1992.
4. Calverley PM, Howatson R, Flenley DC, Lamb D: Clinicopathological correlations in cor pulmonale, *Thorax* 47:494, 1992.
5. Fishman AP: Pulmonary hypertension: beyond vasodilator therapy, *N Engl J Med* 338:321, 1998.
6. Goldhaber SZ: Pulmonary embolism, *N Engl J Med* 339:93, 1998.
7. Goldhaber SZ: Pulmonary embolism thrombolysis: broadening the paradigm, *Circulation* 96:716, 1997.
8. Hansson PO, Welin L, Tibblin G, Eriksson H: Deep vein thrombosis and pulmonary embolism in the general population, *Arch Intern Med* 157:1665, 1997.
9. Kasper W, Konstantinides S, Geibel A, et al: Management strategies and determinants of outcome in acute major pulmonary embolism: results of a multicenter registry, *J Am Coll Cardiol* 30:1165, 1997.
10. PIOPED Investigators: Value of ventilation-perfusion scan in acute pulmonary embolism: results of the prospective investigation of pulmonary embolism diagnosis (PIOPED), *JAMA* 263:2753, 1990.
11. ACCP Consensus Committee on Pulmonary Embolism: Opinions regarding the diagnosis and management of venous thromboembolic disease, *Chest* 113:499, 1998.
12. Simonneau G, Sors H, Charbonnier B, et al: A comparison of low-molecular-weight heparin with unfractionated heparin for acute pulmonary embolism, *N Engl J Med* 337:663, 1997.
13. Weitz JI: Low-molecular-weight heparins, *N Engl J Med* 337:688, 1997.
14. The Columbus Investigators: Low-molecular-weight heparin in the treatment of patients with venous thromboembolism, *N Engl J Med* 337:657, 1997.
15. Decousus H, Leizorovicz A, Parent F, et al: A clinical trial of vena caval filters in the prevention of pulmonary embolism in patients with proximal deep vein thrombosis: prevention du Risque d'Embolie Pulmonaire par Interruption Cave Study Group, *N Engl J Med* 338:409, 1998.
16. Rubin LJ: Primary pulmonary hypertension, *N Engl J Med* 336:111, 1997.
17. McLaughlin VV, Genthner DE, Panella MM, Rich S: Reduction in pulmonary vascular resistance with long-term epoprostenol (prostacyclin) therapy in primary pulmonary hypertension, *N Engl J Med* 338:273, 1998.
18. Maraes D, Loscalzo J: Pulmonary hypertension: newer concepts in diagnosis and management, *Clin Cardiol* 20:676, 1997.

36 Endocrine Disorders and Cardiovascular Disease

Robert C. Bussing
George J. Taylor

DIABETES
Epidemiology[1-5]

The major cause of morbidity and mortality in diabetes is atherosclerosis and its protean manifestations. Myocardial infarction, stroke, and limb loss are all common sequelae of large vessel atherosclerosis. Most deaths in non-insulin-dependent diabetes (NIDDM) are caused by myocardial infarction. With insulin-dependent diabetes (IDDM), younger patients die of renal disease and its complications, and older patients of cardiovascular disease. Coronary artery disease (CAD) is two to four times more common in the diabetic population. Myocardial infarction (MI) has a more complicated course in diabetic patients, with higher mortality and rates of congestive heart failure. Reinfarction is more common, and the results of revascularization are less favorable. More severe and extensive CAD is seen in diabetic patients even though the plaque itself is the same histologically. The protective effects of estrogens are lost in diabetic women, and the MI rate is similar to that of males. The risk of peripheral vascular disease is approximately five times higher in the diabetic population than in the nondiabetic population. Stroke is likewise two to three times higher in diabetic patients.

In addition to atherosclerosis, two other cardiac illnesses merit the consideration of the practitioner: cardiac autonomic neuropathy (which is a major risk factor for so-called silent myocardial infarction and creates an increased risk of sudden cardiac death) and diabetic cardiomyopathy.

Pathophysiology[6-9]

Conventional risk factors for CAD include age, cigarette smoking, hyperlipidemia, hypertension, obesity, and male sex, in addition to diabetes. Diabetes appears to be a particularly potent risk factor. For example, left main coronary disease is more common with diabetes. Generally, the extent of atherosclerosis in diabetic patients is increased when compared with age- and sex-matched controls and after correcting for other risk factors.

Hyperglycemia

Hyperglycemia itself is probably atherogenic. The mechanism is uncertain. Glycosylation of proteins or lipoproteins in the arterial wall, or the toxic effects of hyperglycemia on endothelial function, may have a role. Since uncontrolled diabetes aggravates dyslipidemia and hypertension, it is difficult to sort out the relative contribution of hyperglycemia to atherosclerosis. A WHO Multinational Study[10] published in 1983 found no relation between length and severity of diabetes and subsequent MI. Other studies published since have refuted this. Microvascular disease (including retinopathy and nephropathy) is clearly related to the duration and severity of diabetes. Uncertainty about the relationship of macrovascular disease to glucose control suggests a different pathophysiology.

Hyperinsulinemia

The combination of insulin resistance, hyperinsulinemia, obesity, hypertension, and dyslipidemia (elevated triglycerides and total cholesterol and low HDL cholesterol) has been called *syndrome X*.[11] You may assume that most of your diabetic and hypertensive patients with android obesity have syndrome X, and with it, increased cardiovascular risk (Fig. 36-1).[12] It is a common syndrome in primary care practice.

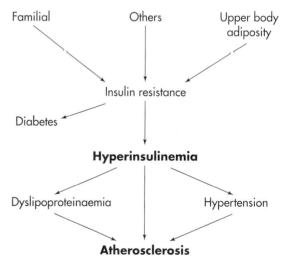

FIG. 36-1
The relationships between hyperinsulinemia, other cardiovascular risk factors, and atherosclerosis.

From Stout RW: *Diabetes and atherosclerosis,* Dordrecht, The Netherlands, 1992, Wolters Kluwer.

Hyperinsulinemia is defined as an inappropriately high insulin level for a given blood glucose, and *insulin resistance* as a reduced effect of insulin at the cellular level. Insulin has a number of vascular effects.[11] It is a growth factor and probably causes smooth muscle cell proliferation in the arterial media. It has a vasoconstricting effect and raises blood pressure. It also blunts lipoprotein lipase (LPL) activity in endothelial cells. Reduced LPL activity is associated with high triglycerides and low HDL cholesterol (see Chapter 12).

Hyperlipidemia

Lipid abnormalities are common in both IDDM and NIDDM and depend on the degree of control of the diabetes[12] (Table 36-1). Primary lipid abnormalities can exist in the diabetic population just as in the nondiabetic population, but some lipid abnormalities are specific to the diabetic state.[13] Poorly controlled insulin-dependent, type I diabetes leads to reduced activity of lipoprotein lipase, required for catabolism of VLDL (see Chapter 12). There is marked elevation of triglycerides and depressed HDL cholesterol. As glucose control improves, LPL efficiency increases, triglycerides fall, and HDL rises.

Uncontrolled non-insulin-dependent, type II diabetes has an adverse effect on reverse cholesterol transport, depressing HDL levels. The patient usually is obese and has overproduction of VLDL and elevated triglycerides.

Both forms of diabetes may affect LDL cholesterol. LDL catabolism is slowed with poor glycemic control, leading to higher levels of LDL. Furthermore, oxidized LDL levels tend to be elevated with poor control. Diabetes leads to increased amounts of smaller and denser LDL, and this type of LDL is more atherogenic. Glycosylation of LDL may reduce its clearance.

With the development of diabetic nephropathy, the lipid abnormalities of the nephrotic syndrome evolve. Total cholesterol, LDL, and VLDL are further elevated.

A patient with type 2 diabetes and no history of MI has a risk of MI that is similar to the risk of *reinfarction* in nondiabetic patients with prior MI.[14] That is the rationale for applying the principles of secondary prevention of MI to all with diabetes (see Chapter 12). That is, an argument can be made for using drug therapy to reduce LDL cholesterol to less than 100 mg/dL in all patients with diabetes, although this approach has not been tested in clinical trails. Correcting hypertriglyceridemia is important as well, the first steps being control of hyperglycemia and weight loss.

Hypertension

Elevated blood pressure compounds the effects of diabetes on the heart and vascular system. Control of hypertension thus becomes even more important if it is complicated by diabetes (see Chapter 31). Two consistent features seem to be present in hypertensive diabetics: increased plasma volume and increased vascular resistance. These two factors provide the rationale for treating hypertensive diabetic patients. All the commonly used antihypertensive drugs may be used, but there are relative advantages and disadvantages (Table 36-2).

| Table 36-1 | Changes in Serum Lipids and Lipoprotein Levels in Diabetes in Either Good or Poor Glycemic Control |

	Insulin-Dependent Diabetes		Non-Insulin-Dependent Diabetes	
	Good Control	**Bad Control**	**Good Control**	**Bad Control**
Serum triglycerides	N	↑↑↑	↑	↑↑↑
Serum cholesterol	↓	↑	↑ (or N)	↑
VLDL	N	↑	↑	↑↑
LDL	↓	↑	N	↑
HDL	↑	↓	↓ (or N)	↓
Apolipoprotein B	↓	↓	N	↑
Apolipoprotein A₁	↑	↓	↓ (or N)	↓

From Trimble ER, McDowell FW: Lipid metabolism and its disorders in diabetes mellitus. *Diabetes and atherosclerosis,* Dordrecht, The Netherlands, 1992, Wolters Kluwer.
N, Same range as nondiabetic subjects.

Table 36-2	Advantages and Disadvantages of Antihypertensive Drugs in Diabetes

Drug	Advantages	Disadvantages
Thiazide diuretics	Combat hypervolemia Synergistic with other agents Inexpensive, usually once daily	May worsen glycemic control May exacerbate hyperlipidemia Electrolyte abnormalities
Beta-blockers	Cardioprotective: reduce the incidence of sudden death and myocardial infarction Inexpensive older agents, once or twice daily dosing	May have adverse effects on lipids May slow insulin release Impotency May reduce peripheral blood flow
Angiotensin-converting enzyme (ACE) inhibitors	Renal protective: reduced intraglomerular pressures, reduced proteinuria Useful in heart failure Insulin sensitivity increased	May induce renal failure if there is renal artery stenosis Hyperkalemia is possible Expensive
Calcium channel blockers	No deleterious effects on organ blood flow Effective in elderly patients with stiff arteries No adverse effect on glucose or lipids Once daily administration	More expensive May increase the risk of myocardial infarction (short-acting nifedipine) May aggravate heart failure or heart block (diltiazem or verapamil) Edema
Angiotensin blocking agents	Same as ACE inhibitors Do not cause cough	Expensive Have not yet proven renal protective or beneficial in heart failure Hyperkalemia
Alpha-blockers	No adverse effects on lipids or glucose control May enhance organ blood flow	Orthostatic hypotension Incontinence in women

The effects of various antihypertensive agents on glucose and lipid metabolism is a concern of practitioners who manage hypertension in diabetic patients. Diuretics and beta-blockers can have adverse effects on both lipids and glucose, although the effects have been minor. The overstated risk of these compounds has reduced their usage. This is unfortunate because the cardioprotective effects of beta-blockers apply to diabetic patients.[15]

Angiotensin-converting enzyme (ACE) inhibitors have beneficial effects on renal function in diabetics with negligible effect on lipids. ACE inhibition has also been associated with increased survival in congestive heart failure patients and after MI. Clearly these compounds have been shown to have beneficial effects in diabetic patients. The calcium channel blockers have been extensively studied and are effective antihypertensives, although short-acting dihydropiridines may increase the risk of MI (see Chapter 31).[16]

Clinical Features of Arteriosclerotic Heart Disease in Diabetes

The historical presentation of a diabetic patient with coronary artery disease in most cases is similar to that of a nondiabetic patient, although there are some differences. Because of autonomic dysfunction and nociceptive dysfunction, silent MI is more common in a diabetic patient. Ischemic cardiomyopathy may occur with no prior history to indicate CAD. Be alert for atypical symptoms of ischemia: vague "gastrointestinal" complaints, exertional dyspnea, or exercise-induced fatigue. Similarly, in a diabetic patient with known CAD, the absence of clinical symptoms does not imply a stable condition. A survey for symptoms is worthwhile but may give a false sense of security.

ECG changes in a diabetic patient may be present without an associated clinical history to indicate CAD. A follow-up ECG should be periodically obtained to be sure no new Q waves have developed. Exercise stress

testing and pharmacologic stress testing are appropriate in the investigation of a diabetic patient with suspected coronary artery disease. These do not require special preparation or precautions because of the diabetes (see Chapters 6 and 9).

Diagnostic coronary angiography does require some special precautions in diabetic patients. Renal function should be monitored if contrast media is injected, even if renal function is normal. Hydration is important to help prevent renal toxicity. Avoiding hypertonic contrast agents and pretreating with theophylline lower the risk of renal toxicity in this setting (see Chapter 10).

Management of Coronary Artery Disease in Diabetic Patients

Diabetes does not alter the treatment of acute MI. Thrombolytic therapy is appropriate, although in-hospital and 5-year mortality are higher.[17, 18] This may be the result of more extensive CAD and more rapid progression of disease in diabetic patients. There is no increase in bleeding complications with thrombolysis.

After MI, diabetic patients do show benefits from long-term beta-blocker and aspirin therapy. Some believe that the dose of aspirin needs to be higher for diabetic subjects (160 mg rather than 85 mg daily).

The medical treatment of angina pectoris (see Chapter 13) is minimally influenced by diabetes. Beta-blockers can mask hypoglycemic symptoms and should be used with caution by insulin-dependent patients with a history of hypoglycemia. However, long-term safety and cardioprotective effects of beta-blockers have been established, and they are not contraindicated.[15]

Coronary bypass surgery is superior to angioplasty for diabetic patients with multivessel CAD[19] (see Chapter 13). With bypass surgery there is lower mortality, less perioperative infarction, and a reduced need for future revascularization. Single-vessel CAD may be treated with angioplasty, although some have found a slightly higher risk of restenosis.

Cardiac Denervation Syndrome

Autonomic neuropathy may cause nociceptive dysfunction, masking the pain of myocardial ischemia with many possible consequences (Box 36-1). There is no specific treatment, but recognition of this problem should increase vigilance in those caring for diabetic patients. In the earlier stages of diabetes, parasympathetic activity is reduced, leading to resting tachycardia or loss of sinus arrhythmia[20] (see Chapter 2). Later, sympathetic innervation is impaired, and heart rate falls. The neuropathy tends to parallel the severity and the length of diabetes. Microalbuminuria may be a marker of neuropathy, as they often coexist.

Diagnostic criteria are summarized in Table 36-3. Two of these features are necessary for establishing a diagnosis of autonomic neuropathy. Heart rate variability

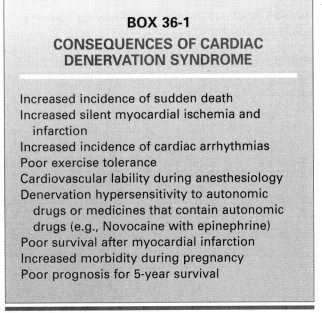

BOX 36-1
CONSEQUENCES OF CARDIAC DENERVATION SYNDROME

Increased incidence of sudden death
Increased silent myocardial ischemia and infarction
Increased incidence of cardiac arrhythmias
Poor exercise tolerance
Cardiovascular lability during anesthesiology
Denervation hypersensitivity to autonomic drugs or medicines that contain autonomic drugs (e.g., Novocaine with epinephrine)
Poor survival after myocardial infarction
Increased morbidity during pregnancy
Poor prognosis for 5-year survival

From Pfeiffer M, Schumer M: Cardiac denervation syndrome. In Lebovitz HE, editor: *Therapy for diabetes mellitus and related disorders*, ed 3, Alexandria, Va, 1998, American Diabetes Association.

is measured while the patient breathes at a fixed rate of five to six breaths/min for 5 minutes. The normal variability is >10 beats/min. The Valsalva maneuver is performed by having a patient blow against a standard pressure. A ratio is formulated comparing the longest R-R after Valsalva to the shortest R-R during Valsalva. The ratio should be greater than 1:1.

Be mindful that patients with cardiac denervation have an increased risk for silent ischemia. Identification of autonomic neuropathy is especially important for a patient having general anesthesia and surgery. There is an increased sensitivity to catecholamines, which may intensify the surgical stress response and requires careful monitoring (see Chapter 48).

Diabetic Cardiomyopathy[21, 22]

Cardiomyopathy may develop in the absence of CAD. Most patients also have autonomic neuropathy. Both systolic and diastolic dysfunction may occur. The pathologic correlate is myocardial hypertrophy and fibrosis. There may be mildly thickened walls in small vessels, but ischemia does not appear to be the cause. The usual clinical pattern is typical congestive heart failure. It is important to exclude CAD even in the absence of chest pain; otherwise the treatment is the same as for a nondiabetic patient with congestive heart failure (see Chapters 22 and 23).

Summary

Box 36-2 reviews general recommendations for the management of patients with diabetes who are at risk for heart disease.

Table 36-3	*Diagnostic Criteria for Cardiac Autonomic Neuropathy*

Test	Abnormal Response
Resting heart rate (HR) after 15 min supine	≥100 beats/min
Beat-to-beat variability. The difference between minimum and maximum HR is determined from ECG obtained during inspiration and expiration with patient breathing 6/min.	≤10 beats/min
Valsalva maneuver. The ratio of longest R-R after Valsalva to shortest R-R during Valsalva is determined from ECG, with patient blowing into a manometer at 40 mm Hg for 15 sec.	≤1.10
HR response to standing. During ECG monitoring the ratio of R-R at the thirtieth beat after standing to R-R at the fifteenth beat is determined.	≤1.00
Blood pressure (BP) response to standing. The fall in systolic BP after 1 min of standing is determined by cuff.	≥30 mm Hg

From Fein FS, Scheuer J: Heart disease in diabetes. In Porte D Jr, Sherwin RS, editors: *Ellenberg and Rifkin's diabetes mellitus*, ed 5, Stamford, Conn, 1996, Appleton & Lange.

BOX 36-2

WAYS TO MONITOR PATIENTS WITH DIABETES FOR THE DEVELOPMENT OF HEART DISEASE

Risk factor modification
1. Optimal control of glucose (glycosylated hemoglobin <8, fasting glucose 70-110)
2. Monitor blood pressure and aggressively treat hypertension
3. Measure lipids at regular intervals, and maintain LDL ≤ 100 mg/dL
4. Check homocysteine levels at least once (see Chapters 12 and 44)
5. Treat smoking aggressively

Screen for atypical symptoms of myocardial ischemia (angina equivalents) and maintain a high index of suspicion for asymptomatic coronary disease

Repeat the ECG periodically

Observe the heart rate response to the Valsalva maneuver. Cardiac denervation may be accompanied by cardiomyopathy or silent ischemia, and there may be an increased risk of sudden death.

THYROID DISEASE AND THE HEART[23-25]

Thyroid hormone has direct and indirect cardiovascular effects (Table 36-4). It increases myocardial contractility and also increases heart rate. Deficiency has both negative inotropic and chronotropic effects. Hyperthyroidism has been shown to adversely effect heart rate and rhythm (causing atrial tachyarrhythmias), and it may also have adverse effects on myocardial function, inducing congestive heart failure and cardiomyopathy.

The effects of thyroid hormone on vascular tone have been studied extensively. Hypothyroidism has been associated with increased systemic vascular resistance, and hyperthyroidism has been shown to do just the opposite.

The indirect cardiovascular actions of thyroid hormone are through its effects on lipid metabolism. Hypothyroidism causes hypercholesterolemia and hypertriglyceridemia and increases the risk of atherosclerosis. The opposite phenomena occur with hyperthyroidism.

Hyperthyroidism

Excessive thyroid hormone causes sinus tachycardia or atrial fibrillation (AF). It rarely provokes ventricular arrhythmias. Less commonly, hyperthyroidism may cause cardiomyopathy that can be reversed by correcting the thyroid abnormalities. If the toxic state is present for some time, prolonged tachycardia or rapid AF may contribute to ventricular dysfunction (tachycardia-induced cardiomyopathy, see Chapter 25). On the other hand, thyroxine decreases systemic vascular resistance and has been suggested as treatment of congestive heart failure.

| Table 36-4 | *Cardiovascular Hemodynamics in Thyrotoxicosis* |

	Hyperthyroidism		Hypothyroidism	
	Change	Comment	Change	Comment
Systemic vascular resistance	↓	50%-70% lower, similar to exercise	↑	50%-60% higher
Cardiac output	↑	200%-300% increase	↓	50% decreased
Blood pressure Systolic Diastolic	↑ ↓	Especially in elderly	↓ (or normal) ↑ (or normal)	Narrowed pulse pressure 20% prevalence of diastolic hypertension
Heart rate	↑	Most often sinus tachycardia; 10%-15% of patients have atrial fibrillation	↓ (or normal)	
Cardiac contractililty	↑	Systolic and diastolic function both enhanced	↓	Systolic and diastolic function both subnormal
Cardiac mass	↑	Hypertrophy from increased cardiac work	↓	Pericardial effusion may suggest cardiomegaly
Blood volume	↑	Increased serum erythropoietin and sodium reabsorption	↓	

Adapted from Klein I, Levery G: The cardiovascular system in thyrotoxicosis; and from Klein I, Ojamaa K: The cardiovascular system in hypothyroidism. In Braverman LE, Utiger RD, editors: *Werner and Ingbar's the thyroid: a fundamental and clinical text, ed 7*, Philadelphia, 1996, Lippincott-Raven.

Table 36-4 lists the common cardiovascular symptoms in thyrotoxicosis. Keep in mind the possibility of "apathetic hyperthyroidism" in elderly patients with new-onset atrial fibrillation. Although thyrotoxicosis is present, the common symptoms of hyperthyroidism are absent. These patients may have an apathetic, dull affect, bordering on somnolence.

Management

Beta-blockers are given acutely to control heart rate and rhythm. The dose is titrated to the patient's heart rate. Definitive treatment of thyrotoxicosis leads to more permanent resolution of cardiovascular problems.

Hypothyroidism

There is reduced heart rate and contractility (Table 36-4). The pulse pressure narrows, cardiac output declines, and systemic vascular resistance increases. ECG abnormalities include sinus bradycardia, prolonged PR interval, and low voltage. Repolarization abnormalities are sometimes present. Decreased blood flow to the extremities is one reason that these patients feel cold.

The cardiovascular effects of hypothyroidism are summarized in Table 36-4. Both systolic and diastolic

cardiac dysfunction may occur. Systemic vascular resistance is increased, possibly aggravating heart failure. There may be hypertension with mild hypothyroidism, but blood pressure usually is low with severe myxedema. Bradycardia, pericardial effusion, hyperlipidemia, and accelerated atherosclerosis may all develop with prolonged hypothyroidism. With thyroid hormone replacement, it is common for total cholesterol to fall from the 260 to 300 range to below 200 mg/dL.

Although left ventricular function may be depressed, congestive heart failure is rarely caused by hypothyroidism in the absence of other cardiac disease. Bradycardia and increased peripheral vascular resistance may aggravate heart failure. Cardiac function improves with hormone replacement.

If coronary artery disease is present, thyroid replacement must be done cautiously, using much lower doses of thyroxine. There is a risk of provoking unstable angina or myocardial infarction by increasing heart rate and contractility. The full replacement dose of levothyroxine is 1.7 µg/kg/day (or 120 µg for a 70 kg person), although older patients require less; full replacement is signified by normalization of the TSH. In the presence of CAD, we begin treatment with 25 µg levothyroxine

per day. The dose is increased each month by 25 μ/day until the TSH is normalized.

If angina worsens with hormone replacement, the dose of levothyroxine should be reduced and the coronary disease evaluated. A patient with severe CAD may need revascularization to tolerate hormone replacement. Some patients are unable to tolerate a full replacement dose and are left with some degree of hypothyroidism and elevation of TSH, although symptoms are usually better.

Hypothyroidism is a common cause of large, yet asymptomatic pericardial effusion. It occurs in one third of patients with myxedema. At times the thyroid condition is missed. Consider the diagnosis in a patient who has massive and unanticipated cardiomegaly on chest x-ray, clear lung fields, and no clinical findings to indicate heart failure. The echocardiogram shows the effusion and confirms normal heart size. As the pericardial effusion develops slowly, the pericardium has time to stretch, and tamponade is unusual. (Such chronic effusions occur with primary pericardial disease in < 5% of cases.) Treatment of hypothyroidism leads to resolution of the effusion, and constrictive pericarditis is rare.

Table 36-5	*Cardiovascular Effects of Common Endocrine Disorders**

Condition	Endocrine Abnormality	Cardiovascular Effects
Diabetes insipidus (DI)	Failure to produce (central DI) or respond to (nephrogenic DI) vasopressin	Polyuria and polydipsia, an inability to concentrate the urine If the patient is unable to drink (coma, anesthesia, and so forth) there may be volume depletion and hypotension.
Cushing's syndrome	Increased cortisol production	Hypertension in 80% of cases
Hyperaldosteronism	Adrenal adenoma (Conn's syndrome) or adrenal hyperplasia	Moderate diastolic hypertension (expanded extracellular volume), hypokalemia resistant to therapy Magnesium often low
Adrenocortical deficiency	Progressive adrenocortical destruction (Addison's disease) or acute destruction of the cortex (Waterhouse-Friderichsen syndrome that may occur with sepsis)	*Chronic:* Asthenia, fatigue, hypotension, small heart on chest x-ray *Acute:* shock
Pheochromocytoma	Catecholamine-producing tumor of the adrenal medulla; rare and related tumors are carotid body and sympathetic ganglion tumors.	Hypertension. It is sustained in 60% of cases, although with blood pressure lability. Paroxysms occur in over half of patients, occasionally resembling anxiety attacks (see Chapter 31).
Hypoglycemia	When acute, release of epinephrine (the most common cause is insulin reaction)	Tachycardia and palpitations Air hunger
Hyperparathyroidism	Excess hormone causes hypercalcemia and hyperphosphatemia	Hypertension is common in elderly patients, but cause and effect is uncertain. Thiazides may aggravate hypercalcemia.
Chronic hypocalcemia	Causes: renal failure, hypoparathyroidism, vitamin D deficiency, hypomagnesemia (malnutrition states or malabsorption)	Long QT interval on ECG Reduced effectiveness of digitalis

*Does not include diabetes and thyroid disease (reviewed in greater depth in Chapter 36) or changes with pregnancy (see Chapter 40) or menopause (see Chapter 41).

CARDIAC EFFECTS OF OTHER ENDOCRINE SYNDROMES

These are less common than diabetes and thyroid disorders and are summarized in Table 36-5.

REFERENCES

1. Donahue RP, Orchard TJ: Diabetes mellitus and macrovascular complications: an epidemiological perspective, *Diabetes Care* 15:1141, 1992.
2. Miettinen H, Lehto S, Salomaa V, et al: Impact of diabetes on mortality after the first myocardial infarction: The FIN-MONICA Myocardial Infarction Register Study Group, *Diabetes Care* 21:69, 1998.
3. Mautner SL, Linn F, Prberts WC: Composition of atherosclerotic plaques in the epicardial coronary arteries in juvenile (type 1) diabetes mellitus, *Am J Cardiol* 70:1264, 1992.
4. Barrett-Connor EL, Cohn BA, Wingard DL, Edelstein SL: Why is diabetes mellitus a stronger risk factor for fatal ischemic heart disease in women than in men? *JAMA* 265:627, 1991.
5. Levine GN, Jacobs AK, Keeler GP, et al: Impact of diabetes mellitus on percutaneous revascularization (CAVEAT-I): CAVEAT I Investigators. Coronary Angioplasty Versus Excisional Atherectomy Trial, *Am J Cardiol* 79:748, 1997.
6. Steiner G: Risk factors for macrovascular disease in type 2 diabetes: classic lipid abnormalities, *Diabetes Care* 22:6, 1999.
7. Haffner SM: Diabetes, hyperlipidemia, and coronary artery disease, *Am J Cardiol* 83:17, 1999.
8. O'Keefe JH Jr, Miles JM, Harris WH, et al: Improving the adverse cardiovascular prognosis of type 2 diabetes, *Mayo Clin Proc* 74:171, 1999.
9. Bohannon NJ: Coronary artery disease and diabetes, *Postgrad Med* 105:66, 1999.
10. West KM, Ahuja MMS, Bennett PH, et al: The role of circulating glucose and triglyceride concentrations and their interactions with other risk factors as determinants of arterial disease in nine diabetic population samples from the WHO Multinational Study, *Diabetes Care* 6:361, 1983.
11. Reaven GM: Role of insulin resistance in human disease, *Diabetes* 37:1595, 1998.
12. Stout RW: *Diabetes and atherosclerosis*, Dordrecht, The Netherlands, 1992, Wolters Kluwer.
13. Howard B: Lipoprotein metabolism in diabetes mellitus, *J Lipid Res* 28:613, 1987.
14. Haffner SM, Lehto S, Ronnemaa T, et al: Mortality from coronary heart disease in subjects with type 2 diabetes and in nondiabetic subjects with and without prior myocardial infarction, *N Engl J Med* 339:229, 1998.
15. Kjekshus J, Gilpin E, Cali G, et al: Diabetic patients and beta-blockers after acute myocardial infarction, *Eur Heart J* 11:43, 1990.
16. Estacio RO, Barrett WJ, Hiatt WR, et al: The effect of nisoldipine as compared with enalapril on cardiovascular outcomes in patients with non-insulin-dependent diabetes and hypertension, *N Engl J Med* 338:645, 1998.
17. Taylor GJ, Moses HW, Katholi RE, et al: Six-year survival after coronary thrombolysis and early revascularization for acute myocardial infarction, *Am J Cardiol* 70:26, 1992.
18. Granger CB, Califf RM, Young S, et al: Outcome of patients with diabetes mellitus and acute myocardial infarction treated with thrombolytic agents: the Thrombolysis and Angioplasty in Myocardial Infarction (TAMI) Study Group, *J Am Coll Cardiol* 21:920, 1993.
19. The BARI Investigators: Influence of diabetes on 5-year mortality and morbidity in a randomized trial comparing CABG and PTCA in patients with multivessel disease: the Bypass Angioplasty Revascularization Investigation, *Circulation* 96:1761, 1997.
20. Ziegler D, Dannelh K, Volksw D, et al: Prevalence of cardiovascular autonomic dysfunction assessed by spectral analysis and standard tests of heart-rate variation in newly diagnosed IDDM patients, *Diabetes Care* 15:908, 1992.
21. Irace L, Iarussi D, Guadagno, et al: Left ventricular performance and autonomic dysfunction in patients with long-term insulin-dependent diabetes mellitus, *Acta Diabetol* 33:269, 1996.
22. Mustonen JN, Uusitupa MIJ, Laakso M, et al: Left ventricular systolic function in middle aged patients with diabetes mellitus, *Am J Cardiol* 73:1202, 1994.
23. Gomberg-Maitland M, Frishman WH: Thyroid hormone and cardiovascular disease, *Am Heart J* 135:187, 1998.
24. Sundaram V, Hanna AN, Koneru L, et al: Both hypothyroidism and hyperthyroidism enhance low density lipoprotein oxidation, *J Clin Endocrinol Metab* 82:3421, 1997.
25. Umpierrez GE, Challapalli S, Patterson C: Congestive heart failure due to reversible cardiomyopathy in patients with hyperthyroidism, *Am J Med Sci* 310:99, 1995.

37 Cardiac Manifestations of Connective Tissue Disease

William M. Simpson, Jr.
George J. Taylor

IMMUNE-MEDIATED INFLAMMATORY DISORDERS

Systemic Lupus Erythematosus

Systemic lupus erythematosus (SLE) is one of the more common rheumatologic diseases, affecting 20/100,000. It is 10 times more common in women than in men and may occur at any age, with the onset most often in the second to third decades. Its etiology is unknown, but a genetic predisposition is strongly suspected. The natural history is variable, with some having only mild symptoms and others following a severe or even lethal course.

SLE is an autoimmune or hypersensitivity disorder. The sterile inflammatory process of SLE involves multiple organ systems (skin, joints, kidneys, brain, and heart) and virtually all serous membranes. Its clinical manifestations depend on the organs involved.

Cardiac Manifestations

Primary cardiac involvement may include abnormalities of the pericardium, endocardium, myocardium, and the coronary arteries. Pericarditis is the most common.[1] Over half of patients with SLE have a pericardial effusion at some point during their clinical course.[1] Pericardial involvement is clinically silent in most of these patients. Rarely pericardial constriction and tamponade occur.[2] Fibrinous pericarditis is typically associated with SLE, but immunosuppressed patients or those with renal failure are at greater risk for purulent pericarditis, the most life-threatening of the pericardial lesions.[3]

The endocarditis of SLE was first described as "atypical verrucous endocarditis" by Libman and Sacks long before lupus was recognized as a clinical entity.[4] The vegetations may develop on any of the four valves but most commonly affect left-sided valves, particularly the mitral. The endocarditis of SLE is usually not associated with valve dysfunction or clinical symptoms and is found in up to 40% of patients with SLE at autopsy.[5] The valvular lesions predispose to infective endocarditis, particularly in patients with immunosuppression.

Overt myocarditis is uncommon in SLE, but ventricular arrhythmias, heart block, and heart failure may rarely occur. Subclinical cardiomyopathy has been associated in some recent reports with SLE. In most cases it is difficult to separate abnormalities due to an autoimmune myocarditis from those caused by manifestations of SLE (e.g., hypertension and pericarditis).

Coronary artery disease is an infrequent manifestation of SLE. Fibrinoid necrosis and thromboembolic occlusion can be seen in the intramural vessels of the heart but are rarely associated with myocardial necrosis or fibrosis.

Lupus in Infancy

Neonatal lupus occurs when anti-Ro (SS-A) autoantibodies (mostly IgG) form and circulate in a pregnant patient who has SLE. These antibodies cross the placenta. A lupus-like illness is produced in the newborn, and it tends to resolve as the maternal antibodies are cleared. One aspect that commonly does not resolve is congenital complete heart block. Lesser degrees of block that generally improve have been described. Other heart lesions (e.g., patent ductus arteriosus, patent foramen ovale, coarctation of the aorta, ASD, tetralogy of Fallot, VSD, and others) have been reported in patients with neonatal lupus, but their connection, if any, to the autoimmune process is unknown.

Management

No laboratory findings can predict cardiac involvement. Serum complement is decreased in most patients with SLE. Since complement is normal or increased in other connective tissue diseases (e.g., rheumatoid arthritis, polyarteritis nodosa, scleroderma, and disseminated infections), this test may be useful in diagnosis of SLE.

Pregnant women with SLE should have a serum anti-Ro (SS-A) antibody measurement as early as possible. Women who are anti-Ro positive should be closely monitored in a high-risk obstetric setting, as should the subsequent pregnancies of mothers whose babies are born with congenital complete heart block.[6]

Treatment

Management of cardiovascular lupus consists of treating the underlying disease, including nonsteroidal antiinflammatory agents, corticosteroids, and in severe cases cytotoxic agents. Arrhythmias, congestive failure, and hypertension should be treated with standard cardiovascular agents. Pericardial effusions occasionally require pericardiocentesis, and lupus valvulitis may rarely require valve replacement.

Polyarteritis Nodosa

Accurate incidence figures of polyarteritis nodosa (PN) are difficult to obtain, since most reports have included diseases other than the classic syndrome. It is believed to be "uncommon" but not "rare." Mean age at onset is 48. The male:female ratio is 1.6:1. The prognosis for patients with untreated PN is extremely poor. Five-year survival is 15% or less; with treatment, this figure increases to over 40%.

PN is characterized by segmental necrotizing inflammation of small- to medium-sized arteries throughout the body, with multiorgan system involvement. The heart, gastrointestinal tract, skin, kidneys, central nervous, and reticuloendothelial and musculoskeletal systems are most commonly involved.

Since necrotizing arteritis can be found in a number of other disorders, PN is normally a diagnosis of exclusion. Other specific arteritises, distinct from PN, include granulomatous arteritis, hypersensitivity arteritis, temporal arteritis, and arteritis involving the aorta or its major branches.

Cardiac Manifestations

The coronary arteries are frequently affected by PN just as they penetrate the myocardium. Early lesions show inflammatory infiltration of the media and adventitia. Later lesions have full-thickness necrosis and inflammation of the vessel wall including the intima and perivascular connective tissue. Still more advanced lesions are associated with aneurysmal dilation and thrombosis. The aneurysms are responsible for the nodular appearance of the arteries, giving this disease its name. The healing phase of intimal damage leads to coronary artery luminal narrowing that may subsequently lead to myocardial infarction.[7]

Conduction system abnormalities are also common in PN, since the arteries supplying the SA and AV nodes are of the size and location to make them prime targets for polyarteritis.[7]

The most frequent cardiovascular manifestation of PN is not related to coronary disease but to the combination of hypertension and chronic renal failure that ultimately causes congestive heart failure (the clinical course of 60% of patients with the disease). PN patients may also present with acute myocardial infarction.

Management

Cytoplasmic antibody with perinuclear staining (p-ANCA) is usually positive in PN. Some authorities consider the p-ANCA a diagnostic study; others require a biopsy or an angiogram to make a diagnosis of PN (since p-ANCA can be positive, although rarely, in inflammatory bowel disease, Kawasaki's disease and tuberculosis).

Therapy for the cardiovascular disease of PN is directed at the specific cardiac dysfunction. Corticosteroids and other antiinflammatory agents are used to treat the underlying disease. Anticoagulation is controversial.

Rheumatoid Arthritis

Rheumatoid arthritis (RA), the most common of the connective tissue diseases, affects women twice as often as men and tends to run in families. However, cardiac involvement in RA is uncommon.

Extraarticular manifestations of RA tend to occur in individuals with high titers of autoantibodies to the Fc component of immunoglobulin G (rheumatoid factors). These autoantibodies apparently incite the inflammatory process in the vascular system that leads to the clinical presentations discussed below.

Cardiac Manifestations

About 30% of RA patients have a diffuse fibrinous pericarditis, but it is clinically silent more than half the time.[8] The clinical course tends to be benign, but large effusions may require pericardicentesis, and pericardial constriction may require pericardiectomy. Symptomatic pericarditis may require a course of corticosteroid therapy.

Rheumatoid nodules may rarely infiltrate the myocardium and heart valves. Most produce no symptoms, but nodules on the valve leaflets have caused valvular insufficiency. If the nodules become necrotic, perforation of the leaflet may lead to severe regurgitation.

Rheumatoid myocarditis may rarely produce arrhythmias, conduction disturbances, and congestive heart failure.

Management

The usual laboratory studies associated with RA are also found in RA with cardiac involvement. No laboratory findings are consistently associated with specific cardiac lesions.

Since most of the cardiac lesions of RA are silent, it is not known whether traditional therapies for RA have any effect on these lesions. Usual treatments for pericarditis, arrhythmias, and conduction disturbances are used when these disorders produce symptoms.

Ankylosing Spondylitis

Ankylosing spondylitis usually affects men early in life and has a chronic, progressive course over 20 to 30 or more years. Identification of the HLA-B27 histocompatibility antigen in nearly all patients with the disease confirms its relationship to other connective tissue diagnoses with a high prevalence of this antigen and its genetic base. It is characterized by progressive inflammatory changes in the spine leading to back pain, dorsal kyphosis, and eventually fusion of costovertebral and sacroiliac joints with immobilization of the spine.

Cardiac Manifestations

The usual lesion is inflammation, then sclerosis of the aortic root, typically causing aortic regurgitation. Extension of fibrosis into the interventricular septum leads to conduction abnormalities. In some cases there is sclerosis of the basal portion of the mitral valve and mitral regurgitation.[9]

Aortic regurgitation occurs in up to 10% of patients, usually after many years of ankylosing spondylitis. It is never a presenting feature of the disease (2% of patients with ankylosing spondylitis for 10 years have aortic regurgitation, 10% after 30 years).

Management

The diagnosis of ankylosing spondylitis is made by the combination of typical lower back disorder plus HLA-B27 positivity.

Treatment is symptomatic, primarily relief of back pain with nonsteroidal antiinflammatory medications. Corticosteroids are generally not used unless iritis is present. The inflammatory lesions of the heart are generally clinically silent until aortic insufficiency develops. By that time so little inflammation remains that steroids are of little benefit.[5] Valve replacement may be necessitated if insufficiency is severe (Chapter 19).

Systemic Sclerosis (Scleroderma)

Systemic sclerosis was first identified over 200 years ago and named for its prominent skin manifestation, scleroderma. The systemic nature of the disease and its ability to affect the heart were recognized much later. Soma Weiss described a pattern of cardiac dysfunction in nine patients with scleroderma and recognized that the cardiac disease was a manifestation of an underlying collagen vascular disease.[10] Females with systemic sclerosis outnumber males 4:1. The prevalence is approximately 1/100,000 patient-years. Symptoms usually appear in the third to fifth decade.

Systemic sclerosis is characterized by fibrous thickening of the skin and fibrous and degenerative alterations of the fingers and certain target organs, especially the esophagus, bowel, kidneys, lung, and heart. Small and medium size arteries and arterioles show intimal proliferation and adventitial scarring. These changes lead to focal vascular lesions and parenchymal necrosis and fibrosis.

Myocardial fibrosis occurs if scleroderma directly involves the heart. The fibrosis tends to be patchy, involving all levels of the myocardium and both ventricles, and is unrelated to large or small vessel occlusions. Focal, patchy myocardial cell necrosis is also present. The appearance of the lesions suggests that fibrosis is the result of ischemic necrosis.[11] It may be the consequence of coronary vasospasm, which may occur with or without angina pectoris.

Cardiac Manifestations

Raynaud's phenomena is the first symptom in most patients. Cardiac involvement is either due to primary involvement of the heart by the sclerosing process or to disease in the lungs or kidneys.

Myocardial systemic sclerosis may present as biventricular heart failure, atrial or ventricular arrhythmias, angina, or sudden cardiac death. Approximately 50% of patients with systemic sclerosis at autopsy have increased myocardial scar tissue. Some clinical cardiac abnormality (heart failure, abnormal rhythm, or conduction) occurs in 30% to 40%. Angina pectoris with normal coronary arteries is possible, and coronary vasospasm is the presumed mechanism.

Pericarditis occurs in 20% or more of patients with systemic sclerosis, but in more than half of cases the pericarditis is caused by renal failure. Constrictive pericarditis and pericardial effusions can occur. Systemic sclerosis rarely, if ever, affects cardiac valves.

Since scleroderma most frequently causes renal and pulmonary parenchymal disease with pulmonary and systemic hypertension, hypertension, heart disease, or cor pulmonale may develop.

There may be "primary pulmonary hypertension" with systemic sclerosis, unrelated to pulmonary fibrosis. Patients with this lesion develop rapidly progressive dyspnea and right-sided congestive failure with clear lungs. Arterial vasospasm is believed to be the major cause of these findings. Sudden unexpected death is common in these patients, as is death from what is usually a benign procedure, such as pericardiocentesis or cardiac catheterization.[5]

Management

There is no specific diagnostic test for systemic sclerosis. Antinuclear antibodies are present in 95% of patients with the disease but are also present in patients with other connective tissue diseases. The diagnosis is usually made on the basis of the clinical syndrome.

No effective therapy is currently available for cardiovascular disease caused by systemic sclerosis. Standard therapy for congestive failure and dysrhythmias should be used. Calcium channel blockers (nifedipine in particular) have been shown to help alleviate Raynaud's events in the fingers. Vasospasm elsewhere—heart, lungs, and kidneys—may also respond to calcium channel blockade, but no controlled studies are available.[12]

Polymyositis and Dermatomyositis

Polymyositis (PM) and dermatomyositis (DM) are idiopathic autoimmune inflammatory myopathies. The annual incidence is 10-30/million in the United States, and the female:male ratio is 2:1. The disease may begin at any age, although there tend to be two peaks in on-

set— ages 5 to 15 years and 40 to 60 years. Overall mortality of patients with PM/DM is about four times that of the general population. Females, blacks, those treated after long delays, and others severely affected at presentation have a poor prognosis.

Changes occur principally in skeletal muscle with infiltrates of inflammatory cells and destruction of muscle fibers with a phagocytic reaction. Perivascular (usually perivenular) inflammatory cell infiltration is the hallmark of PM.

Cardiac Manifestations

A typical heliotrope rash occurs in dermatomyositis. Both PM and DM cause periorbital edema and proximal muscle weakness. In addition to skeletal muscle involvement, 40% of patients have a cardiac manifestation (e.g., atrioventricular conduction abnormalities, tachyarrhythmias, pericarditis with effusion, or dilated cardiomyopathy).[13] A type of myocarditis leading to congestive heart failure has been found on autopsy. Coronary arteritis is possible but rare.

Management

Typical laboratory abnormalities include elevated CPK and aldolase, reflecting muscle breakdown as a result of inflammation. The EMG is abnormal in 40% of cases with markedly increased insertional activity together with the myopathic triad of motor unit action potentials, which are of low amplitude, polyphasic, and have abnormally early recruitment. Myopathic changes are noted in only 40%.

Because some patients benefit from high-dose oral or intravenous corticosteroids, these are usually tried first. Intravenous immunoglobulin also appears promising, but remains second line treatment at present.

Therapy for cardiovascular manifestations of PM/DM includes steroids for underlying inflammation plus symptomatic therapy for the particular cardiac condition.

Temporal (Giant Cell) Arteritis

Temporal arteritis is inflammation of medium and large arteries. It usually involves one or more branches of the external carotid artery, but can involve arteries in many locations. It is an uncommon disease (24/100,000 patient-years) that usually occurs in older people, although it can occur in patients in their forties and younger. TA is rare in blacks and twice as common in women as in men.

Patients with cranial symptoms often have vasculitis of other medium- and large-sized arteries that is not recognized. The disease is a panarteritis with inflammatory mononuclear cell infiltrates and frequent giant cell formation. Pathophysiologic findings in organs are related to the ischemia produced by the involved arteries.

Cardiac Manifestations

Common early symptoms include jaw claudication, headaches, scalp tenderness, and visual disturbance, including blindness. The classic complex is symptoms plus fever, anemia, and an elevated sedimentation rate in an elderly patient. Cardiovascular manifestations include chest pain from aortitis or myocardial ischemia, aortic aneurysm, limb claudication, aortic regurgitation, and stroke. Typically the temporal artery is tender to palpation, or there may be nodularity of the artery or scalp tenderness instead.

Management

In addition to an elevated sedimentation rate, a normochromic or slightly hypochromic anemia is usually present. Abnormal liver-associated enzymes (particularly alkaline phosphatase) and elevated IgG and complement are also common. Diagnosis is confirmed by temporal artery biopsy. Skip lesions make serial sections of an adequate (4 to 6 cm) specimen necessary.

Temporal arteritis and its associated symptoms respond well to corticosteroid therapy. Begin treatment with 60 mg of prednisone per day and taper as symptoms abate (while monitoring the sedimentation rate). It is necessary to continue low dose therapy for at least 12 months to decrease the possibility of relapse.

NONINFLAMMATORY HERITABLE TYPE CONNECTIVE TISSUE DISEASES
Ehlers-Danlos Syndrome

There are 10 forms of Ehlers-Danlos syndrome (EDS), and cardiovascular defects are prominent in only a few of these. The illness occurs in approximately 1 in 5000 births, although it may be twice as prevalent in black populations. The cause is genetically based, but because of overlapping signs and symptoms, many patients and families cannot be assigned to any of the recognized types of EDS.

The natural history of the disease depends on the type. Types I, II, IV, V, and VI have cardiovascular manifestations.[14] The molecular defects in types I-III, V, and VIII are unknown, and type IV has abnormal procollagen. Type VI is caused by a deficiency of lysyl hydroxylase, leading to collagen that is deficient in hydroxylysine, causing formation of unstable cross-links.

Clinical Presentation and Cardiac Manifestations

Type I EDS is an autosomal dominant condition characterized by velvety-textured, fragile, hyperextensible skin that splits easily and heals poorly. The joints are hyperextensible. Small blood vessel involvement produces easy bruisability. Mitral valve prolapse occurs in 50% of patients. Dilation of the aortic root or pulmonary artery and tricuspid valve prolapse can occur.

Type II, also an autosomal dominant disorder, is similar to type I but milder. Mitral valve prolapse is also common in this type. Type III has no significant cardiac manifestations. Type IV is the most severe form of EDS, characterized by rupture of the large arteries, colon, or the gravid uterus. Mitral valve prolapse is frequent. Angiography may cause vascular or organ rupture. Type IV has both autosomal dominant and recessive forms. In Type V, skin hyperextensibility is prominent, but joint hypermobility is mild to moderate. Mitral and tricuspid valve prolapse or insufficiency can occur. Type VI is called the *ocular* type of EDS, but aortic rupture can occur, as well as severe scoliosis, recurrent joint dislocations, and gastrointestinal hemorrhage.

Management

Biochemical and gene analyses for known molecular defects in EDS are possible, but since they are expensive and time consuming, diagnosis is primarily established on the basis of clinical criteria.

There is no specific therapy. Patients with type IV EDS should probably have serial aortic ultrasound studies to screen for asymptomatic dilation or aneurysm formation.[15]

Marfan's Syndrome

Marfan's syndrome has an incidence of 1:10,000-20,000. It is an autosomal dominant disorder with variable penetrance. Approximately 20% arise by spontaneous mutation, which occurs more frequently with advanced paternal age.

The severe form is caused by a single allele mutation of the fibrillin gene. Fibrillin is a major component of the microfibrils, which are abundant in the media of large blood vessels and the suspensory ligaments of the lens.

Clinical Presentation and Cardiac Manifestations

The disease involves the musculoskeletal, cardiovascular, and ocular systems. Patients are tall with long limbs and have scoliosis or kyphosis and pectus deformities. The face is usually long and thin with a high-arched palate. Lens dislocation occurs in 50% to 80% of patients. The most common cardiovascular manifestation is mitral valve prolapse with or without regurgitation. Ascending aortic dilation is the next most common cardiovascular lesion. Aortic rupture, aortic regurgitation, or dissecting aneurysm may result from the dilation.

There is a "form fruste" of Marfan's syndrome, with a marfanoid aorta despite normal body habitus. These patients often have a family history, and therefore a screening echocardiogram is indicated for the children of patients with Marfan's syndrome.

The prevalence of aortic root dilation is greater in males than in females. The risk of cardiovascular complications during pregnancy is a special problem for women with Marfan's syndrome. Aortic dissection may occur before, during, or after labor. Most authorities advise patients with aortic root dilation to avoid pregnancy. Since traumatic aortic rupture can occur, contact sports should be avoided.

Management

Diagnosis is easily established if the patient and other family members have dislocated lens, aortic root dilation, and the marfanoid habitus. All patients in whom the diagnosis is suspected should have a slit-lamp evaluation and an echocardiogram. Homocystinuria should be ruled out by a negative cyanide-nitroprusside test for disulfides in the urine.

There is no specific therapy for the connective tissue disorder. Beta blockade sufficient to lower the resting heart rate to ≤60 beats/min is recommended to delay or prevent aortic dilation. Patients should be followed with serial echocardiograms so that aortic changes can be recognized early. With marked or progressive aortic root dilation, resection of the ascending aortic aneurysm plus aortic valve replacement (Edward's procedure) is commonly recommended. The risk of surgery is markedly greater if you wait until dissection occurs. Marfan's syndrome is the usual cause of dissection of the aorta in young patients, and it is one of the more common causes of aortic insufficiency.

Osteogenesis Imperfecta

There are five types of osteogenesis imperfecta (OI). The overall incidence is approximately 1:12,000. It is a heritable disease that makes bone brittle because of a generalized decrease in bone mass. The most severe forms of OI result in death in utero or shortly after birth. The mild and moderate forms have more variable clinical effects.

Most patients with OI have a defect in one of the two genes for type I procollagen. The abnormal collagen produced as a result leads to the clinical findings outlined below.

Clinical Presentation and Cardiac Manifestations

Silence developed the most commonly used classification structure for OI.[16] Type I is inherited as an autosomal dominant trait and is the mildest form of the disease. Blue sclerae are present, but bone fragility is mild. Type II has extreme bone fragility and blue sclerae and is lethal in utero or shortly after birth. Types III and IV are intermediate in severity, between types I and II. The sclerae are only slightly blue at birth and become white in adulthood. Type III tends to progress with aging, but type IV does not. Type IV is always autosomal dominant; type III may be inherited as either a dominant or recessive trait. All types of OI may affect the heart, although rarely. The severity of cardiac disease parallels

that of OI. Aortic and mitral regurgitation, mitral valve prolapse, and fragility of large blood vessels have all been reported.

Management

There are no practical laboratory tests. Blue sclerae, abnormalities of dentition, and family history along with bone fragility are clinically useful. The cardiovascular changes are usually diagnosed by standard echocardiography and guided by physical findings.

Treatment of the underlying disease is ineffective. Repair of symptomatic cardiac defects has been attempted, but experience is limited and complication rates high.

Pseudoxanthoma Elasticum

The incidence of pseudoxanthoma elasticum (PXE) is uncertain, but it is a rare illness. There are apparently four forms of the disease, two with autosomal dominant and two with autosomal recessive inheritance. The involvement of skin and vessels varies depending on the type.

The basic defect in PXE is not known, but it results in abnormal deposition of calcium on the elastic fibers of the skin, eye, and blood vessels.

The natural history depends on the severity of vascular complications: hypertension, angina, and claudication. Valvular deformity may result from endocardial thickening, and calcification in the conduction system may produce arrhythmias. All the cardiovascular complications may manifest as early as adolescence.

The most obvious clinical finding is "chicken skin"—yellow skin papules often found on the neck and in flexural creases. Angioid streaks and choroiditis are seen in the retina in most cases. The incidence of cardiovascular complications is uncertain, but in one series of patients with PXE approximately one fifth had angina, one fifth had intermittent claudication, and one sixth had calcification of peripheral arteries.[17]

Management

Clinical findings establish the diagnosis. There are no specific laboratory abnormalities. No treatment is available for the basic defect in elastin. Treatment for the cardiovascular complications using standard therapy can delay morbidity and mortality.

REFERENCES

1. Moder KG, Miller TD, Tazelaar HD: Cardiac involvement in systemic lupus erythematosis, *Mayo Clinic Proc* 74:275, 1999.
2. Ansari A, Larson PH, Bates HD: Cardiovascular manifestations of systemic lupus erythematosus, *Prog Cardiovasc Dis* 27:421, 1985.
3. Klacsmann PG, Bulkley BH, Hutchins GM: The changed spectrum of purulent pericarditis: an 86-year autopsy experience in 200 patients, *Am J Med* 63:666, 1977.
4. Libman E, Sacks B: A hitherto undescribed form of valvular and mural endocarditis, *Arch Intern Med* 33:701, 1924.
5. Healy BP: The heart and connective tissue disease. In Hurst JW, editor: *The heart*, ed 7, New York, 1990, McGraw-Hill
6. Healy BP et al: The heart and connective tissue diseases. In Schant RC, editor: *The heart*, ed 8, New York, 1994, McGraw-Hill.
7. Schrader ML, Hochman JS, Bulkley BH: The heart in polyarteritis nodosa: a clinicopathologic study, *Am Heart J* 109:1353, 1985.
8. Bacon PA, Gibson DG: Cardiac involvement in rheumatoid arthritis: an echocardiographic study, *Ann Rheum Dis* 33:20, 1974.
9. Kawasuji M, Hetzer R, Oelert H, et al: Aortic valve replacement and ascending aorta replacement with ankylosing spondylitis: report of three surgical cases and review of the literature, *Thorac Cardiovasc Surg* 30:310, 1982.
10. Weiss S et al: Scleroderm heart disease, with a consideration of certain other visceral manifestations of scleroderm, *Arch Intern Med* 71:749, 1943.
11. Bulkey BH: Progressive system sclerosis with cardiac involvement, *Clin Rheum Dis* 5:131, 1979.
12. Deswal A, Follansbee WP: Cardiac involvement in scleroderma, *Rheum Dis Clin North Am* 22:856, 1996.
13. Dalakas MC: Polymyositis dermatomyositis and inclusion-body myositis, *N Engl J Med* 325:1487, 1991.
14. Yeowell HN, Pinnell SR: The Ehlers-Danlos syndromes, *Semin Dermatol* 12:229, 1993.
15. Steinmann B et al: The Ehlers-Danlos syndrome. In Royce PM, Steinmann B, editors: *Connective tissue and its heritable disorders*, New York, 1993, Wiley-Liss.
16. Sillence DO: Osteogenesis imperfecta: an expanding panorama of variance, *Clin Orthop* 191:11, 1981.
17. Michels VV, Driscoll DJ: Genetics of heart disease. In Giuliani ER, et al, editors: *Mayo Clinic practice of cardiology*, St Louis, 1996, Mosby.

38 Neoplastic Disease and the Heart

Wills C. Geils
George J. Taylor

Neoplastic involvement of the heart is a diagnostic challenge, because it is unusual and tends to mimic other, more common diseases. A high index of suspicion is necessary to make the diagnosis. The heart, like any other organ, can be affected by primary or secondary neoplasms.

PRIMARY TUMORS OF THE HEART

Primary tumors are rare, with a reported incidence in autopsy series ranging from 1 in 3000 to 1 in 15,000.[1] Approximately 75% are benign, and the majority are myxomas and rhabdomyomas. The other 25% are malignant and are usually sarcomas (Box 38-1).

Atrial Myxoma

Epidemiology and Clinical Presentation

Myxomas are the most common of the primary cardiac neoplasms, benign or malignant. The peak incidence is ages 40 to 60, but they can occur at almost any age. The familial form is usually diagnosed between the ages of 20 and 30. It is transmitted in an autosomal dominant pattern, accounts for 10% of cases, and affects men and women equally. The nonfamilial form usually occurs in women (70%).

Myxomas occur in the left atrium 75% of the time and are usually attached by a stalk to the interatrial septum in the area of the fossa ovalis. They also can be found in the right atrium (23%) and ventricles (2%). Most myxomas are isolated lesions, but the familial form can involve multiple lesions.[2]

Left atrial (LA) myxoma can present in a variety of ways. Many patients are asymptomatic, and the tumor is an incidental finding on an echocardiogram. There are three possible symptom complexes:

1. LA myxoma in the left atrium can mimic mitral stenosis or regurgitation, as the tumor disrupts mitral valve function. It may actually block the valve. Symptoms include dyspnea, orthopnea, or edema. Onset of symptoms may be sudden, and they may be provoked by a particular body position. In fact, symptoms that occur suddenly, are predictably positional, and are out of proportion to physical findings raise the possibility of a myxoma.
2. The second type of symptom complex results from peripheral embolism, with stroke, myocardial in-

farction, abdominal pain caused by visceral ischemia, or limb pain with pulselessness and pallor. The diagnosis of a myxoma is sometimes made when tumor cells are found in the extracted thrombus following embolectomy. The friable surface of the myxoma includes both tumor and thrombus, and the embolus is a combination of both.

3. A patient may have constitutional symptoms such as fever, weight loss, weakness and fatigue, or arthralgia. The constitutional presentation is analogous to that of infective endocarditis, collagen vascular disease, or malignancy.[3] Approximately 90% of patients with an atrial myxoma have these constitutional symptoms, and a majority have an elevated erythrocyte sedimentation rate.[4]

Patients with right atrial myxoma have similar constitutional symptoms but also may have chest pain as a result of pulmonary embolus. They may have symptoms of right-sided heart failure due to obstruction of the tricuspid valve (hepatomegaly, ascites, and peripheral edema).

Findings of the physical examination in patients with LA myxoma can resemble those of mitral stenosis, with a loud first heart sound, rales, and a diastolic apical rumble. There may be an extra diastolic heart sound, a "tumor plop," that can be difficult to distinguish from the opening snap of mitral stenosis or from a third heart sound. The tumor plop is a low-pitched sound that occurs after S_2 (an opening snap is usually high pitched); it occurs later than the typical opening snap but earlier than the typical third heart sound. The physical findings of an atrial myxoma, like the symptoms, are often positional.

Management

The diagnosis of myxoma is best made with echocardiography. Almost all are easily visualized with transthoracic echocardiography.[1] Transesophageal echocardiography can help further define the anatomic site or position of the stalk. Magnetic resonance imaging can be useful if the echocardiogram is inconclusive.

Treatment of myxoma consists of prompt surgical removal. At surgery, the myxoma is usually covered with thrombus. Care must be taken to avoid dislodging a small thrombus and sending it downstream. Recur-

BOX 38-1
PRIMARY CARDIAC NEOPLASMS

BENIGN
Myxoma
Rhabdomyoma
Lipoma
Papillary fibroelastoma
Fibroma
Hemangioma
Mesothelioma of the AV node

MALIGNANT
Angiosarcoma
Rhabdomyosarcoma
Fibrosarcoma
Mesothelioma

rences are rare, but when they do occur it is usually within 4 years of surgery.[2] Follow-up echocardiography is recommended to exclude recurrence.

Rhabdomyoma

Rhabdomyomas are the most common benign cardiac tumors of childhood. Most patients are younger than 1 year of age. Approximately one third have tuberous sclerosis. The tumor usually is found in multiple areas of the ventricular myocardium and can extend into the ventricular cavity. Syncope or heart failure may result from obstruction of flow in the ventricles, atrioventricular block, or arrhythmias, including ventricular tachycardia. Hypoxic episodes resembling tetralogy of Fallot spells can be the presenting symptom. The tumor usually is diagnosed by echocardiography or magnetic resonance imaging. Treatment is surgical removal of the tumor, even if multiple, and usually is successful.[2]

Malignant Cardiac Tumors
Angiosarcoma

The malignant primary cardiac neoplasms are sarcomas, the most common being angiosarcomas. Angiosarcomas occur two to three times more frequently in men than in women. They occur most often between the ages of 20 and 50. Most arise from the right atrium or pericardium but also may occur in the right ventricle. Seventy-five percent of patients exhibit signs and symptoms of right-sided heart failure. Most patients have precordial chest pain that is often similar in quality to pericarditis. Prognosis is poor. Surgical therapy usually is impossible because of extensive local disease at the time of diagnosis. Chemotherapy and radiation therapy are

briefly palliative, and most patients die within 1 year of the onset of symptoms.[1]

Rhabdomyosarcoma

Like angiosarcomas, rhabdomyosarcomas are more common in men and occur between the ages of 20 and 50. They arise in any cardiac chamber and are multiple in half the cases. The tumor can affect the function of one or more of the cardiac valves. Therefore, symptoms of left or right-sided heart failure can occur. Prognosis is poor. Neither medical nor surgical therapy is effective, and most patients die within 1 year of diagnosis.[4]

METASTATIC TUMORS

Neoplasms that are metastatic to the heart are 20 to 40 times more common than primary cardiac neoplasms. Of patients dying of malignancy, 2% to 22% have cardiac involvement by metastases.[3] The most common malignancies to metastasize to the heart are from lung, breast, lymphoma, and leukemia (Box 38-2). Lung and breast cancer, because of their high prevalence, are the most frequent sources of metastases to the heart. Melanoma, although a less common malignancy, has the highest frequency of secondary involvement of the heart, metastasizing to the heart in almost 60% of cases.[1]

Malignancies can reach the heart by three routes—by direct extension or through the lymphatic system or bloodstream. Lung and breast cancer metastasize through the lymphatic system, and they most often invade the pericardium. Lung cancer can also invade the pulmonary veins and grow into the left atrium. Adrenal metastases from a primary lung cancer may track up the inferior vena cava into the right atrium. Lymphoma often spreads by direct extension from mediastinal lesions to the pericardium. Intramyocardial and endocardial metastases usually result from hematogenous spread of malignant cells. Leukemia and melanoma spread by the hematogenous route.[3]

Signs or symptoms of metastatic cancer involving the heart are not common. Appreciable cardiac dysfunction develops in only about 10% of patients, and of these, 90% are the result of pericardial involvement and about 10% from intracavitary or myocardial involvement.[2]

Pericardial involvement can present in a variety of ways. There may be pericarditis with chest pain, fever, and friction rub. There may be painless accumulation of pericardial effusion leading to cardiac tamponade (see Chapter 29). Of note, cardiac tamponade that is encountered in patients in general medical practice is most likely caused by neoplasm.[4] There may be large, painless pericardial effusion that accumulates so slowly that there is no hemodynamic impairment. Pericardial involvement can also cause pericardial constriction with signs and symptoms of right-sided heart failure.

Myocardial metastasis can have different clinical presentations depending on the location and extent of involvement. Some patients present with congestive heart failure with dyspnea, orthopnea, and peripheral edema. Angina occurs if tumor impinges on the coronary arteries. If the tumor infiltrates the cardiac conduction system, bradyarrhythmias, atrioventricular block, bundle branch block, or tachyarrhythmias can occur.

The electrocardiogram (ECG) can sometimes demonstrate evidence of cardiac metastases. In a study by Cates et al.,[5] ECGs were reviewed of 210 patients who had a premortem and autopsy diagnosis of cancer. Cardiac metastases were present in 47 (22%) patients. The ECGs of these 47 were compared to the group of 163 patients without cardiac metastases. The most frequently encountered ECG abnormality in the group with cardiac metastases was nonspecific ST-T wave abnormalities (49%). Nineteen (40%) patients had ECG changes suggestive of myocardial ischemia or injury with either segmental or diffuse T wave inversions or ST segment elevation. Of those 19, 17 had no evidence of significant coronary artery disease. Other findings were low voltage and atrial arrhythmias, including atrial tachycardia, atrial fibrillation, and atrial flutter. Electrical alternans is another ECG abnormality that can occur in patients with cardiac metastases with large pericardial effusions.

Management

The diagnosis of secondary neoplasms of the heart can be made noninvasively with echocardiography and magnetic resonance imaging. Echocardiography can visualize intracavitary, intramyocardial, and pericardial lesions. Intracavitary lesions usually cannot be distinguished from thrombus. Intramyocardial lesions can give a heterogeneous appearance to the myocardium and cause wall motion abnormalities.

The most common finding suggestive of cardiac involvement by metastatic disease is a pericardial effusion, which often is quite large. At times, debris can be seen floating within the effusion. Echocardiography can assess the hemodynamic significance of a pericardial effusion. Right atrial or right ventricular diastolic collapse provides echocardiographic evidence of cardiac tamponade. Echo-Doppler evaluation of blood flow across the mitral valve is also useful. If mitral valve flow is reduced after inspiration, cardiac tamponade is likely present. When there is a massive amount of pericardial fluid, the heart can be seen swinging back and forth, which signifies tamponade and accounts for the ECG finding of electrical alternans. Echo-Doppler also can be used to diagnose pericardial constriction that can be secondary to malignancy or radiation therapy.

Magnetic resonance imaging is often complementary to echocardiography in diagnosing metastatic disease of the heart. MRI has a wider field of view than echocardiography and can provide spatial orientation of cardiac and paracardiac structures. It can further delineate pericardial abnormalities based on the thickness of the pericardium and identify extension of tumor from mediastinal lymph nodes or lung parenchyma. MRI can also identify tumors that extend up the inferior vena cava and invade the right atrium, including renal cell carcinoma and hepatoma.[6]

Pericardiocentesis with echo guidance is a useful invasive diagnostic procedure for evaluating pericardial effusions in cancer patients. Most malignant effusions are bloody. One study that pooled 93 cases with both pericardial fluid cytology from pericardiocentesis and pericardial tissue for microscopic examination had 41 true positives and 46 true negatives. No false positives occurred. A total of six patients had a false-negative pericardiocentesis and had evidence of malignancy on histopathologic examination. Fluid cytologic study thus had a sensitivity of 87% and a specificity of 100%. The positive predictive value was 100%, and the negative predictive value was 88%.[7] Pericardiocentesis is an accurate way to diagnose secondary malignancies of the heart in patients with pericardial effusions.

If pericardial cytology is negative in a cancer patient, the diagnosis can be challenging. If the fluid is hemorrhagic with a specific gravity greater than 3 mg/dL and a protein count greater than 3 mg/dL in the absence of a myocardial infarction, the diagnosis is neoplastic pericarditis until proved otherwise.[8] The next step is an open biopsy.

Other causes of pericarditis in cancer patients should not be overlooked. Given that many of these patients are immunocompromised as a result of chemotherapy, opportunistic infections including fungi and tuberculosis are possibilities. Therefore pericardial fluid should be sent not only for cytology but also gram stain, acid fast smear, and culture for bacteria, fungi, and mycobacteria. Still another diagnosis to keep in the differential is effusive-constrictive pericarditis secondary to radiation therapy. This is suspected when removal of pericardial fluid does not improve signs and symptoms of right-sided heart failure. Echocardiography, MRI, and right heart catheterization are useful in diagnosing this condition.

Endomyocardial biopsy can occasionally be helpful in diagnosing intramyocardial and endocardial metastases. This procedure is usually performed through the right internal jugular vein under transesophageal or fluoroscopic guidance. On rare occasions, workup of heart failure with endomyocardial biopsy provides the first clue of a primary malignancy that is lurking elsewhere.

Treatment options for secondary tumors of the heart include chemotherapy, radiation therapy, and surgery. If pericardial involvement is first manifested as tamponade, the acute treatment is pericardiocentesis. Subsequent treatment options include local instillation of chemotherapeutic agents into the pericardial space in an attempt to sclerose the visceral and parietal pericardium. Some agents that have been used with some success are nitrogen mustard, 5-fluorouracil, radioactive phosphorus, and tetracycline. Radiation therapy is an option as well. In fact, radiation therapy in combination with radioactive phosphorus has been used.[9] If a symptomatic pericardial effusion recurs, a pericardial window can be performed under local anesthesia. At times, pericardiectomy is required.

Radiation therapy can be useful in the palliation of metastatic cancer of the heart. In a study by Cham et al., 38 patients with secondary malignancy of the heart underwent radiation therapy. The primary site of malignancy was breast, lung, lymphoma, leukemia, and other miscellaneous sites, including ovary, kidney, and melanoma. Thirty-seven had evidence of pericardial involvement. Of 38 patients, 23 (61%) obtained palliation for a period ranging from 1 month to 36 months.[9] This small study concluded that patients with lymphoma and leukemia should receive at least 1500 rads over 10 days. Patients with carcinoma and sarcoma should receive at least 3000 rads over 4 weeks.

Expected Clinical Course

The prognosis of patients with secondary cancer of the heart, particularly of the pericardium, varies. Life expectancy can range from 6 months for patients with solid tumors to 15 months or longer with lymphoma.[7]

Patients with Hodgkin's disease can have significantly prolonged disease-free survival compared with those with the other malignancies.

CARDIAC COMPLICATIONS OF CANCER THERAPY
Radiation

Generally, between 1500 and 3500 rads can be delivered safely to the heart, pericardium, and mediastinal structures. Beyond 3500 rads, radiation heart disease can occur. The most common manifestation of radiation heart disease is pericarditis, pericardial effusion, or both. The mechanism is unclear, but microscopic examination reveals fibrin deposits on the pericardium. Constrictive pericarditis can be a long-term complication of radiation therapy.

The coronary arteries can also be affected. Coronary lesions following radiation are indistinguishable from atherosclerosis. Indeed, myocardial infarction has occurred in young adults as a complication of radiation treatment of childhood malignancies, in particular, Hodgkin's lymphoma.

Radiation to the heart can also cause mural endocardial thickening and interstitial fibrosis. This occurs mainly in the right-sided chambers because of their proximity to the external beam radiation port.[2]

Chemotherapy

Systemic chemotherapy that is used in the course of treating malignancies can have deleterious effects on the heart. Adriamycin (doxorubicin) is effective against a wide spectrum of malignancies and is well known for its cardiac toxicity. Adriamycin has acute, subacute, and chronic effects on the heart. The acute effects of the drug are seen during intravenous infusion and consist of ECG changes including atrial dysrhythmias and ST segment elevation. The subacute effects occur when a large dose is given too quickly and results in a pericarditis-myocarditis syndrome. The chronic toxic effect is related to cumulative dose. A total dose >450 mg/m^2 can lead to refractory heart failure. When approaching this dose, a radionuclide angiogram (RNA) is performed to assess ejection fraction. It is repeated serially with each subsequent dose. If the ejection fraction is declining, further adriamycin therapy is withheld[1,10] (see Chapter 24).

Cyclophosphamide and 5-fluorouracil are other chemotherapeutic agents with cardiac side effects. Cyclophosphamide is used in the treatment of a variety of tumors including breast cancer, leukemia, and lymphoma. In the commonly used doses, hemorrhagic cystitis can occur. Recently, it has been discovered that large doses of cyclophosphamide that are used in preparation for bone marrow transplantation have toxic cardiac effects. Hemorrhagic myopericarditis has been the most

frequently observed toxic effect. Irreversible heart failure has been reported with doses ranging from 180 to 240 mg/kg. 5-Fluorouracil is used in the treatment of adenocarcinoma of the breast, GI tract, and urinary tract. It has been reported to have caused angina and ECG changes that were probably secondary to coronary spasm. The angina was relieved with nitroglycerine.[1]

REFERENCES

1. Lancaster LD, Ewy GA: Cardiac consequences of malignancy and their treatment, Adv Intern Med 30:275, 1984.
2. Roberts WC: Primary and secondary neoplasms of the heart, Am J Cardiol 80:671, 1997.
3. Hillis LD, Lange RA, Winniford M, Page, R: Primary and secondary cardiac tumors. In Manual of clinical problems in cardiology, New York, 1995, Little, Brown.
4. Wilding G, Green HL, Longo DL, Urba WJ: Tumors of the heart and pericardium, Cancer Treat Rev 15:165, 1988.
5. Cates CU, Virmani R, Vaughn WK, Robertson RM: Electrocardiographic markers of cardiac metastasis, Am Heart J 112:1297, 1986.
6. Pohost G, editor: Magnetic resonance imaging for the evaluation of intracardiac masses. In Cardiovascular applications of magnetic resonance, Armonk, NY, 1993, Futura Publishing.
7. Meyers DG, Bouska DJ: Diagnostic usefulness of pericardial fluid cytology, Chest 95:1142, 1989.
8. Kralstein J, Frishman W: Malignant pericardial diseases: diagnosis and treatment, Am Heart J 113:785, 1987.
9. Cham WC, Freiman AH, Carstens PH, Chu FC: Radiation therapy of cardiac and pericardial metastases, Radiology 114:701, 1975.
10. Singal PK, Iliskovic N: Doxorubicin-induced cardiomyopathy, N Engl J Med 339:900, 1998.

39 Neuromuscular and Neurologic Disorders

Jerome J. Epplin
George J. Taylor

HEREDITARY NEUROMUSCULAR DISORDERS

Hereditary neuromuscular disorders affect skeletal muscle primarily, but most also have cardiovascular manifestations (Table 39-1). Genetic abnormalities are being sought and, when found, may offer promise for treatment. The degree of cardiac involvement in most cases does not correlate well with the severity of the neuromuscular disease.

Duchenne Muscular Dystrophy[1-6]

Duchenne muscular dystrophy is an X-linked progressive dystrophy passed by the mother to 50% of her sons as clinical disease and to 50% of her daughters as a carrier state. The prevalence rate is about 3 per 100,000, with the disease usually presenting by age 3 and nearly always being apparent by age 6. Patients with this disease lack the muscle protein dystrophin in both skeletal and cardiac muscle. The onset of weakness is usually before age 5 years, with an inability to walk after age 12 years. There is "pseudohypertrophy" of the calf muscles, which are large and rubbery, yet weak. The usual cause of death is respiratory failure in the second or third decades, often precipitated by pulmonary infection.

Cardiac involvement is common, with cardiomyopathy conduction disturbances, mitral valve prolapse, and wall motion abnormalities being most conspicuous. Other electrocardiographic (ECG) abnormalities include a shortened PR interval, tall R waves and increased R/S ratio in the right precordial leads, and deep and narrow Q waves in leads I, L, and V_{5-6} (the Qs are too narrow to be diagnostic for infarction). Frequently seen is a loss of posterobasal forces with a predominance of anterior forces. Female carriers of Duchenne muscular dystrophy may show larger R/S ratios in leads V_{1-2}. Rhythm disturbances include either persistent or paroxysmal sinus tachycardia, sinus pauses, and ventricular ectopic beats. Atrial flutter is an uncommon arrhythmia in children in general but may be a preterminal arrhythmia in children with Duchenne muscular dystrophy.

Mitral valve prolapse is common and may be caused by dystrophic changes involving the posterior papillary muscle. Regional wall motion abnormalities may occur, with a predilection for the posterobasal wall of the left ventricle. Small, thickened intramural coronary arteries are frequently reported but not necessarily in the areas of the regional wall motion abnormalities.

Recurrent pulmonary infections are the most common cause of death. Cardiomyopathy is present in most if not all patients over age 18, with systemic emboli occasionally arising from a dilated left ventricle. The degree of left ventricular (LV) dysfunction may be unrelated to the severity of skeletal muscle weakness. Congestive heart failure (CHF) is a frequent complication but usually is not the cause of death. Multiple pulmonary emboli may occur in late stages of the disease. Dilated cardiomyopathy has also been reported in female carriers of Duchenne muscular dystrophy.

Certain cardiac medications must be used with caution in patients with Duchenne muscular dystrophy. Phenytoin and procainamide may worsen muscle weakness, and intravenous verapamil may cause respiratory arrest. Malignant hyperthermia and cardiac arrest have occurred after using halothane, suxamethonium, isoflurane, and succinylcholine.

Becker Muscular Dystrophy[7,8]

Becker muscular dystrophy, with an incidence of 3-6 per 100,000 male births, is an X-linked disease and is more slowly progressive and of later onset than Duchenne muscular dystrophy. It also differs in that the dystrophin produced is abnormal or reduced but not absent.

Pseudohypertrophy and other features may suggest Duchenne muscular dystrophy, and it has been called a "benign" form of Duchenne's disease. Both the disease course and cardiac involvement are variable, most likely because of the variability of the quantity and quality of dystrophin produced. Most patients survive past age 30, with subclinical cardiac involvement being common. ECG abnormalities include shortened PQ segment, bundle branch blocks, infranodal conduction abnormalities, and ventricular arrhythmias. Tall R waves and Q waves in the inferolateral leads may be seen but at a much lower incidence compared with Duchenne muscular dystrophy. Cardiomyopathy, with the right ventricle being severely involved at times, may be progressive and fatal. As in Duchenne muscular dystrophy, its severity is not related to age or the amount of skeletal muscle involved.

433

Table 39-1	*Cardiac Involvement in Neuromuscular Disease*

Neuromuscular Disease	Mode of Inheritance	Neuromuscular Involvement	Cardiac Involvement	ECG Changes	Incidence
Duchenne muscular dystrophy	X-linked recessive	Calf pseudohypertrophy; pelvic, femoral, and pectoral muscle weakness; early onset	LV wall motion abnormalities, cardiomyopathy, MVP, progressive CHF	Short PR, increased R/S in right precordium, deep, narrow Q in lateral leads	1/3300 males
Becker muscular dystrophy	X-linked recessive	As above but later onset and more slowly progressive	Mild, often subclinical cardiomyopathy	Short PR, bundle branch blocks, ventricular arrhythmia	6/100,000 males
Myotonic dystrophy	Autosomal dominant	Myotonia of hands, forearms, jaw; atrophy of sternocleidomastoid	His-Purkinje disease, sudden death, diastolic dysfunction	Atrial flutter or fibrillation, ventricular tachycardia, complete heart block	5/100,000
Limb-girdle muscular dystrophy	Variable, most often autosomal recessive	Pelvic and shoulder girdle	MVP, elevated CK-MB	ST-T changes, atrial fibrillation	1/100,000
Emery-Dreifuss muscular dystrophy	X-linked recessive	Arm, pelvic girdle, contractures of elbow; cervical and Achilles	Atrial standstill, sudden death; also seen in female carriers	Prolonged AV conduction, complete heart block	
Facioscapulohumeral muscular dystrophy	Autosomal dominant	Facial, arm, and shoulder weakness	Questionable atrial standstill	Atrial fibrillation and flutter	

MVP, Mitral valve prolapse; *LV,* left ventricle; *CHF,* congestive heart failure, *AV,* atrioventricular.

Myotonic Dystrophy[9-11]

Myotonic dystrophy is the most common dystrophy occurring in adults, with a prevalence of 5 per 100,000. Inheritance is autosomal dominant with a high rate of penetrance. Myotonia (delayed relaxation after muscle contraction) is a predominant feature, and commonly involves the muscles of the hands, forearms, jaw, and tongue. Atrophy and occasionally disappearance of the sternocleidomastoid occurs. Other characteristics are cataracts, premature baldness, testicular atrophy, and mental decline.

Up to 80% of patients have cardiac involvement, most commonly involving the conducting system, with very few having myocardial involvement. His-Purkinje disease is common and manifested by first-degree AV block, left anterior fascicular block, and a widened QRS. The QT interval may be prolonged. Arrhythmias include atrial flutter or fibrillation, premature ventricular beats, and occasionally ventricular tachycardia. Patients with these ECG abnormalities have an increased risk of sudden death as a result of either high grade conduction defects or malignant arrhythmias, and symptoms of presyncope, syncope, or palpitations should be evaluated.

In addition to skeletal muscular myotonia, there has also been evidence of myocardial myotonia resulting in diastolic dysfunction. Significant congestive heart failure is rare.

Limb-Girdle Muscular Dystrophy[12]

Limb-girdle muscular dystrophy is an ill-defined category of dystrophies characterized by variable inheritance, late onset in life, and slow progression. The pelvic muscles are often involved, with thigh weakness being common. Due to the rarity of the disease (1 per 100,000) and difficulty in making a precise diagnosis, the extent of cardiac involvement has been difficult to

determine. The largest reported series found subclinical cardiac disease in 80% of patients, including elevated CK-MB fraction, mitral valve prolapse, sinus bradycardia, intraventricular conduction defects, and atrial fibrillation.

Emery-Dreifuss Muscular Dystrophy[13,14]

This syndrome is a rare X-linked muscular dystrophy with a slowly progressive course and frequent development of contractures at the elbow, Achilles tendon, and posterior cervical muscles. An increased incidence of atrial paralysis and resultant sudden death is the most important reason to make the diagnosis of this syndrome. Permanent ventricular pacing is indicated in patients with atrial standstill. Progressive cardiomyopathy has been reported, and female carriers of this syndrome may exhibit sinus bradycardia, first-degree heart block, or complete heart block and should be monitored with advancing age.

Facioscapulohumeral Muscular Dystrophy[15]

Facioscapulohumeral muscular dystrophy is an autosomal dominant disorder characterized by progressive facial muscle weakness, inability to close the eyes, and weakness of the arms and shoulders. The incidence of atrial fibrillation and flutter is increased. Earlier reports suggested atrial standstill as a complication of this disease, but these reports probably included cases of Emery-Dreifuss syndrome.

Other Neuromuscular Diseases

Of the more common other neurologic diseases, Charcot-Marie-Tooth syndrome, cerebellar ataxias, and myasthenia gravis are rarely associated with significant cardiac disease.[16] Patients with poliomyelitis have a higher incidence of atrial fibrillation, hyperkinetic left ventricular function, and mitral valve prolapse.

Friedreich's Ataxia[17,18]

Friedreich's ataxia is an autosomal recessive spinocerebellar neuromyopathy. The initial change is cell loss in the dorsal root of the spinal cord, with secondary degeneration in the posterior columns, spinocerebellar tracts, and peripheral nerves. Symptoms commonly include truncal and limb ataxia, dysarthria, loss of deep tendon reflexes and proprioceptive senses, pes cavus, and extensor plantar responses. Kyphoscoliosis is seen several years after onset of the disease and may be severe enough to cause respiratory difficulty.

Cardiac involvement is common, with most patients developing heart failure. CHF is the most common cause of death. As with other neuromuscular disorders, the severity of LV dysfunction does not parallel the degree of neurologic involvement. Vascular disease, especially involving the smaller coronary arteries, commonly occurs.

Cardiac muscle disease is not the result of the spinal cord denervation process. Both hypertrophic and dilated cardiomyopathies occur and do not appear to be a continuum of the same disease but rather a difference in the phenotypic expression of the disease. The hypertrophic type is the most common and is manifested by concentric left ventricular hypertrophy, normal systolic function, and only minimal abnormality of diastolic function. The dilated type is more lethal, with progressive ventricular deterioration. Common ECG findings include atrial fibrillation, ST-T wave abnormalities, right axis deviation, and shortened PR interval. Malignant ventricular arrhythmias rarely occur.

CARDIAC EFFECTS OF STROKE (see Chapter 34)
ECG Changes[19,20]

Electrocardiographic changes frequently accompany stroke, occurring in up to 70% of cases of intracranial bleeding, especially subarachnoid hemorrhage, and 15% of ischemic stroke. Commonly seen patterns include pseudoinfarction changes, prolongation of the QT interval, increased amplitude and duration of the T wave, or deeply and symmetrically inverted T waves. These changes usually occur in the absence of coronary artery disease. Mortality rates are not necessarily increased when such ECG changes are seen in association with subarachnoid hemorrhage, but are increased when seen in the presence of an ischemic stroke.

On the other hand, the deep T wave inversion does reflect myocardial changes. A probable mechanism is intense sympathetic discharge leading to subendocardial ischemia. Elevation of CK-MB has been documented, and autopsy studies have documented subendocardial myolysis. A common clinical issue is the risk of anesthesia and neurosurgery in the presence of these ECG changes and "recent infarction." Although no clinical studies have addressed the issue, we have generally recommended proceeding with emergency, potentially lifesaving neurosurgery without evaluation of coronary anatomy, believing that subendocardial injury in the absence of CAD poses less risk than similar ECG changes associated with a tight coronary stenosis.

Arrhythmias[21]

Significant arrhythmias may be seen in up to 40% of cases of stroke. Ventricular arrhythmias, ranging from isolated PVCs to torsade de pointe and sustained ventricular tachycardia, occur and portend an increased mortality rate. New-onset atrial fibrillation is found in up to 10% of strokes, although it is difficult to rule out the pos-

sibility that atrial fibrillation may be the cause of stroke and not its result. Sinus tachycardia and sinus arrhythmias are frequently seen, especially in midbrain lesions.

Hypertension[22]

Severe sustained hypertension may be seen in the initial stages of stroke. This reaction is more common with hemorrhagic than ischemic stroke. However, elevated pressure cannot be used to diagnose a bleed; it is difficult to tell if the hypertension is the cause of or the result of the stroke.

It is also difficult to distinguish between secondary hypertension caused by a stroke and neurologic changes caused by hypertensive encephalopathy. In both cases the neurologic changes may be caused by a breakdown in cerebral autoregulation, with the hypertension being a compensatory mechanism to maintain cerebral perfusion.

It must also be remembered that only a third of patients remain hypertensive 10 days after the stroke. No study has shown improvement in survival with treatment of acute hypertension in stroke. Precise guidelines are not available, but some principles are generally accepted. Significant hypertension (mean arterial pressure >130 mm Hg with mean arterial pressure = diastolic + one third pulse pressure) should be treated. Pressures do not need to be lowered to normal levels and should not be lowered rapidly.

Some clinical situations require more aggressive treatment of acute hypertension. The blood pressure must be acutely lowered if the stroke is caused by an aortic dissection or when concomitant myocardial ischemia is being worsened. Also, the pressure must be lowered if hypertension causes worsening of cerebral edema in the face of a progressing stroke.

Various agents can be used to lower the pressure (see Chapter 34). Most commonly used are short-acting vasodilating agents such as intravenous sodium nitroprusside or labetalol. Beta blockers are preferable in cases of myocardial ischemia or aortic dissection. Hydralazine should be avoided in cases of aortic dissection. Sublingual nifedipine always should be avoided.

Neurogenic Pulmonary Edema[23]

Strokes involving the medulla or hypothalamus, lesions resulting in increased intracranial pressure, head trauma, or grand mal seizures may cause neurogenic pulmonary edema. This edema fluid accumulates rapidly, is protein rich, and is referred to as *noncardiac pulmonary edema,* a variant of the adult respiratory distress syndrome. Increased permeability of the pulmonary capillaries contributes to excess pulmonary fluid. In addition, sympathetic overactivity may cause a shift of fluid from the systemic to the pulmonary circulation. The fluid usually rapidly clears after the cessation of the aggravating insult.

SOURCES OF CARDIOEMBOLISM[24]

It is conservatively estimated that up to 20% of all ischemic strokes are caused by emboli. Internal carotid arteries with a stenosis of >70% are a significant source of these emboli, with the rest originating from the heart or aortic arch. These patients may be evaluated noninvasively by Doppler studies of the carotids. Common sources of emboli are listed in Box 39-1.

Cardiac sources of emboli may be detected in most cases by echocardiography. Transesophageal echocardiography may be necessary to define an embolic source (see Chapter 34). We use this technique when the transthoracic study is negative and we suspect cardiac thromboembolism (e.g., a young patient with stroke and no apparent cause).

It has become increasingly clear that adequate preventive care such as anticoagulation or appropriate antibiotic therapy may prevent emboli. It is even more important to institute appropriate secondary prevention in patients who have already exhibited disease manifestations.

BOX 39-1

SOURCES OF CEREBRAL THROMBOEMBOLISM

Atherosclerotic
  Internal carotid disease
  Aortic arch disease
  Acute anterior wall myocardial infarction
  Ischemic cardiomyopathy (regional LV contraction abnormality)
  Left ventricular aneurysm
Cardiac tumor
Dilated cardiomyopathies
Arrhythmias
  Atrial fibrillation
  Sick sinus syndrome
Paradoxical embolus (through an atrial septal defect or patent foramen ovale)
Valvular disease
  Mitral stenosis
  Calcific aortic stenosis
  Mitral valve prolapse
  Endocarditis
  Prosthetic mechanical valve
Soon after heart surgery (atrial fibrillation, carotid bruit, and a history of stroke or TIA are risk factors for stroke in this setting).

Atrial Fibrillation

The incidence of stroke in patients over age 65 with nonrheumatic atrial fibrillation is 3% per year. With the institution of warfarin therapy keeping the INR between 2 and 3 the incidence falls to less than 0.5% per year with only a slight increase in bleeding events. Recent studies have shown that the efficacy of stroke prevention decreases significantly when the INR is below 2. At the other extreme, the risk of intracranial bleeding significantly rises with the INR ≥4. Aspirin is better than placebo for the prevention of stroke but is less effective than warfarin (see Chapters 25 and 39).

In patients under age 65 with no other risk factors for stroke, so-called lone atrial fibrillation, there is no evidence of increased incidence of stroke. Aspirin, but not warfarin, therapy is indicated.

It is even more important to anticoagulate a patient in atrial fibrillation who has had a prior stroke. The risk of recurrent stroke is as high as 32% in the first year, with a particularly high risk in the first 2 weeks (see Chapter 25). If a patient with atrial fibrillation has had a prior systemic embolus while adequately anticoagulated, several options are available. Aspirin could be added to the warfarin or the INR could be increased to between 3 and 4. Neither approach has been shown superior to the other.

Contraindications to warfarin therapy are listed in Box 39-2. It should be noted that advanced age is not listed, since studies suggest that patients over age 75 receive the most benefit from anticoagulation.

Patients who have been in atrial fibrillation for more that 2 days should have their INR between 2 and 3 for 3 weeks before elective electrical or chemical cardioversion (see Chapter 25). Warfarin should be continued for 4 weeks *after* establishment of sinus rhythm. Warfarin is not indicated before cardioversion for patients with supraventricular tachycardia, or atrial fibrillation of less than 2 days duration. Some studies indicate that, if left atrial thrombi are not found by transesophageal echocardiography, cardioversion can be safely undertaken in patients who are not anticoagulated.

Mitral Stenosis and Atrial Fibrillation

The combination of atrial fibrillation, either chronic or paroxysmal, and mitral stenosis significantly increases the risk of systemic embolism, and warfarin therapy is indicated. If mitral stenosis with sinus rhythm is present but the left atrial diameter is greater than 5.5 cm, anticoagulation is indicated. If embolization occurs in spite of adequate coagulation, either aspirin could be added or the INR could be increased to between 3 and 4.

Aortic Stenosis

Cerebral emboli causing either stroke or transient ischemic attack may originate from a thickened bicuspid aortic valve. Calcium emboli may also travel to distant organs, including the brain. It is not routinely recommended to anticoagulate a patient with calcific aortic stenosis unless there is evidence of embolization.

Mitral Valve Prolapse

Mitral valve prolapse (MVP) is a common finding, occurring in 3% to 5% of the population, with females affected twice as often as males. The prognosis is usually good, with the most frequent complication being progressive mitral regurgitation (occurring in <10%). The most recent studies indicate no increase in the risk of stroke in young patients with MVP (see Chapter 18). Anticoagulation is not indicated.

Prosthetic Heart Valves

After tissue prosthetic valves have been in place for 3 months, which allows endothelialization to take place, anticoagulation is unnecessary unless patients have other indications for anticoagulation. For the first 3 months after surgery, patients should be anticoagulated with warfarin (the INR kept between 2 and 3).

Mechanical valves have a significant risk of thromboembolism, with prostheses in the mitral position having a higher risk than aortic valves. The INR should be kept in the range of 2.5 to 3.5. If the patient has had a prior thromboembolism or is in atrial fibrillation, the INR should be kept at 3 to 4.5. Aspirin may be used with warfarin, particularly after a thromboembolic event despite a therapeutic INR (see Table 52-4).

Endocarditis

Stroke may be the presenting symptom in patients with infective endocarditis (IE). Stroke is a common compli-

---

BOX 39-2

CONTRAINDICATIONS TO WARFARIN THERAPY

Noncompliant patient
Active bleeding
Coagulopathy
Recent CNS or eye surgery
Pregnancy
Ethanol abuse
Prior severe bleeding with anticoagulation
Prior skin necrosis with warfarin
History of frequent falls (relative
    contraindication)

cation, even for patients who have been stable and following appropriate antimicrobial therapy. However, anticoagulation has not been recommended unless other indications for anticoagulation exist. Transesophageal echocardiography has increased the ability to detect valvular vegetations but cannot accurately predict the risk of a vegetation causing an embolus.

Paradoxical Embolus

Cerebral thromboembolus originating from the venous system passing through a patent foramen ovale or an atrial septal defect may be an underrecognized source of stroke, especially in younger patients (see Chapter 34). In patients with no other obvious source of embolus, a contrast echocardiogram with Valsalva maneuver should be carried out. Whether a patent foramen ovale warrants closure, even when there has been an embolic event, is controversial.

Acute Myocardial Infarction

Mural thrombi develop commonly during acute anterior myocardial infarction not treated with thrombolytic therapy (see Chapter 16). They also occur with inferior MI but at a lesser rate. The risk of stroke with an anterior infarction is as high as 6%, especially if the infarct is

large. Anticoagulation with heparin while hospitalized is recommended, followed by warfarin for 3 months (Table 39-2; see also Tables 16-3 and 17-6). If the myocardial infarction is successfully treated with thrombolysis, treatment with aspirin but not warfarin is indicated.

Dilated Cardiomyopathy

Dilated cardiomyopathy is commonly complicated by mural thrombus, a result of intracavitary stasis of blood in the left ventricle. The effect of anticoagulation in these patients is difficult to assess, because many have other risk factors for stroke or other reasons for anticoagulation. Although no data from clinical trials have documented a need, the common clinical practice is long-term anticoagulation in these cases.

Extracardiac Sources of Emboli

Stroke or transient ischemic attacks commonly are caused by atherosclerotic emboli or thrombi originating from the aortic arch or internal carotid arteries. The aortic arch is best evaluated by transesophageal echocardiography, although no definite guidelines exist to determine which patients should be evaluated. The carotid arteries are best evaluated noninvasively by Doppler studies. If stenosis in the internal carotid is shown to be ≥60% and

Table 39-2	Anticoagulation in Certain Conditions*	
Condition	**Treatment**	**Comment**
Atrial fibrillation, age <65	Aspirin	Assumes no valvular heart disease
Atrial fibrillation, age >65	Warfarin INR 2-3	Continued for life
Mitral stenosis with AF or left atrial diameter >5.5cm	Warfarin INR 2-3	Should be treated even if in sinus rhythm
Tissue prosthetic valve	Warfarin INR 2-3 for 3 months after valve is placed	Then stop warfarin unless other indications exist
Mechanical prosthetic valve	Warfarin INR 2.5-3.5	Keep INR 3-4.5 if in atrial fibrillation
Acute anterior myocardial infarction*	Warfarin INR 2-3 for 3 months	Use aspirin only if treated acutely with thrombolysis
Dilated cardiomyopathy	Warfarin INR 2-3	Controversial
Endocarditis with emboli	Antibiotics	Warfarin for other indications
Aortic stenosis with emboli	Aspirin	Emboli often are calcium
Carotid disease	Aspirin if stenosis <70%	Endarterectomy for stenosis >70%

*See also Table 16-3.

if a surgical center has a morbidity and mortality rate of <6%, then carotid endarterectomy is recommended. Asymptomatic patients with bruits who are found to have a stenosis >60% should also be considered for endarterectomy. Aspirin is advised for patients with a stenosis <60%. However, if a patient continues having transient ischemic attacks or small strokes while taking aspirin and has no indications for surgery, ticlopidine could be used. If this fails, warfarin should be added.

Coronary Bypass Surgery

About 1% of coronary artery bypass surgeries are complicated by acute cerebral vascular events. Suggested mechanisms are embolization of atheromatous material from the ascending surgically traumatized aorta or embolization of a postinfarction left ventricular thrombus. On the other hand, transient atrial fibrillation (which complicates 15% to 20% of procedures), prior TIA or stroke, carotid bruit, and advanced age have been identified as risk factors for postoperative stroke and TIA. This would suggest that the usual causes of cerebral ischemia are operating after heart surgery.

SYNCOPE

As many as 3% of adults have syncope in a given year, and about 30% of them have a recurrence. In many, if not most, the cause remains unknown, even after extensive evaluation. Neurogenic syncope and arrhythmias are reviewed in Chapter 27.

A number of structural abnormalities limit forward cardiac output and may cause syncope. For example, cardiac filling may be limited by pericardial disease or tamponade. Inability to empty the right ventricle completely is seen in pulmonary hypertension or pulmonic stenosis. Indirectly this leads to decreased flow to the left ventricle. Almost any other valvular disease may cause either decreased filling or emptying of the left ventricle.

The most important of these, especially in the elderly, is aortic stenosis. As the gradient across the valve increases and flow decreases, the murmur may become softer and more difficult to hear. One should suspect aortic stenosis as the etiology of syncope if the area of the valve as measured by echocardiography is <0.7 cm.^{2} Hypertrophic subaortic stenosis causes syncope, especially under conditions that decrease blood flow to the heart or that increase myocardial contractility (thereby aggravating obstruction). These conditions include therapy with digoxin or beta agonists, dehydration, Valsalva maneuver, or sudden standing after squatting.

Myocardial tumors, either primary or metastatic, may cause syncope if the tumor is in a position to cause obstruction to flow. Left atrial myxoma obstructing the mitral valve is the most common of these (see Chapter 38). The evaluation for possible structural causes of syncope should include an echocardiogram. The transthoracic echo usually is adequate.

REFERENCES

1. Slucka C: The electrocardiogram in Duchenne progressive muscular dystrophy, *Circulation* 38:933, 1968.
2. Lane RJ, Gardner-Medwin D, Roses A: Electrocardiographic abnormalities in carriers of Duchenne muscular dystrophy, *Neurology* 30:497, 1980.
3. Perloff J: Cardiac rhythm and conduction in Duchenne's muscular dystrophy: a prospective study of 20 patients, *J Am Coll Cardiol* 3:1263, 1984.
4. Perloff J, Moise NS, Stevenson W, Gilmour R: Cardiac electrophysiology in Duchenne muscular dystrophy: from basic science to clinical expression, *J Cardiovasc Electrophysiol* 3:394, 1992.
5. Mirabella M, Servidei S, Manfredi G, et al: Cardiomyopathy may be the only clinical manifestation in female carriers of Duchenne muscular dystrophy, *Neurology* 43:2342, 1993.
6. Chalkiadis GA, Branch KG: Cardiac arrest after isoflurane anaesthesia in a patient with Duchenne's muscular dystrophy, *Anaesthesia* 45:22, 1990
7. Nigro G, Comi LI, Politano L, et al: Evaluation of the cardiomyopathy in Becker muscular dystrophy, *Muscle Nerve* 18:283, 1995.
8. Melacini P, Fanin M, Danieli GA, et al: Cardiac involvement in Becker muscular dystrophy, *J Am Coll Cardiol* 22:1927, 1993.
9. Fragola PV, Luzi M, Calo L, et al: Cardiac involvement in myotonic dystrophy, *Am J Cardiol* 74:1070, 1994.
10. Fragola PV, Autore C, Magni G, et al: The natural course of cardiac conduction disturbances in myotonic dystrophy, *Cardiology* 79:93, 1991.
11. Child J, Perloff J: Myocardial myotonia in myotonic muscular dystrophy, *Am Heart J* 129:982, 1995.
12. Stubgen J: Limb-girdle muscular dystrophy: a noninvasive cardiac evaluation, *Cardiology* 83:324, 1993.
13. Marshall T, Huckell V: Atrial paralysis in a patient with Emery-Dreifuss muscular dystrophy, *Pacing Clin Electrophysiol* 15:35, 1992.
14. Bialer M, McDaniel N, Kelly T: Progression of cardiac disease in Emery-Dreifuss muscular dystrophy, *Clin Cardiol* 14:411, 1991.
15. Stevenson WG, Perloff JK, Weiss JN, Anderson TL: Facioscapulohumeral muscular dystrophy: evidence for selective, genetic electrophysiologic cardiac involvement, *J Am Coll Cardiol* 15:292, 1990.
16. Isner JM, Hawley RJ, Weintraub AM, Engel WK: Cardiac findings in Charcot-Marie-Tooth disease, *Arch Intern Med* 139:1161, 1979.
17. James TN, Cobbs BW, Coghlan HC, et al: Coronary disease, cardioneuropathy, and conduction system abnormalities in the cardiomyopathy of Friedreich's ataxia, *Br Heart J* 57:446, 1987.
18. Child JS, Perloff JK, Bach PM, et al: Cardiac involvement in Friedreich's ataxia: a clinical study of 75 patients, *J Am Coll Cardiol* 7:1370, 1986.

19. Caplan L: Brain embolism, revisited, *Neurology* 43:128, 1993.

20. Davis T, Alexander J, Lesch M: Electrocardiographic changes associated with acute cerebrovascular disease: a clinical review, *Prog Cardiovasc Dis* 36:245, 1993.

21. Oppenheimer S, Cechetto D, Hachinski V: Cerebrogenic cardiac arrhythmias, *Arch Neurol* 47:513, 1990.

22. O'Connell J, Gray C: Treating hypertension after stroke, *BMJ* 308:1523, 1994.

23. Malik A: Mechanisms of neurogenic pulmonary edema, *Circ Res* 57:1, 1985.

24. Hart J: Cardiogenic embolism to the brain, *Lancet* 339:589, 1992.

40 Pregnancy and Heart Disease

Sarita Kansal
George J. Taylor

CARDIOVASCULAR PHYSIOLOGY DURING PREGNANCY

Pregnancy leads to hemodynamic changes in the maternal cardiovascular system that increase the workload of the heart. The maternal blood volume increases by about 40%, and cardiac output increases 1.3-1.5 times the nonpregnant output by the time of delivery.[1] Since the demand on the cardiorespiratory system increases during pregnancy, heart failure may develop in a pregnant woman with cardiovascular disease who is otherwise stable in the nonpregnant state. Table 40-1 summarizes the hemodynamic changes that occur during normal pregnancy.

CARDIAC EVALUATION DURING PREGNANCY

An important first step to ensure a successful outcome of pregnancy in a patient with cardiac disease is early diagnosis and assessment of its severity.

History and Physical Examination

Cardiac evaluation is complicated by the hemodynamic changes of normal pregnancy. These result in signs and symptoms that can either simulate or obscure heart disease (Box 40-1). Anasarca, paroxysmal nocturnal dyspnea, syncope, hemoptysis, and chest pain are not normal symptoms of pregnancy and warrant investigation. Similarly, diastolic murmurs are always abnormal. Severity of heart disease during pregnancy is assessed using the New York Heart Association (NYHA) classification (see Chapter 3).

Laboratory Evaluation

Normal findings on electrocardiography (ECG), chest x-ray, and echocardiography are shown in Box 40-2. The pelvic area should be shielded during a chest x-ray.

Stress testing with a submaximal exercise stress test (heart rate increased up to 75% of maximal predicted heart rate) may be carried out during pregnancy if necessary to establish the diagnosis of ischemic heart disease and assess functional capacity.[2] Radionuclide imaging and cardiac catheterization carry the risk of radiation exposure to the fetus and should be avoided during pregnancy. Currently there is no evidence that MRI is hazardous to the fetus, although it is recommended that MRI be avoided in the first trimester of pregnancy.[3]

COUNSELING PREGNANT PATIENTS WITH HEART DISEASE

The risk of perinatal mortality and maternal morbidity and mortality depends on three factors: the underlying cardiac lesion (Box 40-3), the functional derangement

Table 40-1	*Hemodynamic Changes During Normal Pregnancy*		
Parameter	**First Trimester**	**Second Trimester**	**Third Trimester**
Blood volume	↑	↑↑	↑↑↑
Cardiac output	↑	↑↑ to ↑↑↑	↑↑↑ to ↑↑
Stroke volume	↑	↑↑↑	↑, ↔, or ↓
Heart rate	↑	↑↑	↑↑ to ↑↑↑
Systolic blood pressure	↔	↓	↔
Diastolic blood pressure	↓	↓↓	↓
Pulse pressure	↑	↑↑	↔
Systemic vascular resistance	↓	↓↓↓	↓↓

Modified from Elkayam U, Gleicher N:Hemodynamics and cardiac function during normal pregnancy and the puerperium. In Elkayam U, Gleicher N, editors: *Cardiac problems in pregnancy: diagnosis and management of maternal and fetal disease*, ed 2, New York, 1990, Alan R Liss.
↔, No change compared with nonpregnant level; ↑, small increase; ↑↑, moderate increase; ↑↑↑, large increase; ↓, small decrease; ↓↓, moderate decrease; ↓↓↓, large decrease.

BOX 40-1

CARDIAC SYMPTOMS AND SIGNS DURING *NORMAL* PREGNANCY

SYMPTOMS
Decreased exercise capacity
Tiredness
Dyspnea
Orthopnea
Lightheadedness
Syncope

SIGNS
Inspection
Hyperventilation
Peripheral edema
Distended neck veins with prominent A and V waves and brisk X and Y descent
Capillary pulsation

Precordial palpation
Brisk, diffuse, and displaced left ventricular impulse
Palpable right ventricular impulse
Palpable pulmonary trunk impulse

Auscultation
Increased S_1 with exaggerated splitting
Persistent splitting of S_2
Midsystolic ejection-type murmur at lower left sternal edge or over pulmonary area radiating to left side of neck
Continuous murmurs (cervical venous hum, mammary souffle)

Modified from Elkayam U, Gleicher N: Hemodynamics and cardiac function during normal pregnancy and the puerperium. In Elkayam U, Gleichef N, editors: *Cardiac problems in pregnancy: diagnosis and management of maternal and fetal disease,* ed 2, New York, 1990, Alan R Liss.

BOX 40-2

ELECTROCARDIOGRAPHY, CHEST X-RAY, AND ECHOCARDIOGRAPHY-DOPPLER FINDINGS DURING *NORMAL* PREGNANCY

ELECTROCARDIOGRAM
ORS axis deviation
ST segment and T wave changes
Small Q wave and inverted P wave in lead III (abolished by inspiration)
Increased R wave amplitude in lead V_2
Sinus tachycardia

CHEST X-RAY
Straightening of left upper cardiac border
Horizontal position of the heart
Increased lung markings
Small pleural effusion early postpartum

ECHO-DOPPLER
Increased left and right ventricular dimensions
Unchanged or slightly increased size and systolic function of left ventricle
Mild increase in left and right atrial size
Small pericardial effusion
Increased diameter of tricuspid annulus
Functional tricuspid, pulmonary and mitral insufficiency

Modified from Elkayam U, Gleicher N: Hemodynamics and cardiac function during normal pregnancy and the puerperium. In Elkayam U, Gleichef N, editors: *Cardiac problems in pregnancy: diagnosis and management of maternal and fetal disease,* ed 2, New York, 1990, Alan R Liss.

---

produced by the lesion (those with NYHA classes III and IV should be advised against pregnancy), and the development of pregnancy-related complications (e.g., hypertension, hemorrhage, and infection).

A pregnant patient should be counseled about the risks she and her fetus will face during pregnancy. Patients with surgically correctable lesions should undergo surgery before conception. Those with congenital heart disease must be advised about the risk of their offspring inheriting a congenital lesion. The majority of these lesions have a polygenic mode of inheritance with a 7% (2% to 18%) risk of transmission.[1] Important exceptions include Marfan's syndrome and idiopathic hypertrophic subaortic stenosis, which are autosomal dominant.

GENERAL MANAGEMENT OF HEART DISEASE DURING PREGNANCY

Cigarette smoking and alcohol are dangerous to maternal health and fetal development in normal pregnancy and even more so for a pregnant patient with heart disease. Physical activity may need to be limited, using a patient's sense of fatigue, shortness of breath, and palpitations as indicators. Emotional stress, largely related to coping with both the pregnancy and the heart disease, can lead to an increase in heart rate and cardiac output.

The education of the patient and the family may be the decisive point in the successful outcome of the preg-

BOX 40-3

MORTALITY RISK ASSOCIATED WITH CARDIAC DISEASE IN PREGNANCY

LOW RISK (<1 %)
Septal defects
Patent ductus arteriosus
Pulmonic/tricuspid lesions
New York Heart Association classes I and II

MODERATE RISK (5% TO 15%)
NYHA classes III and IV mitral stenosis
Aortic stenosis
Marfan's syndrome with normal aortic root
Uncomplicated coarctation of the aorta
Past history of myocardial infarction

HIGH RISK (25% TO 50%)
Eisenmenger's syndrome
Pulmonary hypertension
Marfan's syndrome with abnormal aortic root
Peripartal cardiomyopathy

Adapted from Clark SL: *Clin Perinatol* 13:697, 1986.

nancy. The physician's attitude should be one of reassurance and optimism. Hot and humid environments (whirlpools and saunas) are contraindicated. Food intake should be divided into multiple small meals, especially in those with severely limiting heart disease. Arrhythmias, anemia, excessive weight gain, infection, and hyperthyroidism are all treatable conditions that increase the burden on the heart during pregnancy.

ETIOLOGY OF HEART DISEASE IN PREGNANCY

With the incidence of rheumatic heart disease decreasing, congenital heart disease has increased in relative importance in the United States. Heart disease has become the principal nonobstetric cause of maternal death, largely because of advances in the treatment of sepsis and hemorrhage.[4]

CONGENITAL HEART DISEASE

The anatomy, physiology, and prognosis vary significantly among the different forms of congenital heart disease, so accurate diagnosis is essential.

Maternal and Fetal Outcome

A good maternal outcome can be expected in most cases of noncyanotic congenital heart disease (CHD), includ-

ing atrial and ventricular septal defect, PDA, coarctation of aorta, and pulmonary stenosis) (see Chapter 30). The nature of the lesion, history of surgical repair, and functional capacity of the patient influence maternal outcome. Patients previously operated on for ASD, VSD, and PDA and who are currently asymptomatic and have normal hemodynamics do not have an increased risk from pregnancy.

Maternal functional capacity and cyanosis also determine fetal outcome. Fetal wastage is seen in 45% of cyanotic mothers compared with 20% in acyanotic patients with CHD. Low birth weight, prematurity, and increased incidence of mental and physical impairments are commonly seen in children born to mothers with CHD. Limitation of activity during fetal organogenesis and oxygen inhalation during the last trimester of pregnancy may encourage intrauterine growth in women with cyanotic CHD.

Eisenmenger's syndrome is associated with a high risk of maternal mortality, and these patients should be advised against pregnancy. Therapeutic abortion is commonly recommended for those already pregnant.

Labor and Delivery

To obtain better monitoring of hemodynamic status and availability of expert personnel, elective induction of labor after fetal maturity is recommended. Cesarean section should be performed primarily for obstetric reasons and is not routinely indicated.

ACQUIRED VALVULAR LESIONS

Maternal morbidity and mortality from valvular disease result from congestive heart failure or arrhythmias. Atrial fibrillation during gestation has a higher incidence of heart failure and embolization than it does in the nonpregnant state.[5] In patients with valvular abnormalities, it is essential to ask the following questions at every visit. Is hemodynamic status optimal? Is antibiotic prophylaxis against endocarditis necessary? Is anticoagulation needed? Could the patient's current symptoms be caused by heart disease? Should therapeutic plans be changed because the patient is pregnant or considering pregnancy?[4] In contrast to patients with congenital deformities, lack of symptoms in patients with valvular disease is indicative of an acceptable hemodynamic state. The exception is aortic stenosis.

Women with valve disease, even in NYHA functional class I or II, deliver infants that are small for gestational age, but there is no evidence of an increased incidence of congenital malformations.

Mitral stenosis (MS) is the most common rheumatic valvular lesion in pregnancy. Most patients with moderate to severe MS have worsening of their clinical condition during gestation. During pregnancy the aim is to

---

BOX 40-4

INTRAPARTUM MANAGEMENT PROTOCOL FOR PATIENTS WITH VALVULAR DISEASE*

1. Admission to hospital at term with favorable cervix
2. Placement of pulmonary artery catheter and optimization of hemodynamics for 24 hours
3. Induction of labor
4. Labor on left side
5. O_2 administration, 4 to 6 L/min
6. IV D5W to keep vein open
7. Epidural anesthesia
8. Intrapartum hemodynamic management
   a. Mitral stenosis; no pulmonary hypertension. Keep heart rate below 90 beats/min with oral/IV propranolol. Diurese to wedge pressure 12 to 14 mm Hg†
   b. Aortic stenosis or pulmonary hypertension: adjust wedge pressure to 16 to 18 mm Hg‡
9. Prophylaxis against bacterial endocarditis (Table 40-2)

Adapted from Clark SL: *Clin Perinatol* 13:697, 1986.

*For patients who have class I or II throughout pregnancy and do not have pulmonary hypertension or prior MI, steps 1 to 3 and 8 may be omitted.

†This must be done with careful attention to maintenance of blood pressure and cardiac output. This optimal level cannot be achieved in some patients.

‡To maintain a margin of safety against unexpected hypotension or blood loss.

---

reduce heart rate and blood volume by restricting activity and salt intake and using elastic support stockings, gentle diuresis, and beta-blockers. Hemodynamic monitoring for pulmonary edema is recommended at the initiation of labor and is continued for several hours postpartum for symptomatic patients with moderate to severe MS (valve area <1.5 cm^2). The entire labor should be conducted with the patient on her side, since this results in the most stable hemodynamics. Vaginal delivery can be permitted in most patients with MS. Bearing down efforts should be avoided in the second stage of labor.

Mitral regurgitation, aortic regurgitation, and aortic stenosis (valve area >1.0 cm^2) are usually well tolerated in pregnancy. Intrapartum management protocol for patients with valvular heart disease is given in Box 40-4.

OTHER CARDIAC CONDITIONS

Mild valve prolapse is common in women of childbearing age. Pregnancy may reduce the incidence of prolapse-related auscultatory and echocardiographic changes as a result of an increase in left ventricular end-diastolic volume. Emphasis should be on reassurance and the avoidance of unnecessary medications. Beta-blockers may be used, if necessary, for chest pain and arrhythmias.

Marfan's syndrome with pregnancy carries the risk of aortic dissection and death, and there is a 50% risk of transmitting the condition to the child. Aortic regurgitation, heart failure, and aortic dissection occur in the later phase of pregnancy. Women who have cardiac involvement should be advised against pregnancy. The risk of pregnancy is significantly lower in patients without cardiac complications. Preconceptual and then periodic echocardiographic assessment of the aorta is recommended every 6 to 8 weeks during pregnancy. Beta-blockers, which reduce the rate of aortic dilation, should be administered.[6] In women with cardiac complications cesarean section is the preferred method of delivery.

Primary pulmonary hypertension (PPH) has a maternal mortality rate of 40% to 50%. PPH is exacerbated by pregnancy, and symptomatic deterioration usually occurs in the second trimester, with fatigue, dyspnea, syncope, and right ventricular failure. Death occurs most often during late gestation or in the early postpartum period. PPH is also associated with high incidence of fetal loss and growth retardation. Women who have PPH should avoid pregnancy. Oral contraceptives should not be recommended for women with PPH, since a causative link between pulmonary hypertension and estrogen-containing oral contraceptives has been suggested.[7] Anticoagulation is recommended throughout pregnancy and the early postpartum phase. As with Eisenmenger's syndrome, the vaginal route of delivery is safer and preferred over cesarean section.

Table 40-2 | *Guidelines for Endocarditis Prophylaxis*

Site of Procedure	Drug	Standard Dose/Route	Reasons	Alternative Drug	Dose/Route
Dental, oral, upper respiratory tract	Amoxicillin	3 g PO 1 hr before procedure, then 1.5 g PO 6 hr later	Penicillin allergy	Erythromycin ethylsuccinate	800 mg PO 2 hr before procedure, then 400 MG 6 hr later
			Unable to take oral medications	Ampicillin	2 g IV/IM 30 min before, then 1 g IV 6 hr later
				Clindamycin	300 mg IV 30 min before, then 150 mg IV/PO 6 hr later
			High risk, penicillin allergic	Vancomycin	1 g IV starting 1 hr before; repeat dose not necessary
Genitourinary/ gastrointestinal tract	Ampicillin plus gentamicin then amoxicillin	Ampicillin 2 g IV plus gentamicin 1.5 mg/kg IV 30 min before, then amoxicillin 1.5 g PO 6 hr later or repeat IV regimen 8 hr later	Penicillin allergic	Vancomycin plus gentamicin	Vancomycin 1 g IV (over 1 hr) starting 1 hr before plus gentamicin 1.5 mg/kg IV 1 hr before; may be repeated 8 hr later
			Low risk	Amoxicillin	3 g PO 1 hr before; 1.5 g PO 6 hr later

These are the recommendations of the American Heart Association (*JAMA* 264:2919, 1990).

CARDIOMYOPATHIES
Hypertrophic Cardiomyopathy

Hypertrophic cardiomyopathy (HC) has a favorable outcome in most cases. Fetal outcome does not seem to be affected by maternal HO. The risk of inheriting the disease may be as high as 50% in familial cases but less in the sporadic ones. In patients with symptoms, hypovolemia and sympathetic stimulation should be avoided to prevent worsening of left ventricular outflow obstruction. Beta-blockers, calcium channel blockers, and diuretics can be used for treatment. Dual-chamber pacing has been tried in patients who have symptoms early in pregnancy (see Chapter 23). Vaginal delivery is safe in women with HC and is not contraindicated even in symptomatic patients.

Peripartum Cardiomyopathy

Peripartum cardiomyopathy (PPCM) is a form of dilated cardiomyopathy that often affects women with no previous cardiac disease. Symptoms usually occur in the last 4 weeks of pregnancy or the first 6 months postpartum. The incidence of PPCM is greater in older, multiparous women. Twin pregnancies increase the risk, and it is more common among blacks. The exact cause of PPCM is unknown. About half of patients show complete recovery of cardiac function within the first 6 months postpartum. A few have continuous deterioration leading to early death or chronic heart failure. Medical treatment includes rest, diuretics, digoxin, and vasodilators. Hydralazine is considered safe during pregnancy. Angiotensin-converting enzyme (ACE) inhibitors are contraindicated because of fetal renal dysfunction. Anticoagulation with heparin is recommended because of the increased incidence of thromboembolism.

Subsequent pregnancies are often associated with relapses and a high risk for maternal mortality and morbidity, even in those in whom left ventricular function is restored after the first episode. For this reason, PPCU is considered a contraindication to future pregnancy.

CORONARY ARTERY DISEASE

Coronary artery disease is rare among women of child-bearing age, but it may occur. The combination of heavy smoking and concurrent use of oral contraceptives may provoke MI, as both promote thrombosis.[8] Peripartum acute MI may also be due to coronary arteries. The use of oxytocin and prostaglandins may provoke spasm. Coronary aneurysm and dissection are other causes of peripartum acute MI.

The general principles of treatment are the same as with other patients with acute MI, except that thrombolytic therapy is contraindicated (see Chapter 14). Primary PTCA is preferable. Nitrates, beta-blockers, and low-dose aspirin have been used without adverse fetal effects. Elective induction of labor within 2 weeks of infarction is contraindicated.

ARRHYTHMIAS

Pregnancy is associated with an increased incidence of arrhythmias in women with and without organic heart disease. Healthy women may have frequent, asymptomatic atrial and ventricular premature contractions. Those with preexisting dysrhythmias usually tolerate pregnancy well. Digoxin, procainamide, quinidine, and beta-blockers may be administered to pregnant patients. Intrauterine growth retardation previously reported with beta-blockers appears to be caused by underlying disease rather than a drug effect.

Onset of arrhythmia during pregnancy requires evaluation for electrolyte imbalance, thyroid disease, and arrhythmogenic effects of drugs, alcohol, caffeine, and cigarette smoking. Drug therapy should be initiated only if the arrhythmia is symptomatic, hemodynamically important, or life threatening. Pregnant patients with atrial fibrillation should be anticoagulated if they fulfill the criteria accepted for nonpregnant patients (see Chapter 30). Patients with supraventricular tachycardia resistant to medical therapy may undergo DC cardioversion during pregnancy, as the fetal risk with low to moderate energy settings appears small. Electrophysiologic evaluation is usually postponed until the postpartum period.

CARDIAC SURGERY DURING PREGNANCY

In general, cardiac surgery in pregnant women is not associated with increased maternal risk but may lead to fetal wastage. Surgery should be recommended only for patients not responding to medical therapy, and procedures not requiring cardiopulmonary bypass are preferred. To minimize the risk of teratogenicity, surgery should be avoided in the first trimester. The optimal time for open-heart procedures during pregnancy is the early part of the second trimester, because there is least risk of teratogenesis and inducing premature labor at this time.

For severe mitral valve stenosis refractory to medical therapy, closed mitral commissurotomy is preferable to the open technique because it carries only minimal risk to the fetus. Percutaneous mitral balloon valvuloplasty would appear a good alternative to surgery, but is best avoided because of fetal exposure to radiation. For severe aortic valve stenosis, balloon valvuloplasty has been used as palliation, allowing pregnancy to continue.

PROSTHETIC HEART VALVES

The choice of a prosthetic valve for a pregnant woman or a woman of childbearing age is an important issue. Mechanical heart valves increase the risk of thromboembolism and infective endocarditis in mothers, whereas the fetus is at increased risk of warfarin (3% to 4% risk if given in the sixth to ninth week of pregnancy). Tissue valves have been recommended to avoid warfarin anticoagulation early in pregnancy.

Most patients with normally functioning mechanical valves tolerate pregnancy well. The incidence of thromboembolism in women taking anticoagulants is increased despite adequate anticoagulation, since gestation predisposes to thrombosis. A recent retrospective survey concluded that warfarin was safe and also that more thromboembolic and bleeding complications were associated with heparin than with warfarin.[9]

Two approaches to anticoagulation have been recommended. The first consists of subcutaneous injection of heparin throughout pregnancy. The second approach involves substituting heparin for warfarin before conception and using it until the end of the first trimester. Warfarin may be used in the second and third trimesters and intravenous heparin used again near term. Heparin is stopped at the onset of labor and restarted 2 hours after delivery. Warfarin is started at 24 hours and overlapped with heparin for 4 days before heparin is stopped. Although this approach might prevent warfarin embryopathy, other fetopathic effects are still possible. Therefore the potential risks should be explained to patients. Although untested, low-molecular-weight heparin, given subcutaneously, may prove a suitable alternative to IV heparin. Breast-feeding an infant while the mother is taking anticoagulants (heparin or warfarin) is safe.

ANTIBIOTIC PROPHYLAXIS

Even though the American Heart Association does not recommend antibiotic prophylaxis for patients undergoing uncomplicated vaginal delivery, because of the difficulties in predicting complicated deliveries and the devastating effects of endocarditis, antibiotic prophylaxis has been commonly used (Table 40-3).[4,10] The AHA guidelines are reviewed in Chapter 21.

Table 40-3	*Antibiotic Prophylaxis in Pregnant Patients with Cardiac Conditions*

Clinical Considerations	Endocarditis Prophylaxis Recommended	Endocarditis Prophylaxis Not Recommended
Cardiac conditions	Prosthetic cardiac valves (including bioprosthetic and homograft valves) Previous bacterial endocarditis Most congenital cardiac defects Rheumatic and other valve dysfunction (even after surgery) Hypertrophic cardiac myopathy Mitral valve prolapse with regurgitation	Previous coronary artery bypass graft Mitral valve prolapse without regurgitation Physiologic heart murmurs Cardiac pacemakers and defribrillators Isolated secundum atrial septal defect Surgical repair without residue After 6 months of ventricular septal defect or patent ductus arteriosus Previous rheumatic heart disease without valve dysfunction
Dental or surgical procedures	Procedures that cause gingival or mucosal bleeding Urethral catheterization if infection is present Vaginal delivery if infection is present	Cardiac catheterization Cesarean section Uncomplicated vaginal delivery Therapeutic abortion Insertion or removal of intrauterine device

These are the recommendations of the American Heart Association (*JAMA* 264:2919, 1990).

PREGNANCY AFTER TRANSPLANT

The outcome of pregnancy in postcardiac transplant patients appears to be encouraging. Maternal mortality is not increased even though the rates of preterm deliveries, fetal growth retardation, and maternal morbidity are somewhat higher. Extremely careful follow-up is required in view of the added hemodynamic burden of pregnancy, risk of immunosuppression to the fetus, and increased likelihood of infection. Antibiotic prophylaxis with penicillin and gentamicin for cesarean section or forceps delivery is recommended.

CARDIAC INDICATIONS FOR THERAPEUTIC ABORTION

An absolute indication for therapeutic abortion is pulmonary hypertension, either primary pulmonary hypertension or Eisenmenger's syndrome. Management is discretionary for thromboembolic pulmonary hypertension, cardiomyopathies, and Marfan's syndrome.[11]

HYPERTENSION IN PREGNANCY

Hypertension in pregnancy is defined as an increase of 30 mm Hg in systolic and 15 mm Hg in diastolic pressure or a diastolic pressure of 90 mm Hg. It is an important cause of maternal morbidity and mortality. It complicates 8% to 10% of all pregnancies. Following are four categories of hypertension in pregnancy:

1. *Chronic hypertension* is defined as high blood pressure that is present before pregnancy or before the twentieth week of gestation and persisting more than 6 weeks postpartum. Drug therapy is recommended for diastolic blood pressure of 100 mm Hg.

2. *Preeclampsia and eclampsia* is characterized by hypertension accompanied by proteinuria, edema, or both. These occur more frequently in nulligravida patients, older multiparas, and women with multiple gestation. It usually regresses within 24 to 48 hours postpartum. Hospitalization is recommended in preeclamptic patients. Magnesium sulfate has become the drug of choice for preventing and treating seizures in preeclamptic patients. In a severely hypertensive patient, uncontrolled despite 24 to 48 hours of drug therapy, the fetus should be delivered regardless of gestational age.

3. *Transient hypertension* is defined as the development of high blood pressure during pregnancy or in the first 24 hours postpartum, without the other signs of preeclampsia. This condition is predictive of future development of hypertension.

4. *Preeclampsia and eclampsia superimposed on chronic hypertension.* Management includes rest, salt restriction, and antihypertensive drugs. Diuretics, beta-blockers, methyldopa, clonidine, and hydralazine have been used safely in pregnancy. ACE inhibitors are contraindicated except in cases of severe hypertension not responsive to other drugs. Drugs used in the treatment of hypertension and other cardiovascular conditions are surveyed in Table 40-4.

Table 40-4 | *Cardiovascular Drugs in Pregnancy*

Agents	Placental Transfer	Transfer to Breast Milk	Maternal Adverse Effects	Fetal Adverse Effects	Risk Factor Classification*
ANTIBIOTICS					
Aminoglycosides	Yes	Yes	Ototoxicity, nephrotoxicity	Ototoxicity (with streptomycin)	C,D
Cephalothin	Yes	Yes	Hypersensitivity		B
Penicillin	Yes	Yes	Hypersensitivity		B
Vancomycin					C
Tetracycline	Yes	Yes		Discoloration of teeth	D
Erythromycin	Yes	Yes			B
DIURETICS					
Thiazides	Yes	Yes	↓K, ↑Glucose, ↑uric acid, ↑Ca, hypovolemia	↓NA, ↓K, ↓glucose, jaundice	D
Furosemide	Yes	Yes	Same as thiazides but more severe hypovolemia	Possibly teratogenic	C
Spironolactone	Yes	Yes		Feminization	D
INOTROPES					
Digoxin	Yes	Yes	Bradyarrhythmias, tachyarrhythmias, nausea, vomiting		C
Dopamine					C
Epinephrine	Yes		Tachycardia		C
VASODILATORS					
Nitrates					C
Hydralazine			4-BP, lupus syndrome	Thrombocytopenia, acute distress	C
Captopril		Yes	4-BP, agranulocytosis		D
Clonidine		Yes	4-BP, bradycardia		C
Minoxidil			Edema, pericardial effusion		C
Alphamethyldopa	Yes	Yes	Hemolytic anemia, liver disorders		C
Diazoxide	Yes		4-BP, edema	Hypoglycemia	C
ANTIARRHYTHMICS					
Quinidine	Yes	Yes	Thrombocytopenia, ↑GI motility, rhythm exacerbation	Thrombocytopenia	C
Procainamide			GI upset, lupus syndrome		C
Disopyramide	Yes	Yes	↑Uterine contractility		C
Lidocaine	Yes		Confusion, seizure	Bradycardia	C
Flecainide	Yes		Dizziness, blurred vision		C
Mexilitine	Yes	Yes	Dizziness		C
Amiodarone	Yes	Yes	Abnormal liver function tests, thyroid dysfunction, pulmonary fibrosis		C
Adenosine					C

Adapted from Metcalfe J, McAnulty J H, Ueland K: Pregnancy and drug therapy. In *Burewell and Metcalfe's heart disease and pregnancy: physiology and management*, ed 2, Boston, 1986, Little, Brown.

Note: Blank spaces indicate lack of information.

*Risk factor classification (the definitions are those used by the FDA): A, Studies demonstrate no risk to fetus; B, animal studies demonstrate no risk to fetus/no controlled studies in pregnant women; C, animal studies have revealed adverse effects on the fetus/no controlled studies in pregnant women; D, positive evidence of human fetal risk, but the benefit may outweigh the risk in a life-threatening situation; X, animal studies and/or human studies have revealed adverse effects on the fetus, and the risks outweigh any benefit.

| Table 40-4 | *Cardiovascular Drugs in Pregnancy—cont'd* |

Agents	Placental Transfer	Transfer to Breast Milk	Maternal Adverse Effects	Fetal Adverse Effects	Risk Factor Classification
BETA-BLOCKERS					
Propranolol	Yes	Yes	Bronchospasm, congestive heart failure, oxytocic effect on myometrium, bradycardia	Growth retardation, prematurity, bradycardia, respiratory depression, hypoglycemia	C
Metoprolol	Yes	Yes	Less aggravation of reactive airway disease		B
Labetolol	Yes	Yes	Less bradycardia		C
CALCIUM CHANNEL BLOCKERS					
Nifedipine			↓ K, pedal edema		C
Verapamil	Yes		↓ 4K, pedal edema ↓ blood pressure		C
Diltiazem		Yes	↓ blood pressure		C
ANTICOAGULANTS					
Wartarin	Yes	Yes	Bleeding	Abortion, warfarin syndrome, teratogenicity	X (in early pregnancy)
Heparin	No	No	Bleeding, osteoporosis, thrombocytopenia	Abortion	C
Aspirin	Yes	Yes	Bleeding	Abortion, stillbirth, ductal closure, teratogenesis	C, D (in third trimester)

Risk factor classification (the definitions are those used by the FDA): *A*, Studies demonstrate no risk to fetus; *B*, animal studies demonstrate no risk to fetus/no controlled studies in pregnant women; *C*, animal studies have revealed adverse effects on the fetus/no controlled studies in pregnant women; *D*, positive evidence of human fetal risk, but the benefit may outweigh the risk in a life-threatening situation; *X*, animal studies and/or human studies have revealed adverse effects on the fetus, and the risks outweigh any benefit.

REFERENCES

1. Bhagwat AR, Peter JE: Heart disease and pregnancy, *Cardiol Clin* 13:163, 1995.
2. Carpenter MW, Sady SP, Hoegsberg B, et al: Fetal heart rate response to maternal exertion, *JAMA* 259:3006, 1998.
3. Underwood R, Firmin D: *An introduction to magnetic resonance of the cardiovascular system,* London, 1988, Current Medical Literature.
4. Metcalfe J, McAnulty JH, Ueland K: *Burwell and Metcalfe's heart disease and pregnancy: physiology and management,* ed 5, Boston, 1986, Little, Brown.
5. Clark SL: Cardiac disease in pregnancy, *Obstet Gynecol Clin North Am* 18:237, 1991.
6. Shores J, Berger KR, Murphy EA, Pyeritz RE: Progression of aortic dilatation and the benefit of long-term beta-adrenergic blockade in Marfan's syndrome, *N Engl J Med* 330:1335, 1994.
7. Wilson NJ, Neutze JM: Adult congenital heart disease: principles and management guidelines. I. *Aust N Z J Med* 23:498, 1993.
8. Croft P, Hannaford PC: Risk factors for acute myocardial infarction in women: evidence from the Royal College of General Practitioners' oral contraceptive study, *BMJ* 298:165, 1989.
9. Sbarouni E, Oakley CM: Outcome of pregnancy in women with valve prosthesis, *Br Heart J* 71:196, 1994.
10. Elkayam U, Gleicher N: *Cardiac problems in pregnancy: diagnosis and management of maternal and fetal disease,* ed 2, New York, 1990, Alan R Liss.
11. Oakley CM: Cardiovascular disease in pregnancy, *Can J Cardiol* 6(suppl):3, 1990.
12. Briggs GG et al: *Drugs in pregnancy and lactation: a reference guide to fetal and neonatal risk,* ed 4, Baltimore, 1994, Williams & Wilkins.

41 Women and Heart Disease

Sarah E. Stapleton
George J. Taylor

Cardiovascular disease is the number one killer of women in the United States today (Fig. 41-1). The statistics are striking; heart disease accounts for the deaths of half a million women per year. This is more than twice the number of women who died of all types of cancer.[1] It is estimated that 6.5 million women have coronary artery disease; an estimated 2.5 million women have had heart attacks. The cost of their medical care in 1997 was $22 billion, but the human costs are certainly even higher.[2] These values will increase as the population ages, since older women will make up a greater proportion of that population.

Despite overwhelming evidence that cardiovascular disease is a significant health risk to women, this is not a common public perception. One survey indicated that women feared breast cancer three times as much as heart disease and saw their own risk of developing heart disease by age 70 as extremely low (less than 1% in some groups).[3] They are much less likely therefore to associate symptoms with heart disease and wait longer to seek help for chest pain than do men.

Until recently, women have been excluded from most clinical trials that investigate prevention and treatment of heart disease. Clearly, several female-specific conditions are not relevant in males, including postpartum cardiomyopathy, toxemia, preeclampsia (see Chapter 40), and oral contraceptive–associated problems of hypertension and myocardial infarction (MI). Also, trials usually exclude women of childbearing years because of the possibility of pregnancy. Women also have (often exclusionary) comorbid conditions by the time they develop heart disease, since they are 10 to 15 years older than men.

CLINICAL PRESENTATION

Because of the exclusion of women from larger trials on heart disease, it was a common practice to apply to women many of the characteristics of coronary artery disease found in men. However, this practice leads to erroneous and inexact conclusions, since there are multiple differences in the presentation, natural history, and outcomes of coronary artery disease between the sexes. Men can present almost equally with angina, sudden death, or myocardial infarction, whereas women are more likely to present with angina. At the time of pre-sentation, women with angina are generally 10 years older than men and up to 20 years older at the time of myocardial infarction[1] (Fig. 41-2). Atypical chest pain is certainly more common in women; even women with known stable angina report more chest pain while resting, sleeping, or while under stress than do men. During an acute MI women are more likely to have neck and shoulder pain, nausea, vomiting, fatigue, or dyspnea, as well as more common chest pain syndromes.[4]

Many theories have sought to explain these differences in clinical presentation, suggesting women have more vasospastic and microvascular angina, as well as a higher prevalence of mitral valve prolapse.[4] Also reported have been higher fibrinogen levels, different endothelial cell reactivities due to estrogen, and different tissue composition of vascular plaque in women.[5]

Because so many women, and even their physicians, do not recognize their own risk of coronary artery disease, they lessen their physician's suspicions of disease. There remains, as well, the stereotype that women are "overemotional." Women's complaints need to be taken seriously, and angina equivalents must be considered. Many patients have told me that they "definitely do not have chest pain." However, if asked, they readily admit to feeling pressure, heaviness, or mild discomfort. Chronic fatigue and unexplained episodes of nausea may need to be explored.

Traditionally, the prognosis for women with angina (atypical or atypical) was thought to be more "benign" than for men, possibly arising from data in some large studies, including the Framingham study, showing that men who presented with angina had a 25% chance of MI within the next 5 years versus 14% for women. Even when women have a history typical of angina, up to 50% had no findings on angiography versus only 17% of men. This perception of a "benign course of angina" may therefore just reflect the higher incidence of noncardiac chest pain in women.

Proven cardiac disease in women is hardly benign, however. Women with proven MI, for example, have a significantly higher morbidity and mortality than do men. In the acute period, they have a higher incidence of heart failure and cardiogenic shock, possibly because they present at least 5 hours later than men.[1] They also have a higher mortality at 6 weeks; at 1 year 45% of

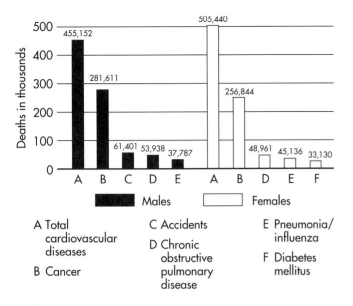

FIG. 41-1

Leading causes of death for all women and men in the United States in 1995 according to the National Center for Health Statistics.

From American Heart Association: Heart and stroke statistical update, 1999. (The statistical update is published yearly and can be obtained from your local AHA office.)

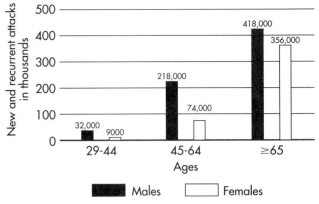

FIG. 41-2

Estimated number of Americans having heart attack in 1995, shown by age and sex. The data were extrapolated from rates in the ARIC community surveillance study of the NHLBI, 1987-1994, and do not include silent myocardial infarction.

From American Heart Association: Heart and stroke statistical update, 1999. (The statistical update is published yearly and can be obtained from your local AHA office.)

women died versus 10% of men.[6] Survivors had higher rates of reinfarction, recurrent angina, and congestive heart failure (Table 41-1).

DIAGNOSTIC TESTING

The low prevalence and atypical features of cardiac disease in women make diagnostic testing for coronary artery disease in women difficult. The exercise electrocardiograph (ECG) has notoriously low specificity. Even the lay press has picked up on this. A woman recently told me that she would not have ECG stress testing because she had read in a women's health magazine that it is "too inaccurate." There is, in fact, some truth to this. The resting ECG shows a higher prevalence of ST-T changes in women.[5] Routine exercise testing does, in fact, have similar sensitivity in both sexes but much lower specificity in women (more false positives). This is especially true in cases of atypical chest pain in young and middle-aged women with a low prevalence of disease.

Patients with a high chance of coronary artery disease, having typical symptoms of angina, cardiac risk factors, and a resting ECG that is normal, should undergo routine exercise testing. It is the woman with a moderate risk of heart disease who provides physicians with the uncertainties about diagnostic testing. These women have up to a 40% false-positive rate on routine exercise testing. Theories to account for this include a lower exercise capacity in

women and the possibility of a gender difference in catecholamine release during exercise, as well as higher incidences of mitral valve prolapse and single-vessel disease in women. It has even been proposed that estrogen has a digitalis-like structure and may produce digitalis-like ECG changes during exercise testing.[7]

Perfusion imaging increases the specificity of exercising testing (see Chapter 8). Some inaccuracy has been attributed to breast attenuation in women, and higher energy isotopes such as technetium-sestamibi have been proposed as alternative perfusion agents to eliminate this artifact. SPECT imaging techniques probably improve accuracy. Others have suggested that stress echocardiography is more accurate for women, but this remains controversial.[8]

Recently proposed is the use of the "QT dispersion" during exercise testing. This is defined as the difference between maximal and minimal QT intervals on the 12-lead ECG. Initial information indicated that a wider stress QT dispersion had a higher sensitivity and specificity than routine exercise testing for the diagnosis of coronary artery disease in women.[9]

Women with typical anginal symptoms should undergo routine exercise stress testing, as should all others, since a negative test does exclude the presence of disease in women. Those with an inconclusive or possibly false-positive test would proceed to exercise testing with perfusion imaging or exercise echocardiography. Practically, this may concern some women who would have to perform a stress test twice. Many of my patients have told me they would rather proceed to the "better test"

Table 41-1	*Gender Differences in Clinical Outcomes for Angina and Myocardial Infarction (MI)*

Variable	Women (%)	Men (%)
PRESENTATION*		
Angina	50	33
Sudden death	<30	33
MI	<30	33
POST-MI, CUMULATIVE MORTALITY †		
In-hospital	6.0	2.0
6 wk	9.0	4.0
1 yr	12.2	6.1
4 yr	36.0	21.0
ACUTE MI		
In-hospital	8.2	8.8
Congestive heart failure	26.8	24.4
Cardiogenic shock	11.1	7.4
Ventricular tachycardia	12.9	10.0

From Villablanca AC: *Postgrad Med* 100:191, 1996.
*Data adapted from the Survival and Ventricular Enlargement (SAVE) trial.
†Data adapted from the Multicenter Investigation of the Limitation of Infarct Size (MILIS) study.

first, and indeed some authors suggest that women with any atypical features to their chest pain should not bother with routine exercise testing[4] (Table 41-2). It is a judgment call, and the cost of testing also must be considered (see Chapter 8).

Women with positive exercise tests are candidates for coronary angiography. However, studies from 10 to 15 years ago show that men were 10 times more likely to be referred for angiography than were women. That number has since declined, but men are still twice as likely as women to have cardiac catheterization.[3]

TREATMENT

Once a woman's coronary artery disease has been diagnosed, however, she may be less likely to be referred for revascularization procedures. The most common reason cited for the less aggressive referral patterns for angioplasty and coronary artery bypass grafting is that women have higher morbidity and mortality rates. They have generally smaller coronary arteries and smaller body size and are usually older with more comorbid illnesses, including diabetes and hypertension.[5]

Coronary artery bypass grafting has some other well-studied gender differences in referral patterns and outcomes. Women are more likely to require emergency surgery by the time of referral, and the complications of heart failure, myocardial infarction, and hemorrhage are higher. Postoperatively, they have a higher incidence of angina and more resultant disability than men. On the other hand, follow-up of patients not sent for aggressive treatment shows a higher incidence of subsequent coronary events. Referral of women for revascularization therefore remains clearly indicated despite the higher morbidity and mortality than in men.[3,10]

Information on medical management of proven coronary artery disease in women is limited. Nitrates, beta-blockers, and calcium antagonists are thought to be equally effective in men and women. Studies show women receive nitrates, calcium-channel blockers, sedatives, diuretics, and other antihypertensives more frequently than men but are less often prescribed aspirin and beta-blockers. A large Nurse's Health Study points to favorable effects of aspirin in reducing the risk of MI in women over the age of 50, but other studies have contradicted these data. Furthermore, it is uncertain whether some of the effects of estrogen on the endothelium influence the antithrombotic effects of aspirin.[5,11]

Thrombolytic therapy is also a topic of controversy. Indications to date are that it benefits men and women equally. However, most trials show more complications associated with its use in women, including recurrent myocardial infarction and bleeding complications, including hemorrhagic stroke.[12] Because of the increased lag time before their arrival at a medical care facility, more advanced age, and related co-morbidities, women often are less favorable candidates for thrombolytic therapy.[13]

After having an MI, women are far less likely than men to undergo cardiac rehabilitation programs. There are few data on the use of ACE inhibitors postinfarction in women, although some studies have shown that they may be more effective in men.[6] Despite the benefits of beta-blockers and aspirin in both sexes after infarction, women have them prescribed less frequently.

RISKS AND PREVENTION OF HEART DISEASE

Clearly, given the uncertainties in diagnosing and treating heart disease in women, it is important to focus on the prevention of heart disease. In general, cardiac risk factors are the same for men and women, but some specific elements deserve slightly different emphasis (see Chapters 12 and 13). Furthermore, a woman's hormonal status is a leading factor in her risk profile.

Smoking remains a significant cardiac risk factor, raising a woman's risk of heart disease two to four times that of nonsmokers. Despite the declining number of smokers in the United States, use among women is ac-

Table 41-2	*Use of Diagnostic Tests in Women with Chest Pain*	

Likelihood of Coronary Heart Disease	Initial Test	Subsequent Test
Low (<20%) No major and ≤1 intermediate or minor determinant	None indicated	None indicated
Moderate (20% to 80%) 1 major or multiple intermediate or minor determinants	Routine ETT Negative Inconclusive Positive Imaging ETT Negative Inconclusive Positive	 None indicated Further testing indicated; selection must be individualized Imaging test or catheterization None indicated Catheterization Catheterization
High (>80%) ≥2 major or 1 major plus inter- mediate and minor determinants	Routine ETT Negative Inconclusive Positive Imaging ETT	 None indicated; observe patient carefully Catheterization Catheterization None indicated

From Douglas PS, Ginsburg GS: *N Engl J Med* 334:1311, 1996.
ETT, Exercise tolerance test.

tually increasing, particularly in younger women. Smoking also may lead to an earlier menopause, introducing another cardiac risk factor. Moreover, smoking also increases the risk of MI in women who are older than 35 years of age and use birth control pills. The good news is that once a woman stops smoking, the risk of heart disease begins to fall almost immediately, and by 3 to 5 years is almost at the level of a nonsmoker's risk.

Diabetes is a more powerful risk factor in women than in men, obliterating the woman's hormonal advantage, possibly by impairing estrogen binding. Mortality rates from heart disease are seven times higher in diabetic versus nondiabetic women and twice as high as in diabetic men. It remains unclear whether tight glycemic control can eliminate this as a risk factor. When other risk factors (e.g., smoking, hypertension, and obesity) are combined with diabetes, the rates of myocardial infarction rise synergistically. Current recommendations therefore emphasize elimination of these other risk factors.

In addition, some have suggested that gestational diabetes may be a marker for increased risk of coronary heart disease, possibly because these women frequently develop non-insulin-dependent diabetes. Women with gestational diabetes are targets for early preventive strategies.[14]

Obesity does not appear to be a primary risk factor for coronary artery disease, but it is associated with hypertension and unfavorable lipid levels. These factors confer on obesity, particularly upper body obesity, an association with coronary artery disease. It is not known whether weight loss reverses this risk.

Hyperlipidemia is a strong risk factor in both men and women. Elevated total cholesterol and LDL levels are not as strongly associated with coronary artery disease in women as in men. Low HDL values and high triglyceride levels seem to be more significant, especially in older women. In some cases, hormone replacement therapy may be preferred therapy for postmenopausal women who have low HDL and high LDL. However, since estrogen can increase triglycerides in 20% to 25% of women, therapy needs to be individualized.

Hypertension also is a significant risk factor in women. In premenopausal women, hypertension increases the death rate from coronary artery disease.[4] Fewer women are hypertensive than men until after the age of 45, when the trend reverses. Blood pressure continues to rise with age and can reach higher levels in women than in men. Nearly 80% of women over age 75 are hypertensive. Drug treatment trials, which have included both men and women, seem to indicate reduction in coronary artery disease with a decrease in blood pressure, although no trials have conducted separate studies on women.

Concern also has been expressed that isolated systolic hypertension, more common in women than in

men, is a particularly strong indicator of cardiac risk. Preeclampsia has been cited as a possible predictor of later coronary disease, thought to be independent of hypertension.[14]

ESTROGEN AS A RISK MODULATOR

Certainly the most unique modifier of cardiac risk factors is the hormonal status of women. As discussed, heart disease tends to develop in women 10 years later than in men; this places them at an age that is usually around the time of menopause. In fact, women who have both ovaries removed, producing surgical menopause, have twice the risk of heart disease. If they receive estrogen-replacement therapy, there is no increased risk. The incidence of heart disease does not suddenly increase for women who undergo natural menopause, probably because menopause is more gradual.[14] A woman spends approximately one third of her life in a postmenopausal state. Approximately 37 million postmenopausal women are living in the United States. As elderly women outnumber elderly men, this number will increase, with the prediction of 50 million postmenopausal women after the year 2000.[1] The question of whether to offer hormone replacement therefore affects many women.

The benefits of estrogen-replacement therapy in coronary artery disease are impressive. From large observational studies, it appears that the risk of coronary artery disease decreases 40% to 50% in postmenopausal women who take estrogen-replacement therapy. There is perhaps an even greater risk reduction for women with known coronary artery disease (up to 70% to 90%).[17] The mechanisms of this protective effect are multifactorial. Estrogen has been shown to have favorable effects on the lipid profile, raising HDL and lowering LDL by 10% to 15%. It decreases the amount of uptake and accumulation of lipid in the vessel wall. There is also thought to be more favorable body fat distribution, a better coagulation profile with an increase in fibrinolytic activity, lower fibrinogen levels, improved vascular reactivity, and less LDL oxidation (Box 41-1).

Beyond heart disease, estrogen combats the uncomfortable symptoms of menopause, specifically vasomotor changes (hot flashes, vaginal dryness, and mood swings). Estrogen is protective against continued bone loss after menopause, which leads to osteoporosis. Drawbacks include a possible increase in triglyceride levels, which, as mentioned, may increase the risk of coronary artery disease in some elderly women. Endometrial cancer is increased by up to six times normal if estrogen is unopposed by progesterone. Gallbladder disease, too, is increased, and the possible risk of in-

---

BOX 41-1

HOW ESTROGEN REPLACEMENT THERAPY MAY PROTECT THE HEART

Increases high-density lipoprotein (HDL) cholesterol
Decreases low-density lipoprotein (LDL) cholesterol
Reduces oxidation of LDL cholesterol
Lowers uptake of LDL cholesterol in blood vessels
Decreases lipoprotein (a)
Binds to vascular estrogen receptors
Reduces vascular tone
Preserves endothelial function
Increases prostaglandin I2 release
Decreases thromboxane A2 formation
Decreases fibrinogen
Reduces plasminogen activator inhibitor
Decreases fasting blood glucose and insulin levels

Adapted from Sullivan JM: *Prog Cardiovasc Dis* 38:211, 1995; from Hennekens CH, Judelson DR, Wenger NK: *Patient Care* 30:116, 1996.

---

creased breast cancer is a major concern. The data linking estrogen replacement and breast cancer are controversial, however. There does appear to be a slightly increased risk, especially among long-term estrogen users, and this possibility is a strong deterrent for many women.

Ongoing trials are investigating the effect of progesterone added to estrogen to negate the risk of endometrial cancer in woman who have not had a hysterectomy. The most prominent study is the postmenopausal estrogen/progestin intervention (or PEPI trial). All the hormone combinations seem to have beneficial lipid effects, although estrogen alone had the greatest effect on HDL levels. The addition of progesterone did not reduce the cardioprotective effect of the postmenopausal estrogen therapy. The investigators were unable to associate the protective effects with the duration of hormone use, but the effects did last fewer than 3 years after discontinuing hormone replacement.[18]

With the generally positive data on estrogen-replacement therapy, the American College of Physicians' Task Force has stated that "all women should consider taking preventive hormone therapy."[17] Only 20% of women who are good candidates for hormone replacement currently receive it. The major reason for this is the fear of

breast cancer. Many women ask me what I would do, and I have no set answer. I usually tell them that it is a personal decision and that they have to balance the benefits and risks in their own case. If their family has a history of heart disease or severe osteoporosis but no family history of breast cancer, the decision is easy. It is more difficult for a patient with a family history of cardiac disease and breast cancer.

There is some hope, however, that a new age is dawning in hormone-replacement therapy with designer estrogens. Raloxifene is classified as a selective estrogen-receptor modulator. It inhibits the growth of estrogen-receptor breast tumors while increasing bone mineral density and lowering total and LDL cholesterol. Although it will not provoke a menstrual period, hot flashes and other vasomotor symptoms associated with menopause may actually increase. Thus it does not mitigate the discomforts of menopause, but it does protect against osteoporosis and probably against heart disease, while avoiding undesirable effects on the breast or the uterus.[19]

REFERENCES

1. Villablanca AC: Coronary heart disease in women, *Post grad Med* 100:191, 1996.
2. Higgins M: How to estimate and reduce coronary heart disease risk in women, *Cardiol Rev* 5:199, 1997.
3. Hennekens CH, Judelson DR, Wenger NK: Coronary disease: the leading killer, *Patient Care* 30:116, 1996.
4. Douglas PS, Ginsbury GS: The evaluation of chest pain in women, *N Engl J Med* 334:1311, 1996.
5. Douglas PS: Coronary artery disease in women. In Braunwald B, editor: *Heart disease: a textbook of cardiovascular medicine,* ed 5, New York, 1996, WB Saunders.
6. Gernard M: Coronary artery disease in women, *Res Staff Phys* 27:31, 1993.
7. Marwick TH, Anderson T, Williams MJ, et al: Exercise echocardiography is an accurate and cost-efficient technique for detection of coronary artery disease in women, *J Am Coll Cardiol* 26:335, 1995.
8. Miller DD: Optimal imaging approaches for the evaluation of chest pain syndromes in women, *Cardiol Rev* 5:279, 1997.
9. Stoletniy LN, Pal RG: Value of QT dispersion in the interpretation of exercise stress test in women, *Circulation* 96:904, 1997.
10. Subramaniam PN: What you should know about heart disease in women, *Int Med* 18:1, 1997.
11. Rosene-Montella K: Coronary artery disease in women, *Int Med* 15:72, 1994.
12. Woodfield SL, Lundergan CF, Reiner JS, et al: Gender and acute myocardial infarction: is there a different response to thrombolysis? *J Am Coll Cardiol* 29:35, 1997.
13. Hochman JS, McCabe CH, Stone PH, et al: Outcome and profile of women and men presenting with acute coronary syndromes: a report from TIIMI III B, *J Am Coll Cardiol* 30:141, 1997.
14. Rich-Edwards JW, Manson YE, Hennekens CH, et al: The primary prevention of coronary heart disease in women, *N Engl J Med* 332:1758, 1995.
15. LaRosa JC: Triglycerides and coronary risk in women and the elderly, *Arch Intern Med* 157:961, 1997.
16. O'Brien T, Nguyen TT: Lipids and lipoproteins in women, *Mayo Clinic Proc* 72:235, 1997.
17. O'Keefe JH, Kim SC, Hall RR: Estrogen replacement therapy after coronary angioplasty in women, *J Am Coll Cardiol* 29:1, 1997.
18. Grodstein F, Stampfer MJ, Manson YE, et al: Postmenopausal estrogen and progestin use and the risk of cardiovascular disease, *N Engl J Med* 335:453, 1996.
19. Delmas PD, Bjarnason NH, Mitlak BH, et al: Effects of raloxifene on bone mineral density, serum cholesterol concentrations, and uterine endometrium in postmenopausal women, *N Engl J Med* 337:1641, 1997.

BIBLIOGRAPHY

Chasan-Taber L, Stampfer MJ: Epidemiology of oral contraceptives and cardiovascular disease, *Ann Intern Med* 128:467, 1998. The best recent summary of a huge volume of data.

Mendelsohn ME, Karas RH: The protective effects of estrogen on the cardiovascular system, *N Engl J Med* 340:1801, 1999. A thorough review.

Vogel RA, Corretti MC: Estrogens, progestins, and heart disease: can endothelial function divine the benefit? *Circulation* 97:1223, 1998. Also reviews trials that are currently in progress.

42 Infections in Patients with Heart Disease

Steven D. O'Marro
Adrian B. Van Bakel

COMMON INFECTIONS ENCOUNTERED IN PATIENTS WITH HEART DISEASE

Nosocomial Infections

A nosocomial infection is acquired in the hospital setting and is not present or incubating at the time of admission. These infections often develop after discharge when length of stay is aggressively shortened.

The most common types of nosocomial infections are urinary tract infections (40%), surgical wound infections (25%), lower respiratory tract infections (16%), and primary bacteremia (3.5%).[1] Sinusitis may occur as a nosocomial infection in patients with nasogastric and nasotracheal tubes, which obstruct sinus drainage.

The endemic rate of nosocomial infections in municipal or academic hospitals is approximately 8%. The rate is lower in private hospitals (2.5% to 3%).[1] Up to one half of all nosocomial infections result from bacteria that are brought into the hospital as part of the patient's own flora. These "autogenous" infections are the result of debilitating effects of illness and its treatment, including the effect of antimicrobial therapy that encourages emergence of resistant gram negative, gram positive, and fungal pathogens.[1,2]

Nosocomial infection also occurs as a consequence of contact spread (i.e., from the hands of hospital personnel). Adequate hand washing significantly reduces this mechanism of infection. Health care workers may also harbor pathogens as part of their normal flora (e.g., nasal carriage of *Staphylococcus aureus* and nasal and rectal carriage of group A beta *Streptococcus*).

Infection also may be acquired in the hospital as a result of contaminated ventilation systems (*Aspergillus*), water (especially *Legionella* spp.), medical devices, and intravenous solutions.

Urinary Tract Infections

Urinary tract infections (UTI) are the most common of all hospital acquired infections and usually are caused by gram negative bacilli or enterococci, usually reflecting the perineal flora. Three fourths are associated with instrumentation, usually a Foley catheter. A single catheterization confers a 1% risk of infection, with the risk increasing for each day that the catheter remains in place (approximately 1% for each extra day). Infection may also occur as a consequence of contamination on the hands of hospital personnel. Underlying illness and female sex increase the risk of nosocomial UTI.[1]

Mechanisms for reducing the risk of nosocomial UTI include appropriate selection of patients for Foley catheterization, separation of catheterized patients, hand washing, shorter duration of catheterization, and maintaining a closed system.[1]

The consequences of nosocomial UTI include prolonged hospitalization and as much as a two- to three-fold increased risk of mortality.[3]

Surgical Wound Infections

Wound infections are usually acquired perioperatively. The pathogens vary depending on the type of surgery. The risk is higher for procedures performed at a contaminated or infected site (8.5% to 13%) than at a clean site (2% to 5%).[1] Additional factors to consider in surgical wound infections include the experience and skill of the surgeon, the duration of the procedure, the severity of illness, reoperation, and failure to use antibiotic prophylaxis.[3]

In clean procedures, including saphenous vein harvest site infections, *S. aureus* and coagulase-negative *Staphylococcus* are important pathogens, presenting 5 to 7 days after the procedure.

Pneumonia

Patients who develop pneumonia while on a ventilator have an unusually high mortality risk.[4] In cardiology patients, pulmonary edema may be confused with obscure pneumonitis, making diagnosis difficult. Often, repeated chest x-rays (after appropriate treatment of the heart failure) are necessary for identifying the infiltrate. One indication of pulmonary artery catheterization is to sort out the cause of a diffuse infiltrate.

In addition to mechanical ventilation, risk factors for pneumonia include underlying illness (especially obstructive lung disease), alteration of consciousness, thoracic and abdominal surgery, the use of broad-spectrum antibiotics, stress ulcer prophylaxis that reduces gastric acidity (a pulmonary defense), and advanced age.[1] Unfortunately, oral flora takes on characteristics of the rectal flora as one ages.

Usual pathogens in nosocomial pneumonia include *Pseudomonas aeruginosa, Enterobacter* spp., and enteric gram negative rods. *Legionella* infections have been associated with hospital water supply. *Aspergillus* infections may result from exposure of an immunocompromised patient to contaminated ventilation equipment or hospital construction.

Bacteremia

Vascular catheter-related infection is heralded by fever and inflammation at the site. Up to 90% of nosocomial bacteremias are associated with central venous and arterial catheters.[1] Peripheral intravenous catheters carry a lower risk of nosocomial infection (about 1%) but account for many cases because they are more commonly used than central lines. Other nosocomial infections are associated with a 2% to 4% risk of secondary bacteremia.[1]

Central venous catheter infection is associated with increased risk at extremes of age, as well as in situations associated with immunodeficiency, loss of skin integrity, or alteration in normal skin flora.[3] Additional risk factors include the severity of illness, size and number of lumens in the catheter, catheter composition, catheter location (femoral catheters are higher risk than other central catheters), and catheter placement more than 72 hours.[5] Although not mandated by practice guidelines, replacement of central lines after 5 to 7 days, using a new vascular site, is a standard policy of many intensive care units. In each case, the risk (and difficulty) of line placement must be weighed against the risk of infection.

The prevalence of catheter-related bacteremias can be lowered by ensuring aseptic technique in placement and maintenance, as well as by reducing the duration of catheterization. New materials (microbe-resistant polymers and antibiotic-impregnated catheters) are expensive, and the cost-to-benefit ratio is uncertain. Replacement of a potentially infected catheter over a guide wire is controversial. The procedure is associated with reduced morbidity (e.g., pneumothorax and hemorrhage) when compared with replacement of the central catheter at a new site; however, the new catheter will be promptly infected if the old catheter was infected. Infection is even more certain if the surgeon does not put on a new pair of sterile gloves after removing the infected line. In performing such a procedure, it may be helpful to do a roll culture of the catheter tip using the method of Maki.[6] If more than 15 CFU of organisms on a plate are found, the new catheter should be removed and appropriate antibiotic therapy instituted.

The most common pathogens associated with devices are *S. aureus* and *S. epidermidis*; however, enteric gram negative rods and yeast may also cause these infections. TPN infusion increases the risk of catheter-related fungemia.[5]

Pseudobacteremia

A common reason for infectious disease consultation is the finding of a positive blood culture in a patient who recently had a fever or an increased white blood cell count. In many cases the reason for obtaining the blood cultures has resolved. The isolated organism often does not correlate with clinical findings. The problem is more complex if the patient has recently had surgery or if fever is caused by something other than infection (e.g., myocardial necrosis, atelectasis, drugs, and postpericardiotomy syndrome). Recent valve replacement heightens concern regarding the significance of the positive culture.

Pseudobacteremia can be caused by contaminated culture medium, contaminated culture collection tubes or devices, a laboratory change to biphasic culture system, contamination by the phlebotomist's flora, and the patient's skin flora. Under the best conditions, 2% to 3% of blood cultures collected from peripheral veins are contaminated by skin flora.[7]

The diagnosis of pseudobacteremia requires repeat blood cultures. True fungemia or bacteremia matching the clinical impression of sepsis can be confirmed by obtaining two or three cultures over a 12- to 24-hour period. If sepsis is not clinically evident but infective endocarditis is a concern, then as many as four to five cultures may be needed to rule out contamination with skin flora. Recent studies suggest transesophageal echocardiography (TEE) is cost effective for excluding valve infections in patients with *S. aureus* bacteremia.[8] The role of this procedure in the setting of positive blood cultures due to usual skin flora is unclear. One must be careful to treat the patient, not the test results, in this setting.

Treatment of Nosocomial Infections

Treatment of nosocomial infections varies depending on the site of the infection and the clinical presentation. Infected foreign material should be removed if possible, including urinary catheters and vascular lines.

Prolonged stay in an intensive care unit raises concern that plasmid rich, gram negative rods such as *Pseudomonas aeruginosa* or *Enterobacter* spp. may cause urinary tract infection. Fungal urinary tract infections also occur in critically ill patients who are taking broad-spectrum antibiotics and in debilitated chronically ill or elderly patients, especially those with indwelling catheters. Failure of treatment should prompt evaluation for prostatitis or a more proximal urinary tract infection, either pyelonephritis or a perinephric abscess.

The treatment of surgical wound infections varies depending on the site of the infection. Debridement should be considered, with cultures and smears obtained at the time of initial evaluation or at debridement. For example, if coagulase-negative staphylococci are suspected in a saphenous vein harvest site infection,

then empiric therapy with vancomycin is recommended until the results of cultures are available to guide therapy. Saphenous vein harvest site infections are often complicated by venous stasis (see below), and diligent wound care is required.

Nosocomial pneumonia is usually caused by *Pseudomonas aeruginosa, Enterobacter,* or *Serratia* species. A gram stain with follow-up culture should guide therapy. Therapeutic bronchoscopy may be necessary. Treatment usually requires multiple antibiotics. Mortality is high, and consultation with the infectious disease service is warranted.

Treatment of nosocomial bacteremia requires identification of the possible source. If the bacteremia is the result of another infection, treatment is designed to resolve this infection. If the bacteremia is related to an infected catheter, the catheter is removed and the tip is cultured quantitatively. Remember that half of the coagulase-negative staphylococci (e.g., *S. epidermidis*) are resistant to methicillin. Thus empiric vancomycin therapy is required until culture data are available to guide treatment. Obtaining two blood cultures and repeating them 4 to 6 hours later is adequate to rule out endovascular infection.[7] A catheter-related infection is treated by removing the catheter and administering an appropriate bactericidal antibiotic for 10 to 14 days. Sustained bacteremia (repeatedly positive blood cultures) implies an endovascular infection and requires prolonged treatment (3 to 4 weeks) and an assessment of the heart valves.

Median Sternotomy Wound Infections

Wound infection complicates median sternotomy in 1% of all patients. This serious complication increases the mortality of bypass surgery to as high as 14% to 47%, and the cost of care is more than threefold higher than usual.[9]

Mediastinal dehiscence may be a sign of sternal wound infection, but it occurs more often in the absence of infection.[10] Infection may be superficial or deep. Superficial infection is confined to the subcutaneous tissue and is associated with a stable osteosynthesis. Deep infection is associated with sternal osteomyelitis. The retrosternal space also may be infected.

Deep infection, or "mediastinitis," may present as early as 4 days or as late as 3 months after surgery. Clinical findings may include fever, leukocytosis, inflammation of the wound, and purulent drainage from the wound. With sternal inflammation the depth and extent of the infection are unclear. Often, only with time and observation can the depth and extent of the infection be determined. Postoperative changes confound attempts at imaging. CT scans, bone gallium scans, and tomograms are misleading. Even patients without infection have elevation of acute-phase reactants after surgery, so the sedimentation rate does not help. Clues to the presence of a deep infection include increasing postoperative pain more than 5 to 7 days after surgery and failure to respond to superficial debridement and antibiotic therapy designed to treat a "superficial" infection.[9]

The risk of mediastinitis is increased by diabetes mellitus, obesity, obstructive lung disease, smoking, a low cardiac output state, remote infections, previous sternotomy, and prolonged hospitalization before heart surgery. Infection is more common with longer, complex operations, excessive use of electrocautery, the use of bone wax, blood transfusions, and the use of both the right and left internal mammary arteries (causing sternal ischemia).[9,10] Postoperative risk factors for infection include the need for reexploration, prolonged stay in the ICU, mechanical ventilation longer than 48 hours, need for a tracheostomy or cardiopulmonary resuscitation, and low flow states. Infections may occur autogenously or as a result of cross contamination from the hands and mucous membranes of hospital personnel.

Suppurative, deep mediastinal infection requires surgical debridement, which consists of an assessment of the vascularity of the tissues, debridement of devitalized cartilage and bone, and irrigation of the mediastinal space if retrosternal infection is found. Closure of the sternum over tubes used for irrigation may be successful if the sternum is viable and the infection presents early after coronary artery bypass graft. It is difficult to predict the success of this technique.

Current surgical practice favors debridement of all nonviable bony and soft tissues, antibiotic therapy to ensure microbiologic control, and subsequent flap closure. Closure may involve the use of a rotated omental flap or rotated rectus abdominis or pectoralis major flaps, or both.

Antimicrobial therapy is directed at the pathogen (usually *S. epidermidis* or *S. aureus*) that is identified in preoperative and operative cultures. A prolonged course of treatment (6 weeks) is recommended, given the presence of sternal osteomyelitis.

Patients who refuse flap closure have a large, open chest wound that will heal secondarily over 3 to 4 months after antibiotic therapy plus saline wet-to-dry dressings. During that time the mediastinum is exposed, and little tissue covers the heart. It sounds bad, but the cosmetic result of diligent wound care and prolonged antibiotic therapy can be superior to flap reconstruction. However, flap reconstruction lowers mortality and morbidity, particularly the chance of forming mediastinal to cutaneous fistulas.

Infectious Complications of Peripheral Vascular Disease

Most infections are caused by organisms colonizing skin ulcers caused by other illnesses, including venous or arterial insufficiency and neuropathy. Patients with

diabetes often have all these conditions, plus microvascular insufficiency and altered immune function (decreased white blood cell chemotaxis and killing).

Illness occurs when pathogens colonizing ulcers invade surrounding healthy tissue. The clinical presentation may be associated with inflammation—redness, warmth, tenderness, and swelling. Pain, which is distinct from claudication, may occur. Patients with venous insufficiency may have increased swelling and drainage. In those with neuropathy, however, the process can be insidious. Microvascular and large vessel disease can obscure the usual signs of inflammation and, more important, interfere with usual host responses and delivery of antibiotic to tissue. Infection may progress rapidly, usually because of a variety of aerobic and anaerobic pathogens (necrotizing synergistic cellulitis).

The clinical approach varies with the underlying illness. With *venous insufficiency,* treatment of complicating diseases is critical (congestive heart failure, liver and renal disease, and poor nutrition). Elevation of the extremities at rest and support stockings (TEDS) help. Patients should be encouraged to exercise at a level consistent with their physical limitations. Weight loss is recommended, but compliance is rare. Diligent wound care is critical. Multiple regimens have been used, and surgical referral may be necessary. Saline wet-to-dry dressings are gentle and effective. In some cases, hydrotherapy may be used for debridement. Occasionally patients will fail to heal and require tissue flaps.

Neuropathic ulcers require special attention to weight bearing and friction. Podiatric referral for construction of a fitted shoe should be considered. Patients should be taught to inspect their shoes prior to use for foreign objects and their feet after use for signs of tissue changes related to pressure.

Patients with arterial insufficiency require thorough study of the circulation to the affected limb (see Chapter 33). The T_cPO_2 is a useful value in diabetic patients; ≤ 30 mm Hg predicts an inability to heal. In such cases revascularization is necessary (see Chapter 33). Local therapy for the ulcer includes debridement and wet-to-dry dressings.

A variety of pathogens may be recovered from skin ulcers, including gram positive cocci, enteric gram negative rods, enterococci and anaerobes (including *Peptostreptococcus, Clostridium* sp., and *Bacteroides*). Antimicrobial therapy should be initiated only after appropriate cultures are obtained and tailored to the microbiology at the time of culture.

Exploration of the ulcer may reveal penetration to bone. This finding confirms osteomyelitis, a common finding in diabetic patients with coincident microvascular disease and neuropathy. It can occur in the upper extremities, the diabetic hand syndrome. A plain x-ray (two views) to rule out underlying bone infection is recommended if the depth of the ulcer is uncertain.

Antimicrobial therapy is preferably postponed until the time of surgical debridement and culture in a clinically stable patient. If acute signs of inflammation, ascending infection, or fever are present, then epidemiology and gram stains guide prompt empiric therapy. One choice of many possible regimens in the setting of arterial insufficiency is a beta-lactamase plus beta-lactamase inhibitor combination and an aminoglycoside. A second-generation cephalosporin with antianaerobic activity also can be used. Patients with venous insufficiency ulcers or neuropathic ulcers may need only a first-generation cephalosporin or antistaphylococcal beta-lactam.

A multidisciplinary approach to the care of these patients is critical. Control of diabetes mellitus and a care plan for vascular reconstruction require multiple specialists. Coincident with the design of antibiotic therapy, the clinician should communicate with colleagues regarding a plan to debride nonviable tissue and to restore the circulation. Control of the infection is important before vascular surgery but may be impossible in the absence of revascularization. Percutaneous angioplasty may offer an alternative to amputation in this scenario and can postpone or obviate the need for surgery (see Chapter 33). After revascularization and debridement, an evaluation of the extremity for occult osteomyelitis with bone and gallium scans or MRI helps to guide the duration of antibiotic therapy. Patients with osteomyelitis require a minimum 6-week course of antibiotic therapy and consideration of a long-term intravenous access (PICC or Groshong).

Postoperative patients should be monitored for the success of vascular reconstruction, wound care, and antibiotic therapy. A physiatry (rehabilitation) care plan is recommended. Postoperative patients also should be monitored for possible prosthetic graft infection.

Infections of Prosthetic Vascular Grafts and Stents

Infections of peripheral prosthetic grafts are associated with a 10% to 30% mortality risk and a 10% to 70% risk of amputation.[11] Infections of abdominal aortic grafts are associated with a 25% to 75% mortality risk and a 10% to 25% risk of amputation. Infections of thoracoabdominal aortic grafts are associated with a poor prognosis, partly because complete graft excision may not be possible. Infections of percutaneously placed endovascular stents are being reported as well, including coronary artery stents.

The clinical presentation of a prosthetic graft infection varies depending on the site of the graft, the extent of tissue injury and anastomotic damage caused by the pathogen, and the inflammatory response to it. Usually,

peripheral graft infections cause inflammation and purulent drainage. Fever, malaise, and weight loss may occur in a patient with a peripheral graft infection. These may be the only symptoms in an aortic graft infection. Localized findings include a tender and pulsatile mass at the site of the graft. This usually implies a pseudoaneurysm (a contained but disrupted anastomosis). More catastrophic presentations include gastrointestinal hemorrhage from an aortoenteric fistula, sepsis, and hemorrhagic shock caused by rupture of the graft.

Most graft infections are caused by gram positive organisms (*S. epidermidis*, *S. aureus*, *Streptococcus viridans*, and enterococci). *Enterobacteriaceae* and *Pseudomonas aeruginosa* are less common causes of these infections.

Diagnosis of a prosthetic graft infection is determined on the basis of the clinical presentation. When it is suspected, blood cultures, imaging of the involved graft, and vascular surgical consultation should be obtained. Imaging the graft can be done by ultrasound or by computed axial tomography. The findings may be confusing if the graft is new, since air and fluid may be present around a graft for 4 to 6 weeks after it is placed. If fluid is found and infection is a concern, then a needle aspiration of the fluid for microbiologic study can be considered.

If a graft infection is likely, empiric therapy is initiated while the surgical care plan is being formulated and while awaiting the results of cultures. An antibiotic regimen consisting of vancomycin plus an aminoglycoside has been suggested. Therapy is later tailored to the cultures and is continued for 4 to 6 weeks, followed by oral antibiotics if the graft cannot be removed.

The surgical approach to prosthetic graft infections varies depending on the location of the graft and the severity of the illness. Surgical goals include controlling hemorrhage, ensuring adequate circulation distal to the graft, and debridement. Patients with acute hemorrhage or sepsis need prompt graft excision. There is an increased risk of amputation and death. Revascularization by creation of an extraanatomic axillofemoral or axillopopliteal graft in another tissue plane is favored for hemodynamically stable patients. This can be accomplished days before the infected graft is resected.

Prosthetic graft infection may be prevented by perioperative antibiotics (cefazolin or vancomycin in cefazolin-allergic patients). Risk of these infections is increased by prolonged operative time, operation at a site of previous surgery, and groin dissections.

INFECTIONS OF THE HEART
Myocarditis

Myocarditis is considered if a patient has unexplained heart failure or a cardiac arrhythmia in the setting of a recent illness. Commonly, the prodromal illness is remote or not recalled. The clinical findings may even mimic myocardial infarction.

Damage to the myocardium may result from 0direct cellular injury, damage to the coronary vasculature, adverse effects of contiguous inflammation, the elaboration of toxins (diphtheria and *Clostridium* sp.), and the effects of cytotoxic T cell clones engendered by the infection. T cell clones react to viral antigen in cell membranes or viral products mimicking self-molecules, resulting in autoimmunity. The exact cause of direct myocyte injury varies with the pathogen.[12,13]

No cause is established in most cases. Recent studies have demonstrated RNA with homology to Coxsackie B virus types 1 to 6 in myocardial specimens of patients with dilated cardiomyopathy and chronic coronary disease. Additional RNA viruses implicated in myocarditis include poliomyelitis virus and other members of the enterovirus group, measles virus, mumps virus, bunyaviruses, toga viruses, and arena viruses.[12]

The role of HIV in causing myocarditis is unclear. Dilated cardiomyopathy subsequently develops in one in five patients with untreated AIDS; no cause is found in 80%. It is suspected that CD_4 helper/suppressor dysfunction may predispose to infection by cardiotropic viruses. An alternative hypothesis is that CD_4 suppressor dysfunction predisposes to an autoimmune myocarditis. Direct toxic effects of HIV have not been demonstrated.[14]

DNA viruses implicated in myocarditis include members of the adenovirus group and herpes virus group (vaccinia, variola, and hepatitis B).

Bacteremia may directly or indirectly cause myocarditis. Pathogens suspected of directly infecting the myocardium include streptococci and staphylococci, *Meningococcus* spp, *Salmonella*, *Brucella*, *Legionella*, *Rickettsia* spp., and *Borrelia burgdorferi* (Lyme disease). *Corynebacterium diphtheriae* indirectly causes myocarditis, because its toxin interferes with myocyte protein synthesis. *C. perfringens* acts both directly (metastatic abscess) and through elaboration of a toxin to produce myocyte and conduction system disease.

Protozoan organisms and parasites also may cause myocarditis. Chagas disease (*Trypanosoma cruzi*) should be considered in a patient with cardiomyopathy and a history of travel to Central and South America. Sleeping sickness (due to *T. gambiense* and *T. rhodesiense*) should be considered if the travel history includes sub-Saharan Africa. *Trichinella* sp. should be considered if there is a history of ingestion of partially cooked pork or bear meat. Toxoplasmosis in its disseminated form is associated with myocarditis and should be considered in a patient with a history of ingestion of partially cooked meat or exposure to outdoor cats.

Fungal myocarditis is limited to the immunocompromised host and may be caused by *Cryptococcus neoformans*, *Candida* spp., and *Aspergillus*.

Susceptibility to myocarditis may be age dependent, with younger patients being more severely affected. There may be a genetic predisposition.

The clinical presentation of myocarditis varies from the asymptomatic patient found to have a dilated heart on chest x-ray, to rapidly fatal cardiomyopathy in a patient with a recent illness. It is one of the causes of sudden cardiac death in young athletes. A young child may present with systemic febrile illness, disseminated intravascular coagulopathy, and diffuse involvement of the lung, liver, and central nervous system, followed by the evolution of cardiac disease.

The ECG may show ST segment elevation and subsequently T wave inversion. QRS changes and the evolution of left bundle branch block are associated with an increased risk of sudden death. Tachycardia out of proportion to the severity of illness is characteristic.

Echocardiography is useful for guiding endomyocardial biopsy and monitoring a patient's clinical course. Regional wall motion abnormalities, which may be reversible, may be demonstrated. Elevations of the CPK-MB and troponin I may occur, mimicking myocardial infarction.

Endomyocardial biopsy confirms the diagnosis of myocarditis in 16% to 100% of cases. Interobserver variability in interpretation, variation in the time of sampling during the disease course, sampling error, and poorly defined histopathologic criteria account for this wide range of results. Early in the infection, there is eosinophilia about myofibers and edema. Later, loss of striation may occur with nuclear degeneration, fragmentation, and acute inflammation, which is subsequently replaced by lymphocytes and plasma cells. The process either resolves or progresses to dilated cardiomyopathy associated with fibrosis and loss of myofibers. The specific cause of myocarditis is rarely found.

In all patients, it is important to consider possible noninfectious causes, including collagen vascular diseases, endocrinopathies, the effect of drugs (including cocaine and alcohol), radiation, the peripartum state, and multiple other illnesses that may depress contractility (see Chapter 24).

Most patients with myocarditis recover completely. Treatment is directed at the suspected etiologic agent. Exercise may worsen the disease and bed rest is recommended. Supportive care including oxygen, hemodynamic support and monitoring and careful attention to volume status is critical. The use of immunosuppressive medications acutely is *contra*indicated. Use of glucocorticoids in chronic coronary disease or dilated cardiomyopathy has no demonstrated efficacy; however, some studies suggest benefits in selected cases.[15]

Pericarditis (see Chapter 29)

The pericardium is a mesothelial structure made up of collagen. The outer portion is the parietal pericardium, which adheres to the great vessels. The portion adherent to the surface of the heart is the visceral pericardium. Normally, there is 15 to 50 ml of fluid in the pericardial sac—the space between the visceral and parietal pericardium.

Pericarditis is inflammation of the pericardium and has both infectious and noninfectious etiologies. Most cases of idiopathic pericarditis are thought to be viral. Patients who suffer myocarditis usually have pericarditis as well ("myopericarditis").

Bacterial pericarditis may result from spreading of a contiguous focus in the chest or heart. The source may be pneumonia, endocarditis, or trauma, including surgical wound infections. Infection may spread hematogenously to the pericardium. Pericarditis associated with pleuropulmonary infections is due to *S. aureus* and *Streptococcus pneumoniae* in more than half of cases. Gram negative bacilli may be found, especially in the elderly. Atypical pneumonia pathogens have been implicated, especially *Mycoplasma pneumoniae* and *Legionella* sp. Fungal pericarditis occurs in approximately 1 in 20 patients with disseminated histoplasmosis. A sterile inflammation of the pericardial space may occur owing to contiguous inflammation in mediastinal lymph nodes.

M. tuberculosis may cause a pericarditis as a consequence of hematogenous spread during a bacillemia, spread through lymphatics from peribronchial, peritracheal, and mediastinal lymph nodes, and from pleuropulmonary infections. With pericarditis caused by tuberculosis, the pain may be vague and major symptoms may include weight loss, night sweats, cough, and shortness of breath. The course of pericarditis in tuberculosis may be insidious.

The physical findings of pericarditis and pericardial effusion are reviewed in Chapter 29. The ECG is abnormal in 9 of 10 patients. ST segment elevation occurs early, and T waves invert after the ST segment returns to baseline. Electrical alternans may occur if there is a large pericardial effusion.

Echocardiography confirms the diagnosis, allows quantitation of size, and can detect impending hemodynamic compromise. It can be used to guide pericardiocentesis. Pericardiocentesis is recommended only in the setting of impending tamponade or if the effusion has been present for more than 3 weeks. Diagnostic yield is higher if pericardial biopsy can be performed. The risk of the procedure is otherwise too high to justify the low yield in most cases, which resolve spontaneously.

Patients with pericarditis who are acutely ill, febrile, and have high white cell counts may have purulent pericarditis. This process is rapidly fatal if not treated aggressively, including pericardiotomy with biopsy and drainage.

Treatment of pericarditis is similar to that recommended for myocarditis and includes treating any underlying disease, bed rest, hemodynamic support, and analgesia. Antiinflammatory therapy with aspirin or indomethacin may relieve pain. A short course of high-dose steroids may be prescribed if pain does not respond to other antiinflammatory therapy (see Chapter 29).

Most patients improve spontaneously. Recurrent pericarditis and progressive inflammation leading to fibrosis and constriction may occur. In pericarditis due to *M. tuberculosis,* up to one half of patients may progress to constriction despite appropriate therapy. Early pericardiotomy may be warranted.

Possible Infectious Causes of Coronary Artery Disease

On the basis of serologic diagnosis, several authors have reported a possible association between both *Chlamydia pneumoniae* infection or *Helicobacter pylori* infection and coronary artery disease.[16-19] *C. pneumoniae* has been isolated from atherosclerotic plaque.[17] No association between coronary disease and cytomegalovirus (CMV) infection was found in explanted hearts before cardiac transplantation, but an association has been made between CMV disease and rapid evolution of cardiac allograft vasculopathy.[20-22]

REFERENCES

1. Weinstein RA: Risk factors for nosocomial infections. American Hospital Association/Centers for Disease Control Training Course in Hospital Epidemiology, Chicago, May 16, 1991.
2. Platt R, Goldman D, Hopkins C: Epidemiology of nosocomial infections. In Gorbach SL, Bartlett JG, Blacklow NR, editors: *Infectious diseases,* Philadelphia, 1992, WB Saunders.
3. Platt R, Polk BF, Murdock B, Rosner B: Mortality associated with nosocomial urinary tract infection, *N Engl J Med* 307:637, 1982.
4. Celis R, Torres A, Gatell TM, et al: Nosocomial pneumonia: a multivariate analysis of risk and prognosis, *Chest* 93:318, 1988.
5. Henderson DK: Bacteremia due to percutaneous intravascular devices. In Mandell GL, Douglas RG Jr, Bennett JE, editors: *Principles and practice of infectious diseases,* New York, 1990, Churchill Livingstone.
6. Maki DG, Weise CE, Sarafin HW: A semi-quantitative method for identifying intravenous catheter-related infections, *N Engl J Med* 296:1305, 1997.
7. Wilson ML: Clinically relevant, cost-effective clinical microbiology strategies to decrease unnecessary testing, *Am J Clin Pathol* 107:154, 1997.
8. Fowler VG Jr, Li J, Corey GR, et al: Role of echocardiography in evaluation of patients with *Staphylococcus aureus* bacteremia: experience in 103 patients, *J Am Coll Cardiol* 30:1072, 1997.
9. Gottlieb LJ, Beahm EK, Krizek TJ, Karp RB: Approaches to sternal wound infections, *Adv Cardiac Surg* 7:147, 1996.
10. Oakley EL, Reida M, Wright JE: Postoperative mediastinitis: classification and management, *Ann Thorac Surg* 61:1030, 1996.
11. Calligaro KD, DeLaurentis DA, Veigh FR: An overview of the treatment of infected prosthetic vascular grafts, *Adv Surg* 29:3, 1996.
12. Martino T, Liu Pr, Sole MJ: Viral infection and pathogenesis of dilated cardiomyopathy, *Circ Res* 74:182, 1994.
13. Sole MJ, Liu P: Viral myocarditis: a paradigm for understanding the pathogenesis and treatment of dilated cardiomyopathy, *J Am Coll Cardiol* 22(suppl):99, 1993.
14. Epstein J, Eichbaum Q, Lipschultz SE: Cardiovascular manifestations of HIV infection, *Compr Ther* 22:485, 1996.
15. Mason JW, O'Connell JB, Herskowitz A, et al: A clinical trial of immunosuppressive therapy for myocarditis, *N Engl J Med* 333:269, 1995.
16. Patel P, Mendall MA, Carrington D, et al: Association of *Helicobacter pylori* and *Chlamydia pneumoniae* infections with coronary heart disease and cardiovascular risk factors, *BMJ* 311:711, 1995.
17. Ramirez JA: Isolation of *Chlamydia pneumoniae* from the coronary artery of a patient with coronary atherosclerosis, *Ann Intern Med* 125:979, 1996.
18. Mendall MA, Carrington D, Strachan D, et al: *Chlamydia pneumoniae:* risk factors for seropositivity and association with coronary heart disease, *J Infect* 30:121, 1995.
19. Whincup PH, Mendall MA, Perry IJ, et al: Prospective relations between *Helicobacter pylori* infection, coronary heart disease, and stroke in middle-aged men, *Heart* 75:568, 1996.
20. Kol A, Sperti G, Shani J, et al: Cytomegalovirus replication is not a cause of instability in unstable angina, *Circulation* 91:1910, 1995.
21. Dummer S, Lee A, Breinig MK, et al: Investigation of cytomegalovirus infection as a risk factor for coronary atherosclerosis in the explanted hearts of patients undergoing heart transplantation, *J Med Urol* 44:305, 1994.
22. Koskinen PK, Nieminin MS, Krogerus LA, et al: Cytomegalovirus infection and accelerated cardiac allograft vasculopathy in human cardiac allografts, *J Heart Lung Transplant* 12:724, 1993.

43 Nutritional Disorders, Obesity, and Alcoholism

Robert Kushner
Alex Lickerman

Diet and excessive alcohol consumption are associated with 8 of the 10 leading causes of death, including heart diseases, stroke, and atherosclerosis. After tobacco use, the combination of diet and sedentary activity accounts for an estimated 300,000 deaths each year. Obesity alone is a risk factor for coronary heart disease, high blood pressure, diabetes, and some forms of cancer, all leading to higher mortality. Lifestyle counseling remains one of our most productive activities in primary care medicine.

In the United States the two most important nutritionally related disorders associated with cardiovascular disease are obesity and excessive alcohol use. The role of dietary saturated fat and cholesterol is discussed elsewhere in Chapter 12. Other nutritional disorders, such as beriberi heart disease from thiamine deficiency and cardiac cachexia from protein-calorie malnutrition, are seen less frequently. The role of hyperhomocystinemia as a risk factor for cardiovascular disease, resulting from low levels of dietary folate, vitamin B_6, and vitamin B_{12}, has only recently been recognized.

OBESITY

If your practice reflects national statistics, then at least one third of your patients are obese.[1] Among African-American and Mexican-American female patients the prevalence is about one in two. The cause for this obesity epidemic is multifactorial, including rapid changes in technology that lessen the need for everyday physical activity and the overabundance of high-calorie and fatty convenience foods. These environmental forces act on a diversity of ill-defined genetic, metabolic, and biologic factors that determine which individuals will develop obesity.

Since obesity is often associated with cardiovascular disease, your first step is to identify which patients are at high risk. This categorization of risk includes the same elements of a history, physical examination, and selective laboratory work as for any other patient, plus two determinations: the patient's body mass index (BMI) and waist circumference.

Body Mass Index

BMI, calculated as weight in kilograms divided by the height in meters squared, has replaced the traditional ideal body weight calculations. BMI is simple (it is not necessary to determine frame size and gender to read the table) and is directly related to the risk for morbidity and mortality. As shown in Figure 43-1, a healthy BMI is a value between 18.5 and 25. Risk begins to rise thereafter as an asymptotic curve. Rates of all-cause and cardiovascular mortality increase as BMI rises.[2] The classification in Table 43-1 has been recommended by the National Institutes of Health Expert Panel on the Identification, Evaluation, and Treatment of Overweight and Obesity in Adults.[3]

Body Fat Distribution

The second risk criterion for the assessment of obesity is waist circumference. This measurement is recommended as part of the initial physical examination by the Joint National Committee (JNC) VI. The preferential deposition of fat in the upper body and abdomen, so-called android distribution, poses a significantly higher risk for atherosclerotic diseases compared with lower body fat distribution, called *gynoid obesity*. The elevated risk is thought to result from an accumulation of metabolically active intraabdominal visceral fat. Since this fat depot can be accurately measured only by computed tomographic (CT) scan or magnetic resonance imaging (MRI), the single best surrogate determination is measurement of the waist circumference. By convention, this is performed at the level of the iliac crests. A circumference of 102 cm (40 inches) for men and 88 cm (35 inches) for women is associated with increased risk for hyperinsulinemia, glucose intolerance, diabetes, dyslipidemia, and hypertension.[3] A single waist measurement is now considered superior to measuring the waist-hip ratio (WHR), although both can be performed if desired.

Obesity and Cardiovascular Disease
Hypertension

One of the most important clinical effects of obesity is increased blood pressure. Multiple cross-sectional and longitudinal studies have demonstrated the following observations:

1. A strong correlation exists between body weight and blood pressure in normotensive and hypertensive individuals.

2. Weight gain increases blood pressure, whereas weight loss produces a corresponding decrease.
3. The frequency of hypertension is greater in obese individuals, with prevalence rates about twice those among persons of normal weight.
4. The risk of hypertension appears to parallel the degree of obesity.
5. Obesity is an independent risk factor for hypertension.

These studies also show that the relationship between obesity and hypertension is strongest for younger adults (ages 20 to 39 years) and then gradually decreases for persons of older age.[4]

The pathogenesis of obesity-induced hypertension is not entirely understood but appears to result from underlying hemodynamic alterations, renal dysfunction, and an increase in sympathetic nervous system activity, possibly as a result of insulin resistance. The hemodynamic changes seen in obesity are fundamentally caused by the increase in adipose tissue and lean body mass that accompany weight gain. Because adipose tissue consists of about 14% water, an accumulation of body fat is also accompanied by an expansion of extracellular water and total blood volume. The increase in lean body mass (representing about one fourth of the total weight gain) is associated with an increase in oxygen consumption. The net result of these two metabolic demands is an increase in cardiac output proportional to body size. Since resting heart rate usually remains within a normal range, the increased cardiac demand is met by an increase in stroke volume. Mean arterial pressure may remain normal or only slightly increased because of a reciprocal reduction in systemic vascular resistance.

In the kidney this increased flow state is associated with renal hyperperfusion and hyperfiltration. The initiation of obesity-related hypertension is thought to result from abnormal renal sodium and water handling. An altered "pressure natriuresis" has been observed that is characterized by increased renal tubular sodium reabsorption and further expansion of the extracellular fluid volume. When maintained, the inevitable consequence is a rise in blood pressure.

The mechanisms responsible for renal dysregulation have not been clearly elucidated but appear to be mediated by increased sympathetic nervous system activity, activation of the renin-angiotensin system, and altered intrarenal physical forces that compress the renal medulla.[5] The mechanisms by which obesity activates the sympathetic nervous system are unknown; however, insulin resistance and hyperinsulinemia have been suggested as possible etiologic factors.

Physical Examination

The primary consideration when checking the blood pressure of an obese patient is that a proper cuff is used. A bladder of inappropriate width for the patient's arm circumference causes a systematic error in blood pressure measurement. If the bladder is too narrow, the pressure will be overestimated and lead to a false diagnosis of hypertension. To prevent errors, the bladder width should be 40% to 50% of upper arm circumference. Therefore a large adult cuff (15 cm wide) should be chosen for patients with mild to moderate obesity, and a thigh cuff (18 cm wide) should be used for patients whose arm circumference is greater than 16 inches.

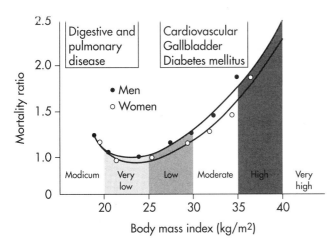

FIG. 43-1
Relationship of BMI to risk. A healthy or good body weight range is between 20 and 25 kg/m².
From Bray GA: *Am J Clin Nutr* 55:488,1992.

	Table 43-1	Classification of Overweight and Obesity in Adults

BMI Category	Health Risk Based on BMI	Risk Adjusted for Presence of Comorbid Conditions or Other Risk Factors
<25	Minimal	Low
25 to <27	Low	Moderate
27 to <30	Moderate	High
30 to <35	High	Very high
35 to <40	Very high	Extremely high
>40	Extremely high	Extremely high

From Expert Panel on the Identification, Evaluation, and Treatment of Overweight and Obesity in Adults, National Institutes of Health, June 1998.

Left Ventricular Hypertrophy[6,8]

As already reviewed, metabolic demands are increased in obesity because of the increase in total body oxygen consumption and circulatory volume. Cardiac output and cardiac work load increase in proportion to body weight. The expanded intravascular volume increases venous return and the preload of the left ventricle. As a consequence, left ventricular (LV) and atrial chamber volumes increase. The rise in LV filling pressure and end-diastolic diameter increases wall tension (in accordance to the law of Laplace, see Chapter 2), causing the LV wall to thicken or hypertrophy. This adaptation to LV wall stress produces *eccentric* LV hypertrophy, wherein LV cavity size and wall mass both increase. A pure afterload state (aortic stenosis or hypertension without an increase in intravascular volume) causes *concentric* LV hypertrophy, or thickened muscle with a small LV cavity.

Echocardiographic studies have shown a positive correlation between both LV wall thickness and internal dimension with the degree of obesity even in the absence of hypertension. Among the severely obese, duration of obesity is associated with higher LV mass, poorer LV systolic function, and greater impairment of LV diastolic filling. Depressed cardiac performance may already be present in a moderately to severely obese patient, even if the patient is normotensive and has no signs of cardiac disease.

With a rise in arterial pressure, cardiac afterload is heightened, which further increases LV wall stress, causing the LV hypertrophy to increase. At this point, cardiac adaptation is of the *concentric* type, with little or no additional chamber dilation (Fig. 43-2). Echocardiographic studies from the Framingham study have shown that LV mass increases consistently across increasing tertiles of systolic pressure and BMI, both separately and jointly.[7] If sustained, these alterations in LV loading predispose to further impairment in LV systolic function and ultimately to congestive heart failure.[4]

Examination and Testing

Mildly to moderately obese patients with LV hypertrophy remain asymptomatic as long as LV function is maintained. The earliest symptom is typically dyspnea on exertion.

The chest x-ray is often normal at this stage, although an enlarged cardiac silhouette may be seen. The electrocardiogram (ECG) has poor sensitivity for LV hypertrophy in obese individuals for several reasons, including the attenuating effect of excessive adipose tissue on precordial QRS voltage amplitudes and a shift toward the left in the electrical axis as a result of a change in the anatomic position of the heart. These effects lead to an underestimation of LV hypertrophy by most standard ECG diagnostic scoring criteria. Although specificity for LV hypertrophy generally remains above 95%, sensitivity is very low (usually under 15%) and drops further with increasing BMI. If you want to screen for LV hypertrophy in your office, the most sensitive criterion for this population is the Cornell voltage method (R wave in lead aVL plus S wave in lead V_3) or its derivative, the Cornell product (Cornell voltage times the QRS duration).[9] Voltage criteria for these methods are shown in Table 43-2.

The gold standard for detecting LV hypertrophy is the transthoracic echocardiogram (TTE). A TTE should be obtained in patients suspected of having LV hypertrophy for assessment of LV function. For patients with severe obesity in whom images are difficult to obtain because of increased chest wall thickness, a transesophageal echocardiogram (TEE) may be indicated.

Cardiomyopathy of Obesity

Congestive heart failure (CHF) is the end result of chronic and persistent abnormal cardiac loading. As volume overload continues, hypertrophy fails to adequately offset chamber dilation. The high cardiac output of obesity is maintained at the expense of elevated LV filling pressures. Wall stress increases and eventually leads to myocardial decompensation. Thus CHF in severe obesity most commonly occurs as a sequela of long-standing eccentric LV hypertrophy and in the absence of other organic heart disease. Although systemic hypertension aggravates LV failure, the cardiomyopathy of obesity may develop in normotensive patients.

Compared with those of weight-matched obese patients without CHF, echocardiographic studies demonstrate that CHF patients have significantly greater LV cavity size, end-systolic wall stress, and LV mass. In addition, right heart and pulmonary artery pressures are significantly elevated (these may be assessed by right-sided cardiac catheterization or noninvasively using echo-Doppler techniques).

Over three quarters of severely obese patients with CHF are diagnosed with idiopathic dilated cardiomyopathy. In contrast to the previous belief that obesity cardiomyopathy results from an accumulation of fat in the myocardium, the increased cardiac weight is actually associated with thickened and hypertrophied ventricles.

The Clinical Syndrome

Patients with cardiomyopathy are typically severely obese, with BMIs greater than 40 kg/m². In a recent study by Alpert et al.[10] the duration of severe obesity was identified as the strongest predictor of CHF. They found that the odds of CHF increased by 1.46 per year, so the probability of CHF is 66% for a person who is severely obese for 20 years.

Typically, patients have recurrent exacerbations of CHF symptoms over several years. They often report recent weight gain with progressively increasing dyspnea,

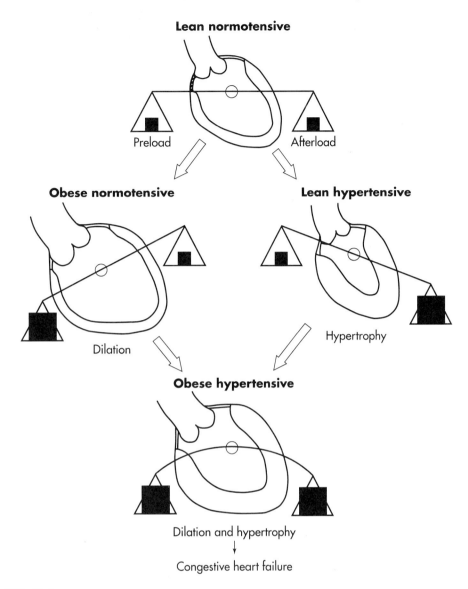

FIG. 43-2
Cardiac adaptation to obesity and hypertension. Obesity increases blood volume and preload, leading to dilation. Hypertension is a pure afterload state, causing LV hypertrophy. The two together cause both dilation and LV hypertrophy.
From Messerli FH: *Lancet* 1:1165, 1982.

Table 43-2	*Electrocardiographic Voltage Criteria for Left Ventricular Hypertrophy*			
	Cornell Method (mV) (RaVL + SV₃)		**Cornell Product Method (mV-ms) [(RaVL + SV₃) × QRS duration]**	
	Men	**Women**	**Men**	**Women**
Sensitivity 50%	1.96	1.58	1976	1453
Specificity 95%	2.53	2.03	2529	1847

Data from Norman JE, Levy D: *J Am Coll Cardiol* 26:1022, 1995.

orthopnea, and leg edema. Chest x-ray shows the usual findings of CHF with cardiomegaly and pulmonary vascular congestion. An echocardiogram should be obtained for assessment of LV and right ventricular (RV) wall function and thickness, chamber size, ejection fraction, and the presence of other causes of cardiomyopathy, such as valvular or pericardial disease.

Obesity Hypoventilation Syndrome and Obstructive Sleep Apnea

Obesity is associated with multiple pulmonary function abnormalities, including reduced functional residual capacity (FRC), end-expiratory reserve volume (ERV), vital capacity (VC), and compliance of the lung and chest wall. These changes increase the mechanical work of breathing, and they make it difficult to meet the increased demands of exercise or stress. With advancing severity and duration of obesity, ventilatory insufficiency may develop, as evidenced by progressive hypercapnia, hypoxemia, and polycythemia. This condition is called the obesity hypoventilation syndrome (OHS).

Obesity also predisposes to obstruction of the airway at the palatal or hypopharyngeal level. Increased fat deposition adjacent to the pharyngeal airway, in the soft palate and uvula, along with relaxation of the upper airway dilating muscles, causes increased upper airway resistance and temporary cessation of airflow during sleep. This results in recurrent episodes of apnea and hypopnea, brief awakenings from sleep, and sleep disruption. Consequently, the patient experiences excessive daytime hypersomnolence, referred to as *obstructive sleep apnea (OSA)*.

The presence of both respiratory abnormalities—OHS and OSA—in a severely obese patient is called *Pickwickian syndrome,* after Joe, the "fat and red-faced boy in a state of somnolency," described by Charles Dickens in *The Pickwick Papers.* Both conditions produce serious effects on the cardiovascular system and contribute to increased morbidity and mortality. The cardiovascular complications include pulmonary hypertension, cor pulmonale, congestive heart failure, cardiac arrhythmias, and sudden death. Hypoxemia causes vasoconstriction of the pulmonary arteries and muscularization of pulmonary arterioles, a process aggravated by hypercapnic acidosis. With vasoconstriction, pulmonary arterial diastolic pressure rises. Sustained increases in pulmonary vascular resistance and pressure increase RV workload. The development of RV hypertrophy and dilation may result in cor pulmonale. The prevalence of pulmonary hypertension or cor pulmonale in OSA patients has been reported to range from 17% to 42%. The pathogenesis of LV and RV failure in patients with severe obesity is summarized in Figure 43-3.

Obese persons with OSA are five times more likely to have hypertension than similarly obese persons without

sleep-disordered breathing. The apnea-hypertension association is thought to be mediated by chemoreceptor activation and increased or prolonged sympathetic nerve activity brought about by hypoxic stimulation. Plasma catecholamine levels rise markedly throughout the course of apnea and correlate with overnight oxygen desaturation. The mechanisms by which nightly recurrent blood pressure elevations lead to sustained daytime systemic hypertension are not clearly understood but may involve central or peripheral resetting of neural control mechanisms, or vascular remodeling.[11] Hypoxia-induced increases in systemic vascular resistance and afterload

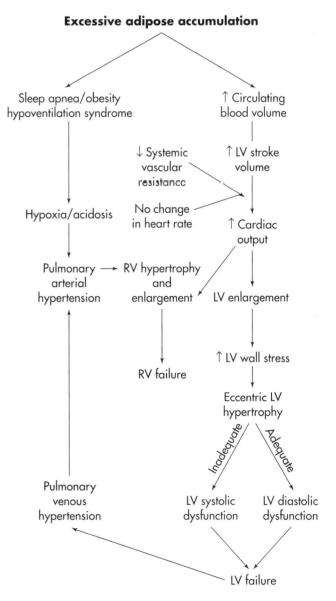

FIG. 43-3

Pathogenesis of congestive heart failure in morbidly obese individuals with and without the OSA/OHS syndrome. *LV,* Left ventricle; *RV,* right ventricle.

From Alpert MA, Hashimi MW: *Am J Med Sci* 306:117, 1993.

also have been linked to a higher prevalence of LV hypertrophy in this population. In one study of 51 middle-aged men with OSA, the prevalence of LV hypertrophy among those with severe OSA and hypertension was 70%, a complication rate considerably higher than that found with essential hypertension alone.[12]

Cardiac rhythm and conduction abnormalities are additional effects of sleep apnea. Cyclic bradyarrhythmias and tachyarrhythmias have been reported in more than 75% of patients with OSA. Sinus arrhythmia, sinus bradycardia, and transient atrioventricular (AV) block is caused by increased vagal tone in response to vigorous respiratory efforts during obstruction. On arousal, a sudden sympathetic discharge triggers tachycardia and ventricular arrhythmia. The associated hypoxia, hypercapnia, and acidoses also contribute to arrhythmias. The frequency of apnea-associated arrhythmias is proportional to the severity of oxyhemoglobin desaturation.

Examination and Testing

Patients with severe obesity and OHS typically have signs and symptoms consistent with CHF, including pulmonary rales, extensive peripheral edema, sinus tachycardia, gallop rhythm, cyanosis, and somnolence. Diagnostic evaluation shows cardiac enlargement and pulmonary congestion on chest x-ray, right axis deviation on ECG, polycythemia, and hypoxia, hypercapnia, and respiratory acidosis on arterial blood gas analysis. These patients must be treated immediately.

Unlike OHS, the presentation of OSA may be more subtle. Loud snoring and fatigue are frequently the only symptoms. Since 60% to 90% of OSA patients evaluated in sleep clinics are obese, this population demands a more focused history and physical examination.

The following key signs and symptoms point to OSA[13]:

- Apnea observed by a bed partner
- Habitual snoring
- Nocturnal gasping, choking, or resuscitative snorting
- History of systemic hypertension
- Daytime somnolence
- Periods of irresistible sleep
- Unrefreshing sleep
- Morning headaches
- Cognitive impairment
- Depression

Common physical findings are male gender, increased neck circumference, upper body fat distribution, oropharyngeal crowding, and tonsillar hypertrophy. Do not wait for your patient to fall asleep while driving (or in your examining room) before suspecting this illness.

A sleep study (polysomnography) should be performed to confirm the presence of OSA and to assess the patient's level of risk. Sleep studies are conducted overnight by recording multiple respiratory and cardio-vascular measurements, including respiratory effort, heart rate and rhythm, airflow, and blood oxygen levels. Test results usually are presented as an apnea-hypopnea index (AHI) score, where an AHI of 5 (five or more episodes per hour of sleep) defines the disease. Pertinent information to look for is the AHI score, duration of apneas/hypopneas, lowest SO_2 recorded, and type of cardiac events. Many sleep laboratories conduct "split-night studies," in which a therapeutic trial of continuous positive airway pressure (CPAP) is applied during the second half of the night if OSA is diagnosed.

Coronary Artery Disease

The relationship between obesity and coronary heart disease is well established. Obesity is a major risk factor for atherosclerotic cardiovascular disease (ASCVD), and ASCVD is the primary cause for obesity-related increased mortality. Age-adjusted relative risk for ASCVD mortality has generally been noted to increase by a factor of 1.20 to 1.75, depending on the population and age studied. Several long-term epidemiologic studies have shown that coronary artery disease (CAD) mortality increases an average 4% to 6% for every 1 BMI unit (kg/m^2) starting at a BMI of about 20 to 24 kg/m^2.[14] Although this relationship is striking, the question of whether obesity is an *independent* risk factor for CAD is still debated. The controversy arises because the observed BMI-associated risk of CAD is always attenuated, but not entirely removed, when other cardiovascular disease risk factors are included in multivariate analysis. The most important fact for the clinician, however, is that obesity aggravates other risk factors (Box 43-1). In addition, obesity may function as a surrogate marker of other lifestyle factors that are directly or indirectly re-

---

BOX 43-1

CARDIOVASCULAR RISK FACTORS ASSOCIATED WITH OBESITY

Hypertension
Impaired glucose tolerance
Insulin resistance and hyperinsulinemia
Type 2 diabetes mellitus
Hypercholesterolemia (low-density lipoprotein subparticles pattern B)
Hypertriglyceridemia
Low levels of high-density lipoprotein cholesterol
Plasminogen activator inhibitor-1 (PAI-1)
Tissue-type plasminogen activator (t-PA)
Factor VII

lated to health, such as increased intake of total calories, physical inactivity, and smoking.

Regional fat distribution has also emerged as a risk factor for CAD. Many of the metabolic complications of obesity, including hyperinsulinemia, glucose intolerance, insulin resistance, elevated blood pressure, and dyslipoproteinemia, are correlated with the level of visceral adipose tissue. The clustering of these metabolic abnormalities has been called *syndrome X*, or the insulin resistance syndrome. Multiple epidemiologic studies have shown that an elevated WHR, a surrogate marker for excess abdominal visceral fat, accounts for a significant portion of the link between obesity and CAD mortality. Thus upper body fat distribution (android obesity) identifies a subgroup of obese individuals with the highest risk for CVD.

Examination and Testing

Evaluation for CAD is reviewed elsewhere in Chapter 13. Obesity does not appear to increase the incidence of silent myocardial ischemia and therefore is not an indication for CAD screening in the absence of symptoms or other risk factors. When perfusion imaging is planned, sestamibi is preferred over thallium because it is less affected by soft tissue attenuation.

Sudden Death and Mortality

As noted by Hippocrates, "sudden death is more common in those who are naturally fat than in the lean." A striking increase in mortality risk was demonstrated by Drenick et al.[15] in a prospective study of 200 severely obese men (average weight, 316 pounds) followed for a mean period of $7\frac{1}{2}$ years. A twelvefold excess in mortality was observed for those 25 to 34 years old and a sixfold excess in those 35 to 44 years of age. Cardiovascular disease accounted for over half of all deaths, with an incidence 30% higher than for age-matched men.

The patients at highest risk for sudden death are those with severe obesity and OHS or OSA. The major cardiopulmonary findings on autopsy are biventricular heart failure with LV and RV hypertrophy and dilation and severe pulmonary congestion. Some studies have shown increased fat and fibrosis throughout the cardiac conduction system. CAD is a less frequent finding.

The cause of death is most often a cardiac arrhythmia. Various factors predispose to ventricular dysrhythmia in obesity-cardiomyopathy, including stretching of the myocardium, myositic hypertrophy, fibrosis and fat infiltration of the conduction system, increased myocardial oxygen demands, and hypoxia. An obese patient with eccentric LV hypertrophy alone also is at increased risk for ventricular ectopy. Identification of ventricular ectopy or a prolonged QT interval on routine ECG or 24-hour Holter monitoring may signify a higher risk for sudden death in this population.

Management of Obesity

General Concepts of Diet, Physical Activity, and Behavioral Counseling

Obesity studies have repeatedly shown that the most commonly associated chronic diseases, such as hypertension, type 2 diabetes, and dyslipidemia, are improved with as little as a 10% loss in weight. This amount of weight loss is not only realistic but also achievable and sustainable. The information presented here regarding behavioral modification, dietary counseling, and physical activity guidance is best delivered by a team approach using physicians, dietitians, nurses, and exercise specialists. You cannot make patients lose weight; they must be interested in taking control and participating in the process. Your role is to provide information, guidance, and direction.

Stages of Change Model. One of the most useful tools for determining if the patient is ready to participate is the Stages of Change Model (also known as the Transtheoretical Model of Behavior Change), which was originally developed during efforts to effect behavioral change in smoking cessation.[16] The different stages and appropriate actions for both practitioner and patient are shown in Table 43-3.

Determining the patient's stage of change provides an appropriate starting point at which to address weight concerns. Patients are often able to identify which stage of change is the best match for their current level of commitment, if given a brief description of attitudes typical of each. In addition to determining how interested or ready patients are to begin making lifestyle changes, it is also necessary to ascertain their current diet and activity patterns. This is most conveniently accomplished by asking patients to keep food and activity diaries for several days to a week, either before coming in for a first visit or after the first visit. Food and activity diaries are invaluable as a tool for targeting problem areas related either to eating or to exercise behaviors.

Dietary Counseling. The first goal of all diet information must be nutritionally sound eating. A brief review of the dietary records by yourself, a dietitian, or a trained office nurse can alert you to any major deficiencies that exist (typically, lack of fruits, vegetables, and whole grains), irregular meal patterns (e.g., nighttime eating), or excessive intake of high-calorie items (e.g., fried foods, dressings, and desserts). Two new strategies that have emerged in nutritional counseling are (1) to view the diet in qualitative terms and (2) to encourage inclusion rather than preach exclusion.

Many patients "turn off" or are unable to fully comprehend the concepts of calorie counting, fat gram counting, or exchange groups. Although these skills are useful when mastered, they often complicate or confuse the principal message: eat a balanced diet modified in total fat and calories. An additional positive counseling

Table 43-3	Stages of Change: Appropriate Methods for Effecting Lifestyle Change	

Stage	Characteristics of Stage	Appropriate Treatment Approach
Precontemplation	Not thinking about change or just beginning to consider change	Provide information
Contemplation	Recognizing need to change, thinking about doing so	Help to solve ambivalence through information; help patient to see discrepancies in beliefs
Preparation	Taking initial steps to change, developing plan Starting to make small changes	Start teaching behavior modification techniques; continue education
Action	Taking specific steps, gaining control over problem	Continue with cognitive and behavior change efforts; traditional programs most effective at this point; identify areas of resistance and treat
Maintenance	Achieving initial goals, consolidating changes into new lifestyle, working to prevent relapse	Relapse control (monitoring, lapse prevention)

technique is to encourage the *inclusion* of missing food groups, such as fruits, vegetables, or whole grain products, rather than lecturing the patient on avoiding, excluding, or banning a favorite dessert. An extremely useful visual teaching tool is the USDA food pyramid. Patients can compare their own food records to the pyramid, noting any deficiencies or excesses. In this way you can begin to "shape" patients' diets.

Physical Activity Counseling. Similar to dietary goals, it is important to communicate a simple message about physical activity. Many patients still believe that unless they are willing to devote at least 20 minutes to vigorous exercise at least three times a week they might as well not bother at all. A revised goal has been recommended by the Surgeon General's Report on Physical Activity and Health, which concludes that cardiovascular health can be improved and maintained on a regimen of 30 minutes of *accumulated* activity each day.[17] It does not have to be continuous or vigorous. Physicians who can devote even 5 minutes of office time to educate patients about the importance of exercise and who convey an attitude that expresses concern about patients' exercise level have been able to increase their patients' activity levels.

Use of Modified Diets. There are three types of modified diets: very-low calorie diets (VLCDs), protein-sparing modified fast (PSMF), and over-the-counter (OTC) meal replacements. The primary purpose of prescribing one of these diets is to promote a rapid and significant short-term weight loss. VLCDs are specific foods or liquid formulas that generally supply ≤800 kcal , 50 to 80 g protein, and 100% of the recommended daily allowance (RDA) for vitamins and minerals. Examples include Optifast, HMR, and Nutrimed; these must be purchased from the manufacturer.

PSMFs are hypocaloric, high-protein, low-carbohydrate diets that use table foods. The prescription calls for 1.5 g of high-biologic-value protein per kilogram of IBW per day in two or three meals, supplemented with 25 mEq of potassium, 800 mg of calcium, a multiple vitamin/mineral capsule, and ≥1.5 L of fluid.

OTC products such as Slimfast and Sweet Success are prescribed to replace two out of three meals per day. Each of these plans effects rapid weight loss and requires close medical monitoring for dehydration and electrolyte imbalance. These treatments are usually reserved for patients with an immediate need for improved metabolic control or diuresis (e.g., poorly controlled diabetes, hypertension, or congestive heart failure). This short-term beneficial treatment must be weighed against the scattered reports of sudden death occurring as a complication of rapid dieting. Although modern VLCDs are considered safer because they use high-quality sources of protein from soy, egg, and milk instead of hydrolyzed collagen, the definitive cause of the reported sudden deaths has not been determined. Currently, their use should be restricted to 16 weeks with close monitoring of electrolyte levels. The development of any complications or prolongation of the QT complex on serial ECGs is an indication to discontinue the diet immediately.

Pharmacotherapy. Antiobesity medications can greatly benefit patients who are unable to control their body weight by changing lifestyle alone. Two anorexiant

medications, fenfluramine and dexfenfluramine, were voluntarily removed from the market in 1997 because of safety concerns related to unexplained valvulopathy. The newest anorexiant was approved in 1998. Sibutramine hydrochloride monohydrate (Meridia) acts through serotonin and norepinephrine reuptake inhibition (SNRI). When combined with lifestyle modification, patients can expect to achieve a 5% to 10% reduction in body weight over 6 to 12 months. Side effects are primarily cardiovascular, with a small increase in mean blood pressure (1 to 2 mm Hg) and a small increase in heart rate (4 beats/min). Sibutramine should not be used in patients with a history of CAD, congestive heart failure, arrhythmias, or stroke.

Orlistat (Xenical) is a gastrointestinal lipase inhibitor with clinically insignificant absorption into the body. It acts by competitively inhibiting the absorption of approximately one third of dietary fat. In addition to modest weight loss, the drug decreases elevated blood lipid levels. Its major side effect is gastrointestinal, causing diarrhea and oily stools as a result of the passage of unabsorbed dietary fat.

Surgery. A gastric restrictive surgical procedure, either vertical banding gastroplasty (VBG) or gastric stapling with roux-en-Y intestinal bypass (GIB), is the most effective treatment for patients with clinically severe obesity (BMI >40 kg/m^2). When performed as part of an overall comprehensive treatment plan, average weight losses of 50% of excess weight are routinely achieved and maintained.[3] Concomitant improvements in metabolic and cardiovascular comorbidities are also seen. This treatment can be lifesaving for patients with OHS, OSA, or Pickwickian syndrome; however, long-term success requires dedication on the part of the patient and finding a highly skilled surgeon and obesity team to provide support and guidance.

Effects of Obesity Treatment on Cardiovascular Complications. The first recommendation to any patient with obesity should be to lose weight, since weight loss has been demonstrated to reverse many of the coexisting cardiovascular risk factors (Fig. 43-4). Almost all metabolic abnormalities, with the exception of Lp(a), can be improved by modest weight reduction (5 to 10 kg), although gender differences have been noted.[18] Even though weight loss alone is beneficial, this represents only one of multiple recommendations you should be making to your patients (see Chapter 11).

The take-home message from weight reduction trials is that relatively small amounts of weight loss lead to substantial beneficial effects on blood pressure, LV hypertrophy, heart failure, pulmonary disease (OHS and OSA), and probably mortality.[19,20] It is not necessary to reach ideal body weight to achieve a clinically meaningful effect. For example, an 8 to 10 kg reduction in weight has been shown to lower blood pressure, blood volume, oxygen consumption, and stroke volume in

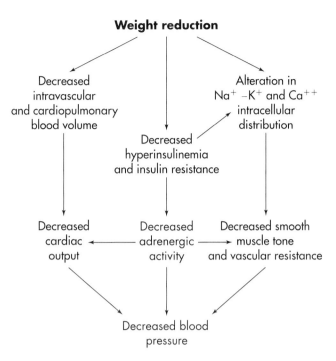

FIG. 43-4
Physiologic changes with weight reduction.

From Reisin E: Obesity hypertension: nonpharmacologic and pharmacologic therapeutic modalities. In Laragh JH, Brenner BM, editors: *Hypertension: pathophysiology, diagnosis, and management,* ed 2, New York, 1995, Raven.

those with cardiac dysfunction and to reduce the number and severity of apneic spells in those with OSA.

It may seem unusual to devote this much space in a cardiology text to the treatment of obesity. However, there is little that we can do as primary care physicians that has as much influence on our patients' cardiovascular health as working with them on weight management.

ALCOHOLISM
Epidemiology and Natural History

Alcoholism is broadly defined as a chronic illness characterized by continued drinking in the face of adverse consequences. It is often progressive and fatal. Alcoholics can be identified by their preoccupation with alcohol, inability to control drinking behavior, and denial. As with other addictions, tolerance to the effects of alcohol develops; the patient must consume progressively greater amounts to achieve intoxication.

Alcoholism is estimated to affect 10% of adult Americans and ranks as the third leading cause of death in the United States. Prospective studies have shown that alcoholics have two to four times the mortality of nonalcoholic controls.[21] Notably, alcoholic patients who succeed in achieving and maintaining long-term abstinence have identical mortality as nonalcoholic patients. Unfortunately, it is also estimated that over three quarters of alcoholics never receive treatment.

The etiology of alcoholism remains poorly understood. A predisposition to alcoholism seems to be inherited in approximately half of all cases. Other risk factors include social conditioning, close friends or family who exhibit enabling behavior, and being the child of a dysfunctional family.

The natural history of alcoholism can be broken down into four stages that characterize 75% of male alcoholics (Table 43-4). Throughout the course of the disease brief periods of abstinence or successful moderation are typical. Patients should not be lulled into the false belief that these periods represent a cure of their disease, because an eventual return of uncontrolled drinking is the rule.

Cardiovascular Effects

Although mortality from cardiovascular causes has been observed to decrease in association with moderate alcohol consumption, cardiovascular morbidity has been shown to increase.

Hypertension. In observational studies, alcohol intake correlates with an increased risk for hypertension.[22] In addition, blood pressure is more difficult to control in hypertensive patients who consume alcohol. Reduction of intake often improves control of blood pressure.

Arrhythmias. "Holiday heart" refers to the association between binge drinking and arrhythmias. It is common in nonalcoholics. Atrial fibrillation is the usual arrhythmia. Spontaneous reversion to normal sinus rhythm is the norm; a minority of patients require cardioversion. The incidence of sudden cardiac death is also increased in alcoholics, suggesting a predisposition in these patients to ventricular arrhythmias as well.

Cardiomyopathy. Alcohol is recognized as a frequent cause of nonischemic cardiomyopathy. The prevalence of cardiomyopathy in alcoholics is between 11% and 40%. The risk is increased after drinking approximately 80 g (3 oz) of alcohol per day for more than 10 years (six beers, one pint of whiskey, or one and a half bottles of wine per day). On the other hand, we have observed that it often occurs in young alcoholics, in their early 20s, whereas many older alcoholics with much higher total consumption are spared. There is more to the illness than just exposure. It has been theorized that in addition to years of heavy consumption some genetic or environmental predisposition is required to develop alcoholic cardiomyopathy. Interestingly, alcoholics who develop cardiomyopathy often do not have other sequelae of chronic alcohol abuse (cirrhosis or neuropathy).

Evidence that alcohol and its metabolites directly cause alcoholic cardiomyopathy is largely circumstantial. Dilated sarcoplasmic reticulum has been noted on electron micrographs of heart tissue in patients with alcoholic cardiomyopathy. Dysfunction of tubular membranes may limit the availability of calcium to contractile proteins and thereby diminish ventricular performance.

ECG abnormalities are nonspecific and generally unhelpful in making the diagnosis of alcohol-induced cardiomyopathy. The echocardiogram reveals either systolic or diastolic dysfunction. Mild ventricular hypertrophy also may be present, most likely as a result of comorbid conditions such as hypertension. Clinical signs and symptoms are what you would expect for cardiomyopathy due to other causes (see Chapters 22 and 23).

The 4-year mortality for patients with alcoholic cardiomyopathy who continue to drink has been found in some series to be as high as 50%. For those who abstain, however, it drops to 9%. Standard therapies for heart failure apply. At one time prolonged bed rest was recommended, but its efficacy was probably produced by enforced abstention.

Cardiovascular Benefits of Moderate Alcohol Use

Ischemic Heart Disease. The incidence of death from CAD in France is one third that of the United States despite a dietary intake among the French containing three times as much saturated fat. This observation has become popularized as "the French paradox."

Table 43-4	Phases of Alcoholism

Phase	Clinical Picture	Consequences
I	Alcohol is used to relieve tension; lasts months to years	Tolerance develops
II	Increasing preoccupation with obtaining alcohol; loss of control over use	Blackouts occur
III	Psychologic consequences occur (grandiosity, rationalization, aggressive behavior)	Disruption of interpersonal relationships
IV	Chronic intoxication	Deterioration of health and social functioning

The survival advantage enjoyed by the French has been attributed to their increased consumption of wine. Multiple observational studies have shown that mild to moderate alcohol consumption (e.g., two drinks per day) is correlated with a 40% risk reduction in cardiovascular mortality. Fifty percent of this survival advantage is believed to result from increases in high-density lipoprotein cholesterol levels. There is no effect produced by mild to moderate levels of alcohol consumption on low-density lipoprotein cholesterol. Evidence showing an advantage of one type of alcoholic beverage over another has been inconsistent. Whether antioxidants (flavonoids), which are present in some types of alcoholic beverages, contribute to a decreased risk of cardiovascular mortality is unknown.

We do not generally recommend that patients who do not drink start to do so. Patients should be encouraged to begin a program of regular exercise, which has also been shown to be associated with decreased cardiovascular mortality, rather than a regular program of drinking. The risk that patients who are advised to begin drinking alcohol might begin drinking heavily (thereby assuming the attendant health risks of overindulgence) seems to outweigh the potential benefit to be gained from such advice. In patients who already drink, it is recommended that they cut down to one drink per day.

Clinical Presentation

The diagnosis of alcoholism is predicated on the presence of two features: the inability to control alcohol use despite adverse consequences coupled with denial that a problem with alcohol exists. Watch for rituals patients use to control their drinking as possible indicators of alcoholism ("I drink only on weekends after 6 o'clock."). Denial comes in many forms. Outright lying about consumption is rare. Classic denial in which the patient simply refuses to recognize he or she is not in control of the drinking is most common. Memory blackouts produced by drinking represent another form of denial. Euphoric recall refers to the process by which alcoholics can remember only good times associated with alcohol use. Denial also may take the form of genuine confusion. Patients may readily acknowledge a serious problem exists in their lives but have no idea that alcohol is the cause.

The CAGE questions (Table 43-5) are derived from the Michigan Alcoholic Screening Test (MAST). They are 70% to 90% sensitive and 80% to 90% specific for diagnosing alcoholism.[23]

Management of Alcoholism

You may find yourself immediately discouraged and pessimistic about the prognosis once you diagnose a patient as an alcoholic, but you should recognize that alcoholism is a highly treatable illness, although one that is likely to include periods of relapse and recovery like other chronic diseases. With therapy the prognosis is favorable. Seventy percent of alcoholic patients achieve long-term abstinence after treatment for 3 years. "Spontaneous" recovery, or recovery achieved without specific therapy, occurs in an estimated 4% to 26% of patients.

Confrontation

Denial is the main obstacle to achieving long-term abstinence. You must confront your patient with his or her diagnosis of alcoholism. You should be nonjudgmental, persistent, firm, and, above all, clear in explaining the reasons why you believe your patient is alcoholic. Prescribe total abstinence. Your patient likely will meet your confrontation with more denial, perhaps even anger. This should neither surprise nor alarm you. Remember that denial is as much a part of alcoholism as chest pain is a part of CAD. In addition, prospective data suggest physician advice alone to cut down on drinking or to quit drinking altogether is effective in decreasing the mean number of drinks per week, the episodes of binge drinking, and the frequency of excessive drinking.[24]

Showing Empathy

Do not underestimate the power of empathetic statements in allaying fear and anxiety. Emphasize to your patient that alcoholism is a disease and not his or her fault any more than CAD would be. On the other hand, encourage your patient to accept responsibility for his or her behavior. Reassure your patient you will support the endeavor to establish long-term abstinence.

Table 43-5	CAGE Questions	
Letter	**Question**	**Implication**
C	Do you ever feel the need to **C**ut down on your drinking?	Inability to control drinking
A	Do you get **A**nnoyed when people criticize your drinking?	Interpersonal problems caused by drinking
G	Do you ever feel **G**uilty about your drinking?	Negative feelings about drinking-related behavior
E	Do you ever need an **E**ye-opener in the morning to steady your nerves?	Physiologic dependence

Offering Hope

It is also difficult to overemphasize the importance of offering hope. Although it probably will never be effectively studied in randomized, prospective trials, it is a well-recognized principle of psychology that action will occur only if there is hope for success. You must offer a way out—abstinence—and help your patient believe it can be achieved.

The Process of Change

Prochaska and DiClemente's model[16] delineates four stages leading to long-term changes in behavior (see Table 43-3). Similar to making lifestyle change recommendations, make sure your expectations regarding alcohol counseling are realistic in accord with the stage in which you find your patient. Believing that a patient who is in the "precontemplative" stage will behave as if he or she is in the "action" stage is counterproductive and usually results in failure and frustration. At this stage, making the diagnosis of alcoholism known to the patient is the appropriate message. Likewise, explaining the consequences of continuing to drink would be appropriate for a patient in the "contemplative" stage. You must continually reassess the stage in which your patient remains and facilitate passage to the next.

Therapeutic Options

Once you have helped your patient to accept this illness, you are ready to prescribe treatment.

Support Groups. Alcoholics Anonymous (AA) and other similar support groups are available nationwide. Studies have shown that regular attendance at groups like AA is correlated with long-term abstinence.[25] You should strongly encourage your patient to take advantage of one of these programs.

Formal Interventions. If you are meeting resistance in breaking down your patient's denial, a formal intervention may be necessary. The people who are closest to the alcoholic patient are identified and brought together to stage a group confrontation with the patient. The confrontation should be rehearsed. Each person involved should begin with a statement of concern for the alcoholic patient and then list the times and situations in which he or she was made to feel anger, pain, or embarrassment as a result of the alcoholic patient's drinking. The purpose of the intervention is to create a crisis situation in which continued denial becomes overwhelmingly difficult and a plan for treatment is accepted. When done well, such interventions can be extremely successful.

Insight-oriented psychotherapy has been shown repeatedly to be ineffective in achieving long-term abstinence and should not be used except to treat a comorbid psychiatric illness.

Managing Withdrawal

Symptoms of minor withdrawal are not life threatening (Table 43-6) and in general require hospitalization only when severe. Symptoms of major withdrawal may be life threatening and require hospitalization. An estimated 10% of alcoholics fall into this latter category. There is no appreciable difference in success rate for long-term abstinence for inpatient compared to outpatient programs.

Benzodiazepines are indicated for both minor withdrawal symptoms, if severe, and major withdrawal symptoms, if present. They have no role in maintaining chronic abstinence. Long-acting sedative-hypnotics are best. Librium is most frequently used on a tapered schedule.

Follow-up and Expected Clinical Course

If relapse is to occur, it is most likely to do so in the first 6 weeks. It is recommended that you see the patient at frequent intervals during that time, once or even twice weekly if possible. Also, extra visits during especially stressful times (e.g., holidays, birthdays, anniversaries) may be useful in preventing relapses. Although relapse is recognized as a part of the natural history of alcoholism, patients do not need to be informed of this fact. It is potentially damaging to the instillation of hope.

Factors associated with prognosis are listed in Box 43-2. If you are committed to your patient's recovery, if you view alcoholism as a chronic disease with a well-described natural history, and if you embark on a clear plan of treatment, your interactions with your alcoholic patients can be as rewarding as those with your patients who have other chronic diseases.

Table 43-6	*Alcohol Withdrawal Symptoms*	
	Symptom	**Time to Appearance**
Minor	Anorexia, nausea, vomiting, tachycardia, hypertension, diaphoresis, weakness, tinnitus, hyperacusis, pruritus, muscle cramps, mood/sleep disorder	12 to 24 hours
Major	Tremor	8 to 12 hours
	Seizures	8 to 24 hours
	Hallucinations	48 hours
	Delirium tremens	48 to 96 hours

PROTEIN-CALORIE MALNUTRITION

A decrease of 25% of body weight in adults produces decrements in heart size, blood pressure, and venous pressure. Bradycardia occurs in association with QT interval prolongation. In patients with anorexia nervosa, despite a decrease in LV chamber size and mass, no echocardiographic evidence of systolic or diastolic dysfunction at rest or with exercise has been found. However, cardiac output is reduced as a result of reduced stroke volume and heart rate. Ventricular arrhythmias have occurred, probably as a result of accompanying electrolyte disturbances. With dietary repletion, heart function returns to normal within 6 to 8 months.

MISCELLANEOUS NUTRITIONAL DISORDERS

Several nutrients can influence the cardiovascular system; Table 43-7 summarizes their effects. Thiamine deficiency has long been recognized as a major cause of high-output congestive heart failure in the malnourished (those with "wet" beriberi, referring to pulmonary and peripheral congestion). Not commonly appreciated is the fact that thiamine excretion is increased with di-

---

BOX 43-2

FACTORS AFFECTING PROGNOSIS IN ALCOHOLISM

FAVORABLE	UNFAVORABLE
Committed clinician	No perceived threat of loss
Motivated patient	Cognitive impairment present
Crisis situations occur	Presence of enablers
Intact family, job, health	Presence of self-destructive behaviors
Family members also in therapy	Acceptance of derelict subculture class

---

Table 43-7 | *Miscellaneous Nutritional Disorders*

	Thiamine	Selenium	Homocysteine
Epidemiology, etiology, natural history	Rare; more common in the malnourished (e.g., alcoholics) or with diuretics	Syndrome of deficiency described in China (Keshan's disease)	Levels >9 are correlated with an increased risk of venous and arterial thrombosis; a risk factor for ASCVD
Pathophysiology	1. Peripheral vasodilation 2. Biventricular failure 3. Edema	Cardiomyopathy with myocardial necrosis and fibrosis	May reduce the resistance of endothelium to thrombosis
Clinical presentation	*History:* fatigue, dyspnea, palpitations pain/paresthesias in the extremities *Physical:* respiratory distress, low diastolic blood pressure, peripheral, and pulmonary edema, decreased reflexes	Signs and symptoms of congestive heart failure	Levels should be measured in all patients with CAD, cerebrovascular accident, or hypercoagulable states
Therapy	Thiamine 100 mg IV for one dose, then 50 mg po daily	Selenium	Folate 1 mg po daily and/or pyridoxine 25 mg po daily will lower homocysteine levels and may reduce risk of thrombosis

uretic therapy, and thiamine deficiency may parallel deficiencies of potassium and magnesium. With a normal diet, that is rarely a problem. It may become a problem for a frail, elderly person who does not eat well. A multivitamin containing 50 mg thiamine is sufficient to prevent deficiency. We have observed improvements in LV ejection fraction with thiamine supplementation in such cases. Thiamine deficiency should be assumed in the chronic alcoholic and treated.

Selenium deficiency is so rare that it is unlikely you will ever encounter it in clinical practice. Hyperhomocystinemia is increasingly being recognized as contributing a degree of risk for cardiovascular morbidity and mortality; we may one day consider it to be as significant a risk factor as hypercholesterolemia[26] (see Chapters 12 and 44).

REFERENCES

1. Bray GA: Pathophysiology of obesity, *Am J Clin Nutr* 55:488, 1992.
2. Troiano RP, Frongillo EA Jr, Sobal J, Levitsky DA: The relationship between body weight and mortality: a quantitative analysis of combined information from existing studies, *Int J Obesity* 20:63, 1996.
3. Expert Panel on the Identification, Evaluation, and Treatment of Overweight and Obesity in Adults, National Institutes of Health, June 1998.
4. Krieger DR, Landsberg L: Obesity and hypertension modalities. In Laragh JH, Brenner BM, editors: *Hypertension: pathophysiology, diagnosis, and management*, ed 2, New York, 1995, Raven.
5. Hall JE: Mechanisms of abnormal renal sodium handling in obesity hypertension, *Am J Hypertension* 10:49, 1997.
6. Messerli FH: Cardiovascular effects of obesity and hypertension, *Lancet* 1:1165, 1982.
7. Savage DD, Levy D, Dannenberg AL, et al: Association of echocardiographic left ventricular mass with body size, blood pressure, and physical activity (The Framingham Study), *Am J Cardiol* 65:371, 1990.
8. Alpert MA, Hashimi MW: Obesity and the heart, *Am J Med Sci* 306:117, 1993
9. Norman JE, Levy D: Improved electrocardiographic detection of echocardiographic left ventricular hypertrophy: results of a correlated data base approach, *J Am Coll Cardiol* 26:1022, 1995.
10. Alpert MA, Terry BE, Mulekar M, et al: Cardiac morphology and left ventricular function in normotensive morbidly obese patients with and without congestive heart failure and effect of weight loss, *Am J Cardiol* 80:736, 1997.
11. Fletcher EC: The relationship between systemic hypertension and obstructive sleep apnea: facts and theory, *Am J Med* 98:118, 1995.
12. Noda A, Okada T, Yasuma F, et al: Cardiac hypertrophy in obstructive sleep apnea syndrome, *Chest* 107:1538, 1995.
13. Strohl KP, Redline S: Recognition of obstructive sleep apnea, *Am J Respir Crit Care Med* 154:279, 1996.
14. Jousilahti P, Tuomilehto J, Vartiainen E, et al: Body weight, cardiovascular risk factors, and coronary mortality: 15-year follow-up of middle-aged men and women in eastern Finland, *Circulation* 93:1372, 1996.
15. Drenick EJ, Bale GS, Seltzer F, Johnson DG: Excessive mortality and causes of death in morbidly obese men, *JAMA* 243:443, 1980.
16. Prochaska JO, DiClemente CC: Transtheoretical therapy: toward a more integrative model of change, *Psychother Theory Res Pract* 19:276, 1982.
17. US Department of Health and Human Services, Centers for Disease Control and Prevention, National Center for Chronic Disease Prevention and Health Promotion: *Physical activity and health: a report of the Surgeon General*, Washington, DC, 1996, US Government Printing Office.
18. Van Gaal LF, De Leeuw IH: The beneficial effects of modest weight loss on cardiovascular risk factors, *Int J Obesity* 21(suppl):5, 1997.
19. Reisin E: Obesity hypertension: nonpharmacologic and pharmacologic therapeutic modalities. In Laragh JH, Brenner BM, editors: *Hypertension: pathophysiology, diagnosis, and management*, ed 2, New York, 1995, Raven.
20. Grundy SM, Balady GJ, Criqui MH, et al: Guide to primary prevention of cardiovascular diseases. A statement for healthcare professionals from the Task Force on Risk Reduction. American Heart Association Science Advisory and Coordinating Committee, *Circulation* 95:2329, 1997.
21. Klatsky AL, Armstrong MA, Friedman GD: Alcohol and mortality, *Ann Intern Med* 117:646, 1992.
22. Klatsky AL, Friedman GD, Siegelaub AB, Gerard MJ: Alcohol consumption and blood pressure. Kaiser-Permanente Health Examination Data, *N Engl J Med* 296:1154, 1977.
23. Hays JT, Spickard WA Jr: Alcoholism: early diagnosis and intervention, *J Gen Intern Med* 2:420, 1987.
24. Fleming MF, Barry KL, Manwell LB, et al: Brief physician advice for problem alcohol drinkers: a randomized controlled trial in community-based primary care practices, *JAMA* 277:1039, 1997.
25. Hoffman NG, Harrison PA, Belille CA: Alcoholics Anonymous after treatment: attendance and abstinence, *Int J Addict* 18:311, 1983.
26. Nygard O, Nordrehaug JE, Refsum H, et al: Plasma homocysteine levels and mortality in patients with coronary artery disease, *N Engl J Med* 337:230, 1997.

BIBLIOGRAPHY

Alexander JK: The heart and obesity. In Hurst JW, editor: *The heart: arteries and veins*, ed 7, New York, 1990, McGraw-Hill.
Eckel RH: Obesity in heart disease. A statement for healthcare professionals from the nutrition committee, American Heart Association, *Circulation* 96:3248, 1997.
Fingerhood MI, Barker LR: Alcoholism and associated problems. In Barker LR, editor: *Principles of ambulatory medicine*, ed 4, Baltimore, 1995, Williams & Wilkins.
Hirsch J, Leibel RL: The genetics of obesity, *Hosp Pract (Off Ed)* 33.55, 1998.
Pearson TA: Alcohol and heart disease, *Circulation* 94:3023, 1996.
Regan TJ: The heart, alcoholism, and nutritional disease. In Hurst JW, editor: *The heart: arteries and veins*, ed 7, New York, 1990, McGraw-Hill.

44 Effects of Renal Disease on the Heart

Richard E. Katholi
J. Antonio G. Lopez
Richard T. Bilinsky

Renal dysfunction has several cardiac effects. When renal disease is in its end stage and is being treated with dialysis, cardiovascular disease is a principal cause of mortality, with heart failure causing 15% of deaths, myocardial infarction 10%, and pericarditis 3%.[1]

CONSEQUENCES OF RENAL FAILURE— HYPERTENSION

Hypertension develops in most patients with progressive renal failure. Whatever the cause of the progressive renal failure, three factors can contribute to the hypertensive process, including sodium reduction, increased activity of the renin-angiotensin system, and increased activity of the sympathetic nervous system. Hemodynamic studies in patients with end-stage renal disease have shown elevated cardiac output and mean arterial pressure but normal systemic vascular resistance.[1] The elevated cardiac output and normal systemic vascular resistance are usually caused by anemia. When anemia is corrected, the cardiac output falls and mean arterial pressure and systemic vascular resistance rise. Many patients with end-stage renal disease who are treated with erythropoietin have elevated blood pressure that is related to the increase in peripheral vascular resistance and blood viscosity when the hematocrit rises to normal levels.

With end-stage renal failure, arterial pressure is dependent on blood volume, and blood pressure may be controlled by ultrafiltration through dialysis, with control of salt and water intake in the interdialysis interval.

A minority of patients with chronic renal failure have hypertension that is related less to volume than to an elevation in the activity of the renin-angiotensin system. This hypertension may not be controlled by lowering blood volume but does respond to "medical nephrectomy," with angiotensin-converting enzyme inhibitor or angiotensin II receptor blocker therapy, or to surgical removal of the kidneys.[1] A third mechanism contributing to hypertension in patients with chronic renal insufficiency is increased sympathetic nervous system activity. Contributing factors include reduced baroreceptor activity with resultant increased central sympathetic outflow and intrarenal adenosine-mediated increased renal afferent nerve activity, which leads to sympathoadrenal activity.[2] The long-term consequences of hypertension caused by renal failure are similar to those of essential hypertension (see Chapter 31).

HEART FAILURE IN PATIENTS WITH CHRONIC RENAL DISEASE

As shown in Table 44-1, chronic renal failure can impair cardiac performance by various mechanisms. Left ventricular (LV) stroke work index, end-diastolic pressure, and size are increased in many patients with end-stage renal disease. LV hypertrophy is also a frequent finding. In addition, impairment of cardiac performance may result from ischemic heart disease. Dialysis may lead to depletion of essential substances, including thiamine, and thiamine depletion can lead to systolic dysfunction (beriberi heart disease). This improves with thiamine replacement.

Although the presence of cardiomyopathy in uremic patients has been suggested, its existence as a specific entity has been difficult to document in view of the many other possible causes of cardiac dysfunction in patients with chronic renal failure. In a study of dialysis patients carefully selected for the absence of coronary artery disease, valvular abnormalities, diabetes, or hypertension, LV dilation and hypertrophy were both present. Furthermore, the ratio of LV radius to LV wall thickness was higher in dialysis patients as compared with controls. This observation suggested an impaired ability of the uremic myocardium to hypertrophy, resulting in a ventricular mass inadequately adapted to chamber size and pressure. In this regard, there is suggestive evidence that uremic myocardial dysfunction may be reversible, since hemodialysis has been found to improve the LV ejection fraction, both acutely and chronically, with the greatest improvement occurring in patients with dilated hearts.

Chronic anemia is another important factor contributing to myocardial dysfunction in dialysis patients. Studies of human erythropoietin treatment of hemodialysis patients have shown decreases in LV diameter and improved contractility as hematocrit increases.

After kidney transplantation, serial echocardiograms have documented the regression of LV hypertrophy. Finally, dialysis patients with dilated nonischemic car-

Table 44-1	*Treatable Causes of Heart Failure in Renal Insufficiency*

Abnormality	Mechanism
Hypertension	Increased ventricular afterload
Hypervolemia	Increased ventricular preload
Anemia	Increased cardiac work (high-output state)
Lipid abnormalities	Increased atherogenesis
Hyperhomocystinemia	Negative inotropic effect
Pericarditis	Pericardial constriction, tamponade

Ionic alterations
  Hyperkalemia
  Hypocalcemia
  Hypermagnesemia
  Metabolic acidosis
	Negative inotropic effect

Disordered calcium and vitamin D metabolism	Metastatic calcification (cardiac vascular); possible vitamin D–deficiency cardiomyopathy
Arteriovenous shunt for hemodialysis	Increased cardiac work (high-output state)
Thiamine depletion by dialysis or chronic diuresis	Thiamine deficiency causing beriberi heart
Uremic toxins	Possible direct myocardial depressant effects

Modified from Braunwald E, editor: *Heart disease: a textbook of cardiovascular medicine*, ed 4, Philadelphia, 1992, WB Saunders.

diomyopathy in class III or IV heart failure have shown symptomatic improvement as well as increases in ejection fraction after kidney transplantation. Therefore patients should not necessarily be denied kidney transplantation because of congestive heart failure if they are otherwise good transplant candidates.

In patients with renal failure the dosage of cardiac medications excreted by the kidneys must be adjusted. Nitrates and calcium channel antagonists, nifedipine, diltiazem, and verapamil, are metabolized by the liver, so no dosage adjustment is necessary.

CORONARY ATHEROSCLEROSIS

Numerous risk factors for coronary atherosclerosis have been identified in patients with end-stage renal disease. Of these, hypertension is the most important. Coronary atherosclerosis appears to accelerate in uremic patients. The National Cooperative Dialysis Study demonstrated a significant increase in cardiovascular morbidity in patients who received shorter dialysis treatments or who ran higher blood urea nitrogen concentrations.[3] These observations imply that the adequacy of a dialysis routine has a significant effect on cardiovascular mortality.

Coronary artery bypass surgery has been carried out successfully in patients with renal failure and symptomatic coronary artery disease refractory to medical therapy, although postoperative mortality is increased compared with that of patients without renal disease.[4] Although the short-term results of coronary angioplasty are satisfactory in patients being treated with long-term dialysis, these patients have a higher incidence (greater than 60%) of restenosis than patients with normal renal function, so coronary artery bypass surgery appears to be the preferred therapy for patients treated with long-term renal dialysis. In addition, angina unassociated with coronary atherosclerosis is being increasingly recognized in patients with chronic renal failure, presumably related to the combination of severe hypertension, LV hypertrophy, anemia, and coronary endothelial dysfunction.

Lipid Abnormalities and Hyperhomocystinemia

Homocysteine is a demethylated derivative of the essential sulfur-containing amino acid methionine. Methionine is the principal methyl donor in almost all methylation reactions and is derived from dietary protein. Elevated blood levels of homocysteine have recently re-

ceived attention as an important risk factor for vascular disease, including coronary atherosclerosis, peripheral vascular disease, and cerebrovascular disease. Prospective studies demonstrate that there is a threefold increase in the development of coronary artery disease with homocysteine levels exceeding the 95th percentile. In the rare syndrome of homocystinuria, which is an autosomal recessive condition associated with premature atherosclerotic and thromboembolic disease, hyperhomocystinemia is unusually severe. In this metabolic disorder caused by homozygosity for defective genes, the fasting homocysteine concentration is greater than 400 μmol/L. The majority of cases of hyperhomocystinemia are caused by defects in gene encoding for homocysteine-metabolizing enzymes or by deficiencies in vitamins that are involved in the metabolism of homocysteine.

Hyperhomocystinemia appears to aggravate atherosclerosis by at least three general mechanisms: (1) endothelial cell toxicity, (2) increased platelet adhesiveness, and (3) modification of clotting factors. Two thirds of patients with elevated homocysteine levels have an insufficiency of cofactors (vitamin B_6, vitamin B_{12}, and folate) involved in homocysteine metabolism. Increased plasma homocysteine levels are found in patients with renal dysfunction and correlate inversely with the glomerular filtration rate.[5-8] Plasma levels of homocysteine may decrease by 40% during chronic hemodialysis but continue to remain elevated above normal levels. Plasma homocysteine levels among peritoneal dialysis patients are lower than in patients on chronic hemodialysis but still remain above normal levels. The mechanism of hyperhomocystinemia in patients with chronic renal failure is still under investigation. Reduced excretion of homocysteine does not appear to be the cause. It is currently believed that reduced metabolism, which accounts for 70% of daily homocysteine elimination from plasma, plays a major role.

Since event rates for myocardial infarction or stroke are fivefold to tenfold higher in patients with end-stage renal disease who also have significantly elevated homocysteine levels, this amino acid may contribute independently to these fatal and nonfatal cardiovascular disease outcomes.[9,10] Clinical studies are in progress to determine whether normalizing homocysteine levels will decrease cardiovascular events and what doses of vitamin B_6, vitamin B_{12}, and folate will be required.[10]

We now believe that all patients with renal insufficiency should have a fasting plasma homocysteine level measured. Homocysteine levels greater than the 95th percentile (greater than 16 μmol/L for men and postmenopausal women and greater than 14 μmol/L for premenopausal women) are considered elevated. The next step in the evaluation of a patient with hyperhomocystinemia is to measure fasting levels of vitamin B_6, vitamin B_{12}, and folate to exclude a vitamin deficiency as the cause. If blood testing indicates a vitamin deficiency, then replacement therapy with the deficient vit-

amin should be instituted with either folic acid 1 mg, vitamin B_6 12.5 mg, or vitamin B_{12} 0.5 mg orally daily. If vitamin levels are normal and hyperhomocystinemia is evident, then homocysteine-lowering therapy should be instituted with daily oral doses of folic acid 1 mg, vitamin B_6 12.5 mg, and vitamin B_{12} 0.5 mg. Goal homocysteine levels are less than 10 μmol/L. After renal transplantation, or with immunosuppressive therapy, higher doses of folic acid are necessary, possibly 5 to 15 mg orally, together with the usual doses of vitamins B_6 and B_{12}.

No clinical trials have demonstrated a benefit of homocysteine-lowering therapy. However, while clinical trials are in progress, it appears reasonable to treat these high-risk patients. Treatment is innocuous, inexpensive, and effective, and normalization of levels may occur after approximately 2 weeks. Repeat measurement of homocysteine concentration is recommended 6 to 8 weeks after initiating vitamin therapy to determine whether recommended goals have been accomplished.

UREMIC PERICARDITIS

Pericarditis is a frequent and serious complication of chronic renal failure. Before the advent of dialysis, pericarditis was detected in about half of the patients with chronic renal failure and was usually a harbinger of death. It now occurs in 20% of uremic patients on chronic dialysis.[1] Pericarditis often develops before the initiation of dialysis or during the first few months of therapy.

The pathophysiology is uncertain. A viral cause has been proposed. Toxic catabolic nitrogen metabolites and secondary hyperparathyroidism have also been suggested as mechanisms. This is supported by the observations that uremic pericarditis is rare in patients with acute renal failure and that uremic pericarditis often improves with the initiation of dialysis in previously untreated patients. On the other hand, no correlation exists between pericarditis and the levels of catabolic metabolites in uremic patients. It has also been proposed that pericarditis in dialysis patients may reflect an immunologic response.

Acute uremic pericarditis is characterized by the appearance of hemorrhagic, fibrinous exudate involving both parietal and visceral pericardial surfaces, with little acute inflammatory cellular reaction. In some patients the friable pericardial surface may bleed, leading to hemorrhagic effusion. The effusion often organizes and forms thick adhesions within the pericardial space.

Chest pain usually develops in patients with uremic pericarditis. A pericardial rub is heard in 90% of patients. Tamponade is possible.

A small pericardial effusion is common in uremic patients. In the absence of typical pain and friction rub, a small effusion is not diagnostic of pericarditis. Asymptomatic effusions occur in 36% to 62% of uremic pa-

tients who require dialysis and appear to be related to volume overload and clinical congestive heart failure. On the other hand, a large effusion with pericarditis that persists after 10 days of intensive dialysis carries a high risk of tamponade. It should be remembered that pulsus paradoxicus may be absent in uremic patients with pericardial tamponade and coexisting LV systolic dysfunction with elevated LV filling pressures.

Vigorous dialysis is the treatment for uremic pericarditis. If pericarditis develops before the initiation of dialysis, patients usually respond to dialysis. When there is an effusion, a period of 10 days to 3 weeks of intensive dialysis is usually required for resolution of the effusion. Whether pericardiocentesis or pericardial window should be the initial therapy has been debated. If there is hemodynamic evidence of pericardial tamponade, our initial approach is percutaneous catheter pericardiocentesis with continuous catheter drainage of the pericardial sac for 24 to 48 hours. Subxiphoid pericardiectomy or limited pericardiotomy is reserved for patients with hemodynamic instability or recurrent pericardial effusion after pericardiocentesis. A loculated pericardial effusion may necessitate surgical drainage.

ULTRAFILTRATION AS A TREATMENT FOR CONGESTIVE HEART FAILURE IN PATIENTS WITH RENAL INSUFFICIENCY

In patients with renal insufficiency who develop congestive heart failure, expansion of extracellular fluid volume and renal retention of sodium are exaggerated. Electrolyte abnormalities are common. When diuretics are effective, the azotemia frequently worsens. If they are not effective, congestion worsens.

Peritoneal dialysis has been tried in patients with congestive heart failure and renal insufficiency. However, this approach may be complicated by significant protein loss in the dialysate effluent, variable hyperglycemia, and the hyperosmolar syndrome. Hemodialysis has also been employed in patients with congestive heart failure and renal insufficiency, but hypotension is a frequent complication as a result of a decrease in total peripheral resistance.

To circumvent this problem, ultrafiltration has been used successfully.[11] This approach affords greater hemodynamic stability than hemodialysis. Vascular volume is held constant and cardiac output remains stable, despite a decrease in total extracellular fluid volume.

Ultrafiltration removes plasma free water to achieve the desired fluid balance and control. The usual rate of fluid removal is 1.5 to 2.0 L/hr, and the usual treatment regimen is 2 hours daily, or every other day, until a target "dry weight" is reached. The benefits of ultrafiltration therapy are compensation of congestive heart failure, reduction in oral medications, fewer hospitalizations, and a significant decrease in the overall cost of treatment. It also allows corrections of electrolyte abnormalities. The benefits are counterbalanced by tradeoffs, including the need for establishing vascular access, adherence to a regular treatment schedule, and possible further loss of renal function.

The ultrafiltration schedule is variable once the reference "dry weight" has been achieved. It can range from 2 or 3 hours two or three times per week to an intermittent, "as needed" schedule based on the patient's ability to restrict oral fluid intake. Whether ultrafiltration significantly and persistently improves LV ejection fraction is undetermined.

REFERENCES

1. Braunwald E, editor: *Heart disease: a textbook of cardiovascular medicine*, ed 4, Philadelphia, 1992, WB Saunders.
2. Katholi RE: Renal nerves in the pathogenesis of hypertension in experimental animals and humans, *Am J Physiol* 245:1, 1983.
3. Sreepada R et al: Hemodynamic and cardiac correlates of different hemodialysis regimens: The National Cooperative Dialysis Study, *Kidney Int* 23(suppl 13):89, 1983.
4. Jahangiri M, Wright J, Edmondson S, Magee P: Coronary artery bypass grafting in dialysis patients, *Heart* 78:343, 1997.
5. Bostom AG, Lathrop L: Hyperhomocystinemia in end-stage renal disease: prevalence, etiology, and potential relationship to arteriosclerotic outcomes, *Kidney Int* 52:10, 1997.
6. Bostom AG, Shemin D, Verhoef P, et al: Elevated fasting total plasma homocysteine levels and cardiovascular disease outcomes in maintenance dialysis patients: a prospective study, *Arterioscler Thromb* 17:2554, 1997.
7. Gupta A, Robinson K: Hyperhomocysteinaemia and end-stage renal disease, *J Nephrol* 10:77, 1997.
8. Moustapha A, Naso A, Nahlawi M, et al: Prospective study of hyperhomocystinemia as an adverse cardiovascular risk factor in end-stage renal disease, *Circulation* 97:138, 1998.
9. Nygard O, Nordrehaug JE, Refsum H, et al: Plasma homocysteine levels and mortality in patients with coronary artery disease, *N Engl J Med* 337:230, 1997.
10. Bostom AG, Gohh RY, Beaulieu AJ, et al: Treatment of hyperhomocystinemia in renal transplant recipients: a randomized, placebo-controlled trial, *Ann Intern Med* 127:1089, 1997.
11. Fonarow GC, Stevenson LW, Walden JA, et al: Impact of a comprehensive heart failure management program on hospital readmission and functional status of patients with advanced heart failure, *J Am Coll Cardiol* 30:725, 1997.

45 Cardiovascular Genetic Diseases

Jerry T. Thompson
Terrence X. O'Brien

Cardiovascular disease is a complex process influenced by at least three factors: (1) genetic background, (2) genetic mutation, and (3) environment. Two individuals with the same genetic mutation may not develop the same disease because of the influence of the other factors. This chapter explains how genetic disorders are analyzed, illustrates how this analysis can affect treatment and potential cure, and describes the known genetic cardiovascular disorders. It is not a comprehensive review on genetics. Instead we rely on the reader's background in basic genetics and biology. Several excellent references are provided in the bibliography.

MOLECULAR GENETICS

Cardiovascular disorders have a putative genetic component that, in interaction with a greater or lesser degree with the overall genetic background of an individual as well as with environmental factors, is responsible for disease. Genetic traits may be additive or synergistic with environmental interactions, leading to a complex Gaussian distribution of disease in the population; an individual patient may be aligned with another patient who has acquired disease from a different combination of factors yet has reached the same disease end point. The advantage of a genetic approach in research is that it can potentially identify the primary cause(s) of a disease. The discovery of new genetic causes and contributions to cardiovascular disease increases monthly.

For the practicing clinician a fundamental grasp of the methods used to identify genes related to cardiovascular disease is essential to understanding clinical applications being continuously advanced in the literature. Currently these are mainly diagnostic and prognostic applications. However, rapid progress being made in exogenous gene expression and delivery promises novel gene therapies in the future based on the specific identification of genes and gene products involved in complex cardiovascular pathology. The tables presented in this chapter succinctly list the current known genetic causes of cardiovascular diseases to illustrate the kind of information that will become increasingly available to primary care providers. Just as one cannot make a diagnosis not considered in the differential diagnosis, one cannot look up the latest in-formation on a genetic disease if it is not recognized as such. The demand for genetic testing will increase as physicians and patients learn how results affect clinical care, disease progression, and disease susceptibility, which may affect family planning. Ethical considerations concerning the use and acquisition of genetic applications, like any medical information, will require continuous vigilance and reassessment.

How Molecular Genetic Abnormalities Are Found

Each somatic human nucleus has 23 pairs of chromosomes (44 autosomal and two sex-linked chromosomes). One chromosome from each pair is inherited from each parent. When deoxyribonucleic acid (DNA) replication occurs within a meiocyte (germ cell replication), homologous chromosomes have regional crossovers with each other that result in the rearrangement of neighboring groups of alleles (that is, single copies of genes, of which every individual gets two copies, one from each autosomal chromosome). Each chromosome then segregates into individual germ cells. In this process, genetic diversity is created both by varying the assortment of whole chromosomes available in germ cells and by homologous recombination between chromosome pairs that produce chromosomes different from the parental ones. This is illustrated in Figure 45-1. The probability of a recombination occurring between two points on a chromosome is proportional to the amount of DNA between them. This relationship is the basis for genetic linkage studies.

Linkage Analysis

The first step in identifying a disease state as genetic is to demonstrate that the disease shows inheritance and involves having an affected family for genetic study. The phenotype of every available member of the kindred is carefully determined. Then members are genotyped by "restriction fragment length polymorphism" (RFLP) or, more recently, by "variable number of tandem repeats" (VNTR) using DNA isolated from each person's leukocytes (discussed later). Depending on the gene, transmission may be autosomal dominant, autosomal recessive, sex-linked, or mitochondrial. An allele of a gene

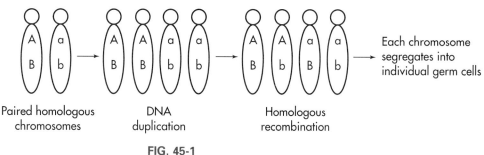

FIG. 45-1
Genetic recombination (see text).

that produces the same phenotype in homozygous individuals (two identical alleles) as well as in heterozygous individuals (two different alleles) is termed *dominant*. If a phenotype is present only in homozygotes, the abnormality is considered *recessive*. The ratio of family members with a particular gene mutation who express at least some of the clinical features is termed the *penetrance*. Penetrance may be incomplete and may vary with age, environment, and the rest of an individual's genetic makeup.

A heritable disease may arise from single-gene, multigene, or chromosomal abnormalities. Chromosomal abnormalities are generally the most clinically severe, whereas single-gene abnormalities are the most susceptible to deciphering by molecular genetics. In a family the inheritance of a marker with the disease phenotype increases the probability that the marker is physically near the culprit gene. For example, two loci separated by a few thousand nucleotides rarely recombine, yet two loci on the same chromosome separated by 10 million nucleotides may recombine frequently, perhaps 10% of the time. Each phenotype and genotype is analyzed to determine the statistical odds of a DNA marker being near a disease gene. This is termed a LOD score, which is a logarithmic scale where +3 (i.e., 1000:1 odds) is considered good evidence for linkage to a genetic trait associated with the disease phenotype in question. For example, the long QT syndrome (sudden death from ventricular arrhythmias associated with a baseline prolonged QT interval on electrocardiography) was found to be linked to chromosome 11p15.5 in several families with a combined LOD score of 5.25, or greater than 100,000:1 odds of association. In the case of the Holt-Oram (heart-hand) syndrome there is a LOD score of 25, or 10^{25}:1 odds of association to chromosome 12q24.1.

DNA Polymorphism

The key to figuring out what part of a chromosome might be associated with a disease is to have regions of DNA that are identifiably different between different chromosomes. DNA is composed of coding regions as well as vast noncoding regions of DNA between genes. In fact, actual genes compose only about 5% of the hu-

man genome. These huge regions of DNA are not subject to as much evolutionary pressure and are quite variable. Originally the genomic markers used to take advantage of this fact involved points where DNA-cleaving (restriction) enzyme sites happened to vary in different members of the population. DNA digestion could then yield distinctive patterns of DNA fragments that could be analyzed for any relationship to a particular phenotype, termed *RFLP*. The genes responsible for several cardiovascular diseases were determined in this way, including familial hypertrophic cardiomyopathy and supravalvular aortic stenosis. Although this method is common clinical genetic analysis, these unique enzymatic sites are relatively few and far between and have forced the development of other techniques.

Human DNA has innumerable sequences that are tandemly repeated throughout the genome. Although the purpose of these tandem repeats is largely unknown, they can be used for linkage analysis because the number and exact sequences of these repeats are quite variable, detectable, and inheritable. DNA marker probes can be made to these VNTR that are usually in 11- to 60-nucleotide units, greatly increasing the sensitivity and chance for disease linkage in a kindred. A further technologic advance is the use of clusters of repeated DNA sequences termed *small tandemly repeated* (STR) or *microsatellite* polymorphisms that occur frequently and variably enough throughout the human genome to provide high-resolution gene maps. Common STRs may contain just two to six nucleotides in their repeating units (e.g., $[CA]_n$) and thus can be amplified by the polymerase chain reaction (PCR), which can amplify specific DNA segments millions-fold for further analysis using published nucleotide primers. This allows one to display the fragments by running them out on polyacrylamide-urea gels, as shown in Figure 45-2. Both of these analyses link a specific DNA pattern (RFLP, VNTR, or STR) to the disease phenotype compared to the DNA pattern of "normal" kindred.

Functional and Positional Gene Analysis

Gene identification and cloning strategies have determined the cause of several inheritable cardiovascular

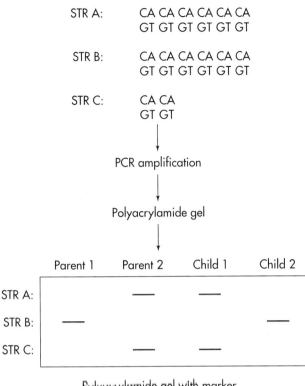

STR A: CA CA CA CA CA CA
          GT GT GT GT GT GT

STR B: CA CA CA CA CA CA
          GT GT GT GT GT GT

STR C: CA CA
          GT GT

          PCR amplification

          Polyacrylamide gel

	Parent 1	Parent 2	Child 1	Child 2
STR A:		—	—	
STR B:	—			—
STR C:		—	—	

Polyacrylamide gel with marker
STR inheritance pattern

FIG. 45-2
STR amplification by the PCR.

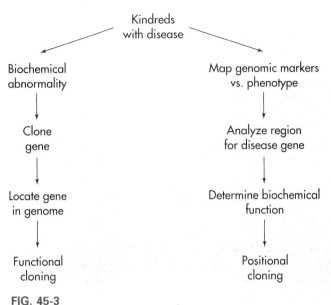

FIG. 45-3
Functional versus positional genetic analysis.

diseases. The approach of "functional cloning" is based on knowing an abnormal gene product (e.g., protein), then using its amino acid sequence and deduced nucleotide (DNA) sequence to design probes to find the relevant gene(s). This is also termed the *candidate gene* approach. Examples where this has been successful include several abnormalities in lipid metabolism and, outside of cardiovascular disease, phenylketonuria and G6PD deficiency. This approach can be limited by the often insufficient understanding of the biochemistry of most cardiovascular diseases within the context of complex environmental interactions. Therefore contemporary approaches also take advantage of hundreds of known, sequenced genes along each human chromosome that act like "road signs." Once there is linkage between a polymorphic marker and a phenotype, potentially making use of RFLPs or STRs, genes known to be in the region may become candidates for the disease. This is called *positional cloning*. Further analysis of the DNA may also identify novel genes in the region that may be involved in the disease process. These strategies are sketched in Figure 45-3.

Of course, one must keep in mind that a chromosomal marker is just that, a marker, and it itself has nothing to do with the disease but rather determines the position of a gene associated with the phenotype. Genetic markers identify a chromosomal region, termed *locus*, that often includes potentially hundreds of known and unknown genes, including the gene responsible for (or associated with) the phenotype in question. The beauty of this process is that no prior knowledge of the protein or biochemistry of the disease is required—just a phenotype with some degree of heritability. Therefore once such a genomic region is identified, the disease gene and its defining mutation can be systematically sought from within that region. For example, this approach led to the identification of two gene mutations in ion channels that can cause the long QT syndrome, SCN5A, and HERG (see also Table 45-1).

CARDIAC GENETIC DISORDERS

Most of the genetically defined known cardiovascular diseases are relatively rare and have usually been discovered through the availability of an appropriate kindred. Literature in this field is burgeoning, and Table 45-1 is constructed to summarize the major known disorders. The reader is referred to the general references at the end of this chapter for further information on particular disorders. Also, the medical literature and computer databases can provide current information and indicate where contacts can be made for current diagnostic studies, referral, or therapy.

Inherited Vascular Disorders

Since so many biochemical processes can contribute to atherosclerosis and each involves many related pathways, it is not surprising that many different combinations of genetic factors interact with environmental factors, leading to such varying degrees of disease in a

| Table 45-1 | *Cardiac Genetic Disorders* |

Disease	Genetic Defect	Clinical Syndrome
Arrhythmogenic right ventricular dysplasia	Autosomal dominant Apoptosis probably involved Heterogeneous chromosomal locations	Right ventricle dilated with fibrofatty replacement Ventricular arrhythmias
Atrial myxoma (Carney complex)	Autosomal dominant Heterogeneous, but linked to chromosome 2p	7% have familial history May recur in intracardiac or extracardiac locations with associated lentiginosis and endocrine dysfunction
Dilated cardiomyopathy	Heterogeneous—may be autosomal dominant, recessive, or X-linked Associated with mutations in dystrophin gene, other associated loci with no known responsible gene	20% of cardiomyopathies have a genetic component, present in second or third decade Ventricular dilation, decreased systolic function lead to congestive heart failure, arrhythmias Conduction defects in some forms
Hypertrophic cardiomyopathy	Mutations in various sarcomeric contractile proteins: • β-cardiac myosin heavy chain • α-tropomyosin • Cardiac troponin T • Cardiac myosin binding protein C Myosin light chains 2 and 3 Incomplete penetrance	Increased left ventricular mass, especially septal Screen by echocardiography Systolic, diastolic dysfunction Myofibrillar disarray 3% to 5% annual mortality, commonly by sudden death
Hemostatic factors and myocardial infarction (MI)	Coagulation factor VII polymorphisms Fibrinogen mutations Plasminogen activator inhibitor type I polymorphisms	Increased MI risk or association with certain genotypes
Long QT syndrome • Romano-Ward syndrome • Jervell and Lange-Nielson syndrome	Voltage-gated potassium channels (HERG, KCNE1 and KVLQT1) Cardiac sodium channel (SCN5A) Autosomal dominant Autosomal recessive	Prolonged QT complex ECG interval Syncope and/or sudden death from polymorphic ventricular tachycardia Also with congenital neural deafness Found in 1% of deaf children
Mitochondrial cardiomyopathy	Point mutations in mitochondrial DNA, especially of tRNA	Extremely rare Various syndromes that can develop cardiomyopathy: MELAS (mitochondrial encephalomyopathy, lactic acidosis, and stroke) MERFE (myoclonic epilepsy with ragged red fibers) Kearns-Sayre syndrome MIMyCA (maternally inherited myopathy and cardiomyopathy) NADH-coenzyme Q reductase deficiency

Table 45-1	*Cardiac Genetic Disorders—cont'd*

Disease	Genetic Defect	Clinical Syndrome
MI and angiotensin-converting enzyme polymorphisms	Insertion (I)/deletion (D) polymorphism in intron 16	Controversial association with MI
Muscular dystrophies: • Duchenne and Becker dystrophies	X-linked Dystrophin protein defect (different mutations of the same gene)	Incidence 1:3500 males Myocyte necrosis, fatty replacement, fibrosis Diagnosis by syndrome muscle biopsy, molecular testing Elevated CPK (creatinine phosphokinase), muscle wasting Cardiomyopathy with congestive heart failure Earlier cardiac involvement with Duchenne's
• Emery-Dreifuss	X-linked or autosomal dominant Emerin protein defect	Cardiomyopathy with conduction system abnormalities, arrhythmias Childhood onset, scapuloperoneal weakness
• Myotonic	Autosomal dominant Myotonin protein kinase	Congenital, classic, minimal forms based on severity, age Most common muscular dystrophy of adulthood Conduction system abnormalities, arrhythmias common
• X-linked dilated cardiomyopathy	X-linked Cardiac dystrophin defect	Rare, cardiomyopathy with early congestive heart failure No or less skeletal involvement

population. For example, lipoprotein genetic patterns using twin and family studies suggest heritability contributes greater than 50% of the disease risk. Common genetic factors contributing to atherosclerosis include lipoprotein metabolism, homocystine levels, and hemostatic factor production. Genetically based classifications of atherosclerotic risk factors are used increasingly to target therapy and provide risk counseling. Major gene identifications and their disease associations are listed in Table 45-2.

Congenital Heart Disease Genetics

The heart is the first organ to form in vertebrates and requires a sophisticated and largely unknown genetic program to form successfully. Since congenital cardiac abnormalities can occur in about 2% of live births and often appear heritable, research efforts have focused on identifying underlying molecular mechanisms. The consequence may be present at birth or may not manifest until adulthood or until after poorly understood

and complex environmental interactions. The major genetic defects known or highly suspected to be associated with several congenital cardiac defects are listed in Table 45-3.

MOLECULAR BIOLOGY AND UNDERSTANDING CARDIOVASCULAR DISEASE

The revolutionary progress in molecular biology over the past several years has contributed a new level of basic understanding of human disease. It is important for clinicians to be familiar with the general concepts and terms used in molecular biology so that they can read and assess the modern medical literature.

The main dogma of molecular biology is that double-stranded DNA stores genetic information that is, in a regulated way, transcribed into single-stranded ribonucleic acid (RNA) and then translated into protein. During DNA replication, each strand serves as a tem-

Table 45-2	Inherited Vascular Disorders

Disease	Genetic Defect	Clinical Syndrome
Ehlers-Danlos syndrome IV	Type III procollagen Autosomal dominant	Rare Aneurysms and rupture of large arteries, skin elasticity, mitral valve prolapse, reduced collagen synthesis
Familial aortic aneurysm	Unknown	Heterogeneous; often associated with other cardiovascular and connective tissue abnormalities
Familial combined hyperlipidemia	Unknown Autosomal dominant	Common, found in 1% of population Increased low-density lipoprotein (LDL), very low-density lipoprotein (VLDL), apo B Premature myocardial infarction
Familial defective apo B 100	Apo B 100	Rare Defective LDL clearance
Familial hypercholesterolemia	LDL receptor deficiency	Incidence 1:100,000 (homozygous) Markedly elevated cholesterol levels, xanthomas, early coronary disease
Homocystinuria	Cystathionine B-synthase or methylenetetrahydrofolate reductase mutations Autosomal dominant	Elevated homocysteine levels associated with occlusive vascular disease
Hypertension, essential	Unknown, complex Angiotensinogen polymorphisms linked in some populations	Inherited risk factors interacting with complex environmental factors
Hypertension, monogenic forms:	Autosomal dominant	Rare
• Glucocorticoid suppressible hypertension	11-β-hydroxylase/aldosterone synthase	Abnormal aldosterone production
• Liddle's syndrome	Epithelial amiloride-sensitive sodium ion channel	Abnormal sodium ion resorption in distal renal tubule
Osler-Rendu-Weber syndrome	Endoglin gene (receptor for transforming growth factor β)	Epistaxis, telangiectasia, and visceral vascular abnormalities
Type III hyperlipidemia	Apo E allele Autosomal recessive	1:5000 persons Often seen with type 2 diabetes

plate for specialized enzymes that insert complementary nucleotides serially to produce two identical double-stranded helices.

In rare instances during the replication process or by some environmental factor, the DNA coding sequence is altered, generating a mutation. If a mutation occurs in a germ line cell, then the mutation can be passed to the individual's offspring. Genes may be found to be mutated by deletions, additions, or substitutions of one or more of the nucleotides in the DNA sequence, which may or may not produce disease, depending on what the effects are on the protein produced. It is the abnormal function of expressed proteins that contributes to a clinical phenotype.

Messenger RNA (mRNA) is transcribed from DNA, processed to remove introns, and then transported from

Table 45-3	*Congenital Heart Disease Genetics*

Disease	Genetic Defect	Clinical Syndrome
Bicuspid aortic valve	Unknown	0.9% incidence 17% of cases familial
DiGeorge syndrome and velocardiofacial syndrome	Deletions or translocations at chromosome 22q11 Autosomal dominant Genetic heterogenicity for both syndromes	Associated with conotruncal defects (e.g., truncus arteriosus, tetralogy of Fallot or conal ventricular septal defects) with multiple manifestations Abnormal facies 1:4000 birth incidence
Down syndrome	Trisomy 21	Accounts for many atrial septal defects, well-described phenotype
Ellis-van Creveld syndrome	Autosomal recessive Linkage to chromosome 4p16.1	Atrial septal defects Short stature, bony defects and polydactyly, dental deformities
Familial total anomalous pulmonary venous return	Autosomal dominant Chromosome 4 location	Familial form a rare cause May have septal defects
Holt-Oram (heart-hand) syndrome	Autosomal dominant Variable expression Inactivated TBX5 gene	Secundum atrial septal defect most common heart defect, next ventricular septal defect 32% with ECG abnormalities only (conduction disease) Limb abnormalities, especially upper body and hand 0.95:100,000 incidence
Marfan's syndrome	Fibrillin-1 mutation Autosomal dominant	Cardiovascular, skeletal, and ocular abnormalities, especially of aortic valve and root
Supravalvular aortic stenosis	Often elastin mutations Linkage to chromosome 7q11.2	Incidence 1:25,000 births May be isolated or part of William's syndrome (retardation, hypercalcemia, connective tissue defects)
Mitral valve prolapse	Unknown	Familial form rare (although MVP common) and more associated with sudden death
Noonan's syndrome	Linkage to chromosome 12q2	Pulmonic valve degeneration among other cardiac abnormalities Lymphedema, facial and skeletal abnormalities
Tetralogy of Fallot	Complex transmission, may be autosomal dominant May have chromosome 22q11 microdeletions	10% of congenital heart disease Ventral septal defect with pulmonic stenosis, overriding aorta, right ventricular hypertrophy

the nucleus to the cytoplasm, where it is translated into protein at the ribosomes. This collinear expression of the genetic material facilitates complex regulation at many levels: DNA (via introns and exons), transcription, pretranscription and posttranscription, translation, posttranslation, and during degradation of mRNA and protein. The complex regulation of proteins could also result in genetic disorders. For example, a protein may be produced at a lower rate than normal because of a mutation in a specific regulating protein (the protein

is then said to be *underexpressed*). The lower cellular concentration of the cardiac-specific protein may lead to a phenotypic trait; however, detection of regulatory mutations is much more difficult. None of the identified cardiovascular diseases listed in Tables 45-1 to 45-3 have been linked to this type of abnormality.

What Is Gene Therapy?

Gene therapy in its simplest of forms is the introduction of DNA that specifies a protein of interest into cells. Once in the cell, the DNA integrates into a chromosome and is transcribed and translated by the cellular machinery to produce the protein. Today, researchers can introduce the DNA into most cells in vitro; however, the efficiency for most cell types is extremely low.

The challenge of the clinical use of gene therapy is to get the DNA into the correct cells of a living organism and have it expressed only in those cells. The location on the chromosome where the introduced DNA integrates cannot be tightly controlled. This leads to the potential of insertional mutations, which could be as detrimental as the original mutation.

One type of gene therapy uses cells modified in vitro to be transplanted to the organism, thus bypassing the need for specific in vivo delivery of the DNA. However, this method will not work for most, if not all, of the cardiovascular diseases. Major technical problems must be overcome before gene therapy becomes a common clinical practice.

THE HUMAN GENOME PROJECT

The concept of the Human Genome Project is to produce a complete genomic and physical map (largely existent currently) of the human genome and to sequence the approximately 80,000 to 100,000 human genes within the next 10 years. Such a resource would define the position of each gene and facilitate study of putative disease-causing genes and their expression and/or mutations as well as the protein product. This will improve the ability to test candidate disease genes, as well as the precision of positional cloning.

The Future

The importance of a genetic approach in understanding a complex disease is that it has the potential to identify the disease's primary causes and thereby direct more specific and, in many cases, novel therapy. Eventually, molecular biology will revolutionize medical therapy far beyond genetically engineered and produced natural substances such as rtPA, erythropoietin, and insulin, the examples we have today. Most of the available kindreds with heritable cardiovascular disease have been investigated. The difficult challenge for the future is deciphering more complex and prevalent pathologies with mul-

tiple, varying genetic and environmental components, such as atherosclerosis, hypertension, and congenital heart disease.

BIBLIOGRAPHY

Basson CT, Seidman CE: Genetic studies of myocardial and vascular disease. In Topol EJ editor: *Textbook of cardiovascular medicine,* Philadelphia, 1998, Lippincott-Raven.

Caskey CT: Muscular dystrophies affecting the heart. In Willerson JT, Cohn JN, editors: *Cardiovascular medicine,* New York, 1995, Churchill Livingstone.

Chien KR, Grace AA: Broader perspectives on heart disease and cardiologic practice. In Braunwald E, editor: *Heart disease: a textbook of cardiovascular medicine,* ed 5, Philadelphia, 1997, WB Saunders.

Chien KR, Zhu H, Knowlton KU, et al: Transcriptional regulation during cardiac growth and development, *Annu Rev Physiol* 55:77, 1993.

Consevage M, Cyran S: Basic elements of gene mapping and identification, *Curr Opin Cardiol* 12:288, 1997.

Corvol P, Jeunemaitre X: Genetics of hypertension. In Topol EJ, editor: *Textbook of cardiovascular medicine,* Philadelphia, 1998, Lippincott-Raven.

Gelb BD: Molecular genetics of congenital heart disease, *Curr Opin Cardiol* 12:321, 1997.

Iacoviello L, Di Castelnuovo A, de Knijff P, et al: Polymorphisms in the coagulation factor VII gene and the risk of myocardial infarction, *N Engl J Med* 338:79, 1998.

Keating MT, Atkinson D, Dunn C, et al: Consistent linkage of the long QT syndrome to the Harvey ras-1 locus on chromosome 11, *Am J Hum Genet* 49:1335, 1991.

Lewin B: *Genes V,* Oxford, 1994, Oxford University Press.

Lusis AJ, Weinreb A, Drake TA: Genetics of atherosclerosis. In Topol EJ, editor: *Textbook of cardiovascular medicine,* Philadelphia, 1998, Lippincott-Raven.

Miewicz D: Genetic aspects of congenital heart disease. In Willerson JT, Cohn JN, editors: *Cardiovascular medicine,* New York, 1995, Churchill Livingstone.

Pyeritz RE: Genetics and cardiovascular disease. In Braunwald E, editor: *Heart disease: a textbook of cardiovascular medicine,* ed 5, Philadelphia, 1997, WB Saunders.

Wang Q, Chen Q, Li H, Towbin JA: Molecular genetics of long QT syndrome from genes to patients, *Curr Opin Cardiol* 12:310, 1997.

Watson JD, Hopkins NH, Roberts JW, Steitz JA: *Molecular biology of the gene,* ed 4, Menlo Park, Calif, 1994, Benjamin Cummings.

ACKNOWLEDGMENTS

This work was supported by the Office of Research and Development, Medical Research Service, Ralph H. Johnson Department of Veteran Affairs Medical Center, Charleston, South Carolina, where Dr. O'Brien is a Research Associate, and by National Heart, Lung, and Blood Institute Grant HL-55284 (TXO) as well as National Institute of Health Training Grant T32-HL-07260-19 (JTT). The secretarial expertise of Mrs. Fe Matutina is gratefully acknowledged.

46 Psychologic Disorders, Stress, Drugs, and Drug Abuse

Michael G. Huber
George J. Taylor

That a special relationship exists between the mind and body has been suspected for centuries. The folk saying that one can "die from a broken heart" supports the long-held belief that mood and the heart are interconnected. Songwriters, poets, and philosophers espoused this theory long before medical investigators substantiated it. It is imperative that altered emotional states, their treatments, and the use of mood-altering substances be assessed and factored into the care of patients who have or are at risk for heart disease.

DEPRESSION

Depression is a term used to describe various emotional states. It has commonly been used by the public and press to describe feelings of disappointment, dejection, or grief. Public education to make people aware that depression is a form of mental illness has not eliminated the confusion. A recent survey of the general population about mental illness revealed some alarming misconceptions: 71% believe mental illness is caused by emotional weakness, 45% believe it is the patient's fault, 35% believe it is the result of sinful behavior, and only 10% believe it involves the brain and has a biologic basis.[1] We will use the term *depression* to refer to a number of syndromes that have as a key feature an abnormally low mood. Specific diagnostic criteria exist for the various depressive disorders, but the main point here is that depression is pathologic, has a variety of symptoms, is biologically based, and is often disabling.

Epidemiology, Etiology, and Natural History of Depression

Major depression is common. Lifetime prevalence in the United States is approximately 10%. Females are twice as likely as males to be affected (Box 46-1). The exact cause of depression is unclear. An overly simplified way of explaining potential causes is that genetically vulnerable individuals experience stressful life events that adversely affect the functioning of neurotransmitter systems involving serotonin and norepinephrine. Over half of patients who experience major depression have a recurrence later in life. People with dysthymia or "minor depression" (2 years or more of chronic, mild depres-

sion) may be at increased risk for development of major depression, and roughly 25% of patients have persistent residual symptoms with social or occupational impairment between episodes.[2] Approximately 1% of the population have a manic or hypomanic episode and are diagnosed as having bipolar disorder.

Relationship to Heart Disease

The relationship between depression and heart disease has been the focus of numerous studies over the past two decades. There are several basic questions regarding this relationship. For example, are people who are depressed but do not have heart disease more likely to develop heart disease? Several studies show that otherwise healthy patients who are depressed have an increased risk of cardiovascular morbidity and mortality (Box 46-2). Depressed individuals are 1.5 to 2.0 times more likely than nondepressed individuals to suffer a myocardial infarction.[3]

Another issue is how depression affects those who already have cardiovascular disease. A strong body of evidence has linked depression to cardiovascular mortality (Box 46-3). The mortality of depressed patients after myocardial infarction may be as high as 3.5 times that of the nondepressed. Do not take comfort knowing that a patient has only minor depression. Almost half of patients with minor depression were found to have developed major depression in the year after myocardial infarction.[4]

What is the basis for this relationship between cardiovascular disease and depression? No definitive causal relationship has been found. One hypothesis is that platelet abnormalities exist in depressed individuals.[3] Other studies have suggested that abnormalities of lipid metabolism in depressed patients may increase cardiovascular risk. Depression that occurs late in life may be the result of vascular changes in the central nervous system, and it is conceivable that in certain cases ischemic heart disease and depression are sequelae of atherosclerosis.

Clinical Presentation

The clinical presentation of depressed patients varies greatly. Occasionally patients report being depressed. Unfortunately this is the exception rather than the rule.

489

BOX 46-1
MAJOR DEPRESSION

Lifetime prevalence	5% to 12% in the United States
Age of onset	Usually late twenties but may occur at any age
Sex	Female:male ratio approximately 2:1
Length of episode	If untreated, 6 months to several years
Family history	1.5 to 3 times greater risk if first-degree biologic relative affected
Recurrence rate	Greater than 50% lifetime recurrence; risk increases with each recurrence

---

BOX 46-2
DEPRESSION AND CARDIOVASCULAR MORBIDITY AND MORTALITY

Healthy individuals with elevated depression ratings were more likely to develop and die of ischemic heart disease.

Depressed men had a higher relative risk of myocardial infarction (relative risk = 1.68).

Men without a history of angina or myocardial infarction who had higher levels of depression were more likely to suffer a first infarction and had an elevated risk of cardiovascular mortality.

Individuals with elevated depression scores were 65% more likely to develop ischemic heart disease.

Major depression increased the risk of myocardial infarction more than fourfold. Dysphoric individuals not meeting criteria for major depression were at intermediate risk for myocardial infarction.

From Glassman AH, Shapiro PA: *Am J Psychiatry* 155:1, 1998.

BOX 46-3
DEPRESSION AND THE OUTCOME OF CARDIAC PATIENTS

Approximately 20% of patients with coronary artery disease had major depression. This group was 2.5 times more likely to develop a serious cardiac complication over the next 12 months.

Postinfarction survivors at 1 year had lower baseline depression ratings than nonsurvivors. Neither anger nor anxiety was associated with increased mortality.

At 6 months after index myocardial infarction, 17% of the depressed patients had died compared with 3% of the nondepressed group.

Minor depression after infarction was associated with increased mortality at 12 and 18 months.

From Glassman AH, Shapiro PA: *Am J Psychiatry* 155:1, 1998.

BOX 46-4
COMPLAINTS THAT MAY INDICATE DEPRESSION

Insomnia
Memory problems
Chronic pain
Boredom
Weight loss
Sleeping too much
Diminished energy
Restlessness
Irritability

Weight gain
Change in appetite (increased or decreased)
Poor concentration
Numerous unexplained physical complaints
Anxiety
Easily fatigability

Box 46-4 lists common complaints that may indicate an underlying depression. Often patients visit a primary care provider in search of an explanation for their distress.

Clinical Evaluation of Depression

It is up to the clinician to inquire about depression. There is a wide spectrum of depressive illnesses. The diagnostic criteria are listed in the *Diagnostic and Statistical Manual of Mental Disorders* (DSM).[5] These depressive disorders range from transient depressive symptoms in response to a stressor called *adjustment disorder with depressed mood* to *major depressive episode*, a syndrome of five or more depressive symptoms present nearly every day for at least 2 weeks that causes clinically significant distress, functional impairment, or both. A chronic condition of depressed mood more days than not, accompanied by at least two other depressive symptoms persisting for at least 2 years is known as *dysthymia*. A useful screening tool for a variety of mental disorders is the PRIME-MD, which consists of a patient questionnaire to guide a structured interview. When used regularly, it can identify cases of depression that are likely to be missed by the clinician, and it requires fewer than 10 minutes to administer.[6] Suicidal ideations, plans, and intention should be routinely assessed.

A number of medications may induce depression. Box 46-5 lists some of the more common ones.

Management of Depression

The first step is patient education. Let the patient know that depression is common, has a biologic basis, and is treatable. The next step is choosing an antidepressant. In general the various antidepressants are equally effective but have different safety and side effect profiles. The tricyclic antidepressants are sedating, anticholinergic, cause orthostatic hypotension, and prolong the QT interval. They can be lethal in overdose in quantities as small as 2 g. The selective serotonin reuptake inhibitors (SSRIs) are commonly prescribed and have a higher therapeutic index and more favorable side effect profile

than tricyclic agents. Table 46-1 lists typical starting and maintenance doses of common antidepressants.

Side effects are most frequent at the initiation of therapy or after dosage increases. The SSRIs can cause gastrointestinal (GI) disturbances, anorgasmia, insomnia, or restlessness. For mild to moderate side effects it is helpful to reassure the patient that they are usually transient. More bothersome side effects warrant a dose reduction or a change to another agent. Patients who are anxious may notice an exacerbation of their anxiety and may benefit from a 2- to 4-week course of a benzodiazepine.

Follow-up and Expected Clinical Course

Antidepressants require 4 to 6 weeks to take effect. Patients should be told this and should be given resources to use if their condition worsens, such as phone numbers to the clinic, emergency after-hours services, and help lines. Seeing a patient back in the office at 2 weeks can help to manage side effects and improve compliance. Once the patient responds, visits can be less frequent. Be aware that patients may look better before they feel better, and the risk of suicide must be reassessed as the patient improves. Patients taking tricyclic agents may need to be seen more frequently to individualize the dose and dispense smaller quantities to reduce the chances of a lethal overdose. Failure to respond to an adequate dose of an antidepressant after 6 weeks, intolerable side effects, the emergence of manic symptoms (abnormally elevated mood, racing thoughts, pressured speech, or decreased need for sleep), psychosis, or intensification of suicidal ideation necessitate prompt referral to a psychiatrist. Patients who respond to antidepressant medication should continue taking a maintenance dose at least 6 months after resolution of the depressive symptoms. Discontinuation should not coincide with stressors. Indefinite continuation should be considered for geriatric patients, those with a history of dysthymia, or those who have had more than one episode of major depression.

ANXIETY

Anxiety can be an adaptive, normal emotion. The evolutionary advantage of the "fight-or-flight" response to a threat is obvious. There is a well-known relationship between anxiety and test-taking performance that shows that performance increases with anxiety up to a certain point. Levels of anxiety exceeding this point result in a decline in performance. At times, anxiety can be inappropriate, maladaptive, and distressing. A host of disorders share the core symptom of excessive and distressing levels of anxiety. There are several specific anxiety disorders. We will focus attention on panic disorder and specific phobia resulting from the overlap with cardiac symptoms, as well as on the implications for management.

BOX 46-5

MEDICATIONS REPORTED TO INDUCE DEPRESSION

Propanolol	Cimetidine
Reserpine	Levodopa
NSAIDs	Oral contraceptives
Benzodiazepines	Metoclopramide
Clonidine	Ranitidine
Digitalis	Glucocorticoids

| Table 46-1 | *Antidepressant Starting and Maintenance Doses (mg/day)* |

	Initial Dose (mg)	Maintenance Dose (mg)	Comments
TRICYCLICS			
Amitriptyline	25 to 50	100 to 300	Avoid in elderly
Imipramine	25 to 50	100 to 300	Moderate tricyclic side effects
Nortriptyline	10 to 25	50 to 150	Fewer tricyclic side effects
SSRIs			
Paroxetine	10 to 20	20 to 50	Short half-life
Sertraline	25 to 50	50 to 200	Short half-life, give q am or q hs
Fluoxetine	10 to 20	20 to 40	Long half-life, doses to 80 mg/day for obsessive-compulsive disorder or eating disorders
ATYPICAL ANTIDEPRESSANTS			
Venlafaxine	37.5 to 75	300	May increase blood pressure
Nefazodone	100 to 200	300 to 600	Sedating, fewer sexual side effects
Bupropion	75 to 150	300 to 450	Avoid if eating disorder or seizure disorder present

Epidemiology and Natural History

The lifetime prevalence of panic disorder is approximately 2%. Another 3% to 4% have had a panic attack but do not meet criteria for panic disorder. Women are twice as likely as men to be affected. The typical age of onset is late adolescence or early adulthood. A smaller peak also occurs in the 35- to 40-year-old age group. Roughly one third of patients with panic disorder develop agoraphobia, which is a fear and avoidance of situations and places where escape would be impossible and embarrassment likely in the event of a panic attack. Substance abuse is often a comorbid condition that may result from attempts at self-medication. Depression may share biologic underpinnings with panic disorder and can also result from the demoralizing effects of chronic anxiety. The combination of panic disorder and depression increases the risk of suicide.

Specific phobia is the most common anxiety disorder and is typified by excessive and persistent fear of specific objects and situations. Adults recognize their fear as being unreasonable or excessive.

Relationship to Cardiovascular Disease

Panic attacks often result in emergency room visits. They involve a discrete period of intense fear and are associated with at least four other symptoms that develop abruptly and reach a peak within 10 minutes. Symptoms involving the cardiovascular system include chest pain or discomfort, palpitations, a racing heart, shortness of breath, or a smothering sensation. These patients also may have a distinct fear of imminent death. In a study of patients who had chest pain and were referred for coronary angiography, 46% of those with normal arteries met criteria for panic disorder, compared with only 6.5% with positive studies.[7] As many as half of cardiology outpatients with atypical chest pain actually have panic disorder.[7]

Panic disorder and phobic anxiety increase the risk of cardiovascular mortality. Persons with a lifetime history of panic disorder have double the risk of stroke compared with patients who have other psychiatric disorders. Phobic anxiety has also been found to be a predictor of sudden death.[7]

Clinical Presentation

Patients with panic disorder often come to the emergency room or urgent care settings. They may complain of chest pain, shortness of breath, or a fear of imminent death. A hallmark of panic disorder is the crescendo of anxiety and physical symptoms, which reach their peak in under 10 minutes. Self-medication with alcohol is common, and the symptoms of panic disorder may become more pronounced when a patient decreases alcohol use. Phobic anxiety is unlikely to be mentioned by patients in the clinic unless they fear receiving an injection. This is because the feared object or situation is simply avoided. A person with a fear of snakes is unlikely to take a job in the reptile house at the zoo. There are times when career changes necessitate involvement in the stressing situation, such as air travel, and phobic patients may then request treatment.

Clinical Evaluation

The PRIME-MD may be used to screen for panic disorder. It is important to consider the medical conditions listed in Box 46-6, which may mimic the symptoms of

BOX 46-6
MEDICAL CONDITIONS THAT MAY MIMIC PANIC DISORDER

Thyroid dysfunction	Both hyperthyroidism and hypothyroidism may present as anxiety. Check thyroid-stimulating hormone level.
Adrenal dysfunction	Pheochromocytoma is rare but check 24-hour urinary catecholamine metabolite concentrations if suspected.
Parathyroid dysfunction	Hyperparathyroidism may present as panic disorder. Check serum calcium level.
Vestibular dysfunction	Anxiety can be associated with ataxia, nausea, and vomiting.
Hypoglycemia	Anxiety may be associated with sedation, slurred speech, visual changes, and hunger.
Intoxication	Caffeine, amphetamines, or cocaine
Withdrawal	Alcohol, barbiturates, or benzodiazepines

From Kaplan HI, Sadock BJ: *Comprehensive textbook of psychiatry*, ed 6, Baltimore, 1995, Williams & Wilkins.

a panic attack. Patients should also be evaluated for co-morbid depression and substance abuse. The risk of suicide is elevated in patients with both panic disorder and depression and should be routinely assessed. Patients should be directly questioned about places or situations that they avoid. Agoraphobia may be problematic as patients learn to avoid situations or locations where a panic attack may be humiliating or a quick escape may not be possible.

Management of Anxiety

The optimal treatment of panic disorder combines medications and psychotherapy. The SSRIs sertraline and paroxetine have received Food and Drug Administration approval for the treatment of panic disorder. Other antidepressants have been used by clinicians. Dosages are similar to those used to treat depression. However, patients may experience an intensification of their anxiety with the initial doses. This can be managed by patient education and by starting with a very low dose, such as a daily oral dose of sertraline 25 mg or paroxetine 10 mg. Concomitant use of a benzodiazepine such as lorazepam or clonazepam may be helpful. Patients with a history of substance abuse may be at risk of abusing benzodiazepines. Benzodiazepines should be gradually tapered to avoid withdrawal symptoms. A referral for psychotherapy should be considered. Patients with agoraphobia may benefit from cognitive behavioral therapy or systematic desensitization.

Specific phobias are rarely treated. Treatment is indicated if the phobia interferes with a patient's functioning. Systematic desensitization and flooding have been used to expose patients to the feared stimulus while they learn to modulate their level of distress. Recent advances in virtual reality technology may make treatment of the fear of heights and the fear of flying more available and cost effective.

Follow-up and Expected Clinical Course

The onset of the therapeutic effects of an SSRI may take 4 to 8 weeks. A return appointment the week after initiating treatment can be helpful to monitor for side effects and compliance. Patients often report a gradual decrease in the frequency and intensity of panic attacks over time. Substance use, depression, and suicidal ideation should be reassessed periodically. Patients who have remained in stable condition may ask to discontinue medications. A slow and gradual taper over many months allows the identification of reemerging symptoms. A slow taper over 6 months or more can help to avoid confusing benzodiazepine withdrawal symptoms with symptoms caused by the primary disorder.

STRESS

Stress has long been considered a risk factor for illness. Not all stressful events are unwanted. Job promotions, the birth of a child, and winning the lottery may be very

desirable, but they alter an existing equilibrium. Individuals react differently to stress. Identifying specific patterns of reaction to stress can allow for behavioral changes, which in turn may alter the development and progression of disease.

Relationship to Cardiovascular Disease

Type A behavior is typified by a sense of time urgency and competitive hostility. This behavior pattern has been shown to be a predictor of angina but not necessarily myocardial infarction.[8] Hostility alone increases mortality from coronary heart disease, as well as mortality from all causes. A possible mechanism is that hostile individuals have exaggerated hemostatic and cardiovascular reactivity when faced with stressful events. Other factors may include platelet hyperreactivity during acute stress and chronic increases in the activity of the sympathetic nervous system. The risk of myocardial infarction is significantly elevated 2 hours after an episode of expressed anger and up to 24 hours after a psychologically stressful event.[8]

The time of day can also influence the risk of infarction and sudden death. The risk is highest within 2 hours of awakening. It is interesting that cortisol, which is released during periods of acute stress, displays a diurnal variation with significantly higher levels in the morning.

Management Issues

Patients who are facing difficult socioeconomic stressors should be referred to a social worker for evaluation and identification of available resources. Primary care clinics have pursued the formation of stress management groups to teach patients coping skills. Unfortunately, many patients who would benefit the most are not motivated to seek treatment until they have an ischemic event. Patient education groups such as parenting classes, wellness seminars, and self-relaxation training can be used to teach basic techniques, and these appeal to many patients and have less stigma than referral to a mental health care provider. Patients who are motivated can benefit from biofeedback and can learn to alter their physiologic responses as measured by heart rate, blood pressure, and electromyographic recordings. Referral for psychotherapy can be beneficial by teaching the patient cognitive reframing and behavioral modification. Underlying mood or anxiety disorders should be ruled out because they are often more responsive to treatment than personality traits.

DRUGS USED TO TREAT PSYCHIATRIC DISORDERS

Effective pharmacologic treatment is available for mood disorders, anxiety disorders, and psychosis. Progress is being made in the development of drugs that act more specifically, have fewer side effects, and show a more favorable safety profile.

Tricyclic Antidepressants

The tricyclic antidepressants (TCAs) have been used to treat depression since the early 1950s. Initial studies reported response rates as high as 80% for depressed patients. The availability of an effective treatment with a relatively low therapeutic index has posed a unique challenge to clinicians providing care to depressed patients.

Cardiovascular Effects

TCAs can cause orthostatic hypotension. Alterations in cardiac conduction, rate, rhythm, and contractility have also been found. These agents have class IA antiarrhythmic properties like quinidine. They can exacerbate preexisting cardiac conduction delays.

Management Issues

All patients with a history of cardiac symptoms or who are over 40 years of age should have an electrocardiogram before beginning treatment with a TCA. First-degree heart block does not preclude treatment with a TCA. However, patients with right bundle branch block or intraventricular conduction delay are at increased risk for sudden death. Other side effects include orthostatic hypotension, sedation, and anticholinergic side effects such as tachycardia, urinary retention, and constipation. In general, amitriptyline produces the most severe side effects, and nortriptyline and desipramine are the least offensive. Imipramine has a side effect profile that is intermediate. Serum levels of TCAs can vary widely from patient to patient. Close monitoring of response, side effects, and blood levels may be necessary to determine the optimal dose. Patients should be informed that it may take up to 6 weeks before they notice improvement. Patients with anxious features should be started on the lowest possible dose with a gradual titration to follow.

Overdose

Cardiac complications are the leading cause of death in the 2% to 3% of TCA overdoses that are fatal.[9] Ingestion of 2 g of a TCA can be lethal. TCAs are concentrated in the myocardium and have profound cardiotoxic effects.[9] The drugs inhibit the fast sodium channels, resulting in conduction delays and various dysrhythmias, including refractory ventricular tachycardia and fibrillation. Box 46-7 summarizes the treatment of TCA overdose.

Selective Serotonin Reuptake Inhibitors

Although the TCAs are effective antidepressants, they have many side effects. A newer class of antidepressants is the SSRIs. Fluoxetine was the earliest of these agents

BOX 46-7
MANAGEMENT OF TRICYCLIC ANTIDEPRESSANT (TCA) OVERDOSE

SUPPORTIVE

Secure the airway, supplemental oxygen, continuous cardiac monitoring, pulse oximetry, intravenous access, and baseline ECG

LABORATORY VALUES

Electrolytes, blood urea nitrogen, creatinine, glucose, acetaminophen level, and complete blood cell count (CBC). Add arterial blood gas and chest x-ray if alkalinization is necessary. TCA level does not closely correlate with prognosis or alter treatment.

GASTRIC DECONTAMINATION

Gastric evacuation up to 12 hours after ingestion. Administer activated charcoal with a cathartic such as sorbitol. Avoid syrup of ipecac.

TREATMENT OF CARDIAC TOXICITY

Hyperventilation, intravenous sodium bicarbonate as indicated by acidosis, refractory hypotension, prolonged cardiac conduction with QRS >0.16 sec, ventricular dysrhythmias, or cardiac arrest.

TREATMENT OF DYSRHYTHMIAS

Correction of hypoxia, hypotension, and acidosis. Sodium bicarbonate is indicated before initiating other antiarrhythmic drugs. Class IA and IC agents are absolutely contraindicated. Lidocaine is the standard antiarrhythmic after sodium bicarbonate fails. Complete heart block,
Mobitz type II heart block, and refractory symptomatic bradycardia are indications for insertion of a temporary pacemaker. Isoproterenol, magnesium, and atrial overdrive pacing can be used in cases of torsade de pointes.

CARDIAC ARREST

Per standard ACLS protocol; however: (1) sodium bicarbonate should be administered early; (2) avoid type IA and IC antiarrhythmic drugs; and (3) continue resuscitation efforts for at least 1 hour.

HYPOTENSION

Intravascular volume repletion, sodium bicarbonate, and vasopressors.

CENTRAL NERVOUS SYSTEM TOXICITY

Administer thiamine, dextrose, and naloxone for altered mental status. Avoid flumazenil because of risk of precipitating seizures. Treat seizures with intravenous diazepam or phenobarbitol.

DISPOSITION

Admit to a critical care unit if one of the following is observed within 6 hours of emergency room admission: coma, seizure, hypotension, respiratory depression, dysrhythmia requiring treatment, or conduction delay.

From Pimentel L, Trommer L: *Emerg Med Clin North Am* 12:533, 1994.

to be used in this country. This class also includes sertraline, paroxetine, and fluvoxamine. Their effectiveness in treating depression is comparable to that of the TCAs. The pharmacy cost may be higher for an SSRI, but when additional costs such as physician visits to manage side effects, obtaining serum drug levels, and monitoring by ECGs are factored in, they may be more cost effective.

Cardiovascular Effects

The SSRIs do not have the direct cardiotoxic properties of the TCAs. Case reports of SSRI use by patients with preexisting heart disease and reports of overdoses have associated SSRIs with various arrhythmias and heart block. The incidence is extremely low and of questionable clinical significance. All of the SSRIs inhibit the

P450 isoenzyme IID6 to some degree, and this can lead to elevated levels of various drugs, including type IC antiarrhythmics and beta-blockers. Life-threatening arrhythmias have been reported with the combination of the antihistamines terfenadine or astemizole with the SSRIs nefazodone or fluvoxamine because of the inhibition of the cytochrome P450 IIIA4 isoenzyme.

Overdose

The most common features of an SSRI overdose are nausea, vomiting, tremor, and a decreased level of consciousness.[10] Cardiac toxicity is rare but can occur in patients who have ingested other drugs. Treatment of overdose is supportive. A single dose of activated charcoal is indicated. Seizures may occur and are usually self-limited.

Lithium

Lithium is an element found to have a calming effect on animals and humans. It has been effective in the treatment of acute mania. It has antidepressant properties but is less effective than other antidepressants at treating unipolar depression.

Cardiovascular Effects

Lithium can cause benign electrocardiographic changes such as T wave flattening or inversion. Various arrhythmias have been associated with lithium use in patients with underlying cardiac disease. Palpitations, dizziness, and syncope can result from lithium-induced sinoatrial (SA) node dysfunction. Patients with underlying SA node dysfunction such as sick sinus syndrome may require a pacemaker to be treated safely with lithium.[11]

Management Issues

Lithium is excreted by the kidneys and can cause reversible renal impairment. Hypothyroidism develops in about 5% of patients taking lithium. Side effects can include weight gain, polyuria, tremor, and a worsening of dermatologic conditions, including acne and psoriasis. A young, healthy patient may require a lithium level of 1.0 to 1.4 mmol/L for acute mania and may be maintained with a level of 0.6 to 1.0 mmol/L. Elderly patients generally require levels 50% lower. Signs and symptoms of toxicity include nausea, vomiting, and diarrhea. With higher blood levels, neurologic signs may include tremor, ataxia, dysarthria, and confusion. Patients should be instructed to avoid salt restriction, diuretics, and nonsteroidal antiinflammatory drugs (NSAIDs), because they may elevate lithium levels.

Overdose

Lithium toxicity is a medical emergency. Gastric lavage should be performed if an overdose is suspected. Supportive measures such airway and cardiovascular support should be undertaken. In the absence of renal failure or congestive heart failure, vigorous hydration with normal saline solution should be instituted. Hemodialysis should be used if the lithium level is greater than 3.0 mmol/L, if signs of toxicity are severe, or if there is renal failure or poor urine output. Lithium levels that remain elevated despite treatment should raise the suspicion of a lithium bezoar.

Anticonvulsants

Several anticonvulsants have been effective in the treatment of bipolar disorder. Carbamazepine and valproic acid have been well studied. Gabapentin and lamotrigine are currently under investigation for potential mood-stabilizing properties.

Cardiovascular Effects

Carbamazepine has been associated with symptomatic bradycardias in the elderly. It has also been shown to cause cardiac conduction delays but to a lesser degree than the TCAs.[10] Valproic acid, gabapentin, and lamotrigine are not known to have specific cardiovascular effects.

Management Issues

Carbamazepine can induce hepatic microsomal enzymes, causing a decrease in the level of many drugs, including warfarin, TCAs, and antipsychotics. It can augment the action of digitalis, resulting in bradycardia.[11] Patients who have toxic levels appear drunk.

Overdose

Patients who have taken an overdose of carbamazepine may exhibit an altered mental status, nystagmus, clonus, or ataxia. Laboratory findings can include hyponatremia, hypokalemia, hyperglycemia, and elevations in transaminase levels. Cardiac arrhythmias and widening of the QRS complex have been reported but are rarely problematic in uncomplicated carbamazepine overdoses.[10] Management of an overdose involves repeated doses of activated charcoal along with supportive measures.

Benzodiazepines

Benzodiazepines are sedative hypnotics and have a higher therapeutic index than barbiturates. They bind to receptors linked to the GABA receptors and chloride channels in the central nervous system to potentiate the action of the inhibitory neurotransmitter GABA.

Cardiovascular Effects

There are no clinically significant direct cardiovascular effects. A withdrawal state can result from abrupt discontinuation or dose reduction. Features of withdrawal include tachycardia, hypertension, tremor, and possibly seizures.

Antipsychotics

Antipsychotics have also been known as neuroleptics or major tranquilizers. They have complex actions but can be thought of as blocking postsynaptic dopamine receptors. Several novel or atypical antipsychotics have recently become available that have improved side effect profiles and are possibly more effective for refractory cases of psychosis.

Cardiovascular effects

Tachycardia and orthostatic hypotension are more commonly associated with the low-potency agents such as thioridazine and chlorpromazine. These agents also can slow cardiac conduction and lead to heart block or torsade de pointes. Side effects of neuroleptics include sedation, anticholinergic side effects, and orthostatic hypotension. These are managed by reducing the dose or changing to a higher potency agent such as haloperidol. The novel antipsychotic clozapine commonly causes tachycardia and orthostatic hypotension.

Overdose

Ingestion of toxic amounts of antipsychotics usually results in central nervous system depression and cardiovascular toxicity. Hypotension, tachycardia, atrioventricular block, intraventricular conduction delay, and various arrhythmias have been demonstrated and are usually evident within the first few hours after overdose. Treatment measures are supportive. Activated charcoal should be administered. Type IA, IC, II, and possibly III antiarrhythmic agents should be avoided.[10] Seizures should be treated with intravenous diazepam or lorazepam. Patients with seizures, arrhythmias, hypotension, or severe central nervous system depression should be admitted, possibly to a critical care unit. Asymptomatic patients should be monitored for 4 to 6 hours before seeking a psychiatric disposition.

DRUG ABUSE

Human use of intoxicants dates back at least 10,000 years. The use and abuse of substances persist despite episodic shifts in social policy and cultural mores. It is estimated that the abuse of substances costs the United States over $300 billion annually in direct and indirect costs.[12] When does the use of a substance constitute abuse? Generally speaking, substance abuse is when a patient's social or occupational functioning is impaired by substance use, when the substance is used in hazardous situations, or when use results in recurrent legal troubles. Hallmarks of substance dependence are the development of tolerance to the intoxicating effects, the presence of a characteristic withdrawal state with discontinuation, and compulsive use, often seen as numerous unsuccessful attempts to reduce substance use. Specific diagnostic criteria are listed in DSM-IV.[5]

Specific Drugs of Abuse

Nicotine

Approximately 25% of American adults smoke. The percentage of young people who smoke has increased despite aggressive public education efforts. Each year 20% of the deaths in the United States are smoking related.[13] Smokers are more likely than nonsmokers to be heavy drinkers or users of illicit drugs.

Nicotine may lead to cardiovascular disease by several different mechanisms, including increased sympathetic activity, platelet aggregation, alterations in lipid metabolism, and hypercoagulability.[13] Treatment of nicotine dependence is reviewed in Chapter 11 and Table 46-2.

Alcohol

The cardiovascular effects of alcohol are reviewed in Chapter 43. Over half of the total alcohol consumption is by 6.5% of the population in the United States. Roughly 13% of men and 3% of American women consume two or more alcoholic beverages per day.[13] Women tend to begin heavy drinking later in life, and generally their medical deterioration is more rapid. A simple screening tool described in Table 43-6 is the acronym "CAGE." One positive response should raise suspicion. Two or more positive responses correlate highly with alcoholism.

Treatment. Alcohol withdrawal is associated with significant morbidity and mortality. The best predictor of alcohol withdrawal is a previous history of withdrawal. The clinician should inquire about any previous history of "shakes," seizures, or delirium associated with withdrawal. If a patient has a history of seizures or altered mental status, or if he or she has severe medical comorbidity, you should undertake detoxification of the patient as an inpatient. Alcohol withdrawal usually begins 12 hours after the last drink and peaks at 48 to 72 hours. This time frame may be delayed in the elderly. A tapering dose of benzodiazepine such as lorazepam 2 mg orally three or four times daily can be used as a starting point. Tachycardia, hypertension, and tremor are indications for increasing the dose. The addition of an anticonvulsant such as carbamazepine 200 mg orally four times a day for up to 1 week should be considered in patients with a history of withdrawal seizures. Thiamine should be given 100 mg intramuscularly, then as 100 mg orally each day. Alcoholic patients often have low magnesium stores and supplementation can reduce the risk of seizures and arrhythmias.

Cocaine

Over 5 million Americans use cocaine regularly. The predominant cardiovascular effects are mediated by alpha-adrenergic stimulation, resulting in an increased heart rate, increased systemic blood pressure, and in-

Table 46-2	*Pharmacologic Treatments for Smoking Cessation*	
Agent	**Dose**	**Contraindications**
Nicotine gum	2 or 4 mg chewed at 1- to 2-hour intervals, not to exceed 80 mg in 24 hours. Taper by 12 weeks.	Unstable arrhythmia, worsening angina, or in the early recovery phase after myocardial infarction. Use cautiously in cases of hyperthyroidism, hypertension, or pheochromocytoma.
Nicotine patch	Apply 21 mg patch qd for 4 to 12 weeks, then taper. Start with lower dose if weight less than 45 kg, if smoking fewer than 10 cigarettes a day, or if cardiovascular disease is present.	Same as above
Bupropion SR (Zyban)	150 mg PO qd for 4 days, then 150 mg PO bid for up to 12 weeks.	History of seizures or eating disorder

creased coronary artery tone. The resulting increase in myocardial oxygen demand and decrease in myocardial oxygen supply account for the occurrence of angina pectoris, myocardial infarction, or sudden death in young, otherwise healthy patients, including first-time users.[14] Chronic cocaine users may have multiple subendocardial infarctions that result in congestive heart failure. Sinus tachycardia is the most common arrhythmia seen with cocaine use; however, ventricular fibrillation may occur. The concomitant use of alcohol or tobacco can significantly increase the risk of myocardial ischemia.

Treatment. Rapid oxygenation and sedation with a benzodiazepine are the first steps in managing cocaine-associated chest pain. Beta-blockers should be avoided, because unopposed alpha-adrenergic stimulation could result in coronary arterial vasospasm.[15] Nitroglycerin and verapamil can reduce both hypertension and coronary vasoconstriction and are the drugs of choice for cocaine-associated chest pain. Furosemide and digoxin may be the drugs of choice for congestive heart failure. Ventricular fibrillation may be treated with verapamil 5 to 10 mg intravenously over 2 minutes.[16] Patients who are abusing cocaine should be counseled about the drug's deleterious effects and referred to a substance abuse program and Narcotics Anonymous.

Marijuana

Marijuana use is commonplace in American culture. Roughly one in three high school students reports having used it in the past year. Despite being illegal, marijuana has become more popular in the past decade. Many of the previous theories about the hazards of cannabis have been debunked. However, smoking marijuana is particularly hazardous to patients with angina.

It has been demonstrated to decrease myocardial oxygen supply, increase myocardial oxygen demand, and decrease the amount of exercise time preceding anginal pain.[17]

Treatment. The management of acute intoxication is usually reassurance. Patients with angina should be informed that marijuana use is contraindicated. Urine drug screens are helpful if use is suspected. However, the ability to detect marijuana use varies with the frequency of use. Infrequent users test positive for a few days, and regular users test positive for several weeks after discontinuing use. Referral to a treatment program is indicated for those who continue to use this substance. Narcotics Anonymous is also available.

Opiates

Opiate abuse in the United States has increased in the past decade. The glamorization of this class of drugs is reflected by the term *heroin chic*. Although various routes of administration are used, intravenous use is responsible for the most adverse health consequences.

The spread of hepatitis and human immunodeficiency virus (HIV) is of concern. Over 25% of new AIDS cases occur in intravenous drug users.[13] Endocarditis can result from organisms from various sources, including the injected drug, skin contaminants, an underlying cellulitis, or "cleansing" solutions such as saliva or tap water. Other cardiovascular complications include arrhythmia, mycotic aneurysm, and thrombophlebitis.

Treatment. Treatment of an acute opiate overdose consists of naloxone 2 mg intravenously in 5 minutes followed by 2 mg intravenously every 20 to 60 minutes. Endocarditis can be difficult to diagnose in this population. The majority of cases of drug-related endocarditis

occur on the right side of the heart. Classic findings such as petechiae, peripheral emboli, and hemorrhage may be absent in right-sided endocarditis. All febrile intravenous drug users should be hospitalized and evaluated for endocarditis.

Detoxification can be accomplished by administering oral or parenteral opiates and gradually tapering the dose. Clonidine 0.1 to 0.3 mg orally three times daily can be used adjunctively to treat drug craving, piloerection, sweating, and anxiety. The opiate antagonist naltrexone has been used to hasten detoxification and to maintain abstinence once detoxification has been completed.

REFERENCES

1. Stahl SM: *Essential psychopharmacology*, New York, 1996, Cambridge University Press.
2. American Psychiatric Association: *Practice guideline for major depressive disorder in adults*, Washington, DC, 1993, The Association.
3. Glassman AH, Shapiro PA: Depression and the course of coronary artery disease, *Am J Psychiatry* 155:1, 1998.
4. Hance M, Carney RM, Freedland KE, Skala J: Depression in patients with coronary heart disease: a 12-month follow-up, *Gen Hosp Psychiatry* 18:61, 1996.
5. American Psychiatric Association: *Diagnostic and statistical manual of mental disorders*, ed 4, Washington, DC, 1994, The Association.
6. Spitzer RL, Williams JB, Kroenke K, et al: Utility of a new procedure for diagnosing mental disorders in primary care: The PRIME-MD 1000 study, *JAMA* 272:1749, 1994.
7. Fleet RP, Beitman BD: Unexplained chest pain: when is it panic disorder? *Clin Cardiol* 20:187, 1997.
8. Allan R, Scheidt S, editors: *Heart & mind: the practice of cardiac psychology*, ed 1, Washington, DC, 1996, American Psychological Association.
9. Pimentel L, Trommer L: Cyclic antidepressant overdoses, *Emerg Med Clin North Am* 12:533, 1994.
10. Haddad LM, Shannon MW, Winchester JF, editors: *Clinical management of poisoning and drug overdose*, ed 3, Philadelphia, 1998, WB Saunders.
11. Arana GW, Hyman SE: *Handbook of psychiatric drug therapy*, ed 2, Boston, 1991, Little, Brown.
12. American Psychiatric Association: Practice guideline for the treatment of patients with substance use disorders: alcohol, cocaine, opioids, *Am J Psychiatry* (suppl) 155:11, 1995.
13. Lowinson JH et al, editors: *Substance abuse: a comprehensive textbook*, ed 3, Baltimore, 1997, Williams & Wilkins.
14. Pitts WR, Lange RA, Cigarroa JE, Hillis LD: Cocaine-induced myocardial ischemia and infarction: pathophysiology, recognition, and management, *Prog Cardiovasc Dis* 40:65, 1997.
15. Shih RD, Hollander JE: Management of cocaine-associated chest pain, *Hosp Physician* 11:45, 1996.
16. Fleming MF, Barry K, editors: *Addictive disorders: a practical guide to treatment*, St Louis, 1992, Mosby.
17. Gottschalk LA, Aronow WS, Prakash R: Effect of marijuana and placebo-marijuana smoking on psychological state and psychophysiologic cardiovascular functioning in anginal patients, *Biol Psychiatry* 12:2, 1977.

47 Advanced Age and Heart Disease

Leslye C. Pennypacker
George J. Taylor

Although the exact chronologic age at which a person becomes "elderly" is debated, the U.S. population is undoubtedly aging rapidly. Current demographic projections suggest a doubling of our population over age 65 by the year 2030. Moreover, the "oldest old" sector—those over age 85—is the single fastest growing sector of our population. The "graying of America," coupled with the fact that heart disease is the most frequent reason for hospitalization and death in the elderly, underscores the importance of understanding the effect of aging on heart disease.

AGING OF THE CARDIOVASCULAR SYSTEM

As with virtually all areas of investigation of cellular aging, the debate between what is normal aging and what is disease rages on in the field of cardiovascular physiology. Particularly difficult to decipher is the effect of lifestyle, occult disease, and intrinsic aging on the cardiovascular system.[1,2] Because of the difficulty in controlling for lifestyle variables and occult disease, much of what we know about aging in the cardiovascular system is extrapolated from animal models. In addition, longitudinal data on humans are scant, and the results can be difficult to interpret because of variable patient selection criteria. Nonetheless, some clinically relevant, albeit broad, generalizations should be remembered:

1. The heterogeneity in the aging process increases with increasing age (i.e., "Not all 80-year-olds are created equal!").
2. With advancing age, most of the important changes in cardiovascular physiology are more pronounced with stress and exercise.
3. Assessment of "functional cardiac status" may be much more meaningful than determination of other objective physiologic measures such as ejection fraction.[3]

Table 47-1 summarizes some of the physiologic changes that occur with advancing age. Many of these are not clinically relevant in healthy elderly subjects and may be noted only in settings of cardiovascular stress. An exception to this is the fairly predictable increase in age-associated conduction system disturbances seen both at rest and during stress. These appear to result from progressive fibrosis of the sinoatrial node, ventric-

ular septum, and mitral and aortic valve rings and leaflets. The clinical consequences include an increase in ectopic beats, intraventricular conduction defects, tachyarrhythmias, and bradyarrhythmias.

The reliance on increasing stroke volume (as opposed to heart rate, as is seen in younger subjects) to maintain cardiac output in response to stress can be quite significant in elderly patients with or without diminished pump function. Deconditioning can exacerbate these problems, and this improves with exercise training. Even frail elderly patients can benefit from graded exercise programs, with an increase in VO_2max (see Chapter 17).

SPECIFIC DISEASES

There are two axioms of geriatric medicine that warrant emphasis, particularly when considering the possibility of cardiovascular disease in elderly patients:

1. The *atypical presentation of typical disease* should always be considered.
2. *Occum's razor dulls with age* (i.e., there may be more than one diagnosis associated with any given sign or symptom).

As the experienced clinician knows, diagnosing and managing common illnesses in elderly patients are often humbling and challenging tasks. This chapter offers some specific suggestions on how best to approach major cardiovascular disorders in geriatric patients.

Coronary Artery Disease
Epidemiology

The prevalence of coronary artery disease (CAD) in the elderly is difficult to determine because the method of calculation influences the result. Clinical studies indicate that up to 30% of persons more than 60 years old have symptomatic CAD.[2] Autopsy studies, on the other hand, demonstrate CAD in as many as 60%.[4] This large discrepancy most likely results from the common occurrence of occult, or "silent," CAD in the elderly. Interestingly, although CAD is common, only 10% to 12% of elderly patients report that their heart disease limits their activities of daily living (ADL).[5] Usually ADL impairments are attributed to joint or bone disorders, which may limit the person's ability to exercise, thus

Table 47-1 *Changes in Cardiac Function with Aging*

	Resting state (Young vs Old)	During Exercise or Stress Young	Old
Heart rate	No difference	Increase	Less increase
Preload	No difference	No change or fall	Increase
Afterload	Increase with age	No change	Increase
Stroke volume	No difference	Little change	Increase
Left ventricular ejection fraction	No difference	Marked increase	Variable

preventing the symptoms of CAD. This is worth remembering when deciding how aggressively to pursue a diagnostic evaluation for occult CAD. Is CAD going to limit the patient, or will arthritis or other illnesses protect the person from experiencing CAD-related symptoms? This is not to say that "silent ischemia" is benign, but the functional status of the patient should be considered when making diagnostic and therapeutic decisions for elderly or frail patients.

Clinical Presentation

More than half of elderly patients with significant CAD do not have classic symptoms of exertional substernal chest pain (see Chapter 13). Dyspnea and dry cough often are anginal equivalents. In addition, because the single most common presenting symptom for acute myocardial infarction (MI) in elderly patients is new-onset shortness of breath, the recognition of CAD can be particularly challenging in patients with coexisting lung disease.[6] In these patients, our index of suspicion must remain high for CAD, and diagnostic evaluation should generally include electrocardiogram (ECG) and possibly cardiac enzyme measurements if symptoms worsen rapidly. Similarly, falls and syncope may also be the presenting symptom for an elderly patient with acute MI.

Management and Recommendations

As already noted, it is vital to consider a patient's overall functional status when making decisions regarding how best to manage CAD. Certainly chronologic age, as an isolated predictor, is of little value in anticipating how a patient will respond to treatment. A healthy, active, functionally independent 80-year-old patient should be approached much the same as one would approach a patient 15 or 20 years younger. Many are living into their eighth and ninth decades with remarkable preservation of quality of life. Conversely, frail, functionally limited 65-year-old patients may not benefit from aggressive diagnostic and therapeutic interventions. Before recom-

mending cardiac catheterization, you should carefully assess whether the benefits of angioplasty or bypass surgery outweigh the risks. Elderly patients are much more likely to have concurrent diseases (e.g., hypertension, peripheral vascular disease, and cerebrovascular disease) that may compound perioperative and long-term postsurgical complications.[7-11] Therefore a thorough assessment of a patient's overall status is warranted before proceeding with cardiac catheterization.

Another note of caution: establishing a patient's baseline mental status should be a priority in the diagnostic workup of all elderly CAD patients. Unfortunately, if this is omitted from the evaluation, it may be difficult to know whether the "altered mental status" seen after catheterization or heart surgery is new or old. This can be problematic, since unrecognized delirium—not uncommon in the ICU setting—carries a remarkably high mortality in elderly hospitalized patients.

Thrombolytic therapy for acute MI may outweigh the risks of treatment when used in carefully selected patients (see Chapter 15). Clinical difficulties with reperfusion therapy in elderly patients include the following:

1. Symptoms of MI may be nonspecific or atypical.
2. The risk of bleeding (particularly intracranial) is higher with thrombolysis.
3. Mental status changes may impede the consent process.
4. The presentation is often delayed (more than 6 hours after the onset of MI).
5. Underlying ECG changes may confound the diagnosis of MI.
6. Elderly patients more often have contraindications to therapy.

Many clinicians consider errors of commission worse than errors of omission. As a result, even when selection criteria are met, they are hesitant to use thrombolytics in elderly patients.[12] A large multicenter trial examining the efficacy of thrombolytics in the elderly population was attempted (the Thrombolytic Therapy in an Older

Patient Population [TTOPP] study) but was aborted early because of low patient recruitment rates.

In the absence of contraindications, elderly patients meeting the usual selection criteria for coronary thrombolysis who come within 6 hours of symptom onset should be offered reperfusion therapy (see Chapter 15). Because older patients are also the ones with the greatest chance for benefit, clinicians should strive to remove chronologic age as a factor weighing against the use of this treatment.

Congestive Heart Failure

Epidemiology

The Medicare and National Health and Nutrition Examination Survey (NHANES-1) data have documented increasing congestive heart failure (CHF) with advanced age[13,14]:

1. The prevalence of CHF doubles with each decade from age 45 to age 85 years.
2. Mortality from CHF increases with increasing age, so 90% of CHF deaths occur in those at least 65 years old.
3. CHF is the most common reason for hospitalization and repeat admission for elderly patients (more than 50% are readmitted within 3 to 6 months after index admission).
4. Although in-hospital mortality from CHF has declined slightly over the past decade, a higher proportion of CHF patients are requiring discharge to chronic care facilities after hospitalization.

The overall cost of managing CHF in the United States is estimated to be between $10 and $30 billion annually (exceeding the combined HCFA hospitalization costs for cancer and MI).[15] With an aging population, these figures will not likely decline despite advances in treatment.

Clinical Presentation and Evaluation

Old patients with CHF may have more subtle symptoms such as a dry cough (due to elevated pulmonary artery pressures) and progressive confusion (due to poor cerebral perfusion).[16] Like angina pectoris, the multiple other illnesses that limit exercise tolerance can mask the exertional dyspnea of early heart failure. Other symptoms such as fatigue and weakness are easily overlooked or mistakenly attributed to "just getting old."

The physical examination may also be misleading.[15,16] For example, elderly patients with CHF may not have an S_3 gallop because diastolic dysfunction is more common. They may not have compensatory tachycardia because of conduction disease. Murmurs may be soft or absent despite significant valvular disease. Rales may be surprisingly absent even when the chest x-ray shows pulmonary congestion. Peripheral edema may be caused by venous insufficiency rather than CHF.

Noninvasive evaluation is helpful, especially echocardiography. Not only is it safe, but information regarding wall motion, ejection fraction (differentiating systolic from diastolic dysfunction), and valvular function usually provides a guide to management[15-19] (see Chapters 22 and 23). The ECG and chest x-ray are also useful elements of the evaluation but rarely provide information that makes an echocardiogram unnecessary. Remember that diastolic dysfunction is a more common cause of heart failure in elderly patients, and measurement of left ventricular ejection fraction is necessary for making that diagnosis (see Chapter 23). Cardiac catheterization is rarely indicated in the diagnostic evaluation of CHF in an elderly patient unless there is concern about potentially reversible CAD.

Management

Many older patients with CHF are already at an advanced stage of the disease when they come for evaluation. They may require aggressive nonpharmacologic and medical management early in their course. If the patient is relatively independent, there may be an opportunity for compliance with nonpharmacologic interventions such as sodium and fluid restriction. However, more functionally dependent individuals must rely on others for food selection and preparation, and dietary changes may be difficult. To maximize compliance, efforts should be made to carefully explain these recommendations to patients and care givers.

Drug therapy depends on whether there is systolic or diastolic dysfunction. Management of the two different classes of heart failure is reviewed in Chapters 22 and 23. Because increased diastolic stiffness is so common, there tends to be increased sensitivity to diuretics (note Fig. 23-4). It may be better to try thiazides before more potent loop diuretics. Always start with a low dose and carefully monitor electrolyte levels. Even the milder thiazide diuretics can increase urinary output enough to hinder functional independence in elderly patients with continence problems. It is not uncommon for patients to intermittently omit or discontinue their diuretic therapy if the increased urinary output makes it impossible for them to manage their ADL.

ACE inhibition is the first choice of treatment for CHF caused by systolic dysfunction for both elderly and younger patients. Contraindications to their use are similar, but the elderly are more likely to suffer from symptomatic hypotension. Prescribe an appropriately low starting dose and monitor blood pressure, electrolyte levels, and renal function more carefully.

Digoxin has a narrow therapeutic window in the elderly population and should therefore be used with greater caution than in younger patients. Most agree that digoxin should be used in elderly patients with CHF and atrial fibrillation to help decrease rapid ven-

tricular rates, but debate continues regarding its use in elderly patients in sinus rhythm. We prescribe digoxin for confirmed systolic dysfunction if response to diuretics plus ACE inhibitors is inadequate, or for those who cannot tolerate afterload reduction therapy. All elderly patients who are taking digoxin should be monitored carefully for signs and symptoms of digoxin toxicity, and clinicians should not rely on "normal" serum digoxin levels to exclude clinical toxicity. Confusion or altered vision may be symptomatic of toxicity despite a level that is in the high therapeutic range.

Other therapies for CHF, including beta blockade, may be considered for older patients, but with the caveat that side effects are more common (see Chapter 22).

Valvular Heart Disease

The prevalence of isolated valvular heart disease caused by rheumatic fever declines with increasing age in the United States. However, we are still surprised by the occasional elderly woman with heart failure who turns out to have mitral stenosis. Exclusion of occult valvular disease is one more reason to obtain an echocardiogram when there is new-onset CHF. Degenerative valve disease is the usual problem in old patients. Calcific aortic stenosis is the most common valvular lesion that requires valve replacement in the elderly.[20]

As with other heart conditions, other illnesses may mask symptoms of valvular heart disease. Physical findings, including heart murmurs, may not fit the classic description. For example, murmurs of valvular stenosis may be soft or absent if cardiac output is low. Keep occult valvular disease in mind when evaluating apparently noncardiac problems such as bronchitis (mitral stenosis), falls or syncope (aortic stenosis), and weakness (most valvular lesions).

"Incidental" valvular abnormalities detected on echocardiography may not require intervention if the patient is truly asymptomatic and hemodynamically stable. However, these patients need careful follow-up and surveillance for impending symptom onset, since it is best to intervene surgically before impaired valvular function leads to deterioration in ventricular pump function (see Chapters 18 to 20).

Conversely, "expectant management" is not an ideal strategy in elderly patients with *symptomatic* valvular heart disease. Since the treatment of choice for many of them is surgical, immediate attention to determining a patient's operative risk is essential. The following are well-defined markers of increased operative mortality and poor functional outcome:

- Ventricular dysfunction
- Inoperable CAD
- Moderate to severe heart failure
- Pulmonary hypertension
- Need for preoperative pacemaker placement

- Poor baseline functional or nutritional status
- Comorbid conditions, including lung, renal, or vascular disease

Aortic balloon valvuloplasty has been disappointing, because repeat stenosis of dilated valves is common. It is used occasionally as a method of stabilizing a patient in cardiogenic shock before surgery or as a palliative procedure for nonoperative candidates. Chronologic age alone has not been shown to correlate with higher perioperative complications. Functional status and "physiologic age" determine the risk:benefit ratio of surgical intervention in these patients.

Arrhythmias

As a result of age-related changes in the cardiac conduction system, the prevalence of cardiac arrhythmias increases with age. Symptomatic ventricular arrhythmias are uncommon unless there is coronary artery disease or left ventricular dysfunction. However, atrial arrhythmias and bradyarrhythmias may occur without coexisting structural heart disease.

Palpitations, lightheadedness, or syncope raises the possibility of occult arrhythmias.[21] However, geriatric patients also may present atypically with new-onset confusion, agitation, or a decline in functional status. In addition to standard evaluation and treatment of arrhythmias (see Chapters 25 to 28), here are a few suggestions regarding elderly patients:

1. Hyperthyroidism should be considered in all elderly patients who present with new-onset supraventricular arrhythmias, since the arrhythmia may be the only symptom.
2. If a patient gives a history of any premonitory symptoms (dizziness, palpitations, chest pain, and so forth) before a fall or syncopal episode, the yield of Holter monitoring is much greater than when these symptoms are lacking.[21]
3. Sick sinus syndrome (tachybrady syndrome) is particularly common in elderly patients and may require dual treatment, pacemaker plus drug therapy, to control symptoms.
4. If a pacemaker is indicated, atrioventricular sequential pacing should be strongly considered in the elderly because of the greater relative contribution of the "atrial kick" to cardiac output in these patients (because of diastolic dysfunction, Fig. 23-4).
5. Periodic monitoring of both potassium and magnesium levels in elderly patients who are taking diuretics should be done, since both hypokalemia and hypomagnesemia can exacerbate atrial and ventricular arrhythmias.
6. Because the risk of embolic events secondary to atrial fibrillation increases with increasing age, anticoagulation is critical; old age alone does not contraindicate warfarin therapy.

Hypertension

The wealth of cross-sectional and longitudinal data now available demonstrates a progressive rise in the incidence and prevalence of hypertension with increasing age. [22,33] Most commonly this is demonstrated by a disproportionate rise in systolic blood pressure, and isolated systolic hypertension (ISH) appears to be even more predictive of cardiovascular risk than diastolic hypertension in elderly patients. [22-24] Large population analyses demonstrate that more than 50% of the U.S. population over age 65 have ISH, but interestingly this trend does not exist in nonindustrialized societies.

Because of the strong and continuous relationship between hypertension, CAD, stroke, and cardiovascular death, the importance of treating HTN may be greater in the elderly population. The relative risk reduction with treatment is similar comparing younger and older hypertensive patients, but the absolute benefit of treatment in the elderly is estimated to be two to four times greater because of the higher prevalence of cardiovascular disease in this age group. Table 47-2 summarizes data from three clinical trials of treatment of hypertension in elderly patients: the Systolic Hypertension in the Elderly Program (SHEP), the Swedish Trial in Old Patients with Hypertension (STOP-H), and the Medical Research Council (MRC) studies. [25-27]

Because of these convincing data, revised World Health Organization (WHO) and Joint National Committee (JNC VI) recommendations urge the treatment of both combined (SBP/DBP) and isolated systolic hypertension in the elderly. However, it is still worth remembering that few patients older than 75 years were studied in these trials, and most of those represented were the "healthy elderly" who had minimal comorbid disease.

Clinical Presentation

Hypertension is no more likely to cause symptoms in elderly than in younger patients, so the diagnosis is most often made based on screening blood pressure readings. A few suggestions are as follows:

1. Home (or "out-of-office") blood pressure readings may be more reliable than those taken in the office ("white coat" hypertension).
2. Repeated measures of blood pressure are suggested, since some evidence shows that elderly patients have more lability of pressure.
3. Always check orthostatic pressures. The decision to treat, and the subsequent response, should be based on the lower readings to avoid postural hypotension, a common complication of treatment in the elderly.

Table 47-2	Clinical Trials of Hypertension in the Elderly		
	SHEP[25]	**STOP-H**[26]	**MRC**[27]
Number randomized	4736	1627	4396
Mean age (range)	72 (60-80)	76 (70-84)	70 (65-74)
Blood pressure inclusion criteria (mm Hg)			
Systolic	160-219	180-230	160-209
Diastolic	<90	>90	<115
Treatment(s)	Chlorthalidone (with atenolol)	Atenolol or metoprolol or pindolol or Moduretic*	Atenolol or Moduretic*
Mean follow-up (yr)	4.5	2.1	5.8
Results (therapy vs placebo) Mean reduction in blood pressure (mm Hg)	12/4	20/8	14/6
Reduction % in:			
Total mortality	13	43	3
Stroke (all)	37	47	25
Coronary artery disease	25	13	19
Cardiovascular events (all)	32	40	17

*Moduretic = hydrochlorothiazide + amiloride.

4. Pseudohypertension, or artificially higher cuff pressure readings caused by arterial stiffening, should be suspected if the pressure readings are out of proportion to the clinical findings (specifically retinal findings) or if a patient develops profound postural hypotension despite low-dose, cautious therapy. A positive Osler's maneuver (a palpable brachial artery despite inflation of the cuff above the systolic pressure) may suggest this diagnosis.

5. Renovascular hypertension is common in elderly patients and should be suspected if moderate to severe diastolic hypertension develops de novo or if previously controlled hypertension becomes uncontrollable.

Management

In otherwise healthy elderly patients with well-documented hypertension, it is reasonable to begin with lifestyle modification. There is a growing body of evidence that "you can teach an old dog new tricks," because many elderly patients are motivated to make such changes. The response to these interventions is as potent as that seen in younger individuals.

The recommendations of experts outlined in the JNC VI are certainly reasonable for most healthy elderly patients (see Chapter 31); however, we still have few data to guide us in the management of our oldest, and perhaps frailest, patients. Caution should be exercised because of an increased likelihood of comorbid conditions, concurrent drug therapies, and narrower therapeutic windows for most medications. Following are a few specific suggestions and words of caution:

1. If antihypertensive agents are needed, make an effort whenever possible to "double up" therapeutic interventions (e.g., using an alpha-blocker in an elderly hypertensive man with prostatic hypertrophy or an ACE inhibitor in a patient with CHF or diabetes).[25]

2. Consider whether other drugs might be contributing to hypertension (e.g., nonsteroidal antiinflammatory drugs, over-the-counter sinus remedies with alpha-adrenergic activity, and ethanol).

3. Combination preparations or lower doses of more than one class of drugs may successfully control blood pressure and have fewer side effects.

4. Although diuretics remain the cornerstone of effective, affordable therapy, elderly patients with borderline or overt incontinence can have significant declines in functional independence when given diuretics.

5. Initial starting doses of antihypertensive agents should be as low as possible despite high pressure readings. Unless there are clinical signs of hypertensive crisis, lowering blood pressure rapidly has no benefit. The side effects induced by overly aggressive therapy may convince a patient not to continue with medications at all.

Hyperlipidemia in the Elderly

Available population data (Framingham study) reveal that approximately 25% of men and 42% of women over age 65 years have total serum cholesterol levels greater than 240 mg/dL, the commonly accepted threshold for initiation of treatment. Interestingly, men have higher cholesterol levels on average than women up until age 50, at which point women begin to catch up.[25] The rise in serum low-density lipoprotein (LDL) cholesterol levels after menopause points to the role of estrogen in the metabolism of lipids. The clinical relevance of this is obvious, as the risk of CAD mirrors these trends. Postmenopausal women have as high a CAD risk as age-matched men.

On the other hand, it appears that hyperlipidemia is a less potent risk factor for heart disease in elderly patients (older than 70 years of age) when compared with younger individuals. In fact, the value of LDL and high-density lipoprotein (HDL) levels as predictors of the relative risk of CAD *decreases* with increasing age in both men and women (although absolute risk continues to rise).[29,30]

No clinical trials support the treatment of hyperlipidemia in elderly patients. Therefore the current National Cholesterol Education Program (NCEP) guidelines make no specific recommendations for persons older than 65 years of age. In addition to the recommendations outlined in Chapter 12, we make these suggestions:

1. Aggressive screening and treatment of hyperlipidemia in frail elderly patients with multiple comorbid conditions is probably not warranted despite the higher risk of CAD .

2. Dietary measures to reduce serum lipid levels may be worth recommending to elderly patients, but any restrictions should be made in the context of the patient's overall health and nutritional status. Beware of overly aggressive caloric reduction.

3. Elderly patients with documented cardiovascular disease and a lower burden of concomitant illnesses may benefit from cholesterol-lowering therapy if closely monitored to avoid toxicity.

4. The protective effect of estrogen may be substantial in postmenopausal women, and hormone replacement should be considered a treatment option for those with other risk factors for CAD (see Chapter 41).

REFERENCES

1. Wei JY: Age and the cardiovascular system, *N Engl J Med* 327:1735, 1992.

2. Lakatta EG, Gerstenblith G: Alterations in circulatory function. In Hazzard WR: *Principles of geriatric medicine and gerontology,* ed 2, New York, 1990, McGraw-Hill.

3. Larson EB, Bruce RA: Health benefits of exercising in an aging society, *Arch Intern Med* 147:353, 1987.

4. Elveback L, Lie JT: Continued high incidence of coronary artery disease at autopsy in Olmstead County, Minnesota, 1950-1979, *Circulation* 70:345, 1984.

5. Belsky JK: Disability and health care. In Belsky JK, editor: *Here today: making the most of life after fifty,* New York, 1988, Ballantine Books.

6. Aronow WS: Prevalence of presenting symptoms of recognized acute myocardial infarction and of unrecognized healed myocardial infarction in elderly patients, *Am J Cardiol* 60:1182, 188, 1987.

7. Cheitlin MD: Coronary bypass surgery in the elderly, *Clin Geriatr Med* 12:195, 1996.

8. Stemmer EA, Aronow WS: Surgical treatment of coronary artery disease in the elderly, *Clin Geriatr* 5:19, 1997.

9. Krumholz HM, Forman DE, Kuntz RE, et al: Coronary revascularization after myocardial infarction in the very elderly: outcomes and long-term follow-up, *Ann Intern Med* 119:1084, 1993.

10. Tuman KJ, McCarthy RJ, Najafi H, Ivankovich AD: Differential effects of advanced age on neurologic and cardiac risks of coronary artery operations, *J Thorac Cardiovasc Surg* 104:1510, 1992.

11. Roach GW, Kanchuger M, Mangano CM, et al: Adverse cerebral outcomes after coronary bypass surgery: multicenter study of Perioperative Ischemia Research Group and the Ischemia Research and Education Foundation Investigators, *N Engl J Med* 335:1857, 1996.

12. Krumholz HM, Murillo JE, Chen J, et al: Thrombolytic therapy for eligible elderly patients with acute myocardial infarction, *JAMA* 277:1683, 1997.

13. Croft JB, Giles WH, Pollard RA, et al: National trends in the initial hospitalization for heart failure, *J Am Geriatr Soc* 45:270, 1997.

14. Schocken DD, Arrieta MI, Leaverton PE, Ross EA: Prevalence and mortality rate of congestive heart failure in the United States, *J Am Coll Cardiol* 20:301, 1992.

15. Senni M, Redfield MM: Congestive heart failure in elderly patients, *Mayo Clin Proc* 72:453, 1997.

16. Tresch DD: The clinical diagnosis of heart failure in older patients, *J Am Geriatr Soc* 45:1128, 1997.

17. Aronow WS: Treatment of congestive heart failure in older persons, *J Am Geriatr Soc* 45:1252, 1997.

18. Doughty R, Andersen V, Sharpe N: Optimal treatment of heart failure in the elderly, *Drugs Aging* 10:435, 1997.

19. Rich MW, Bosner MS, Chung MK, et al: A multidisciplinary intervention to prevent the readmission of elderly patients with congestive heart failure, *N Engl J Med* 33:1190, 1995.

20. Vliestra RE, Gaxiiola E: Aortic stenosis in the elderly: a decade of changing concepts, *Am J Geriatr Cardiol* 6:26, 1997.

21. Cordon M, Huang M, Gryfe CI: An evaluation of falls, syncope, and dizziness by prolonged ambulatory cardiographic monitoring in a geriatric institutional setting, *J Am Geriatr Soc* 30:6, 1982.

22. Hansson L: Hypertension in the elderly, *J Hypertens* 14(suppl 3):17, 1996.

23. Fletcher A, Bulpitt C: Epidemiology of hypertension in the elderly, *J Hypertens* 12(suppl 6):3, 1994.

24. Insua JT et al: Drug treatment of hypertension in the elderly: a meta-analysis, *Ann Intern Med* 121:355, 1994.

25. SHEP Cooperative Research Group: Prevention of stroke by antihypertensive treatment in older persons with isolated systolic hypertension, *JAMA* 265:3255, 1991.

26. Dahlof B, Lindholm LH, Hansson L, et al: Morbidity and mortality in the Swedish Trial in Old Patients with Hypertension (STOP-Hypertension), *Lancet* 338:1281, 1991.

27. MRC Working Party: Medical Research Council trial on treatment of hypertension in older adults: principal results, *Br Med J* 304:405, 1992.

28. Sowers JR, Farrow SL: Treatment of elderly hypertensive patients with diabetes, renal disease, and coronary artery disease, *Am J Geriatr Cardiol* 5:57, 1996.

29. LaRosa JC: Treating cholesterol in the elderly—is it useful? *Clin Geriatr* 5:28, 1997.

30. Kannel WB, Wilson PWF: Update on hyperlipidemia in the elderly: is this a risk factor for heart disease? *Am J Geriatr Cardiol* 5:9, 1996.

31. Adult Treatment Panel II: National Cholesterol Education Program: second report of the expert panel on detection, evaluation, and treatment of high blood cholesterol in adults, *Circulation* 89:1333, 1994.

48 Cardiac Risks of Noncardiac Surgery and Perioperative Management

Quentin A. Pletsch
George J. Taylor

Roughly 1 million of the 25 million people who have noncardiac surgery each year in the United States have underlying coronary artery disease (CAD). More than half of those having vascular surgery also have CAD. The most common cause of death after general surgery is myocardial ischemia. Cardiologists are often asked to define the cardiac risks of anesthesia and surgery and to provide "medical clearance." This evaluation is properly the role of the primary care physician, reserving cardiology consultation for the patient identified as high risk. The primary care physician is also frequently asked to help the surgeon with the management of common cardiac problems before and after surgery.

ASSESSMENT OF CARDIAC RISKS OF NONCARDIAC SURGERY

Identification of high- or low-risk patients is straightforward because it is evidence based. A number of prospective studies carefully gathered clinical data before surgery, then monitored patients for cardiac complications during and after the operation. The findings of these studies are generally in agreement and form the basis of the risk assessment protocols offered by the American College of Physicians (ACP) and by the American Heart Association and American College of Cardiology.[1-3] We particularly like the streamlined organization of the ACP practice guidelines and outline them for your use.

The Patient's Risk

Almost all the data used to define the patient's risk profile come from the history and physical examination (Fig. 48-1, Table 48-1, and Box 48-1). There are two levels of screening. The first uses the cardiac risk index (Box 48-1) to identify those at high risk, who have a 10% to 15% chance of a postoperative cardiac event (including MI and cardiac death). The second level of screening is applied to the remaining patients using the low risk variables (Table 48-1), which allow clinical classification into low- (0 to 3%) and intermediate-risk (3% to 10%) groups.

Level 1 Screen

The modified cardiac risk index uses a point system to rank clinical features that predicted MI or cardiac death

in the multicenter trials (Table 48-1). Thus either class IV angina or critical aortic stenosis indicates higher risk than MI more than 6 months ago. Note that risk factors for premature atherosclerosis, including hypertension, elevated cholesterol, cigarette smoking, obesity, and diabetes, do *not* appear in this box because they were not statistically significant predictors of postoperative complications. Risk is quantified using a point system (Box 48-1). Class II or III patients with at least 20 points have surgery postponed until they are further evaluated and treated (Fig. 48-2).

Level 2 Screen

After the initial screening, non-high-risk patients with 0 to 15 points (class I) are subjected to a second level of screening using "low-risk variables," which are used to screen patients at lower risk (Table 48-1). This list of clinical variables includes diabetes and hypertension plus left ventricular hypertrophy but none of the other risk factors for early CAD (e.g., family history, obesity, dyslipidemia, or cigarette smoking). A patient with none or just one of these findings is classified as truly "low risk" and has less than 3% chance of a cardiac complication of anesthesia and surgery. Noninvasive screening studies for CAD do not refine risk assessment for these lowest risk patients, and the ACP guidelines indicate that any benefit of testing is overshadowed by risks (including unnecessary interventions as well as cost).[2]

The intermediate-risk patient, with two or more of the low-risk variables, has a 3% to 15% chance of a cardiac complication. At this point in the protocol the type of surgery has a role. The evidence supports a diagnostic test for CAD when the patient is to have vascular surgery. There is high incidence of CAD in those with peripheral vascular disease, and prospective studies have shown a benefit from noninvasive testing.

There is uncertainty about the intermediate-risk patient who is having *nonvascular surgery*. The incidence of underlying CAD is lower than it is with vascular disease, and studies have not identified a benefit from noninvasive screening for ischemia.[2] Thus Figure 48-1 suggests surgery without further testing, but hedges by pointing out that the evidence is weak. The American Heart Asso-

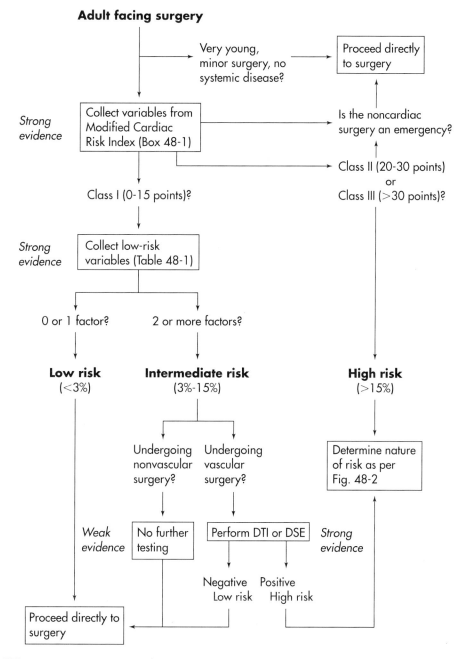

FIG. 48-1

An algorithm for the cardiac risk assessment of patients having noncardiac surgery. Boxed phrases indicate recommended actions. *Italicized* words beside the boxes indicate the level of evidence supporting the recommendation. If no italicized word is present, no evidence exists for or against use. Percentages indicate the chance of a cardiac complication of surgery, usually MI or cardiac death. *DTI,* Dipyridamole thallium imaging; *DSE,* dobutamine stress echocardiography.

From American College of Physicians: *Ann Intern Med* 127:309, 1997.

Table 48-1 | *Low-Risk Variables*

Criteria of Eagle et al.[4]	Criteria of Vanzetto et al.[5]
Age >70 years	Age >70 years
History of angina	History of angina
Diabetes mellitus	Diabetes mellitus
Q waves on ECG	Q waves on ECG
History of ventricular ectopy	History of myocardial infarction
	Ischemic ST segment changes on resting ECG
	Hypertension plus LV hypertrophy on ECG
	History of congestive heart failure

From American College of Physicians: *Ann Intern Med* 127:309, 1997.

BOX 48-1
MODIFIED CARDIAC RISK INDEX*

VARIABLE	POINTS, *n*
Coronary artery disease	
Myocardial infarction <6 months earlier	10
Myocardial infarction >6 months earlier	5
Canadian Cardiovascular Society angina classification†	
Class III	10
Class IV	20
Alveolar pulmonary edema	
Within 1 week	10
Ever	5
Suspected critical aortic stenosis	20
Arrhythmias	
Rhythm other than sinus or sinus plus atrial premature beats on ECG	5
>5 premature ventricular contractions on ECG	5
Poor general medical status, defined as any of the following: Po₂ <60 mm Hg, Pco₂ >50 mm Hg, K⁺ level <3 mmol/L, blood urea nitrogen level >50 mmol/L, creatinine level >260 μmol/L, bedridden	5
Age >70 years	5
Emergency surgery	10

From American College of Physicians: *Ann Intern Med* 127:309, 1997.
*Class 1 = 0 to 15 points; class II = 20 to 30 points; class III = more than 30 points.
†Canadian Cardiovascular Society classification of angina (2): 0 = asymptomatic; I = angina with strenuous exercise; II = angina with moderate exertion; III = angina with walking 1 to 2 level blocks or climbing 1 flight of stairs or less at a normal pace; IV = inability to perform any physical activity without development of angina.

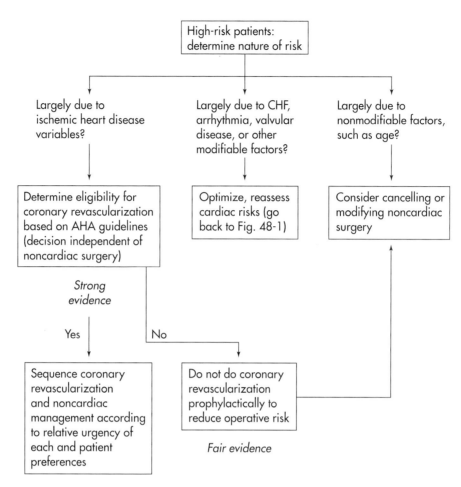

FIG. 48-2

An algorithm for the management of patients at high risk for perioperative cardiac complications. Boxed phrases indicate recommended actions, and *italicized* words below the boxes indicate the level of evidence supporting the recommendation. If no italicized word is present, no evidence exists for or against use. *AHA,* American Heart Association; *CHF,* congestive heart failure.

From American College of Physicians: *Ann Intern Med* 127:309, 1997.

ciation (AHA) guidelines use exercise tolerance to stratify patients; a person with poor functional capacity (an inability to exercise at the 4 MET level or to walk up stairs to the second floor) who is having a high-risk operation might have noninvasive screening for ischemia. With normal exercise tolerance, testing is not recommended.[3]

Risk of the Operation

As noted, MI is more common after vascular than nonvascular surgery, probably because of the incidence of underlying CAD rather than the stress of the operation. The risk of a cardiac event is highest with vascular and orthopedic procedures (13% risk of a cardiac complication) and is followed by abdominal and thoracic (8%), head and neck, and ophthalmic or prostate operations (3%). Emergency surgery, prolonged operations (lasting over 5 hours), and procedures that are hemodynamically stressful are higher risk.[3] Thus resection of a dissecting aortic aneurysm would be considerably riskier than femoral artery bypass surgery. As Box 48-1 acknowledges, emergency surgery precludes screening for CAD, contributing to higher risk.

Comment

Algorithms like the one in Figure 48-1 look complicated and can be intimidating, but this is an especially good algorithm. The clinical data used to make decisions are easily obtained from the history and physical examination. Using the table, the box, and the figure allows prompt assessment of cardiac risk with surgery.

Laboratory Screening for Ischemia

Highest and lowest risk patients are readily identified using clinical variables. It is the intermediate-risk patient who benefits from noninvasive screening, especially when facing vascular surgery.

The stress electrocardiogram (ECG) is of uncertain usefulness. The ACP guideline points out that half or more of those with vascular or orthopedic illness cannot exercise to target heart rate or work load. Its review of clinical trials concludes that exercise testing is not reliable even when a diagnostic test is achieved.[2] On the other hand, the AHA practice guideline indicates that in "most ambulatory patients, the test of choice is exercise ECG testing."[3] Stress imaging studies would be reserved for those who cannot exercise or those who may not have an interpretable ECG. Despite this recommendation, the AHA review indicated that those with a negative stress ECG tended to have a higher complication rate than those with a negative imaging study, so imaging appears to be a more powerful screening tool.

Pharmacologic stress imaging has the largest and best record of performance, and dipyridamole (or adenosine) perfusion scanning and dobutamine stress echocardiography are both effective. One study of intermediate-risk patients found a 1% incidence of MI or cardiac death with a negative perfusion scan and a 23% incidence when the scan was positive for reversible ischemia.[4] With a negative imaging study, no further cardiac evaluation is indicated. However, remind the patient and family that low risk does not mean zero risk. After we have done the best we can do, there remains a finite risk with any operation.

Measurement of left ventricular ejection fraction (LVEF) generally is not useful and is not an element of routine screening. It is worth doing for a patient with heart failure who has not had left ventricular (LV) function documented previously or if there has been a change in clinical status. It may be helpful in sorting out dyspnea of uncertain etiology.

Cardiology Consultation

In some metropolitan areas it has become routine for middle-aged patients to visit a cardiologist before general surgery. We consider this an excessive response to an apparently litigious environment. There is no medical justification for automatic consultation; it is not supported by the American College of Cardiology practice guidelines, and it is not the standard of care.[3] Primary care doctors and surgeons are capable of applying the screening protocol. The high-risk patient, identified by clinical criteria or by a screening study for ischemia, may benefit from cardiology referral, and that is based on the specific needs of the patient and the judgment of his or her doctor.

PREOPERATIVE AND POSTOPERATIVE MANAGEMENT ISSUES

Figure 48-2 outlines the ACP guideline for high-risk patients. Those with clinical or laboratory evidence of uncontrolled ischemia need coronary angiography and possibly revascularization. The risk of noncardiac surgery is lower after coronary revascularization. However, getting the patient through a noncardiac operation is rarely the only indication for bypass surgery or angioplasty. Instead, noncardiac surgery is just one variable within the total clinical picture that is considered when recommending coronary revascularization.[3]

Other cardiac conditions also need to be "tuned up" before surgery. Patients with heart failure should be at dry weight and following optimal afterload-reducing therapy. Arrhythmias should be controlled. Electrolyte levels, including magnesium, should be normalized, an especially important issue for those treated with diuretics.

Beta-Adrenergic Blockade

Those with CAD or those who have risk factors for CAD may be treated with beta-blockers. The Multicenter Study of Perioperative Ischemia Research found that atenolol given throughout hospitalization resulted in an 8% reduction in mortality and a 15% reduction in combined rates of MI, unstable angina, or heart failure requiring hospitalization during a 6-month follow-up.[6] Patient selection for treatment included established CAD or two risk factors for CAD (age at least 65 years, current smoking, hypertension, diabetes, or cholesterol at or exceeding 240 mg/dL) and no contraindications to beta blockade. The result is consistent with other studies that have shown reduced intraoperative ischemia and blood pressure with beta blockade.[2]

This was a relatively small study, but it *suggests* a new standard of care for perioperative management. Further study is needed to confirm the result and to refine patient selection. For example, it is unlikely that beta blockade is needed after revascularization or for other patients with CAD at low risk for active ischemia (e.g., single-vessel CAD and completed MI).

Treatment Protocol

Barring contraindications, for those with a heart rate of at least 55 beats/min and systolic blood pressure greater than 100 mm Hg, give intravenous atenolol 5 mg 30 minutes before surgery and again just after surgery. After surgery, give oral atenolol 50 mg (for heart rate 55 to 64 beats/min) or 100 mg (for heart rate exceeding 65 beats/min) daily until hospital discharge. If the patient is not able to take oral medications, the daily intravenous dose of atenolol is 5 to 10 mg every 12 hours.

Hypertension

Moderate hypertension is not an independent risk factor for cardiac complications.[3] When associated with severe LV hypertrophy, it is a low-risk variable (Table 48-1). Mild to moderate elevation of blood pressure is not an indication to delay surgery. Uncontrolled hypertension, defined by the AHA guidelines as diastolic pres-

sure of at least 110 mm Hg, is a reason to delay elective surgery.[3]

Parenteral beta blockade, as described earlier, is a good way to control blood pressure during surgery. Transdermal clonidine and other intravenous vasodilators may also be used. Because of its heart rate—lowering effect, we also like intravenous diltiazem for mild or moderate hypertension. Severe hypertension that is not easily controlled may require intravenous nitroprusside.

Congestive Heart Failure

It is important to identify heart failure preoperatively because it alters the prognosis and changes postoperative management. If there are symptoms, physical findings, or changes on the ECG or chest x-ray that raise a possibility of LV dysfunction, obtain an echocardiogram. Severe depression of LV function and clinical heart failure are indications for hemodynamic monitoring with a pulmonary artery catheter. The most common cause of postoperative congestion is iatrogenic fluid overload, and the patient with LV dysfunction is more susceptible. Furthermore, salt and water retention are components of the surgical stress response (see later discussion). More careful monitoring of fluid status is necessary. Especially useful are daily weights in addition to intake and output monitoring.

The cause of heart failure also influences management. For example, hypertrophic cardiomyopathy and reduced LV compliance produces a preload-sensitive condition. A loss of atrial contraction with postoperative atrial fibrillation would be poorly tolerated and require urgent cardioversion.

Valvular Heart Disease

Critical aortic stenosis should be repaired before elective noncardiac surgery. Mitral stenosis does not require surgical correction, but careful attention to heart rate is necessary, since tachycardia may lead to pulmonary edema. The stress of surgery may precipitate atrial fibrillation in patients with mitral valve disease and left atrial enlargement.

Endocarditis prophylaxis is the other major consideration for patients with valvular disease and congenital heart disease. Antibiotic coverage is indicated for drainage of an infected site or for oral, lower gastrointestinal, gallbladder, and genitourinary procedures (see Chapter 21).

Atrial Fibrillation and Flutter

Atrial fibrillation and flutter are common "cardiac events" after cardiac and noncardiac surgery, especially in elderly patients. Remember that atrial flutter may be a sign of occult pulmonary embolus. Atrial arrhythmias are commonly precipitated by electrolyte abnormalities, particularly low levels of magnesium. When the magnesium ion (Mg^{+2}) level is below 2.0 mg/dL, our first treatment is replacement so that the level rises to about 2.5 mg/dL, which often requires 6 to 8 g of magnesium sulfate intravenously.

Prompt cardioversion is indicated. Do not wait a couple of days for spontaneous conversion. By then you must worry about peripheral embolization during conversion to sinus rhythm. If correction of electrolyte levels does not work, our next step is ibutilide. More than half of those patients with postoperative atrial fibrillation respond to intravenous ibutilide 1 mg infused over 10 minutes intravenously, with a repeat dose 10 minutes later if atrial fibrillation persists. Ibutilide is a class III agent. Proarrhythmia is possible, with torsade de pointes more likely when the QT interval is prolonged. Most drug trials excluded patients with QT complexes exceeding 440 msec, and that is a relative contraindication. Proarrhythmia risk is also higher with depressed LV function. Those given ibutilide should remain on telemetry for at least 6 hours after treatment.

Concomitant treatment for atrial tachyarrhythmias includes control of the ventricular rate with digoxin, beta blockade, or calcium blocking agents (see Chapter 25). Other drugs may be used for cardioversion. *However, if the rapid heart rate causes hemodynamic instability or unstable angina, do not hesitate to cardiovert immediately using DC countershock.*

A patient with atrial fibrillation before surgery should have good control of ventricular rate (see Chapter 25). Prophylactic digitalization has been suggested (without evidence-based support) for patients in sinus rhythm at high risk for postoperative atrial fibrillation, including the elderly and others with subcritical mitral valve disease, a history of supraventricular arrhythmias, or known left atrial enlargement. Chest surgery provokes atrial fibrillation more than other operations.

Anticoagulants

No clinical trial data have clarified the perioperative management of anticoagulation. Practice varies widely. Kearon and Hirsh[7] have reviewed the available evidence and make sensible and conservative recommendations (Table 48-2).

High Risk for Embolism

During the first month after a thromboembolic event the risk of recurrence is highest (40% recurrence of venous and 15% recurrence of arterial thromboembolism).[7] Thus it is best to delay elective surgery for at least 1 month after any thromboembolic event, since surgery always requires interruption of warfarin therapy. If surgery must be done in the first, high-risk month, warfarin may be stopped 4 days before surgery, and intravenous heparin started 2 days *before* surgery, while the INR is normalizing. *Postoperative* heparin has a net ben-

Table 48-2	Recommendations for Preoperative and Postoperative Anticoagulation in Patients Who Are Taking Oral Anticoagulants*		
Indication		**Before Surgery**	**After Surgery**
Acute venous thromboembolism			
Month 1		IV heparin†	IV heparin†
Months 2 and 3		No change‡	IV heparin
Recurrent venous thromboembolism§		No change‡	SC heparin
Acute arterial embolism			
Month 1		IV heparin	IV heparin¶
Mechanical heart valve		No change‡	SC heparin
Nonvalvular atrial fibrillation		No change‡	SC heparin

From Kearon C, Hirsh J: *N Engl J Med* 336:1506, 1997.

*IV heparin denotes intravenous heparin at therapeutic doses, and SC heparin subcutaneous unfractionated or low-molecular-weight heparin in doses recommended for prophylaxis against venous thromboembolism in high-risk patients.

†A vena caval filter may be considered if acute venous thromboembolism has occurred within 2 weeks or if the risk of bleeding during intravenous heparin therapy is high.

‡Intravenous heparin is not substituted for warfarin. If convenient, subcutaneous heparin may be used (e.g., if patient is in hospital).

§The term refers to patients whose last episode of venous thromboembolism occurred more than 3 months before evaluation but who require long-term anticoagulation because of a high risk of recurrence.

¶Intravenous heparin should be used after surgery only if the risk of bleeding is low.

efit for those with recent venous thrombosis and probably for patients with recent arterial embolus, despite an increase in bleeding. It is usually started 12 hours after surgery if there is no active bleeding (timing is the surgeon's decision). It is continued for about 3 days and is stopped once the INR is above 2.0.

Lower Risk for Embolism

The usual indications for chronic warfarin therapy are recurrent venous thromboembolism (the risk of repeat embolus is 15% per year) and as prophylaxis for those with nonvalvular atrial fibrillation (4.5% per year risk of embolism) or a mechanical heart valve (8% per year risk).[7] Reviewing available data, Kearon and Hirsh[6] suggest that full-dose, intravenous heparin increases overall morbidity for chronically anticoagulated patients who have not had a recent embolism. The increase in bleeding with heparin overshadows the small benefit from reduced embolism, since the absolute risk of embolism is so low (Table 48-2).

There is a spectrum of risk within this group. A patient with nonvalvular atrial fibrillation with a remote history of arterial embolus has a 12% per year risk of recurrence. The risk of embolization is higher for atrial fibrillation plus mitral valve disease or LV dilation and dysfunction. Mechanical prostheses in the mitral valve position are more prone to thrombosis than aortic valve prostheses. If such issues, or their combination, raise particular concern for a patient, you may decide to treat with intravenous heparin for 2 days before surgery, but the risks of intravenous heparin *after* surgery exceed any benefit.[7] Instead, resume the maintenance dose of warfarin 1 to 3 days after surgery, depending on the operation and clinical course.

No evidence indicates that *subcutaneous* heparin prevents arterial thromboembolism in patients with atrial fibrillation or mechanical heart valves. Nevertheless, it appears sensible to prescribe it in the usual fashion as prophylaxis against postoperative venous thrombosis.[7] You may be killing two birds with one stone.

MANAGEMENT DURING SURGERY: THE ANESTHESIOLOGIST'S PERSPECTIVE

Surgical mortality and morbidity have decreased despite the fact that elderly patients with significant concomitant diseases represent an increasingly greater percentage of patients having surgery. Better outcomes can be attributed to several factors, including improvements in anesthesia, preoperative cardiovascular tuning, intraoperative and postoperative monitoring and management, and advances in surgical techniques.

General versus Regional Anesthesia

General and regional anesthesia are compared in Box 48-2. Regional anesthesia includes spinal and epidural anesthesia administered either as a "single shot" or as a continuous infusion of local anesthetics through a catheter.

General Anesthetic Agents

Significant properties of nitrous oxide and of the potent volatile anesthetic agents are listed in Table 48-3. Nitrous oxide is not sufficiently potent to be used alone as an inhalation anesthetic and thus is usually used in combination with a second agent to achieve surgical anesthesia. Administering nitrous oxide reduces the dose requirement of the second agent and thus decreases the undesirable side effects of the second agent. Nitrous oxide stimulates the sympathetic nervous system, resulting in increased sympathetic tone that counteracts the hypotensive effect of the second agent. Compared with the potent anesthetic agents, nitrous oxide alone has minimal respiratory depressant effects. Although nitrous oxide does not undergo significant biotransformation and thus is

---

BOX 48-2
COMPARISON OF REGIONAL AND GENERAL ANESTHESIA

REGIONAL ANESTHESIA	GENERAL ANESTHESIA
Primary anesthetic is a local anesthetic (e.g., bupivacaine or lidocaine)	Primary anesthetic is a potent, volatile agent (e.g., halothane or isoflurane)
No cardiac depression	Direct myocardial depression
Spontaneous respiration without respiratory depression	Respiratory depression requiring assisted or controlled ventilation
Protective airway reflexes maintained	Loss of protective airway reflexes
No organ toxicity	Slight risk of hepatic or renal toxicity
Compromised sympathetic nervous system resulting in hypotension*	Most agents depress the sympathetic nervous system
Local anesthetic drugs not associated with malignant hyperthermia	Minimal effect on surgical stress response
Greatly attenuates the stress response to surgery	All potent, volatile agents can trigger malignant hyperthermia

---

*The hypotensive effect of regional anesthesia may be more difficult to control than hypotension with general anesthesia. For this reason, regional anesthesia is often not used in patients with aortic stenosis.

relatively free of organ toxicity, there is evidence that chronic exposure of operating room personnel results in an increased incidence of spontaneous abortions, decreased fertility, and neuropathies.

The potent anesthetic agents have several properties in common (Table 48-3). All produce dose-dependent respiratory depression that blunts ventilatory drive in response to hypercapnia and hypoxemia. All agents are pungent, although halothane and sevoflurane are relatively less so and will allow a smooth inhalation induction of anesthesia. Pungent vapors irritate the respiratory tract, resulting in coughing, breath holding, laryngospasm, and increased secretions. All agents cause arterial hypotension as a result of direct myocardial depression and vasodilation; however, cardiac output may or may not be maintained, depending on the extent of vasodilation and the increase in heart rate. The depression in systemic blood pressure is partially offset by surgical stress (see later discussion). The volatile agents disrupt autoregulation of cerebral blood flow with a resulting increase in intracranial pressure. Generally, blood flow to the liver and kidneys is reduced, and liver and renal toxicity may be significant, especially in patients with preexisting hepatic or renal dysfunction. Postoperative nausea and vomiting are commonly associated with all agents, although the site of the surgical procedure and the administration of narcotics also plays a role. Finally, all agents can trigger malignant hyperthermia in susceptible patients.

Halothane was introduced into clinical practice more than 40 years ago. Although it is still commonly used in pediatric patients because of its rapid, smooth induction of anesthesia and lack of airway irritation, newer agents have largely replaced its use in adults (Table 48-3). Isoflurane is now the most commonly used inhalation agent in the United States. In contrast to halothane, cardiac output is generally maintained during isoflurane anesthesia. The maintenance of cardiac output can be explained by peripheral arterial vasodilation that reduces systemic vascular resistance and slightly increases heart rate. Isoflurane causes a dose-dependent depression of ventilation, and it blocks hypoxic pulmonary vasoconstriction, which leads to the development of hypercapnia and ventilation-perfusion mismatching during anesthesia. Only approximately 0.2% of isoflurane is metabolized, resulting in the low toxicity seen with this agent. Newer agents, desflurane and sevoflurane, have special properties that may make

Table 48-3	Clinical Advantages and Disadvantages of Selected Inhalational Anesthetics	

Anesthetic	Advantages	Disadvantages
Nitrous oxide	Analgesia Rapid uptake and elimination Little cardiac or respiratory depression Nonpungent	Sympathetic stimulation Expansion of closed air spaces Requires high concentration Interferes with vitamin B_{12} metabolism
Halothane	Inexpensive Effective in low concentrations Nonpungent	Chemically less stable Slow uptake and elimination Susceptible to biotransformation Idiosyncratic hepatic toxicity Decreases cardiac output Catecholamine-induced ventricular ectopy
Isoflurane	Good muscle relaxation Decreases cerebral metabolic rate Minimal biotransformation* Maintains cardiac output	Pungent odor Potent vasodilator
Desflurane	Rapid uptake and elimination Stable molecule Minimal biotransformation	Airway irritant Low boiling point Sympathetic stimulation Pungent odor
Sevoflurane	Rapid uptake and elimination Nonpungent	Susceptible to biotransformation Reacts with soda lima and Baralyme Increases serum fluoride concentrations
Enflurane	Good muscle relaxation Stable heart rate	Pungent odor Seizure activity on EEG Decreases cardiac output (myocardial depression)

*Agents with minimal biotransformation and that are eliminated by the lungs have less renal and hepatic toxicity.

them good choices for selected patients. Enflurane is used with less frequency (Table 48-3).

Regional Anesthesia

Although the physiologic advantages of a regional anesthetic in patients with significant heart disease have been well-documented, significant differences in cardiac complications between regional and general anesthesia have not been reported. For example, a recent study by Bode et al.[8] involving 423 patients with vascular disease undergoing peripheral vascular surgery demonstrated that the choice of anesthetic technique (general, spinal, epidural) did not significantly affect cardiac complications or hospital length of stay.

Box 48-3 describes commonly used regional anesthetic techniques, and Table 48-4 describes practical considerations used in choosing a technique. Patient factors such as mental status, ability to communicate, anxiety level, and ability to cooperate are important when administering regional anesthesia. Duration and type of surgery and patient positioning are important. An inadequate regional anesthetic or a surgical procedure that outlasts the regional anesthetic may require conversion to a general anesthetic technique, and studies have demonstrated that the combination increases the risk for cardiac complications when compared with successful regional or general anesthesia alone. Operations such as transurethral resections of the prostate, which may be complicated by bladder perforation, can be more easily monitored under regional anesthesia because the patient can indicate abdominal pain. Since regional anesthetics cause a partial sympathetic blockade, there is a diminished ability to compensate for acute blood loss, and significant hypotension may occur during the procedure. Patients with hyperactive airways, such as those with asthma or obstructive pulmonary disease, may avoid the stimulus of endotracheal intubation if a regional technique is used. In healthy obstetric patients for whom outcomes are similar for both regional and general anesthetics, patients often have

BOX 48-3
COMPARISON OF SPINAL AND EPIDURAL ANESTHESIA

SPINAL	EPIDURAL
Rapid onset	More gradual onset
Lower concentration of drug	Lower incidence of hypotension
More profound (dense) block	Possible to selectively block different levels of spinal cord
Greater incidence of postdural puncture headache	

SPINAL AND EPIDURAL

Awake patient with protective airway reflexes

Sympathetic block with resulting afterload reduction

Continuous infusion possible for postoperative analgesia

strong preferences for the ability to be awake for the delivery and to interact with their spouse and infant.

The induction of general anesthesia can be associated with myocardial depression and hypotension, which may not be well tolerated by patients with significant cardiac disease. Vasodilation and myocardial depression can usually be treated with intravenous fluids and vasoactive drugs.

Advantages of a general anesthetic include the establishment of a secure airway, the establishment and maintenance of a relatively stable blood pressure in most patients, the ability to match the duration of the anesthetic to the duration of the procedure, and the ability to accommodate the wishes of many patients who prefer to be "asleep."

Surgical Stress Response

We are beginning to have a greater understanding of the importance of physiologic changes that occur in response to the trauma of surgical stimulation and how these changes affect perioperative morbidity and mortality. The stress response to surgery involves changes in the autonomic nervous system and endocrine system, many of which persist for several days (Table 48-5). Regional anesthetic techniques decrease the stress response. This

---

Table 48-4 | *Practical Considerations in Choosing an Anesthetic Technique*

Anesthesia Type	Desirable	Undesirable
Regional	Cardiac contractility maintained	Vasodilation from sympathetic block may lead to hypotension
	Reduction in afterload may improve left ventricular function	Reduction in preload may reduce ventricular filling pressures
	Patient awake with spontaneous respirations	Oversedation of restless patient may lead to respiratory depression and airway obstruction
	Decrease in stress response	
	Avoids endotracheal intubation	
	Low organ toxicity	
	Preferred by obstetric patients	
General	Airway secure	Myocardial depression and hypotension
	Unlimited duration	Decreased pulmonary mechanics such as decreased compliance and functional residual capacity
	Often patient preference	Higher incidence of postoperative nausea and vomiting
	Good blood pressure control	Hepatic and renal toxicity (rare)

advantage of regional anesthesia is more pronounced in surgical procedures performed below the level of the umbilicus (T10) and less so for operations performed on the upper half of the body.

Notably, regional anesthetics reduce the incidence of postoperative arterial thromboembolism in patients with peripheral vascular disease, probably by blocking secretion of plasminogen activator inhibitor-1 (PAI-1). Patients undergoing major orthopedic surgery, such as total hip replacement, using epidural anesthesia have a decreased incidence of deep vein thrombosis and pulmonary embolism. Selective blockade by thoracic epidural anesthesia of sympathetic innervation to the heart at the level of T1-T4 would theoretically decrease myocardial oxygen demand, improve hemodynamics, and increase coronary blood flow to ischemic regions of the heart. However, regional anesthesia has not been found to lessen the incidence of postoperative MI in patients with CAD.

Although blunting the stress response seems desirable, equally apparent is the necessity of this response for the body to survive the stressful event successfully. Activation of the sympathetic nervous system along with the many hormonal changes help maintain blood pressure, increase central venous pressure, maintain perfusion of vital organs, promote hemostasis, and enhance the metabolic pathways for energy requirements.

Postoperative Analgesia

Numerous studies have confirmed that postoperative pain relief is better with the administration of local anesthetics and analgesics through an epidural catheter than with systemic opioids. The stress response to surgery involving the humoral, metabolic, and sympathetic changes reaches its maximal effect after surgery, and the continuation of local anesthetic administration into the immediate postoperative period can modify the extent of the response. Systemic administration of opioids alone is not adequate to attenuate the stress response even when adequate analgesia is achieved. Continuous infusion of local anesthetics and opioids through an epidural catheter has several distinct advantages over intermittent administration of systemic opioids by intramuscular injection, patient-controlled analgesia (PCA) infusion, or oral administration. For example, continuous infusion of narcotics keeps patients in a steady-state condition of analgesia, avoiding variance in blood levels. In addition, the amount of narcotics administered can be greatly decreased if administered through the epidural catheter, thereby decreasing the incidence of side effects like nausea and vomiting, respiratory depression, urinary retention, and pruritus. Although some studies have suggested that patients receiving epidural narcotics are able to walk sooner, have lowered morbidity, and are hospitalized for less time, it is not clear whether improved postoperative analgesia improves outcomes.

Table 48-5 | *The Surgical Stress Response*

Stress Hormone or Effect*	Physiologic Change
Catecholamines (both epinephrine and norepinephrine)	Increased heart rate, peripheral vascular resistance, blood pressure, myocardial contractility and oxygen consumption; gluconeogenesis
Vasopressin	Fluid retention
Corticotropin and cortisol	Increased blood glucose (gluconeogenesis)
Aldosterone	Sodium (fluid) retention
Increased glucagon, decreased insulin	Increased blood glucose
Decreased thyroid-stimulating hormone	Lower thyroid hormone (lower metabolic rate)
Plasminogen activator inhibitor (PAI)-1	Decreased fibrinolysis, higher fibrinogen, and a hypercoagulable state
Increased platelet aggregation	Hypercoagulable state

* A number of these effects persist for a week after surgery.

REFERENCES

1. American College of Physicians: Guidelines for assessing and managing the perioperative risk from coronary artery disease associated with major noncardiac surgery, *Ann Intern Med* 127:309, 1997.
2. Palda VA, Detsky AS: Perioperative assessment and management of risk from coronary artery disease, *Ann Intern Med* 127:313, 1997.
3. Eagle KA, Brundage BH, Chaitman BR, et al: Guidelines for perioperative cardiovascular evaluation for noncardiac surgery: report of the American College of Cardiology/American Heart Association Task Force on Practice Guidelines (Committee on Perioperative Cardiovascular Evaluation for Noncardiac Surgery), *J Am Coll Cardiol* 27:910, 1996.
4. Eagle KA, Coley CM, Newell JB, et al: Combining clinical and thallium data optimizes preoperative assessment of cardiac risk before major vascular surgery, *Ann Intern Med* 110:859, 1989.
5. Vanzetto G, Machecourt J, Blendea D, et al: Additive value of thallium single-photon emission computed tomography myocardial imaging for prediction of perioperative events in clinically selected high cardiac risk patients having abdominal aortic surgery, *Am J Cardiol* 77:143, 1996.
6. Mangano DT, Layug EL, Wallace A, Tareo I: Effects of atenolol on mortality and cardiovascular morbidity after non cardiac surgery. The Multicenter Study of Perioperative Ischemia Research Group, *N Engl J Med* 335:1713, 1996.
7. Kearon C, Hirsh J: Management of anticoagulation before and after elective surgery, *N Engl J Med* 336:1506, 1997.
8. Bode RH et al: Cardiac outcome after peripheral vascular surgery, *Anesthesiology* 84:3, 1996.

BIBLIOGRAPHY

Carpenter RL: Does outcome change with pain management? *Refresher Courses in Anesthesiology* 23:29, 1995.

Roy RC: General versus regional anesthesia for the elderly patient, *Refresher Courses in Anesthesiology* 24:233, 1996.

Wiklund RA, Rosenbaum SH: Anesthesiology (two parts), *N Engl J Med* 337:1132, 1997.

49 Insurance, Disability, and Other Legal Issues

Charles L. Lucore
Mark E. Hansen

DISABILITY DUE TO ESTABLISHED OR PRESUMED CARDIOVASCULAR DISEASE

Considerable attention has been focused on the interrelationships between cardiovascular disease, long-term health, and employment. The cost associated with cardiovascular disease and disability includes the cost of medical care for patients with acute and chronic disease, as well as the indirect cost associated with loss of productivity and permanent loss of employment. Equally important is that a person's self-esteem is related to performance in the workplace. Premature disability may contribute not only to economic hardship but also to diminished self-esteem and, in some cases, psychiatric illness.

Disability with Coronary Artery Disease

Mark et al.[1] published an excellent study evaluating factors responsible for disability in patients with coronary disease. Patients referred for diagnostic catheterization were evaluated at that time and at follow-up. Medical, functional, psychologic, economic, and job-related variables were evaluated. One-year follow-up was 91% of the initial cohort (1252 patients). Patients who were no longer working at 1 year generally were older, female, or African-American. Diabetes and hypertension were more prevalent among patients not working at 1 year. Patients who were disabled had more severe functional impairment from angina at initial evaluation or had a history of heart failure. Co-morbid conditions such as cerebrovascular and peripheral vascular disease were also more common. As confirmed by logistic regression analysis, independent variables predicting disability at 1 year after catheterization included age, race, congestive heart failure, and extracardiac vascular disease.[1]

Physically demanding employment also was associated with more disability at 1 year. However, psychosocial demands and job stress were not predictive of employment status; 84% of patients having percutaneous transluminal angioplasty (PTCA) and 79% of patients receiving coronary artery bypass grafting (CABG) were still working at 1 year. Although the most powerful predictors of lack of employment at 1 year were congestive heart failure or evidence of extracardiac vascular disease, demographic and socioeconomic factors such as age, race, and education were responsible for 45% of the predictive information allowing assessment of return to work. Interestingly, left ventricular ejection fraction and extent of coronary disease (number of diseased vessels), the two most powerful predictors of mortality in coronary disease, were not predictive of 1 year employment based on multivariate logistic regression analysis. In this selected, nonrandomized population, it did not appear that coronary revascularization in this study ultimately improved return to work rates as compared with medical therapy.[1]

Disability and Return to Work after Coronary Revascularization

Several studies have evaluated the effects of CABG and PTCA on angina, employment status, and self-perception of health. An early report from Hammermeister et al.[2] indicated that work status 3 months after surgery or catheterization was the best predictor of continued employment 15 months later. Mark et al.[3] evaluated the effects of PTCA, CABG, or medical therapy on unemployment at 1 year in patients with coronary disease. Patients who had coronary angioplasty returned to work earlier than those who had bypass surgery, but at 1 year no significant differences in employment rates were noted. Patients selected for medical therapy had rates of return to work similar to patients who underwent revascularization. However, these were selected groups and not randomized.

The most recent evaluation is from the randomized intervention, treatment of angina (RITA) trial.[4] This study found that patients who had undergone angioplasty returned to work more rapidly than patients who had bypass surgery, but at 2 years no significant difference was noted in employment rates between groups with either revascularization strategy. Both revascularization strategies were effective for relief of angina, although patients undergoing angioplasty were more likely to require repeat intervention within 1 year to further relieve recurrent angina (33% versus 3.4%). Angina did appear to contribute to impairment of health and of self-esteem in these patients. A predictor of well-being included relief of angina with successful revascularization.[4]

Another study by Fitzgerald et al.[5] identified that, although patients after PTCA may return to work sooner

519

than those having coronary artery bypass grafting (59% at 1 month and 87% at 6 months), many patients still lacked the confidence in their ability to return to work even when they appeared to be physically capable of doing so. Patients with physically demanding jobs (blue collar), low levels of self-confidence, and fewer than 12 years of education were less likely than other patients to resume work over the 2-year study period.

All these studies emphasize that social, educational, and psychologic factors have similar importance to physical disability in determining return to employment following the identification of ischemic heart disease.

Return to Work after Acute Myocardial Infarction

These concepts also apply to return to work following myocardial infarction. Although length of hospital stay for treatment of myocardial infarction has dramatically decreased over the past 15 years, the timing of return to work has not changed substantially. [6] Return to work appeared to be affected by physician recommendation, patient independence, and perception of adequate support to return to work. Riegel et al.[7] reported that 60% of those initially employed returned to work at 1 month, and almost 90% returned to work at 4 months after myocardial infarction. Predictors of return to work at 1 month were younger age, absence of extracardiac medical problems, better health perceptions, and adequate socioeconomic support. Dennis et al.[8] reported that the early return to work of individuals deemed at "low risk" on the basis of an occupational evaluation was associated with important economic benefits. The study suggested that occupational evaluation may facilitate return to work and also expedite the physician's recommendations for return to work. [8]

Chest Pain and Its Psychosocial Aspects

Specific factors leading to disability in patients with documented ischemic heart disease have been identified.[1] However, patients who have chronic chest pain may or may not have underlying ischemic heart disease. Numerous studies have shown that patients with chest pain, whether they have coronary disease or not, often have psychiatric disorders including panic disorder, hypochondriasis, depression, or phobias. The effect of these psychiatric illnesses on disability has been well documented by Chernen et al.[9] It is important to note that patients with noncardiac chest pain have an excellent prognosis.[10,11] However, maintenance of social and occupational productivity remains as challenging for patients with chest pain without identifiable coronary disease as it does for patients with documented coronary disease.

Although psychiatric disorders, namely generalized anxiety, depression, and somatic neuroticism, have been observed in patients with chronic coronary dis-

ease, exceptionally high rates of these illnesses are also found in patients with chest pain and no significant coronary disease. These patients have a particularly high rate of health care facility use and an inability to return to work. One study of a cohort of 570 patients with chest pain and normal coronary angiograms found that 43% had panic disorder and another 26% had a generalized anxiety disorder.[12] To more effectively manage these patients whose disability levels may rival those of patients having coronary artery disease, behavioral and psychiatric evaluation may be helpful, as may psychopharmacologic therapy.

Disability Due to Life-Threatening Arrhythmias

The use of automatic implantable cardiac defibrillators (AICD) has been increasing in patients with life-threatening ventricular arrhythmias and sudden death.[13] These arrhythmias are characterized by their unpredictability, rapidity of onset, and potential for severe incapacitation. AICDs, although life-sustaining, do not eradicate arrhythmias. The AICD invariably imposes psychologic stress. Physician awareness of state and federal regulations concerning driving and the use of heavy machinery by patients with serious ventricular arrhythmias or sudden death may be limited. In fact, as recently as 1994 only eight states had specific regulations addressing motor vehicle operation by patients with syncope caused by cardiac arrhythmias.[14] Most physicians in these areas—even electrophysiologists—were not aware of the local regulations.

Anderson and Camm[14] suggested a tentative structure for regulations pertaining to driving and work by patients with AICDs. They stressed that their recommendations were excessively cautious. Patients who had not received DC countershock from their device within 12 to 24 months and who had significant LV dysfunction could be considered for return to driving. Those with higher ejection fractions who were without symptomatic arrhythmias could return to driving within 6 months of AICD placement. For patients who have been shocked by their device, the data are insufficient at this point to conclude when it may be safe to resume driving. The authors felt that patients with AICDs should not resume driving as an occupation nor should they engage in others where syncope would create public risk.

Beauregard et al.[15] recently reviewed actual driving risks in patients with arrhythmia control devices. They emphasized that *patients* believed that their risk of a significant disabling arrhythmic event while driving was quite low. There may be some clinical experience to support this. Since few states have regulations concerning driving by individuals with arrhythmia and AICDs, the authors recommended that the risk of driving should be carefully considered for all patients with AICDs. Driving

restrictions might be based on the type of arrhythmia. For recurrent sustained ventricular tachycardia, indefinite driving prohibition might be reasonable. However, for patients with ventricular fibrillation without recurrence, 1 year of prohibition may allow an estimation of risk for recurrent episodes, and if there are no further episodes in 1 year, the risk may be lower than in patients with frequent discharges or recurrent arrhythmia. Whatever the physician recommends should be done with knowledge of state and federal guidelines, if any, and with adequate documentation. [15]

Employment, Insurability, and Congenital Heart Disease

Truesdell and McGrath[16] documented the problems encountered by adults with congenital heart disease in the workforce. Even patients with mild congenital cardiac anomalies were refused employment 50% more often than those with no cardiac disability. Those with moderate to severe disability were denied employment four times as often as normal individuals, and unemployment rates are three times the national average. More recently, employment rates among patients with mild congenital heart disease are improving, but employment rates for patients with ventricular septal defect, pulmonic stenosis, and aortic stenosis have not increased.

Truesdell and McGrath[16] indicate that young adults with congenital heart disease who appear limited occupationally by their handicaps should be considered for vocational rehabilitation. The American Heart Association has classified activity recommendations for young patients with heart disease based on anatomic lesion and its severity (Boxes 49-1 and 49-2).

Although federal regulations favor employment for these individuals, and guidelines are available for the extent and intensity of occupations depending on the disorder, patients typically meet resistance in the job market. [16] Much of the misunderstanding is related to the inability of employers to assess the true severity of even mild congenital abnormalities. However, some patients may also perceive themselves to be more disabled than their physician's assessment. This erroneous view

---

BOX 49-1

CLASSIFICATION OF OCCUPATIONAL ACTIVITY—FOR USE WITH OCCUPATIONAL RECOMMENDATIONS

CATEGORY I
Very heavy work: Peak load of 7.6 cal/min and above. Involves lifting objects in excess of 100 lb, with frequent lifting or carrying of objects weighing 50 lb or more.

CATEGORY II
Heavy work: Peak load of 7.6 cal/min and above. Involves lifting 100 lb maximum and frequent lifting or carrying of objects weighing up to 50 lb.

CATEGORY III
Medium work: Peak load of 5 to 7.5 cal/min. Involves lifting 50 lb maximum, with frequent lifting or carrying of objects weighing up to 25 lb.

CATEGORY IV
Light work: Peak load of 2.6 to 4.9 cal/min. Involves lifting 20 lb maximum, with frequent lifting and carrying of objects weighing up to 10 lb. Even though the weight may be negligible, a job is also in this category if it requires considerable walking or standing, or if it involves sitting most of the time with some pushing and pulling of arm or leg controls.

CATEGORY V
Sedentary work: Peak load of 2.5 cal/min and below. Involves lifting 10 lb maximum and occasionally lifting or carrying such articles as dockets, ledgers, and small tools. Although a sedentary job is defined as one that involves sitting, a certain amount of walking and standing is often necessary. Jobs are sedentary if walking and standing are required only occasionally and other sedentary criteria are met.

Data from Gutgesell HP, Gessner IH, Vetter VL, et al: *Circulation* 74:5, 1986, American Heart Association. In McGrath KA, Truesdell SC: *Nurs Clin North Am* 29:319, 1994.

BOX 49-2

OCCUPATIONAL RECOMMENDATIONS FOR YOUNG PATIENTS WITH HEART DISEASE

DIAGNOSIS	OCCUPATIONAL	DIAGNOSIS	OCCUPATIONAL
Aortic insufficiency		Pulmonary stenosis	
Mild	II	Mild	I
Moderate	III	Moderate	III
Severe	IV	Severe	IV
Aortic stenosis		Pulmonary hypertension	
Mild	II	(idiopathic)	
Moderate	III	PA pressure < 0.5 systemic	IV
Severe	IV	PA pressure ≥ 0.5 systemic	V
Atrial septal defect		Tetralogy of Fallot, postoperative	
No PVOD	I	RV pressure < 50 mm Hg*	II
Mild to moderate PVOD	III	RV pressure ≥ 50 mm Hg	III
Moderate PVOD	IV	or cardiomegaly	
Cardiomyopathy		Ventricular septal defect	
Congestive (dilated)	V	No PVOD	I
Hypertrophic	IV	Mild to moderate PVOD	III
Coarctation of aorta		Moderate to severe PVOD	IV
Operated, normal BP	I	Other major defects†	
Hypertensive	III	(unoperated or palliated only)	IV
Hypertension		Other major defects†	
Mild	II	(postoperative intracardiac	
Moderate or severe	III	repair)	III
Mitral insufficiency		Cardiac arrhythmias	
Mild, no cardiomegaly	II	Complete heart block	II
Moderate	III	Pacemaker (artificial)	II
Severe (+/− atrial fibrillation)	V	Premature atrial contractions	I
Mitral stenosis		Premature ventricular	
Mild	III	contractions with	
Moderate	IV	Normal heart	I
Severe (+/− atrial fibrillation)	V	Congenital or acquired heart	III
Mitral valve prolapse		disease	
Mild, no symptoms	I	Supraventricular tachycardia	II
Patent ductus arteriosus		Ventricular tachycardia with	
No PVOD	I	Normal heart	II
Mild to moderate PVOD	III	Congenital or acquired heart	IV
Moderate to severe PVOD	IV	disease	
		Wolff-Parkinson-White	I

Data from Gutgesell HP, Gessner IH, Vetter VL, et al: *Circulation* 74:5, 1986, American Heart Association. In McGrath KA, Truesdell SC: *Nurs Clin North Am* 29:319, 1994.
*Exercise testing recommended before athletic competition.
†Marked individual variation exists for these categories. Recommendations should be adjusted for individual requirements.
PVOD, Pulmonary vascular occlusive disease (pulmonary hypertension).

could lead to disability and many times can be alleviated or at least addressed by second opinions or long-term counseling and support.

Deanfield and Celermajer[17] evaluated the employability of young adults with congenital heart disease. Regardless of whether the defect was corrected, they found inconsistencies in job policies, because of the lack of appropriate guidelines limiting employment opportunities for young adults with congenital heart disease. In Great Britain, patients with complex congenital heart lesions

Table 49-1	*Objective Criteria for SSA Disability**

Illness	Test	Objective Functional Criteria
Coronary artery disease (angina pectoris)	1. Stress electrocardiogram, stress perfusion scan, stress echocardiogram, stress radionuclide angiogram 2. Coronary angiogram	1. A positive test documenting stress-induced ischemia at a workload $\leq$5 METS (must have the ECG tracings, not just the report) 2. Flow-restricting stenosis and a clinical history indicating that exercise testing "presents a risk to the individual" (e.g., unstable angina pectoris; see Chapter 13)
Congestive heart failure	Cardiac imaging study	1. CT radio >0.5 on chest x-ray, or 2. LV diastolic size >5.5 cm on echo, or 3. LV ejection fraction $\leq$30%
Peripheral artery disease	Doppler studies	Ankle-brachial systolic blood pressure ratio <0.5. Exercise studies may be done if the ratio is >0.5.
Arrhythmias	Ambulatory monitoring	Arrhythmia coincident with syncope or near-syncope despite best therapy
Cyanotic congenital heart disease		1. Hematocrit $\geq$55%, or arterial O_2 saturation <90% on room air, or PO_2 $\leq$60, or 2. Exercise-induced cyanosis with PO_2 $\leq$60 at an exercise level $\leq$5 METS, or 3. Heart failure with ventricular dysfunction (as described above)
Cardiac transplant		Considered disabled for 1 year, then evaluated with the above criteria

*To be used in addition to clinical findings indicating functional limitation. From the Social Security Administration: Disability evaluation under Social Security, SSA pub no 64-039, 1998.

were uninsurable, and those with mild lesions were insured at a very high rates. Significant inconsistencies were noted between various insurance companies.[17]

Disability and Congestive Heart Failure

The advent of angiotensin-converting enzyme inhibitors and angiotensin II blocking agents have contributed to improved functional capacity in patients with heart failure. However, heart failure remains a significant contributor to disability in patients with and without coronary disease.[1] The 1990 Americans with Disabilities Act mandates that an employer cannot prohibit employees from returning to work after an episode of congestive heart failure if they can perform the essential functions of their jobs with and without reasonable accommodations.

Writing the Disability Application Letter

We are commonly asked to write a letter supporting a patient's application for disability benefits. The physi-

cian often recoils from this important service for a variety of reasons. A physician may believe the patient is not truly disabled and therefore does not qualify for benefits. The physician feels uncomfortable about having to disagree with the patient (in medicine we rarely find ourselves in a adversarial position). Physicians also may be uncertain about how to write such a letter.

The biggest mistake is to argue with your patient about his or her disability status. By doing so, you suggest to the patient that you have some control over the process, when you do not. *Instead, you should point out that the doctor does not make the disability determination;* that is done by the relevant agency (Social Security Administration, SSA, or the insurance company). All the doctor does is supply the data. One benefit of this system is that the doctor can remain the patient's friend and advocate, gathering supportive data and presenting it in as favorable light as possible. If the chance of a favorable ruling is small, you may point this out to the patient, yet still assert that you will do your best to help.

SSA disability benefits for heart disease usually require objective evidence of cardiac dysfunction (Table 49-1). The criteria are found in SSA Publication No. 64-039, *Disability Evaluation Under Social Security*, also known as the "blue book." (The state department of vocational rehabilitation is the best place to find a copy; calling the SSA information number did not work for us.)

We construct the disability letter in three sections. The first is a description of the medical history including specific information about exercise-limiting symptoms. The second, and most important, is a presentation of objective evidence of cardiac disability (Table 49-1). The third is a description of your work recommendations based on clinical and laboratory evidence. For example: "Because of angina with mild exertion and a positive stress ECG at low workloads, I have recommended that the patient lift and carry no more than 15 pounds (about one bag of groceries)."

Patients usually are unfamiliar with the disability application process. Many believe that any episode of cardiac illness disables them. An honest description of how the process works, and of the required objective evidence, may convince some not to waste time with a futile effort. Thus a patient who has no demonstrable ischemia and normal LV function after bypass surgery usually decides not to apply for SSA disability.

On the other hand, we frequently encounter patients who obviously qualify for disability benefits but who give up after the initial rejection by SSA. Such rejections often are the result of the SSA having inadequate data. Your job is to collect the functional data needed by the SSA and to present your patient's case clearly. When you do it correctly, you may expect a fair result.

Insurance and Access to Cardiovascular Care

The effect of insurance type on access to cardiovascular care is currently intensively being evaluated. Certain managed care organizations have attempted to use a gate keeper approach to reduce unnecessary subspecialty consultations and to establish protocols to preclude self-referral to specialists. Many primary care–based protocols and guidelines mandate an initial primary care evaluation and possibly even testing and subsequent referral to cardiologists for specific problems or procedures. Currently, evaluation of the access to subspecialty care in regions with heavy managed care penetration is being assessed. In one large survey, this access was rated as inadequate by as many as 30% of consumers.[18]

Another insurance issue involves access and quality indicators for treatment of specific acute cardiovascular illnesses. Since many managed care organizations may temper enthusiasm for emergency room visits, concerns have arisen pertaining to delayed presentation of patients with myocardial infarction to emergency rooms. At least one recent study documented differences between outcomes for treatment of myocardial infarction in patients with fee-for-service versus managed care plans.[19] However, an earlier study found no difference in outcome after infarction associated with type of insurance.[20] Every et al.[21] reported that HMO patients had similar in-hospital outcomes after myocardial infarction but longer lengths of stay. Capitation strategies limiting the incentive of physicians to supply diagnostic and therapeutic interventions based on reimbursement may also influence health care quality and outcomes. This area is actively being studied.[18]

LEGAL ISSUES IN PRACTICE

Medicolegal issues of cardiovascular care are nicely summarized by Cheney in a recent textbook of cardiovascular medicine.[22] A comprehensive body of law has been developed to help the legal system and professional liability insurers determine whether a particular patient's poor outcome was a result of negligence and what the compensation should be. The establishment of a physician/patient relationship provides an obligation of care by the physician to the patient. Despite the common trend for specialists like cardiologists to have limited relationships and contact with patients and their families in managed care situations, the legal system continues to expand the situations in which cardiologists are considered to have a legal obligation to patients. A physician's duty to his or her patient is to apply the care and skill that is ordinarily exercised by an average physician. A certain standard of care is usually applicable to a situation, although it can be the subject of debate. For the standard of care to be established in a legal action, it requires expert testimony. These witnesses educate jurors concerning the standard of care in a particular case and identify whether a physician has violated this standard. The physician's negligence must clearly contribute to the poor outcome to be the basis for recovery in a malpractice suit.

The areas of concern regarding medical malpractice risk include diagnostic errors, informed consent, withdrawing or withholding medical intervention, and lack of documentation for drug- and device-related claims. The patient's medical record is the primary evidence for plaintiff attorneys and their experts concerning medical malpractice suits. All health care providers involved in patient care should document and communicate to each other the relevant aspects of their own participation, and they must make entries in the patient's chart as necessary. Appropriate documentation is the physician's most important resource in court; inappropriate or lack of documentation is understandably damaging. Subsequent alteration of medical records to improve documentation is unacceptable and can contribute to punishment that extends beyond negligence.

As the population ages, advanced directives become increasingly more important to allow patients to main-

tain their rights to prevent prolongation of life by extraordinary means. The health care power of attorney is a signed and witnessed document that appoints an agent to make decisions concerning health care provision in the event the individual does not have the capacity to make his or her own decisions. A living will is a document that specifically addresses prolongation of life by extraordinary means. Many states have enacted natural death legislation that allows a natural process of dying for persons who are comatose or who have no reasonable probability of returning to a productive, cognitive state. If the physician confirms this state and meets the legal prerequisites, extraordinary means of support including tube feeding may be withheld or discontinued. This is usually done with the concurrence of the patient's health care power of attorney, spouse, guardian, or a majority of the first-degree relatives. As always, good documentation is the strongest defense against frivolous legal action.

REFERENCES

1. Mark DB, Lam LC, Lee KL, et al: Identification of patients with coronary disease at high risk for loss of employment: a prospective validation study, *Circulation* 86.1485, 1992.
2. Hammermeister KE, DeRouen TA, English MT, Dodge HT: Effect of surgical versus medical therapy on return to work in patients with coronary artery disease, *Am J Cardiol* 44:105,1979.
3. Mark DB, Lam LC, Lee KL, et al: Effects of coronary angioplasty, coronary bypass surgery, and medical therapy on employment in patients with coronary artery disease: a prospective comparison study, *Ann Intern Med* 120:111, 1994.
4. Pocock SJ, Henderson RA, Seed P, et al: Quality of life, employment status, and anginal symptoms after coronary angioplasty or bypass surgery: 3-year follow-up in the Randomized Intervention Treatment of Angina (RITA) Trial, *Circulation* 94:135, 1996.
5. Fitzgerald ST, Becker DM, Celentano DD, et al: Return to work after percutaneous transluminal coronary angioplasty, *Am J Cardiol* 64:1108, 1989.
6. Lusk SL: Linking practice and research: return to work following myocardial infarction, *AAOHN* 43:155, 1995.
7. Riegel BJ, Dracup KA: Does overprotection cause cardiac invalidism after acute myocardial infarction? *Heart Lung* 21:529, 1992.
8. Dennis C, Houston-Miller N, Schwartz RG, et al: Early return to work after uncomplicated myocardial infarction: results of a randomized trial, *JAMA* 260:214, 1988.
9. Chernen L, Friedman S, Goldberg N, et al: Cardiac disease and nonorganic chest pain: factors leading to disability, *Cardiology* 86:15, 1995.
10. Bass C, Cawley R, Wade C, et al: Unexplained breathlessness and psychiatric morbidity in patients with normal and abnormal coronary arteries, *Lancet* 1:605, 1983.
11. Kemp HG, Kronmal RA, Vlietstra RE, Frye R: Seven-year survival of patients with normal or near normal coronary arteriograms: A CASS Registry study, *J Am Coll Cardiol* 7:479, 1986.
12. Vitaliano PP: Coping in chest pain patients with and without psychiatric disorders, *J Consult Clin Psychol* 57:338, 1989.
13. Pinski SL, Chen P: Implantable cardioverter-defibrillators, *Textbook of Cardiovascular Medicine* 69:1913, 1998.
14. Anderson MH, Camm AJ: Legal and ethical aspects of driving and working in patients with an implantable cardioverter-defibrillator, *Am Heart J* 127:1185, 1994.
15. Beauregard LA, Barnard PW, Russo AM, Waxman HL: Perceived and actual risks of driving in patients with arrhythmia control devices, *Arch Intern Med* 155:609, 1995.
16. McGrath KA, Truesdell SC: Employability and career counseling for adolescents and adults with congenital heart disease, *Nurs Clin North Am* 29:319, 1994.
17. Celermajer DS, Deanfield JE: Employment and insurance for young adults with congenital heart disease, *Br Heart J* 69:539, 1993.
18. Van Tassel RA et al: Cardiovascular care in the managed care era, *Textbook of Cardiovascular Medicine* 42:1135, 1998.
19. Casale PN et al: Patients enrolled in a health maintenance organization have higher in-hospital mortality when admitted with an acute myocardial infarction, *Circulation* (suppl I) 96:1, 1997.
20. Kreindel S, Rosetti R, Goldberg R, et al: Health insurance coverage and outcome following acute myocardial infarction, *Arch Intern Med* 157:758, 1997.
21. Every NR, Fihn SD, Maynard C, et al: Resource utilization in treatment of acute myocardial infarction: staff-model health maintenance organization versus fee-for-service hospitals, *J Am Coll Cardiol* 26:401, 1995.
22. Cheney ML: Medicolegal issues, *Textbook of Cardiovascular Medicine* 40:1107, 1998.

50 Cardiac Emergencies Including Cardiac Arrest, Resuscitation, and Trauma

Bruce W. Usher, Jr.
George J. Taylor

HYPERTENSIVE CRISES
Epidemiology and Etiology

The epidemiology and etiology of hypertension are discussed in Chapter 31. Because of effective therapy, hypertensive crises are now seen in less than 1% of all Americans with hypertension.[1] However, given the prevalence of hypertension in our society, primary care physicians must learn to manage this complication.

Hypertensive crises can be classified as *hypertensive urgencies* and *hypertensive emergencies*. Hypertensive urgencies are characterized by elevated blood pressure without end-organ damage; they often can be managed with oral medications on an outpatient basis. Hypertensive emergencies, on the other hand, involve end-organ damage and require prompt lowering of blood pressure (within hours) using intravenous medications.

Table 50-1 lists some of the more common causes of hypertensive crises. It is important to realize that a majority of patients with crises have underlying essential hypertension that may be worsened by either medical noncompliance or the concomitant use of other medications or drugs.

Pathophysiology

As blood pressure rises and persists above certain critical levels, a cascade of local and systemic effects initiate a cycle of further increases in blood pressure, vascular damage, and ultimately tissue ischemia and death. These include endothelial damage, platelet activation, local accumulation of free radicals and prostaglandins, pressure natriuresis, hypovolemia, and activation of the renin-angiotensin system.[2]

Clinical Presentation

Although patients with hypertensive crises occasionally are asymptomatic, the presentation usually is quite dramatic. After documenting extreme elevation of blood pressure, look for evidence of end-organ damage that defines a hypertensive emergency and necessitates prompt treatment. Table 50-2 outlines the particular clinical findings that define hypertensive crises; they serve as baseline measures that are important to follow during treatment. Always look for concomitant conditions or complications that may need individualized treatment including dissecting aneurysms, myocardial ischemia and infarction, hypertensive encephalopathy, and cerebrovascular accidents.

Laboratory Evaluation

Although laboratory results help confirm suspicions of end-organ damage and serve as guides for both immediate and long-term management, do not delay treatment while waiting for test results to come back. Routine laboratory work is summarized in Table 50-3.

Management

The initial goal of therapy is not to immediately achieve a normal blood pressure, but rather to carefully lower mean arterial pressure in hopes of avoiding the risk of hypoperfusion leading to end-organ ischemia or infarction.

All patients with hypertensive crises should be admitted to an intensive care setting. These patients need prompt yet controlled reduction of their blood pressure with parenteral antihypertensive agents (be careful not to overshoot and create dangerous hypotension). Intravenous access must be established. Additionally, the placement of an arterial line helps with titration of blood pressure, given the potency and rapid action of these agents.

A sensible goal for most patients with a hypertensive emergency is reduction of mean arterial pressure by approximately 25%, or a reduction of diastolic blood pressure to 100 to 110 mm Hg over 1 to 2 hours.[1] We try to maintain this level for the next day or two as oral therapy is instituted and the parenteral agents are tapered off. We do not know of any definite time courses for return to a normotensive state, but within 2 to 4 weeks seems to be a safe guideline to follow.

Table 50-4 provides a summary of the most commonly used parenteral agents along with dosing regimens, rapidity of action, and some special indications for use.

An important concept often not appreciated is that many patients with hypertensive emergencies are volume depleted on presentation. This is believed to result from a pressure diuresis; these patients actually need volume infusions to control their blood pressure.[1]

Table 50-1	*Causes of Hypertensive Crises*

Cause	Comment
Essential hypertension	No obvious cause of crisis
Cessation of hypertension therapy	A rebound phenomenon
Drug abuse	Cocaine, amphetamines, diet pills, and others; drug screen if suspicious
Sympathomimetic or anticholinergic drugs	Decongestants, tricyclic antidepressants
Renal artery stenosis	Superimposed on essential hypertension; consider if older person has worsening of hypertension or crisis
Renal parenchymal disease	Most commonly glomerulonephritis (look for red cell casts in the urine)
Preeclampsia or eclampsia	Hypertension plus proteinuria and/or edema. Treat severe hypertension near term or during labor with hydralazine or calcium blockers (if not on magnesium infusion, which potentiates hypotension). Diazoxide and labetalol are also used. Avoid ACE inhibitors (fetal renal failure) and nitroprusside (fetal cyanide poisoning).

Table 50-2	*Important Clinical Findings in Patients with Hypertensive Crises—Definition of the Syndrome*

Blood pressure	Usually >120-130 mm Hg diastolic
Funduscopic examination	Hemorrhages, exudates, papilledema
Neurologic examination	Headaches, confusion, somnolence, focal deficits, seizures, nausea and vomiting
Cardiopulmonary status	Rales, gallops, pulse deficits (suggesting dissection), murmurs, chest pain, and/or ECG changes of ischemia
Body fluid status	*Volume depletion* (poor skin turgor, dry mucous membranes, orthostasis, elevated BUN:Cr ratio) vs *overload* rales, edema, neck vein distention, characteristic chest x-ray)

Drug Therapy

Nitroprusside

Nitroprusside remains one of the most commonly used agents in the management of hypertensive emergencies. It is a potent arteriolar and venous dilator, relaxing vascular smooth muscle by stimulating the formation of cyclic guanosine monophosphate. It is light sensitive and thus requires a covered infusion reservoir. Nitroprusside is metabolized to thiocyanate, which is excreted in the urine. Patients with renal insufficiency are at increased risk to develop cyanide toxicity, which usually takes several days to develop unless a high-dose infusion is required.[3] In combination with beta-adrenergic antagonists, nitroprusside effectively manages dissecting aneurysms, since it lowers pressure and blunts the rate of rise in pressure [dp/dt].

Nitroglycerine

Nitroglycerine has a limited role in hypertensive emergencies because its effect on blood pressure is less pre-

Table 50-3	Initial Laboratory Evaluation of Hypertensive Crisis

Test	Comment
Chem-7	Renal function, K$^+$ (important if taking diuretics)
Mg^{++}	Important if taking diuretics; Mg will improve response to antihypertensive treatment
CBC and smear	Exclude hemolysis
Urinalysis	Proteinuria, casts, red cells
Drug screen	If suspicious of illicit drug use
ECG	Exclude myocardial ischemia or infarction
Chest x-ray	Pulmonary congestion, exclude aortic dissection
CT scan or MRI	Exclude other intracranial pathology if altered mental status or abnormal neurologic findings present.

Do not delay initiation of blood pressure–lowering therapy while waiting for laboratory results.

dictable than that of nitroprusside. Use it for myocardial ischemia or congestive heart failure.

Nicardipine

Nicardipine is a calcium channel blocker that has been approved for treatment of severe hypertension. It is a dihydropyridine derivative that is more water soluble, making it useful parenterally. Nicardipine has been found to be as effective as nitroprusside when compared in a multicenter, prospective, randomized trial of postoperative patients with severe hypertension.[4] Its advantages include reduction of both cardiac and cerebral ischemia, and its dosing is not weight dependent.

Hydralazine

Hydralazine is an arteriolar vasodilator used mainly in pregnancy-induced hypertensive emergencies. Hydralazine may cause reflex tachycardia and increase myocardial oxygen demand, thus exacerbating anginal symptoms in patients with coronary artery disease.

Enalaprilat (Vasotec)

As the only parenteral angiotensin-converting enzyme inhibitor, enalaprilat is used in patients with left ven-

tricular failure. Be careful with patients with known or suspected high renin states, since this may precipitate dramatic hypotension.

Trimethaphan

Trimethaphan is a ganglionic blocker that blocks transmission of impulses at the sympathetic and parasympathetic ganglia. Its use is limited by numerous side effects and by the lack of familiarity with the drug. Trimethaphan has a special value in patients with dissecting aneurysms owing to its ability to reduce [dp]/[dt], similar to the combination of nitroprusside and beta blockade.

Phentolamine

Phentolamine is a pure alpha-adrenergic blocker used primarily in hypertensive emergencies associated with catecholamine excess. It may cause tachyarrhythmias and thus may precipitate angina in patients with coronary artery disease.

Esmolol

Esmolol is a pure beta-blocking agent with an extremely short half-life and rapid onset of action. It is useful in treating patients with myocardial ischemia and dissecting aneurysms. It should be avoided if a pheochromocytoma or illicit drug use is suspected. Hypertension may worsen with unopposed alpha activity.

Labetalol

Labetalol is a combination alpha- and beta-blocker that effectively maintains blood pressure reduction in most hypertensive emergencies. The fall in blood pressure results from a combined drop in systemic vascular resistance and cardiac output. It is useful in conditions of catecholamine excess, but should not be used in patients with left ventricular failure. Labetalol is given intravenously in the emergency setting and can be subsequently replaced with oral preparations.

In contrast to hypertensive emergencies, the management of hypertensive urgencies can be managed on an outpatient basis. You must be able to lower mean arterial pressure by 20% or diastolic blood pressure to less than 120 mm Hg. The patient must be seen in follow-up the next day. Oral antihypertensive therapy is reviewed in Chapter 31. For urgent cases, consider oral clonidine, which provides a fairly rapid and predictable reduction in blood pressure. Avoid short-acting nifedipine, especially sublingually, since it may cause precipitous lowering of blood pressure and may provoke coronary or cerebral ischemia. For patients whose blood pressure does not fall within a day, we admit them to the hospital for inpatient management.

Follow-up and Clinical Course

Before effective pharmacologic therapy, the annual survival rate for patients with hypertensive emergencies was

| Table 50-4 | | *Intravenous Drugs Used To Treat Hypertensive Crisis* | | |

Drug	Intravenous Dosage	Onset of Action	Side Effects	Specific Indications
Nitroprusside	0.25-10 µg/kg/min	Instant	Nausea, vomiting, cyanide toxicity	Most all HTN emergencies (careful with azotemia)
Nitroglycerine	5-100 mg/min	2-5 min	Tachycardia, flushing, headache, vomiting	Coronary ischemia
Nicardipine	2-10 mg/hr	5-10 min	Tachycardia, flushing, headache, phlebitis	Most all HTN emergencies except acute left heart failure
Hydralazine	10-20 mg	10-20 min	Tachycardia, nausea, headache, worsening of angina	Preeclampsia and eclampsia
Enalaprilat	1.25-5 mg q6hr	15 min	Hypotension in high renin states	Acute left ventricular failure
Phentolamine	5-10 mg	1-2 min	Tachycardia, flushing	Catecholamine excess
Trimethaphan	0.5-5 mg/min	1-5 min	Orthostasis, dry mouth, blurred vision, bowel/bladder dysfunction	Aortic dissection
Esmolol	500 µg/kg/min over 4 min bolus then 150-300 µg/kg/min	1-2 min	Hypotension	Aortic dissection in combination with nitroprusside
Labetalol	20-80 mg bolus q10 min then 2mg/min	5-10 min	Vomiting, dizziness, scalp tingling	Most all HTN emergencies except heart failure

less than 25%, and only 1% of patients were alive at 5 years. Today, 80% of these patients are alive at 5 years.[5] Late mortality is usually caused by renal failure and stroke.[6] After initial management, it is imperative to (1) exclude a correctable cause of hypertensive emergency and (2) effectively control blood pressure (see Chapter 31).

CARDIAC TAMPONADE
Etiology
Compression of the heart by fluid within the pericardial sac limits diastolic filling of the cardiac chambers, causing cardiac output to drop. Table 50-5 lists some of the more common causes of pericardial effusions requiring drainage.

Pathophysiology
The rise of pressure within the pericardial space is related to several factors, including the volume of fluid, the rate at which the fluid accumulates, and the relative compliance of the pericardial sac itself.[7] The peri-

cardium takes time to stretch. With slow accumulation of fluid over weeks to months (as with malignant effusions or hypothyroidism), a few liters of fluid may have accumulated before hemodynamic compromise becomes evident. With acute tamponade (as seen with trauma or myocardial rupture), as little as a few hundred milliliters of fluid raises pericardial pressure.

As intrapericardial pressure approaches the diastolic filling pressure in the cardiac chambers, filling of the heart is limited and stroke volume falls (see Chapter 2). Initially, cardiac output and blood pressure are maintained by compensatory tachycardia and vasoconstriction. Progressive impairment of filling causes hypotension and shock.

Clinical Presentation
It is the fall in cardiac output and rise in systemic venous pressure that leads to many of the clinical manifestations of cardiac tamponade. Most patients are symptomatic on presentation, but it is a difficult diagnosis to make unless you think of it.

| Table 50-5 | *Causes of Pericardial Effusion That May Lead to Tamponade* |

Cause	Comment
Trauma	Penetrating, blunt, or iatrogenic (perforation of the heart by catheter). Bloody effusion, but the association with trauma points to the cause.
Malignancy	Most common: lung and breast cancer, leukemia/lymphoma. Effusion usually bloody and cytology usually positive. Also a complication of radiation therapy.
Infection	Tuberculosis, bacterial, fungal, or viral, often in patients with AIDS.
Uremia	Patient usually on dialysis. Effusion may be loculated, hard to tap.
Postcardiotomy syndrome	A history of heart or chest surgery within 2 months. High sedimentation rate.
Post myocardial infarction	Dressler's syndrome; usually within 2 months of MI. High sedimentation rate. In the acute setting, consider cardiac rupture.
Connective tissue disease	Systemic lupus, rheumatoid arthritis. Pericardial fluid often has positive serology. Drug-induced lupus may also cause it.
Idiopathic pericarditis	Tamponade is possible with viral pericarditis.
Anticoagulant therapy	Consider this in patients with myocardial infarction or cardiomyopathy.

The "classic" triad—hypotension, elevated jugular venous pressure, and a small, quiet heart—may be present only with abrupt development of tamponade, as seen in trauma cases.[8] More commonly, symptoms of dyspnea, orthopnea, fatigue, and abdominal complaints secondary to hepatic engorgement predominate. The patient's general appearance varies in degree of discomfort; blood pressure may be normal, and the appreciation of elevated jugular venous pressure is often difficult.

The presence of a paradoxical pulse, although not specific for pericardial tamponade, is important in the initial assessment, as it is always present in these patients (see Chapter 4). On the other hand, Kussmaul's sign is not seen in pure, uncomplicated tamponade but can be seen in constrictive pericarditis or effusive-constrictive cases.

Laboratory Diagnosis

A chest x-ray showing the characteristic "water bottle" configuration does not indicate cardiac tamponade but should raise suspicion of pericardial effusions. The electrocardiogram may reveal electrical alternans, but this finding is not common nor specific for cardiac tamponade.

An echocardiogram should be performed if time permits. The echo confirms the presence of pericardial effusions; no effusion rules out tamponade. Although certain echocardiographic features suggest cardiac tam-

ponade, including right atrial and ventricular collapse, swinging motion of the heart, and abnormal inspiratory increases in right ventricular and decreases in left ventricular dimensions, the combination of a moderate to large pericardial effusion in the setting of dyspnea, jugular venous distension, and a paradoxical pulse points toward the diagnosis of tamponade and the need for pericardiocentesis.

Management

Definitive therapy is drainage of the pericardial fluid. While preparations are being made for pericardiocentesis, a few temporizing measures may be useful. Rapid volume infusion promotes ventricular filling and improves stroke volume. Isoproterenol increases heart rate and myocardial contractility and lowers systemic vascular resistance, which may help augment stroke volume in the setting of tamponade. Again, these measures are only temporizing and often are not helpful, so drainage must be performed as soon as possible.

Pericardiocentesis

Needle pericardiocentesis should be performed by skilled and experienced physicians using the standard subxiphoid approach, which avoids the pleura and the large epicardial coronary arteries and is considered the safest. Necessary equipment includes a long, 16 to 18 gauge needle, a 30 to 60 ml syringe, and a sterile alliga-

tor clip to a V-lead ECG monitor. Additionally, a stopcock helps with drainage of large effusions.

1. Position the patient with the head and thorax elevated 30 to 45 degrees. This allows gravity to work for you, pooling the fluid inferiorly and anteriorly.
2. Carefully prepare and drape the skin.
3. Locally anesthetize the area with 1% lidocaine.
4. Make a small stab incision just to the left and below the xiphoid process.
5. Attach the needle to the syringe partially filled with lidocaine. Attach the sterile alligator clip to the needle hub and hook it to the V-lead of the ECG machine or monitor (being careful to ensure appropriate grounding). You can also attach the needle to a stopcock with tubing for drainage of fluid or measurement of intrapericardial pressures.
6. Direct the needle posteriorly until the tip is just behind the rib cage. Flatten the needle toward the abdomen and advance it slowly toward the left shoulder. Aspirate repeatedly while injecting lidocaine to clear the needle and provide adequate anesthesia.
7. Advance the needle until *fluid is obtained* or *ST elevation* is noted on the ECG monitor, indicating contact with the epicardium. When this injury pattern is seen, smoothly withdraw the needle while aspirating until fluid withdrawn. If no fluid returns, remove the needle, flush, and repeat above steps, slightly changing the direction of the needle.
8. If bloody fluid is withdrawn and it is uncertain whether it is pericardial fluid or blood from a cardiac chamber, drop a bit on a gauze or in a bedside container. Pericardial blood should not clot owing to various antithrombotic constituents of pericardial fluid.
9. Withdraw fluid as long as it comes easily. Continue monitoring the pericardial-lead ECG. Relief of tamponade with a rise in blood pressure may occur after withdrawing 50 to 100 ml of fluid.

With relief of acute tamponade, you have bought time for the patient's transfer to the cardiac center. Further management may require surgery and a pericardial window.

Complications and Expected Clinical Course

The major complications of needle pericardiocentesis are laceration of coronary vessels and perforation of the myocardium. Other problems that may arise include arrhythmias, reflex hypotension (for which atropine can be effective), or pneumothorax. Even in the most experienced hands, needle pericardiocentesis is associated with morbidity and occasional mortality, both of which may be reduced with echocardiographic localization of the pericardial fluid.[7] For these reasons, you want the

procedure done by an experienced operator. On the other hand, this often is a medical emergency, and recognition of tamponade and emergency drainage by an "inexperienced" family physician may be lifesaving.

The clinical course is largely dictated by the underlying cause of tamponade. It is essential to monitor the patient after drainage for evidence of reaccumulation, which can be confirmed by echocardiographic imaging. Constrictive pericarditis may play a significant role down the road, and the primary care physician should always keep this diagnosis in mind when taking care of patients with a history of effusion or pericarditis.

ACUTE PULMONARY EDEMA

Chronic congestive heart failure is discussed in Chapters 22 and 24. Acute (flash) pulmonary edema is a true cardiac emergency characterized by a dramatic presentation that is often as frightening to the physician as it is to the patient. This review of treatment for pulmonary congestion applies to most cardiac causes of acute pulmonary edema.

Pathophysiology

The hallmark of cardiogenic pulmonary edema is elevated pulmonary vascular pressure, which is in distinct contrast to noncardiogenic pulmonary edema in which vascular pressure is normal but vascular permeability is altered.[9] A rapid increase in left atrial pressure is transmitted to pulmonary capillaries and leads to filtration of fluid across the pulmonary endothelium into the interstitial space, ultimately flooding the alveolar space. This causes impaired oxygen exchange, decrease in lung compliance, a sensation of suffocation with the increased work of breathing, and higher heart rate and blood pressure.[10] There may be increased cardiac work load, worsening of hypoxia, and further myocardial depression. If not interrupted in a timely fashion, it may be fatal.

Clinical Presentation

Patients with acute pulmonary edema are in marked respiratory distress and feel a sense of drowning. They appear agitated and restless and often are sitting upright. They use their accessory muscles of respiration, have flared nasal alae, may be diaphoretic and cyanotic, and may be coughing pink, frothy sputum. The diagnosis is straightforward.

Management

Once acute pulmonary edema is recognized clinically, treatment includes supplemental oxygen, establishment of intravenous access and cardiac monitoring, and use of morphine sulfate, diuretics, and vasodilators. These measures should be instituted while further history is

Table 50-6	*Treatment of Acute Pulmonary Edema**

Treatment	Comment
90%-100% oxygen by face mask	Use continuous oximetry if possible. If there is hypercapnia (with Pco_2 >50) or respiratory effort is failing, intubate and use positive pressure ventilation. Positive end-expiratory pressure lowers both preload and afterload.
Diuretics: furosemide 20-80 mg IV (or double the usual home dose given IV)	Onset of action <5 min, peak effect at 20 min, duration of action 2hr. Works as a preload reducer (venodilator) as well as a diuretic. Repeat dose in 10 min if no response.
Morphine sulfate, 2-5mg IV at 10-min intervals	Morphine reduces sympathetic flow, causes vasodilation (preload reduction), and reduces work of breathing. Watch for respiratory depression (although this is rarely a problem).
Vasodilators: IV nitroglycerine (for dose, see Table 50-4)	Use if blood pressure is >100 mmHg, and watch carefully for hypotension. Both preload and afterload reduction with IV use. Sublingual nitroglycerine reduces preload; use for less severe congestion and for those with known CAD or angina.
Aminophylline 150 mg IV, then 0.2 mg/kg/hr	A bronchodilator with mild diuretic activity. Consider it when there is significant wheezing (common with pulmonary edema).
Rotating tourniquets	Reduces venous return to the heart (lowering preload). An old-fashioned, rarely used treatment, but think of it if the situation is desperate.
Phlebotomy	Abrupt preload reduction. Do only after documenting a normal hematocrit (recall that anemia may precipitate heart failure). Use bags from the blood bank and take off two units (the red cells may be readministered later). This is used only when all else has failed.

*To be administered concurrently.

taken, appropriate laboratory work is drawn, and chest x-rays and electrocardiograms are obtained. If the initial blood pressure is below 90 to 100 mm Hg systolic, a dopamine infusion should be started at 2.5 to 5.0 µg/kg/min and titrated to achieve an optimal perfusion pressure. Table 50-6 summarizes the treatments, which are administered concurrently.

All patients should be admitted to a hospital and closely monitored as the pulmonary edema resolves and condition stabilizes. Further evaluation depends on results of initial workup, with therapy aimed at the underlying cause.

CARDIAC TRAUMA
Epidemiology and Etiology

Cardiac trauma is one of the leading causes of death in the United States in persons under the age of 40.[10] These injuries may follow motor vehicle accidents, gun shot wounds, stabbings, falls, cardiac resuscitative procedures, and even iatrogenically medically related inci-

dents involving catheter insertion procedures. Obviously, patients with major chest trauma are initially managed by specialized physicians including trauma surgeons and emergency personnel. Less severe injury may affect cardiac structures and may be overlooked (Table 50-7), only to cause difficulty later. As indicated in the table, new ECG changes, heart failure, or murmurs are indications for evaluation by a cardiologist.[11,12]

Prognosis for recovery from myocardial contusion is quite good. In contrast to patients with myocardial infarctions who are older, have diffuse coronary artery disease, and have multiple co-morbidities, a young patient with no underlying heart disease usually does well. Late complications, although rare, include ventricular arrhythmias, formation of both true and false aneurysms, acquired valvular disease, and subsequent cardiac rupture.

Commotio Cordis (Cardiac Concussion)

A number of cases of sudden death have been caused by a sharp but apparently minor blow to the left chest.[13]

Table 50-7	*Injury of the Heart, Pericardium, and Great Vessels*

Injury	Diagnosis and Management
Pericardium	A variety of syndromes: (1) acute pericarditis, presentation and management no different from other causes of pericarditis (see Chapter 29); (2) pericardial hemorrhage and tamponade; (3) postcardiotomy syndrome or pericardial constriction (see Chapter 29).
Myocardium	Contusion (with ECG changes), laceration, or rupture with tamponade, pseudo-aneurysm, or aneurysm (also with ECG changes). New ECG changes indicate a need for cardiology evaluation (beginning with an echocardiogram). Contusion may cause ST-T wave changes or Q wave on the ECG. It may also cause chest pain, difficult to separate from the chest wall pain caused by the trauma. Arrhythmias may complicate contusion, and atrial fibrillation indicates poor outcome.[11] Avoid nonsteroidal agents that may interfere with myocardial healing. Prognosis is good in the absence of coexisting CAD.[12]
New heart murmur	Most are associated with severe heart failure and are surgical emergencies. Lesions: septal perforation with VSD (there may be new heart failure without a murmur), rupture of a papillary muscle or chordae tendineae (with mitral regurgitation), or rupture of a semilunar valve (aortic or pulmonic valve regurgitation). Any new murmur or the development of heart failure necessitates cardiologic evaluation.
Coronary artery Injury	Thrombosis, laceration, and fistula formation are possible. New ECG changes or symptoms of ischemia are indications for cardiologic evaluation.
Injury to the aorta	Dislocation of the aorta at the level of the aortic root is one cause of death with chest trauma. Dissection and/or aneurysm or injury to the aortic valve may appear as a "late" complication (see Chapter 32).

Victims are usually young and are usually injured while playing baseball, softball, or hockey. The impact of the ball or puck is low-energy, insufficient to cause contusion. At autopsy there is no apparent injury. Victims do not have the illnesses associated with sudden cardiac death in young athletes (hypertrophic cardiomyopathy, arrhythmogenic RV dysplasia, congenital coronary artery anomaly, or myocarditis).

The probable mechanism is ventricular fibrillation (VF). Studies in pigs show that a moderate blow to the precordium delivered between 30 and 15 msec before the peak of the T wave may induce VF.[14] The vulnerable period in the cardiac cycle is about 1/100 of a second, explaining the rarity of this event. VF occurs with the next beat and is not preceded by ventricular ectopic beats or ventricular tachycardia.

The incidence of this newly recognized condition is uncertain. Maron's registry of sudden deaths recently recorded 69 cases.[13] There may be nonfatal cases with self-terminating arrhythmia (clinically, the player who is hit and has a brief loss of consciousness).

Treatment includes a precordial thump, rapid application of CPR, and defibrillation. Left chest protectors are being developed for those participating in higher risk sports, and safety baseballs have been proposed for Little League baseball.

SUDDEN CARDIAC DEATH
Epidemiology and Etiology

Sudden cardiac death continues to account for approximately 50% of all cardiovascular-related deaths.[15,16] Most episodes of sudden cardiac death occur outside the hospital, and the initial rhythm usually is VF. Pulseless ventricular tachycardia is managed identically to VF and carries a somewhat better prognosis. Asystole as the initial rhythm is ominous and has a very low rate of successful resuscitation. Pulseless electrical activity (PEA), formerly called *electromechanical dissociation* (EMD), also may cause sudden cardiac death, and success of resuscitation depends on whether there is a reversible cause such as hypovolemia, tamponade, tension pneumothorax, severe acidosis or hyperkalemia, hypothermia, drug overdose, or massive pulmonary embolism. Sudden cardiac death is the first manifestation of underlying CAD in 20% of patients.[16]

Physiology of CPR

As mentioned previously, the earlier a patient is diagnosed and resuscitative measures are initiated, the better the outcome. The basic premise behind CPR is generation of enough blood flow to the heart and brain to allow for successful defibrillation and preservation of organ viability. Two mechanisms control blood flow and organ perfusion: *vascular compression,* which squeezes the heart and vascular structures between the sternum and vertebral column, and the *thoracic pump,* which is the more important mechanism. Chest compression generates an abrupt rise in intrathoracic pressure, and this is transmitted to all blood-containing structures. This explains the success of CPR in patients with emphysema and barrel-chest deformity.[17]

The most important aspect of CPR physiology is coronary perfusion pressure (CPP), defined as aortic diastolic pressure minus right atrial diastolic pressure. This positive aorta to right atrial pressure gradient leads to increased coronary and myocardial perfusion. As CPP increases, myocardial perfusion improves and the ultimate success of the resuscitative effort is enhanced.[17] Methods used to increase CPP include (1) increasing the compression rate (explaining why the AHA now recommends 80 to 100 compressions per minute),[13] (2) increasing the force of compression, which is difficult to measure and can lead to increased resuscitative-induced trauma, and (3) administering epinephrine, which has been shown to elevate aortic diastolic pressure with minimal changes in right atrial pressures. Prolonged compression duration may boost flow to the periphery.

Management

CPR

Cardiopulmonary resuscitation encompasses both basic life support (BLS) and advanced cardiac life support (ACLS). Following the *ABCs* and calling for emergency care personnel are the initial actions to be performed. Once the airway is opened, ventilation is initiated, and chest compressions begun per standard BLS protocol; these efforts are continued until emergency personnel arrive. An initial 200 J countershock should be delivered as soon as possible (with automatic external defibrillators if out-of-hospital arrest), and the patient should be hooked up to a cardiac monitor. While CPR is continued, a large-bore peripheral venous catheter should be placed for delivery of drugs during the resuscitative effort. Endotracheal intubation provides the most effective way of ensuring adequate ventilation and should be performed as soon as possible, allowing for no more than 30 seconds per attempt while chest compressions are held. Once ventilation (parameters set to deliver 10 to 12 breaths per minute with tidal volume of ~1000 ml) and peripheral venous access are established, ACLS is continued on the basis of the underlying rhythm. If a patient has been intubated but venous access cannot be obtained, epinephrine, lidocaine, and atropine are drugs that can be administered through the endotracheal tube. Doses 2 to 2.5 times the recommended intravenous dose diluted in 10 ml distilled water or normal saline are sprayed with a catheter down the tube while chest compressions are held.[18]

Electrical Defibrillation

Electrical defibrillation is the most important treatment for patients with sudden cardiac death due to ventricular fibrillation or pulseless ventricular tachycardia. The widespread use of automatic external defibrillators has allowed for more rapid delivery of shocks, which is most important in terms of the ultimate success rate of resuscitative efforts. Initial energy delivered is 200 J, followed by 200 to 300 J, and finally 360 J in rapid succession for VF/VT. It has been shown that 90% of successful defibrillation attempts occur with 200 J in patients weighing less than 90 kg.[10] Positioning of the electrodes and paddles is important (right of upper sternum and below the left nipple in the midaxillary line with hand-held paddles). Alternatively, adhesive electrodes can be placed anteriorly over the left precordium and posteriorly behind the heart in the right infrascapular region. If VF/VT is successfully terminated with electrical shock but recurs, defibrillation should be reinitiated at the energy level that was previously successful. With persistent VF/VT, subsequent shocks should be delivered 30 to 60 seconds after each dose of medication given (drug-shock, drug-shock pattern).

Precordial Thump

Precordial thump is considered a class IIb recommendation (acceptable, possibly helpful) in a witnessed cardiac arrest in which the patient is pulseless and a defibrillator is not readily available.[16] Ventricular tachycardia can deteriorate into ventricular fibrillation, asystole, and pulseless electrical activity with a precordial thump, thus this method should not be used in patients with VT and a pulse unless a defibrillator and pacemaker are available.[18]

Epinephrine

Epinephrine remains the initial drug to use for cardiac arrest associated with VF/VT, pulseless electrical activity, and asystole. Through its alpha-adrenergic effect, myocardial and cerebral perfusion are increased. The dosage used is 1 mg (1:10,000 solution) intravenous push every 3 to 5 minutes followed by a 10 to 20 ml intravenous flush to ensure delivery into the central circulation. Several studies have evaluated higher doses of epinephrine (0.07 to 0.2 mg/kg) and found increased rates of return of spontaneous circulation but no change in overall survival.[19,20] There was no evidence of increased harm to the patient with high-dose epinephrine, and thus the AHA considers its use as a IIb recommendation (acceptable, possibly helpful).[18]

Lidocaine

Lidocaine remains the antiarrhythmic of choice for treatment of VF/VT cardiac arrest if initial defibrillation and epinephrine have failed. The initial bolus is 1.0 to 1.5 mg/kg intravenously, which can be repeated every 5 to 10 minutes up to a total 3.0 mg/kg (remember to follow each bolus with a 360 J shock within 30 seconds). If perfusion is restored, a continuous infusion at 1 to 4 mg/min can be started. Remember to monitor closely for toxicity in patients on maintenance infusions given the relatively narrow toxic-therapeutic balance. The dosages should be reduced in the elderly, in patients with low cardiac output states, and in patients with hepatic dysfunction.

Bretylium

In refractory VF/VT after lidocaine fails, bretylium is a good second-line antiarrhythmic. Initial dosage is 5 mg/kg intravenous bolus (followed by 360 J shock) and can be increased to 10 mg/kg and repeated every 5 minutes. Maximal dosage is 30 to 35 mg/kg. If perfusion is restored, a continuous infusion can be started at 1 to 2 mg/min.

Other Drugs

Procainamide is another antiarrhythmic that can be used in refractory VF/VT cardiac arrest patients. It should be used as a third-line agent, since it is difficult to deliver an optimal load in a relatively short period of time (as opposed to both lidocaine and bretylium). The chance of successful resuscitation at this point is extremely low, and one should consider ceasing efforts. Intravenous amiodarone has been shown to be potentially useful as a last resort in the setting of refractory VF/VT. Williams et al.[21] studied the efficacy of intravenous amiodarone in the setting of prolonged in-hospital resuscitation from cardiac arrest, reporting a 57% (8 of 14) initial survival to hospital discharge in a select group of patients. Amiodarone may have a role in resuscitative efforts in the future but currently is not recommended by the standard ACLS protocol. The use of sodium bicarbonate can be potentially harmful (causing hyperosmolarity, hypernatremia, alkalosis, and worsening central venous acidosis) and should be used only in patients with known hyperkalemia, severe acidosis, or tricyclic overdose, all of which may be reversible causes of pulseless electrical activity. Magnesium sulfate can be used in a patient with refractory VF/VT, since it is known to prevent these arrhythmias and is relatively safe. It remains the treatment of choice in patients with torsade de pointes. Calcium is considered class IIA (probably helpful) in cardiac arrest associated with hyperkalemia, hypocalcemia, or calcium channel blocker overdose and toxicity.[18]

REFERENCES

1. Calhoun DA, Oparil S: Treatment of hypertensive crisis, *N Engl J Med* 323:1177, 1990.
2. Kaplan NM: *Clinical hypertension*, ed 6, Baltimore, 1994, Williams & Wilkins.
3. Varon J, Fromm RE Jr: Hypertensive crises: the need for urgent management, *Postgrad Med* 99:189, 1996.
4. Halpern NA, Goldberg M, Neely C, et al: Postoperative hypertension: a multicenter, prospective, randomized comparison between intravenous nicardipine and sodium nitroprusside, *Crit Care Med* 20:1637, 1992.
5. Kaplan NM: Management of hypertensive emergencies, *Lancet* 344:1335, 1994.
6. Webster J, Petrie JC, Jeffers TA, Lovell HG: Accelerated hypertension: patterns of mortality and clinical factors affecting outcome in treated patients, *Q J Med* 86:485, 1993.
7. Spodick DH: *The pericardium: a comprehensive textbook*, New York, 1997, Marcel Dekker.
8. Beck CS: Two cardiac compression triads, *JAMA* 104:714, 1935.
9. Gropper MA, Wiener-Kronish JP, Hashimoto S: Acute cardiogenic pulmonary edema, *Clin Chest Med* 15:501, 1994.
10. Braunwald E, editor: *Heart disease: a textbook of cardiovascular medicine*, ed 5, Philadelphia, 1997, WB Saunders.
11. McLean RF, Devitt JH, McLellan BA, et al: Significance of myocardial contusion following blunt chest trauma, *J Trauma* 33:240, 1992.
12. Cachecho R, Grindlinger GA, Lee VW: The clinical significance of myocardial contusion, *J Trauma* 33:68, 1992.
13. Curfman GD: Fatal impact: concussion of the heart, *N Engl J Med* 338:1841, 1998.
14. Link MS, Wang PJ, Pandian NG, et al: An experimental model of sudden death due to low-energy chest-wall impact (commotio cordis), *N Engl J Med* 338:1805, 1998.
15. Domanski MJ, Zipes DP, Schron E: Treatment of sudden cardiac death: current understandings from randomized trials and future directions, *Circulation* 95:2694, 1997.
16. Myerburg RJ, Kessler KM, Castellanos A: Sudden cardiac death: epidemiology, transient risk, and intervention assessment, *Ann Intern Med* 119:1187, 1993.
17. Kern K: Cardiopulmonary resuscitation physiology, *ACC Current Journal Review* 6:11, 1997.
18. Emergency Cardiac Care Committee and Subcommittees, American Heart Association, *JAMA* 268:2171, 1992.
19. Stiell IG, Hebert PC, Weitzman BN, et al: High-dose epinephrine in adult cardiac arrest, *N Engl J Med* 327:1045, 1992.
20. Brown CG, Martin DR, Pepe PE, et al: A comparison of standard-dose and high-dose epinephrine in cardiac arrest outside the hospital, *N Engl J Med* 327:1051, 1992.
21. Williams ML, Woelfel A, Cascio WE, et al: Intravenous amiodarone during prolonged resuscitation from cardiac arrest, *Ann Intern Med* 110:839, 1989.

51

Technical Aspects of ICU-CCU Care

Angela J. Caldieraro-Bentley
George J. Taylor

A number of places in the hospital are mildly disorienting for doctors and staff who do not work there daily. The operating rooms, catheterization laboratory, and morgue come to mind. The intensive care unit (ICU) and coronary care unit (CCU) share this characteristic as they have become the locus of highly technical medical practices, somewhat intimidating to those unfamiliar with them. An overview of a few of the technical operations of the ICU should improve your level of comfort and understanding and enable you to discuss management with the technical insiders (especially the nurses) responsible for patient care.

OXYGENATION AND VENTILATION
Oxygen Therapy

Supplemental oxygen is common on the cardiac service. It is routinely given during acute myocardial infarction (MI) (see Chapter 14) and to patients with unstable coronary syndromes and congestive heart failure. In many of these cases it is not indicated, since the patient has a normal PaO_2 and arterial oxygen saturation.

Table 51-1 outlines common methods of oxygen delivery. A major concern is the risk of depressing ventilatory drive. A patient with obstructive lung disease and chronic hypercapnia may have a nonfunctional CO_2 receptor and therefore depends on the central hypoxic receptor. An excessively high FIO_2 can push the arterial oxygen content above the threshold needed to stimulate breathing, resulting in hypoventilation, CO_2 retention, respiratory acidosis, and possibly respiratory arrest. A precise titration of FIO_2 using a Venturi mask resolves the situation. The goal of treatment is a PaO_2 in the mid-50 range.

Mechanical Ventilation

The usual indication for ventilator therapy is respiratory failure, which is a clinical diagnosis; you can tell that the patient is wearing out and that the ventilatory effort is fading. Sensorium is often clouded. Arterial blood gases confirm a rising $PaCO_2$ and respiratory acidosis (remember that $CO_2 + H_2O \rightarrow H_2CO_3^- + H^+$). PaO_2 is usually low but is a less reliable indicator of respiratory fatigue. Patients with obstructive airway disease, including asthma, reach a point at which they do not have the energy necessary for the increased work of breathing. The work of breathing is increased for those with pulmonary congestion as well, since wet, heavy lungs are harder to move.

Objective measurements that help with the decision to intubate and ventilate include respiratory rate >30/min, PaO_2 <60mm Hg (with FIO_2>60%), $PaCO_2$ >50 mm Hg plus pH <7.35, inspiratory force <-25 cm H_2O, and an absent gag or cough reflex. Demonstration of a rising $PaCO_2$ plus low pH is more important than the absolute $PaCO_2$, because many with obstructive lung disease have chronic hypercapnia. A failure to respond to intensive medical therapy (e.g., bronchodilators, diuretics, and so on) often figures in the decision to intubate.

Methods of Ventilation

Table 51-2 summarizes the choices available for most modern ventilators. A patient requiring total ventilator support usually uses the assist control mode and, during the weaning process, synchronous intermittent mandatory ventilation (SIMV). Spontaneous breathing through the ventilator circuit during SIMV requires greater effort than normal respiration. The endotracheal tube, for example, increases total airway resistance. Some of this may be overcome by adding a small amount of pressure support.[1]

Ventilator Settings

A patient in respiratory arrest needs maximal support. Assist control ventilation at an FIO_2 of 90% to 100% is appropriate, with the settings changed according to blood gas measurement. Ventilatory rate is usually set at 10 to 15 breaths/min. For severe airway obstruction, 12 breaths/min or less allows adequate time for exhalation.

Tidal volume (TV) has traditionally been set at 10 to 12 ml/kg body weight. The risk of barotrauma may be lessened with lower TVs. Patients with pulmonary congestion and low lung compliance (wet lungs are stiff lungs) may develop much higher peak airway pressure with "normal" TV. Reducing the TV to 6 to 8 ml/kg may avoid mechanical complications such as pneumothorax. On the other hand, reduced TV means a lower minute ventilation and a potentially higher $PaCO_2$. Balancing this in favor of lower airway pressure and higher $PaCO_2$ is called *permissive hypercapnia*.[2] This approach re-

Table 51-1	Methods of Oxygen Delivery

Method	Comment
Nasal prongs	Most convenient for the patient Exact concentration of inspired oxygen is uncertain. A rough guide: 1 L/min = 24% O_2; FIO_2 increases by 4% with each additional 1 L/min.
Venturi (venti) mask	Allows precise delivery of oxygen with masks set for FIO_2 of 24, 28, 31, 35, 40, or 50% Preferred for patients with obstructive lung disease
Rebreather, partial rebreather masks	Allows patient to rebreathe exhaled CO_2. Used for hyperventilating patients to prevent respiratory alkalosis
Nonrebreather mask	A one-way valve prevents exhaled air from entering the reservoir bag, increasing FIO_2 to about 90%. Used for patients requiring high FIO_2
Continuous positive airway pressure (CPAP)	An alternative to intubation and mechanical ventilation with PEEP; for alert and cooperative patients

Table 51-2	Methods of Mechanical Ventilation

Continuous mandatory ventilation (CMV)	Rate and tidal volume (TV) are fixed.	Used during general anesthesia, rarely by an awake patient.
Assist control (AC)	Patient triggers each breath; there is a backup rate (when there is a failure to breathe, the machine delivers breaths at a set rate).	The advantage is a degree of respiratory muscle exercise. The sensitivity of the ventilator is set so that the patient's normal inspiratory effort triggers the machine.
Intermittent mandatory ventilation (IMV)	Allows the patient to breathe independently of the machine, without assistance; the machine delivers breaths at a predetermined rate.	Rarely used now, as SIMV is available. Would "stack" breaths, delivering a breath at any time in the respiratory cycle.
Synchronized IMV (SIMV)	The machine delivers breaths at a predetermined rate, but synchronizes them with spontaneous breaths.	Used during weaning, as the patient is breathing independently and with partial assistance. The extra breaths provided by the machine represent partial support (e.g., set it to deliver 4-8 breaths/min).
Pressure support (PS)	Augments patient-triggered breaths, delivering air at a preset pressure; TV is determined not by the machine but by lung mechanics and patient effort.	A small amount of PS is often used during SIMV to overcome the added resistance of the endotracheal tube while the patient is breathing spontaneously. Infrequently used as the primary form of ventilation, since changes in airway resistance, lung compliance, and patient effort may drastically change minute ventilation.
Positive end-expiratory pressure (PEEP)	Positive airway pressure throughout the respiratory cycle keeps airways open.	Primary use is hypoxic respiratory failure (e.g., ARDS, pulmonary edema). It is used together with other ventilator modes.

quires careful monitoring of pH to avoid respiratory acidosis. It has been applied in patients with status asthmaticus, as well as pulmonary congestion.

Barotrauma includes injury to endothelium, epithelium, and basement membrane, as well as rupture and pneumothorax. It is useful to monitor airway pressure, since *plateau* pressures in the 40 to 50 cm H_2O range are associated with trauma. Alarms for p*eak* airway pressure are set for pressures >50 cm H_2O.

Although not a ventilator setting, the *patient's position* plays a role in complications. Pooling of secretions and nosocomial pneumonia are more common if a patient is always supine. Our long-term ventilator patients now spend at least 2 hours per day in the prone position, which often improves oxygenation.

Positive end-expiratory pressure (PEEP) may be added to improve oxygenation for patients with severe pulmonary congestion (e.g., cardiogenic pulmonary edema or adult respiratory distress syndrome, ARDS).[3] PEEP prevents the collapse of alveoli and small airways at the end of expiration and forces fluid from the alveolar to the interstitial space. This reduces intrapulmonary "shunting" (that is, all blood circulates past open and ventilated airways) and may dramatically raise PaO_2.

PEEP is potentially dangerous. Higher airway pressure may be traumatic. Barotrauma—both pneumothorax and alveolar injury—is more common when PEEP and continuous positive pressure ventilation are combined. By increasing intrathoracic pressure, PEEP decreases venous return to the heart, and cardiac output may fall. It may help to monitor LV filling pressure with a pulmonary artery catheter if high levels of PEEP are used or if patients have depressed cardiac function.

Fighting the Ventilator and Sedation

If a previously stable ventilator patient becomes acutely distressed, a new problem may have developed. Disconnect and manually ventilate with 100% O_2 while searching for the cause (e.g., pneumothorax, a change in airway resistance, mucus plug or increased secretions, poor coordination of the patient's effort with the rhythm of the ventilator, change in the position of the endotracheal tube or cuff leak, and many others).

Patient anxiety is a common problem, and sedation often is necessary. Short-acting benzodiazepines may be preferable to long-acting agents, especially if there is liver dysfunction (which delays clearance). Long-acting drugs may substantially delay weaning. If respiratory drive and air hunger are excessive, neuromuscular blockade may be added to sedation to reduce respiratory muscle fatigue and myocardial oxygen demand and to prevent high airway pressures.

Weaning

A number of goals should be met before discontinuing mechanical ventilation (Box 51-1). The patient must be ready before making any attempt. There are a number of weaning techniques, and most require the patient to work with the ventilator. Changing the mode from assist-control to SIMV allows the patient to breathe without assistance. Gradually decreasing the SIMV rate (the number of breaths delivered by the machine) has the patient gradually work more. For a patient who has been ventilator dependent for some time, a trial of SIMV for 30 minutes three times a day is a good start.

HEMODYNAMIC MONITORING
Technical Considerations

The pressure transducer should be positioned at the level of the right atrium with all vascular monitoring systems. This so-called phlebostatic axis is located in the fourth intercostal space at the midaxillary line. This is the correct level regardless of the patient's position. A carpenter's level should be used for accurate positioning. Do not underestimate the importance of meticulous positioning. Recall that 1 cm H_2O = 2.63 mm Hg. Thus a transducer that is positioned 4 cm below the phlebostatic axis results in pressure measurements that are falsely elevated by more than 10 mm Hg. Raising the patient 4 cm without raising the transducer would have the same effect.

Good quality pressure recording requires a system that is well flushed and free of air (with special attention to the dome of the transducer and stopcocks). When reported pressure measurements do not make sense, it is best to start at the beginning: flush the system and rebalance and reposition the transducer.

Arterial Pressure Line

Most arterial lines are placed in the radial artery using a percutaneous technique that is similar to the method

---

BOX 51-1

GOALS TO MEET BEFORE WEANING A PATIENT FROM THE VENTILATOR

Correction of the underlying process (pneumonia, congestion, and so forth)
Stable hemodynamics
Adequate respiratory strength (a negative inspiratory force of at least 20 cm H_2O, and vital capacity 10-15 ml/kg body weight)
Compliant, dry lungs
Normal laboratory results (acid-base balance, electrolytes, hemoglobin)
No respiratory depressants on board
Adequate nutritional status
Adequate sleep and rest

used for inserting a short intravenous catheter. The radial artery is safe to use, and circulation to the hand is rarely jeopardized. An alternative is the brachial artery, which has greater risk because collateral circulation is not as reliable. Arterial lines are kept free of thrombus with a slow, pressurized, continuous heparin drip, but distal pulses should be carefully monitored.

Pulmonary Artery Pressure Monitoring

The typical flotation pulmonary artery (PA) catheter has four lumens: a distal port (beyond the balloon), a balloon inflation port, a proximal, right atrial port, and a thermistor probe with an electrical connector for measuring cardiac output. Medicine and fluid can be infused through the proximal port but not through the distal, PA port. Catheters with an extra, proximal infusion port are available.

The PA catheter is inserted through a venous introducer sheath from the internal jugular, subclavian, brachial, or femoral veins. The balloon floats once it is filled with air, following the venous current through the right atrium and ventricle and into the pulmonary artery (Fig. 51-1). In practice, advancing the catheter to the PA usually is not that simple and requires catheter manipulation. It is another of those techniques in medicine that seems easy for an experienced operator.

Apart from complications associated with insertion (e.g., venous injury, pneumothorax, retroperitoneal bleeding, arrhythmias including ventricular tachycardia or heart block as the line passes through the heart), the major risk of an indwelling catheter is infection. The risk increases with femoral vein insertion and with time. Catheters impregnated with antimicrobial agents appear to lower the risk and may be considered when a lengthy period of monitoring appears necessary.

Indications and Interpretation

The usual indication for PA catheterization is to determine a patient's volume, or preload, status (see Chapter 2). Preload is also known as *LV filling (diastolic) pressure*. LV diastolic pressure may be directly measured in the catheterization laboratory. The PA catheter is an alternative method that may be used in the ICU for continuous monitoring of LV filling pressure (see Fig. 51-1). When the balloon is inflated and the catheter is wedged into position, the distal lumen of the PA catheter is in open contact with the LV during diastole. This so-called pulmonary wedge pressure (PWP) is identical to LV diastolic pressure unless the patient has mitral valve stenosis (see Chapter 18). The normal PWP is 10 to 15 mm Hg. Patients with heart failure or increased LV stiffness have pressures above 20 mm Hg. When the hydrostatic pressure in the pulmonary capillary bed is above 25 mm Hg, fluid is forced into the interstitial space, causing the symptoms and physical signs of pulmonary congestion. In contrast, a patient who is hypotensive and

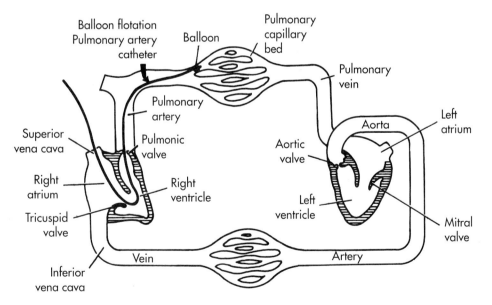

FIG. 51-1
Pulmonary artery catheterization. With the balloon inflated at the tip of the flotation catheter, the catheter is "wedged" into a pulmonary artery branch to measure downstream pressure. During diastole a channel is open from the end of the catheter through the pulmonary capillary bed, pulmonary veins, and left atrium to the left ventricle. This allows measurement of left ventricular diastolic, or "filling," pressure.

From Taylor GJ: *Thrombolytic therapy for acute myocardial infarction,* Cambridge, Mass, 1992, Blackwell Scientific.

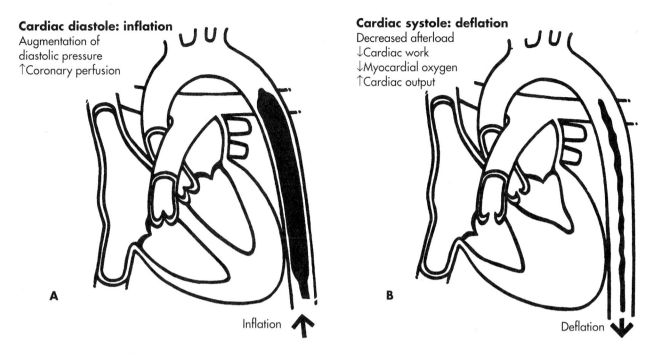

Cardiac diastole: inflation
Augmentation of
diastolic pressure
↑Coronary perfusion

A

Inflation

Cardiac systole: deflation
Decreased afterload
↓Cardiac work
↓Myocardial oxygen
↑Cardiac output

B

Deflation

FIG. 51-2
The intraaortic balloon pump (IABP). The balloon catheter is positioned in the descending aorta, above the renal artery and distal to the subclavian artery. **A,** During diastole the balloon is rapidly inflated, displacing its volume into the peripheral circulation (including the coronary and cerebral beds). **B,** During ventricular systole, the balloon is deflated.

has a PWP <10 to 18 mm Hg may be given normal saline with little risk of pulmonary congestion.

The clinical issues in acutely ill patients that are answered by measuring PWP are common: Is hypotension due to inadequate volume (low PWP) or to poor LV function (normal or high PWP)? Is pulmonary congestion caused by heart failure (high PWP) or by alveolar injury (ARDS, normal PWP)?

The catheter may also be used to measure cardiac output (CO) using a thermodilution technique. Cool saline is injected upstream, and the intensity of the bolus detected downstream by the thermistor is inversely proportional to flow; higher flow dilutes the bolus. CO and preload measurements are the variables that determine the LV function curve (Chapter 2). The data are useful when regulating therapy for unstable patients with heart failure, shock, or ARDS.

INTRAORTIC BALLOON PUMP

The intraaortic balloon pump (IABP) is used to augment cardiac output, usually in patients with cardiogenic shock.[4] In theory it is a simple device. A 40 ml sausage-shaped balloon is positioned in the descending aorta (Fig. 51-2), rapidly inflated, and then deflated between heart beats, while the aortic valve is closed. The

inflated balloon displaces its volume, 40 ml, which is pushed to the peripheral circulation, including the coronary and cerebral beds. The effect of the extra pump is readily apparent from the arterial pressure tracing (Fig. 51-3). Stroke volume may thus increase by 40 ml, and the effect on cardiac output to the periphery is impressive; at a heart rate of 60 beats/min, cardiac output increases by 2.4 L/min (60 beats/min × 40 ml/beat). This may represent a 75% to 100% increase in cardiac output for a patient with LV failure and shock.

The IABP reduces afterload. Moving 40 ml out of the aorta reduces impedance to LV emptying (think of it as creating an empty space, or "vacuum," in the aorta). The IABP thus reduces the work load of the heart in addition to augmenting coronary and peripheral blood flow. Intractable angina usually resolves with balloon pumping.

The biggest problem with the IABP is the size of the balloon catheter. It is inserted through the femoral artery, which is partially occluded by the device. It cannot be used in patients with severe peripheral artery disease or disease of the aorta. Leg ischemia distal to the insertion site is a common complication.

A specific cardiac contraindication to its use is severe aortic valve regurgitation. Inflation of the balloon pushes blood back across the incompetent aortic valve. Experience has also taught us to avoid the IABP for those

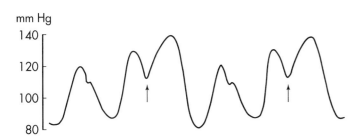

FIG. 51-3
Arterial pressure tracing from a patient who is using the intraaortic balloon pump (IABP) with 1:2 pumping (the balloon inflates with every other beat). The arrows mark the beginning of balloon inflation, and the second hump of the pressure curve is generated by balloon inflation, which displaces 40 ml blood from the aorta. Blood flow is proportional to the area under the pressure curve. In this patient cardiac output increased by 35% with the IABP.

with end-stage heart disease, since IABP dependency is a clinical disaster. The IABP can be used only temporarily and should be used to treat an underlying problem that will improve (e.g., stunned heart muscle after surgery) or can be corrected (e.g., coronary revascularization).

When first inserted, the balloon is inflated with each heart beat (1:1 pumping). As the patient improves, inflation may be decreased to every second or third beat. This is the usual method for weaning the patient from the IABP.

LEFT VENTRICULAR ASSIST DEVICE

The left ventricular assist device (LVAD) is the closest thing we have to a mechanical heart, and there are a number of them on the market. A common design has the implantable LVAD pump connected to the LV, which stops contracting (Fig. 51-4).[5] Blood returning to the LV is pumped by the machine to the ascending aorta. Initially, the HeartMate device was used as a bridge to cardiac transplantation. With the LVAD working, congestive heart failure resolves, and patients are able to walk and exercise. Overall clinical status improves, and the results of transplantation after LVAD support are excellent. With current technology, the risk of peripheral embolus is about 2%.[5]

Because of the good results, there is speculation that the LVAD will be implanted as permanent therapy for heart failure. The breakthrough needed for this to be possible is improved battery technology, making the device portable.

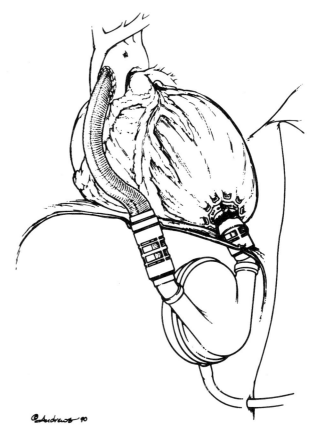

FIG. 51-4
The HeartMate left ventricular assist device. The pump is implanted in the left upper quadrant of the abdomen. The inlet conduit is sewn to the apex of the left ventricle. Output from the pump is routed to the ascending aorta.

From Radovancevic B, Frazier OH, Duncan JM: *J Cardiac Surg* 7:203, 1992.

REFERENCES

1. Tobin MJ: Mechanical ventilation, *N Engl J Med* 330:1056, 1994.
2. Orebuagh SL: Initiation of mechanical ventilation in the emergency department, *Am J Emerg Med* 14:59, 1996.
3. Kirkpatrick AW, Meade RA, Mustard RA, Stewart TE: Strategies of invasive ventilatory support in ARDS, *Shock* 6:17, 1996.
4. Hanlon-Pena PM, Ziegler JC, Stewart R: Management of the intra-aortic balloon pump patient, *Crit Care Nurs Clin North Am* 8:389, 1996.
5. McCarthy PM: HeartMate implantable left ventricular assist device: bridge to transplantation and future applications, *Ann Thorac Surg* 59:46, 1995.

52 Heart Surgery

Joel A. Schneider
George J. Taylor

Surgery of the heart has probably reached the limit set by nature to all surgery: no new method and no new discovery can overcome the natural difficulties that attend.

STEPHEN PAGE, *The Surgery of the Chest*, 1896

HISTORICAL OVERVIEW[1]

Borrowing terms of geological time, the "Eocene age" of heart surgery predated the development of the heart-lung bypass machine in 1954. During this age, bold physicians made daring and sensational attempts to remedy hitherto unapproachable mechanical lesions. In 1897 Rend first sutured a laceration of the heart, and the patient survived. Souttar did the first successful mitral valve commissurotomy in 1925, but more than 20 years passed before Harken and Baily demonstrated a clear benefit from the procedure. In 1955 Lillehei successfully corrected congenital lesions by "cross circulation" with an anesthetized parent so that the child's heart could be opened for repair. At about the same time, Vineberg implanted the internal mammary artery directly into a myocardial tunnel in the beating left ventricle for the purpose of myocardial revascularization. Claude Beck "reversed" the coronary circulation by grafting a nonarterial conduit to the coronary sinus, and Zen experimented with myocardial channels, hoping to promote neovascularization in patients with coronary artery disease (CAD).

The period from 1954 to 1967 was the "Jurassic age" of cardiac surgery. In 1954 Gibbon successfully closed an atrial septal defect using his newly invented heart-lung bypass device, the culmination of two decades of work. Interestingly, his subsequent patients died, and he abandoned its use. Others quickly adopted the new technology and used it to repair atrial and ventricular septal defects, tetralogy of Fallot, transposition of the great vessels, and pulmonic valve stenosis. Albert Star used the first artificial heart valve in 1960, and it is not rare to see one of his original 1260 model valves still working after 30 years.

The modern era of heart surgery began in 1967, when coronary bypass was popularized by Favalaro at the Cleveland Clinic.[1] The number of patients having heart surgery mushroomed, and there was progressive simplification and improvement in heart-lung bypass technology. Earlier pump oxygenators required 14 units of blood to prime the pump, yet by 1980 bloodless prime was the rule.

Our frontiers are very much an assimilation of our own past. Many of the experimental models of earlier ages are being revisited. The myocardial channeling studies of Zen in 1960 are being continued with transmyocardial laser revascularization (now approved by the FDA), and we are trying to match the excellent results of coronary bypass surgery using heart-lung bypass by reinventing coronary bypass with the beating heart.

TECHNICAL ISSUES THAT APPLY TO MOST CARDIAC SURGICAL PROCEDURES

Like many highly specialized areas in medicine, cardiac surgery has its own vernacular. A glossary of frequently used terms is appended to the end of this chapter, This is not rocket science, and the terms refer to straightforward plumbing issues. Some of the terms are arcane, and the glossary may help you interpret a letter that you receive from your surgical or cardiology consultants.

Heart-Lung Bypass

During cardiopulmonary bypass, the heart is stopped (arrested), giving the surgeon a still and relatively bloodless operative field. Vital organs, especially the brain, cannot tolerate prolonged hypoxia. Blood flow and oxygen supply are provided by the heart-lung bypass machine. With the typical bypass circuit, blood is drained from the right atrium into a reservoir. It then passes through an oxygenator, is filtered, and is pumped back into the arterial system, usually the ascending aorta. The pump is adjusted so that pressure is adequate to maintain cerebral blood flow. Blood from surgical field suction may also be filtered, oxygenated, and returned to the arterial circulation (the so-called cell-saver technology).

Cardioplegia

Cross clamping of the aorta essentially prevents blood flow to the heart muscle. Maintaining myocardial via-

bility is a technical problem that is just as critical as the perfusion of other vital organs during surgery. In earlier times the heart was stopped by inducing ventricular fibrillation; however, mechanical activity persists with fibrillation, and without ventricular decompression, ischemic injury may develop during fibrillation.

Prevention of ischemic injury is the goal of cardioplegia, the current approach to placing the heart at rest and preserving cellular function and viability during the operation. The heart is arrested in diastole by infusing a solution high in potassium. Excess potassium depolarizes the cell membrane, preventing contraction. Cardioplegia solutions may have a number of other components, including magnesium, procaine, mannitol, and adenosine. In addition, the solution and the heart are cooled to about 10° C, further reducing the metabolic demands of the resting heart muscle. After surgery, the heart is warmed and the potassium solution is washed out, at which time myocardial excitation and contraction resume.

Monitoring During Surgery

As with other major surgical procedures, ECG and hemodynamic monitoring are used. Patients with cardiac dysfunction routinely have pulmonary artery pressure, venous saturation, and cardiac indices monitored during and after surgery (see Chapters 2 and 51).

The transesophageal echocardiogram is commonly used to be sure that no air remains in the cardiac chambers at the end of the operation and to assess left ventricular function. In addition, it allows detection and quantification of valvular regurgitation after valve repair while the patient is still in the operating room. If repair seems inadequate, it is relatively easy to go back on pump and either revise the repair or insert a valve prosthesis.

Cardiac-Assist Devices

Heart surgery for patients with advanced left ventricular dysfunction has become commonplace. In borderline cases there often is uncertainty preoperatively about the patient's ability to tolerate surgery. Despite our sophisticated methods for measuring cardiac function, the operation itself is the ultimate test. Coming off bypass is the critical test of the heart's ability to support blood pressure and organ perfusion.

Cardiac dysfunction at this time may be temporary. Hemodynamic support for a day or two may allow the heart time to recover from the stress of surgery. Catecholamine or phosphodiesterase inhibitor (e.g., milrinone) infusion may be used to stimulate myocardial contractility and support blood pressure. The intraaortic balloon pump (IABP) is the next step for those who cannot generate sufficient cardiac output after surgery (see Chapter 51). If the heart fails to recover, a ventricular-assist device may be used longer term and is usually a bridge to cardiac transplantation. It is rarely used for temporary support after surgery.

RISKS OF HEART SURGERY

The choice of any therapy boils down to the balance between benefit and risk. With normal ventricular function, an otherwise healthy person having coronary bypass surgery may have a mortality risk as low as 1-2/1000. But in the real world of cardiac surgery, patients are not selected just because they would benefit from surgery, but rather because they are likely to do worse without it.

As our surgical patient population becomes older and has more concomitant illness, the chance of an intraoperative or postoperative complication increases. This change in demographics parallels an aging population. In addition, angioplasty has taken our lowest-risk patients—those who are young and with limited disease—out of the surgery cohort.

Because of the large volume of procedures, coronary surgery has the best derived statistics.[2,3] Thus, a 75-year-old woman having emergency re-do CABG with a low ejection fraction would have a mortality risk as much as 17 times that of a 55-year-old man with normal ejection fraction having a first, elective procedure. Other comorbidities that increase the risk of surgery include angioplasty during admission (necessitating emergency surgery), recent myocardial infarction, ventricular arrhythmias, diabetes, cerebral vascular disease, obstructive lung disease and elevated creatinine.

COMPLICATIONS OF HEART SURGERY

The major concern is death during or soon after surgery. (In most studies an operative mortality is defined as death within 30 days of surgery.) The risks have been described above and are largely determined by patient selection. You may encounter a number of other complications, especially as patients are being discharged so early after surgery.

Stroke

Patients with CAD not infrequently have vascular disease elsewhere. Stroke is a complication in 1% to 2 % of cardiac operations.[4,5] It is more common in elderly patients, those with a prior history of stroke or transient ischemic attack, and those who develop postoperative atrial fibrillation. A carotid bruit and known extracranial carotid disease indicate a higher risk. Carotid endarterectomy may be considered before coronary bypass or as an adjunctive procedure in an attempt to prevent postoperative stroke. Knowledge of a severely atheromatous aorta may prompt a change in cross-clamp technique.

Even with our best efforts to prevent stroke, it remains a finite (1% to 2%) and potentially devastating complication of surgery. In most cases it is out of the control of the surgeon and surgical team, since it is not related to surgical technique or skill. We consider it an unavoidable risk of surgery that must be understood and accepted by patients and their families (and the primary care physician).

Stroke usually occurs within 4 days of surgery and rarely after discharge. Those with embolic stroke in a setting of atrial fibrillation often recover immediately. Others with large, fixed neurologic deficits may die or be severely disabled.

Atrial Fibrillation

Atrial fibrillation (AF) develops during the week after surgery in as many as 15% to 20% of patients having heart surgery. It may occur as late as 7 days and thus is not uncommon after hospital discharge. There do not appear to be cardiac "risk factors" for this complication; it is not a function of the severity of heart disease. However, it may be preventable; prophylactic therapy with beta-blockers reduces the incidence by almost half. Maintaining normal serum magnesium may also help. (Low serum magnesium is often associated with AF after noncardiac operations as well.)

There usually are no serious clinical consequences of postoperative AF. Although it has been identified as a risk factor for postoperative stroke, only a small percentage of patients with AF develop stroke.[5] Patients are alarmed by the rapid pulse and associated fatigue and by the notion that it is a cardiac complication of surgery. Reassurance is in order: AF is easy to treat, has few long-term consequences, and rarely recurs. Most patients spontaneously convert to sinus rhythm.

The usual treatment principles apply (see Chapter 25). The ventricular rate may be controlled with digoxin, beta-blockers, or calcium channel blockers. Ibutilide (Corvert) is our first choice for cardioversion, although electrical cardioversion is highly effective and safe. Other membrane-active agents may be used including quinidine, procainamide, and sotalol. If AF persists for more than 48 hours, anticoagulation is necessary. Immediate correction of hypokalemia and hypomagnesemia is imperative; without this, cardioversion may be unsuccessful.

After cardioversion, we usually continue drug therapy for 1 month, and have noted little risk of AF recurring. The pathophysiology of AF in this setting is uncertain. We tell patients that it seems related to the normal inflammatory process of healing. Once that has passed, AF does not return. If it does, it is the result of the underlying cardiac condition, not the surgery.

Postpericardiotomy Syndrome

This autoimmune reaction after heart surgery is pleuropericarditis with fever that develops more than 1 week after the operation.[6-8] Any mechanical manipulation of the pericardium can cause it, including cardiac trauma or perforation of the heart by a pacemaker wire. The serositis is like that of Dressler's syndrome. The incidence is about 10% with heart surgery, with mild cases largely unrecognized; some estimate an incidence as high as 30%.[7]

It is an easy condition to diagnose when you are aware of it. The problem is that primary care physicians, who send just a few patients for heart surgery, do not encounter this problem that often even though it is relatively common. The usual clinical picture is fever plus pleurisy or pericarditis during the month after surgery. The patient may feel poorly out of proportion to physical findings. Patchy pneumonitis is common, and it is commonly mistaken for culture-negative pneumonia. There may be a pericardial friction rub, and ECG and echocardiographic results demonstrate pericarditis (see Chapter 29). There may be lymphocytosis with mild elevation of the white cell count, but granulocytosis is unusual. All patients have marked elevation of the sedimentation rate, and this may be monitored to follow the course of the illness. *If you suspect postpericardiotomy, order a sedimentation rate.*

When we see patients with this in the clinic we rarely admit them to hospital, but follow them with frequent outpatient visits. For mild cases, nonsteroidal antiinflammatory drugs work, and indomethacin has been used traditionally. More severe cases respond dramatically to a short course of steroids with a tapering dose (e.g., a Medrol dose-pack). Patients who require longer and higher dose therapy probably should be followed up by a cardiologist.

Most patients have a single episode with no recurrence. As with Dressler's syndrome, some patients have intermittent recurrences, with episodes as late as 1 year after surgery. Recurrence is easily identified by symptoms and an elevated sedimentation rate. Postcardiotomy tends to "burn out," with later flare-ups less severe and farther apart. Although possible, pericardial fibrosis and constriction are rare. We reassure patients that the inflammatory condition does not hurt the heart and that they may expect to do well long term.

Wound Infection and Dehiscence

Deep wound infection is fortunately rare, with mediastinitis occurring in less than 1%. It is devastating when it occurs, resulting in months-long hospitalization for antibiotic therapy and wound care. Unexplained fever, elevated white count, or fluctuance or excessive mobility of the sternotomy should prompt an immediate return of the patient to the heart surgeon. Spontaneous drainage of a large amount of fluid from the incision indicates sternal dehiscence.

Superficial dehiscence of a portion of the sternotomy incision or, more commonly, of the vein harvest site in

the leg is managed at home with debridement and appropriate dressing changes. The heart surgeon and the surgeon's nurse are skilled in managing this common problem, with the cardiologist and primary care doctors providing moral support. While an aggravation, local wound problems are not serious and the outlook is good.

Pleural Effusion

The "postpump" chest x-ray always shows changes, including sternal wires, atelectasis, some widening of the mediastinum, and pleural effusion. Postoperative effusion usually is on the left side, whereas pleural effusion with heart failure tends to be on the right. Large effusion may necessitate thoracentesis, and the fluid is bloody. It is not necessary to send it for laboratory examination. Repeat drainage of pleural fluid is uncommon.

Elevated Left Hemidiaphragm

Routine chest x-ray after surgery may reveal an elevated left hemidiaphragm indicating phrenic nerve injury and resultant paralysis of the left hemidiaphragm. It is thought to result from a variety of insults, including cold injury accompanying myocardial preservation, dissection of the internal thoracic artery, or direct mechanical trauma. The diagnosis is confirmed with fluoroscopic observation of the diaphragm while the patient sniffs (the "sniff test"). This is another of the complications of thoracotomy that is out of the surgeon's control, and its occurrence does not signify a breach of the standard of surgical care. Spontaneous recovery is common but may take months.

Indications for Heart Surgery

Heart surgery is no longer considered a last resort when all available medical therapies have failed. Instead it is recommended whenever it may provide the most direct and greatest improvement in a patient's functional ability, longevity, and freedom from future medical needs and interventions. Conversely, cardiac surgery should not be recommended just because no satisfactory medical therapy is available.

An abundance of evidence-based medicine guides our selection of treatment for most cardiac conditions. Clinical trials and practice guidelines for surgery have been reviewed for coronary artery disease (see Chapters 13 and 17), valvular disease (see Chapters 18 to 21), congenital heart disease (see Chapter 30), cardiac arrhythmias (see Chapters 25 to 28), heart failure (see Chapters 22 and 23), and pericardial disease (see Chapter 29). Box 52-1 provides an overview of heart conditions that may or may not be reparable using a surgical approach.

BOX 52-1

A SURVEY OF HEART CONDITIONS AND APPLICABILITY OF MECHANICAL (SURGICAL) TREATMENT

HEART SURGERY MAY HELP
Coronary artery disease
Valve stenosis or insufficiency
Infected cardiac valves
Congenital heart disease
Ventricular aneurysm
Myxoma of the heart
Some cardiac arrhythmias (e.g., atrial fibrillation, preexcitation syndrome)

HEART SURGERY (OTHER THAN TRANSPLANTATION) USUALLY DOES NOT HELP
Eisenmenger's complex
Primary muscle disease (cardiomyopathy)
Coronary artery disease with inadequate distal (target) vessels
Cancer of the heart
Heart disease in the setting of multisystem failure

TECHNICAL CONSIDERATIONS FOR SPECIFIC CARDIAC OPERATIONS

Coronary Artery Bypass Grafting

Coronary artery atheroma tends to be focal and located in the proximal third of the involved coronary artery. A relatively disease-free distal vessel makes coronary artery bypass grafting (CABG) possible.

The most commonly used and original bypass conduit is the saphenous vein, reversed so that the venous valves do not obstruct flow. With time, the vein thickens in response to arterial pressure, becoming "arterialized." Vein grafts are particularly susceptible to atherosclerosis. The lesion is somewhat different from plaque in native arteries, as it is softer and has a surface that crumbles easily. Late angiographic studies, 10 years after CABG, have demonstrated occlusion in at least 30% of vein grafts. High flow through the graft seems protective, because grafts to large vessels have better longevity than grafts to small, lower flow coronary branches. Diseased vein grafts are frustrating to deal with, since the soft and friable plaque responds poorly to angioplasty.

The most important single advance in bypass grafting has been the use of the internal mammary artery (IMA).[1,9] The left IMA (LIMA) easily reaches the left anterior descending artery, which supplies the anterior wall of the left ventricle. This region of myocardium is particularly important: losing it with anterior infarction

often is devastating, and preservation of anterior wall viability tends to confer a good prognosis (regardless of what is happening to other coronary vascular distributions). In addition to supplying the most important region of the heart, the LIMA seems to endure, with patency rates at 10 years approaching 95%. For unknown reasons, atherosclerosis rarely develops in the LIMA. If stenosis occurs, it is more like the plaque encountered in native arteries than that in the crumbly, soft vein graft lesion; it usually can be fixed with angioplasty. We estimate that experienced surgeons use the LIMA for more than 95% of LADs grafted, especially for patients younger than 70 years old.

Right IMA grafts are occasionally used for the right coronary artery. The long-term patency rate of this system is not as good as the LIMA to the LAD, but is more like that of vein grafts. When possible, doing a bypass operation with both IMAs and no vein grafts is appealing, because the patient will have no leg incision. The downside of this approach is that diverting both IMAs compromises blood flow to the sternum. This is a possible (and debatable) risk for sternal wound infection after surgery, especially in diabetic patients.

Most CABG procedures are done using heart-lung bypass. New technology allows "beating heart" surgery, in which a device stabilizes the heart in the operative field while the graft is sewn into the distal coronary artery.[10] Relative advantages and disadvantages of the beating heart technique are summarized in Box 52-2. The choice of approach depends on the coronary anatomy, extent of disease, quality of distal "target" vessels, and how well the patient tolerates having the beating heart lifted from the pericardium and rotated.

Follow-up after CABG

Most patients are asked to see the primary care doctor 1 to 2 weeks after discharge. The patient is still uncomfortable and needs reassurance that, with time and exercise, symptoms will resolve and normal level of vigor will return. Although many are ready to return to sedentary jobs 6 weeks after surgery, few are back to normal. Most, especially older, patients have continued fatigue for at least 6 weeks. Knowing this is normal helps them get through it.

A majority of our patients participate in formal cardiac rehabilitation programs. Those who do have a more rapid recovery of exercise tolerance. They also do better with risk factor modification.

Many drugs used after heart surgery are needed only temporarily, including iron replacement and antiarrhythmic therapy. Lifelong treatment with aspirin is indicated after CABG. An important goal is reduction of LDL cholesterol to <100 mg/dL, which requires drug therapy for most of our patients (see Chapter 12). Once CAD is recognized, one thing the primary care physician can do to improve prognosis is to ensure that elevated cholesterol does not "slip through the cracks."

Modifying other risk factors is also important. It seems that heart surgery is a good way to stop smoking. But with time, many patients forget what they have been through and return to old patterns of behavior. The primary care physician—and the clinic staff—should relentlessly pursue smoking cessation, weight management, and exercise during the year after CABG. It is well established that just asking about cigarettes during clinic visits has a favorable effect (see Chapter 11).

VALVULAR HEART DISEASE

In the 1970s some speculated that surgery for valvular disease would diminish with the decline in rheumatic fever. This has not proven to be the case. Currently there are about 4000 valve replacements and an equal number of valve repairs in the United States. Many of these patients have degenerative disease of either the mitral or aortic valves and are typically much older than patients in the past.

BOX 52-2

POTENTIAL ADVANTAGES OF "BEATING HEART" CABG VERSUS SURGERY USING HEART-LUNG BYPASS*

ISSUES FAVORING BEATING HEART SURGERY
Avoids the systemic inflammatory response attributed to cardiopulmonary bypass
Less hemodilution, since the pump is not primed
Avoids the cost of cardiopulmonary bypass
Less postoperative bleeding (avoids the platelet effects of bypass on platelet function, and heparin is unnecessary)

ISSUES FAVORING CARDIOPULMONARY BYPASS
Bloodless and motionless operating field, allowing greater technical precision
An ability to decompress and rotate the heart, allowing better visualization of arteries
Relieves the heart of its work load while its own blood supply is being repaired

---

*These should be considered patient selection issues. The question is not "which operation is better," but rather "which operation is better for this patient." Thus a patient with stenosis in a difficult to reach location would be better off with cardiopulmonary bypass. Another with more accessible target vessels could have a beating heart procedure.

Valve replacement for calcific aortic stenosis is the most common valve operation in adults. Despite the advanced age of most of these patients, surgical mortality has fallen to less than 5%. The hypertrophied left ventricle is quite susceptible to ischemic injury. Improved myocardial preservation (cardioplegia) during surgery and more rapid operations account for improved outcome.

The major advance in mitral valve surgery is the recognition that valve repair and preservation of papillary muscle function lead to better LV function after surgery (see Chapter 18). Repair is often possible for those with mitral prolapse, papillary muscle dysfunction, or cordal rupture. It is contraindicated if there is valve infection, annular or leaflet calcification, or an inability to tolerate a more prolonged operation. As noted above, the transesophageal echocardiograph is used during and after surgery to evaluate the functional result of valve repair.

Choice of Valve Prosthesis

The broad choice is between mechanical and tissue prostheses. We will not discuss the relative merits of different mechanical valves. The commonly used bioprosthesis is the porcine heterograft; others include cadaveric valves, bovine pericardial valves, and the patient's own pulmonic valve transplanted to the aortic position.

Valve selection issues are summarized in Box 52-3. The disadvantage of mechanical valves is the need for lifelong anticoagulation using warfarin.[11] Without anticoagulation, the risk of embolic stroke is as high as 20% per year. The risk of valve thrombosis, and therefore embolism, is especially high with mechanical valves in the mitral position, and more aggressive anticoagulation is necessary (Table 52-1). There is no standard protocol

---

BOX 52-3
SELECTION OF VALVE PROSTHESIS

YOUNG PATIENT (<45 YEARS OLD)
Mechanical valve (risk of valve degeneration exceeds risk of anticoagulation)*

OLDER PATIENT
Can tolerate anticoagulation: mechanical valve
Cannot tolerate anticoagulation: tissue valve

VERY OLD PATIENT
Tissue valve (risk of anticoagulation exceeds risk of valve degeneration)

---

*Another possibility is the Ross procedure, in which the patient's pulmonic valve is transferred to the aortic position, and another prosthesis is placed in the pulmonic position. This is a long and difficult operation and is reserved for younger patients who cannot tolerate anticoagulation.

Table 52-1 | *Anticoagulation Guidelines for Patients with Prosthetic Heart Valves: The Mayo Clinic Protocol*

Clinical Issue	Target INR	Aspirin (mg/day)
AORTIC VALVES		
Bileaflet mechanical (e.g., St. Jude)	2.5	81
Other mechanical	3.0	81
Bioprosthetic valve: low risk*	2.5 for 3 mo	325 indefinitely
Bioprosthetic: high risk*	2.5 indefinitely	81
MITRAL VALVES		
Mechanical valves	3.0	81
Bioprosthetic valve	2.5 indefinitely†	81
Bioprosthetic valve and high bleeding risk	2.5 for 3-6 mo	325 indefinitely
MITRAL VALVE REPAIR		
Low risk*	2.5 for 3 mo	325 indefinitely
High risk*	2.5 indefinitely	81

Modified from Tiede DJ, Nishimura RA, Gastineau DA, et al: *Mayo Clin Proc* 73:665, 1998.
*Clinical factors indicating *high risk* for thromboembolism include a first-generation tilting disc (Bjork-Shiley) or ball-cage (Starr-Edwards) valve in the mitral position, a double-position prosthetic valve, atrial fibrillation, severe left ventricular dysfunction, prior embolic event, and a hypercoagulable state. The absence of any of these indicates *low risk*. In practice, many surgeons do not use warfarin after tissue valve replacement.
†At many medical centers, warfarin is given for just 3 months to patients who are at low risk for thromboembolism, and they are treated with 325 mg aspirin.

for prosthetic valve anticoagulation. The one used by the Mayo Clinic is sensible, and their review is a thorough summary of available clinical trials (Table 52-1).[11] It is now common to add low-dose aspirin to warfarin for patients younger than 70 years old.[11]

Note that anticoagulation does not bring the risk of embolism to zero. One study documented systemic embolism in 15% to 17% of men followed 11 years with both mechanical and tissue valves.[12]

The major disadvantage of tissue valves is structural valve failure. In a randomized trial about 15% of tissue valves in the aortic position failed within 11 years, and in the mitral position the failure rate was 36%.[12]

In some studies the failure rate of tissue valves exceeds 50% by the fifteenth postoperative year. Calcific degeneration of tissue valves is especially common in young people and those with renal dysfunction. For these reasons, tissue valves are usually reserved for older patients, for whom the tradeoff between lower valve longevity and avoiding anticoagulation seems reasonable. Other circumstances that would favor a tissue valve include an inability to take anticoagulants, including difficulties with compliance.

Follow-up after Valve Replacement

Routine echocardiography is not indicated. A change in the murmur across the valve, a new murmur suggesting perivalvular or valvular regurgitation, and new symptoms are indications for an echocardiogram. Any of these issues should prompt referral to a cardiologist, who usually plans to see the patient at 1- to 2-year intervals in any case.

A major responsibility of the primary care doctor is monitoring anticoagulation. The routine follow-up physical examination should include careful auscultation of valve sounds and listening for the murmur of aortic regurgitation in patients with an aortic valve prosthesis. I always record, "crisp valve sounds and no diastolic murmur" in my clinic notes. Crisp mechanical valve sounds should remain crisp. Muffled sounds and new symptoms may indicate a valve thrombosis. A new diastolic murmur usually identifies a perivalvular leak.

Mechanical valves often cause low-grade, though clinically insignificant, hemolysis. More severe hemolysis and anemia are usually the result of a perivalvular leak.

REFERENCES

1. Favaloro RG: Critical analysis of coronary artery bypass graft surgery: a 30-year journey, *J Am Coll Cardiol* 31:1, 1998.
2. Jones RH, Hannan EL, Hammermeister KE, et al: Identification of perioperative variables needed for risk adjustment of short-term mortality after coronary artery bypass graft surgery, *J Am Coll Cardiol* 28:1478, 1996.
3. Edwards FH, Carey JS, Grover FL, et al: Impact of gender on coronary bypass operative mortality, *Ann Thorac Surg* 66:125, 1998.
4. Lazar HL, Menzoian JO: Coronary artery bypass grafting in patients with cerebrovascular disease, *Ann Thorac Surg* 66:968, 1998.
5. Taylor GJ, Malik SA, Collier JA, et al: Usefulness of atrial fibrillation as a predictor of stroke after isolated coronary artery bypass grafting, *Am J Cardiol* 1987; 60:905,.
6. Davenport J: Postpericardiotomy syndrome, *Am Fam Physician* 39:185, 1989.
7. Engle MA, Gay WA, Zabriskie JB, Senterfit LB: The postpericardiotomy syndrome: 25 years' experience, *J Cardiovasc Med* 4:321, 1984.
8. Kahn AH: The postcardiac delayed injury syndromes, *Clin Cardiol* 15:67, 1992.
9. Sergeant PT, Blackstone EH, Meyns BP: Does arterial revascularization decrease the risk of infarction after coronary artery bypass grafting? *Ann Thorac Surg* 66:1, 1998.
10. Talwalkar NG, Cooley DA: Minimally invasive coronary artery bypass grafting, *Cardiol Rev* 6:345, 1998.
11. Tiede DJ, Nishimura RA, Gastineau DA, et al: Modern management of prosthetic valve anticoagulation, *Mayo Clin Proc* 73:665, 1998.
12. Hammermeister KE, Sethi GK, Henderson WG, et al: A comparison of outcomes in men 11 years after heart-valve replacement with a mechanical valve or bioprosthesis, *N Engl J Med* 328:1289, 1993.

BIBLIOGRAPHY

Frazier OH, Kadipasaoglu KA, Cooley DA: Transmyocardial laser revascularization, *Tex Heart Inst J* 25:24, 1998.
Tam JW, Masters RG, Burwash IG, et al: Management of patients with mild aortic stenosis undergoing coronary artery bypass grafting, *Ann Thorac Surg* 65:1215, 1998.

APPENDIX

A Glossary of Cardiac Surgical Terms Commonly Found in Operative Notes and Discharge Summaries

Balloon pump—A sausage-shaped, 40 ml balloon placed through the femoral artery and positioned in the descending aorta. Rapid and sequential inflation and deflation is timed with the cardiac cycle to improve cardiac output (see Chapter 51).

"Cabbage," or *CABG (coronary artery bypass graft)*—The most common open heart operation, in which a graft is routed from the proximal aorta to the coronary artery distal to the stenosing or obstructing lesion.

Cannulate—placement of the arterial and venous tubing lines into the aorta (usually) and the right atrium (usually, less often the vena cavae) for the purpose of going "on pump."

Cardioplegia—a solution used to stop and preserve the heart during cardiopulmonary bypass; there are a number of recipes, but the essential elements are high potassium to depolarize the cells and stop the heart in diastole and cold ($\leq 10^\circ$ C) to reduce metabolic demand.

Catheter—preshaped plastic line used to engage the coronary artery ostium during angiography.

Cross clamp, cross clamp time—application of an occlusive vascular clamp across the ascending aorta at the time cardioplegic solution is given and the heart stopped. The length of time that the heart is stopped during surgery.

Decannulate—removal of the arterial and venous lines used for cardiopulmonary bypass.

Free IMA graft—an internal mammary that is dissected free of its subclavian artery origin and is then connected to the proximal aorta like a saphenous graft.

Homograft valve—a cadaver valve.

Internal mammary artery graft (IMA)—The right and left IMAs are branches of the subclavian artery that run along the inner surface of the ribs, parallel and to each side of the sternum. When used as a bypass graft, the proximal connection of the IMA is not disturbed and the distal vessel is dissected free and side branches ligated. It is then inserted into the distal coronary artery. Long-term patency of the left IMA (LIMA) to the anterior descending artery is unusually good (see text).

Mechanical valve—an artificial valve made using pyralyte carbon discs that tilt (e.g., the St. Jude valve, the most commonly used prosthesis world-wide) or a mobile ball that floats in a metal ring and stent (the Star-Edwards valve).

Open heart surgery—a general term for procedures using the heart-lung bypass machine. Notwithstanding that coronary artery bypass surgery is performed on the surface of the heart and that the heart chambers are not opened, CABG is usually called "open heart surgery."

Pericardial valve—a bovine xenograft (a graft from another species) prosthesis.

Porcine, or pig, valve—a bioprosthetic (xenograft) valve made from the fixed (essentially a tanning process) aortic valve of a pig that is mounted in a metal and fabric stent.

Proline—a monofilament polyethylene suture material that is a favorite for sewing bypass grafts.

Pump sucker—a suction device that returns shed blood to the heart-lung bypass machine.

Pump—the heart-lung bypass machine including a roller, or centrifugal pump, an oxygenator, and venous blood reservoir.

Reversed saphenous vein graft (RSV)—a commonly used conduit for coronary artery bypass.

Sequential graft—a bypass graft that supplies more than one target vessel. Usually smaller branches have side-to-side anastomoses, and the distal end of the graft is inserted into the largest of the targets. By convention, the *number of bypass grafts* refers to the number of target vessels bypassed and not the number of grafts that are used. Thus a five-vessel bypass procedure might include a LIMA sequentially to two anterior descending artery branches and a vein graft sequentially to three circumflex branches.

Target—used when referring to the coronary artery distal to the stenosing lesion. The quality of the target vessel refers to its size (bigger is much better) and the presence or absence of atherosclerosis in the distal vessel.

Ventricular-assist device (VAD)—the LVAD is a pump placed between a left atrial line and the aorta, and the RVAD is positioned between the right atrium and pulmonary artery. The VAD essentially replaces the chamber, doing all its work (see Chapter 51).

53 Palliative Care and End-of-Life Decisions

George J. Taylor
Bert Keller
Leslye C. Pennypacker

PALLIATIVE CARE FOR PATIENTS WITH HEART DISEASE

Cardiovascular disease is the most common cause of death in the United States. Consequently, primary care physicians frequently care for patients with fatal heart disease. Terminal heart disease seems different from other inevitably fatal illnesses. With lung cancer, for example, we know and accept the prognosis, and the timing of death is relatively predictable. The patient and family quickly know what the doctor knows, that the end of life is just months away, and all prepare to shift into a palliative mode. With heart disease, however, it invariably seems that there is "one more thing" to do or try. The timing of death may not be predictable; a patient with end-stage heart failure may live just months but may also stabilize and live for years. As a result, most patients with heart disease frequently receive "maximal medical therapy until death."[1] A minority of patients with chronic heart disease decide against further aggressive or interventional treatment. Hopefully with the support of family and their doctors, they decide to pursue a course of palliative therapy, and that is the subject of this chapter.

Do not despair or lose interest if a patient declines treatment. The care of a seriously ill patient at the end of life is among our most satisfying experiences in medicine when we do it well. This requires understanding and acceptance of the patient's decision and acceptance of the inevitable. At this juncture, the doctor must eschew the notion that prolongation of survival is the goal of that patient's medical care. Instead, relief of suffering and a peaceful death become the goals.

This is an uncertain time for patients and families. Most of us are uncomfortable with unfamiliar situations and do not want to do or say the wrong thing. Spending time with the patient and family, helping them understand their roles and what is appropriate, relieves one element of our suffering and theirs. We are all comforted when we know what to expect and what is expected of us.

Terminal care is a clinical skill, as important for your patient as the proper choice of curative therapy. To do it well requires clinical knowledge. Best at it is the doctor who sees this aspect of practice as a positive experience, approaching it with equanimity and grace.

Congestive Heart Failure

The treatment of congestive heart failure (CHF) is reviewed in Chapters 22 and 23. All the drugs are given to relieve congestion and are thus palliative. Angiotensin-converting enzyme (ACE) inhibitors improve survival, but they have an even more dramatic effect on symptoms. An interesting difference between the generalist and the heart failure specialist is that the latter has learned to *maximize the dose of ACE inhibitors* to optimally control symptoms (see Chapter 22). Digoxin has not been found to change prognosis, but it relieves symptoms and reduces the need for hospitalization (see Chapter 22).

Diuretic Resistance

The patient with end-stage CHF is usually taking the maximal tolerated dose of ACE inhibitors, as well as digoxin and diuretics, yet still has recurrence of pulmonary congestion. Fine tuning volume becomes the major issue and requires adjustment of the diuretic dose, as well as salt and fluid intake.

Thiazide diuretics are effective in the early phase of CHF but have usually been replaced by loop diuretics in the later stage of the disease, most commonly furosemide (Lasix). It has been around a long time, we all have experience with it, and it is inexpensive.

There are, however, problems with Lasix, and resistance to its actions is common. The bioavailability of furosemide is variable. On average, about 50% is absorbed, but the range is 10% to 100%, making it difficult to know how much a particular patient is getting.[2] This is solved by gradually increasing the dose until diuresis is achieved. The rate of absorption is slowed in heart failure, prolonging the half-life but not changing the amount of furosemide that reaches the distal tubule. Another problem is that renal responsiveness to all of the loop diuretics is reduced in patients with CHF, by as much as 60% to 70% when compared with normals.[2] This may be compounded by renal insufficiency, which impairs delivery of furosemide to the site of action (there is reduced secretion of drug into urine in the

proximal tubule, so delivery to the distal tubule is reduced). The net effect of all this is "diuretic tolerance"; higher than usual doses of furosemide are needed.

What is the highest dose of furosemide that can be given, beyond which there is no additional benefit? It seems that the maximal effect is achieved with an intravenous bolus injection of 160 to 200 mg furosemide.[2] At higher doses, there is no increase in natriuresis, but the risk of tinnitus increases. A hospitalized patient with severe pulmonary congestion may need this high intravenous dose several times a day. The maximal *oral dose* is about twice the intravenous dose when renal function is normal, but higher still with renal insufficiency. Occasionally a patient is unresponsive to high doses of furosemide because of poor absorption. Before giving up and committing the patient to dialysis for control of volume, you might try an especially high oral dose of furosemide, perhaps 600 mg.

A better decision would be a trial of torsemide (Demadex) or bumetanide (Bumex). These newer loop diuretics have a mechanism of action that is identical to furosemide: they are secreted into urine in the proximal tubule and act on the distal tubule. *The big difference is that bioavailability with oral dosing is much better,* with 80% to 100% of both drugs absorbed even in the presence of splanchnic congestion or renal insufficiency. Both are metabolized and excreted by the liver, and the elimination half-life is not affected by renal insufficiency. However, renal insufficiency does reduce the secretion of drug into the proximal tubule, so higher doses are needed.

If you are treating a patient with intravenous medicine there is not much advantage of torsemide or bumetanide over furosemide. However, with oral therapy, better absorption of the newer agents makes them almost as effective as they would be if given intravenously.

When comparing the newer loop diuretics, the major difference is elimination half-life, which is longer for Demadex (Table 53-1). This may be advantageous, since there is some evidence for rebound sodium retention between diuretic doses for severely ill patients.[2] For this reason, continuous infusion furosemide has been advocated for severe congestion and diuretic resistance (a loading dose of 40 mg, then 10 to 40 mg/hr, with the higher dose given when creatinine clearance is less than 25 ml/hr). The cost of Demadex and Bumex is similar, and therefore Demadex is our usual choice if a patient has been resistant to furosemide. The comparable oral dose of Demadex is one half the furosemide dose.

Another issue is whether to give loop diuretics once or twice a day. Early in the course of CHF, when congestion is effectively controlled with once-daily dosing, there is no reason to give the drug more frequently. Active diuresis restricts the patient's activities. With more resistant congestion, twice-daily dosing is usually necessary. With furosemide, morning and noon dosing frees the evening for other activities. With Demadex, the oral doses should be separated by 6 hours.

Multiple Drug Therapy

If a patient is taking maximal doses of a loop diuretic and congestion is poorly controlled, an effective strategy may be the addition of an oral thiazide (Table 53-2). Thiazides work more distally in the nephron, blocking the absorption of sodium that escaped the loop of Henle (and the action of the loop diuretic). Thus there is a synergistic effect of thiazide and loop diuretics[2] (Table 53-2).

Metolazone (Zaroxolyn and others) has been marketed for this purpose in the United States and is widely used. Hydrochlorothiazide (HCTZ) is more rapidly absorbed, has a shorter half-life (hours rather than 2 days), and therefore does not accumulate in the body, and is much cheaper. For these reasons, HCTZ may be the preferable drug.[2] With severe heart failure the dose is 100 to 200 mg/day given in two doses. The dose of HCTZ must be increased when there is renal insufficiency.

An occasional patient resistant to loop and thiazide diuretics will respond to a potassium-sparing diuretic, such as spironolactone, that acts on the distal nephron

Table 53-1	Diuretic Drugs

| Drug | Oral Absorption (% | Elimination Half-Life (Hr) | | CHF |
		Normal	Renal Insufficiency	
Furosemide	10-100*	1.5-2	2.8	2.7
Bumetanide	80-100	1	1.6	1.3
Torsemide	80-100	3-4	4-5	6
Hydrochlorothiazide	65-75	2.5	Increased	Uncertain

*Absorption may be at the low end of this range with CHF and splanchnic congestion.

Table 53-2	*An Approach to Diuretic Therapy with Advanced CHF*
First step: Loop diuretic	1. Titrate the dose to effective diuresis 2. Give often enough to maintain a response, depending on the severity of congestive symptoms 3. Substitute torsemide for furosemide if there is resistance to therapy (for more reliable absorption and increased half-life) 4. Consider intravenous and possibly continuous infusion furosemide if there is resistance to oral therapy
Second step: Add a thiazide diuretic based on renal function	Cl_{cr} >50 ml/hr, give HCTZ 25-50 mg/day Cl_{cr} =20-50 ml/hr, give HCTZ 50-100 mg/day Cl_{cr} <20 ml/hr, give HCTZ 100-200 mg/day
Third step: Add or substitute a distal diuretic (spironolactone, triamterene, amiloride).	Consider this if hypokalemia has been a problem or for added natriuresis (see text). The distal agents are most effective when renal function is normal.

(Table 53-2). It is given in combination with the loop diuretic. Our clinical impression is that this often works for those with peripheral edema, although this has not been tested. The clinical responsiveness can be predicted by measuring urine electrolytes. Low urinary sodium and high potassium suggests that potassium is being exchanged for sodium in the distal nephron (the aldosterone mechanism), and spironolactone should work. If urinary potassium is low, spironolactone probably will not be effective. The half-life of spironolactone is sufficient for once-daily dosing to be adequate (50 to 200 mg/day). It may take a couple of weeks before diuresis begins.

Another drug to consider when the loop-thiazide diuretic combination fails is acetazolamide plus the loop diuretic. It is especially effective if there is metabolic alkalosis. The dose is 500 mg intravenously in addition to continuous infusion of the loop diuretic.

Dopamine As a "Diuretic"

At low dose, <3 µg/kg/min, dopamine improves renal hemodynamics and is thought to promote diuresis. We still try it, but at least one study failed to document a measurable benefit in patients with CHF.[2,3]

Salt and Fluid Restriction

Salt restriction is critical, even though we have effective diuretics. Our heart failure clinic tends to use lower doses of diuretics for patients with advanced CHF, and we attribute this to more effective management of dietary sodium. This clinic has a dietitian who works with each patient to reduce salt intake to less than 2 g/day. As a rule, doctors are less effective than dietitians in effecting real changes in diet.

Fluid restriction has become common practice, although there are no studies documenting efficacy. Our heart failure clinic suggests restriction of fluids to less than 1.5 to 2 L/day for patients who need more than 80 mg/day of furosemide.

Ultrafiltration

When other efforts have failed, ultrafiltration almost always relieves congestive symptoms. It is minimally invasive but does require treatment in a dialysis unit (see Chapter 44). Patients with end-stage disease often do not wish to pursue this.

Palliation for Terminal Heart Failure

Many with CHF and advanced LV depression die suddenly with ventricular arrhythmias. Others develop severe congestion that is poorly controlled despite maximal medical therapy. Because of poor exercise tolerance, they need help with even simple activities of daily living. Home oxygen may provide some relief. Outpatient dobutamine therapy may help (see Chapter 22). Additional bed rest—recumbency—may contribute to diuresis.

Even those with terminal CHF are candidates for aggressive medical management, and they tend to receive maximal therapy until death. The prevalence of do-not-resuscitate orders has been estimated at less than 5%, despite the findings of a study that one quarter of patients with end-stage disease wished to avoid resuscitation.[1,4] This study also found a poor correlation between the patient's desire and the doctor's perception of it. When compared with fatal illnesses such as AIDS and cancer, resuscitation was addressed less commonly with heart failure patients.

Hospice Care

A person with end-stage CHF who is frequently admitted to the hospital for diuresis and who has declining quality of life may reasonably elect to avoid aggressive treatment, including cardiopulmonary resuscitation. At this stage we find it helpful to enroll the patient in a

Table 53-3	*Effects of Opioids in Congestive Heart Failure*

Effect	Comment
Reduced anxiety	
Reduced sensitivity to hypercapnia	There may be a "resetting" of the receptor, providing one mechanism for relief of dyspnea. (The patient tolerates a larger amount of respiratory fatigue—a higher $PaCO_2$— without sensing it.) There is less effect on the hypoxemia receptor, so it is unusual for patients to stop breathing.
Effect on airway receptors	Blocking airway irritant receptors may reduce bronchospasm, an action that has been demonstrated in obstructive lung disease.
Venodilation	Peripheral pooling of blood reduces venous return to the heart (preload; see Chapter 2). There is reduced left atrial and pulmonary capillary pressures and prompt relief of congestion.
Depression of respiration	A possibility with higher doses, but this is an infrequent effect of morphine therapy. It may be used without hesitation in advanced CHF and obstructive lung disease. Appropriate monitoring is important, particularly when initiating therapy.
Direct myocardial effects	None; there is little danger of myocardial depression and worsening of heart failure (which is why morphine is commonly used in cardiac anesthesia).

hospice. Current federal regulations provide for hospice care if survival is estimated to be less than 6 months, and such patients with advanced CHF meet this criterion. The hospice nurse is able to administer intravenous diuretics and in some cases may be able to give intravenous dobutamine. Management of dietary sodium often improves with special attention. Such measures may enable the patient to remain at home, out of the hospital. We have been struck by how often symptoms resolve once regular hospice visits begin.

Morphine

Do not underestimate the usefulness of morphine to relieve suffering for a patient with intermittent, severe pulmonary congestion (Table 53-3). It is a venodilator, reducing blood return to the heart. Pulmonary capillary pressure and symptoms of congestion are promptly reduced. In addition, it blunts the anxiety that comes with severe dyspnea. You are used to seeing this response in the emergency room when treating pulmonary edema, and you may expect the same effect in a congested patient at home.

There is concern that morphine may depress respiration. In practice, with all but extreme doses, this is rare in patients with pulmonary edema (or with severe dyspnea in advanced lung disease, for that matter). Although respiratory depression is possible, the usually observed effect is relief of dyspnea, as well as anxiety and agitation.

Outpatient, parenteral morphine is difficult to administer and control. It is best accomplished in a hospice setting. Hospice nurses have significant experience with narcotic analgesia—more than most physicians— and can competently regulate its use in patients with heart failure. A brief inpatient stay may help with selection of an effective dose of morphine.

A reasonable initial oral dose of morphine (Roxanol) is 2.5 to 5 mg, given at 1- to 4-hour intervals. The dose may be increased by as much as 50% at 4- to 12-hour intervals as needed to control symptoms. It may be preferable to use the medicine as needed (prn) rather than throughout the day, especially if attacks of dyspnea are intermittent. Within reason, there is no maximum allowable dose. Our hospice experience has taught us to raise the dose until congestion is effectively controlled or until intolerable side effects occur (e.g., excessive somnolence or a change in respiration). The hospice nursing and physician staff provides a useful resource when using higher dose opiates. Constipation may limit the tolerable dose of morphine, especially in elderly patients. The hospice team has experience dealing with it.

Nebulized and inhaled morphine, 5 to 25 mg (the equivalent of 2.5 to 12.5 mg intravenously) is a good alternative to oral or parenteral dosing. Morphine recep-

tors are present in the airway, and there may be a direct pulmonary effect depending on the cause of dyspnea. The onset of action with nebulized morphine is more rapid than with an oral dose, with mental relaxation occurring within 2 to 5 minutes. In addition, inhalation drug delivery may be more convenient than parenteral therapy, depending on the abilities of the home caregiver. A nebulizer can be prepared within minutes of an attack of dyspnea and administered by the patient or caregiver.

We have had experience with a number of patients with CHF who reached the stage of illness requiring frequent hospital admission and who were admitted to a hospice program for home treatment with morphine and intravenous diuretics. The usual result has been improved symptoms, less anxiety for the patient and home caregivers, and an interruption of the cycle of repeated hospitalization.

Occasionally we hear a physician argue that potent drugs that might affect the level of consciousness should be avoided at the end of life so that "the patient can interact with the family." Experience shows the contrary. Morphine, by relieving congestion and blunting anxiety, often improves mental status. Both the patient and family are relieved.

Coronary Artery Disease

The principles of treatment for angina pectoris are reviewed in Chapter 13. The treatment of end-stage CAD will become a more prevalent issue with the aging population. It is now common to see the patient who has had two or more revascularization procedures. Eventually, every patient reaches a point at which nothing more can be fixed, and medical therapy is the only option. We are often surprised how well medical treatment controls symptoms. Many improve with time, probably because collateral circulation develops.

Those with stenosis of large coronary arteries often die suddenly or in the setting of myocardial infarction. Worse angina that is poorly controlled with medicine develops in a small percentage of those with CAD.

Home oxygen may help with control of symptoms. We have not found hospice care as useful for angina as it is for CHF. We less commonly prescribe narcotic analgesics for those with poorly controlled angina, although some with end-stage ischemic cardiomyopathy use it to relieve pain and control congestion.

Rest Therapy

One of our teachers, Julian Beckwith, taught us that one option for those with uncontrollable angina is reduced activity, a "bed-to-chair" lifestyle. This was a common approach before the 1960s and at times it is still appropriate. Do not get us wrong; we are strong believers in the value of exercise and exercise therapy for CAD. But

there comes a time when it does not work, and reduced activity offers the best palliation. Some elderly patients prefer this alternative to open heart surgery.

ETHICAL ISSUES AT END OF LIFE
The New Medical Ethics

During the past two decades of this century, practice standards have shifted in favor of patient autonomy. Previously, the central ethic in the practice of medicine was beneficence. The all-knowing and beneficent physician was trusted to know, and then to do, what was in the patient's best interest. With this model, the physician viewed the patient as a passive recipient of care. Disagreeing with the doctor was considered inappropriate. We all know doctors who view any disagreement as an affront to their authority.

The change to a "patient autonomy" model does not minimize the moral responsibility of the physician. On the other hand, the doctor's unquestioned control over what happens to the patient has been altered. Now the emphasis is on our obligation to inform, to carefully review and recommend alternatives, and then to respect and support the patient's wishes. What this means to all of us—as future patients—is that when we are old and sick, we retain control of decision making. No one can make us do something we do not want. That is what we want for ourselves and our families, and it should be what we want for our patients.

End-of-Life Decisions

We noted the general reluctance to give up on the patient with heart disease. There is always the possibility of one more interventional procedure. We are trained to prolong life whenever possible, and aggressive therapy may be life prolonging.

But at what cost? An elderly person offered heart surgery may object that it is not worth the expense of the procedure. The young doctor then points to Medicare and supplemental insurance and argues that "it's paid for." But that may not be the cost the patient means. Suffering is another expense that must be factored. An octogenarian may recognize that there is limited time ahead and knows that the recovery time from surgery is prolonged and morbidity higher at that age. The decision that a small increment in survival is not worth what must be endured to purchase it is often a rational one. The patient may decide that it is not worth the monetary expense either. Even when "it is paid for," an older person often understands that the expense is borne by the younger generation, including one's children and grandchildren.

Whether to choose life-prolonging treatment is thus a value decision. It involves the patient's assessment of the probable quality of extra time, as well as all the

"costs" of therapy. No one is qualified to make that value decision for another person, and we should not try to make it for our patients.

A survey of elderly patients and their families has documented concern about inappropriate and aggressive care at the end of life.[5] Subjects of the study felt they often were convinced to choose procedures or aggressive care they did not want. A major issue for elderly or chronically ill people is whether modern, scientific medicine will allow them a peaceful death.

The proper solution to the old or chronically ill person's dilemma is adherence to the principle of autonomy, including a willingness of the doctor to accept and support a patient's decision to avoid aggressive therapy and to provide effective palliative care. You may feel that the patient has decided to give up too early and stands to lose years of good life unnecessarily. You may certainly point this out, and it is your duty to give your best advice. But you must stop short of arm twisting. It is the patient's right to refuse therapy, even when you believe it is a mistake.

Such decisions are not always straightforward. A patient may decide that it is easier to die of heart disease than of some other degenerative illnesses of old age. A survey of the families of 18,000 patients who died after age 65 years found that only 14% were fully functional in the last year of life.[6] Most of the natural causes of death were preceded by disability and dependency in the last year of life. A prominent exception was death from acute MI, where older patients "were far more likely to be fully functional in the year before death."[6]

The trend of scientific medicine has been the elimination of illnesses that are rapidly fatal. What remains are conditions like dementia, stroke, and heart failure. A person who has been chronically ill or who is experiencing the decline of old age may elect to refuse treatment for a curable acute illnesses, and reclaim such "old man's friends" as pneumonia, heart attack, or urosepsis. An autonomous person has that right, just as there is a right to refuse life-prolonging chemotherapy. This principle would apply to a patient with coronary artery disease or aortic stenosis, both amenable to surgical repair despite advanced age.

Some will mistakenly interpret this as an argument against life-prolonging therapy for old people. That is not our intent. We would agree that age should *not* disqualify a person for any treatment.[7] Treatment shown to prolong life by clinical trials should be applied irrespective of age, *if that is what the patient wants.* Our purpose is to provide support for patients who have decided to avoid possibly life-prolonging but *unwanted* therapy.

Are We (Doctors) in Control?

Doctors, particularly inexperienced ones, often overestimate their influence at the end of life. Patients who are in intensive care units may be dependent on life-support devices. Withdrawal of support results in death. In such cases the doctor may believe that "the patient only dies when I allow it." Pursuing this logic, the doctor thus has control over life and death, a patently silly notion.

It also suggests that the doctor has more responsibility for death than is the case. It is a matter of fact that a terminally ill patient *dies of a disease.* Our intervention affects only the timing and the amount of suffering. By withdrawing life-prolonging support at the patient's direction, the doctor is not responsible for death, nor is the patient. (Daniel Callahan develops this line of reasoning in *The Troubled Dream of Life.*[8] We recommend it for you as well as your patients. It has been useful as a focus for community-based study groups.)

When to Make End-of-Life Decisions

The worst time to make end-of-life decisions is during an acute illness such as myocardial infarction or pulmonary edema. It is difficult for a patient and family to make rational decisions while the patient is in pain. Often they are dealing with an unfamiliar doctor in the emergency room.

Instead, decisions about the goals and limits of medical care should be made with the primary care physician when a patient is stable. Such decisions may evolve over the course of multiple office visits. The patient and family have ample time to understand as much as possible about ongoing illness and possible clinical developments. It should be made clear that final decisions about care rest with the patient and that the doctor can be counted on to support the patient regardless of the decision. The importance of advanced directives cannot be overestimated, including a living will and durable power of attorney for health care.[9-12] The patient should identify a surrogate decision maker and have detailed discussion about the goals of medical care and its limits. The doctor, patient, and the patient's surrogate should be aware that the power to make decisions passes undiminished to the surrogate if the patient becomes incompetent. The surrogate's role is thus a critical one and requires availability in the event of a crisis, a clear understanding of the patient's wishes, and a willingness to do the job.[10]

Decisions about end-of-life care can be changed. Declining heart surgery may be an exception, and the patient should be aware of this. There may be a window of opportunity for the surgical repair of valvular or coronary artery disease, and delay beyond a certain point may mean deterioration of ventricular function, rendering surgery unfeasible.

These big picture discussions are the responsibility of the primary care physician who has an ongoing relationship with the patient and family. A cardiology consultant may help with clarification of clinical issues. It is

important to select a sensible and experienced consultant, and one who does not have a reputation for bending patients to his or her will. We are concerned that subspecialists may focus on the illness rather than the patient and may feel an obligation to sell a potentially curative procedure (e.g., the surgical repair of aortic stenosis for an octogenarian). Primary care doctors may suffer from the same shortcoming, but the nature of primary care increases the chance of an approach that recognizes that the power to decide is shared by the patient and doctor.[13]

Extreme Symptoms in the Terminal Patient

What do we do for a patient with end-stage heart disease who comes to the emergency room in a near terminal condition but with extreme symptoms? A common issue is pulmonary edema unresponsive to intravenous diuretics. It is unfortunate that doctors often tell the patient and family that intubation and ventilation is the only hope for relieving symptoms. Despite a previous decision to avoid ventilator therapy, a desperate patient and family may have a change of mind, especially when this seems the only chance for relief.

An effective alternative that should be considered is higher dose morphine, titrated to relieve dyspnea. There may be depression of respiration with a dose sufficient to relieve symptoms. In this case the moral imperative is to provide relief of suffering for the dying patient, even if high-dose opiates contribute to more rapid death. There is no culpability.[14,15] This is not assisted suicide or euthanasia, but rather necessary therapy for extreme symptoms.

REFERENCES

1. Krumholz HM, Phillips RS, Hamel MB, et al: Resuscitation preferences among patients with severe congestive heart failure: results from the SUPPORT project, *Circulation* 98:648, 1998.
2. Brater DC: Diuretic therapy, *N Engl J Med* 339:387, 1998.
3. Vargo DL, Brater DC, Rudy DW, Swan SK: Dopamine does not enhance furosemide-induced natriuresis in patients with congestive heart failure, *J Am Soc Nephrol* 7:1032, 1996.
4. Stevenson LW: Rites and responsibility for resuscitation in heart failure, *Circulation* 98:619, 1998.
5. Lynn J, Teno, J, Phillips R, et al: Perceptions by family members of the dying experience of older and seriously ill patients, *Ann Intern Med* 126:97, 1997.
6. Lentzner H, Pamuk E, Rhodenhiser E, et al: The quality of life in the year before death, *Am J Public Health* 82:1093, 1992.
7. King III SB, Ullyot DJ, Basta L, et al: Application of medical and surgical interventions near the end of life, *J Am Coll Cardiol* 31:933, 1998.
8. Callahan D: *The troubled dream of life,* New York, 1993, Simon & Schuster.
9. Annas G: The health care proxy and the living will, *N Engl J Med* 324:1210, 1991.
10. Meisel A: Legal myths about terminating life support, *Arch Intern Med* 151:1497, 1991.
11. Emanuel E, Emanuel L: Proxy decision making for incompetent patients: an ethical and empirical analysis, *JAMA* 267:2067, 1992.
12. Menikoff J, Sachs G, Siegler M: Beyond advance directives—health care surrogate laws, *N Engl J Med* 327:1165, 1992.
13. Brody H: *The healer's power,* New Haven, Conn, 1992, Yale University Press.
14. Johnson-Neely K, Krammer LM: End-of-life care: palliative strategies for vomiting and dyspnea, *Fam Pract Recertification* 20:13, 1998.
15. Sachs GA, Ahronheim J, Rhymes J, et al: Good care of dying patients: the alternative to physician-assisted suicide and euthanasia, *J Am Geriatr Soc* 43:553, 1995.

PART THREE

Cardiology Drug Reference

Cardiology Drug Reference*

Compiled by Julie D. Lawrence and George J. Taylor

INSTRUCTIONS FOR USE

The drug entries that follow are organized in a uniform fashion as follows (when there is no information in a category applicable to a given drug, the category has been deleted entirely):

Drug name (generic)

Pronunciation (phonetic)

Trade names (Canadian trade names marked with; including combination drugs and prescription vs. over-the-counter designation)

Chemical Class

Therapeutic Class

Clinical Pharmacology (including information about the mechanism of action and pharmacokinetics of the drug)

Indications and Uses (uses not approved by the FDA marked with *)

Dosage

Available Forms/Cost of Therapy (average wholesale prices of brands are given)

Contraindications (if the only contraindication is hypersensitivity, this category has been deleted)

Precautions

Pregnancy and Lactation

Side Effects/Adverse Reactions (listed by organ system; *common side effects* [greater than 5% incidence] are *italicized*; ***potentially life-threatening side effects*** are ***bold and italicized***)

Drug Interactions (if applicable). (The clinical significance of each drug interaction is derived from data presented in Hansten PD, Horn JR: *Drug interactions analysis and management,* Vancouver, Wash, 1997, Applied Therapeutics.) Interactions are classified by potential severity as: ▲ Avoid combination, risk always outweighs benefit; ❷ Usually avoid combination, use combination only under special circumstances; or ❸ Minimize risk, take action as necessary to reduce risk of adverse outcome due to drug interaction. Interactions of lesser significance, either because they are minor or poorly documented, are not included. If no drug interactions are known, or if the interactions are of minimal risk, this category has been deleted.

Lab Test Interactions (if applicable). (Only laboratory interactions that are well documented and are analytical in nature are included. Changes in lab results that reflect the physiologic action of the drug or an adverse metabolic effect of the drug are not included. If no lab interactions are known, this category has been deleted.)

Special Considerations (if applicable), such as patient education or monitoring or information about the place of the drug in therapy.

Every possible effort has been made to ensure the accuracy and currency of the information. However, drug information is constantly changing and is subject to interpretation. Neither the authors, editors, nor publishers can be responsible for information that has either changed or been erroneously published, or for the consequences of such errors. Decisions regarding drug therapy for a specific patient must be based on the independent judgment of the clinician.

ABBREVIATIONS

ABG	arterial blood gas
ac	before meals
ACE	angiotensin-converting enzyme
ACTH	adrenocorticotropic hormone
ADH	antidiuretic hormone
aer	aerosol
ALT	alanine aminotransferase, serum
ANA	antinuclear antibody
aPTT	activated partial thromboplastin time
AST	aspartate aminotransferase, serum
AV	atrioventricular
bid	twice a day
BP	blood pressure
BUN	blood urea nitrogen
c-AMP	cyclic adenosine monophosphate
cap	capsule
Ca	calcium
CAD	coronary artery disease
cath	catheterize
CBC	complete blood count
chew tab	tablet, chewable
CHF	congestive heart failure
Cl	chloride
cm	centimeter
CMV	cytomegalovirus
CNS	central nervous system
CO₂	carbon dioxide
COPD	chronic obstructive pulmonary disease
CPAP	continuous positive airway pressure
CPK	creatine phosphokinase
CrCl	creatinine clearance
cre	cream
Creat	creatinine
CSF	cerebrospinal fluid
CV	cardiovascular
CVA	cerebrovascular accident
CVP	central venous pressure
D5W	5% dextrose in water
DIC	disseminated intravascular coagulation
dL	deciliter
DLCO	diffusing capacity of carbon monoxide
DNA	deoxyribonucleic acid
DUB	dysfunctional uterine bleeding

ECG	electrocardiogram
EDTA	ethylenediaminetetraacetic acid
EEG	electroencephalogram
EENT	eye, ear, nose, throat
elix	elixir
ESR	erythrocyte sedimentation rate
ET	via endotracheal tube
EXT REL	extended release
FEV1	forced expiratory volume in 1 second
FSH	follicle- stimulating hormone
g	gram
G6PD	glucose-6-phosphate dehydrogenase
GGTP	gamma glutamyl transpeptidase
GI	gastrointestinal
gtt	drop
GU	genitourinary
H2	histamine$_2$
Hct	hematocrit
HCG	human chorionic gonadotropin
HEME	hematologic
Hgb	hemoglobin
5-HIAA	5-hydroxyindoleacetic acid
HIV	human immunodeficiency virus
H$_2$O	water
HMG CoA	3-hydroxy-3-methylglutaryl coenzyme A
HPA	hypothalamic-pituitary-adrenal
hr	hour
hs	at bedtime
HSV	Herpes simplex virus
IgG	immunoglobulin G
IM	intramuscular
in	inch
INF	infusion
INH	inhalation
inj	injection
INR	international normalized ratio
IO	intraosseous
IPPB	intermittent positive pressure breathing
IV	intravenous
K	potassium
kg	kilogram
L	liter
L-A	long acting
lb	pound
LDH	lactate dehydrogenase
LDL	low density lipoprotein
LFT	liver function tests
LH	luteinizing hormone
liq	liquid
LMP	last menstrual period
loz	lozenge
lyphl	lyophilized
m	meter
m²	square meter
MAOI	monoamine oxidase inhibitor
MDI	metered dose inhaler
mEq	milliequivalent
mg	milligram
Mg	magnesium
MI	myocardial infarction
min	minute
ml (mL)	milliliter
mm	millimeter
mmol	millimole
mo	month
MS	musculoskeletal
Na	sodium

neb	nebulizer
NPO	nothing by mouth
NS	normal saline
NSAID	nonsteroidal antiinflammatory drug
O$_2$	oxygen
oint	ointment
OTC	over the counter
oz	ounce
PaCO$_2$	arterial partial pressure of carbon dioxide
PaO$_2$	arterial partial pressure of oxygen
pc	after meals
PCWP	pulmonary capillary wedge pressure
PO	by mouth
pr	per rectum
prn	as needed
PT	prothrombin time
PTH	parathyroid hormone
PTT	partial thromboplastin time
PVC	premature ventricular contraction
q	every
qAM	every morning
qd	every day
qh	every hour
qid	four times a day
qod	every other day
qPM	every night
q2h	every 2 hours
q3h	every 3 hours
q4h	every 4 hours
q6h	every 6 hours
q8h	every 8 hours
q12h	every 12 hours
RAIU	radioactive iodine uptake
RBC	red blood cell or count
RESP	respiratory
RNA	ribonucleic acid
sc	subcutaneous
sl	sublingual
sol	solution
SO$_4$	sulfate
ss	one half
supp	suppository
sus rel	sustained release
susp	suspension
sust	sustained
syr	syrup
T$_3$	triiodothyronine
T$_4$	thyroxine
tab	tablet
tid	three times a day
tinc	tincture
top	topical
trans	transdermal
TSH	thyroid stimulating hormone
TT	thrombin time
U	unit
UA	urinalysis
URI	upper respiratory tract infection
UTI	urinary tract infection
UV	ultraviolet
vag	vaginal
VMA	vanillylmandelic acid
vol	volume
VS	vital signs
WBC	white blood cell or count
wk	week
yr	year

FEDERAL CONTROLLED SUBSTANCES ACT SCHEDULES

SCHEDULE I: No accepted medical use in the United States and a high abuse potential. Examples include heroin, marijuana, LSD, peyote, mescaline, psilocybin, and methaqualone.

SCHEDULE II: High abuse potential with severe dependence liability. Examples include opium, morphine, codeine, fentanyl, hydromorphone, methadone, meperidine, oxycodone, oxymorphone, cocaine, amphetamine, methamphetamine, phenmetrazine, methylphenidate, phencyclidine, amobarbital, pentobarbital, and secobarbital.

SCHEDULE III: Lesser abuse potential with moderate dependence liability. Examples include compounds containing limited quantities of certain narcotic or nonnarcotic drugs, such as barbiturates, glutethimide, methyprylon, nalorphine, benzphetamine, chlorphentermine, clortermine, phendimetrazine, and paregoric; suppository dosage form containing amobarbital, secobarbital, or pentobarbital.

SCHEDULE IV: Low abuse potential. Examples include barbital, phenobarbital, mephobarbital, chloral hydrate, ethchlorvynol, ethinamate, meprobamate, paraldehyde, methohexital, fenfluramine, diethylpropion, phentermine, chlordiazepoxide, diazepam, oxazepam, clorazepate, flurazepam, clonazepam, prazepam, lorazepam, alprazolam, halazepam, temazepam, triazolam, mebutamate, dextropropoxyphene, and pentazocine.

SCHEDULE V: Low abuse potential. These products contain limited quantities of certain narcotic drugs generally for antitussive or antidiarrheal purposes.

FDA PREGNANCY CATEGORIES

A: Adequate studies in pregnant women have not demonstrated a risk to the fetus in the first trimester of pregnancy, and there is no evidence of risk in later trimesters.

B: Animal studies have not demonstrated a risk to the fetus, but there are no adequate studies in pregnant women; **OR** animal studies have shown an adverse effect, but adequate studies in pregnant women have not demonstrated a risk to the fetus during the first trimester of pregnancy, and there is no evidence of risk in later trimesters.

C: Animal studies have shown an adverse effect on the fetus, but there are no adequate studies in humans; **OR** there are no animal reproduction studies and no adequate studies in humans.

D: There is evidence of human fetal risk, but the potential benefits from the use of the drug in pregnant women may be acceptable despite its potential risks.

X: Studies in animals or humans demonstrate fetal abnormalities or adverse reaction; reports indicate evidence of fetal risk. The risk of use in a pregnant woman clearly outweighs any possible benefit.

abciximab

(ab-six´-i-mab)
Rx: ReoPro
Chemical Class: Platelet glycoprotein IIb/IIIa receptor antagonist
Therapeutic Class: Antiplatelet

CLINICAL PHARMACOLOGY

Mechanism of Action: Inhibits platelet aggregation by preventing binding of fibrinogen, von Willebrand factor, and other adhesive molecules to GP IIb/IIIa receptor sites on activated platelets, thus inhibiting platelet aggregation. Also binds to vitronectin receptor, a separate mechanism for blocking clot formation.

italic = common side effects

Pharmacokinetics
IV: After IV bolus, free plasma concentrations decrease initially with a $t_{1/2} <10$ min, followed by second $t_{1/2} \sim 30$ min; platelet function recovers over course of 48 hr, although abciximab remains in circulation for about 15 days; greater than 80% GP IIb/IIIa receptor inhibition after continuous infusion

INDICATIONS AND USES: An adjunct to percutaneous coronary intervention for prevention of cardiac ischemic complications in patients undergoing percutaneous coronary intervention and in patients with unstable angina not responding to conventional medical therapy when percutaneous coronary intervention is planned within 24 hr. Intended for use with aspirin and heparin.

DOSAGE
Adult
IV: Bolus of 0.25 mg/kg administered 10-60 min before start of percutaneous coronary interventions, followed by continuous infusion of 0.125 µg/kg/min (to maximum of 10 µg/min) for 12 hr. Patients with unstable angina not responding to conventional medical therapy and who plan to undergo percutaneous coronary intervention within 24 hr may be treated with 0.25 mg/kg IV bolus followed by 18- to 24-hour infusion of 10 µg/min, concluding 1 hr after percutaneous coronary intervention.

$ AVAILABLE FORMS/COST OF THERAPY
• 2mg/ml is supplied in 5 ml vials containg 10 mg: **$450.00**

CONTRAINDICATIONS: Active internal bleeding; GI or GU bleeding of clinical significance in past 6 wk; history of CVA within 2 yr, or CVA with significant residual neurologic deficit; bleeding diathesis; administration of oral anticoagulants within 7 days unless PT is ≤1.2 times control, thrombocytopenia (<100,000 cells/mcl); major surgery or trauma within 6 wk; intracranial neoplasm, arteriovenous malformation or aneurysm; severe, uncontrolled hypertension; presumed or documented history of vasculitis; use of IV dextran before percutaneous coronary intervention, or intent to use it during an intervention; hypersensitivity to any component of product or murine proteins.

PRECAUTIONS: Bleeding precautions; minimize vascular and other trauma; use of thrombolytics, anticoagulants, and other antiplatelet agents; thrombocytopenia; readministration of abciximab

PREGNANCY AND LACTATION: Pregnancy category C; animal studies have not been conducted; should be given to pregnant women only if clearly needed; not known if excreted in human milk

SIDE EFFECTS/ADVERSE REACTIONS
CNS: ***intracranial hemorrhage, stroke***
CV: ***ventricular tachycardia, complete AV block, embolism, hypotension, bradycardia***
GI: dyspepsia, diarrhea, ileus, gastroesophageal reflux, nausea, vomiting, abdominal pain
GU: urinary retention, dysuria
*HEME: bleeding, **thrombocytopenia, anemia, leukocytosis***
MS: myalgia
RESP: pneumonia
MISC: ***anaphylaxis,*** back pain, chest pain, headache, puncture site pain, peripheral edema

DRUG INTERACTIONS
❷ *Anticoagulants:* May increase bleeding time, use caution
❷ *Antiplatelet agents:* May increase bleeding time, use caution
❷ *Thrombolytics:* May increase bleeding time, use caution

bold italic = life-threatening reactions

SPECIAL CONSIDERATIONS

• Shown to decrease death, MI, or need for urgent intervention for recurrent ischemia within 30 days of percutaneous coronary intervention

• Readministration of abciximab may result in human antichimeric antibody formation that could cause allergic or hypersensitivity reactions, thrombocytopenia, or diminished benefit

MONITORING PARAMETERS

• Monitor platelet count, PTT, SCT, and aPTT before infusion

---

acebutolol
(a-ce-bute'oh-lol)

Rx: Monitan ✤, Rhotral ✤, Sectral

Chemical Class: β_1-selective (cardioselective) adrenoreceptor blocker with intrinsic sympathomimetic activity

Therapeutic Class: Antihypertensive; antidysrhythmic (class II)

CLINICAL PHARMACOLOGY

Mechanism of Action: Blocks β_1-adrenergic receptors; produces negative chronotropic and inotropic effects; slows conduction of AV node; decreases renin-aldosterone-angiotensin system activity at high doses; inhibits β_2-receptors in bronchial system at high doses

Pharmacokinetics

PO: Onset $1-1\frac{1}{2}$ hr, peak 2-4 hr, duration 10-12 hr, $t_{1/2}$ 6-7 hr; excreted unchanged in urine; protein binding 5%-15%

INDICATIONS AND USES: Hypertension, ventricular premature beats

DOSAGE

Adult

• Hypertension: PO 400 mg qd or in 2 divided doses; increase to desired response; usual range 400-800 mg/day

• *Ventricular premature beats:* PO 200 mg bid, may increase gradually; usual range 600-1200 mg daily

$ AVAILABLE FORMS/COST OF THERAPY

• Cap, Gel—Oral: 200 mg, 100's: **$105.98-$109.49;** 400 mg, 100's: **$130.53-$140.90**

CONTRAINDICATIONS: Cardiogenic shock, heart block (2nd, 3rd degree), sinus bradycardia, CHF

PRECAUTIONS: Major surgery, diabetes mellitus, renal disease, thyroid disease, COPD, asthma, well-compensated CHF, aortic, mitral valve disease

PREGNANCY AND LACTATION: Pregnancy category B; acebutolol and diacetolol metabolite cross placenta and appear in breast milk with a milk:plasma ratio of 7.1 and 12.2; use in nursing mothers not recommended

SIDE EFFECTS/ADVERSE REACTIONS

CNS: Catatonia, depression, *dizziness,* drowsiness, *fatigue,* hallucinations, *headache,* insomnia, lethargy, memory loss, strange dreams

CV: Bradycardia, *CHF,* cold extremities, postural hypotension, *2nd or 3rd degree heart block, shock*

EENT: Dry, burning eyes, sore throat

GI: Diarrhea, elevated transaminases, *ischemic colitis, mesenteric arterial thrombosis,* nausea, vomiting

GU: Impotence

HEME: Agranulocytosis, positive ANA, *purpura, thrombocytopenia*

METAB: Hyperglycemia, increased hypoglycemic response to insulin

RESP: Bronchospasm, dyspnea, wheezing

SKIN: Alopecia, fever, rash

DRUG INTERACTIONS

Drugs

▪ *Amiodarone:* Bradycardia/ventricular dysrhythmia

▪ *Ampicillin:* Reduced β-blocker effect

▪ *Anesthetics, local:* Enhanced sympathomimetic effects, hypertension due to unopposed α-receptor stimulation

▪ *Antacids:* May reduce β-blocker absorption

▪ *Antidiabetics:* Delayed recovery from hypoglycemia, hyperglycemia, attenuated tachycardia during hypoglycemia, hypertension during hypoglycemia

▪ *Digoxin:* Bradycardia

▪ *Dipyridamole:* Bradycardia

▪ *Epinephrine:* Enhanced pressor response resulting in hypertension

▪ *Neostigmine:* Bradycardia

▪ *Neuroleptics:* Increased serum levels of both resulting in accentuated pharmacologic response to both drugs

▪ *NSAIDs:* Reduced hypotensive effects

▪ *Phenylephrine:* Acute hypertensive episodes

▪ *Prazosin:* First-dose hypotensive response enhanced

▪ *Tacrine:* Additive bradycardia

▪ *Theophylline:* Antagonist pharmacodynamics

SPECIAL CONSIDERATIONS

PATIENT/FAMILY EDUCATION

Don't discontinue abruptly, taper over 2 wk; may precipitate angina if stopped abruptly

---

acetazolamide
(a-set-a-zole'a-mide)

Rx: Acetazolam ✤, Dazamide, Diamox, Diamox Sequels

Chemical Class: Sulfonamide derivative; carbonic anhydrase inhibitor

Therapeutic Class: Diuretic, anticonvulsant; antiglaucoma agent; mountain sickness

---

CLINICAL PHARMACOLOGY

Mechanism of Action: Inhibits carbonic anhydrase activity. In kidney results in alkaline diuresis, retards excessive neuronal discharge in CNS, reduces aqueous humor formation in eye. Metabolic acidosis enhances ventilatory oxygenation at high altitude.

Pharmacokinetics

PO: Onset $1-1\frac{1}{2}$ hr, peak 2-4 hr, duration 6-12 hr

PO-SUS REL: Onset 2 hr, peak 8-12 hr, duration 18-24 hr

IV: Onset 2 min, peak 15 min, duration 4-5 hr

65% absorbed if fasting (oral), 75% absorbed if given with food; $t_{1/2}$ $2\frac{1}{2}-5\frac{1}{2}$ hr; excreted unchanged by kidneys (80% within 24 hr); crosses placenta

INDICATIONS AND USES: Open-angle glaucoma, narrow-angle glaucoma (preoperatively, if surgery delayed), epilepsy (petit mal, grand mal, mixed), edema in CHF, drug-induced edema, acute mountain sickness (prevention and treatment)

DOSAGE

Adult

• *Narrow-angle glaucoma:* PO/IV 250 mg q4h or 250 mg bid, to be used for short-term therapy

• *Open-angle glaucoma:* PO/IV 250-1000 mg/day in divided doses for amounts over 250 mg

• *Edema:* IV 250-375 mg/day in AM

• *Seizures:* PO/IV 8-30 mg/kg/day, usual range 375-1000 mg/day

---

* = non FDA-approved use

• *Mountain sickness:* Treatment: PO 250 mg q8-12h; Prophylaxis: PO 125 mg bid; Periodic breathing at altitude: PO 62.5-125 mg with dinner or hs

Child

• *Edema:* IV 5 mg/kg/day in AM

• *Seizures:* PO/IV 8-30 mg/kg/day in divided doses tid or qid, or 300-900 mg/m²/day, not to exceed 1.5 g/day

Ⓢ AVAILABLE FORMS/COST OF THERAPY

• Tab, Uncoated—Oral: 125 mg, 100's: **$6.70-$30.06;** 250 mg, 100's: **$5.95-$44.89**

• Cap, Gel, Sus Action—Oral: 500 mg, 100's: **$96.30**

• Inj, Lyphl-Sol—500 mg/5ml, 5 ml: **$31.20-$36.59**

CONTRAINDICATIONS: Hypersensitivity to sulfonamides, severe renal disease, severe hepatic disease, electrolyte imbalances (hyponatremia, hypokalemia), hyperchloremic acidosis, Addison's disease, long-term use in narrow-angle glaucoma, COPD

PRECAUTIONS: Hypercalciuria

PREGNANCY AND LACTATION: Pregnancy category D; premature delivery and congenital anomalies in humans; teratogenic (defects of the limbs) in mice, rats, hamsters, and rabbits; not recommended for nursing mothers

SIDE EFFECTS/ADVERSE REACTIONS

CNS: Anxiety, confusion, depression, dizziness, drowsiness, fatigue, headache, nervousness, paresthesia, sedation, *seizures,* stimulation

EENT: Myopia, tinnitus

GI: Anorexia, constipation, diarrhea, *hepatic insufficiency,* melena, nausea, taste alterations, *vomiting,* weight loss

GU: Crystalluria, glucosuria, *hypokalemia,* polyuria, renal calculi, *uremia*

HEME: Agranulocytosis, aplastic anemia, hemolytic anemia, leukopenia, pancytopenia, purpura, thrombocytopenia

METAB: Hyperglycemia

SKIN: Fever, photosensitivity, pruritus, *rash, Stevens-Johnson syndrome,* urticaria

MISC: Loss of taste of carbonated beverages

DRUG INTERACTIONS

Drugs

▣ Methenamine compounds: Alkalinization of urine decreases antibacterial effects

▣ Phenytoin: Increased risk of osteomalacia

▣ Primidone: Decreased primidone levels

▣ Flecainide quinidine: Alkalinization of urine increases quinidine serum levels

❷ Salicylates: Increased serum levels of acetazolamide—CNS toxicity

Labs

False increase: 17 hydroxysteroid

SPECIAL CONSIDERATIONS

PATIENT/FAMILY EDUCATION

Carbonated beverages taste flat

---

adenosine

(ah-den'oh-seen)

Rx: Adenocard, Adenoscan

Chemical Class: Endogenous nucleoside

Therapeutic Class: Antidysrhythmic

CLINICAL PHARMACOLOGY

Mechanism of Action: Slows conduction through AV node; interrupts reentry pathways through AV node

Pharmacokinetic

IV: Cleared from plasma in <30 sec, $t_{1/2}$ 10 sec

INDICATIONS AND USES: PSVT, including PSVT associated with Wolff-Parkinson-White syndrome; does not convert atrial flutter, atrial fibrillation, or ventricular tachycardia to normal sinus rhythm; symptomatic relief of varicose vein complications with stasis dermatitis

DOSAGE

Adult

• *PSVT:* IV bolus 6 mg; if conversion to normal sinus rhythm does not occur within 1-2 min, give 12 mg by rapid IV bolus; may repeat 12 mg dose again in 1-2 min

• *Varicose veins:* IM 25 mg once or twice daily until relief is obtained and then 25 mg 2 or 3 times weekly for maintenance

Child

• *PSVT:* IV bolus 0.05 mg/kg; if not effective within 2 min, increase dose in 0.05 mg/kg increments every 2 min to a maximum of 0.25 mg/kg or until termination of PSVT; median dose, 0.15 mg/kg; do not exceed 12 mg/dose

Ⓢ AVAILABLE FORMS/COST OF THERAPY

• Inj, Sol—IM: 25 mg/ml, 10 ml:**$5.60-$18.50**

• Inj, Sol—IV: 3 mg/ml, 2 ml: **$26.36-$30.43**

CONTRAINDICATIONS: 2nd or 3rd degree heart block, AV block, sick sinus syndrome, atrial flutter, atrial fibrillation, ventricular tachycardia

PRECAUTIONS: Asthma

PREGNANCY AND LACTATION: Pregnancy category C; fetal effects unlikely

SIDE EFFECTS/ADVERSE REACTIONS

CNS: Apprehension, arm tingling, blurred vision, dizziness, headache, lightheadedness, numbness

CV: Atrial tachydysrhythmia, chest pain, *facial flushing (18%),* hypotension, palpitations, sweating

GI: Groin pressure, metallic taste, nausea, throat tightness

RESP: Chest pressure, dyspnea, hyperventilation

DRUG INTERACTIONS

Drugs

▣ β-blockers: Bradycardia

▣ *Dipyridamole:* Increased serum adenosine levels, potentiates pharmacologic effects of adenosine

▣ *Nicotine:* Greater hemodynamic response to adenosine (hypotension, chest pain)

▣ *Theophylline/caffeine:* Inhibits hemodynamic effects of adenosine

---

alteplase

(al-teep'lase)

Rx: Activase

Chemical Class: Tissue plasminogen activator (TPA)

Therapeutic Class: Thrombolytic

CLINICAL PHARMACOLOGY

Mechanism of Action: Promotes fibrin conversion of plasminogen to plasmin; able to bind to fibrin, convert plasminogen in thrombus to plasmin, which leads to local fibrinolysis, limited systemic proteolysis

Pharmacokinetics

IV: Cleared by liver, 80% cleared within 10 min of drug termination

INDICATIONS AND USES: Acute MI: for lysis of thrombi obstructing coronary arteries, improvement of ventricular function,

---

and reduction in incidence of CHF; pulmonary embolism; acute ischemic stroke within 3h of onset; unstable angina pectoris*

DOSAGE

Adult

• *Acute MI:* IV 15 mg bolus, then 0.75 mg/kg over 30 min (max 50 mg), then 0.5 mg/kg over 60 min (max 35 mg)

• *Pulmonary embolism:* IV 100 mg over 2 hr

S AVAILABLE FORMS/COST OF THERAPY

• Inj, Lyphl-Sol—IV: 1 mg/ml, 20 mg: **$550.00**; 1 mg/ml, 50 mg: **$1375.00**; 1 mg/ml, 100 mg: **$2750.00**

CONTRAINDICATIONS: Active bleeding, hemorrhagic stroke, severe uncontrolled hypertension, intracranial/intraspinal surgery/trauma, aneurysm, arteriovenous malformation, brain tumor

PRECAUTIONS: Recent (within 10 days) major surgery (e.g., coronary artery bypass graft, obstetric delivery, organ biopsy); previous puncture of noncompressible vessels; cerebrovascular disease; recent gastrointestinal or genitourinary bleeding (within 10 days); recent trauma (within 10 days); hypertension (systolic BP 180 mm Hg and/or diastolic BP 110 mm Hg); high likelihood of left heart thrombus (e.g., mitral stenosis with atrial fibrillation); acute pericarditis; bacterial endocarditis; hemostatic defects including those secondary to severe hepatic or renal disease; significant liver dysfunction; pregnancy; diabetic hemorrhagic retinopathy, or other hemorrhagic ophthalmic conditions; septic thrombophlebitis or occluded arteriovenous cannula at seriously infected site; advanced age (>75 yr); patients currently receiving oral anticoagulants (e.g., warfarin); any other condition in which bleeding constitutes a significant hazard or would be particularly difficult to manage because of its location; readministration

PREGNANCY AND LACTATION: Pregnancy category C. Unknown if excreted in breast milk

SIDE EFFECTS/ADVERSE REACTIONS

CV: Accelerated idioventricular rhythm, sinus bradycardia, ventricular tachycardia

HEME: Intracranial, retroperitoneal, surface, GI, GU bleeding; increased PT, APIT, TT

SKIN: Rash, urticaria

DRUG INTERACTIONS

Drugs

⬛ *Heparin, acetylsalicylic acid, dipyridamole: Increased bleeding*

Labs

Decrease: Fibrinogen (mitigated by collecting blood in presence of aprotinin)

SPECIAL CONSIDERATIONS

Compress arterial puncture sites at least 30 min

MONITORING PARAMETERS

• *Before initiation of therapy:* coagulation tests, hematocrit, platelet count

• *During therapy:* ECG, mental status, neurologic status, vital signs; heparin (in doses sufficient to prolong the APTT to 1.5-2 times control value) is usually administered in conjunction with thrombolytic therapy; aspirin may also be administered to inhibit platelet aggregation during and/or following postthrombolytic therapy

---

amiloride

(a-mill'oh-ride)

Rx: Midamor

Chemical Class: Pyrazine

Therapeutic Class: Potassium-sparing diuretic

CLINICAL PHARMACOLOGY

Mechanism of Action: Inhibits renal sodium reabsorption, reduces both potassium and hydrogen secretion and their subsequent excretion

Pharmacokinetics

PO: Onset 2 hr, peak 6-10 hr, duration 24 hr; excreted unchanged in urine (60%), feces (40%); $t_{1/2}$ 6-9 hr

INDICATIONS AND USES: Adjunctive treatment with thiazide or loop diuretics in congestive heart failure or hypertension to help restore potassium balance; lithium-induced polyuria*; aerosolized administration (drug dissolved in 0.3% saline delivered by nebulizer) in cystic fibrosis*

DOSAGE

Adult

• PO 5 mg qd, may be increased to 10-20 mg qd if needed

S AVAILABLE FORMS/COST OF THERAPY

• Tab, Uncoated—Oral: 5 mg, 100's: **$25.50-$46.08**

CONTRAINDICATIONS: Hyperkalemia (serum potassium >5.5 mEq/L), impaired renal function

PRECAUTIONS: Dehydration, diabetes, acidosis, hepatic function impairment, children

PREGNANCY AND LACTATION: Pregnancy category B; excretion into breast milk unknown; use caution in nursing mothers

SIDE EFFECTS/ADVERSE REACTIONS

CNS: Anxiety, decreased libido, depression, dizziness, encephalopathy, fatigue, *headache,* insomnia, mental confusion, nervousness, paresthesias, tremor, vertigo, weakness

CV: Angina, *dysrhythmias,* orthostatic hypotension

EENT: Blurred vision, increased intraocular pressure, loss of hearing, nasal congestion, tinnitus

GI: Abdominal pain, anorexia, constipation, cramps, *diarrhea,* dry mouth, dyspepsia, flatulence, GI bleeding, jaundice, *nausea, vomiting*

GU: Dysuria, frequency, impotence, polyuria

HEME: Agranulocytopenia, leukopenia, thrombocytopenia (rare)

METAB: Acidosis, hyperkalemia, hypochloremia, hyponatremia

MS: Cramps, joint pain

SKIN: Alopecia, pruritus, rash, urticaria

DRUG INTERACTIONS

Drugs

⬛ *ACE inhibitors:* Hyperkalemia in predisposed patients

❷ *Potassium:* Hyperkalemia in predisposed patients

⬛ *Quinidine:* Increased ventricular arrhythmias

SPECIAL CONSIDERATIONS

PATIENT/FAMILY EDUCATION

• Notify clinician of muscle weakness, fatigue, flaccid paralysis

• Take with food or milk for GI symptoms

• Take early in day to prevent nocturia

• Avoid large quantities of potassium-rich foods: oranges, bananas,

• salt substitutes

MONITORING PARAMETERS

• BP: postural hypotension may occur

• Electrolytes

• Glucose (serum), BUN, serum creatinine

---

* = non FDA-approved use

amiodarone
(a-mee'oh-da-rone)
Rx: Cordarone
Chemical Class: Iodinated benzofuran derivative
Therapeutic Class: Antidysrhythmic (class III)

CLINICAL PHARMACOLOGY
Mechanism of Action: Prolongs action potential duration and effective refractory period; noncompetitive α- and β-adrenergic inhibition

Pharmacokinetics
PO: Slowly and variably absorbed, onset 1-3 wk; extensive distribution; $t_{1/2}$ 26-107 days; eliminated via hepatic excretion into bile

INDICATIONS AND USES: Life-threatening recurrent ventricular fibrillation and hemodynamically unstable ventricular tachycardia unresponsive to adequate doses of other antiarrhythmics; refractory-sustained or paroxysmal atrial fibrillation and paroxysmal supraventricular tachycardia,* symptomatic atrial flutter,* CHF (low dose)*

DOSAGE
Adult
• PO loading dose 800-1600 mg/day for 1-3 wk; then 600-800 mg/day for 1 mo; maintenance 200-600 mg/day (lower doses effective for supraventricular arrhythmias)

Child
• PO loading dose 10-15 mg/kg/day or 600-800 mg/1.73 m²/day for 4-14 days or until adequate control of dysrhythmia or prominent adverse effects occur; maintenance 5 mg/kg/day or 200-400 mg/1.73 m²/day qd for several weeks; reduce to lowest effective dosage possible
• IV 5 mg/kg over 30 min followed by PO 800 mg qd × 7 days, then 600 mg qd × 3 days, then 200-400 mg qd maintenance; IV load allows shorter time to arrhythmic control than PO load; or IV 5 mg/kg bolus followed 15 min later by continuous IV infusion of 20 mg/kg/day for 3-5 days

ⓈAVAILABLE FORMS/COST OF THERAPY
• Tab, Uncoated—Oral: 200 mg, 100's: **$306.95**
• Inj, Sol—intravenous-50 mg/ml, 3 ml: **$68.75**

CONTRAINDICATIONS: Severe sinus-node dysfunction, with resultant marked sinus bradycardia; 2nd and 3rd degree AV block; syncope caused by episodes of bradycardia (except when used in conjunction with a pacemaker); hypersensitivity

PRECAUTIONS: Thyroid disease, 2nd or 3rd degree AV block, electrolyte imbalances, bradycardia, pulmonary disease (poorer prognosis should pulmonary toxicity develop)

PREGNANCY AND LACTATION: Pregnancy category D; due to a very long $t_{1/2}$, amiodarone should be discontinued several months before conception to avoid early gestational exposure, reserve for refractory dysrhythmias; newborns exposed to amiodarone should have TFTs; excreted into breast milk; contains high proportions of iodine; breast feeding not recommended

SIDE EFFECTS/ADVERSE REACTIONS
Adverse reactions occur in about 75% of patients receiving doses 400 mg/day and cause discontinuation of drug in 7%-18% of patients
CNS: Ataxia, *dizziness,* fatigue, *headache,* insomnia, involuntary movements, lack of coordination, malaise, paresthesias, peripheral neuropathy, tremors
CV: Bradycardia, **cardiac conduction abnormalities,** CHF, ***dysrhythmias,*** hypotension, **sinoatrial node dysfunction, sinus arrest**
EENT: Blurred vision, corneal microdeposits, dry eyes, halos, loss of vision, optic neuritis, optic neuropathy, photophobia

GI: Abdominal pain, anorexia, constipation, diarrhea, hepatotoxicity, nausea, vomiting
METAB: Hyperthyroidism or hypothyroidism
MS: Pain in extremities, weakness
RESP: Cough, dyspnea, ***pulmonary fibrosis(1/1000),*** pulmonary inflammation
SKIN: Alopecia, angioedema, blue-gray skin discoloration, photosensitivity, rash, spontaneous ecchymosis
MISC: Abnormal salivation, abnormal taste or smell, coagulation abnormalities, edema, flushing

DRUG INTERACTIONS
Drugs
⬛ *Aprinidine:* Increased aprinidine concentrations
⬛ *β-adrenergic blockers:* Bradycardia, cardiac arrest, or ventricular arrhythmia shortly after initiation of β-adrenergic blockers that undergo extensive hepatic metabolism (propranolol, sotalol, metoprolol)
⬛ *Calcium channel blockers:* Cardiotoxicity with bradycardia and decreased cardiac output with diltiazem and, potentially, verapamil
⬛ *Cholestyramine, Colestipol:* Decreased amiodarone plasma concentrations
⬛ *Cimetidine:* Increased amiodarone plasma concentrations (other H₂ blockers likely have no effect)
⬛ *Cyclosporine, Tacrolimus:* Increased cyclosporine, tacrolimus concentrations
⬛ *Digitalis glycosides:* Accumulation of digoxin
⬛ *Flecainide, Ecainide:* Increased flecainide, ecainide serum concentrations
⬛ *Oral anticoagulants:* Enhanced hypoprothrombinemic response to warfarin
⬛ *Phenytoin:* Increased serum phenytoin concentrations, decreased amiodarone concentrations
⬛ *Procainamide:* Increased procainamide concentrations
⬛ *Quinidine:* Increased quinidine plasma concentrations
⬛ *Theophylline:* Increased theophylline levels
Labs
Increase: Serum T4 and serum reverse T3
Decrease: Serum T3

SPECIAL CONSIDERATIONS

Should be administered only by clinicians experienced in treatment of life-threatening dysrhythmias who are thoroughly familiar with the risks and benefits of amiodarone therapy
PATIENT/FAMILY EDUCATION
• Take with food and/or divide doses if GI intolerance occurs
• Use sunscreen or stay out of sun to prevent burns
• Report side effects immediately
• Skin discoloration is usually reversible
MONITORING PARAMETERS
• Chest x-ray and PFTs (baseline and q3 mo)
• Electrolytes
• LFTs
• ECG (measure PR, QRS, QT intervals; check for PVCs, other dysrhythmias); QT interval prolongation of 10%-15% suggests therapeutic effect
• TFTs
• CNS symptoms

---

italic = common side effects

bold italic = life-threatening reactions

amlodipine
(am-loh' dih-peen)
Rx: Norvasc
Combinations
  Rx: with benazepril (Lotrel)
Chemical Class: Dihydropyridine; calcium channel blocker
Therapeutic Class: Antihypertensive; antianginal

CLINICAL PHARMACOLOGY
Mechanism of Action: Inhibits calcium ion influx across cell membrane in vascular smooth muscle and cardiac muscle; produces relaxation of coronary vascular smooth muscle, peripheral vascular smooth muscle; reduces total peripheral resistance (afterload); increases myocardial oxygen delivery
Pharmacokinetics
PO: Onset undetermined (ionized at physiologic pH resulting in gradual association and disassociation with receptor binding site and gradual onset of action), peak 6-12 hr, $t_{1/2}$ 30-50 hr, metabolized by liver, excreted in urine (90% as metabolites)
INDICATIONS AND USES: Chronic stable angina pectoris, hypertension, vasospastic (Prinzmetal's or variant) angina, CHF
DOSAGE
Adult
• *Angina:* PO 5-10 mg qd
• *Hypertension:* PO 5 mg qd initially, may increase up to 10 mg/day (small, fragile, or elderly patients or patients with hepatic insufficiency may be started on 2.5 mg qd)
$ AVAILABLE FORMS/COST OF THERAPY
• Tab, Uncoated—Oral: 2.5 mg, 100's: **$125.66;** 5 mg, 100's: **$125.66;** 10 mg, 100's: **$217.45**
PRECAUTIONS: CHF, hypotension, hepatic insufficiency, aortic stenosis, elderly
PREGNANCY AND LACTATION: Pregnancy category C; unknown if excreted into milk; use caution in nursing mothers
SIDE EFFECTS/ADVERSE REACTIONS
CNS: Anxiety, asthenia, depression, dizziness, fatigue, headache, insomnia, malaise, nervousness, paresthesia, somnolence, tremor
CV: Bradycardia, *dysrhythmia,* hypotension, palpitations, *peripheral edema,* syncope, tachycardia
GI: Abdominal cramps, constipation, diarrhea, dry mouth, flatulence, gastric upset, nausea, vomiting
GU: Nocturia, polyuria
SKIN: Hair loss, pruritus, rash, urticaria
MISC: Cough, epistaxis, flushing, muscle cramps, nasal congestion, sexual dysfunction, shortness of breath, sweating, tinnitus, weight gain
DRUG INTERACTIONS
Drugs
▪ *Barbiturates:* Reduced plasma concentrations of amlodipine
▪ *β-adrenergic blockers:* Enhanced effects of β-adrenergic blockers; reduced clearance of amlodipine
▪ *Calcium:* May reduce response
▪ *Carbamazepine:* Reduced plasma concentrations of amlodipine
▪ *Diltiazem:* Reduced clearance of amlodipine
▪ *Erythromycin:* Reduced clearance of amlodipine
▪ *Grapefruit juice:* Reduced clearance of amlodipine
▪ *H_2 blockers:* Increased plasma concentration of amlodipine possible
▪ *Proton pump inhibitors:* Increased plasma concentration of amlodipine possible
▪ *Quinidine:* Increased plasma concentration of amlodipine; reduced plasma quinidine level

▪ *Rifampin:* Reduced plasma concentration of amlodipine
▪ *Vincristine:* Reduced vincristine clearance

SPECIAL CONSIDERATIONS
PATIENT/FAMILY EDUCATION
Notify clinician of irregular heart beat, shortness of breath, swelling of feet and hands, pronounced dizziness, hypotension

amrinone
(am'ri-none)
Rx: Inocor
Chemical Class: Bipyrimidine derivative
Therapeutic Class: Cardiac inotropic agent

CLINICAL PHARMACOLOGY
Mechanism of Action: Cardiac inotrope distinct from digitalis glycosides or catecholamines; direct vasodilator, which reduces preload and afterload; not a β-adrenergic agonist; dose-related increases in cardiac output occur (28% at 0.75 mg/kg to about 61% at 3 mg/kg IV bolus); pulmonary capillary wedge pressure, total peripheral resistance, and diastolic and mean arterial pressures show dose-related decreases; heart rate generally unchanged
Pharmacokinetics
Onset of action 2-5 min, peak 10 min, duration variable, $t_{1/2}$ 4-6 hr; metabolized in liver, 60%-90% excreted in urine as drug and metabolites; in patients with compromised renal and hepatic perfusion, plasma levels of amrinone may rise during the infusion period
INDICATIONS AND USES: Short-term management of congestive heart failure unresponsive to other medication
DOSAGE
Adult
• IV bolus 0.75 mg/kg over 2-3 min; start infusion of 5-10 μg/kg/min; may give another 0.75 μg/kg bolus 30 min after start of therapy; daily dose should not exceed 10 mg/kg; the above dosing regimen will yield a plasma concentration of amrinone of 3 μg/ml; increases in cardiac index show a linear relationship to plasma concentration in a range of 0.5 μg/ml to 7 μg/ml
$ AVAILABLE FORMS/COST OF THERAPY
• Inj, Sol—IV: 5 mg/ml, 20 ml vial: **$67.63**
CONTRAINDICATIONS: Hypersensitivity to bisulfites, severe aortic or pulmonic obstructive valvular disease, acute MI
PRECAUTIONS: Diuretic therapy (decreased cardiac filling pressure may cause decreased response to amrinone), arrhythmias
PREGNANCY AND LACTATION: Pregnancy category C
SIDE EFFECTS/ADVERSE REACTIONS
CV: Chest pain, *dysrhythmias (3%),* headache, hypotension (1.3%)
GI: Abdominal pain, anorexia, hepatotoxicity, hiccups, nausea, vomiting
HEME: Thrombocytopenia (2.4%); dose dependent
RESP: Pleuritis
SKIN: Allergic reactions, burning at injection site
MISC: Fever, hypersensitivity reaction manifested by pleuritis, pericarditis, myositis, or interstitial pulmonary infiltrates
DRUG INTERACTIONS
Drugs
• *Furosemide:* Precipitates when furosemide is injected into an IV line infusing amrinone
Labs
• *Increase:* Serum digoxin (Abbott TdX method)

---

* = non FDA-approved use

SPECIAL CONSIDERATIONS
MONITORING PARAMETERS
• BP and pulse q5 min during infusion; if BP drops 30 mm Hg, stop infusion
• Cardiac output and pulmonary capillary wedge pressure
• Monitor platelet count and serum K, Na, Cl, Ca, BUN, creatinine, ALT, AST, and bilirubin daily

anagrelide
(ah-na′ greh-lide)
Rx: Argylin
Chemical Class: Not available
Therapeutic Class: Antiplatelet agent

CLINICAL PHARMACOLOGY
Mechanism of Action: Reduces blood platelet count, perhaps via a dose-related reduction in platelet production resulting from a decrease in megakaryocyte hypermaturation
Pharmacokinetic
PO: Peak 1 hr, bioavailability reduced by food; extensively metabolized; metabolites eliminated in urine (> 70%) and feces (10%); t$_{1/2}$ 1.3 hr, terminal elimination t$_{1/2}$ approximately 3 days
INDICATIONS AND USES: Essential thrombocythemia
DOSAGE
Adult
• PO 0.5 mg qid or 1 mg bid; dose may be adjusted after at least 1 wk to the lowest amount required to maintain platelet count <600,000; do not increase dose by >0.5 mg/day in any 1 wk period; do not exceed 10 mg/day or 2.5 in a single dose
$ AVAILABLE FORMS/COST OF THERAPY
• Cap, opaque—Oral: 0.5 mg, 100's: **$NA;** 1 mg, 100's: **$NA**
PRECAUTIONS: Known or suspected heart disease; renal or hepatic function impairment
PREGNANCY AND LACTATION: Pregnancy category C; not recommended in women who are or may become pregnant; excretion into breast milk unknown
SIDE EFFECTS/ADVERSE REACTIONS
CNS: Dizziness, headache (44.5%)
*CV: **Arrhythmia, cerebrovascular accident,** chest pain, **CHF,** edema, hemorrhage, palpitations, postural hypotension, syncope, tachycardia, vasodilation*
EENT: Abnormal vision, amblyopia, diplopia, epistaxis, rhinitis, sinusitis, tinnitus
*GI: Abdominal pain, anorexia, aphthous stomatitis, constipation, diarrhea (24.3%), dyspepsia, elevated liver enzymes, flatulence, gastritis, **GI hemorrhage,** melena, nausea, vomiting*
GU: Dysuria, hematuria
HEME: Anemia, ecchymosis, lymphadenoma, **thrombocytopenia**
MS: Arthralgia, back pain, leg cramps, myalgia
RESP: Asthma, dyspnea
SKIN: Alopecia, photosensitivity, pruritus, rash
MISC: Asthenia, chills, fever, flu symptoms, malaise, neck pain, pain, paresthesia
MONITORING PARAMETERS
Platelet count q2 days during first wk, then weekly thereafter until maintenance dose reached

ardeparin
(ar-da-pare′ in)
Rx: Normiflo
Chemical Class: Depolymerized heparin derivative (low molecular weight heparin)
Therapeutic Class: Anticoagulant

CLINICAL PHARMACOLOGY
Mechanism of Action: Inhibits thrombosis by inactivating factor Xa and inhibiting the conversion of prothrombin to thrombin; has higher ratio of anti-factor Xa to antithrombin activity (1.7:2.0) than does unfractionated heparin (1.22); does not significantly influence bleeding time, platelet function, prothrombin time (PT), or activated partial thromboplastin time (aPTT) at recommended doses
Pharmacokinetics
SC: Absolute bioavailability 92%, peak 2.4-3 hr, duration 8-12 hr; likely undergoes saturable elimination; t$_{1/2}$ 2.5-3.3 hr
INDICATIONS AND USES: Prevention of deep vein thrombosis (DVT), which may lead to pulmonary embolism following knee replacement surgery
DOSAGE
Adult
• SC 50 anti-Xa units/kg q12h for up to 14 days or until fully ambulatory; begin therapy the evening after surgery or the following morning; for patients 100 kg use the 5000 anti-Xa unit/0.5 ml solution (dose in ml = patient weight [kg] × 0.005 ml/kg); for patients >100 kg use the 10,000 anti-Xa unit/0.5 ml solution (dose in ml = patient weight [kg] × 0.0025 ml/kg)
$ AVAILABLE FORMS/COST OF THERAPY
Sol, inj—SC: 5000 units/0.5 ml: **$15.45;** 10,000 units/0.5 ml: **$24.50**
CONTRAINDICATIONS: Active major bleeding; hypersensitivity to pork products; thrombocytopenia associated with a positive in vitro test for antiplatelet antibody in the presence of ardeparin
PRECAUTIONS: History of heparin-induced thrombocytopenia; increased risk for hemorrhage; hypersensitivity to methylparaben or propylparaben, or sulfite sensitivity
PREGNANCY AND LACTATION: Pregnancy category C; teratogenic effects observed following administration of high doses IV in rats and rabbits; excretion in breast milk unknown but likely minimal
SIDE EFFECTS/ADVERSE REACTIONS
CNS: Confusion
CV: Hemorrhage
GI: Constipation, increased AST and/or ALT, nausea, vomiting
*HEME: Anemia, **thrombocytopenia***
SKIN: Ecchymosis, pruritus, rash
MISC: Fever

SPECIAL CONSIDERATIONS
Not interchangeable with other low molecular weight heparins
PATIENT/FAMILY EDUCATION
• Administer by deep SC inj into abdominal wall; alternate inj sites
• Report any unusual bruising or bleeding to clinician
MONITORING PARAMETERS
• CBC with platelets, stool occult blood, urinalysis

italic = common side effects   ***bold italic*** = life-threatening reactions

aspirin
(as´pir-in)
Rx: Easprin, ZORprin
OTC: A.S.A., Ancasal ✢, Aspergum, Bayer, Bayer Children's Aspirin, Ecotrin, Ecotrin Maximum Strength, 8-Hour Bayer Timed Release, Empirin, Genprin, Maximum Bayer, Norwich Extra-Strength, St. Joseph Children's, Supasa ✢, Therapy Bayer
Combinations
   Rx: with butalbital (Fiorinal); with codeine (Empirin); with dihydrocodeine (Synalgos DC); with hydrocodone (Azdone); with oxycodone (Percodan); with propoxyphene (Darvon)
   OTC: with antacids (Ascriptin, Bufferin, Magnaprin)
Chemical Class: Salicylate derivative
Therapeutic Class: Nonnarcotic analgesic; antiinflammatory; antiplatelet agent; antipyretic

CLINICAL PHARMACOLOGY
Mechanism of Action: Inhibits prostaglandin synthesis and release; acts on the hypothalamus heat-regulating center to reduce fever; blocks prostaglandin synthetase action, which prevents formation of the platelet-aggregating substance thromboxane A_2
Pharmacokinetics
PO: Well-absorbed, enteric coated product may exhibit erratic absorption, onset 15-30 min (delayed with enteric coated), peak 1-2 hr, duration 4-6 hr
PR: Absorption erratic, onset slow, duration 4-6 hr
Metabolized by liver, metabolites excreted by kidneys; $t_{1/2}$ 3 hr at lower doses (300-600 mg), 5-6 hr (1000 mg) up to 30 hr in larger doses (due to saturable metabolic pathways)
INDICATIONS AND USES: Mild to moderate pain and fever; inflammatory conditions such as rheumatic fever, rheumatoid arthritis, and osteoarthritis; thromboembolic disorders; reducing risk of recurrent transient ischemic attacks; reducing the risk of death or nonfatal MI in patients with previous MI or unstable angina; low doses may be useful in preventing toxemia of pregnancy*
DOSAGE
Adult
• *Arthritis:* PO 2.6-5.2 g/day in divided doses q4-6h
• *Pain/fever:* PO/PR 325-650 mg q4h prn, not to exceed 4 g/day
• *Transient ischemic attacks:* PO 325-650 mg qd or bid (325 mg/day may be as effective as larger doses and associated with fewer side effects)
• *MI prophylaxis:* PO 165-325 mg/day
Child
• Arthritis: PO 60-90 mg/kg/day in divided doses; usual maintenance dose 80-100 mg/kg/day divided q6-8h; maintain serum salicylate level of 150-300 mg/ml
• *Pain/fever:* PO/PR 10-15 mg/kg/dose q4-6h prn
S AVAILABLE FORMS/COST OF THERAPY
• Tab, Chewable—Oral: 81 mg, 36's: **$1.00-$2.25**
• Tab, Enteric Coated—Oral: 81 mg, 100's: **$6.89;** 325 mg, 100's: **$1.15-$13.60;** 500 mg, 60's: **$1.55-$6.26;** 650 mg, 100's: **$3.70-$4.51**
• Gum Tab, Chewable—Oral: 227 mg, 16's: **$2.26**
• Tab, Film Coated—Oral: 325 mg, 100's: **$0.80-$3.70;** 500 mg, 100's: **$1.29-$3.50;** 600 mg, 100's: **$3.50**
• Tab, Enteric Coated, Sus Action—Oral: 800 mg, 100's: **$9.00-$32.80;** 975 mg, 100's: **$11.48-$36.64**
• Supp—Rect: 120 mg, 12's: **$1.80-$3.60;** 300 mg, 12's: **$2.39-$3.59;** 600 mg, 12's: **$2.60-$3.89**

CONTRAINDICATIONS: Hypersensitivity to salicylates, NSAIDs, or tartrazine (FDC yellow dye #5); GI bleeding; hemophilia; hemorrhagic states
PRECAUTIONS: Anemia, asthma, nasal polyps, nasal allergies, hepatic disease, renal disease, Hodgkin's disease, pre/postoperatively, children or teenagers with flulike symptoms (may be associated with the development of Reye's syndrome), gout, history of coagulation defects, bleeding disorders
PREGNANCY AND LACTATION: Pregnancy category C (category D if full doses used in 3rd trimester); use in pregnancy should generally be avoided; in pregnancies at risk for the development of pregnancy-induced hypertension and preeclampsia, and in fetuses with intrauterine growth retardation, low-dose aspirin (40-150 mg/day) may be beneficial; excreted into breast milk in low concentrations
SIDE EFFECTS/ADVERSE REACTIONS
CNS: Confusion, dizziness, drowsiness, headache
EENT: Dimness of vision, reversible hearing loss, tinnitus
GI: Acute reversible hepatotoxicity, anorexia, cholestasis, diarrhea, *dyspepsia,* epigastric discomfort, GI bleeding, heartburn, increased transaminase levels, *nausea*
HEME: Decreased plasma iron concentration, hyperuricemia (low dose), hyperuricosuria (high dose), *leukopenia,* prolonged bleeding time, shortened erythrocyte survival time, *thrombocytopenia*
METAB: Hypoglycemia, hypokalemia, hyponatremia
RESP: Hyperpnea, wheezing
SKIN: Angioedema, bruising, hives, rash, urticaria
MISC: Fever, thirst
DRUG INTERACTIONS
Drugs
🖪 *ACE inhibitors:* Reduced antihypertensive effect
❷ *Acetazolamide:* Increased concentrations of acetazolamide, possibly leading to CNS toxicity
🖪 *Antacids:* Decreased serum salicylate concentrations; high dose salicylates only
🖪 *Corticosteroids:* Increased incidence and/or severity of GI ulceration; enhanced salicylate excretion
🖪 *Diltiazem:* Enhanced antiplatelet effect of aspirin
🖪 *Ethanol:* Enhanced aspirin-induced GI mucosal damage and aspirin-induced prolongation of bleeding time
🖪 *Griseofulvin:* Reduced serum salicylate level
🖪 *Intrauterine contraceptive device:* May reduce contraceptive effectiveness
❷ *Methotrexate:* Increased serum methotrexate concentrations and enhanced methotrexate toxicity
❷ *Oral anticoagulants:* Increased risk of bleeding by inhibiting platelet function and possibly by producing gastric erosions
🖪 *Probenecid:* Salicylates inhibit the uricosuric activity of probenecid
🖪 *Sulfinpyrazone:* Salicylates inhibit the uricosuric activity of sulfinpyrazone
🖪 *Sulfonylureas:* Enhanced hypoglycemic response to sulfonylureas
🖪 *Warfarin:* Enhanced hypoprothrombinemic effect of warfarin
Labs
• *Increase:* Serum acetaminophen (Glynn-Kendal method), urine acetoacetate (Gerhardt ferric chloride procedure), urine glucose (Ames Clinitest method), serum HbAlc (chromatographic and electrophoretic, but not colorimetric methods), urine hippuric acid, urine homogentisic acid, urine homovanillic acid, urine ketones (Gerhardt's test), urine phenyl ketones, CSF and urine protein (Folin-Ciocalteu method), serum and urine uric acid (nonspecific methods only)
• *Decrease:* Serum albumin, urine glucose (glucose oxidase methods), total serum phenytoin (but not free serum phenytoin)

---

* = non FDA-approved use

SPECIAL CONSIDERATIONS

PATIENT/FAMILY EDUCATION
• Administer with food
• Do not exceed recommended doses
• Read label on other OTC drugs, many contain aspirin
• Therapeutic response may take 2 wk (arthritis)
• Avoid alcohol ingestion, GI bleeding may occur
Not to be given to children with flulike symptoms, Reye's syndrome may develop

MONITORING PARAMETERS
• AST, ALT, bilirubin, creatinine, CBC, hematocrit if patient is on long-term therapy

---

atenolol
(a-ten'oh-lol)
Rx: Tenormin
Combinations
  Rx: with chlorthalidone (Tenoretic)
Chemical Class: β_1-selective (cardioselective) adrenoreceptor blocking agent
Therapeutic Class: Antihypertensive; antianginal; antidysrhythmic (class II)

CLINICAL PHARMACOLOGY
Mechanism of Action: Competes with β-adrenergic agonists for β_1-receptor sites, inhibiting chronotropic and inotropic responses to β_1-adrenergic stimulation (cardioselective); slows conduction of AV node, decreases heart rate, decreases O_2 consumption in myocardium, decreases renin-aldosterone-angiotensin system at higher doses; blocks β_2-receptors in bronchial system at higher doses; no membrane stabilizing or intrinsic sympathomimetic (partial agonist) activities
Pharmacokinetics
PO: Peak 2-4 hr, $t_{1/2}$ 6-7 hr; excreted unchanged in urine; protein binding 6%-16%

INDICATIONS AND USES: Angina pectoris due to coronary atherosclerosis; hypertension; acute MI; migraine headache prophylaxis*; alcohol withdrawal syndrome*; esophageal varices in cirrhotic patients*; situational anxiety*; ventricular dysrhythmias*; rate control in atrial fibrillation*

DOSAGE
Adult
• IV 5 mg over 5 min, repeat in 10 min if initial dose is well tolerated, then start PO dose 10 min after last IV dose; PO 50 mg qd, increasing q1-2 wk to 100 mg qd, may increase to 200 mg qd for angina
Child
• PO Initial 1-1.2 mg/kg/dose given daily, maximum 2 mg/kg/day
• Renal impairment:

Creatinine Clearance	Maximum Dose	Dosing Interval
15-35 ml/min	50 mg or 1 mg/kg/dose	Daily
<15 ml/min	50 mg or 1 mg/kg/dose	Every other day

⑤AVAILABLE FORMS/COST OF THERAPY
• Tab, Uncoated—Oral: 25 mg, 100's: **$9.09-$95.62;** 50 mg, 100's: **$4.64-$97.57;** 100 mg, 100's: **$9.45-$146.35**
• Inj, Sol—IV, Buffered: 5 mg/10 ml, 10 ml: **$6.38**

CONTRAINDICATIONS: Cardiogenic shock, 2nd or 3rd degree heart block, sinus bradycardia, CHF unless secondary to a tachyarrhythmia treatable with β-blockers, overt cardiac failure
PRECAUTIONS: Major surgery, diabetes mellitus, renal disease, thyroid disease, COPD, asthma, well-compensated heart failure, abrupt withdrawal, peripheral vascular disease
PREGNANCY AND LACTATION: Pregnancy category C; safe use for treatment of hypertension in pregnant women has been demonstrated; no fetal malformations reported, but experience during the first trimester is lacking; excreted into breast milk; monitor nursing infants closely for bradycardia and other signs and symptoms of β-blockade

SIDE EFFECTS/ADVERSE REACTIONS
CNS: Depression, *dizziness,* drowsiness, *fatigue,* hallucinations, insomnia, *lethargy,* memory loss, mental changes, strange dreams
CV: Bradycardia, CHF, cold extremities, postural hypotension, profound hypotension, **2nd or 3rd degree heart block**
EENT: Dry burning eyes, sore throat, visual disturbances
GI: Diarrhea, dry mouth, **ischemic colitis, mesenteric arterial thrombosis,** *nausea,* vomiting
GU: Impotence, sexual dysfunction
HEME: **Agranulocytosis, thrombocytopenia**
METAB: Hyperglycemia, hyperlipidemia (increase TG, total cholesterol, LDL; decrease HDL), **masked hypoglycemic response** (sweating excepted)
RESP: Bronchospasm, dyspnea, wheezing
SKIN: Alopecia, pruritus, rash

DRUG INTERACTIONS
Drugs
◪ *Adenosine:* Bradycardia aggravated
◪ *Amoxicillin, Ampicillin:* Reduced atenolol bioavailability
◪ *Antacids:* Reduced atenolol absorption
◪ *Calcium channel blockers:* See dihydropyridine and verapamil
◪ *Clonidine:* Exacerbation of rebound hypertension upon discontinuation of clonidine
◪ *Dihydropyridines:* Additive hemodynamic effects; increased serum concentration of atenolol
◪ *Dipyridamole:* Bradycardia aggravated
◪ *Lidocaine:* Increased serum lidocaine concentrations possible
◪ *Neostigmine:* Bradycardia aggravated
◪ *NSAIDs:* Reduced antihypertensive effects of atenolol
◪ *Physostigmine:* Bradycardia aggravated
◪ *Prazosin:* First-dose response to prazosin may be enhanced by β-blockade
◪ *Tacrine:* Bradycardia aggravated
  Theophylline: Antagonistic pharmacodynamic effects
❷ *Verapamil:* Enhanced effects of both drugs, particularly AV node conduction slowing; reduced atenolol clearance

SPECIAL CONSIDERATIONS

PATIENT/FAMILY EDUCATION
• Do not discontinue drug abruptly, may precipitate angina
• Report bradycardia, dizziness, confusion, depression, fever, shortness of breath, swelling of the extremities
• Take pulse at home, notify clinician if <50 beats/min
• Avoid hazardous activities if dizziness, drowsiness, lightheadedness are present
• May mask the symptoms of hypoglycemia, except for sweating, in diabetic patients

MONITORING PARAMETERS
Blood pressure, pulse

---

italic = common side effects

bold italic = life-threatening reactions

atorvastatin
(a-tor'va-sta-tin)
Rx: Lipitor
Chemical Class: HMG-CoA reductase inhibitor
Therapeutic Class: Antilipemic

CLINICAL PHARMACOLOGY
Mechanism of Action: Inhibits HMG-CoA reductase, necessary enzyme for cholesterol synthesis; reduces total cholesterol, LDL-cholesterol, triglycerides, apo B; produces variable increases in HDL-cholesterol and apo A1
Pharmacokinetics
PO: Peak 1-2 hours; 12% bioavailability; food decreases absorption 30% (not clinically significant); (98% protein bound; metabolized via CYP-3A4; $t_{1/2}$ 14 hours
INDICATIONS AND USES: Adjunctive treatment to diet for elevated total cholesterol, LDL-cholesterol, apo B, and triglycerides levels; primary hypercholesterolemia and mixed lipidemias
DOSAGE
Adult
• PO: 10-80 mg qd; dose can be administered any time of day without regard to meals
S **AVAILABLE FORMS/COST OF THERAPY**
• Tablet, film-coated—Oral: 10 mg, 90's: **$164.16;** 20 mg, 90's: **$253.80;** 40 mg, 90's: **$305.64**
CONTRAINDICATIONS: Active liver disease; unexplained persistent elevations of serum transaminases; pregnancy and lactation
PRECAUTIONS: Liver dysfunction
PREGNANCY AND LACTATION: Pregnancy category X; not recommended for nursing mothers
SIDE EFFECTS/ADVERSE REACTIONS
CNS: Headache
CV: Migraine, palpitation, postural hypotension, syncope, vasodilation
EENT: Amblyopia, dry eyes, taste disturbances, tinnitus
GI: Abdominal pain, constipation, diarrhea, dyspepsia, flatulence, gastroenteritis, LFT abnormalities
HEME: Anemia, ecchymosis, petechia, thrombocytopenia
METAB: Hyperglycemia, increased creatinine phosphokinase
MS: Arthralgia, leg cramps, *myalgia*
SKIN: Pruritus, rash
MISC: Face edema, fever, flulike syndrome, malaise, photosensitivity
DRUG INTERACTIONS
Drugs
S Azole antifungals (fluconazole, itraconazole, ketoconazole, miconazole): Increased atorvastatin levels; increased risk of rhabdomyolysis
S Erythromycin: Increased atorvastatin concentrations (approximately 40%); increased risk of rhabdomyolysis
S Nefazodone: Increased atorvastatin levels; increased risk of rhabdomyolysis

SPECIAL CONSIDERATIONS
• Potency and ability to lower serum triglycerides is unique among the HMG-CoA reductase inhibitors
• No outcome data available

benazepril
(ben-a-ze'pril)
Rx: Lotensin
Combinations
  Rx: with hydrochlorothiazide (Lotensin HCT)
Chemical Class: Angiotensin-converting enzyme (ACE) inhibitor
Therapeutic Class: Antihypertensive

CLINICAL PHARMACOLOGY
Mechanism of Action: Selectively suppresses renin-angiotensin-aldosterone system; inhibits ACE, preventing the conversion of angiotensin I to angiotensin II; results in dilation of arterial, venous vessels
Pharmacokinetics
PO: Peak $1/2$-1 hr, serum protein binding 97%, $t_{1/2}$ 10-11 hr; metabolized by liver to active metabolite (benazeprilat), which is excreted by the kidneys
INDICATIONS AND USES: Hypertension, CHF,* diabetic nephropathy*
DOSAGE
Adult
• PO 10 mg qd initially, increase as needed to 20-40 mg/day divided bid or qd
• Renal impairment: PO 5 mg qd with CrCl 30 ml/min/1.73 m²; increase as needed to maximum of 40 mg/day
S **AVAILABLE FORMS/COST OF THERAPY**
• Tab, Uncoated—Oral: 5 mg, 100's: **$69.48;** 10 mg, 100's: **$69.48;** 20 mg, 100's: **$69.48;** 40 mg, 100's: **$69.48**
PRECAUTIONS: Impaired renal and liver function, dialysis patients, hypovolemia, diuretic therapy, collagen-vascular diseases, CHF, elderly, bilateral renal artery stenosis
PREGNANCY AND LACTATION: Pregnancy category C (1st trimester), category D (2nd and 3rd trimesters); ACE inhibitors can cause fetal and neonatal morbidity and death when administered to pregnant women; detectable in breast milk in trace amounts, a newborn would receive 0.1% of the mg/kg maternal dose; effect on nursing infant has not been determined
SIDE EFFECTS/ADVERSE REACTIONS
CNS: Anxiety, *dizziness, fatigue, headache,* insomnia, paresthesia
CV: Angina, hypotension, palpitations, postural hypotension, syncope (especially with first dose)
GI: Abdominal pain, constipation, melena, nausea, vomiting
GU: Decreased libido, impotence, increased BUN/creatinine, urinary tract infection
HEME: **Agranulocytosis, neutropenia**
METAB: Hyperkalemia, hyponatremia
MS: Arthralgia, arthritis, myalgia
RESP: Asthma, bronchitis, *cough,* dyspnea, sinusitis
SKIN: Angioedema, flushing, rash, sweating
DRUG INTERACTIONS
Drugs
❷ *Allopurinol:* Combination may predispose to hypersensitivity reactions
S *α-adrenergic blockers:* Exaggerated first dose hypotensive response when added to benazepril
S *Aspirin:* May reduce hemodynamic effects of benazepril; less likely at doses under 236 mg; less likely with nonacetylated salicylates
S *Cyclosporine:* Combination may cause renal insufficiency
Insulin: Benazepril may enhance insulin sensitivity
S *Iron:* Benazepril may increase chance of systemic reaction to IV iron
S *Lithium:* Reduced lithium clearance

---

* = non FDA-approved use

▪ *Loop diuretics:* Initiation of benazepril may cause hypotension and renal insufficiency in patients taking loop diuretics
▪ *NSAIDs:* May reduce hemodynamic effects of benazepril
Potassium-sparing diuretics: Increased risk of hyperkalemia

SPECIAL CONSIDERATIONS

PATIENT/FAMILY EDUCATION
• Do not use salt substitutes containing potassium without consulting clinician
• Rise slowly to sitting or standing position to minimize orthostatic hypotension
• Notify clinician of mouth sores, sore throat, fever, swelling of hands or feet, irregular heartbeat, chest pain
• Dizziness, fainting, lightheadedness may occur during 1st few days of therapy

MONITORING PARAMETERS
• BUN, creatinine (watch for increased levels that may indicate acute renal failure)
• Potassium levels, although hyperkalemia rarely occurs

---

bepridil
(beh'prih-dill)
Rx: Vascor
Chemical Class: Calcium channel blocker
Therapeutic Class: Antianginal

CLINICAL PHARMACOLOGY
Mechanism of Action: Inhibits both slow calcium and fast sodium inward currents across the cell membrane during cardiac depolarization; produces relaxation of coronary vascular smooth muscle; dilates coronary arteries; decreases SA/AV node conduction; dilates peripheral arteries

Pharmacokinetics
PO: Peak 2-3 hr, 99% bound to plasma proteins, $t_{1/2}$ 24 hr; completely metabolized in the liver, excreted in urine and feces

INDICATIONS AND USES: Chronic stable angina; because of potential side effects (ventricular arrhythmias, agranulocytosis), should be reserved for patients who are unresponsive to, or intolerant of, other antianginal medication; may be used alone or in combination with β-blockers and/or nitrates

DOSAGE
Adult
• PO 200 mg qd initially, increase after 10 days depending on response, max 400 mg/day; most patients maintained on 300 mg/day

⑤ AVAILABLE FORMS/COST OF THERAPY
• Tab, Plain Coated—Oral: 200 mg, 100's: **$291.12;** 300 mg, 100's: **$355.08;** 400 mg, 100's: **$400.46**

CONTRAINDICATIONS: Sick sinus syndrome, 2nd or 3rd degree heart block, Wolff-Parkinson-White syndrome, hypotension 90 mm Hg systolic, uncompensated cardiac insufficiency, history of serious ventricular dysrhythmias, congenital QT interval prolongation or taking other drugs that prolong QT interval

PRECAUTIONS: CHF, renal disease, hepatic disease, children, hypokalemia, left bundle branch block, sinus bradycardia, recent MI

PREGNANCY AND LACTATION: Pregnancy category C; excreted in breast milk; use caution in nursing mothers

SIDE EFFECTS/ADVERSE REACTIONS
CNS: Anxiety, *asthenia,* confusion, depression, *dizziness,* drowsiness, fatigue, *headache,* insomnia, lightheadedness, nervousness, tremor, weakness

CV: **AV block,** bradycardia, CHF, **dysrhythmia (torsades de pointes, ventricular tachycardia),** edema, hypotension, palpitations
EENT: Blurred vision, tinnitus
GI: Constipation, *diarrhea,* dry mouth, *gastric upset,* increased liver function studies, *nausea,* vomiting
GU: Nocturia, polyuria
HEME: **Agranulocytosis** (rare)
RESP: Shortness of breath
SKIN: Rash

DRUG INTERACTIONS
Drugs
▪ *Digitoxin:* Reduced clearance; increased digitoxin levels; potential toxicity
▪ *Digoxin:* Increased serum digoxin concentrations

SPECIAL CONSIDERATIONS

PATIENT/FAMILY EDUCATION
• ECGs will be necessary during initiation of therapy and after dosage changes
• Notify provider immediately for irregular heartbeat, shortness of breath, pronounced dizziness, constipation, or hypotension
• May be taken with food or meals

MONITORING PARAMETERS
• Blood pressure, pulse, respiration, ECG intervals (PR, QRS, QT) at initiation of therapy and again after dosage increases
• Serum potassium

---

betaxolol
(bay-tax'oh-lol)
Rx: Kerlone, Betoptic, Betoptic S
Combinations
   Rx: with pilocarpine (Betoptic Pilo)
Chemical Class: β₁-selective (cardioselective) adrenoreceptor blocker
Therapeutic Class: Antihypertensive; antiglaucoma agent

CLINICAL PHARMACOLOGY
Mechanism of Action: Preferentially competes with β-adrenergic agonists for available β₁-receptor sites inhibiting the chronotropic and inotropic responses to β₁-adrenergic stimulation (cardioselective); blocks β₂-receptors in bronchial system at higher doses; weak membrane stabilizing activity; lacks intrinsic sympathomimetic (partial agonist) activity; the exact mechanism of ocular antihypertensive action is not established, but appears to be a reduction of aqueous production; does not produce miosis or accommodative spasm, which are frequently seen with miotic agents

Pharmacokinetics
PO: Peak 1.5-6 hr
OPHTH:
Onset 30 min, duration 12 hr
50% protein bound; metabolized by liver, excreted in urine as metabolites and unchanged drug; $t_{1/2}$ 14-22 hr

INDICATIONS AND USES: Hypertension; chronic open-angle glaucoma

DOSAGE
Adult
• PO 10 mg qd, increased to 20 mg qd after 7-14 days if desired response is not achieved; doses 20 mg/day have not produced additional antihypertensive effect
• OPHTH 1 gtt bid

---

italic = common side effects

bold italic = life-threatening reactions

Elderly
• PO reduce initial dose to 5 mg qd
$ AVAILABLE FORMS/COST OF THERAPY
• Susp—Ophth: 0.25%, 2.5, 5, 10, 15 ml: **$20.63**/5 ml
• Sol—Ophth: 0.5%, 2.5, 5, 10, 15 ml: **$20.63**/5 ml
• Tab, Plain Coated—Oral: 10 mg, 100's: **$79.43**; 20 mg, 100's: **$119.11**
CONTRAINDICATIONS: Cardiogenic shock, 2nd or 3rd degree heart block, sinus bradycardia, CHF unless secondary to a tachydysrhythmia treatable with β-blockers
PRECAUTIONS: Major surgery, diabetes mellitus, renal disease, thyroid disease, COPD, asthma, well-compensated heart failure, abrupt withdrawal, peripheral vascular disease; ophthalmic preparations can be absorbed systemically
PREGNANCY AND LACTATION: Pregnancy category C; excretion into breast milk unknown; use caution in nursing mothers
SIDE EFFECTS/ADVERSE REACTIONS
CNS: Depression, *dizziness,* drowsiness, *fatigue,* hallucinations, insomnia, *lethargy,* memory loss, mental changes, strange dreams
CV: Bradycardia, **CHF,** cold extremities, profound hypotension, **2nd or 3rd degree heart block**
EENT: Blepharoptosis, diplopia, dry burning eyes, keratitis, ptosis, sore throat, visual disturbances
GI: Diarrhea, dry mouth, ***ischemic colitis, mesenteric arterial thrombosis,*** *nausea,* vomiting
GU: Impotence, sexual dysfunction
HEME: ***Agranulocytosis, thrombocytopenia***
METAB: Hyperlipidemia (increase TG, total cholesterol, LDL; decrease HDL), masked hypoglycemic response to insulin (sweating excepted)
RESP: ***Bronchospasm,*** dyspnea
SKIN: Alopecia, pruritus, rash
DRUG INTERACTIONS
Drugs
▣ *Adenosine:* Increased risk of bradycardic response
▣ *Antacids:* Decreased absorption of oral betaxolol
▣ *Antidiabetics:* Altered response to hypoglycemia, prolonged recovery of normoglycemia, hypertension, blockade of tachycardia; may increase blood glucose and impair peripheral circulation
▣ *Dipyridamole:* Bradycardia
▣ *Neostigmine:* Additive risk of bradycardia
▣ *NSAIDs:* Reduced hypotensive effects of β-blockers
▣ *Tacrine:* Additive bradycardia
▣ *Theophylline:* Antagonistic pharmacodynamic effects
▣ *Verapamil:* Enhanced effects of both drugs, particularly atrioventricular conduction slowings

SPECIAL CONSIDERATIONS
• Do not discontinue drug abruptly, may precipitate angina or MI
• May mask the symptoms of hypoglycemia, except for sweating or dizziness, in diabetic patients
• Anaphylactic reactions may be more severe and not be as responsive to usual doses of epinephrine
• Transient stinging/discomfort is relatively common with ophthalmic preparations, notify clinician if severe
MONITORING PARAMETERS
• Blood pressure, pulse, intraocular pressure (ophth)

---

bisoprolol
(bis-o-prole′lole)
Rx: Zebeta
Combinations
   Rx: with hydrochlorothiazide: (Ziac)
Chemical Class: β₁-selective (cardioselective) adrenoreceptor blocker
Therapeutic Class: Antihypertensive

CLINICAL PHARMACOLOGY
Mechanism of Action: Selective β₁-adrenergic blocker; blocks β₂-receptors at doses above 20 mg per day
Pharmacokinetics
PO: Peak plasma level 2-4 hr, plasma $t_{1/2}$ 9-12 hr; 50% excreted unchanged in urine; protein binding 30%; metabolized in liver to inactive metabolites; full antihypertensive effect after 1 wk of therapy; if creatinine clearance 40 ml/min, plasma $t_{1/2}$ tripled; in cirrhotics, plasma $t_{1/2}$ is 8.3 to 21.7 hours
INDICATIONS AND USES: Mild to moderate hypertension
DOSAGE
Adult
• PO 2.5-5.0 mg qd, max dose 20 mg qd; reduce dose in renal or hepatic impairment
$ AVAILABLE FORMS/COST OF THERAPY
• Tab, Plain Coated—Oral: 5 mg, 30's: **$29.11**; 10 mg, 30's: **$29.11**
• Tab, Plain Coated—Oral: with hydrochlorothiazide: 2.5 mg/6.25 mg, 100's: **$97.06**; 5 mg/6.25 mg, 100's: **$97.06**; 10 mg/6.25 mg, 30's: **$29.11**
CONTRAINDICATIONS: Cardiogenic shock, heart block (2nd, 3rd degree), sinus bradycardia, overt cardiac failure
PRECAUTIONS: Major surgery, diabetes mellitus, renal or hepatic disease, thyroid disease, COPD, asthma, well-compensated heart failure, aortic or mitral valve disease, peripheral vascular disease, myasthenia gravis; do not stop therapy abruptly, taper over 2 wk
PREGNANCY AND LACTATION: Pregnancy category C; excreted in breast milk
SIDE EFFECTS/ADVERSE REACTIONS
CNS: Catatonia, depression, dizziness, drowsiness, *fatigue,* hallucinations, headache, insomnia, lethargy, memory loss, mental changes, peripheral neuropathy, strange dreams, vertigo
CV: Bradycardia, **CHF,** cold extremities, postural hypotension, ***profound hypotension, 2nd or 3rd degree heart block, ventricular dysrhythmias***
EENT: Dry burning eyes, rhinitis, sinusitis, sore throat
GI: Diarrhea, flatulence, gastric pain, gastritis, increased AST/ALT (1-2 times normal in 4%), ischemic colitis, mesenteric arterial thrombosis, nausea, vomiting
GU: Decreased libido, impotence
HEME: Purpura
METAB: Azotemia, hyperglycemia, hyperkalemia, hypertriglyceridemia, hyperuricemia, increased hypoglycemic response to insulin
MS: Arthralgia, joint pain
RESP: ***Bronchospasm,*** cough, dyspnea, wheezing
SKIN: Alopecia, fever, pruritus, rash, sweating
MISC: Decreased exercise tolerance, edema, facial swelling, weight gain
DRUG INTERACTIONS
Drugs
▣ *Adenosine:* Additive bradycardia
▣ *Amiodarone:* Increased bradycardic effect of bisoprolol

---

3 *Antidiabetics:* Reduced response to hypoglycemia (sweating persists)

3 *Barbiturates:* Enhanced bisoprolol metabolism

3 *Cimetidine:* Plasma levels of β-blocker may be elevated

3 *Cocaine:* Bisoprolol potentiates cocaine-induced coronary vasoconstriction

3 *Contrast media:* Increased risk for anaphylaxis

3 *Digoxin, digitoxin:* Potentiation of bradycardia

3 *Dipyridamole:* Additive bradycardia

3 *Fluoxetine:* Fluoxetine inhibits CYPD26, partially responsible for bisoprolol metabolism; increased β-blocker effects

3 *Lidocaine:* β-blocker-induced reductions in cardiac output and hepatic blood flow may yield increased lidocaine concentrations

3 *Neostigmine:* Additive bradycardia

3 *Neuroleptics:* Decreased bisoprolol metabolism; decreased neuroleptic metabolism

3 *NSAIDs:* Reduced antihypertensive effect

3 *Physostigmine:* Additive bradycardia

3 *Prazosin:* Enhanced 1st-dose response to prazosin

3 *Rifampin:* Increases clearance by 51%, reduced β-blocker effects

3 *Tacrine:* Additive bradycardia

2 *Theophylline:* Bisoprolol reduces clearance of theophylline; antagonistic pharmacodynamics

SPECIAL CONSIDERATIONS
PATIENT/FAMILY EDUCATION
• Do not stop drug abruptly (may cause/precipitate angina); taper over 2 wk

---

bretylium
(bre-til'ee-um)
Rx: Bretylate ♦, Bretylol
Chemical Class: Quaternary ammonium derivative
Therapeutic Class: Antidysrhythmic (class III)

CLINICAL PHARMACOLOGY
Mechanism of Action: Causes an early release of norepinephrine from postganglionic nerve terminals, then selectively accumulates in sympathetic ganglia and their postganglionic adrenergic neurons where it inhibits norepinephrine release; suppresses ventricular fibrillation and ventricular dysrhythmias; increases action potential duration and effective refractory period without changes in heart rate

Pharmacokinetics
IV: Onset 5 min for suppression of ventricular fibrillation, onset 20-120 min for suppression of ventricular tachycardia

IM: Onset 20-120 min for suppression of ventricular tachycardia, duration 6-24 hr; 80% excreted unchanged by kidneys in 24 hr

INDICATIONS AND USES: Ventricular tachycardia and other life-threatening ventricular dysrhythmias that have failed to respond to 1st-line agents; ventricular fibrillation

DOSAGES
Adult
• Ventricular fibrillation: IV bolus 5 mg/kg, then 10 mg/kg repeated q15 min, up to total 30-35 mg/kg; maintenance therapy is IV INF 1-2 mg/min or 5-10 mg/kg over 10 min q6h
• *Ventricular dysrhythmias:* IV INF 500 mg diluted in 50 ml D₅W or NS, infuse over 10-30 min, may repeat in 1 hr, maintain with 1-2 mg/min or 5-10 mg/kg over 10-30 min q6h; IM 5-10 mg/kg undiluted, repeat in 1-2 hr if needed, maintain with same dose q6-8h

Child
• Ventricular fibrillation: IV bolus 5 mg/kg, then 10 mg/kg if ventricular fibrillation persists

$ AVAILABLE FORMS/COST OF THERAPY
• Inj, Sol—IM, IV: 50 mg/ml, 10 ml: **$21.38-$35.01**

CONTRAINDICATIONS: Digitalis toxicity (initial release of norepinephrine caused by bretylium may aggravate digitalis toxicity)

PRECAUTIONS: Renal disease; postural hypotension, hypertension or increased frequency of PVCs and other dysrhythmias may occur transiently in some patients; aortic stenosis, pulmonary hypertension

PREGNANCY AND LACTATION: Pregnancy category C

SIDE EFFECTS/ADVERSE REACTIONS
CNS: Anxiety, confusion, dizziness, psychosis, syncope
CV: Angina, bradycardia, *hypotension, postural hypotension (50%),* PVCs, transient hypertension
GI: Nausea, vomiting
RESP: ***Respiratory depression***

---

bumetanide
(byoo-met'a-nide)
Rx: Bumex, Burinex ♦
Chemical Class: Sulfonamide derivative
Therapeutic Class: Loop diuretic

CLINICAL PHARMACOLOGY
Mechanism of Action: Inhibits sodium and chloride reabsorption in the ascending limb of the loop of Henle; potassium excretion is increased in a dose related fashion; may have an additional action in the proximal tubule

Pharmacokinetics
PO: Onset ½-1 hr, duration 4 hr
IM: Onset 40 min, duration 4 hr
IV: Onset 5 min, duration 2-3 hr 94-96% bound to plasma proteins; excreted by kidneys; t₁/₂ 1-1½ hr

INDICATIONS AND USES: Edema associated with congestive heart failure, hepatic and renal disease, including the nephrotic syndrome; hypertension; adult nocturia*

DOSAGE
Adult
• PO 0.5-2.0 mg qd, may give 2nd or 3rd dose at 4-5 hr intervals up to max of 20 mg/day, may be given on alternate days or intermittently; IV/IM 0.5-1.0 mg/day, may give 2nd or 3rd dose at 2-3 hr intervals up to max of 10 mg/day

Child >6 months
• PO/IM/IV 0.015 mg/kg/dose qd or qod, maximum 0.1 mg/kg/day or 10 mg

$ AVAILABLE FORMS/COST OF THERAPY
• Inj, Sol—IM, IV: 0.25 mg/ml, 2 ml: **$1.62-$1.83**
• Tab, Uncoated—Oral: 0.5 mg, 100's: **$27.18-$31.13;** 1 mg, 100's: **$38.15-$43.71;** 2 mg, 100's: **$64.53-$73.90**

CONTRAINDICATIONS: Anuria, hepatic coma, severe electrolyte depletion

PRECAUTIONS: Dehydration, ascites, severe renal disease, hepatic cirrhosis, volume depletion, allergy to sulfonamides, thrombocytopenia, diabetes

PREGNANCY AND LACTATION: Pregnancy category C; excretion into breast milk unknown

SIDE EFFECTS/ADVERSE REACTIONS
CNS: Dizziness, fatigue, headache, vertigo, weakness
CV: ECG changes, *hypotension*
EENT: Blurred vision, ear pain, ototoxicity, tinnitus

---

italic = common side effects   ***bold italic*** = life-threatening reactions

GI: Abdominal pain, anorexia, cramps, diarrhea, dry mouth, *nausea,* upset stomach, vomiting
GU: Glycosuria, *polyuria,* **renal failure,** sexual dysfunction
*HEME: **Thrombocytopenia***
METAB: Hyperglycemia, hyperuricemia, hypocalcemia, hypochloremic alkalosis, *hypokalemia,* hypomagnesemia, hyponatremia
MS: Arthritis, hyperuricemia, *muscular cramps,* stiffness, tenderness
SKIN: Photosensitivity, pruritus, purpura, rash, ***Stevens-Johnson syndrome,*** sweating
DRUG INTERACTIONS
Drugs
🔟 *ACE inhibitors:* Hypotension, renal insufficiency
🔟 *Digitalis glycosides:* Diuretic-induced hypokalemia may increase the risk of digitalis toxicity
🔟 *Indomethacin:* Reduced diuretic and antihypertensive efficacy of bumetanide

SPECIAL CONSIDERATIONS
Cross-sensitivity with furosemide rare; may substitute bumetanide at a 1:40 ratio with furosemide in patients allergic to furosemide; may show cross-hypersensitivity to sulfonamides
PATIENT/FAMILY EDUCATION
Take early in the day
MONITORING PARAMETERS
Electrolytes: potassium, sodium, chloride
BUN, glucose, CBC, serum creatinine
Uric acid, calcium, magnesium
Weight, I&O

---

candesartan cilexetil
(can'-da-sartin sil-ex'-a-til)
Rx: Atacand
Chemical Class: Angiotensin II receptor antagonist
Therapeutic Class: Antihypertensive

CLINICAL PHARMACOLOGY
Mechanism of Action: Blocks vasoconstrictor and aldosterone-secreting effects of angiotensin II by blocking binding of angiotensin II
Pharmacokinetics: Converted in GI tract to active form; peak serum concentrations occur after 3-4 hr; highly bound to plasma protein; eliminated in urine, bile, and feces; $t_{1/2} \sim 9$ hr
INDICATIONS AND USES: Hypertension
DOSAGE
Adults >18 years
• PO 2-32 mg qd, usual starting dose 16 mg daily; may divide into bid if necessary; use lower doses in volume depletion and impaired renal function
💲 **AVAILABLE FORMS/COST OF THERAPY**
• Tab, Uncoated—Oral: 4 mg, 8 mg, 16 mg, 30's: **$30.00;** 32 mg tab, 30's: **$42.00**
CONTRAINDICATIONS: Hypersensitivity to any component of product
PRECAUTIONS: Hypotension, hyperkalemia, impaired renal function, volume-depleted patients
PREGNANCY AND LACTATION: Pregnancy category C (1st trimester) and D (2nd and 3rd trimesters); may cause fetal morbidity and death; not known if excreted into human milk
SIDE EFFECTS/ADVERSE REACTIONS
CNS: headache, dizziness
CV: hypotension

EENT: pharyngitis, rhinitis
GI: dyspepsia, elevated liver enzymes
GU: hematuria, increased serum creatinine and BUN
HEME: decreased Hgb and Hct
METAB: hyperuricemia, increased potassium
MS: myalgia
RESP: dyspnea
MISC: back pain, angiodema
DRUG INTERACTIONS
Drugs
🔟 *Diuretics:* concurrent volume depletion caused by diuretic therapy may result in hypotension or elevated serum creatinine and BUN

SPECIAL CONSIDERATIONS
• Exact role of this chemical class for treatment of CHF and diabetic nephropathy is not known

---

captopril
(kap'toe-pril)
Rx: Capoten
Chemical Class: Angiotensin-converting enzyme (ACE) inhibitor
Therapeutic Class: Antihypertensive; congestive heart failure agent; renal protectant

CLINICAL PHARMACOLOGY
Mechanism of Action: Selectively suppresses renin-angiotensin-aldosterone system; inhibits angiotensin-converting enzyme (ACE); prevents conversion of angiotensin I to angiotensin II; results in dilation of arterial and venous vessels
Pharmacokinetics
PO: Peak 1 hr (presence of food reduces absorption by 3%-40%), duration 2-6 hr, $t_{1/2}$ 2-3 hr; metabolized by liver, excreted in urine (40%-50% unchanged); crosses placenta; excreted in breast milk
INDICATIONS AND USES: Hypertension, heart failure, left ventricular dysfunction after MI, diabetic nephropathy (proteinuria 500 mg/day) in type I patients; hypertensive crises,* neonatal and childhood hypertension,* rheumatoid arthritis,* diagnosis of anatomic renal artery stenosis,* diagnosis of primary aldosteronism,* idiopathic edema,* Barter's syndrome (improves K metabolism and corrects hypokalemia),* Raynaud's syndrome
DOSAGE
Adult
• *Hypertensive crisis:* PO 25 mg increasing q2h until desired response; not to exceed 450 mg/day
• *Hypertension:* PO initial dose 12.5 mg bid-tid (consider discontinuing previous antihypertensive therapy, especially diuretics before starting); may increase to 50 mg bid-tid at 1-2 wk intervals; usual range 25-150 mg bid-tid; max 450 mg/day
• *Diabetic nephropathy:* PO 25 mg tid
• *Congestive heart failure:* PO 12.5 mg bid-tid (consider smaller doses in patients vigorously pretreated with diuretics and who may be hyponatremic and/or hypovolemic, i.e., a starting dose of 6.25); may increase to 50 mg bid-tid; after 14 days, may increase to 150 mg tid if needed
Child
• *Hypertension:* Initiate 0.15 mg/kg/dose; double at intervals of approx. 2 hr until BP controlled (max 6 mg/kg/24 hr)
💲 **AVAILABLE FORMS/COST OF THERAPY**
• Tab, Uncoated—Oral: 12.5 mg, 100's: **$4.43-$72.56;** 25 mg, 100's: **$6.66-$78.44;** 50 mg, 100's: **$11.63-$134.53;** 100 mg, 100's: **$20.82-$179.14**

---

* = non FDA-approved use

CONTRAINDICATIONS: Heart block, bilateral renal artery stenosis

PRECAUTIONS: Dialysis patients, hypovolemia, leukemia, scleroderma, lupus erythematosus, blood dyscrasias, thyroid disease, COPD, asthma, impaired renal function, severe renal artery stenosis, CHF, hyperkalemia, potassium-sparing diuretics, cough, aortic stenosis, pediatric use (limited experience; infants, especially newborns, may be more susceptible to the adverse hemodynamic effects)

PREGNANCY AND LACTATION: Pregnancy category C (1st trimester) and D (2nd and 3rd trimesters—fetal and neonatal hypotension, neonatal skull hypoplasia, anuria, reversible or irreversible renal failure, death, oligohydramnios); excreted into breast milk in small amounts; compatible with breast feeding

SIDE EFFECTS/ADVERSE REACTIONS

CNS: Chills, fever

CV: Chest pain, hypotension, palpitations, postural hypotension, tachycardia

GI: Loss of taste

GU: **Acute reversible renal failure,** dysuria, frequency, impotence, nephrotic syndrome, nocturia, oliguria, polyuria, proteinuria

HEME: **Agranulocytosis, neutropenia**

METAB: Hyperkalemia, hyponatremia

RESP: Angioedema, **bronchospasm,** *cough,* dyspnea

SKIN: Rash

DRUG INTERACTIONS

Drugs

❷ *Allopurinol:* Increased risk of hypersensitivity reactions including Stevens-Johnson syndrome, skin eruptions, fever, and arthralgias

🔢 *α-blockers:* Possible exaggerated "first dose" response

🔢 *Aspirin:* Reduced hemodynamic effects of captopril; less likely at doses <236 mg qd

🔢 *Azathioprine:* Increased risk of neutropenia

🔢 *Cyclosporine:* Increased nephrotoxicity

🔢 *Indomethacin:* Inhibits the antihypertensive response to ACE inhibition; other NSAIDs probably have similar effect

🔢 *Insulin:* ACE inhibitors enhance insulin sensitivity; hypoglycemia possible

🔢 *Iron:* Increased risk of systemic reaction (GI symptoms, hypotension) with parenteral iron

🔢 *Lithium:* Increased risk of lithium toxicity

🔢 *Loop diuretics:* Initiation of ACE inhibition therapy with concurrent intensive diuretic therapy may cause significant hypotension, renal insufficiency

🔢 *Mercaptopurine:* Increased risk of neutropenia

🔢 *Potassium, Potassium-sparing diuretics:* ACE inhibition tends to increase potassium; increased risk of hyperkalemia in predisposed patients

Labs

• Blood in urine: Decreased reactivity with occult blood test

• Fructosamine: Captopril interferes with assay increasing serum fructosamine

• Ketones in urine: False positive dip-sticks

• False positive: Urine acetone

SPECIAL CONSIDERATIONS

• ACE inhibition can account for approximately 0.5 mEq/L rise in serum potassium

• Consider for initiation and titration of ACE inhibition in severe CHF to stability before prescribing less expensive, qd ACE inhibitors for treatment long term

---

carteolol

(kar-tee'oe-lole)

Rx: Cartrol, Ocupress

Chemical Class: Nonselective β-adrenergic blocker with intrinsic sympathomimetic activity

Therapeutic Class: Antihypertensive; antiglaucoma agent

CLINICAL PHARMACOLOGY

Mechanism of Action: Nonselective β-adrenergic blocker with intrinsic sympathomimetic activity

Pharmacokinetics

PO: Onset 1-2 hr, peak 2-4 hr, duration 8-12 hr, $t_{1/2}$ 6-8 hr, food slows absorption but does not lower total absorption; metabolized by liver (metabolites inactive), excreted in urine, bile; crosses placenta

INDICATIONS AND USES: Chronic open-angle glaucoma, hypertension (does not alter serum cholesterol or triglycerides)

DOSAGE

Adult

• *Hypertension:* PO 2.5-10 mg qd; in renal impairment: CrCl 20-60 ml/min, dosage interval is 48 hr; CrCl 20 ml/min, dosage interval is 72 hr

• *Chronic open-angle glaucoma:* Ophth sol, 1%, 1 gtt in affected eye bid

💲 **AVAILABLE FORMS/COST OF THERAPY**

• Sol—Ophth: 1%, 5 ml: **$18.17**; 1%, 10 ml: **$34.28**

• Tab, Plain Coated—Oral: 2.5 mg, 100's: **$106.18**; 5 mg, 100's: **$106.18**

CONTRAINDICATIONS: Hypersensitivity to β-blockers, heart block (2nd or 3rd degree), sinus bradycardia, overt CHF, bronchial asthma

PRECAUTIONS: Major surgery, diabetes mellitus, renal disease, thyroid disease, COPD, well-compensated heart failure, nonallergic bronchospasm; exacerbation of angina or MI may occur following abrupt discontinuation of β-blockers; ophth carteolol may be absorbed systemically; adverse reactions found with systemic administration may occur with ophth administration

PREGNANCY AND LACTATION: Pregnancy category C; excreted in breast milk

SIDE EFFECTS/ADVERSE REACTIONS

CNS: Anxiety, catatonia, decreased concentration, depression, dizziness, drowsiness, *fatigue (7%),* headache, insomnia, lethargy, mental changes, nightmares, paresthesia

CV: **AV block,** bradycardia, chest pain, **CHF,** orthostatic hypotension, palpitations, peripheral vascular insufficiency, **ventricular dysrhythmias**

EENT: Double vision; dry, burning eyes; sore throat, tinnitus, visual changes

GI: Anorexia, constipation, diarrhea, dry mouth, flatulence, nausea, vomiting

GU: Dysuria, ejaculatory failure, impotence, urinary retention

HEME: **Agranulocytosis, thrombocytopenic purpura (rare)**

MS: Arthralgia, joint pain, muscle cramps

RESP: **Bronchospasm,** dyspnea, nasal stuffiness, pharyngitis, wheezing

SKIN: Alopecia, fever, pruritus, rash, urticaria

MISC: Decreased exercise tolerance, facial swelling, Raynaud's syndrome, weight change

DRUG INTERACTIONS

Drugs

🔢 *Adenosine:* Increased risk of bradycardic response

🔢 *Amiodarone:* Increased bradycardic effect of carteolol

---

italic = common side effects

bold italic = life-threatening reactions

◨ *Antacids:* Decreased absorption of oral carteolol

◨ *Antidiabetics:* Carteolol reduces response to hypoglycemia (sweating excepted)

◨ *Antipyrine:* Many β-blockers increase serum concentrations of antipyrine; though antipyrine is not used therapeutically, this interaction has implications by other drugs whose metabolism is similarly inhibited

◨ *Barbiturates, rifampin:* Enhanced carteolol metabolism

◨ *Bupivacaine:* Potentiates cardiodepression and heart block

◨ *Cimetidine, Propafenone, Propoxyphene, Quinidine:* Decreased carteolol metabolism

◨ *Cocaine:* β-Blockade increases angina-inducing potential of cocaine

◨ *Contrast media:* Increased risk of anaphylaxis

◨ *Digoxin, digitoxin:* Bradycardia potentiated

◨ *Dipyridamole:* Bradycardia

◨ *Epinephrine:* Enhanced pressor response resulting in hypertension and bradycardia

◨ *Fluoxetine:* Fluoxetine inhibits CYP2D6 responsible for hepatic metabolism; increased β-blocking activity

◨ *Isoproterenol:* Reduced effectiveness of isoproterenol in the treatment of asthma

◨ *Neuroleptics:* Decreased carteolol metabolism; decreased neuroleptic metabolism

◨ *Nonsteroidal antiinflammatory drugs:* Reduced antihypertensive effect

◨ *Physostigmine:* Additive bradycardia

◨ *Prazosin, terazosin:* Enhanced 1st-dose response to prazosin

◨ *Tacrine:* Additive bradycardia

◨ *Theophylline:* Decreased metabolism of theophylline

SPECIAL CONSIDERATIONS
PATIENT/FAMILY EDUCATION
• Do not stop drug abruptly; taper over 2 wk
• Do not use OTC products containing α-adrenergic stimulants (nasal decongestants, cold remedies) unless directed by physician

---

carvedilol
(kar-vay'da-lole)
Rx: Coreg
Chemical Class: α- and β-blocker
Therapeutic Class: Antihypertensive; congestive heart failure agent

---

CLINICAL PHARMACOLOGY
Mechanism of Action: Racemic mixture with nonselective β-adrenoreceptor and α-adrenergic blocking activity; no intrinsic sympathomimetic activity; reduces cardiac output, reduces tachycardia, causes vasodilation and reduces peripheral vascular resistance, leading to decreased blood pressure; reduces plasma renin activity when given for at least 4 wk

Pharmacokinetics
PO: Extensive first pass metabolism, 25% to 35% bioavailable; β-blocker effects seen in 30-60 min; terminal elimination $t_{1/2}$ 7-10 hr; 98% protein bound; extensive hepatic metabolism, metabolite 13 times more potent β-blocker than parent drug, 2% excreted unchanged in urine; metabolites excreted in bile and feces

INDICATIONS AND USES: Hypertension (alone or in combination with other antihypertensives, especially thiazides); CHF*; angina pectoris*; idiopathic cardiomyopathy*

DOSAGE
Adult
• PO 6.25-50 mg bid (dosage must be individualized; start at 3.125 bid; increase every 7-14 days as tolerated)

$ AVAILABLE FORMS/COST OF THERAPY
• Tab—Oral: 3.125 mg, 6.25 mg, 12.5 mg, 25 mg, 100's: **$99.84**

CONTRAINDICATIONS: Significant hepatic dysfunction, NYHA class IV decompensated cardiac failure, bronchial asthma, 2nd or 3rd degree AV block, cardiogenic shock, severe bradycardia

PRECAUTIONS: CHF, peripheral vascular disease, diabetes (masking of hypoglycemic symptoms, potentiation of insulin-induced hypoglycemia), hypoglycemia, thyrotoxicosis (abrupt withdrawal may exacerbate symptoms, precipitate thyroid storm), elderly, renal impairment, mild hepatic dysfunction, history of severe allergies with anaphylaxis (increased sensitivity to allergen, less responsive to epinephrine)

PREGNANCY AND LACTATION: Pregnancy category C; increased spontaneous abortion in animal studies; unknown if excreted in human breast milk; because of potential risk not recommended in lactation

SIDE EFFECTS/ADVERSE REACTIONS
CNS: Dizziness
CV: **AV block,** bradycardia (2%), **CHF,** postural hypotension (1.8%), syncope (0.1%)
GI: Elevated LFTs (1.1%)
RESP: **Bronchospasm**
DRUG INTERACTIONS
Drugs
◨ *Benzodiazepines:* Increased benzodiazepine activity
◨ *Cimetidine:* Via inhibition of hepatic metabolism, cimetidine increases many β-blocker serum concentrations
◨ *Digoxin:* Concurrent carvedilol increases digoxin serum conc. and AUC.
◨ *Nonsteroidal antiinflammatory drugs:* Reduced antihypertensive effect
◨ *Rifampin:* 70% decrease in carvedilol concentrations

SPECIAL CONSIDERATIONS
• Do not discontinue abruptly, taper over 1-2 wk
• If heart rate drops below 55 beats/min, reduce dosage
• Initiate therapy with 3.125 mg dosage to decrease risk of syncope
• Take with food
• Careful monitoring essential when initiating therapy to detect and correct worsening heart failure
• Avoid driving, hazardous tasks during initiation of therapy
• Response less in blacks

---

cerivastatin
(se-reev' a-stat-in)
Rx: Baycol
Chemical Class: HMG-CoA reductase inhibitor (statin)
Therapeutic Class: Antilipemic

CLINICAL PHARMACOLOGY
Mechanism of Action: Competitively inhibits HMG-CoA reductase enzyme, which catalyzes the rate-limiting step in cholesterol biosynthesis (increases HDL-cholesterol, decreases total cholesterol, apolipoprotein B, triglycerides, and LDL-cholesterol)

Pharmacokinetics
PO: Peak 2½ hr; well absorbed (PO bioavailability 60%); 99% protein bound; moderately distributed into tissues; metabolized by liver, CYP3A4 and others (two major metabolites, 50, 100% as ac-

---

tive as parent); low clearance drug; metabolites excreted in feces; $t_{1/2}$ 2-3 hr

INDICATIONS AND USES: Adjunct to diet in hypercholesterolemia (Types IIa and IIb) when response to dietary restriction of saturated fat and cholesterol and other nonpharmacologic measures alone have been inadequate

DOSAGE

Adult

• PO 0.3 mg qd in the evening; may be taken with or without food; no dosage adjustments necessary for renal function as low as CrCl 60 ml/min; for CrCl (60 ml/min, start with 0.2 mg qd

$ AVAILABLE FORMS/COST OF THERAPY

• Tab—Oral: 0.2 mg, 100's: **$132.00**; 0.3 mg, 100's: **$132.00**

CONTRAINDICATIONS: Active liver disease; unexplained persistent elevations of serum transaminases

PRECAUTIONS: Liver dysfunction or heavy alcohol ingestion; renal insufficiency; conditions predisposing to renal failure secondary to rhabdomyolysis (e.g., sepsis, hypotension, trauma, metabolic, endocrine, or electrolyte disorders), or uncontrolled epilepsy

PREGNANCY AND LACTATION: Pregnancy category X; not recommended for nursing mothers

SIDE EFFECTS/ADVERSE REACTIONS

CNS: Insomnia
CV: Peripheral edema
GI: Diarrhea, dyspepsia, *transaminasemia*
GU: Urinary tract infection
MS: Arthralgia, myalgia
RESP: Cough, pharyngitis, rhinitis, sinusitis
SKIN: Rash

DRUG INTERACTIONS

Drugs

▪ *Azole antifungals (fluconazole, itraconazole, ketoconazole, miconazole):* Increased cerivastatin levels; increased risk of rhabdomyolysis

▪ *Erythromycin:* Increased cerivastatin concentrations; increased risk of rhabdomyolysis

▪ *Fibric acid derivatives:* Increased risk of myopathy

▪ *Cyclosporine:* Increased cyclosporine concentrations; increased risk of rhabdomyolysis

▪ *Nefazodone:* Increased cerivastatin levels; increased risk of rhabdomyolysis

▪ *Niacin:* Isolated cases of myopathy and rhabdomyolysis have occurred in patients receiving other "statins" and niacin

SPECIAL CONSIDERATIONS

• Base statin selection on cost and formulary availability; may have advantage over lovastatin, simvastatin, atorvastatin for drug interactions and risk of rhabdomyolysis

PATIENT/FAMILY EDUCATION

• Take with evening meal or at bedtime; report muscle pain, tenderness, or weakness; adherence to diet, exercise, and weight loss recommendations

MONITORING PARAMETERS

• Cholesterol levels; creatine phosphokinase levels with symptoms of myalgia and consider withdrawal of drug; regular monitoring of hepatic function tests (ALT) during the first year of therapy, with periodic monitoring thereafter suggested by the manufacturer

---

chlorothiazide

(klor-oh-thye'a-zide)
Rx: Diurigen, Diuril
Combinations
　Rx: with methyldopa (Aldoclor, Supres ♣); with reserpine (Diaserp, Diupres)
Chemical Class: Sulfonamide derivative
Therapeutic Class: Antihypertensive; thiazide diuretic

CLINICAL PHARMACOLOGY

Mechanism of Action: Acts on distal tubule, increasing excretion of water, sodium, chloride, potassium, magnesium

Pharmacokinetics

PO: Onset 2 hr, peak 4 hr, duration 6-12 hr, not well absorbed
IV: Onset 15 min, maximal action 30 min
Eliminated unchanged by the kidneys; crosses placenta, but not blood-brain barrier; excreted in breast milk; $t_{1/2}$ 45-120 min

INDICATIONS AND USES: Edema, hypertension, diuresis

DOSAGE

Adult

• *Edema:* PO/IV 500 mg-1 g/day in 1-2 divided doses
• *Hypertension:* PO 500 mg-1 g/day in 1-2 divided doses; max 2 g/day in divided doses

Child

• *Diuresis/hypertension:* PO 10-20 mg/kg/day in 2 divided doses, not to exceed 375 mg per day in infants up to 2 yr of age or 1 g per day in children 2 to 12 yr of age; infants less than 6 mo of age, up to 30 mg/kg/day in 2 divided doses; IV use generally not recommended

$ AVAILABLE FORMS/COST OF THERAPY

• Tab, Uncoated—Oral: 250 mg, 100's: **$4.98-$13.96**; 500 mg, 100's: **$5.76-$22.14**
• Susp—Oral: 250 mg/5 ml, 237 ml: **$10.19**
• Inj—IV: 500 mg: **$9.18**

CONTRAINDICATIONS: Anuria, renal decompensation

PRECAUTIONS: Fluid or electrolyte imbalance (including sodium, potassium, magnesium, calcium), hyperuricemia, renal disease, hepatic disease, gout, COPD, lupus erythematosus, diabetes mellitus, elderly, postsympathectomy, hyperparathyroidism, elevated cholesterol/triglycerides

PREGNANCY AND LACTATION: Pregnancy category D; excreted in low concentrations in breast milk; compatible with breast feeding

SIDE EFFECTS/ADVERSE REACTIONS

CNS: Anxiety, depression, *dizziness,* drowsiness, fatigue, headache, paresthesia, weakness
CV: Irregular pulse, orthostatic hypotension, palpitations, volume depletion
EENT: Blurred vision
GI: Anorexia, constipation, cramps, diarrhea, GI irritation, hepatitis, *nausea,* pancreatitis, vomiting
GU: Frequency, glucosuria, polyuria, uremia
HEME: **Agranulocytosis, aplastic anemia, hemolytic anemia, leukopenia, neutropenia, thrombocytopenia**
METAB: Hypercalcemia, hyperglycemia, *hyperuricemia;* hypochloremia, *hypokalemia,* hypomagnesemia, hyponatremia, hypophosphatemia, increased creatinine, BUN
SKIN: Fever, photosensitivity, purpura, rash, urticaria

DRUG INTERACTIONS

Drugs

▪ *Digitalis glycosides:* Diuretic-induced hypokalemia may increase the risk of digitalis toxicity

---

italic = common side effects　　　**bold italic** = life-threatening reactions

Labs
Interference: Urine 17-hydroxycorticosteroids

SPECIAL CONSIDERATIONS
MONITORING PARAMETERS
• Electrolytes, i.e., sodium, chloride, potassium, BUN, creatinine, glucose, magnesium
• Minimal doses (125-250 mg qd) may provide optimal blood pressure control without added metabolic and electrolyte disturbance

---

chlorthalidone
(klor-thal'i-done)
Rx: Hygroton, Thalitone
Combinations
Rx: with atenolol (Tenoretic); with clonidine (Combipres); with reserpine (Regroton)
Chemical Class: Phthalimidine derivative
Therapeutic Class: Antihypertensive; thiazide diuretic

CLINICAL PHARMACOLOGY
Mechanism of Action: Blocks sodium/water reabsorption in distal tubule; increases excretion of water, sodium, chloride, potassium, magnesium, bicarbonate
Pharmacokinetics
PO: Onset 2 hr, peak 6 hr, duration 48-72 hr, excreted unchanged by kidneys; crosses placenta; $t_{1/2}$ 40 hr
INDICATIONS AND USES: Edema associated with CHF, hepatic cirrhosis, renal dysfunction (i.e., nephrotic syndrome, acute glomerulonephritis) and corticosteroid and estrogen therapy; hypertension; calcium nephrolithiasis*; osteoporosis*; diabetes insipidus*
DOSAGE
Adult
• PO 15-100 mg/day or 100 mg every other day
Child
• PO 2 mg/kg 3×/wk
S AVAILABLE FORMS/COST OF THERAPY
• Tab, Uncoated—Oral: 25 mg, 100's: **$3.90-$72.21;** 50 mg, 100's: **$4.34-$89.05;** 100 mg, 100's: **$10.40-$148.86**
CONTRAINDICATIONS: Anuria, renal decompensation
PRECAUTIONS: Hypokalemia, renal disease (CrCl (35 ml/min), hepatic disease, gout, diabetes mellitus, elderly
PREGNANCY AND LACTATION: Pregnancy category D; compatible with breast feeding
SIDE EFFECTS/ADVERSE REACTIONS
CNS. Anxiety, depression, *dizziness,* drowsiness, *fatigue,* headache, paresthesia, *weakness*
CV: Irregular pulse, orthostatic hypotension, palpitations, volume depletion
EENT: Blurred vision
GI: Anorexia, constipation, cramps, diarrhea, GI irritation, hepatitis, *nausea,* pancreatitis, *vomiting*
GU: Frequency, glucosuria, impotence, polyuria, **uremia**
HEME: **Agranulocytosis, aplastic anemia, hemolytic anemia, leukopenia, neutropenia, thrombocytopenia**
METAB: Gout, hypercalcemia, hyperglycemia, hyperuremia; hypochloremia, *hypokalemia,* hypomagnesemia, hyponatremia, increased creatinine, BUN
SKIN: Fever, photosensitivity, purpura, rash, urticaria
DRUG INTERACTIONS
Drugs
▪ *Antidiabetics:* Increased dosage requirements due to increased glucose levels

▪ *Calcium:* Increased risk of milk-alkali syndrome
▪ *Carbenoxolone:* Additive potassium wasting, severe hypokalemia
▪ *Cholestyramine, Colestipol:* Reduced absorption
▪ *Diazoxide:* Hyperglycemia
▪ *Digitalis glycosides:* Diuretic-induced hypokalemia increases risk of digitalis toxicity
▪ *Lithium:* Increased lithium levels, potential toxicity
▪ *Methotrexate:* Increased risk of bone marrow depression

SPECIAL CONSIDERATIONS
• Doses 25 mg/day are likely to potentiate potassium excretion, but provide no further benefit in sodium excretion or blood pressure reduction

---

cholestyramine
(koe-less-tir'a-meen)
Rx: Questran, Questran Light
Chemical Class: Bile acid sequestrant
Therapeutic Class: Antilipemic

CLINICAL PHARMACOLOGY
Mechanism of Action: Absorbs, combines with bile acids to form insoluble complex that is excreted via feces; loss of bile acids lowers cholesterol levels
Pharmacokinetics
PO: Excreted in feces, max effect in 2 wk
INDICATIONS AND USES: Primary hypercholesterolemia, pruritus associated with partial biliary obstruction, diarrhea caused by excess bile acid or *Clostridium difficile* toxin,* digitalis toxicity*
DOSAGE
Adult
• PO 4 g 1-6 × daily (recommended schedule is bid), not to exceed 32 g/day
Child
• PO 240 mg/kg/day in 3 divided doses
S AVAILABLE FORMS/COST OF THERAPY
• Powder—Oral: 4 g/9 g, 60 pkts: **$70.00-$89.33;** 378 g: **$35.35-$39.13** (Questran)
• Powder, Reconst—Oral: 4 g/5 g, 60 pkts: **$70.00-$89.33;** 210 g: **$35.35-$39.13** (Questran Light)
CONTRAINDICATIONS: Complete biliary obstruction
PRECAUTIONS: Children, constipation
PREGNANCY AND LACTATION: Pregnancy category C
SIDE EFFECTS/ADVERSE REACTIONS
CNS: Dizziness, drowsiness, headache, tinnitus, vertigo
GI: Abdominal pain, constipation, fecal impaction, flatulence, hemorrhoids, *nausea,* peptic ulcer, steatorrhea, vomiting
HEME: Bleeding, decreased pro-time, decreased vitamin A, D, K, red cell folate content, hyperchloremic acidosis
MS: Joint pain, muscle
SKIN: Irritation of perianal area, tongue, skin; rash
DRUG INTERACTIONS
Drugs
▪ *Acetaminophen, Amiodarone, Corticosteroids, Diclofenac, Digitalis glycosides, Furosemide, Methotrexate, Metronidazole, Thiazide diuretics, Thyroid hormones, Valproic acid:* Cholestyramine reduces interacting drug concentrations and probably subsequent therapeutic response
▪ *Oral anticoagulants:* Inhibition of hypoprothrombinemic response; colestipol might be less likely to interact

---

* = non FDA-approved use

SPECIAL CONSIDERATIONS
Avoid use in patients with elevated triglycerides
PATIENT/FAMILY EDUCATION
• Give all other medications 1 hr before or 4 hr after cholestyramine to avoid poor absorption
• Mix drug with applesauce or noncarbonated beverage (2-6 oz), let stand for 2 min; do not take dry

---

clonidine
(klon'i-deen)
Rx: Catapres, Catapres-TTS, Dixarit ✦, Duraclon
Combinations
  Rx: with chlorthalidone (Combipres)
Chemical Class: Imidazoline derivative
Therapeutic Class: Antihypertensive

CLINICAL PHARMACOLOGY
Mechanism of Action: Stimulates α_2-adrenergic receptors in the brain stem, resulting in reduced sympathetic outflow from the CNS and a decrease in peripheral resistance
Pharmacokinetics
PO: Peak 3-5 hr
TOP: Therapeutic plasma levels 2-3 days after initial application, drug released at constant rate for approximately 7 days; following removal, plasma levels persist for 8 hr then decline slowly over several days
Metabolized in liver, excreted in urine (50% unchanged); $t_{1/2}$ 12-16 hr
INDICATIONS AND USES: Hypertension, alcohol withdrawal,* diabetic diarrhea,* Gilles de la Tourette syndrome,* hypertensive urgencies,* menopausal flushing,* opiate detoxification,* postherpetic neuralgia,* smoking cessation,* ulcerative colitis*; in combination with opiates for severe pain in cancer patients (inj)
DOSAGE
Adult
• PO 0.1 mg bid initially, increase 0.1-0.2 mg/day if needed, max 2.4 mg/day (minimize sedation by giving majority of daily dose hs); TOP apply patch to hairless area of intact skin on upper arm or torso once q7d, rotate sites, start with TTS-1 (0.1 mg/24 hr) and increase after 1-2 wk if needed (using (2 TTS-3 systems usually does not improve efficacy)
• *Severe cancer pain:* 30 µg/hr via continuous epidural infusion; use caution with infusion rates (40 µg/hr
Child
• PO 5-25 µg/kg/day in divided doses q6h, increase at 5-7 day intervals
AVAILABLE FORMS/COST OF THERAPY
• Tab, Uncoated—Oral: 0.1 mg, 100's: **$2.40-$57.82;** 0.2 mg, 100's: **$2.70-$88.46;** 0.3 mg, 100's: **$3.38-$111.02**
• Film, cont rel—Percutaneous: 2.5 mg/unit (TTS-1): **$7.73** 5 mg/unit (TTS-2): **$13.02;** 7.5 mg/unit (TTS-3): **$18.07**
• Inj—Epidural: 100 µg/ml, 10 ml: **$51.00**
PRECAUTIONS: Severe coronary insufficiency, recent MI, cerebrovascular disease, chronic renal failure, abrupt discontinuation (PO)
PREGNANCY AND LACTATION: Pregnancy category C; secreted into breast milk; hypotension has not been observed in nursing infants, although clonidine was found in the serum of the infants

SIDE EFFECTS/ADVERSE REACTIONS
Less severe with transdermal systems
CNS: Agitation, anxiety, delirium, depression, *dizziness,* dreams or nightmares, *drowsiness,* hallucinations, headache, insomnia, nervousness, restlessness, sedation
CV: Bradycardia, **CHF, dysrhythmias,** orthostatic hypotension, palpitations, Raynaud's phenomenon, rebound hypertension, tachycardia
GI: Anorexia, *constipation, dry mouth,* nausea, parotid pain, transient LFT elevations, vomiting
GU: Impotence, loss of libido, nocturia, urinary retention
METAB: Gynecomastia, transient elevation of blood glucose, weight gain
MS: Cramps of the lower limbs, fatigue, muscle or joint pain, weakness
SKIN: Alopecia, angioedema, hair thinning, pruritus, rash, transient localized skin reactions (TOP), urticaria
DRUG INTERACTIONS
Drugs
3 *β-blockers:* Rebound hypertension from clonidine withdrawal exacerbated by noncardioselective β-blockers
2 *Cyclic antidepressants:* Cyclic antidepressants may inhibit the antihypertensive response to clonidine
3 *Cyclosporine, tacrolimus:* Increased cyclosporine or tacrolimus concentrations
3 *Insulin:* Diminished symptoms of hypoglycemia
3 *Neuroleptics, nitroprusside:* Severe hypotension possible

SPECIAL CONSIDERATIONS
PATIENT/FAMILY EDUCATION
• Avoid hazardous activities, since drug may cause drowsiness
• Do not discontinue oral drug abruptly or withdrawal symptoms may occur (anxiety, increased BP, headache, insomnia, increased pulse, tremors, nausea, sweating)
• Response may take 2-3 days if drug is given transdermally

---

clopidogrel
(clo-pid'o-grill)
Rx: Plavix
Chemical Class: Thienopyridine
Therapeutic Class: Platelet aggregation inhibitor

CLINICAL PHARMACOLOGY
Mechanism of Action: Selectively and irreversibly inhibits ADP-induced platelet aggregation by inhibiting the binding of ADP to its receptors on platelets, thereby affecting ADP-dependent activation of the glycoprotein IIb/IIIa complex, the major receptor for fibrinogen
Pharmacokinetics
PO: Peak 1 hr; (significant antiaggregating activity in 2 hr); steady-state effect on bleeding time (1-2 × baseline), 3-7 days; following discontinuation, baseline values return in 5 days 50% absorbed (PO); clopidogrel is a prodrug that is activated by hepatic metabolism (CYP1A), to the major circulating metabolite, a carboxylic acid derivative, which is a CYP2C9 inhibitor; metabolite excreted in both feces and urine; $t_{1/2}$ of major metabolite, 8 hr
INDICATIONS AND USES: Reduction of atherosclerotic events (myocardial infarction, stroke, and vascular death) in patients with atherosclerosis documented by recent stroke, myocardial infarction, or established peripheral arterial disease

---

italic = common side effects

bold italic = life-threatening reactions

DOSAGE

Adult

• Antiplatelet effects: 75 mg qd (no dosage adjustments for elderly patients or those with renal impairment)

$ AVAILABLE FORMS/COST OF THERAPY

• Tab, Film-coated—Oral: 75 mg, 100's: **$289.15**

CONTRAINDICATIONS: Active pathologic bleeding; coagulation disorders; patients receiving anticoagulants or other antiplatelet agents

PRECAUTIONS: Previous hypersensitivity or other untoward effects related to ticlopidine; hypertension; hepatic or renal impairment; history of bleeding or hemostatic disorders; history of drug-related hematologic disorders; patients scheduled for major surgery; pregnancy

PREGNANCY AND LACTATION: Pregnancy category B; excreted into breast milk in rats

SIDE EFFECTS/ADVERSE REACTIONS

CNS: Dizziness, headache, intracranial bleeding

CV: Hypertension

GI: Abdominal pain, diarrhea, dyspepsia, *GI ulceration and hemorrhage,* nausea

GU: Liver enzyme elevation

HEME: Neutropenia (uncommon), prolonged bleeding time, purpura

SKIN: Pruritus, rash, urticaria

DRUG INTERACTIONS

Drugs

▣ *Fluvastatin:* Inhibition of hepatic metabolism (CYP2C9) of fluvastatin with increased risk of rhabdomyolysis

▣ *Nonsteroidal antiinflammatory agents:* Increased nonsteroidal antiinflammatory levels and effects

▣ *Phenytoin:* Inhibition of hepatic metabolism (CYP2C9) of phenytoin and increased risk of toxicity; in vitro data

▣ *Tamoxifen:* Inhibition of hepatic metabolism (CYP2C9) and increased tamoxifen effects

▣ *Tolbutamide:* Inhibition of hepatic metabolism (CYP2C9) of tolbutamide with increased risk of hypoglycemia; in vitro data

▣ *Torsemide:* Inhibition of hepatic metabolism (CYP2C9) of torsemide with enhanced diuretic effects; in vitro data

▣ *Warfarin:* Inhibition of hepatic metabolism (CYP2C9) of warfarin with enhanced hypoprothrombinemic effects; in vitro data

SPECIAL CONSIDERATIONS

• Comparative studies indicate that the drug is at least effective as aspirin; comparisons with ticlopidine lacking, however, no frequent CBC monitoring necessary; given the alternative mechanism to aspirin, perhaps combination therapy will be useful (studies unavailable)

PATIENT/FAMILY EDUCATION

• Inform clinician of signs and symptoms of bleeding, before surgery, dental work; inform clinician of sore throat, fever, etc. (consider neutropenia)

---

colestipol
(koe-les'ti-pole)
Rx: Colestid
Chemical Class: Bile acid sequestrant
Therapeutic Class: Antilipemic

CLINICAL PHARMACOLOGY

Mechanism of Action: Combines with bile acids to form insoluble complex that is excreted through feces; increased fecal loss of bile acids leads to increased oxidation of cholesterol to bile acids, in-

creased hepatic uptake of LDLs, and decreased serum LDL levels; serum triglyceride levels may increase or remain unchanged

Pharmacokinetics

PO: Not absorbed; excreted in feces

INDICATIONS AND USES: Primary hypercholesterolemia, xanthomas, pruritus due to biliary obstruction,* diarrhea due to bile acids*

DOSAGE

Adult

• PO 5-30 g qd in 2-4 divided doses, ac and hs; increase dose by 5 g at 1-2 mo intervals

$ AVAILABLE FORMS/COST OF THERAPY

• Granule—Oral: 5 g/scoop, 500 g: **$85.71**

• Packet—Oral: 5 g/plot, 90's: **$120.86**

• Tab, Uncoated—Oral: 1 g, 120's: **$37.96**

CONTRAINDICATIONS: Biliary obstruction

PRECAUTIONS: Lactation; children; bleeding disorders; may prevent absorption of fat-soluble vitamins such as A, D, E, and K; prolonged use may lead to the development of hyperchloremic acidosis;

PREGNANCY AND LACTATION: Pregnancy category B

SIDE EFFECTS/ADVERSE REACTIONS

CNS: Dizziness, headache

GI: Abdominal pain, constipation, fecal impaction, flatulence, hemorrhoids, nausea, peptic ulcer, steatorrhea, vomiting

HEME: Bleeding

METAB: Decreased vitamin A, D, E, K absorption; hyperchloremic acidosis

SKIN: Irritation of perianal area, rash

DRUG INTERACTIONS

Drugs

▣ *Acetaminophen, Amiodarone, Corticosteroids, Diclofenac, Digitalis glycosides, Furosemide, Methotrexate, Metronidazole, Thiazide diuretics, Thyroid hormones, Valproic acid:* Cholestyramine reduces interacting drug concentrations and probably subsequent therapeutic response

▣ *Oral anticoagulants:* Inhibition of hypoprothrombinemic response; colestipol might be less likely to interact

SPECIAL CONSIDERATIONS

• Bile acid sequestrant choice should be based on cost and patient acceptability

• Give all other medications 1 hr before colestipol or 4 hr after colestipol to avoid poor absorption

---

dalteparin
(doll'teh-pare-in)
Rx: Fragmin
Chemical Class: Low molecular weight heparin
Therapeutic Class: Anticoagulant

CLINICAL PHARMACOLOGY

Mechanism of Action: Enhances the inhibition of factor Xa and thrombin by antithrombin; potentiates preferentially the inhibition of coagulation factor Xa, while only slightly affecting clotting time, e.g., activated partial thromboplastin time (APTT)

Pharmacokinetics

SC: Peak levels of plasma anti–factor Xa activity in about 4 hr; absolute bioavailability 87%; $t_{1/2}$ 1.47-2.5 hr (prolonged in renal failure)

INDICATIONS AND USES: Prophylaxis against deep vein thrombosis, which may lead to pulmonary embolism, in patients undergoing abdominal surgery who are at risk for thromboembolic complications (40 yr of age, obese, undergoing surgery under general

---

* = non FDA-approved use

anesthesia lasting longer than 30 min, malignancy, history of deep vein thrombosis or pulmonary embolism); treatment of venous thromboembolism*

DOSAGE

Adult

SC 2500 IU qd starting 1-2 hr before surgery and for 5 to 10 days postoperatively

$ AVAILABLE FORMS/COST OF THERAPY
• Sol—SC: 2500 anti–Factor Xa/0.2 ml: **$13.95;** 5000 anti–factor Xa/0.2 ml: **$23.71**

CONTRAINDICATIONS: Active major bleeding, thrombocytopenia associated with positive in vitro tests for antiplatelet antibody in the presence of dalteparin, known hypersensitivity to pork products

PRECAUTIONS: History of heparin-induced thrombocytopenia; severe uncontrolled hypertension, bacterial endocarditis, congenital or acquired bleeding disorders, active ulceration and angiodysplastic gastrointestinal disease, hemorrhagic stroke or shortly after brain, spinal, or ophthalmologic surgery; bleeding diathesis, thrombocytopenia or platelet defects; severe liver or kidney insufficiency; hypertensive or diabetic retinopathy; recent gastrointestinal bleeding

PREGNANCY AND LACTATION: Pregnancy category B

SIDE EFFECTS/ADVERSE REACTIONS

HEME: Hemorrhage, ***thrombocytopenia***

SKIN: Pain at injection site, skin necrosis

DRUG INTERACTIONS

Drugs

◼ *Aspirin:* Increased risk of hemorrhage
◼ *Oral anticoagulants:* Additive anticoagulant effects

SPECIAL CONSIDERATIONS
• Cannot be used interchangeably (unit for unit) with unfractionated heparin or other low molecular weight heparins

MONITORING PARAMETERS
• CBC; stool occult blood tests; no special monitoring of blood clotting times (e.g., APTT) is needed

---

diazoxide
(dye-az-ox′ide)
Rx: Hyperstat (IV), Proglycem (PO)
Chemical Class: Benzothiadiazine derivative
Therapeutic Class: Antihypertensive; antihypoglycemic

CLINICAL PHARMACOLOGY

Mechanism of Action: Vasodilates arteriolar smooth muscle by direct relaxation; reduction in blood pressure with concomitant increases in heart rate, cardiac output; decreases release of insulin from β-cells in pancreas, resulting in an increase in blood glucose

Pharmacokinetics

PO: Onset 1 hr, duration 8 hr

IV: Onset 1-2 min, peak 5 min, duration 3-12 hr

$t_{1/2}$ 20-36 hr; excreted slowly in urine; crosses blood-brain barrier, placenta

INDICATIONS AND USES: Hypertensive crisis when urgent decrease of diastolic pressure required; increase blood glucose levels in hyperinsulinism

DOSAGE

Adult

• *Hypertension:* IV bolus 1-3 mg/kg rapidly up to a max of 150 mg in a single inj; dose may be repeated at 5-15 min intervals until desired response is achieved; give IV in 30 sec or less

• *Hypoglycemia:* PO initial 1 mg/kg q8h, adjusted prn according to response; maintenance 3-8 mg/kg/day given bid-tid (max 15 mg/kg/day)

Child

• *Hypertension:* IV bolus 1-2 mg/kg rapidly; administration same as adult; not to exceed 150 mg

• *Hypoglycemia:* PO initial 3.3 mg/kg q8h, adjusted prn; maintenance 8-15 mg/kg/day given bid-tid

$ AVAILABLE FORMS/COST OF THERAPY
• Inj, Sol—IV: 15 mg/ml, 20 ml: **$97.90**
• Cap—Oral: 50 mg, 100's: **$317.63**
• Susp—Oral: 50 mg/ml, 30 ml: **$105.88**

CONTRAINDICATIONS: Hypersensitivity to thiazides, sulfonamides; hypertension associated with aortic coarctation or AV shunt; pheochromocytoma; dissecting aortic aneurysm; functional hypoglycemia

PRECAUTIONS: Tachycardia; fluid, electrolyte imbalances; lactation; impaired cerebral or cardiac circulation; gout; diabetes mellitus

PREGNANCY AND LACTATION: Pregnancy category C

SIDE EFFECTS/ADVERSE REACTIONS

CNS: Anxiety, blurred vision, confusion, dizziness, EPS, euphoria, headache, insomnia, malaise, paresthesia, sleepiness, TIAs, weakness

CV: Angina pectoris, edema, hypotension, palpitations, rebound hypertension, ***supraventricular tachycardia,*** T-wave changes

EENT: Cataracts, diplopia, lacrimation, ring scotoma, subconjunctival hemorrhage, tinnitus

GI: Changes in ability to taste, dry mouth, nausea, vomiting

GU: Decreased urinary output, hematuria, increased BUN, reversible nephrotic syndrome

HEME: Decreased hemoglobin/hematocrit, ***thrombocytopenia***

METAB: Hyperglycemia, hyperuricemia

SKIN: Hypertrichosis, rash

MISC: Breast tenderness, allergic reactions

DRUG INTERACTIONS

Drugs

• *Carboplatin, cisplatin:* Increased risk of nephrotoxicity
• *Hydralazine:* Severe hypotensive reactions
• *Phenytoin:* Decreased phenytoin levels in children, probably due to enhanced metabolism
• *Thiazide diuretics:* Hyperglycemia

SPECIAL CONSIDERATIONS
• Often administered concurrently with a diuretic to prevent congestive heart failure due to fluid retention
• Oral susp dosage form produces higher concentration than cap form
• Hyperglycemia transient (24-48 hr) after IV administration
• If not effective within 2-3 wk of treatment of hypoglycemia, reevaluate

---

digitoxin
(di-ji-tox′in)
Rx: Crystodigin, Digitaline ✦
Chemical Class: Digitalis derivative
Therapeutic Class: Antidysrhythmic; cardiac glycoside

CLINICAL PHARMACOLOGY

Mechanism of Action: Increases influx of calcium ions into intracellular cytoplasm, resulting in increased cardiac muscle contractility (positive inotropic effect); decreases SA and AV node conduction (negative chronotropic effect)

---

italic = common side effects

bold italic = life-threatening reactions

Pharmacokinetics
PO: Onset 1-4 hr, peak 8-12 hr, $t_{1/2}$ 168-192 hr, 90%-97% bound to plasma proteins; metabolized by the liver, excreted via the kidneys (metabolites)
INDICATIONS AND USES: Congestive heart failure (CHF), atrial fibrillation, atrial flutter, paroxysmal atrial tachycardia (PAT), cardiogenic shock
DOSAGE
Adult
• Loading dose PO (rapid) 0.6 mg, followed by 0.4 mg, then 0.2 mg at q4-6h intervals; (slow) 0.2 mg bid for 4 days; maintenance dose
• PO 0.05-0.3 mg qd. Dosage reduction not needed in renal function impairment
Child
• Loading dose PO <1 yr 0.045 mg/kg, 1-2 yr 0.04 mg/kg, >2 yr 0.03 mg/kg divided into 3, 4, or more portions with >6 hr between doses; maintenance dose PO 1/10 loading dose
$ AVAILABLE FORMS/COST OF THERAPY
• Tab, Uncoated—Oral: 0.05 mg, 100's: **$2.92;** 0.1 mg, 100's: **$5.14**
CONTRAINDICATIONS: Ventricular tachycardia, ventricular fibrillation
PRECAUTIONS: Hypokalemia, hypomagnesemia, hypercalcemia, hypothyroidism, severe pulmonary disease, sick sinus syndrome, hepatic disease, acute MI, AV block, elderly, Wolff-Parkinson-White syndrome
PREGNANCY AND LACTATION: Pregnancy category C; passes readily to fetus; excretion into breast milk unknown; digoxin, a related cardiac glycoside, is considered compatible with breast feeding
SIDE EFFECTS/ADVERSE REACTIONS
CNS: Anorexia, apathy, confusion, delirium, disorientation, drowsiness, EEG abnormalities, hallucinations, headache, mental depression, neuralgia, psychosis, restlessness, seizures, weakness
CV: Atrial fibrillation, AV block, bradycardia, premature ventricular contractions (PVCs), ventricular fibrillation, ventricular tachycardia
EENT: Visual disturbances (blurred, yellow or green vision, halo effect)
GI: Abdominal discomfort, diarrhea, hemorrhagic necrosis of the intestines, nausea, vomiting
HEME: Eosinophilia, thrombocytopenia
SKIN: Rash
DRUG INTERACTIONS
Drugs
▣ *Alprazolam, amiodarone, diltiazem, verapamil, bepridil, nitrendipine, quinidine, carvedilol, cyclosporine, erythromycin and tetracyclines (change in bacterial flora causing effect may persist for months), hydroxychloroquine, NSAIDs, azole antifungals, omeprazole, lansoprazole, propafenone, quinine, spironolactone, tacrolimus:* Increased digoxin levels
▣ *Amphotericin B diuretics:* Enhanced digitalis toxicity secondary to drug-induced hypokalemia
▣ *β-blockers:* Potentiation of bradycardia
▣ *Calcium (IV):* Digitalis toxicity
❷ *Charcoal:* Reduced digitalis levels
▣ *Cholestyramine, Kaolo-pectin (digoxin tablets only), neomycin, penicillamine, rifampin, sulfasalazine:* Reduced digitalis levels
▣ *Metoclopramide, cisapride:* Reduced digitalis levels by slowly dissolving digoxin tablets only (Lanoxin tablets and capsules not affected)
▣ *Succinylcholine:* Increased arrhythmias
Labs
• False increase: Urine 17-hydroxycorticosteroids

SPECIAL CONSIDERATIONS
• When digitalis indicated digoxin is 1st line drug because of its shorter $t_{1/2}$ and faster clearance in the event toxicity develops
• Rule out digitalis toxicity if nausea, vomiting, arrhythmias develop
• Listed adverse effects are mostly signs of toxicity
MONITORING PARAMETERS
• Heart rate and rhythm, periodic ECGs
• Serum potassium, magnesium, calcium, creatinine
• Serum digitoxin levels when compliance, effectiveness, or systemic availability is questioned or toxicity suspected; therapeutic range 9-25 ng/ml

---

digoxin
(di-jox'in)
Rx: Lanoxicaps, Lanoxin
Chemical Class: Digitalis derivative
Therapeutic Class: Antidysrhythmic; cardiac glycoside

CLINICAL PHARMACOLOGY
Mechanism of Action: Increases influx of calcium ions into intracellular cytoplasm, resulting in increased cardiac muscle contractility (positive inotropic effect); decreases SA and AV node conduction (negative chronotropic effect)
Pharmacokinetics
IV: Onset 5-30 min, peak 1-5 hr
PO: Onset 30-120 min, peak 2-6 hr, $t_{1/2}$ 30-40 hr, 20%-25% bound to plasma proteins; excreted mainly by kidneys
INDICATIONS AND USES: Congestive heart failure in patients receiving diuretics or diuretics and ACE inhibitors (CHF), control of ventricular response rate in atrial fibrillation, atrial flutter, paroxysmal atrial tachycardia (PAT), cardiogenic shock
DOSAGE
Administer IV slowly over 5 min; IM route not recommended due to local irritation, pain, and tissue damage
Adult
• Loading dose (give 1/2 total dose initially, then 1/4 total dose in each of 2 subsequent doses at 8-12 hr intervals); IV 0.5-1 mg; PO 0.75-1.5 mg; maintenance dose IV 0.1-0.4 mg qd; PO 0.125-0.5 mg qd
Child >10 yr
• Loading dose (administered as for adult); IV 8-12 μg/kg; PO 10-15 μg/kg; maintenance dose IV 2-3 μg/kg qd; PO 2.5-5 μg/kg qd
Child 5-10 yr
• Loading dose (administered as for adult); IV 15-30 μg/kg; PO 20-35 μg/kg; maintenance dose IV 4-8 μg/kg divided q12h; PO 5-10 μg/kg divided q12h
• *Child 2-5 yr*
Loading dose (administered as for adult); IV 25-35 μg/kg; IV 30-40 μg/kg; maintenance dose IV 6-9 μg/kg divided q12h; PO 7.5-10 μg/kg divided q12h
Child 1-24 mo
• Loading dose (administered as for adult); IV 30-50 μg/kg; PO 35-60 μg/kg; maintenance dose IV 7.5-12 μg/kg divided q12h; PO 10-15 μg/kg divided q12h
Full-term infant
• Loading dose (administered as for adult); IV 20-30 μg/kg; PO 25-35 μg/kg; maintenance dose IV 5-8 μg/kg divided q12h; PO 6-10 μg/kg divided q12h
Preterm infant
• Loading dose (administered as for adult); IV 15-25 μg/kg; PO 20-30 μg/kg; maintenance dose: IV 4-6 μg/kg divided q12h, PO 5-7.5 μg/kg divided q12h

⑤ AVAILABLE FORMS/COST OF THERAPY

• Inj, Sol—IM, IV: 0.1 mg/ml, 1 ml: **$5.66;** 0.25 mg/ml, 2 ml: **$1.04-$2.36**
• Elixir—Oral: 0.05 mg/ml, 60 ml: **$10.40-$21.26**
• Cap, Elastic—Oral: 0.05 mg, 100's: **$17.04;** 0.1 mg, 100's: **$18.60;** 0.2 mg, 100's: **$21.64**
• Tab, Uncoated—Oral: 0.125 mg, 100's: **$3.19-$19.58;** 0.25 mg, 100's: **$7.54-$19.58;** 0.5 mg, 100's: **$25.00**

CONTRAINDICATIONS: Ventricular tachycardia, ventricular fibrillation

PRECAUTIONS: Hypokalemia, hypomagnesemia, hypercalcemia, hypothyroidism, severe pulmonary disease, sick sinus syndrome, hepatic disease, acute MI, AV block, elderly, Wolff-Parkinson-White syndrome

PREGNANCY AND LACTATION: Pregnancy category C, passes readily to fetus; excreted into breast milk; considered compatible with breast feeding

SIDE EFFECTS/ADVERSE REACTIONS

CNS: Anorexia, apathy, confusion, delirium, disorientation, drowsiness, EEG abnormalities, hallucinations, headache, mental depression, neuralgia, psychosis, restlessness, *seizures,* weakness
*CV: **Atrial fibrillation, AV block,*** bradycardia, premature ventricular contractions (PVCs), ***ventricular fibrillation, ventricular tachycardia***
EENT: Visual disturbances (blurred, yellow or green vision, halo effect)
GI: Abdominal discomfort, *diarrhea, **hemorrhagic necrosis of the intestines,*** *nausea, vomiting*
*HEME: Eosinophilia, **thrombocytopenia***
SKIN: Rash

DRUG INTERACTIONS

Drugs

③ *Alprazolam, amiodarone, diltiazem, verapamil, bepridil, nitrendipine, quinidine, carvedilol, cyclosporine, erythromycin and tetracyclines (change in bacterial flora causing effect may persist for months), hydroxychloroquine, NSAIDs, azole antifungals, omeprazole, lansoprazole, propafenone, quinine, spironolactone, tacrolimus:* Increased digoxin levels

③ *Amphotericin B diuretics:* Enhanced digitalis toxicity secondary to drug-induced hypokalemia

③ *β-blockers:* Potentiation of bradycardia

③ *Calcium (IV):* Digitalis toxicity

③ *Charcoal:* Reduced digitalis levels

③ *Cholestyramine, Kaolo-pectin (digoxin tablets only) neomycin, penicillamine, rifampin, sulfasalazine:* Reduced digitalis levels

③ *Cyclophosphamide:* Impaired digoxin (especially tablets) absorption; digitoxin not affected

③ *Metoclopramide, cisapride:* Reduced digitalis levels by slowly dissolving digoxin tablets only (Lanoxin tablets and capsules not affected)

③ *Succinylcholine:* Increased arrhythmias

Labs

• False increase: Urine 17-hydroxycorticosteroids

SPECIAL CONSIDERATIONS

• Preferred digitalis glycoside
• Rule out digitalis toxicity if nausea, vomiting, arrhythmias develop
• Listed adverse effects are mostly signs of toxicity

MONITORING PARAMETERS

• Heart rate and rhythm, periodic ECGs
• Serum potassium, magnesium, calcium, creatinine
• Serum digoxin levels when compliance, effectiveness, or systemic availability is questioned or toxicity suspected

• Obtain serum drug concentrations at least 8-12 hr after a dose (preferably before next scheduled dose); therapeutic range 0.5-2.0 ng/ml

---

diltiazem

(dil-tye′a-zem)
Rx: Cardizem, Cardizem CD, Cardizem SR, Dilacor XR, Nu-Diltiaz ✦
Combinations
   Rx: with enalapril (Tiazac)
Chemical Class: Benzothiazepine calcium channel blocker
Therapeutic Class: Antianginal; antihypertensive; antidysrhythmic (class IV)

CLINICAL PHARMACOLOGY

Mechanism of Action: Inhibits calcium ion influx across cell membrane during cardiac depolarization; produces relaxation of coronary vascular smooth muscle, dilates coronary arteries, slows SA/AV node conduction times, dilates peripheral arteries

Pharmacokinetics
PO: Peak 2-3 hr
PO SUS REL: Peak 6-11 hr
PO QD CAP: Peak 10-14 hr
$t_{1/2}$ 3.5-8 hr, 70%-80% bound to plasma proteins; metabolized by liver, excreted in urine (96% as metabolites)

INDICATIONS AND USES: *Oral:* Angina pectoris due to coronary artery spasm, chronic stable angina, essential hypertension (SR only). *Parenteral:* Atrial fibrillation or flutter (IV), paroxysmal supraventricular tachycardia (IV). Also prevention of reinfarction of non-Q-wave MI,* tardive dyskinesia,* Raynaud's syndrome,* migraine headache prophylaxis*

DOSAGE

Adult

• *IMMED REL PO* 30 mg qid, gradually increase to 180-360 mg/day divided tid-qid until optimal response is obtained; *SUS REL* (Cardizem SR) PO 60-120 mg bid, adjust at 14 day intervals until optimal response obtained, optimum range 240-350 mg/day; *SUS REL* (Cardizem CD, Dilacor XR) once daily cap PO 180-240 mg qd, max 540 mg/day; *IV* 0.25 mg/kg as a bolus over 2 min (a second 0.35 mg/kg bolus dose may be administered after 15 min if response is inadequate), then continuous INF of 5-15 mg/hr for up to 24 hr; conversion from IV to PO, start PO approximately 3 hr after bolus dose; PO (mg/day) = 10 × {[rate (mg/hr) × 3] +3}; 3 mg/hr = 120 mg/day; 5 mg/hr = 180 mg/day; 7 mg/hr = 240 mg/day; 11 mg/hr = 360 mg/day

⑤ AVAILABLE FORMS/COST OF THERAPY

• Cap, Gel, Sus Action—Oral: 60 mg, 100's: **$69.20-$91.50;** 90 mg, 100's: **$79.20-$104.81;** 120 mg, 100's: **$96.48-$136.44;** 180 mg, 100's: **$108.19-$122.64;** 240 mg, 100's: **$116.84-$174.30;** 300 mg, 100's: **$224.70**
• Tab, Plain Coated—Oral: 30 mg, 100's: **$10.85-$50.13;** 60 mg, 100's: **$16.89-$78.44;** 90 mg, 100's: **$23.09-$110.44;** 120 mg, 100's: **$30.20-$143.63**
• Inj, Sol—IV: 5 mg/ml, 5 ml: **$13.22**

CONTRAINDICATIONS: Sick sinus syndrome or 2nd or 3rd degree heart block (except with a functioning pacemaker), hypotension (90 mm Hg systolic, acute MI with pulmonary congestion, atrial fibrillation or atrial flutter associated with an accessory bypass tract such as in WPW syndrome or short PR syndrome (IV), ventricular tachycardia (IV)

PRECAUTIONS: CHF, hypotension, hepatic injury, children, impaired renal or hepatic function

---

italic = common side effects

bold italic = life-threatening reactions

PREGNANCY AND LACTATION: Pregnancy category C; excreted into breast milk in concentrations that may approximate those in maternal serum; use caution in nursing mothers

SIDE EFFECTS/ADVERSE REACTIONS

CNS: Abnormal dreams, amnesia, depression, *dizziness,* gait abnormality, hallucinations, *headache,* insomnia, nervousness, paresthesia, personality change, somnolence, tremor

CV: Angina, ***arrhythmia, AV block (1st degree), AV block (2nd or 3rd degree),*** bradycardia, bundle branch block, ***congestive heart failure,*** *edema,* flushing, hypotension, palpitations, syncope, tachycardia

GI: Anorexia, constipation, diarrhea, dysgeusia, dyspepsia, GERD; mild elevations of LFTs; *nausea,* thirst, vomiting, weight increase

METAB: Metabolic acidosis

SKIN: Petechiae, photosensitivity, pruritus, rash, urticaria

DRUG INTERACTIONS

Drugs

■ *α-blockers:* Possible increased antihypertensive effect

■ *Amiodarone:* Cardiotoxicity with bradycardia and decreased cardiac output

■ *Antipyrine:* Increased antipyrine concentrations

■ *Aspirin:* Enhanced antiplatelet activity

■ *Azole antifungals:* Possible increased calcium channel blocker effects

■ *β-blockers:* Inhibition of metabolism of propranolol and metoprolol (not atenolol); additive effects on cardiac conduction and hypotension

■ *Calcium (large doses):* Inhibition of diltiazem activity

■ *Calcium channel blockers:* Increased nifedipine concentrations

❷ *Carbamazepine:* Increase in carbamazepine toxicity

■ *Cyclosporine, tacrolimus:* Increased blood concentrations, renal toxicity

■ *Digitalis glycosides:* Reduced elimination, increased digitalis levels, toxicity

■ *Ecainide:* Increased ecainide levels

■ *Erythromycin, troleandomycin:* Increased levels calcium channel blocker

■ *H₂-receptor antagonists:* Serum diltiazem concentrations increased

■ *Lithium:* Neurotoxicity

■ *Neuromuscular blockers:* Prolonged blockade by vecuronium and pancuronium

■ *Nitroprusside:* Enhanced hypotension

■ *Phenobarbital:* Reduced calcium channel blocker concentration

■ *Phenytoin:* Increased phenytoin levels

■ *Rifampin:* Decreased diltiazem concentrations

■ *Tricyclic antidepressants:* Increased TCA levels

Labs

• *False positive:* Urine ketones

---

dipyridamole

(dye-peer-id'a-mole)

Rx: Persantine

Chemical Class: Substituted pyrimidine derivative

Therapeutic Class: Coronary vasodilator, antiplatelet agent

CLINICAL PHARMACOLOGY

Mechanism of Action: Inhibits platelet adhesion, likely by inhibiting thromboxane A₂ formation and inhibiting phosphodiesterase

Pharmacokinetics

PO: Onset 30 min, peak 2-2½ hr, duration 6 hr

IV: Onset 1 min, peak 7 min, duration 30 min

Protein binding 91%-99%, conjugated in liver to glucuronide, excreted in bile, undergoes enterohepatic recirculation

INDICATIONS AND USES: With warfarin to prevent thromboembolic complications of cardiac valve replacement; with aspirin to prevent coronary bypass graft occlusion* or transient ischemic attack*; as diagnostic aid in thallium myocardial perfusion imaging for the evaluation of CAD

DOSAGE

Adult

• *Transient ischemic attack:* PO 50 mg tid, 1 hr ac, not to exceed 400 mg qd

• *Inhibition of platelet adhesion:* PO 50-75 mg qid in combination with aspirin or warfarin

• *Diagnostic aid in myocardial perfusion studies:* IV 0.14 mg/kg/min for 4 min, max dose 60 mg

Child

• *Inhibition of platelet adhesion:* PO 3-6 mg/kg/day in 3 divided doses

$ AVAILABLE FORMS/COST OF THERAPY

• Tab, Coated—Oral: 25 mg, 100's: **$2.25-$33.85;** 50 mg, 100's: **$4.13-$54.54;** 75 mg, 100's: **$5.93-$72.96**

• Inj, Sol—IV: 5 mg/ml, 10 ml: **$144.00**

PRECAUTIONS: Ischemic heart disease, bleeding disorders, hypotension

PREGNANCY AND LACTATION: Pregnancy category C; excreted in breast milk

SIDE EFFECTS/ADVERSE REACTIONS

CNS: Dizziness, headache

GI: Abdominal distress, anorexia, diarrhea, nausea, vomiting

SKIN: Flushing, rash

DRUG INTERACTIONS

Drugs

■ *Adenosine:* Dipyridamole reduces adenosine metabolism

■ *β-blockers:* Dipyridamole promotes bradycardia due to β-blockers

SPECIAL CONSIDERATIONS

• Contributes little to the antithrombotic effect of aspirin

---

disopyramide

(dye-soe-peer'a-mide)

Rx: Disopyramide, Norpace, Norpace CR, Rythmodan ✽, Rythmodan-LA ✽

Chemical Class: Substituted pyramide derivative

Therapeutic Class: Antidysrhythmic (class IA)

CLINICAL PHARMACOLOGY

Mechanism of Action: Type I antidysrhythmic drug; lengthens effective refractory period of the atrium and ventricle; decreases conduction velocity; has minimal effect on effective refractory period of the AV node; decreases the disparity in refractoriness between infarcted and adjacent normal myocardium; has anticholinergic actions

Pharmacokinetics

PO: Peak 30 min-3 hr, duration 6-12 hr, t₁/₂ 4-10 hr; metabolized in liver, excreted unchanged in urine (50%) and feces (10%); crosses placenta; protein binding concentration dependent (50%-65% at plasma levels of 2-4 μg/ml)

INDICATIONS AND USES: Life-threatening ventricular dysrhythmias such as sustained ventricular tachycardia; supraventricular tachycardia*

DOSAGE
Adult
• PO 100-200 mg q6h; in renal dysfunction, if CrCl 30-40 ml/min, dose should be 100 mg q8h, if CrCl 15-30 ml/min, dose should be 100 mg q12h, if CrCl <15 ml/min, dose should be 100 mg q24h; may give loading dose of 300 mg for rapid effect; PO (SUS REL CAP) 200-300 mg q12h; not recommended in renal dysfunction

Child
• PO age 12-18 yr: 6-15 mg/kg/day in divided doses q6h; age 4-12 yr: 10-15 mg/kg/day in divided doses q6h; age 1-4 yr: 10-20 mg/kg/day in divided doses q6h; age <1 yr: 10-30 mg/kg/day in divided doses q6h

$ AVAILABLE FORMS/COST OF THERAPY
• Cap, Gel—Oral: 100 mg, 100's: **$10.43-$54.55**; 150 mg, 100's: **$11.93-$64.43**
• Cap, Gel, Sus Action—Oral: 100 mg, 100's: **$53.10-$65.69**; 150 mg, 100's: **$39.75-$77.64**

CONTRAINDICATIONS: 2nd or 3rd degree block, cardiogenic shock, CHF (uncompensated), sick sinus syndrome, QT prolongation

PRECAUTIONS: Children, diabetes mellitus, renal disease, hepatic disease, myasthenia gravis, narrow-angle glaucoma, cardiomyopathy, conduction abnormalities (including accessory pathways)

PREGNANCY AND LACTATION: Pregnancy category C; excreted in breast milk

SIDE EFFECTS/ADVERSE REACTIONS
CNS: Anxiety, depression, *dizziness,* fatigue, *headache,* insomnia, paresthesias, psychosis
CV: Angina, **AV block,** *bradycardia,* **cardiac arrest, CHF,** chest pain, edema, *hypotension,* increased QRS or QT duration, PVCs, syncope, tachycardia
EENT: Blurred vision; *dry nose, throat, eyes;* narrow-angle glaucoma
GI: Anorexia, *constipation (11%),* diarrhea, *dry mouth (32%),* flatulence, nausea, vomiting
GU: Hesitancy *(14%),* impotence, *retention,* urinary frequency, urgency
HEME: **Agranulocytosis,** anemia (rare), **thrombocytopenia**
METAB: Hypoglycemia
MS: Pain in extremities, weakness
SKIN: Pruritus, rash, urticaria

DRUG INTERACTIONS
Drugs
3 *Barbiturates, phenytoin, rifampin:* Reduced disopyramide level via induction
3 *β-blockers:* Enhanced negative inotropy
3 *Clarithromycin, erythromycin, troleandromycin:* Macrolide increased disopyramide-serum concentration resulting in dysrhythmias
3 *Lidocaine:* Arrhythmias or heart failure in predisposed patients
3 *Potassium, potassium-sparing diuretics:* Increased potassium concentration can enhance disopyramide effects on myocardial conduction

Labs
• *Increase:* Liver enzymes, lipids, BUN, creatinine
• *Decrease:* Hgb/Hct, blood glucose

SPECIAL CONSIDERATIONS
• Due to potential for prodysrhythmic effects, use for asymptomatic PVCs or lesser dysrhythmias should be avoided

MONITORING PARAMETERS
• Monitor ECG closely; if PR, QRS, or QT interval increase by 25%, stop drug
• Therapeutic plasma levels are 2-4 μg/ml

---

dobutamine
(doe-byoo′ta-meen)
Rx: Dobutrex
Chemical Class: Catecholamine
Therapeutic Class: Sympathomimetic

CLINICAL PHARMACOLOGY
Mechanism of Action: Causes increased contractility, increased coronary blood flow and heart rate by direct action on β_1-receptors in heart; reduces systemic vascular resistance
Pharmacokinetics
IV: Onset 1-2 min, peak 10 min, $t_{1/2}$ 2 min; metabolized in liver (inactive metabolites); metabolites excreted in urine

INDICATIONS AND USES: Short-term treatment of adults with cardiac decompensation due to depressed myocardial contractility; diagnostic aid for ischemic heart disease*

DOSAGE
Adult
• IV INF 2.5-15 μg/kg/min, max dose 40 μg/kg/min

$ AVAILABLE FORMS/COST OF THERAPY
• Inj, Dry-Sol—IV: 12.5 mg/ml, 20 ml: **$7.50-$12.00**

CONTRAINDICATIONS: Hypertrophic cardiomyopathy, uncontrolled atrial fibrillation or flutter (unless a digitalis preparation is used before starting therapy with dobutamine)

PRECAUTIONS: Children, hypertension, sulfite sensitivity (preparation may contain sulfite)

PREGNANCY AND LACTATION: Pregnancy category C; excreted in breast milk

SIDE EFFECTS/ADVERSE REACTIONS
CNS: Anxiety, dizziness, headache, paresthesia
CV: Angina, **dysrhythmia,** hypertension, palpitations, PVCs, *tachycardia*
GI: Heartburn, nausea, vomiting
METAB: Hypokalemia
MS: Leg cramps

DRUG INTERACTIONS
Drugs
• *Sodium bicarbonate:* Alkalinizing substances inactivate dobutamine

SPECIAL CONSIDERATIONS
MONITORING PARAMETERS
• Continuously monitor ECG, BP, and PCWP

---

dopamine
(doe′pa-meen)
Rx: Intropin
Chemical Class: Catecholamine
Therapeutic Class: Vasopressor; sympathomimetic

CLINICAL PHARMACOLOGY
Mechanism of Action: Stimulates both adrenergic and dopaminergic receptors in a dose-dependent manner; low doses (1-5 μg/kg/min) stimulate mainly dopaminergic receptors producing renal and mesenteric vasodilation; intermediate doses (5-15 μg/kg/min) stimulate both dopaminergic and β_1-adrenergic recep-

---

italic = common side effects

bold italic = life-threatening reactions

tors producing cardiac stimulation and renal vasodilation; large doses (15 μg/kg/min) stimulate α-adrenergic receptors producing vasoconstriction and increases in peripheral vascular resistance and blood pressure

Pharmacokinetics

IV: Onset 5 min, duration <10 min; metabolized in plasma, kidneys, and liver by MAO (75% to inactive metabolites, 25% to norepinephrine); $t_{1/2}$ 2 min

INDICATIONS AND USES: Correction of hemodynamic imbalances in shock syndromes (e.g., MI, trauma, septicemia, renal failure, CHF); COPD*; CHF*; respiratory distress syndrome (RDS) in infants*

DOSAGE

Adult and Child

• IV INF 1-20 μg/kg/min, titrated to desired response; do not exceed 50 μg/kg/min

⑤ AVAILABLE FORMS/COST OF THERAPY

• Inj, Conc-Sol—IV: 40 mg/ml, 5 ml: **$1.07-$25.92;** 80 mg/ml, 5 ml: **$1.24-$41.50;** 160 mg/ml, 5 ml: **$1.96-$8.13**

CONTRAINDICATIONS: Pheochromocytoma, uncorrected tachydysrhythmia or ventricular fibrillation

PRECAUTIONS: Hypovolemia, arterial embolism, occlusive vascular disease, abrupt discontinuation, sulfite sensitivity, concurrent use of MAOIs

PREGNANCY AND LACTATION: Pregnancy category C; because dopamine is indicated only in life-threatening situations, chronic use would not be expected; no data available regarding use in breast feeding

SIDE EFFECTS/ADVERSE REACTIONS

CNS: Headache

CV: Aberrant conduction, *anginal pain,* bradycardia, *ectopic beats,* hypertension, *palpitation, tachycardia, vasoconstriction,* widened QRS complex

EENT: Dilated pupils (high doses)

GI: Nausea, vomiting

GU: Azotemia

RESP: Dyspnea

SKIN: Gangrene (high doses for prolonged periods of time), necrosis, piloerection, tissue sloughing with extravasation

DRUG INTERACTIONS

Drugs

⬛ *Ergot alkaloids:* Gangrene has been reported

⬛ *Phenytoin:* Increased risk of hypotension with IV phenytoin administration

Labs

• *False increase:* Urine amino acids; urine catecholamines; serum creatinine

• *False decrease:* Serum creatinine

SPECIAL CONSIDERATIONS

• *Dilute before use if not prediluted;* antidote for extravasation: infiltrate area as soon as possible with 10-15 ml NS containing 5-10 mg phentolamine

MONITORING PARAMETERS

• Urine flow, cardiac output, blood pressure, pulmonary wedge pressure

---

doxazosin

(dox-ay'zoe-sin)

Rx: Cardura

Chemical Class: Quinazoline derivative

Therapeutic Class: Antihypertensive; benign prostatic hypertrophy agent

CLINICAL PHARMACOLOGY

Mechanism of Action: Selectively blocks postsynaptic α_1-adrenergic receptors; dilates both arterioles and veins; relaxes smooth muscle in bladder neck and prostate

Pharmacokinetics

PO: Onset 2 hr, peak 2-3 hr; 98% bound to plasma proteins; extensively metabolized in liver, excreted via bile, feces, and urine; $t_{1/2}$ 22 hr

INDICATIONS AND USES: Hypertension, benign prostatic hyperplasia (BPH), CHF*

DOSAGE

Adult

• PO 1 mg qd, increasing to 16 mg qd if required; usual range 4-16 mg/day

⑤ AVAILABLE FORMS/COST OF THERAPY

• Tab, Uncoated—Oral: 1 mg, 100's: **$94.54;** 2 mg, 100's: **$94.54;** 4 mg, 100's: **$99.24;** 8 mg, 100's: **$104.21**

PRECAUTIONS: Children, hepatic disease

PREGNANCY AND LACTATION: Pregnancy category C; may accumulate in breast milk; use caution in nursing mothers

SIDE EFFECTS/ADVERSE REACTIONS

CNS: Anxiety, asthenia, ataxia, depression, *dizziness,* fever, *headache,* hypertonia, insomnia, nervousness, paresthesia, somnolence

CV: Chest pain, *dysrhythmia,* edema, flushing, palpitations, postural hypotension, tachycardia

EENT: Abnormal vision, tinnitus, vertigo

GI: Abdominal discomfort, constipation, diarrhea, dry mouth, flatulence, nausea, vomiting

GU: Incontinence, polyuria

MS: Arthralgia, myalgia

RESP: Dyspnea

SKIN: Pruritus, rash

DRUG INTERACTIONS

Drugs

⬛ *ACE inhibitors:* Increased potential for first dose hypotension

⬛ *Indomethacin:* Decreased hypotensive effect of doxazosin

⬛ *Verapamil, nifedipine:* Enhanced hypotensive effects of both drugs

SPECIAL CONSIDERATIONS

PATIENT/FAMILY EDUCATION

• Alert patient to the possibility of syncopal and orthostatic symptoms, especially with 1st dose ("1st-dose syncope")

• Initial dose should be administered at bedtime in the smallest possible dose

---

* = non FDA-approved use

enalapril/enalaprilat
(en-al'a-pril)
Rx: Vasotec
Combinations
  Rx: with felodipine (Lexxel); with hydrochlorothiazide (Vaseretic)
Chemical Class: Angiotensin-converting enzyme (ACE) inhibitor
Therapeutic Class: Antihypertensive; congestive heart failure agent; renal protectant

CLINICAL PHARMACOLOGY
Mechanism of Action: Selectively suppresses renin-angiotensin-aldosterone system; inhibits ACE, preventing conversion of angiotensin I to angiotensin II; results in dilation of arterial, venous vessels
Pharmacokinetics
PO: Peak $\frac{1}{2}$-$1\frac{1}{2}$ hr (enalaprilat 3-4 hr), metabolized by liver to active metabolite (enalaprilat), excreted in urine and feces; $t_{1/2}$ $1\frac{1}{2}$ hr (enalaprilat 11 hr)
IV (enalaprilat): Onset 5-15 min
INDICATIONS AND USES: Hypertension, heart failure, left ventricular dysfunction (clinically stable asymptomatic patients, decreases rate of overt heart failure), diabetic nephropathy,* hypertensive emergencies (enalaprilat)*
DOSAGE
Adult
• PO 2.5-5 mg qd, increase prn, usually 10-40 mg/day divided qd-bid; IV (enalaprilat) 0.625-1.25 mg/dose given over 5 min q6h; dosing adjustment in renal impairment: CrCl 10-50 ml/min, 75%-100% of normal dose; CrCl <10 ml/min, 50% of normal dose
Child
• PO 0.1 mg/kg/day initially, increase prn over 2 wk to max of 0.5 mg/kg/day; IV (enalaprilat) 5-10 μg/kg/dose q8-24 hr
$ AVAILABLE FORMS/COST OF THERAPY
• Tab, Uncoated—Oral: 2.5 mg, 100's: **$77.16;** 5 mg, 100's: **$98.04;** 10 mg, 100's: **$102.94;** 20 mg, 100's: **$146.44**
• Inj, Sol—IV: 1.25 mg/ml, 1 ml: **$13.76**
PRECAUTIONS: Impaired renal and liver function, dialysis patients, hypovolemia, diuretic therapy, collagen-vascular diseases, CHF, elderly, bilateral renal artery stenosis
PREGNANCY AND LACTATION: Pregnancy category C (1st trimester), category D (2nd and 3rd trimesters); ACE inhibitors can cause fetal and neonatal morbidity and death when administered to pregnant women; when pregnancy is detected, discontinue ACE inhibitors as soon as possible; detectable in breast milk in trace amounts; effect on nursing infant has not been determined; use with caution in nursing mothers
SIDE EFFECTS/ADVERSE REACTIONS
CNS: Anxiety, dizziness, fatigue, headache, insomnia, paresthesia
CV: Angina, hypotension, palpitations, postural hypotension, syncope (especially with 1st dose)
GI: Abdominal pain, constipation, melena, nausea, vomiting
GU: Decreased libido, impotence, increased BUN/creatinine, UTI
HEME: **Agranulocytosis, neutropenia**
METAB: Hyperkalemia, hyponatremia
MS: Arthralgia, arthritis, myalgia
RESP: Asthma, bronchitis, *cough,* dyspnea, sinusitis
SKIN: **Angioedema,** flushing, rash, sweating
DRUG INTERACTIONS
Drugs
❷ *Allopurinol:* Predisposition to hypersensitivity reactions to ACE inhibitors

🛽 *Aspirin, NSAIDs:* Inhibition of the antihypertensive response to ACE inhibitors
🛽 *Insulin:* Enhanced insulin sensitivity
🛽 *Iron:* Increased risk of anaphylaxis with administration of parenteral (IV) iron
🛽 *Lithium:* Increased risk of serious lithium toxicity
🛽 *Loop diuretics:* Initiation of ACE inhibitor therapy in the presence of intensive diuretic therapy results in a precipitous fall in blood pressure in some patients; ACE inhibitors may induce renal insufficiency in the presence of diuretic-induced sodium depletion
🛽 *Potassium:* Increased risk for hyperkalemia
🛽 *Potassium-sparing diuretics:* Increased risk for hyperkalemia
🛽 *Prazosin, terazosin, doxazosin:* Exaggerated first-dose hypotensive response to α-blockers

SPECIAL CONSIDERATIONS
PATIENT/FAMILY EDUCATION
• Do not use salt substitutes containing potassium without consulting clinician
• Rise slowly to sitting or standing position to minimize orthostatic hypotension
• Notify clinician of mouth sores, sore throat, fever, swelling of hands or feet, irregular heartbeat, chest pain
MONITORING PARAMETERS
• BUN, creatinine (watch for increased levels that may indicate acute renal failure)
• Potassium levels, although hyperkalemia rarely occurs; may account for as much as 0.5 mEq/L rise in serum potassium

enoxaparin
(e-nox-ah-pair'in)
Rx: Lovenox
Chemical Class: Depolymerized heparin derivative (low molecular weight heparin)
Therapeutic Class: Anticoagulant

CLINICAL PHARMACOLOGY
Mechanism of Action: Inhibits thrombosis by inactivating factor Xa and inhibiting the conversion of prothrombin to thrombin; has a higher ratio of anti-factor Xa to antithrombin activity (3.35) than unfractionated heparin (1.22); does not significantly influence bleeding time, platelet function, prothrombin time (PT), or activated partial thromboplastin time (aPTT) at recommended doses
Pharmacokinetics
SC: Peak activity 3-5 hr, $t_{1/2}$ 41/2 hr
INDICATIONS AND USES: Prevention of deep vein thrombosis (DVT), which may lead to pulmonary embolism following hip and knee replacement surgery; treatment of DVT (1 mg/kg q12h until warfarin therapy is therapeutic for over 48 h)*; prevention of deep vein thrombosis (DVT) long term when other modalities inappropriate*
DOSAGE
Adult
• *Prevention:* SC 30 mg bid beginning as soon as possible following surgery for 7-14 days
• *Treatment:* SC 1 mg/kg q12h
$ AVAILABLE FORMS/COST OF THERAPY
• Inj, Sol—SC: 30 mg/0.3 ml: **$16.80**
CONTRAINDICATIONS: Active major bleeding, drug-induced thrombocytopenia
PRECAUTIONS: Bacterial endocarditis, bleeding disorder, active ulceration, angiodysplastic GI disease, hemorrhagic stroke; recent

---

italic = common side effects

bold italic = life-threatening reactions

brain, spinal, or ophthalmologic surgery; history of heparin-induced thrombocytopenia; renal function impairment; elderly; children
PREGNANCY AND LACTATION: Pregnancy category B; excretion into breast milk unknown; use caution in nursing mothers
SIDE EFFECTS/ADVERSE REACTIONS
CNS: Confusion, fever
CV: Edema
GI: Increased ALT, AST; nausea
HEME: Hemorrhage, hypochromic anemia, ***thrombocytopenia***
SKIN: Ecchymosis, erythema at inj site, hematoma, local irritation, pain

SPECIAL CONSIDERATIONS
• Cannot be used interchangeably with other low molecular weight heparins
PATIENT/FAMILY EDUCATION
• Administer by deep SC inj into abdominal wall; alternate inj sites
• Report any unusual bruising or bleeding to clinician
MONITORING PARAMETERS
• Platelets, occult blood, Hgb, Hct, anti-factor Xa activity

---

epinephrine
(ep-i-nef′rin)
Vasopressor: **Rx:** Adrenalin, Sus-Phrine
Bronchodilator: **Rx:** Adrenaline, Racepinephrine, Sus-Phrine: **OTC:** Adrenalin, AsthmaHaler Mist, Asthma-Nefrin, Bronitin Mist, Bronkaid Mist, Medihaler-Epi, microNefrin, Nephron Inhalant, Primatene Mist, S-2, Vaponefrin
Decongestant: **OTC:** Adrenaline
Antiglaucoma agent: **Rx:** Epifrin, Glaucon
Emergency Kit: **Rx:** EpiPen, EpiPen Jr.
Combinations
   Rx: with etidocaine (Duranest with Epinephrine); with prilocaine (Citanest Forte); with lidocaine (Xylocaine with Epinephrine); with pilocarpine (E-Pilo Ophthalmic)
Chemical Class: Catecholamine
Therapeutic Class: Vasopressor; antiglaucoma agent; bronchodilator; decongestant

---

CLINICAL PHARMACOLOGY
Mechanism of Action: Stimulates α-, β_1-, and β_2-adrenergic receptors resulting in bronchodilation, cardiac stimulation, nasal decongestion, and dilation of skeletal muscle vasculature; effects on vasculature are dose dependent, small doses produce vasodilation while large doses produce vasoconstriction; decreases production of aqueous humor and increases aqueous outflow; dilates the pupil by contracting the dilator muscle
Pharmacokinetics
SC: Onset 3-5 min
INH: Onset 1 min
OPHTH: Onset 1 hr
Taken up into the adrenergic neuron and metabolized by monoamine oxidase and catechol-*O*-methyltransferase; circulating drug metabolized by liver; inactive metabolites excreted in urine
INDICATIONS AND USES: Cardiac arrest, acute asthmatic attacks, nasal congestion, open-angle glaucoma, anaphylactic reactions
DOSAGE
Adult
• *Bronchodilator:* IM/SC (1:1000) 0.1-0.5 mg q12-15 min-4 hr; IV 0.1-0.25 mg (single dose max 1 mg); SC susp (1:200) 0.5-1.5 mg (0.1-0.3 ml); NEB instill 8-15 gtt into nebulizer reservoir, adminis-

ter 1-3 inhalations 4-6 times/day; MDI 1-2 puffs at 1st sign of bronchospasm
• *Cardiac arrest:* IV/intracardiac 0.1-1 mg (1-10 ml of 1:10,000 dilution) q3-5 min prn; IV intermediate dose 2-5 mg q3-5 min; escalating dose 1 mg-3 mg-5 mg 3 min apart; high dose 0.1 mg/kg q3-5 min; intratracheal 1 mg q3-5 min (higher doses [e.g., 0.1 mg/kg] should be considered only after 1 mg doses have failed)
• *Hypotension:* IV INF 1-4 µg/min
• *Anaphylactic reaction:* IM/SC 0.2-0.5 mg q20 min-4 hr (single dose max 1 mg)
• *Glaucoma:* Ophth 1 gtt qd-bid
• *Nasal congestion:* Intranasal apply prn; do not use for (3-5 days
Child
• *Bronchodilator:* SC 10 µg/kg (0.01 ml/kg of 1:1000), max single dose 0.5 mg; susp (1:200) 0.005 ml/kg/dose (0.025 mg/kg/dose) q6h, max 0.15 ml (0.75 mg)/dose; NEB 0.25-0.5 ml of 2.25% racemic epinephrine solution diluted in 3 ml NS q1-4h
• *Cardiac arrest:* IV/intratracheal 0.01 mg/kg (0.1 ml/kg) of 1:10,000 sol q3-5 min prn, max 5 ml
• *Refractory hypotension:* IV INF 0.1-4 µg/kg/min
• *Anaphylactic reaction:* SC 0.01 mg/kg q15 min for 2 doses then q4h prn, max 0.5 mg/dose
• *Nasal congestion (>6 yr):* Intranasal apply prn
Neonate
• *Cardiac arrest:* IV/intratracheal 0.01-0.03 mg/kg (0.1-0.3 ml/kg) of 1:10,000 sol q3-5 min prn
$ AVAILABLE FORMS/COST OF THERAPY
• Inj, Sol—IM: 0.15, 0.3 mg/0.3 ml, 1's: **$24.60**
• Inj, Sol—IM, IV, SC: 0.1 mg/ml, 10 ml: **$3.20-$14.46;** 1 mg/ml, 1 ml: **$0.91-$15.00**
• Inj, Sol—IV: 5 mg/ml, 0.3 ml: **$2.82**
• Inj, Susp—SC: 0.5%, 0.3 ml: **$3.60**
• Sol—INH: 1%, 7.5 ml: **$13.19**
• Aer—INH: 0.22 mg/INH, 15 ml: **$9.28;** 0.3 mg/INH, 15 ml: **$8.65**
• Sol—Ophth: 0.5%, 15 ml: **$27.66**
• Sol—Ophth, Top: 1%, 15 ml: **$29.66**
• Sol—Ophth, Top: 2%, 15 ml: **$32.46**
• Sol—Nasal: 1 mg/ml, 30 ml: **$9.82**
CONTRAINDICATIONS: Cardiac dysrhythmias, angle-closure glaucoma, local anesthesia of fingers and toes, general anesthesia with halogenated hydrocarbons or cyclopropane, organic brain damage, labor, coronary insufficiency
PRECAUTIONS: Elderly, cardiovascular disease, hypertension, diabetes, hyperthyroidism, psychoneurotic individuals, thyrotoxicosis, parkinsonism
PREGNANCY AND LACTATION: Pregnancy category C; excreted into breast milk; use caution in nursing mothers
SIDE EFFECTS/ADVERSE REACTIONS
CNS: Anxiety, dizziness, fear, headache, hemiplegia, restlessness, ***subarachnoid hemorrhage,*** *tremor,* weakness
CV: Anginal pain, ***dysrhythmias,*** hypertension, palpitations
GI: Nausea, vomiting
GU: Urinary retention
RESP: Respiratory difficulty
SKIN: Hemorrhage at inj site, pallor, urticaria, wheal
DRUG INTERACTIONS
Drugs
3 *β-blockers:* Noncardioselective β-blockers enhance pressor response to epinephrine resulting in hypertension and bradycardia
3 *Chlorpromazine, clozaril, thioridazine:* Reversal of epinephrine pressor response
2 *Cyclic antidepressants:* Pressor response to IV epinephrine markedly enhanced

---

* = non FDA-approved use

SPECIAL CONSIDERATIONS
PATIENT/FAMILY EDUCATION
• Do not exceed recommended doses
• Wait at least 3-5 min between inhalations with MDI
• Notify clinician of dizziness or chest pain
• Do not use nasal preparations for >3-5 days to prevent rebound congestion
• To avoid contamination of ophth preparations, do not touch tip of container to any surface
• Do not use ophth preparations while wearing soft contact lenses
• Transitory stinging may occur on instillation of ophth preparations
• Report any decrease in visual acuity immediately
MONITORING PARAMETERS
• Blood pressure, heart rate
• Intraocular pressure

---

epoprostenol (prostacyclin)
(e-poe-pros'ten-ol)
Rx: Flolan
Chemical Class: Prostaglandin
Therapeutic Class: Vasodilator

CLINICAL PHARMACOLOGY
Mechanism of Action: Direct vasodilator of pulmonary and systemic arterial vascular beds; reduces right and left ventricular afterload, increases cardiac output and stroke volume, decreases pulmonary vascular resistance and mean systemic arterial pressure, inhibits platelet aggregation; may also induce bronchodilation, inhibit gastric acid secretion, and decrease gastric emptying
Pharmacokinetics
IV INF: Steady state reached in 15 min; extensively hydrolyzed in blood, some metabolites have pharmacologic activity; excreted (82%) in urine; $t_{1/2}$ 6 min
INDICATIONS AND USES: Long-term IV treatment of primary pulmonary hypertension in New York Heart Association Class III and Class IV patients
DOSAGE
Adult
• IV INF, acute: 2 ng/kg/min, increase by 2 ng/kg/min q15 min until limited by adverse effects, mean maximum-tolerated dose in trials was 8.6 ± 0.3 ng/kg/min
• IV INF, chronic: Initiate at 4 ng/kg/min less than maximum-tolerated rate or at 1/2 maximum-tolerated rate if maximum rate (5 ng/kg/min; increases in rate can be made by 1-2 ng/kg/min q 15 min, decreases by 2 ng/kg/min q 15 min
S AVAILABLE FORMS/COST OF THERAPY
• Inj, dry sol—IV: 0.5 mg/vial: **$15.78;** 1.5 mg/vial: **$31.56;** diluent separate: **$9.48**
CONTRAINDICATIONS: CHF secondary to severe left ventricular systolic dysfunction, patients unable to commit to administration and care of indwelling central venous catheter
PRECAUTIONS: Elderly, concurrent vasodilator use
PREGNANCY AND LACTATION: Pregnancy category B; unknown if excreted in breast milk
SIDE EFFECTS/ADVERSE REACTIONS
CNS: Agitation, anxiety, headache, hyperesthesia, hypoesthesia, nervousness, paresthesia, tremor
CV: Bradycardia, chest pain, dizziness, flushing, hypotension, syncope, tachycardia
GI: Abdominal pain, diarrhea, dyspepsia, *nausea, vomiting*
MS: Back pain, jaw pain, musculoskeletal pain, myalgia

RESP: Dyspnea
MISC: Chills, fever, flulike syndrome, sweating

SPECIAL CONSIDERATIONS
• Clinically shown to improve exercise capacity, dyspnea, and fatigue as early as 1st week of therapy
• Drug is administered chronically on an ambulatory basis with a portable infusion pump through a permanent central venous cathether; peripheral IV infusions may be used temporarily until central venous access obtained
• Patients must be taught sterile technique, drug reconstitution, and care of catheter
• Do not interrupt infusion or decrease rate abruptly
• Unless contraindicated, patients should be anticoagulated to reduce risk of pulmonary thromboembolism or systemic embolism through a patent foramen ovale
MONITORING PARAMETERS
• Postural BP and heart rate for several hr following dosage adjustments

---

eptifibatide
(ep-ti'fib-a-tyde)
Rx: Integrilin
Chemical Class: Platelet glycoprotein IIb/IIIa receptor antagonist
Therapeutic Class : Antiplatelet

CLINICAL PHARMACOLOGY
Mechanism of Action: Reversibly antagonizes binding of fibrinogen, von Willebrand factor, and other adhesive ligands to GP IIb/IIIa receptor, a platelet surface receptor, thus inhibiting platelet aggregation
Pharmacokinetics
Range of 40%-90% inhibition of platelet aggregation at steady state; plasma $t_{1/2}$ 2 1/2 hr; protein binding is minimal; renal clearance accounts for about 50% of total body clearance, no major metabolites
INDICATIONS AND USES: For treatment of patients with acute coronary syndrome, including patients who are to be managed medically and those undergoing percutaneous coronary intervention. Also indicated for treatment of patients undergoing percutaneous coronary intervention. Usually administered in combination with heparin and aspirin for both indications
DOSAGE
Adult
• *Acute coronary syndrome:* IV bolus of 180 µg/kg as soon as possible following diagnosis, followed by continuous infusion of 2 µg/kg/min until hospital discharge or initiation of CABG surgery, up to 72 hr. If patient is undergoing percutaneous coronary intervention while receiving eptifibatide, consideration can be given to decreasing infusion rate to 0.5 µg/kg/min. Infusion should be continued for additional 20-24 hr after procedure, allowing for up to 96 hr of therapy. Patients weighing >121 kg have received maximum bolus of 22.6 mg followed by maximum infusion of 15 mg/hr
• *Percutaneous coronary intervention in patients not presenting with acute coronary syndrome:* IV bolus of 135 µg/kg/min administered immediately before initiation of PCI followed by a continuous infusion of 0.5 µg/kg/min for 20-24 hr.
• In patients with serum creatinine levels between 2.0 mg/dl and 4.0 mg/dl, the 135 µg/kg bolus and 0.5 µg/kg/min infusion should be administered. Little experience with patients weighing >143 kg
• Bolus dose should be given IV push over 1-2 min
S AVAILABLE FORMS/COST OF THERAPY
• IV: 2 mg/ml 10 ml vial (for bolus dose): **$50.40;** 0.75 mg/ml 100 ml vial (for infusion): **$157.50**

---

italic = common side effects

bold italic = life-threatening reactions

CONTRAINDICATIONS: History of bleeding diathesis or evidence of active abnormal bleeding within previous 30 days; severe hypertension (systolic blood pressure >200 mm Hg or diastolic blood pressure >110 mm Hg) not adequately controlled; major surgery within preceding 6 wk; history of stroke within 30 days or any history of hemorrhagic stroke; current or planned administration of another parenteral GP IIa/IIIb inhibitor; platelet count <100,000/mm³; serum creatinine ≥4.0 mg/dl (for the 135 μg/kg bolus and the 0.5 μg/kg/min infusion); dependency on renal dialysis; known hypersensitivity to any component of product

PRECAUTIONS: Bleeding precautions; added care of femoral artery access site in patients undergoing percutaneous coronary intervention; use of thrombolytics, anticoagulants, and other antiplatelet agents; minimize vascular and other trauma; renal insufficiency

PREGNANCY AND LACTATION: Pregnancy category B; animal studies revealed no evidence of harm to fetus; no studies in pregnant women; should be used during pregnancy only if clearly needed; not known if present in human milk

SIDE EFFECTS/ADVERSE REACTIONS

*CV: **Hypotension***

*HEME: **Bleeding, intracranial hemorrhage, thrombocytopenia***

MISC: Anaphylaxis

DRUG INTERACTIONS

Drugs

❷ *Thrombolytics:* Increase in bleeding time, use caution

❷ *Oral antiagulants:* Increase in bleeding time, use caution

❷ *NSAIDs:* Increase in bleeding time, use caution

❷ *Dipyridamole:* Increase in bleeding time, use caution

❷ *Ticlopidine:* Increase in bleeding time, use caution

❷ *Clopidogrel:* Increase in bleeding time, use caution

❷ *Platelet receptor GP IIb/IIIa inhibitors:* Concomitant treatment should be avoided

SPECIAL CONSIDERATIONS

• For acute coronary syndrome, shown to decrease rate of combined end point of death or new MI

• For percutaneous coronary intervention, shown to decrease rate of combined end point of death, new MI, or need for urgent intervention

• Patients in the PURSUIT study >75 years had to weigh ≥50 kg to be enrolled

• Should not be administered through same line as furosemide

MONITORING PARAMETERS

• Monitor Htc or Hgb, platelet count, serum creatinine, and PT/aPTT. In patients undergoing percutaneous coronary intervention, monitor activated clotting time as well

---

esmolol

(ess′moe-lol)

Rx: Brevibloc

Chemical Class: β₁-selective (cardioselective) adrenoceptor blocker

Therapeutic Class: Antidysrhythmic (Class II)

CLINICAL PHARMACOLOGY

Mechanism of Action: Preferentially competes with β-adrenergic agonists for available β₁-receptor sites inhibiting the chronotropic and inotropic responses to β₁-adrenergic stimulation (cardioselective); slows conduction of AV node, decreases heart rate, decreases O₂ consumption in myocardium, also decreases renin-aldosterone-angiotensin system at higher doses; blocks β₂-receptors in bronchial system at higher doses; lacks membrane stabilizing or intrinsic sympathomimetic (partial agonist) activities

Pharmacokinetics

IV: Onset very rapid, duration short; 55% bound to plasma proteins; metabolized by hydrolysis of the ester linkage by esterases in the cytosol of red blood cells, excreted via kidneys; $t_{1/2}$ 9 min

INDICATIONS AND USES: Supraventricular tachycardia; noncompensatory sinus tachycardia; angina pectoris*

DOSAGE

Adult

• IV 500 μg/kg loading dose over 1 min, follow with 50 μg/kg/min INF for 4 min; if therapeutic response inadequate, rebolus with 500 μg/kg over 1 min and increase INF by 50 μg/kg/min for 4 min; repeat this process until therapeutic effect achieved or max dose of 200 μg/kg/min

💲 AVAILABLE FORMS/COST OF THERAPY

• Inj, Sol—IV: 10 mg/ml, 10 ml: **$15.48**; 250 mg/ml, 10 ml: **$73.20**

CONTRAINDICATIONS: Sinus bradycardia, heart block greater than 1st degree, cardiogenic shock or overt heart failure

PRECAUTIONS: Hypotension, peripheral vascular disease, diabetes, hypoglycemia, thyrotoxicosis, renal disease, asthma, children

PREGNANCY AND LACTATION: Pregnancy category C; potential for hypotension and subsequent decreased uterine blood flow and fetal hypoxia should be considered; excretion into breast milk unknown; use caution in nursing mothers

SIDE EFFECTS/ADVERSE REACTIONS

CNS: Depression, *dizziness,* drowsiness, *fatigue,* hallucinations, insomnia, *lethargy,* memory loss, mental changes, strange dreams

CV: Bradycardia, **CHF,** cold extremities, *hypotension,* **2nd or 3rd degree heart block**

EENT: Dry, burning eyes; sore throat; visual disturbances

GI: Diarrhea, dry mouth, **ischemic colitis, mesenteric arterial thrombosis,** *nausea,* vomiting

GU: Impotence, sexual dysfunction

HEME: **Agranulocytosis, thrombocytopenia**

METAB: Masked hypoglycemic response to insulin (sweating excepted)

RESP: **Bronchospasm,** dyspnea, wheezing

SKIN: Alopecia, pruritus, rash

SPECIAL CONSIDERATIONS

• Transfer to alternative agent (e.g., propranolol, digoxin, verapamil): ½ hr after 1st dose of alternative agent, reduce esmolol INF rate by 50%; following 2nd dose of alternative agent, monitor patient's response and, if satisfactory control is maintained for the 1st hr, discontinue esmolol INF

MONITORING PARAMETERS

• Blood pressure, ECG, heart rate, respiratory rate, IV site

---

ethacrynic acid

(eth-a-kri′nik)

Rx: Edecrin

Chemical Class: Ketone derivative of aryloxyacetic acid

Therapeutic Class: Loop diuretic

CLINICAL PHARMACOLOGY

Mechanism of Action: Acts on loop of Henle to inhibit resorption of sodium and water

Pharmacokinetics

PO: Onset ½ hr, peak 2 hr, duration 6-8 hr

IV: Onset 5 min, peak 15-30 min, duration 2 hr

Excreted in urine and feces, crosses placenta; $t_{1/2}$ 30-70 min

---

* = non FDA-approved use

INDICATIONS AND USES: Pulmonary edema; edema in CHF, liver disease, renal disease including nephrotic syndrome, ascites; glaucoma*; hypertension (in combination with other agents),* hypercalcemia*
DOSAGE
Adult
• PO 50-200 mg/day; may give up to 200 mg bid, adjust dose in 25-50 mg increments; IV 50 mg or 0.5-1.0 mg/kg given over several min
Child
PO 25 mg, increased by 25 mg/day until desired effect occurs; not established for infants or parenterally
💲 **AVAILABLE FORMS/COST OF THERAPY**
• Inj, Sol—IV: 50 mg/vial: **$19.75**
• Tab, Uncoated—Oral: 25 mg, 100's: **$30.96;** 50 mg, 100's: **$44.13**
CONTRAINDICATIONS: Anuria, hypovolemia, electrolyte depletion, infants
PRECAUTIONS: Dehydration, ascites, severe renal disease, hypoproteinemia, cirrhosis (may precipitate hepatic encephalopathy), concurrent administration of other ototoxic drugs, sulfa allergy
PREGNANCY AND LACTATION: Pregnancy category B; no data on nursing; contraindicated per manufacturer
SIDE EFFECTS/ADVERSE REACTIONS
CNS: Encephalopathy in hepatic disease, fatigue, headache, vertigo, weakness
CV: Chest pain, ***circulatory collapse,*** ECG changes, hypotension
EENT: Blurred vision, ear pain, hearing loss, tinnitus
GI: Abdominal distension, abdominal pain, ***acute pancreatitis,*** anorexia, cramps, dry mouth, ***GI bleeding,*** jaundice, nausea, severe diarrhea, upset stomach, vomiting
GU: Glycosuria, polyuria, ***renal failure,*** sexual dysfunction
HEME: ***Agranulocytosis, leukopenia, neutropenia, thrombocytopenia***
METAB: Decreased glucose tolerance, hyperglycemia, hyperuricemia, hypocalcemia, hypochloremic alkalosis, *hypokalemia,* hypomagnesemia, hyponatremia
MS: Arthritis, cramps, stiffness
SKIN: Photosensitivity, pruritus, purpura, rash, ***Stevens-Johnson syndrome,*** sweating
DRUG INTERACTIONS
Drugs
🔢 *ACE inhibitors:* Renal insufficiency, hypotension
🔢 *Aminoglycosides,* cisplatin: Increased ototoxicity
🔢 *Cephaloridine:* Combination may result in nephrotoxicity
🔢 *Digitalis:* Hypokalemia-induced digitalis toxicity

SPECIAL CONSIDERATIONS
• Reserve for patients not responding to or intolerant of furosemide or bumetanide

---

felodipine
(fell-o'da-peen)
Rx: Plendil, Renedil ✤
Combinations
  Rx: with enalapril (Lexxel)
Chemical Class: Dihydropyridine; calcium channel blocker
Therapeutic Class: Antihypertensive; antianginal

CLINICAL PHARMACOLOGY
Mechanism of Action: Inhibits calcium ion influx across cell membrane, resulting in dilation of peripheral arteries; no effects on cardiac conduction system; generally associated with increased myocardial contractility, cardiac output, and significantly decreased peripheral vascular resistance
Pharmacokinetics
PO: Onset 2-5 hr, peak 2.5-5 hr, well absorbed; 99% protein bound; metabolized in liver, 0.5% excreted unchanged in urine; $t_{1/2}$ 11-16 hr
INDICATIONS AND USES: Essential hypertension, vasospastic angina,* effort-associated angina,* primary pulmonary hypertension,* Raynaud's disease*
DOSAGE
Adult
• *Hypertension:* PO 5 mg qd initially (2.5 mg in elderly and impaired liver function), usual range 5-10 mg qd; do not exceed 20 mg qd; do not adjust dosage at intervals of <2 wk
💲 **AVAILABLE FORMS/COST OF THERAPY**
Tab, Uncoated, SUS Action—Oral: 2.5, 5 mg, 100's: **$90.50;** 10 mg, 100's: **$162.62**
PRECAUTIONS: Hypotension (<90 mm Hg systolic), hepatic injury, children, renal disease, elderly
PREGNANCY AND LACTATION: Pregnancy category C
SIDE EFFECTS/ADVERSE REACTIONS
CNS: Anxiety, depression, dizziness, fatigue, headache, insomnia, lightheadedness, tinnitus
CV: Edema, hypotension, ***MI,*** palpitations, pulmonary edema, tachycardia, syncope
EENT: Cough, epistaxis, nasal congestion
GI: Gastric upset, gingival hyperplasia
GU: Nocturia, polyuria
HEME: Anemia
RESP: Shortness of breath, wheezing
SKIN: Pruritus, rash
MISC: Flushing, sexual difficulties
DRUG INTERACTIONS
Drugs
🔢 *Carbamazepine:* Reduced felodipine bioavailability
🔢 *Erythromycin:* Increased felodipine concentrations
🔢 *Grapefruit juice:* Inhibits felodipine metabolism, 200% increase in AUC
🔢 *Propranolol:* Enhanced hypotension, increased propranolol concentrations

SPECIAL CONSIDERATIONS
• Results of V-HeFT III indicate felodipine may be used safely in patients with left ventricular dysfunction
PATIENT/FAMILY EDUCATION
• Administer as whole tablet (do not crush or chew)
• Avoid grapefruit juice (see drug interactions)

---

fenofibrate, micronized
(phe'-no-fy-brate)
Rx: TriCor
Chemical Class: Fibric acid derivative
Therapeutic Class: Antihyperlipidemic

CLINICAL PHARMACOLOGY
Mechanism of Action: Not well established; lowers plasma triglyceridces by inhibiting triglyceride synthesis; stimulates breakdown of triglyceride-rich lipoprotein
Pharmacokinetics
PO: Peak plasma levels 6-8 hr, absorption increased with food, protein binding 99%, hydrolyzed by esterases to active metabolite, fenofibric acid, metabolites excreted in urine, $t_{1/2}$ 20 hr

---

italic = common side effects

bold italic = life-threatening reactions

INDICATIONS AND USES: Adjunctive therapy to diet for adult patients with very high elevations of serum triglycerides or who are at risk of pancreatitis

DOSAGE

Initial dose is 67 mg/day, titrate to effect. Reduce dose for severe renal impairment (creatinine clearance <50 ml/min). Maximum dose is three 67 mg capsules or one 200 mg capsule per day. The elderly and those with renal impairment should receive 67 mg daily.

S AVAILABLE FORMS/COST OF THERAPY

• Tab—Oral: 67 mg, 90's: **$56.85;** 200 mg, 90's: **$170.55**

CONTRAINDICATIONS: Hypersensitivity to fenofibrate; hepatic or severe renal dysfunction; preexisting gallbladder disease; patients with unexplained persistent liver function abnormality

PRECAUTIONS: Periodic blood counts are recommended; monitor liver function throughout course of therapy; rhabdomyolysis, renal impairment

PREGNANCY AND LACTATION: Pregnancy category C; teratogenic in animals; should not be used in nursing mothers; potential for tumorigenicity

SIDE EFFECTS/ADVERSE REACTIONS

CNS: Decreased libido, dizziness, increased appetite, insomnia, **_paresthesia_**

CV: Arrhythmia

EENT: Eye irritation, blurred vision

GI: Dyspepsia, elevated LFT, cholelithiasis, pancreatitis, nausea, vomiting, diarrhea

GU: Polyuria, vaginitis

*HEME: **Anemia, leukopenia, thrombocytopenia***

MS: Arthralgia, rhabdomyolysis

RESP: Rhinitis, cough, sinusitis

SKIN: Rash, pruritus

MISC: Fatigue, infections, flu syndrome, pain, headache

DRUG INTERACTIONS

Drugs

❷ *Anticoagulants:* Prolonged PT

🔲 *Bile acid sequestrants:* May bind to fenofibrate, impeding its absorption

❷ *Cyclosporine:* Increased risk of nephrotoxicity

❷ *HMG-CoA reductase inhibitors:* Rhabdomyolysis, severe myopathy, acute renal failure

MONITORING PARAMETERS

• Obtain periodic LFTs including ALT for the duration of treatment. Monitor CBC for anemia, thrombocytopenia, signs of rhabdomyolysis. Monitor renal function

---

fenoldopam

(fen-ole'doe-pam)

Rx: Corlopam

Chemical Class: Benzazepine derivative

Therapeutic Class: Antihypertensive

CLINICAL PHARMACOLOGY

Mechanism of Action: Selective agonist at dopamine (DA₁) receptors; exerts hypotensive effects via decrease in peripheral vascular resistance, with increased renal blood flow, diuresis, and natriuresis

Pharmacokinetics

IV: Onset 20 min, duration 1 hr following discontinuation of infusion; metabolized in liver to a variety of sulfate, glucuronide and methoxy metabolites; 80% excreted in urine (metabolites), 20% excreted in feces; elimination $t_{1/2}$ 10 min

INDICATIONS AND USES: Treatment of hypertension in patients during or shortly after surgery, treatment in hypertension in patients unable to take oral medications

DOSAGE

Adult

• IV INF 0.1 μg/kg/min initially with upward titration; average required maintenance dose in clinical studies was 0.5 μg/kg/min; in severe CHF, doses of 0.1-1.5 μg/kg/min have been studied

S AVAILABLE FORMS/COST OF THERAPY

Not available

PRECAUTIONS: History of portal hypertension or previous variceal bleeding; history of dysrhythmia; CAD; angle-closure glaucoma

PREGNANCY AND LACTATION: Pregnancy category not available

SIDE EFFECTS/ADVERSE REACTIONS

CNS: Dizziness, *headache*

CV: Angina, **_dysrhythmia,_** ECG changes, hypotension, peripheral edema, *tachycardia*

EENT: Blurred vision, increased intraocular pressure

GI: Diarrhea, dry mouth, nausea, vomiting

SKIN: Flushing

SPECIAL CONSIDERATIONS

• Equivalent to nitroprusside in head-to-head comparison in patients with severe hypertension; renal function was improved in patients with hypertension and renal dysfunction

• Use should probably be limited to those patients with severe hypertension

MONITORING PARAMETERS

• Blood pressure, heart rate, urine volume, urinary sodium, serum creatinine, and BUN

---

flecainide

(fle'kah-nide)

Rx: Tambocor

Chemical Class: Benzamide derivative

Therapeutic Class: Antidysrhythmic (Class IC)

CLINICAL PHARMACOLOGY

Mechanism of Action: Produces a dose-related decrease in intracardiac conduction in all parts of the heart with the greatest effect on the His-Purkinje system; causes slight prolongation of refractory periods; decreases the rate of rise of the action potential without affecting its duration

Pharmacokinetics

PO: Peak 3 hr, 40%-50% bound to plasma proteins (α₁-glycoprotein), $t_{1/2}$ 12-27 hr; metabolized by liver, excreted by kidneys

INDICATIONS AND USES: Paroxysmal atrial fibrillation (PAF) and paroxysmal supraventricular tachycardias (PSVT) associated with disabling symptoms; documented life-threatening ventricular dysrhythmias

DOSAGE

Adult

• *PSVT and PAF:* PO 50 mg q12h; may increase q4d by 50 mg q12h to desired response; not to exceed 300 mg/day

• *Sustained ventricular tachycardia:* PO 100 mg q12h; may increase q4d by 50 mg q12h to desired response; not to exceed 400 mg/day

Child

• PO 3 mg/kg/day divided tid; may increase up to 11 mg/kg/day for uncontrolled patients with subtherapeutic levels

S AVAILABLE FORMS/COST OF THERAPY

• Tab, Uncoated—Oral: 50 mg, 100's: **$67.20;** 100 mg, 100's: **$122.04;** 150 mg, 100's: **$167.94**

---

* = non FDA-approved use

CONTRAINDICATIONS: Severe heart block, cardiogenic shock, nonsustained ventricular dysrhythmias, frequent PVCs, non-life-threatening dysrhythmias (due to proarrhythmic effects), recent MI
PRECAUTIONS: Children, renal disease, liver disease, CHF, respiratory depression, myasthenia gravis, sick sinus syndrome, electrolyte disturbances
PREGNANCY AND LACTATION: Pregnancy category C; excreted into breast milk with milk-plasma ratios 1.6:3.7, but considered compatible with breast feeding
SIDE EFFECTS/ADVERSE REACTIONS
CNS: Amnesia, anxiety, ataxia, confusion, depression, *dizziness, euphoria, faintness, fatigue, headache,* hypoesthesia, insomnia, *lightheadedness,* malaise, neuropathy, paresis, paresthesia, *seizures,* somnolence, stupor, syncope, tremor, twitching, unsteadiness, vertigo, weakness
CV: Angina pectoris, *AV block, bradycardia,* chest pain, *CHF, dysrhythmia,* edema, hypertension, hypotension, palpitation, *sinus arrest, sinus pause,* tachycardia
EENT: Blurred vision, diplopia; eye pain, irritation; nystagmus, photophobia, visual disturbances
GI: Abdominal pain, anorexia, change in taste, *constipation,* dry mouth, dyspepsia, flatulence, *nausea,* vomiting
GU: Decreased libido, impotence, polyuria, urinary retention
HEME: **Leukopenia, thrombocytopenia**
MS: Arthralgia, myalgia
RESP: **Bronchospasm**
SKIN: Alopecia, **exfoliative dermatitis,** pruritus, rash, urticaria
DRUG INTERACTIONS
Drugs
◧*Acetazolamide, ammonium chloride, antacids, sodium bicarbonate:* Increases in urine pH decreases flecainide urinary clearance
◧*Amiodarone:* Reduced flecainide dosage requirements
◧*Cimetidine:* Inhibits metabolism of flecainide
◧*Propranolol:* Inhibitors of each other's metabolism; additive negative inotropic effects
◧*Sotalol:* Additive myocardial conduction depression; cardiac arrest reported

SPECIAL CONSIDERATIONS
• Not 1st line therapy
• Reserve for resistant arrhythmias due to proarrhythmic effects
MONITORING PARAMETERS
• Monitor trough plasma levels periodically, especially in patients with moderate to severe chronic renal failure or severe hepatic disease and CHF; therapeutic range 0.2-1 µg/ml

---

fluvastatin
(floo'va-sta-tin)
Rx: Lescol
Chemical Class: HMG-CoA reductase inhibitor
Therapeutic Class: Antilipemic

CLINICAL PHARMACOLOGY
Mechanism of Action: Competitively inhibits HMG-CoA reductase, thereby reducing hepatic cholesterol synthesis; this causes an increase in LDL receptors and LDL clearance
Pharmacokinetics
PO: Onset 15 min, peak 30-60 min, duration 3-4 hr; fully absorbed if taken without food; food slows absorption and reduces peak plasma level by 50%-70%; protein binding 98%; $t_{1/2}$ 0.5-1 hr; metabolized in liver, excreted in bile

INDICATIONS AND USES: Primary hypercholesterolemia; slow progression of coronary atherosclerosis in patients with coronary artery disease
DOSAGE
Adult
• PO: 20-40 mg hs, increase to 40 mg bid if necessary
⑤**AVAILABLE FORMS/COST OF THERAPY**
• Cap—Oral: 20 mg, 100's: **$114.90**; 40 mg, 100's: **$128.46**
CONTRAINDICATIONS: Pregnancy, lactation, active liver disease, unexplained transaminase elevations
PRECAUTIONS: History of liver disease, heavy ethanol use, patients at risk for rhabdomyolysis (acute infection, hypotension, major surgery, or trauma)
PREGNANCY AND LACTATION: Pregnancy category X; contraindicated in breast feeding
SIDE EFFECTS/ADVERSE REACTIONS
CNS: **Headache,** insomnia
GI: Diarrhea, dyspepsia, elevated transaminase levels (1%), **hepatotoxicity,** nausea
MS: Myalgia, myopathy, **rhabdomyolysis**
DRUG INTERACTIONS
Drugs
❷*Azole antifungals (fluconazole, itraconazole, ketoconazole, miconazole):* Increased fluvastatin levels via inhibition of metabolism with increased risk of rhabdomyolysis
◧*Cholestyramine, colestipol:* Reduced bioavailability of fluvastatin
◧*Danazol:* Inhibition of metabolism (CYP3A4) thought to yield increased fluvastatin levels with increased risk of rhabdomyolysis
◧*Fluoxetine:* Less likely to inhibit CYP3A4 hepatic metabolism (vs lovastatin) with less risk of rhabdomyolysis
❷*Gemfibrozil:* Small increased risk of myopathy with combination
◧*Isradipine:* Isradipine probably decreases fluvastatin plasma concentrations minimally
◧*Macrolide antibiotics (clarithromycin, erythromycin, troleandomycin):* Increased fluvastatin levels via inhibition of metabolism with increased risk of rhabdomyolysis
◧*Nefazodone:* Less likely to inhibit CYP3A4 hepatic metabolism (vs lovastatin) with less risk of rhabdomyolysis
◧*Terbinafine:* Minimal effect on the metabolism of fluvastatin
◧*Warfarin:* Addition of fluvastatin may increase hypoprothrombinemic response to warfarin via inhibition of metabolism (CYP2C9)

---

fosinopril
(foss-in-o'pril)
Rx: Monopril
Combinations
  Rx: with hydrochlorothiazide (Monopril-HCT)
Chemical Class: Angiotensin-converting enzyme (ACE) inhibitor
Therapeutic Class: Antihypertensive; congestive heart failure; renal protectant

CLINICAL PHARMACOLOGY
Mechanism of Action: Selectively suppresses renin-angiotensin-aldosterone system; inhibits ACE preventing conversion of angiotensin I to angiotensin II; results in dilation of arterial, venous vessels

---

italic = common side effects

bold italic = life-threatening reactions

Pharmacokinetics
PO: Onset 1 hr, duration 24 hr, peak 3 hr; metabolized to active metabolite (fosinoprilat), $t_{1/2}$ (fosinoprilat) 12 hr; excreted in urine (50%) and feces (50%)

INDICATIONS AND USES: Hypertension, CHF,* diabetic nephropathy,* left ventricular dysfunction after MI*

DOSAGE

Adult
• PO 10 mg qd initially, then 20-40 mg/day divided bid or qd, max 80 mg/day

$ AVAILABLE FORMS/COST OF THERAPY
• Tab, Uncoated—Oral: 10 mg, 100's: **$72.98;** 20 mg, 100's: **$78.11;** 40 mg, 30's: **$23.92**

PRECAUTIONS: Impaired renal and liver function, dialysis patients, hypovolemia, diuretic therapy, collagen-vascular diseases, CHF, elderly, bilateral renal artery stenosis

PREGNANCY AND LACTATION: Pregnancy category C (1st trimester), category D (2nd and 3rd trimesters); ACE inhibitors can cause fetal and neonatal morbidity and death when administered to pregnant women; when pregnancy is detected, discontinue ACE inhibitors as soon as possible; detectable in breast milk in trace amounts, a newborn would receive <0.1% of the mg/kg maternal dose; effect on nursing infant has not been determined; use with caution in nursing mothers

SIDE EFFECTS/ADVERSE REACTIONS
CNS: Anxiety, *dizziness, fatigue, headache,* insomnia, paresthesia
CV: Angina, hypotension, palpitations, postural hypotension, syncope (especially with 1st dose)
GI: Abdominal pain, constipation, melena, nausea, vomiting
GU: Decreased libido, impotence, increased BUN, creatinine, UTI
HEME: **Agranulocytosis, neutropenia**
METAB: Hyperkalemia, hyponatremia
MS: Arthralgia, arthritis, myalgia
RESP: Asthma, bronchitis, *cough,* dyspnea, sinusitis
SKIN: **Angioedema,** flushing, rash, sweating

DRUG INTERACTIONS

Drugs
❷ *Allopurinol:* Combination may predispose to hypersensitivity reactions
❸ *α-adrenergic blockers:* Exaggerated first dose hypotensive response when added to fosinopril
❸ *Aspirin:* May reduce hemodynamic effects of fosinopril; less likely at doses under 236 mg; less likely with nonacetylated salicylates
❸ *Cyclosporine:* Combination may cause renal insufficiency
❸ *Insulin:* Fosinopril may enhance insulin sensitivity
❶ *Iron:* Fosinopril may increase chance of systemic reaction to IV iron
❸ *Lithium:* Reduced lithium clearance
❸ *Loop diuretics:* Initiation of fosinopril may cause hypotension and renal insufficiency in patients taking loop diuretics
❸ *NSAIDs:* May reduce hemodynamic effects of fosinopril
❸ *Potassium-sparing diuretics:* Increased risk of hyperkalemia

SPECIAL CONSIDERATIONS

PATIENT/FAMILY EDUCATION
• Do not use salt substitutes containing potassium without consulting clinician

MONITORING PARAMETERS
• BUN, creatinine (watch for increased levels that may indicate acute renal failure)
• Potassium levels, although hyperkalemia rarely occurs

---

furosemide
(fur-oh'se-mide)
Rx: Furoside ♣, Lasix, Myrosemide, Novosemide ♣, Uritol ♣
Chemical Class: Anthranilic acid
Therapeutic Class: Loop diuretic

CLINICAL PHARMACOLOGY
Mechanism of Action: Inhibits the absorption of sodium and chloride not only in the proximal and distal tubules but also in the loop of Henle

Pharmacokinetis
PO: Onset 1 hr, peak 1-2 hr, duration 6-8 hr, 60% bioavailability
IV/IM: Onset 5 min (slightly delayed with IM), peak ½ hr (IM), duration 2 hr; 98% bound to plasma proteins; 50% of PO dose and 80% of IV dose excreted in the urine within 24 hr, remainder eliminated by non-renal pathways (liver metabolism, excreted unchanged in feces); $t_{1/2}$ 30 min (9 hr in renal failure)

INDICATIONS AND USES: Edema associated with CHF, hepatic cirrhosis, renal disease, nephrotic syndrome; hypertension, pulmonary edema, hypercalcemia*

DOSAGE

Adult
• PO 20-80 mg/day in AM; may give another dose in 6 hr; increase in increments of 20-40 mg up to 400 mg/day if response is not satisfactory
• IM/IV 20-40 mg, increased by 20 mg q2h until desired response (rule of thumb: IV dose = ½ PO dose)
• Pulmonary edema: IV 40 mg given over several min, repeated in 1 hr; increase to 80 mg if needed

Child
• PO/IM/IV 1-2 mg/kg/dose up to 6 mg/kg/day in divided doses q6-12h

$ AVAILABLE FORMS/COST OF THERAPY
• Inj, Sol—IM, IV: 10 mg/ml, 2, 4, 8, 10 ml: **$2.36-$6.88**/10 ml
• Sol—Oral: 10 mg/ml, 60, 120 ml: **$6.60-$11.10**/60 ml; 40 mg/5 ml, 500 ml: **$29.04**
• Tab, Uncoated—Oral: 20 mg, 100's: **$2.10-$16.65;** 40 mg, 100's: **$2.54-$23.00;** 80 mg, 100's: **$5.63-$36.55**

CONTRAINDICATIONS: Anuria

PRECAUTIONS: Diabetes mellitus, dehydration, severe renal disease, hepatic cirrhosis, ascites, systemic lupus erythematosus, gout

PREGNANCY AND LACTATION: Pregnancy category C; cardiovascular disorders such as pulmonary edema, severe hypertension, or CHF are probably the only valid indications for this drug during pregnancy; excreted into breast milk; no reports of adverse effects in nursing infants have been found; thiazide diuretics have been used to suppress lactation

SIDE EFFECTS/ADVERSE REACTIONS
CNS: Dizziness, fever, headache, paresthesia, restlessness, vertigo
CV: Chest pain, **circulatory collapse,** ECG changes, orthostatic hypotension
EENT: Blurred vision, ototoxicity
GI: Anorexia, constipation, cramping, diarrhea, dry mouth, ***ischemic hepatitis,*** jaundice, *nausea,* oral and gastric irritation, pancreatitis, vomiting
GU: Glycosuria, hyperuricemia, urinary bladder spasm
HEME: **Agranulocytosis, anemia, aplastic anemia, leukopenia,** purpura, **thrombocytopenia**
METAB: Hyperglycemia
SKIN: Erythema multiforme, ***exfoliative dermatitis,*** interstitial nephritis, necrotizing angiitis, photosensitivity, pruritus, *rash,* urticaria

---

DRUG INTERACTIONS
Drugs
❷ *Aminoglycosides (gentamicin, kanamycin, neomycin, streptomycin):* Additive ototoxicity (ethacrynic acid > furosemide, torsemide, bumetanide)
3 *Angiotensin-converting enzyme inhibitors:* Initiation of ACEI with intensive diuretic therapy may result in precipitous fall in blood pressure; ACEIs may induce renal insufficiency in the presence of diuretic-induced sodium depletion
3 *Barbiturates (phenobarbital):* Reduced diuretic response
3 *Bile acid-binding resins (cholestyramine, colestipol):* Resins markedly reduce the bioavailability and diuretic response of furosemide
3 *Carbenoxolone:* Severe hypokalemia from coadministration
3 *Cephalosporins (cephaloridine, cephalothin):* Enhanced nephrotoxicity with coadministration
❷ *Cisplatin:* Additive ototoxicity (ethacrynic acid > furosemide, torsemide, bumetanide)
3 *Clofibrate:* Enhanced effects of both drugs, especially in hypoalbuminemic patients
3 *Digitalis glycosides (digoxin, digitoxin):* Diuretic-induced hypokalemia may increase risk of digitalis toxicity
3 *Nonsteroidal antiinflammatory drugs (flurbiprofen, ibuprofen, indomethacin, naproxen, piroxicam, sulindac):* Reduced diuretic and antihypertensive effects
3 *Phenytoin:* Reduced diuretic response
3 *Serotonin-reuptake inhibitors (fluoxetine, paroxetine, sertraline):* Case reports of sudden death; enhanced hyponatremia proposed; causal relationships not established
3 *Terbutaline:* Additive hypokalemia
3 *Tubocurarine:* Prolonged neuromuscular blockade
Labs
• *Cortisol:* False increases
• *Glucose:* Falsely low urine tests with Clinistix and diastix
• *Thyroxine:* Increased serum concentration
• *T_3 uptake:* Interference causes increased serum values

SPECIAL CONSIDERATIONS
PATIENT/FAMILY EDUCATION
• May cause GI upset, take with food or milk
• Take early in the day
• Avoid prolonged exposure to sunlight
MONITORING PARAMETERS
• Frequent serum electrolyte, calcium, glucose, uric acid, creatinine, and BUN determinations during 1st months of therapy and periodically thereafter

---

gemfibrozil
(gem-fi'broe-zil)
Rx: Lopid
Chemical Class: Fibric acid derivative
Therapeutic Class: Antilipemic

CLINICAL PHARMACOLOGY
Mechanism of Action: Inhibits peripheral lipolysis and decreases hepatic extraction of free fatty acids, thus reducing hepatic triglyceride production; inhibits synthesis of VLDL carrier apolipoprotein B, leading to a decrease in VLDL production
Pharmacokinetics
PO: Peak 1-2 hr, 90% bound to plasma proteins, $t_{1/2}$ 1½ hr (biologic $t_{1/2}$ considerably longer due to enterohepatic recycling); metabolized in liver, excreted in urine (glucuronide conjugates)

INDICATIONS AND USES: Hypertriglyceridemia (types IV and V hyperlipidemia); type IIb hyperlipidemia
DOSAGE
Adult
• PO 600 mg bid, 30 min before morning and evening meals
⑤ AVAILABLE FORMS/COST OF THERAPY
• Tab, Plain Coated—Oral: 600 mg, 60's: **$10.80-$71.99**
CONTRAINDICATIONS: Severe hepatic disease, preexisting gallbladder disease, severe renal disease, primary biliary cirrhosis
PRECAUTIONS: Children, suspected cholelithiasis
PREGNANCY AND LACTATION: Pregnancy category B; excretion into breast milk unknown; use caution in nursing mothers
SIDE EFFECTS/ADVERSE REACTIONS
CNS: Fatigue, headache, hypesthesia, paresthesia, vertigo
CV: Atrial fibrillation
EENT: Blurred vision, cataracts, retinal edema
GI: Abdominal pain, constipation, diarrhea, *dyspepsia,* nausea, taste perversion, vomiting
GU: Impotence
HEME: **Anemia, bone marrow hypoplasia,** eosinophilia, **leukopenia, thrombocytopenia**
METAB: Increased blood glucose
MS: Arthralgia, myalgia, myasthenia, myopathy, painful extremities, rhabdomyolysis, synovitis
SKIN: Alopecia, dermatitis, **exfoliative dermatitis,** pruritus
MISC: Weight loss
DRUG INTERACTIONS
Drugs
3 *Binding resins:* Reduced bioavailability of gemfibrozil, separate doses by 2 hr
3 *Glyburide:* Increased risk of hypoglycemia
❷ *HMG CoA reductase inhibitors (lovastatin, simvastatin, atorvastatin):* Increased likelihood of drug-induced myopathy
3 *Pravastatin:* Increased likelihood of drug-induced myopathy
❷ *Warfarin:* Increased hypoprothrombinemic, response to warfarin

SPECIAL CONSIDERATIONS
PATIENT/FAMILY EDUCATION
• May cause dizziness or blurred vision; use caution while driving or performing other tasks requiring alertness
• Notify clinician if GI side effects become pronounced
MONITORING PARAMETERS
• Serum CK level in patients complaining of muscle pain, tenderness, or weakness
• Periodic CBC during first 12 mo of therapy
• Periodic LFTs; discontinue therapy if abnormalities persist
• Blood glucose

---

guanabenz
(gwan'a-benz)
Rx: Wytensin
Chemical Class: Dichlorobenzene derivative
Therapeutic Class: Antihypertensive

CLINICAL PHARMACOLOGY
Mechanism of Action: Stimulates central α_2-adrenergic receptors resulting in decreased sympathetic outflow to the heart, kidneys, and peripheral vasculature; decreases systolic and diastolic blood pressure, systemic vascular resistance, and slightly slows pulse

---

italic = common side effects

bold italic = life-threatening reactions

Pharmacokinetics
PO: Extensive 1st-pass metabolism; peak 2-5 hr, onset 1 hr, duration 12 hr; 90% bound to plasma proteins; metabolized (site undetermined) and excreted in urine and feces; $t_{1/2}$ approximately 6 hr
INDICATIONS AND USES: Hypertension
DOSAGE
Adult
• PO 4 mg bid initially, increase in 4-8 mg/day increments q1-2 wk prn, not to exceed 32 mg bid
⑤ **AVAILABLE FORMS/COST OF THERAPY**
• Tab, Uncoated—Oral: 4 mg, 100's: **$53.17-$79.46**; 8 mg, 100's: **$79.80-$119.30**
PRECAUTIONS: Severe coronary insufficiency, recent MI, cerebrovascular disease; severe renal, hepatic failure; sudden discontinuation, diabetes (causes hypoglycemia unawareness)
PREGNANCY AND LACTATION: Pregnancy category C; excretion into breast milk unknown; use caution in nursing mothers
SIDE EFFECTS/ADVERSE REACTIONS
CNS: Anxiety, ataxia, depression, *dizziness, drowsiness, headache, sedation,* sleep disturbance, *weakness*
CV: Chest pain, dysrhythmias, edema, palpitations, ***rebound hypertension with abrupt cessation***
EENT: Blurred vision, nasal congestion
GI: Abdominal discomfort, constipation, diarrhea, *dry mouth,* epigastric pain, nausea, taste disorder, vomiting
GU: Disturbances of sexual function, urinary frequency
METAB: Gynecomastia
MS: Myalgias
RESP: Dyspnea
SKIN: Pruritus, rash
DRUG INTERACTIONS
Drugs
③ *β-adrenergic blockers (noncardioselective):* May promote hypertension upon withdrawal of guanabenz
❷ *Desipramine:* Inhibits antihypertensive effect
③ *Tricyclic antidepressants:* Inhibits antihypertensive effect

SPECIAL CONSIDERATIONS
PATIENT/FAMILY EDUCATION
• Avoid hazardous activities, since drug may cause drowsiness
• Do not discontinue oral drug abruptly, or withdrawal symptoms may occur (anxiety, increased BP, headache, insomnia, increased pulse, tremors, nausea, sweating)
• Do not use OTC (cough, cold, or allergy) products unless directed by clinician
• Rise slowly to sitting or standing position to minimize orthostatic hypotension, especially elderly
• May cause dizziness, fainting, lightheadedness during 1st few days of therapy
• May cause dry mouth; use hard candy, saliva product, or frequent rinsing of mouth

---

guanethidine
(gwahn-eth'i-deen)
Rx: Ismelin
Chemical Class: Guanidine derivative
Therapeutic Class: Antihypertensive

CLINICAL PHARMACOLOGY
Mechanism of Action: Slowly displaces norepinephrine from its storage in nerve endings and thereby blocks the release of norepinephrine normally produced by nerve stimulation; leads to reduced arteriolar vasoconstriction, especially the reflex increase in sympathetic tone that occurs with a change in position
Pharmacokinetics
PO: Oral absorption highly variable (3%-30%), full therapeutic effect can take 1-3 wk; metabolized in liver, excreted in urine (25%-50% as unchanged drug); $t_{1/2}$ 4-8 days
INDICATIONS AND USES: Hypertension (not 1st-line)
DOSAGE
Adult
• Ambulatory patients: PO 10 mg qd, increase at 5-7 day intervals to a max of 25-50 mg/day
• Hospitalized patients: PO 25-50 mg qd; increase by 25-50 mg/day to desired therapeutic response
Child
• PO 0.2 mg/kg/day; increase by 0.2 mg/kg/day at 7-10 day intervals to a max of 3 mg/kg/day
⑤ **AVAILABLE FORMS/COST OF THERAPY**
• Tab, Uncoated—Oral: 10 mg, 100's: **$53.73**; 25 mg, 100's: **$87.80**
CONTRAINDICATIONS: Pheochromocytoma, CHF, concurrent use with or within 1 wk of MAOI
PRECAUTIONS: Elective surgery (discontinue 2 wk before procedure), fever (reduced dosage requirements), asthma, recent MI, CAD, peptic ulcer, elderly
PREGNANCY AND LACTATION: Pregnancy category C; excreted into breast milk in small quantities; problems in humans have not been documented
SIDE EFFECTS/ADVERSE REACTIONS
CNS: Dizziness, fatigue, *lassitude,* mental depression, tremor, weakness
CV: Angina, ***bradycardia, CHF,*** edema, fluid retention, *orthostatic hypotension,* syncope
EENT: Blurred vision, *nasal congestion,* ptosis of the lids
GI: Diarrhea, dry mouth, nausea, parotid tenderness, vomiting
GU: Impotence, *inhibition of ejaculation,* nocturia, priapism, rise in BUN, urinary incontinence
HEME: Anemia, ***leukopenia, thrombocytopenia***
MS: Myalgia, myopathy
RESP: Asthma, dyspnea
SKIN: Alopecia, dermatitis
DRUG INTERACTIONS
Drugs
❷ *Amitriptyline:* Inhibits antihypertensive effect
③ *Dextroamphetamine:* Inhibits antihypertensive effect
③ *Ephedrine:* Inhibits antihypertensive effect
③ *Haloperidol:* Inhibits antihypertensive effect
③ *MAOIs:* Inhibits antihypertensive effect
③ *Methylphenidate:* Inhibits antihypertensive effect
③ *Norepinephrine:* Exaggerated pressor response to norepinephrine
③ *Phenothiazines:* Inhibits antihypertensive effect
③ *Phenylephrine:* Guanethidine enhances pupillary response to phenylephrine
③ *Thiothixene:* Inhibits antihypertensive effect
③ *Tricyclic antidepressants:* Inhibits antihypertensive effect
Labs
• Increase: BUN

SPECIAL CONSIDERATIONS
PATIENT/FAMILY EDUCATION
• Arise slowly from a reclining position, especially in the morning
• Use alcohol with caution

---

* = non FDA-approved use

• Use caution when standing for prolonged periods of time, exercising, and during hot weather (enhanced orthostatic hypotension)
• Avoid OTC medications unless discussed with clinician
• Notify clinician of fever, severe diarrhea
• Do not discontinue abruptly
MONITORING PARAMETERS
• Sitting and standing blood pressure, pulse

guanfacine
(gwahn′fa-seen)
Rx: Tenex
Chemical Class: Dichlorobenzene derivative
Therapeutic Class: Antihypertensive

CLINICAL PHARMACOLOGY
Mechanism of Action: Stimulates central α_2-adrenergic receptors resulting in decreased sympathetic outflow to the heart, kidneys, and peripheral vasculature; decreases systolic and diastolic blood pressure, systemic vascular resistance, and slightly slows pulse
Pharmacokinetics
PO: Peak 1-4 hr, onset (multiple doses) 1 wk, 70% bound to plasma proteins, 50% bound to erythrocytes; metabolized in liver, excreted in urine (40% as unchanged drug); $t_{1/2}$ 17 hr
INDICATIONS AND USES: Hypertension, heroin withdrawal syndrome,* migraine headache*
DOSAGE
Adult
• PO 1 mg qd, increase to 2 mg qd after 3-4 wk prn
S AVAILABLE FORMS/COST OF THERAPY
• Tab, Uncoated—Oral: 1 mg, 100's: **$70.55-$97.09;** 2 mg, 100's: **$96.75-$128.93**
PRECAUTIONS: Chronic renal or hepatic failure, severe coronary insufficiency, recent MI, cerebrovascular disease, children, diabetes (causes hypoglycemia unawareness)
PREGNANCY AND LACTATION: Pregnancy category B; excretion into human breast milk unknown; excreted in the milk of lactating rats; use caution in nursing mothers
SIDE EFFECTS/ADVERSE REACTIONS
CNS: Dizziness, fatigue, headache, somnolence
CV: Bradycardia, chest pain, palpitations
EENT: Nasal congestion, rhinitis, taste change, tinnitus, vision change
GI: Constipation, cramps, diarrhea, *dry mouth,* nausea
GU: Impotence, urinary incontinence
MS: Leg cramps
RESP: Dyspnea
SKIN: Dermatitis, pruritus, purpura
DRUG INTERACTIONS
Drugs
⬛ *β-adrenergic blockers (noncardioselective):* May promote hypertension upon withdrawal of guanfacine
❷ *Desipramine:* Inhibits antihypertensive effect
⬛ *Tricyclic antidepressants:* Inhibit antihypertensive effect

SPECIAL CONSIDERATIONS
PATIENT/FAMILY EDUCATION
• Avoid hazardous activities, since drug may cause drowsiness
• Do not discontinue oral drug abruptly, or withdrawal symptoms may occur after 3-4 days (anxiety, increased BP, headache, insomnia, increased pulse, tremors, nausea, sweating)
• Do not use OTC (cough, cold, or allergy) products unless directed by clinician

• Rise slowly to sitting or standing position to minimize orthostatic hypotension, especially elderly
• Dizziness, fainting, lightheadedness may occur during 1st few days of therapy
• May cause dry mouth; use hard candy, saliva product, or frequent rinsing of mouth

heparin
(hep′a-rin)
Rx: Liquaemin
Chemical Class: Sulfated glycosaminoglycan
Therapeutic Class: Anticoagulant

CLINICAL PHARMACOLOGY
Mechanism of Action: Potentiates inhibitory action of antithrombin III (heparin cofactor) on several activated coagulation factors, including thrombin (factor IIa) and factors IXa, Xa, XIa, and XIIa, by forming a complex with and inducing a conformational change in the antithrombin III molecule
Pharmacokinetics
IV: Onset immediate (if no loading dose is given, onset may depend on rate of INF)
SC: Onset 20-60 min
Highly bound to plasma proteins; primary route of removal from circulation via uptake by the reticuloendothelial system; also metabolized by liver, eliminated in urine usually as metabolites (50% of IV dose may be excreted unchanged); $t_{1/2}$ 90 min
INDICATIONS AND USES: Venous thrombosis, pulmonary embolism, peripheral arterial embolism; coagulopathies (e.g., disseminated intravascular coagulation); DVT/PE prophylaxis; clotting prevention in arterial and heart surgery, blood transfusions, extracorporeal circulation, dialysis and blood samples; prophylaxis of LV thrombi and CVA after MI*; evolving stroke*; adjunctive therapy of coronary occlusion with acute MI*
DOSAGE
Adult
• *DVT/PE:* IV INF 50-100 U/kg initially, then 15-25 U/kg/hr, adjusted based on aPTT results; intermittent IV 10,000 U initially, then 75-125 U/kg q4-6h; SC 10,000-20,000 units initially, then 8000-10,000 U q8h, or 15,000-20,000 U q12h
• *Prevention of DVT/PE:* SC 5000 U q8-12h until patient is ambulatory
Child
• IV INF 50 U/kg initially, then 15-25 U/kg/hr, increase dose by 2-4 U/kg/hr q6-8h based on aPTT results; intermittent IV 50-100 U/kg initially, then 50-100 U/kg q4h
S AVAILABLE FORMS/COST OF THERAPY
• Inj, Sol—IM, SC: 40,000 U/ml: **$3.12-$7.50**/ml
• Inj, Sol—IV, SC: 1000 U/ml, 1, 2, 5, 10 ml: **$0.73-$1.11**/ml; 2500 U/ml, **$1.34**/ml; 5000 U/ml, 1 ml: **$1.03-$1.61**/ml; 10,000 U/ml, 0.5, 1, 2, 4, 5, 10 ml: **$1.71-$4.05**/ml; 20,000 U/ml, 1, 2, 5 ml: **$1.44-$7.61**/ml
CONTRAINDICATIONS: Severe thrombocytopenia, uncontrolled bleeding (except when due to DIC), suspected intracranial hemorrhage, shock, severe hypotension
PRECAUTIONS: IM inj (avoid due to risk for hematoma), elderly, children, diabetes, renal insufficiency, severe hypertension, subacute bacterial endocarditis, acute nephritis, peptic ulcer disease, severe renal disease
PREGNANCY AND LACTATION: Pregnancy category C; does not cross the placenta, has major advantages over oral anticoagulants as the treatment of choice during pregnancy; is not excreted into breast milk due to its high molecular weight

---

italic = common side effects   ***bold italic*** = life-threatening reactions

SIDE EFFECTS/ADVERSE REACTIONS
CNS: Fever, headache
CV: Allergic vasospastic reactions, shock
EENT: Lacrimation, rhinitis
GI: Nausea, vomiting
GU: Hematuria, priapism
HEME: Hemorrhage, thrombocytopenia, white clot syndrome (new thrombus formation associated with heparin administration)
METAB: Rebound hyperlipidemia, suppressed aldosterone synthesis,
MS: Osteoporosis (after long-term, high doses)
RESP: Anaphylactoid reactions, asthma
SKIN: Chills, *cutaneous necrosis,* delayed transient alopecia, erythema, hematoma/ulceration, histamine-like reactions, local irritation, urticaria

DRUG INTERACTIONS
Drugs
🔳 *Salicylates:* Increased risk of bleeding
🔳 *Warfarin:* Warfarin may prolong the aPTT in patients receiving heparin; heparin may prolong the PT in patients receiving warfarin

SPECIAL CONSIDERATIONS

PATIENT/FAMILY EDUCATION
• Use soft-bristle toothbrush to avoid bleeding gums; avoid contact sports; use electric razor; avoid IM inj
• Report any signs of bleeding: gums, under skin, urine, stools

MONITORING PARAMETERS
• aPTT (usual goal is to prolong aPTT to 1.5-2.5 times normal), usually measure 6-8 hr after initiation of IV and 6-8 hr after INF rate changes; increase or decrease INF by 2-4 U/kg/hr dependent on aPTT
• For intermittent inj, measure aPTT 3.5-4 hr after IV inj
• Platelet counts, signs of bleeding, Hgb, Hct

---

hydralazine
(hye-dral′a-zeen)
Rx: Apresoline, Novo-Hylazin ♣, Nu-Hydral ♣
Combinations
  Rx: with hydrochlorothiazide (Apresazide); with hydrochlorothiazide, reserpine (Ser-Ap-Es)
Chemical Class: Phthalazine derivative
Therapeutic Class: Antihypertensive; congestive heart failure agent

---

CLINICAL PHARMACOLOGY
Mechanism of Action: Preferentially dilates arterioles with little effect on veins; interferes with calcium movement within vascular smooth muscle responsible for initiating or maintaining the contractile state; increases cardiac output, decreases systemic resistance, reduces afterload
Pharmacokinetics
PO: Well absorbed; undergoes 1st-pass metabolism; bioavailability 50% (slow acetylators) or 30% (fast acetylators); peak 60 min, onset 45 min, duration 3-8 hr
IM: Onset 5-10 min, peak 1 hr, duration 2-4 hr
IV: Onset 10-20 min, duration 3-8 hr
Metabolized by liver (genetic variation among individuals in rate of acetylation), excreted in urine; $t_{1/2}$ 0.44-0.47 hr (metabolite 2-4 hr)
INDICATIONS AND USES: Hypertension, CHF,* afterload reduction in severe aortic insufficiency and after valve replacement*

DOSAGE
Adult
• PO 10 mg qid, increase by 10-25 mg/dose q2-5 days as needed to max of 300 mg/day; IM/IV 10-20 mg q4-6h, may increase to 40 mg/dose
Child
• PO 0.75-1 mg/kg/day divided bid-qid, increase over 3-4 wk to 7.5 mg/kg/day divided bid-qid if necessary, do not exceed 200 mg/day; IM/IV 0.1-0.2 mg/kg/dose q4-6h, do not exceed 20 mg/dose
💲 **AVAILABLE FORMS/COST OF THERAPY**
• Inj, Sol—IM, IV: 20 mg/ml, 1 ml: **$28.39-$147.85**
• Tab, Uncoated—Oral: 10 mg, 100's: **$1.88-$20.60;** 25 mg, 100's: **$1.68-$29.44;** 50 mg, 100's: **$2.05-$43.90;** 100 mg, 100's: **$4.28-$61.76**
CONTRAINDICATIONS: CAD, mitral valvular rheumatic heart disease
PRECAUTIONS: Advanced renal disease, children, pulmonary hypertension
PREGNANCY AND LACTATION: Pregnancy category C; commonly used in pregnant women; excreted into breast milk; compatible with breast feeding
SIDE EFFECTS/ADVERSE REACTIONS
CNS: Anxiety, dizziness, headache, peripheral neuritis, psychotic reactions, *tremor*
CV: Angina, edema, flushing, hypotension, *palpitations, reflex tachycardia*
EENT: Nasal congestion
GI: Anorexia, constipation, *diarrhea,* hepatitis, *nausea,* paralytic ileus, *vomiting*
GU: Urination difficulty
HEME: Agranulocytosis, anemia, eosinophilia, *leukopenia*
MS: Arthralgia, muscle cramps
RESP: Dyspnea
SKIN: Pruritus, rash, urticaria
MISC: Lupus-like syndrome (arthralgia, dermatoses, fever, splenomegaly, glomerulonephritis)
DRUG INTERACTIONS
Drugs
🔳 *Diazoxide:* Severe hypotension
🔳 *NSAIDs:* Inhibited antihypertensive response to hydralazine
Labs
False increase: Ca^{++} (slight); urine 17-ketogenic steroids; glucose, uric acid
False decrease: Glucose, uric acid
SPECIAL CONSIDERATIONS
• Lupus-like syndrome more common in "slow acetylators" and following higher doses for prolonged periods
PATIENT/FAMILY EDUCATION
• Take with meals
• Notify clinician of any unexplained prolonged general tiredness or fever, muscle or joint aching, or chest pain
• Stools may turn black
MONITORING PARAMETERS
• CBC and ANA titer before and during prolonged therapy

---

* = non FDA-approved use

hydrochlorothiazide
(hye-droe-klor-oh-thye'a-zide)
Rx: Diuchlor H ✽, Esidrix, Ezide, HydroDiuril, Hydro-Par, Microzide, Neo-Codema ✽, Oretic, Urozide ✽
Combinations
hydralazine (Apresazide); lisinopril (Prinzide, Zestoretic); losartan (Hyzaar); methyldopa (Aldoril); metoprolol (Lopressor HCT); propranolol (Inderide); reserpine (Hydro-Reserp, Hydrorex); spironolactone (Aldactazide); timolol (Timolide); triamterene (Dyazide, Maxzide); irbesartan (Irbesartan-HCTZ)
Chemical Class: Sulfonamide derivative
Therapeutic Class: Antihypertensive; thiazide diuretic

CLINICAL PHARMACOLOGY
Mechanism of Action: Initially causes volume depletion by inhibiting sodium reabsorption in distal tubules. Renal compensation occurs but antihypertensive effect continues because of Na and K reabsorption in vascular smooth muscle and decrease in total peripheral resistance
Pharmacokinetics
PO: Peak 4 hr, onset 2 hr, duration 6-12 hr; excreted unchanged in urine; $t_{1/2}$ 5.6-14.8 hr
INDICATIONS AND USES: Edema associated with CHF, hepatic cirrhosis, corticosteroid and estrogen therapy; hypertension; calcium nephrolithiasis*; osteoporosis*; diabetes insipidus*
DOSAGE
Adult
• PO 12.5-50 mg qd, max 200 mg/day; doses >50 mg/day generally not recommended due to increased incidence of hypokalemia and other metabolic disturbances
Child
• PO (<6 mo) 2-3.3 mg/kg/day divided bid; (>6 mo) 2 mg/kg/day divided bid
Ⓢ AVAILABLE FORMS/COST OF THERAPY
• Sol—Oral: 50 mg/5ml, 500 ml: **$15.37**
• Tab, Uncoated—Oral: 12.5 mg, 100's: **$40.45**; 25 mg, 100's: **$1.68-$13.48**; 50 mg, 100's: **$1.01-$21.35**; 100 mg, 100's: **$2.75-$6.87**
CONTRAINDICATIONS: Anuria, renal decompensation
PRECAUTIONS: Hypokalemia, renal disease, hepatic disease, gout, COPD, lupus erythematosus, diabetes mellitus, children, vomiting, diarrhea, hyperlipidemia
PREGNANCY AND LACTATION: Pregnancy category D; 1st trimester use may increase risk of congenital defects, use in later trimesters does not seem to carry this risk; other risks to the fetus or newborn include hypoglycemia, thrombocytopenia, hyponatremia, hypokalemia, and death from maternal complications; excreted into breast milk in small amounts; considered compatible with breast feeding
SIDE EFFECTS/ADVERSE REACTIONS
CNS: Depression, *dizziness,* drowsiness, *fatigue,* headache, paresthesia, *weakness*
CV: Irregular pulse, orthostatic hypotension, palpitations, volume depletion
EENT: Blurred vision
GI: Anorexia, constipation, cramps, diarrhea, *nausea,* pancreatitis, *vomiting*
GU: Frequency, decreased libido, impotence
HEME: **Agranulocytosis, aplastic anemia, hemolytic anemia, leukopenia, neutropenia, thrombocytopenia**

METAB: Hypercalcemia, *hyperglycemia, hyperuricemia,* hypochloremia, *hypokalemia,* hypomagnesemia, hyponatremia, increased creatinine, BUN
SKIN: Fever, photosensitivity, purpura, *rash,* urticaria
DRUG INTERACTIONS
Drugs
Ⓘ *Antidiabetics:* Thiazide diuretics tend to increase blood glucose, may increase dosage requirements of antidiabetic drugs
Ⓘ *Calcium (high doses):* Risk of milk-alkali syndrome monitor for hypercalcemia
Ⓘ *Cholestyramine/colestipol:* Reduced serum concentrations of thiazide diuretics
Ⓘ *Diazoxide:* Hyperglycemia
Ⓘ *Digitalis glycosides:* Diuretic-induced hypokalemia may increase the risk of digitalis toxicity
Ⓘ *Lithium:* Increased serum lithium concentrations, toxicity may occur
Ⓘ *Methotrexate:* Increased bone marrow suppression
Labs
• False decrease: Urine estriol

SPECIAL CONSIDERATIONS
• May protect against osteoporotic hip fractures
• Loop diuretics more effective if CrCl < 40-50 ml/min
• Combinations with triamterene, lisinopril have potassium-sparing effect
PATIENT/FAMILY EDUCATION
• Take with food or milk
• Will increase urination; take early in the day
• May cause sensitivity to sunlight; avoid prolonged exposure to the sun and other ultraviolet light
• May cause gout attacks; notify clinician if sudden joint pain occurs
MONITORING PARAMETERS
• Serum electrolytes, BUN, creatinine, CBC, uric acid, glucose

ibutilide
(eye-byoo'ti-lide)
Rx: Corvert
Chemical Class: Methanesulfonamide derivative
Therapeutic Class: Antidysrhythmic (Class III)

CLINICAL PHARMACOLOGY
Mechanism of Action: Delays repolarization by activation of a slow, inward current (predominantly sodium); prolongs atrial and ventricular action potential duration and refractoriness; produces mild slowing of the sinus rate and AV conduction; produces dose-related prolongation of QT interval
Pharmacokinetics
IV: 40% bound to plasma proteins; metabolized to 8 metabolites (1 active), excreted in urine (~80%) and feces (~19%); $t_{1/2}$ 6 hr
INDICATIONS AND USES: Rapid conversion of atrial fibrillation or atrial flutter of recent onset to sinus rhythm (atrial arrhythmias of longer duration less likely to respond)
DOSAGE
Adult
• IV (≥60 kg) 1 mg (1 vial) infused over 10 min; (<60 kg) 0.01 mg/kg (0.1 ml/kg); if arrhythmia does not terminate within 10 min after end of initial infusion, a 2nd 10 min infusion of equal strength may be administered
Ⓢ AVAILABLE FORMS/COST OF THERAPY
• Sol—IV: 0.1 mg/ml, 10 ml: **$149.69**

italic = common side effects

bold italic = life-threatening reactions

CARDIOLOGY DRUG REFERENCE

PRECAUTIONS: Heart block; can worsen or induce ventricular dysrhythmias (including torsades de pointes)
PREGNANCY AND LACTATION: Pregnancy category C
SIDE EFFECTS/ADVERSE REACTIONS
CNS: Headache
CV: Bradycardia, bundle branch block, *CHF,* hypertension, hypotension, palpitation, postural hypotension, QT segment prolongation, syncope, tachycardia, *ventricular dysrhythmias*
GI: Nausea
DRUG INTERACTIONS
Drugs
◼ *Disopyramide, quinidine, procainamide, amiodarone, sotalol:* Potential to prolong refractoriness
❷ *Phenothiazines, tricyclic antidepressants, terfenadine, astemizole:* Increased potential for prodysrhythmia due to prolongation of QT interval

SPECIAL CONSIDERATIONS

MONITORING PARAMETERS
• Continuous ECG monitoring for at least 4 hr following infusion or until QTc returns to baseline (longer monitoring if dysrhythmic activity noted). Defibrillator must be available

---

indapamide
(in-dap'a-mide)
Rx: Lozide ✤, Lozol
Chemical Class: Indoline derivative
Therapeutic Class: Antihypertensive; thiazide-like diuretic

CLINICAL PHARMACOLOGY
Mechanism of Action: Acts on proximal section of distal renal tubule by inhibiting reabsorption of sodium; may act by direct vasodilation caused by blocking of calcium channel
Pharmacokinetics
PO: Onset 1-2 hr, peak 2 hr, duration up to 36 hr; excreted in urine, feces; $t_{1/2}$ 14-18 hr
INDICATIONS AND USES: Edema, hypertension
DOSAGE
Adult
• PO 2.5-5 mg qd in AM
💲 **AVAILABLE FORMS/COST OF THERAPY**
• Tab, Plain Coated—Oral: 1.25 mg, 100's: **$63.95;** 2.5 mg, 100's: **$65.98-$84.73**
CONTRAINDICATIONS: Hypersensitivity to sulfonamides; anuria
PRECAUTIONS: Hypokalemia, dehydration, ascites, hepatic disease, severe renal disease, diabetes mellitus, gout, hyperuricemia, sympathectomy
PREGNANCY AND LACTATION: Pregnancy category B; not known if excreted in breast milk
SIDE EFFECTS/ADVERSE REACTIONS
CNS: Depression, *dizziness,* fatigue, *headache,* paresthesias, *weakness*
CV: Dysrhythmias, orthostatic hypotension, palpitations, volume depletion
EENT: Blurred vision, increased intraocular pressure, loss of hearing, nasal congestion, tinnitus
GI: Abdominal pain, anorexia, constipation, cramps, diarrhea, dry mouth, hepatitis, jaundice, *nausea,* pancreatitis, vomiting
GU: Decreased libido, frequency, impotence
METAB: Hypercalcemia, hyperglycemia, *hyperuricemia, hypochloremic alkalosis,* hypokalemia, *hypomagnesemia, hyponatremia*

MS: Cramps
SKIN: Photosensitivity, pruritus, rash, urticaria
DRUG INTERACTIONS
Drugs
◼ *Digitalis glycosides:* Risk of hypokalemia less than other diuretics but monitor (risk digitalis toxicity in hypokalemia)
◼ *Lithium:* Manufacturer recommends avoidance (possible lithium toxicity)

---

irbesartan
(erb'ba-sar-tan)
Rx: Avapro
Chemical Class: Imidazole derivative
Therapeutic Class: Angiotensin II receptor (type AT_1) antagonist; antihypertensive

CLINICAL PHARMACOLOGY
Mechanism of Action: Blocks vasoconstrictor and aldosterone-secreting effects of angiotensin II by blocking its binding to angiotensin II (type AT_1) receptors
Pharmacokinetics
PO: Peak concentrations in 1-2 hr (peak therapeutic effects: blood pressure reductions in 2 hr; increases in plasma renin activity and plasma angiotensin II, 2 hr; reductions in plasma aldosterone, 4 to 8 hr); effects persist greater than 24 hr, orally active, does not require biotransformation to active form
Rapid oral absorption (bioavailability, 60%-80%), 90% serum protein bound; hepatic N-glucuronidation (no active metabolite) via CYP2C9 isoenzyme, excreted by both biliary and renal routes; $t_{1/2}$ 11-15 hr
INDICATIONS AND USES: Hypertension; congestive heart failure*; diabetic nephropathy*
DOSAGE
Adult
• PO 150-300 mg qd (volume- or salt-depleted patients should receive an initial dose of 75 mg; no dosage adjustment needed in elderly or renal or hepatic impairment)
💲 **AVAILABLE FORMS/COST OF THERAPY**
• Capsule—Oral: 75 mg, 90's: **$103.03;** 150 mg, 90's: **$108.45;** 300 mg, 90's: **$189.79**
PRECAUTIONS: Hypersensitivity or other untoward effects during therapy with losartan; renal or hepatic impairment; central nervous system disorders, heart failure; hypotension; volume-depleted patients; renal artery stenosis
PREGNANCY AND LACTATION. Pregnancy category C (1st trimester), category D (2nd and 3rd trimesters); may cause fetal death; not known if excreted in breast milk
SIDE EFFECTS/ADVERSE REACTIONS
CNS: Dizziness, fatigue, headache, weakness or tiredness
CV: First dose hypotension, fluid retention
GI: Diarrhea, dyspepsia/heartburn
MS: Trauma
RESP: Cough, upper respiratory infection
MISC: Angioedema
DRUG INTERACTIONS
Drugs
◼ *α-adrenergic blockers:* Exaggerated first dose hypotensive response when added to irbesartan
◼ *Aspirin:* May reduce hemodynamic effects of fosinopril; less likely at doses under 236 mg; less likely with nonacetylated salicylates
◼ *Loop diuretics:* Initiation of irbesartan may cause hypotension and renal insufficiency in patients taking loop diuretics

---

* = non FDA-approved use

⬛ *NSAIDs:* May reduce hemodynamic effects of irbesartan
⬛ *Potassium-sparing diuretics:* Increased risk of hyperkalemia

SPECIAL CONSIDERATIONS

• Place in therapy: hypertensive patients unable to tolerate angiotensin-converting enzyme (ACE) inhibitors due to general effects related to ACE inhibition (e.g., cough, angioedema)

MONITORING PARAMETERS

• Blood pressure; renal function tests, hepatic function tests, and serum electrolytes periodically during therapy, including in the 1st month of initiation

---

isosorbide dinitrate/mononitrate
(eye-soe-sor'bide)
Dinitrate: **Rx:** Cedocard SR ✿, Coradur ✿, Dilatrate-SR, Isordil, Isotrate Timecelles, Sorbitrate
Mononitrate: **Rx:** Imdur, ISMO, Monoket
Chemical Class: Nitrate derivative
Therapeutic Class: Antianginal

CLINICAL PHARMACOLOGY

Mechanism of Action: Relaxes vascular smooth muscle; the venous (capacitance) system is affected to a greater degree than arterial (resistance) system; venous pooling, decreased venous return to the heart (preload), and decreased arterial resistance (afterload) reduce intracardiac pressures and left ventricular size, thereby decreasing myocardial oxygen demand and ischemia; may also improve regional myocardial blood supply

Pharmacokinetics
Dinitrate
PO: Onset 20-40 min, duration 4-6 hr
PO SUS REL: Onset up to 4 hr, duration 6-8 hr
SL: Onset 2-5 min, duration 1-3 hr
Metabolized by liver in urine as metabolites
Mononitrate
PO: Onset 30-60 min
Not subject to 1st-pass metabolism; <4% bound to plasma proteins; metabolized to inactive metabolites; $t_{1/2}$ 5 hr

INDICATIONS AND USES: Prevention of angina pectoris; relief of acute anginal episodes and prophylaxis before events likely to provoke an attack (SL dinitrate formulation only); CHF,* hypertension (acute)*

DOSAGE

• Asymmetric dosing regimens provide a daily nitrate-free interval to minimize the development of tolerance
Adult
• *Dinitrate:* SL 2.5-5 mg initially, titrate upward until angina is relieved or side effects limit the dose; chewable tabs 5 mg initially, titrate upward until angina is relieved or side effects limit the dose; PO 5-20 mg bid-tid initially (last dose no later than 7 PM), maintenance 10-40 mg bid-tid (last dose no later than 7 PM); PO SUS REL 40 mg qd-bid initially (last dose no later than 2 PM), maintenance 40-80 mg qd-bid (last dose no later than 2 PM)
• *Mononitrate:* PO 5-20 mg bid (with the 2 doses 7 hr apart); PO SUS REL 30-60 mg qd initially, titrate to 120-240 mg qd if necessary

💲 AVAILABLE FORMS/COST OF THERAPY
Dinitrate
• Tab, SL—Oral: 2.5 mg, 100's: **$3.68-$25.94**; 5 mg, 100's: **$3.53-$27.74**; 10 mg, 100's: **$32.38**
• Tab, Uncoated—Oral: 5 mg, 100's: **$2.10-$27.84**; 10 mg, 100's: **$2.06-$31.13**; 20 mg, 100's: **$2.18-$50.23**; 30 mg, 100's: **$2.93-$56.53**; 40 mg, 100's: **$42.72-$61.36**

• Tab, Chewable—Oral: 5 mg, 100's: **$19.99**; 10 mg, **$22.96**
• Cap, Gel, SUS Action—Oral: 40 mg, 100's: **$6.31-$59.48**
• Tab, Coated, SUS Action—Oral: 40 mg, 100's: **$8.00-$59.48**
Mononitrate
• Tab, Uncoated—Oral: 10 mg, 100's: **$68.55**; 20 mg, 100's: **$62.85-$75.96**
• Tab, Coated, SUS Action—Oral: 30 mg, 100's: **$108.21**; 60 mg, 100's: **$113.90**; 120 mg, 100's: **$159.45**

CONTRAINDICATIONS: Hypersensitivity to nitrates, severe anemia, closed-angle glaucoma, postural hypotension, head trauma or cerebral hemorrhage (may increase intracranial pressure), acute MI or CHF (mononitrate)
PRECAUTIONS: Acute MI, hypertrophic cardiomyopathy, glaucoma, volume depletion, hypotension, abrupt withdrawal, continuous delivery without nitrate-free interval (tolerance will develop)
PREGNANCY AND LACTATION: Pregnancy category C; excretion into breast milk unknown; use caution in nursing mothers

SIDE EFFECTS/ADVERSE REACTIONS
CNS: Agitation, anxiety, apprehension, confusion, *dizziness,* dyscoordination, *headache,* hypoesthesia, hypokinesia, insomnia, nervousness, nightmares, restlessness, vertigo, weakness
CV: **Atrial fibrillation, cardiovascular collapse, crescendo angina, dysrhythmias,** edema, hypotension (sometimes with paradoxical bradycardia and increased angina), palpitations, *postural hypotension,* premature ventricular contractions, rebound hypertension, retrosternal discomfort, syncope, tachycardia
EENT: Blurred vision, diplopia
GI: Abdominal pain, diarrhea, dyspepsia, involuntary passing of feces, nausea, tenesmus, vomiting
GU: Dysuria, impotence, involuntary passing of urine, urinary frequency
HEME: **Hemolytic anemia, methemoglobinemia**
MS: Arthralgia, muscle twitching
SKIN: Cold sweat, crusty skin lesions, exfoliative dermatitis, *flushing,* pallor, perspiration, pruritus, rash

SPECIAL CONSIDERATIONS

PATIENT/FAMILY EDUCATION
• Headache may be a marker for drug activity; do not try to avoid by altering treatment schedule; contact clinician if severe or persistent; aspirin or acetaminophen may be used for relief
• Dissolve SL tablets under tongue; do not crush, chew, or swallow
• Do not crush chewable tablets before administering
• Avoid alcohol
• Make changes in position slowly to prevent fainting

---

isradipine
(is-rad'i-peen)
Rx: DynaCirc
Chemical Class: Dihydropyridine calcium channel blocker
Therapeutic Class: Antihypertensive; antianginal

CLINICAL PHARMACOLOGY

Mechanism of Action: Inhibits calcium ion influx across cell membrane in vascular smooth muscle and cardiac muscle; produces relaxation of coronary vascular smooth muscle, peripheral vascular smooth muscle; reduces total peripheral resistance (afterload); increases myocardial oxygen delivery

Pharmacokinetics
PO: Peak 1½ hr, onset 2 hr; 95% bound to plasma proteins; metabolized in liver, excreted in urine and feces (metabolites); $t_{1/2}$ 8 hr

INDICATIONS AND USES: Hypertension, chronic stable angina*

---

italic = common side effects

bold italic = life-threatening reactions

DOSAGE

Adult

• PO 2.5 mg bid initially, increase in 2-4 wk intervals prn to max of 10 mg bid; SUS REL PO 5 mg qd, may increase by 5 mg increments at 2-4 wk intervals, max 20 mg/day

S AVAILABLE FORMS/COST OF THERAPY

• Cap, Gel—Oral: 2.5 mg, 100's: **$59.40; 5** mg, 100's: **$87.18**

• Tab, SUS REL—Oral: 5 mg, 100's: **$109.20; 10** mg, 100's: **$174.00**

PRECAUTIONS: CHF, hypotension, hepatic insufficiency, aortic stenosis, elderly, children

PREGNANCY AND LACTATION: Pregnancy category C; excretion into breast milk unknown; use caution in nursing mothers

SIDE EFFECTS/ADVERSE REACTIONS

CNS: Anxiety, asthenia, depression, dizziness, fatigue, headache, insomnia, malaise, nervousness, paresthesia, somnolence, tremor

CV: Bradycardia, *dysrhythmia,* hypotension, palpitations, *peripheral edema,* syncope, tachycardia

EENT: Epistaxis, nasal congestion, tinnitus

GI: Abdominal cramps, constipation, diarrhea, dry mouth, flatulence, gastric upset, nausea, vomiting

GU: Nocturia, polyuria, sexual dysfunction

SKIN: Hair loss, pruritus, rash, urticaria

MISC: Cough, flushing, muscle cramps, shortness of breath, sweating, weight gain

DRUG INTERACTIONS

Drugs

🔢 *β-blockers:* Enhanced effects of β-blockers; hypotension

🔢 *Calcium:* Reduced activity of isradipine

🔢 *Lovastatin:* Decreased lovastatin concentrations

---

labetalol

(la-bet'a-lole)

Rx: Normodyne, Trandate

Chemical Class: Nonselective α-adrenergic blocker; peripheral β-adrenergic blocker

Therapeutic Class: Antihypertensive

CLINICAL PHARMACOLOGY

Mechanism of Action: Combines both selective, competitive postsynaptic α_1-adrenergic blocking and nonselective, competitive β-adrenergic blocking activity

Pharmacokinetics

PO: Onset 20 min-2 hr, peak 1-4 hr, duration 8-24 hr

IV: Onset 5 min, peak 5-15 min, duration 2-4 hr

50% bound to plasma proteins, metabolized in liver, excreted in urine and feces (metabolites); $t_{1/2}$ 5.5-8 hr

INDICATIONS AND USES: Hypertension, hypertensive emergencies (parenteral), pheochromocytoma,* clonidine withdrawal hypertension*

DOSAGE

Adult

• PO 100 mg bid initially, may increase prn q2-3 days by 100 mg until desired response obtained, max 2.4 g/day; IV 20 mg initially, repeated doses of 40-80 mg may be given at 10 min intervals up to 300 mg total dose; IV INF 2 mg/min initially, titrate to response

S AVAILABLE FORMS/COST OF THERAPY

• Inj, Sol—IV: 5 mg/ml, 20 ml: **$32.39-$35.51**

• Tab, Coated—Oral: 100 mg, 100's: **$46.61-$48.89; 200** mg, 100's: **$66.12-$69.36; 300** mg, 100's: **$87.95-$92.26**

CONTRAINDICATIONS: Bronchial asthma, overt cardiac failure, greater than 1st degree heart block, cardiogenic shock, severe bradycardia, hypersensitivity

PRECAUTIONS: Major surgery, diabetes mellitus, renal disease, hepatic disease, thyroid disease, well-compensated heart failure, nonallergic bronchospasm, abrupt discontinuation, children

PREGNANCY AND LACTATION: Pregnancy category C; does not seem to pose a risk to the fetus, except possibly in the 1st trimester; excreted in breast milk; compatible with breast feeding

SIDE EFFECTS/ADVERSE REACTIONS

CNS: Anxiety, catatonia, depression, dizziness, drowsiness, fatigue, headache, lethargy, mental changes, nightmares, paresthesias (scalp tingling)

CV: AV block, bradycardia, chest pain, *CHF,* orthostatic hypotension, *ventricular dysrhythmias*

EENT: Double vision, dry burning eyes, sore throat, tinnitus, visual changes

GI: Diarrhea, nausea, vomiting

GU: Dysuria, ejaculatory failure, impotence, Peyronie's disease

HEME: Agranulocytosis, thrombocytopenic purpura (reported with other β-blockers only) (rare)

MS: Asthenia, muscle cramps, toxic myopathy

RESP: Bronchospasm, dyspnea, wheezing

SKIN: Alopecia, fever, pruritus, rash, urticaria

DRUG INTERACTIONS

Drugs

🔢 *Cimetidine:* Increased plasma labetalol concentrations

🔢 *Epinephrine:* Increased diastolic pressure and bradycardia during epinephrine infusions

🔢 *NSAIDs:* Reduced hypotensive effects of β-blockers

❷ *Theophylline:* Antagonistic pharmacodynamic effects

Labs

• *False positive:* Urine amphetamine

• *False increase:* Urinary catecholamines, plasma epinephrine

SPECIAL CONSIDERATIONS

PATIENT/FAMILY EDUCATION

• Do not discontinue abruptly

• Transient scalp tingling may occur, especially when treatment is initiated

• May mask the symptoms of hypoglycemia, except for sweating, in diabetic patients

---

lidocaine (systemic)

(lye'doe-kane)

Rx: LidoPen Auto-Injector, Xylocaine

Chemical Class: Aminoacyl amide

Therapeutic Class: Antidysrhythmic (Class IB)

CLINICAL PHARMACOLOGY

Mechanism of Action: Decreases depolarization, automaticity, and excitability in the ventricles during the diastolic phase by a direct action on the tissues, especially the Purkinje network, without involvement of the autonomic system; contractility, systolic arterial blood pressure, atrioventricular (AV) conduction velocity, absolute refractory period are not altered by usual therapeutic doses

Pharmacokinetics

IV: Onset immediate, duration 10-20 min

IM: Onset 5-15 min, duration 60-90 min

60%-80% bound to plasma proteins; metabolized by liver to active metabolites, eliminated in urine (10% as unchanged drug); $t_{1/2}$ 1-2 hr

INDICATIONS AND USES: Acute ventricular dysrhythmias

---

* = non FDA-approved use

DOSAGE

Adult

IV bolus 50-100 mg over 2-3 min, repeat q3-5 min, not to exceed 300 mg in 1 hr, begin IV INF; IV INF 20-50 µg/kg/min (1-4 mg/min); decrease the dose in patients with CHF, acute MI, shock, or hepatic disease; IM 200-300 mg in deltoid muscle, additional doses may be given after 60-90 min if necessary; ET 2-2.5 times the IV dose

Child

• IV/ET/IO 1 mg/kg loading dose, repeat if needed in 10-15 min × 2 doses, begin IV INF; IV INF 20-50 µg/kg/min

$ AVAILABLE FORMS/COST OF THERAPY

For direct IV administration:
• Inj, Sol—IV: 1%, 5 ml: **$2.32**; 2%, 5 ml: **$4.32**

For IV admixture:
• Inj, Sol: 4%, 25 ml: **$2.25**; 10%, 10 ml: **$9.07**; 20%, 10 ml: **$12.53**

CONTRAINDICATIONS: Hypersensitivity to amide anesthetics, Stokes-Adams syndrome, Wolff-Parkinson-White syndrome, severe heart block (in absence of a pacemaker)

PRECAUTIONS: Children, renal disease, liver disease, CHF, reduced cardiac output, digitalis toxicity accompanied by AV block, respiratory depression, genetic predisposition to malignant hyperthermia, atrial fibrillation or flutter

PREGNANCY AND LACTATION: Pregnancy category C; compatible with breast feeding

SIDE EFFECTS/ADVERSE REACTIONS

CNS: Apprehension, confusion, *dizziness,* drowsiness, euphoria, hallucinations, lightheadedness, mood changes, nervousness, *seizures,* tremors, twitching, unconsciousness

CV: Bradycardia, **cardiovascular collapse,** edema, **heart block,** *hypotension*

EENT: Blurred or double vision, tinnitus

GI: Vomiting

RESP: **Respiratory depression and arrest**

SKIN: Rash, swelling, urticaria

MISC: Febrile response, **malignant hyperthermia,** phlebitis at inj site

DRUG INTERACTIONS

Drugs

▪ *Disopyramide:* Induction of dysrhythmia or heart failure in predisposed patients

▪ *Metoprolol, nadolol, propranolol, cimetidine:* Increased serum lidocaine concentrations

Labs

• False increase: Serum creatinine, CSF protein

SPECIAL CONSIDERATIONS

MONITORING PARAMETERS

• Constant ECG monitoring, blood pressure
• Therapeutic serum concentrations are 1.5-6 µg/ml (concentrations >6-10 µg/ml are usually associated with toxicity)

---

lisinopril

(lyse-in'oh-pril)
Rx: Prinivil, Zestril
Combinations
   Rx: with hydrochlorothiazide (Prinzide, Zestoretic)
Chemical Class: Angiotensin-converting enzyme (ACE) inhibitor
Therapeutic Class: Antihypertensive; congestive heart failure agent; renal protectant

CLINICAL PHARMACOLOGY

Mechanism of Action: Selectively suppresses renin-angiotensin-aldosterone system; inhibits ACE preventing the conversion of angiotensin I to angiotensin II; results in dilation of arterial, venous vessels

Pharmacokinetics

PO: Peak 7 hr, onset 1 hr, duration 24 hr; excreted unchanged in urine; $t_{1/2}$ 12 hr (prolonged in renal dysfunction)

INDICATIONS AND USES: Hypertension, CHF, acute MI, diabetic nephropathy*

DOSAGE

Adult

• *Hypertension:* PO 10 mg qd; usual dosage range 20-40 mg/day
• *CHF:* PO 5 mg qd; usual dosage range 5-20 mg/day
• *Acute MI:* PO in hemodynamically stable patients with in 24 hr of acute MI, 5 mg followed by 5 mg after 24 hr, 10 mg after 48 hr, then 10 mg qd; continue for 6 wk (or longer if concurrent hypertension or CHF)
• *Renal impairment:* PO initial dose 5 mg qd (serum creatinine ≥3 mg/dl); initial dose 2.5 mg qd (dialysis patients)

$ AVAILABLE FORMS/COST OF THERAPY

• Tab, Uncoated—Oral: 2.5 mg, 100's: **$52.50-$54.60**; 5 mg, 100's: **$78.76-$81.77**; 10 mg, 100's: **$81.29-$84.54**; 20 mg, 100's: **$87.00-$90.48**; 40 mg, 100's: **$127.20-$132.17**

PRECAUTIONS: Impaired renal function, dialysis patients, hypovolemia, diuretic therapy, collagen-vascular diseases, elderly, bilateral renal artery stenosis

PREGNANCY AND LACTATION: Pregnancy category C (1st trimester), category D (2nd and 3rd trimesters); ACE inhibitors can cause fetal and neonatal morbidity and death when administered to pregnant women; when pregnancy is detected, discontinue ACE inhibitors as soon as possible; detectable in breast milk in trace amounts; a newborn would receive <0.1% of the mg/kg maternal dose; effect on nursing infant has not been determined

SIDE EFFECTS/ADVERSE REACTIONS

CNS: Anxiety, *dizziness, fatigue, headache,* insomnia, paresthesia

CV: Angina, hypotension, palpitations, postural hypotension, syncope (especially with 1st dose)

GI: Abdominal pain, constipation, melena, nausea, vomiting

GU: **Acute renal failure,** decreased libido, impotence, increased BUN, creatinine

HEME: **Agranulocytosis, neutropenia**

METAB: Hyperkalemia, hyponatremia

MS: Arthralgia, arthritis, myalgia

RESP: Asthma, bronchitis, *cough,* dyspnea, sinusitis

SKIN: **Angioedema,** flushing, rash, sweating

DRUG INTERACTIONS

Drugs

❷ *Allopurinol:* Predisposition to hypersensitivity reactions to ACE inhibitors

▪ *Aspirin, NSAIDs:* Inhibition of the antihypertensive response to ACE inhibitors

---

italic = common side effects

bold italic = life-threatening reactions

CARDIOLOGY DRUG REFERENCE

◾ *Insulin:* Enhanced insulin sensitivity

◾ *Lithium:* Increased risk of serious lithium toxicity

◾ *Loop diuretics:* Initiation of ACE inhibitor therapy in the presence of intensive diuretic therapy results in a precipitous fall in blood pressure in some patients; ACE inhibitors may induce renal insufficiency in the presence of diuretic-induced sodium depletion

◾ *Potassium-sparing diuretics:* Increased risk for hyperkalemia

◾ *Prazosin, terazosin, doxazosin:* Exaggerated first-dose hypotensive response to α-blockers

SPECIAL CONSIDERATIONS

PATIENT/FAMILY EDUCATION

• Do not use salt substitutes containing potassium without consulting clinician

• Rise slowly to sitting or standing position to minimize orthostatic hypotension

• Dizziness, fainting, lightheadedness may occur during 1st few days of therapy

• Persistent dry cough may occur and usually does not subside unless medication is stopped

MONITORING PARAMETERS

• BUN, creatinine (watch for increased levels that may indicate acute renal failure)

• Potassium levels, although hyperkalemia rarely occurs

---

losartan
(lo-sar'tan)
Rx: Cozaar
Combinations
  Rx: with hydrochlorothiazide (Hyzaar)
Chemical Class: Angiotensin II receptor antagonist
Therapeutic Class: Antihypertensive

CLINICAL PHARMACOLOGY

Mechanism of Action: Blocks vasoconstrictor and aldosterone-secreting effects of angiotensin II by blocking its binding to angiotensin II receptors

Pharmacokinetics

PO: Converted in liver to active metabolite; peak 1 hr, 3-4 hr for metabolite; excreted in urine, bile, feces; max antihypertensive effect occurs in 3-6 wk

INDICATIONS AND USES: Hypertension, CHF*

DOSAGE

Adult >18 yr

• PO 25-50 mg qd, use lower dosage in volume depleted patients, hepatic disease; range 25-100 mg qd; divide bid if effect at trough inadequate

◾ AVAILABLE FORMS/COST OF THERAPY

• Tab, Uncoated—Oral: 25, 50 mg, 100's: **$114.06**

PRECAUTIONS: Hypotension; volume-depleted patients; renal artery stenosis; CHF; liver disease

PREGNANCY AND LACTATION: Pregnancy category C (1st trimester), category D (2nd and 3rd trimesters); may cause fetal death; not known if excreted in breast milk

SIDE EFFECTS/ADVERSE REACTIONS

CNS: Dizziness, insomnia

EENT: Nasal congestion, sinus disorder

GI: Diarrhea, dyspepsia, elevated liver enzymes

GU: Increased BUN, creatinine

HEME: Decreased Hct

MS: Back pain, leg pain, muscle cramps, myalgia

RESP: Cough

DRUG INTERACTIONS

Drugs

◾ *Cimetidine:* Increased levels of losartan

◾ *Phenobarbital:* Decreased levels of losartan

SPECIAL CONSIDERATIONS

• Exact clinical role in treatment of CHF and diabetic nephropathy not completely defined

• Reasonable alternative in patients with systolic dysfunction who are unable to tolerate ACE inhibitors

---

lovastatin
(lo'va-sta-tin)
Rx: Mevacor
Chemical Class: HMG-CoA reductase inhibitor
Therapeutic Class: Antilipemic

CLINICAL PHARMACOLOGY

Mechanism of Action: Inhibits HMG-CoA reductase, a necessary enzyme for cholesterol synthesis; results in lowered total cholesterol levels, decreased LDL levels, modest decrease in triglycerides, and variable increase in HDL levels

Pharmacokinetics

PO: Peak 2-4 hr; metabolized in liver (metabolites); highly protein bound (>95%); excreted in urine (10%), feces (83%); crosses placenta; excreted in breast milk; max effect on lipid levels in 4-6 wk

INDICATIONS AND USES: As an adjunct to diet in primary hypercholesterolemia (types IIa, IIb); coronary artery disease (to slow the progression of coronary atherosclerosis); mixed hyperlipidemia*

DOSAGE

Adult

• PO 10-20 mg qd with evening meal; may increase to 20-80 mg/day in single or divided doses, not to exceed 80 mg/d; dosage adjustments should be made qmo; for cholesterol levels (300 mg/dl initiate at 40 mg/day

◾ AVAILABLE FORMS/COST OF THERAPY

• Tab, Uncoated—Oral: 10 mg, 60's: **$76.55;** 20 mg, 60's: **$134.99;** 40 mg, 60's: **$242.98**

CONTRAINDICATIONS: Active liver disease

PRECAUTIONS: Past liver disease, alcoholics, severe acute infections, trauma, hypotension, uncontrolled seizure disorders, severe metabolic disorders, electrolyte imbalances

PREGNANCY AND LACTATION: Pregnancy category X (may produce skeletal malformations); not recommended in nursing mothers

SIDE EFFECTS/ADVERSE REACTIONS

CNS: Dizziness, headache, insomnia

EENT: Blurred vision, dysgeusia, lens opacities

GI: Abdominal pain, constipation, diarrhea, dyspepsia, flatus, heartburn, hepatotoxicity, increased transaminases, nausea

MS: Muscle cramps, myalgia, myositis, ***rhabdomyolysis***

SKIN: Pruritus, rash

DRUG INTERACTIONS

Drugs

◾ *Cholestyramine, colestipol:* Decreased bioavailability of lovastatin possible, effect likely overcome by additive lipid-lowering effects of concurrent therapy

◾ *Clarithromycin, cyclosporine, danazol, erythromycin, niacin:* Severe myopathy or rhabdomyolysis

❷ *Clofibrate, gemfibrozil, nefazodone:* Severe myopathy or rhabdomyolysis

---

* = non FDA-approved use

❷ *Fluconazole, itraconazole:* Large increases in lovastatin concentration, myopathy or rhabdomyolysis possible

▪ *Isradipine:* Reduction in lovastatin concentration

▪ *Pectin:* Reduced cholesterol-lowering effect of lovastatin

▪ *Warfarin:* Increased prothrombin time

SPECIAL CONSIDERATIONS

• Less effective in homozygous familial hypercholesterolemia (lack of functional LDL receptors); these patients also more likely to have adverse reaction of elevated transaminases

PATIENT/FAMILY EDUCATION

• Report muscle pain to clinician immediately

MONITORING PARAMETERS

• Check SGPT (ALT) before initiating therapy and q4-6 wk during 1st 3 mo of therapy, q6-12 wk during the next year; discontinue drug if elevated >3 times normal

---

mecamylamine
(mek-a-mill'a-meen)
Rx: Inversine
Chemical Class: Ganglionic blocker
Therapeutic Class: Antihypertensive

CLINICAL PHARMACOLOGY

Mechanism of Action: Blocks transmission of impulses at both sympathetic and parasympathetic ganglia; hypotensive effect is due to reduction in sympathetic tone, vasodilation, reduced cardiac output, and is primarily postural

Pharmacokinetics

PO: Onset 0.5-2 hr, duration 6-12 hr; mostly excreted unchanged in urine

INDICATIONS AND USES: Moderate to severe hypertension (not 1st line)

DOSAGE

Adult

• PO 2.5 mg bid initially, may increase in increments of 2.5 mg q2 days until desired response, usual maintenance dose 25 mg/day divided bid-qid

Ⓢ AVAILABLE FORMS/COST OF THERAPY

• Tab, Uncoated—Oral: 2.5 mg, 100's: **$13.03**

CONTRAINDICATIONS: Mild, labile hypertension; coronary insufficiency, recent MI; uremia; glaucoma; organic pyloric stenosis; patients receiving sulfonamides or antibiotics

PRECAUTIONS: Cerebral arteriosclerosis, recent CVA, renal insufficiency, abrupt discontinuation, prostatic hypertrophy, bladder neck obstruction, urethral stricture

PREGNANCY AND LACTATION: Pregnancy category C; not recommended in nursing mothers

SIDE EFFECTS/ADVERSE REACTIONS

CNS: Choreiform movements, *fatigue,* mental aberrations, paresthesia, *sedation,* **seizures,** tremor, weakness

CV: Orthostatic dizziness, syncope

EENT: Blurred vision, dilated pupils

GI: Anorexia, constipation, dry mouth, glossitis, nausea, **paralytic ileus,** vomiting

GU: Decreased libido, impotence, urinary retention

SPECIAL CONSIDERATIONS

PATIENT/FAMILY EDUCATION

• Take after meals

• Arise slowly from reclining position

• Orthostatic changes are exacerbated by alcohol, exercise, hot weather

MONITORING PARAMETERS

• Maintenance doses should be limited to dose that causes slight faintness or dizziness in the standing position

---

methyldopa
(meth-ill-doe'pa)
Rx: Aldomet, Dopamet ✦, Medimet ✦, Novo-Medopa ✦, Nu-Medopa ✦
Combinations
  Rx: with HCTZ (Aldoril); with chlorothiazide (Aldoclor)
Chemical Class: Catecholamine derivative
Therapeutic Class: Antihypertensive

CLINICAL PHARMACOLOGY

Mechanism of Action: Exact mechanism unknown; thought to involve stimulation of central α_2-adrenergic receptors by a metabolite, α-methylnorepinephrine, thus inhibiting sympathetic outflow to the heart, kidneys, and peripheral vasculature; reduced peripheral resistance and plasma renin activity levels may also contribute to its effect

Pharmacokinetics

PO: Peak 3-6 hr

IV (methyldopate): Onset 4-6 hr, duration 10-16 hr

Weakly bound to plasma proteins; extensively metabolized in GI tract and liver, eliminated in urine; $t_{1/2}$ 1-3 hr

INDICATIONS AND USES: Moderate to severe hypertension

DOSAGE

Adult

• PO 250 mg bid-tid, increase q2d prn, usual dose 1-1.5 g/day in 2-4 divided doses, max 3 g/day; IV (methyldopate) 250-1000 mg q68h, max 4 g/day

• *Dosing interval in renal impairment:* CrCl >50 ml/min 8h; CrCl 10-50 ml/min q8-12h; CrCl <10 ml/min q12-24h

Child

• PO 10 mg/kg/day in 2-4 divided doses, increase q2d prn to max dose of 65 mg/kg/day, do not exceed 3 g/day; IV 2-4 mg/kg/dose; if response not seen within 4-6 hr, may increase to 5-10 mg/kg/dose; administer doses q6-8h; max daily dose 65 mg/kg or 3 g, whichever is less

Dosing interval in renal impairment: CrCl 50 ml/min q8h; CrCl 10-50 ml/min q8-12h; CrCl <10 ml/min q12-24h

Ⓢ AVAILABLE FORMS/COST OF THERAPY

• Inj, Sol—IV: 50 mg/ml, 5 ml: **$1.98-$12.53** (methyldopate)

• Susp—Oral: 250 mg/5 ml, 480 ml: **$60.53**

• Tab, Plain Coated—Oral: 125 mg, 100's: **$6.15-$26.89;** 250 mg, 100's: **$6.75-$34.23;** 500 mg, 100's: **$12.15-$62.53**

CONTRAINDICATIONS: Active hepatic disease; previous methyldopa-associated liver abnormalities; direct Coombs positive hemolytic anemia

PRECAUTIONS: History of liver disease, pheochromocytoma, sulfite sensitivity, renal failure

PREGNANCY AND LACTATION: Pregnancy category B (oral); C (IV); no adverse reactions have been reported despite rather wide use during pregnancy; compatible with breast feeding

SIDE EFFECTS/ADVERSE REACTIONS

CNS: Asthenia, Bell's palsy, decreased mental acuity, depression, *dizziness, headache,* involuntary choreoathetotic movements, light-headedness, paresthesias, parkinsonism, psychic disturbances, *sedation,* symptoms of cerebrovascular insufficiency

CV: Aggravation of angina pectoris, bradycardia, edema, myocarditis, orthostatic hypotension, paradoxical pressor response, pericarditis, prolonged carotid sinus hypersensitivity

EENT: Dry mouth, nasal stuffiness

---

italic = common side effects   ***bold italic*** = life-threatening reactions

GI: Abnormal liver function tests, colitis, constipation, diarrhea, distension, flatus, hepatitis, jaundice, nausea, ***pancreatitis,*** sialadenitis, vomiting

GU: Decreased libido, failure to ejaculate, impotence

HEME: **Bone marrow depression,** eosinophilia, ***granulocytopenia, hemolytic anemia,*** *positive Coombs test (10%-20%),* positive tests for antinuclear antibody, LE cells, and rheumatoid factor

METAB: Amenorrhea, breast enlargement, galactorrhea, hyperprolactinemia

MS: Arthralgia, myalgia

SKIN: Rash, ***toxic epidermal necrolysis***

MISC: Fever, lupus-like syndrome

DRUG INTERACTIONS

Drugs

▪ *Iron:* Inhibited antihypertensive response to methyldopa

▪ *Lithium:* Lithium toxicity not necessarily associated with excessive lithium concentrations

Labs

• *Interference:* Plasma and urine catecholamines, serum creatinine, glucose, serum, and urine uric acid

• *False increase:* Urine amino acids, serum bilirubin, urine ferric chloride test, urine ketones, metanephrines, VMA

• *False decrease:* Serum cholesterol, triglycerides

• *False positive:* Guaiacols spot test, urine melanogen, urine Thormählen test

SPECIAL CONSIDERATIONS

• Perform both direct and indirect Coombs test if blood transfusion needed. If indirect Coombs test positive, interference may occur with cross match. Positive direct Coombs test will not interfere

PATIENT/FAMILY EDUCATION

• Urine exposed to air after voiding may darken

• Do not discontinue abruptly

• Initial sedation usually improves

MONITORING PARAMETERS

• >CBC, liver function tests periodically during therapy

• Direct Coombs test before therapy and after 6-12 mo. If positive rule out hemolytic anemia

---

metolazone
(me-tole'a-zone)

Rx: Mykrox (rapid acting), Zaroxolyn (slow acting)

Chemical Class: Quinazoline derivative

Therapeutic Class: Antihypertensive; thiazide diuretic

CLINICAL PHARMACOLOGY

Mechanism of Action: Increases urinary excretion of sodium and water by inhibiting sodium reabsorption in the early distal tubules; may produce diuresis in patients with GFR <20 ml/min

Pharmacokinetics

PO: (Mykrox) peak 2-4 hr, steady state within 4-5 days; (Zaroxolyn) peak 8 hr; 50%-70% bound to erythrocytes, up to 33% bound to plasma proteins; 70%-95% excreted unchanged in urine by glomerular filtration and active tubular secretion; $t_{1/2}$ 8 hr

INDICATIONS AND USES: Zaroxolyn: edema associated with CHF, nephrotic syndrome, hepatic cirrhosis, corticosteroid and estrogen therapy; has been used concomitantly with furosemide to induce diuresis in patients who did not respond to either diuretic alone; hypertension. Mykrox: hypertension (not indicated for diuresis as dosage not established)

DOSAGE

Adult

• *Edema:* PO (Zaroxolyn) 5-10 mg qAM; up to 20 mg qd may be required for edema associated with renal disease

• *Hypertension:* PO (Zaroxolyn) 1.25-5 mg qAM; (Mykrox) 0.5-1 mg qAM

Child

• PO (Zaroxolyn) 0.2-0.4 mg/kg/day divided q12-24h

⑤ AVAILABLE FORMS/COST OF THERAPY

• Tab, Uncoated—Oral: 0.5 mg, 100's: **$73.63** (Mykrox)

• Tab, Uncoated—Oral: 2.5 mg, 100's: **$46.81-$55.64;** 5 mg, 100's: **$53.21-$61.94;** 10 mg, 100's: **$63.68-$71.84** (Zaroxolyn)

CONTRAINDICATIONS: Anuria, hepatic coma or precoma

PRECAUTIONS: Hypokalemia, renal disease, hepatic disease, gout, COPD, lupus erythematosus, diabetes mellitus, children, vomiting, diarrhea, hyperlipidemia

PREGNANCY AND LACTATION: Pregnancy category D; 1st trimester use may increase risk of congenital defects, use in later trimesters does not seem to carry this risk; other risks to the fetus or newborn include hypoglycemia, thrombocytopenia, hyponatremia, hypokalemia, and death from maternal complications; excreted into breast milk in small amounts; considered compatible with breast feeding

SIDE EFFECTS/ADVERSE REACTIONS

CNS: Depression, *dizziness,* drowsiness, *fatigue, headache,* paresthesia, weakness

CV: Chest pain, irregular pulse, orthostatic hypotension, palpitations, volume depletion

EENT: Blurred vision, dry mouth

GI: Abdominal bloating, *anorexia,* cholecystitis, constipation, cramps, diarrhea, GI irritation, hepatitis, *nausea,* **pancreatitis,** *vomiting*

GU: Frequency, glucosuria, impotence, polyuria

HEME: **Agranulocytosis, aplastic anemia, leukopenia, neutropenia**

METAB: Hypercalcemia, hyperglycemia, hyperuricemia, hypochloremia, *hypokalemia,* hypomagnesemia, hyponatremia, increased creatinine, BUN

MS: Muscle cramps

SKIN: Fever, photosensitivity, pruritus, purpura, *rash,* urticaria

DRUG INTERACTIONS

Drugs

▪ *Antidiabetics:* Thiazide diuretics tend to increase blood glucose

▪ *Calcium:* Milk-alkali syndrome

▪ *Carbenoxolone:* Enhanced hypokalemia

▪ *Cholestyramine, colestipol:* Reduced serum concentrations of thiazide diuretics

▪ *Diazoxide:* Hyperglycemia

▪ *Digitalis glycosides:* Diuretic-induced hypokalemia may increase the risk of digitalis toxicity

▪ *Lithium:* Increased serum lithium concentrations, toxicity may occur

▪ *Methotrexate:* Enhanced bone marrow suppression

SPECIAL CONSIDERATIONS

• More effective than other thiazide-type diuretics in patients with impaired renal function

PATIENT/FAMILY EDUCATION

• Take with food or milk

• Drug will increase urination; take early in the day

MONITORING PARAMETERS

• Serum electrolytes, BUN, creatinine, CBC, uric acid, glucose

---

* = non FDA-approved use

metoprolol
(met-oh'proe-lol)

Rx: Betaloc ✤, Lopresor ✤, Lopressor, Nu-Metop ✤, Toprol XL

Chemical Class: β₁-selective (cardioselective) adrenoreceptor blocker

Therapeutic Class: Antihypertensive; antianginal

CLINICAL PHARMACOLOGY

Mechanism of Action: Blocks β₁-receptor sites inhibiting chronotropic and inotropic responses (cardioselective); slows conduction of AV node, decreases heart rate, decreases myocardial O₂ consumption, decreases renin-aldosterone-angiotensin system at higher doses; blocks β₂-receptors in bronchial system at higher doses; lacks intrinsic sympathomimetic (partial agonist) activity

Pharmacokinetics

PO: Peak effect 1½-4 hr, duration 10-20 hr (peak delayed with extended release)

IV: Peak effect 20 min, duration 5-8 hr

8%-12% bound to plasma proteins; extensively metabolized in liver, excreted in urine (3%-10% unchanged); t₁/₂ 3-4 hr

INDICATIONS AND USES: Chronic stable angina pectoris, hypertension, acute MI (immediate release and IV only), multifocal atrial tachycardia,* rate control in atrial fibrillation*; ventricular dysrhythmias, tachycardias*; migraine prophylaxis,* essential tremor,* aggressive behavior,* congestive heart failure*

DOSAGE

Adult

• *Hypertension:* PO 100 mg/day in single or divided doses, max 450 mg/day; SUS REL 50-100 mg qd, max 400 mg/day

• *Angina pectoris:* PO 50 mg bid, max 400 mg/day; SUS REL 100 mg qd, max 400 mg/day

• *MI: (early treatment)* IV 5 mg q2 min times 3 doses, then PO 25-50 mg q6h 15 min after last IV dose, continue for 48 hr; maintenance 100 mg bid; (late treatment) 100 mg bid as soon as clinical condition allows; continue for at least 3 mo

💲 AVAILABLE FORMS/COST OF THERAPY

• Inj, Sol—IV: 5 mg/5 ml, 1's: **$4.58-$22.18**

• Tab, Coated—Oral: 50 mg, 100's: **$8.25-$56.54;** 100 mg, 100's: **$11.85-$82.07**

• Tab, Coated, SUS Action—Oral: 50 mg, 100's: **$44.63;** 100 mg, 100's: **$67.07;** 200 mg, 100's: **$134.14**

CONTRAINDICATIONS: Cardiogenic shock; 2nd or 3rd degree heart block; sinus bradycardia; CHF unless secondary to a tachydysrhythmia treatable with β-blockers; overt cardiac failure; treatment of MI when heart rate <45 bpm, systolic blood pressure <100 mm Hg

PRECAUTIONS: Major surgery, diabetes mellitus, renal disease, hepatic disease, thyroid disease, COPD, asthma, well-compensated heart failure, abrupt withdrawal, peripheral vascular disease, bradycardia

PREGNANCY AND LACTATION: Pregnancy category B; has been used during pregnancy for treatment of maternal hypertension and tachycardia; monitor newborn for 24-48 hr for bradycardia; compatible with breast feeding

SIDE EFFECTS/ADVERSE REACTIONS

CNS: Confusion, depression, *dizziness, fatigue,* headache, insomnia, memory loss, strange dreams

CV: Bradycardia, **CHF,** cold extremities, **heart block,** hypotension

EENT: Tinnitus, visual disturbances

GI: Constipation, *diarrhea,* dry mouth, heartburn, nausea

GU: Impotence, sexual dysfunction

HEME: **Agranulocytosis** (rare)

METAB: Hyperlipidemia (increased TG, total cholesterol, LDL; decreased HDL); masked hypoglycemic response to insulin (sweating excepted)

RESP: **Bronchospasm** (1%), dyspnea

SKIN: Alopecia, pruritus, rash

DRUG INTERACTIONS

Drugs

🔳 *Amiodarone:* Bradycardia, cardiac arrest, or ventricular dysrhythmia

🔳 *Antidiabetics:* Altered response to hypoglycemia, prolonged recovery of normoglycemia, hypertension, blockade of tachycardia; may increase blood glucose and impair peripheral circulation

🔳 *Antipyrine:* Increased antipyrine concentrations

🔳 *Barbiturates:* Reduced β-blocker concentrations

❷ *β-agonists:* Antagonism of bronchodilating effect

🔳 *Bromazepam, diazepam, oxazepam:* Increased benzodiazepine effect (lorazepam and alprazolam unaffected)

🔳 *Cimetidine, etintidine, propafenone, propoxyphene, quinidine:* Increased plasma metoprolol concentration

🔳 *Dihydropyridines (nicardipine, nifedipine, felodipine, isradipine, nisoldipine):* Increased β-blocker effects

🔳 *Diltiazem, verapamil:* Enhanced effects of both drugs, particularly atrioventricular conduction slowing

🔳 *Dipyridamole, tacrine:* Bradycardia

🔳 *Fluoxetine:* Enhanced effect of β-blocker

🔳 *Isoproterenol:* Potential reduction in effectiveness of isoproterenol in the treatment of asthma; less likely with cardioselective agents like metoprolol

🔳 *Local anesthetics:* Use of local anesthetics containing epinephrine may result in hypertensive reactions in patients taking β-blockers

🔳 *NSAIDs:* Reduced hypotensive effects of β-blockers

🔳 *Phenylephrine:* Enhanced pressor response to phenylephrine, particularly when it is administered IV

🔳 *Prazosin:* First-dose response to prazosin may be enhanced by β-blockade

🔳 *Quinolones:* Inhibition of β-blocker metabolism, increased β-blocker effects

🔳 *Rifampin:* Reduced plasma metoprolol concentration

🔳 *Theophylline:* Antagonistic pharmacodynamic effects

SPECIAL CONSIDERATIONS

PATIENT/FAMILY EDUCATION

• Do not discontinue abruptly; may precipitate angina

• Take pulse at home; notify clinician if <50 beats/min

metyrosine
(me-tye'roe-seen)

Rx: Demser

Chemical Class: Catecholamine synthesis inhibitor

Therapeutic Class: Antipheochromocytoma agent

CLINICAL PHARMACOLOGY

Mechanism of Action: Competitively inhibits tyrosine hydroxylase, the rate-limiting step in catecholamine synthesis; decreases endogenous catecholamine concentrations

Pharmacokinetics

PO: Peak 1-3 hr, onset within 1st 2 days of therapy; excreted unchanged in urine; t₁/₂ 3.4-7.2 hr

---

italic = common side effects

bold italic = life-threatening reactions

INDICATIONS AND USES: Pheochromocytoma (preoperative preparation for surgery; patients in whom surgery is contraindicated; chronic treatment in malignant neoplasm), adjunct to neuroleptics in chronic schizophrenia*

DOSAGE

Adult and Child >12 yr

• PO 250 mg qid, may increase by 250-500 mg qd up to max of 4 g/day in divided doses

$ AVAILABLE FORMS/COST OF THERAPY

• Cap, Gel—Oral: 250 mg, 100's: **$142.49**

CONTRAINDICATIONS: Hypertension of unknown etiology

PRECAUTIONS: Impaired hepatic or renal function, children <12 yr

PREGNANCY AND LACTATION: Pregnancy category C

SIDE EFFECTS/ADVERSE REACTIONS

CNS: Anxiety, confusion, depression, disorientation, drooling, hallucinations, headache, insomnia and psychic stimulation upon drug withdrawal, parkinsonism, *sedation, speech difficulty,* tremor, trismus

CV: Peripheral edema

EENT: Nasal stuffiness

GI: Abdominal pain, *diarrhea (10%),* dry mouth, increased AST, nausea, vomiting

GU: Crystalluria, failure to ejaculate, hematuria, impotence, transient dysuria

HEME: Anemia, eosinophilia, ***thrombocytopenia,*** thrombocytosis

METAB: Breast swelling, galactorrhea

MISC: Hypersensitivity reactions (urticaria, pharyngeal edema)

DRUG INTERACTIONS

Drugs

3 *Phenothiazines, haloperidol:* Potentiation of EPS

Labs

• *False increase:* Urinary catecholamines (due to presence of metyrosine metabolites)

SPECIAL CONSIDERATIONS

PATIENT/FAMILY EDUCATION

• Maintain a daily liberal fluid intake

• Avoid alcohol or CNS depressants

MONITORING PARAMETERS

• Blood pressure, ECG

---

mexiletine

(mex-il'e-teen)

Rx: Mexitil

Chemical Class: Lidocaine derivative

Therapeutic Class: Antidysrhythmic (Class IB)

CLINICAL PHARMACOLOGY

Mechanism of Action: Blocks the fast sodium channel in cardiac tissues; reducing rate of rise and amplitude of the action potential, and decreasing the effective refractory period in Purkinje fibers; does not significantly alter sinus node automaticity, left ventricular function, systolic arterial blood pressure, AV conduction velocity, QRS or QT intervals

Pharmacokinetics

PO: Onset 0.5-2 hr, peak 2-3 hr; 60%-75% bound to plasma proteins; metabolized in liver, eliminated via bile and urine; $t_{1/2}$ 10-12 hr (prolonged in hepatic or renal failure, reduced cardiac output, acute MI)

INDICATIONS AND USES: Documented, life-threatening ventricular dysrhythmia; diabetic neuropathy*

DOSAGE

Adult

• PO 200 mg q8h initially, adjust in 50-100 mg increments q2-3 days, do not exceed 1200 mg/day

Child

• PO 1.4-5 mg/kg/dose q8h

• Dosing adjustment in renal impairment: Administer 50%-75% of normal dose if CrCl <10 ml/min

• Dosing adjustment in hepatic disease: Administer 25%-30% of normal dose

$ AVAILABLE FORMS/COST OF THERAPY

• Cap, Gel—Oral: 150 mg, 100's: **$69.05-$82.68;** 200 mg, 100's: **$82.22-$98.34;** 250 mg, 100's: **$95.66-$108.94**

CONTRAINDICATIONS: Cardiogenic shock, preexisting 2nd or 3rd degree AV block (if pacemaker not present)

PRECAUTIONS: Structural heart disease, hepatic disease, renal function impairment, children, 1st degree AV block, preexisting sinus node dysfunction, intraventricular conduction abnormalities, hypotension, severe CHF, seizure disorder

PREGNANCY AND LACTATION: Pregnancy category C; limited data do not suggest significant risk to the fetus; compatible with breast feeding

SIDE EFFECTS/ADVERSE REACTIONS

CNS: Changes in sleep habits, confusion, *coordination difficulties,* depression, *dizziness,* fatigue, fever, hallucinations, headache, *lightheadedness,* nervousness, paresthesias, psychosis, *seizures,* short-term memory loss, speech difficulties, *tremor,* weakness

CV: Angina, atrial dysrhythmias, AV block, bradycardia, ***cardiogenic shock,*** chest pain, ***CHF,*** conduction disturbances, edema, hot flashes, hypertension, hypotension, ***increased ventricular dysrhythmias,*** palpitations, PVCs, syncope

EENT: Blurred vision, tinnitus

GI: Abdominal pain, altered taste, changes in appetite, constipation, diarrhea, dry mouth, dysphagia, esophageal ulceration, hepatitis, oral mucous membrane changes, peptic ulcer, pharyngitis, salivary changes, ***upper GI bleeding,*** upper GI distress *(nausea, vomiting, heartburn, 40%)*

GU: Decreased libido, impotence, urinary hesitancy

HEME: ***Agranulocytosis, leukopenia,*** positive ANA, ***thrombocytopenia*** (rare)

MS: Arthralgia

RESP: Dyspnea, hiccups

SKIN: Diaphoresis, dry skin, ***exfoliative dermatitis,*** hair loss, rash

DRUG INTERACTIONS

Drugs

3 *Acetazolamide, sodium bicarbonate:* Alkalinization of urine retards mexiletine elimination

3 *Phenytoin, rifampin:* Reduced mexiletine concentrations

3 *Quinidine:* Elevated mexiletine concentrations

2 *Theophylline:* Elevated theophylline serum concentrations and toxicity

SPECIAL CONSIDERATIONS

• Because of proarrhythmic effects, not recommended for non-life-threatening arrhythmias

• Antiarrhythmic drugs have not been shown to increase survival of patients with ventricular arrhythmias

PATIENT/FAMILY EDUCATION

• Take with food or antacid

MONITORING PARAMETERS

• Therapeutic mexiletine concentrations 0.5-2 μg/ml

---

* = non FDA-approved use

milrinone
(mill're-none)
Rx: Primacor
Chemical Class: Bipyridine derivative
Therapeutic Class: Congestive heart failure agent

CLINICAL PHARMACOLOGY
Mechanism of Action: Positive inotropic agent with vasodilator properties; selective inhibitor of peak III cAMP phosphodiesterase isozyme in cardiac and vascular muscle; reduces preload and afterload by direct relaxation of vascular smooth muscle
Pharmacokinetics
IV: Onset 2-5 min, peak 10 min, duration variable, $t_{1/2}$ 2-4 hr; metabolized in liver, excreted in urine as drug (83%) and metabolites
INDICATIONS AND USES: Short-term management of CHF not responsive to other medication (can be used with digitalis)
DOSAGE
Adult
• IV bolus 50 µg/kg given over 10 min; start INF of 0.375-0.75 µg/kg/min
• Reduced dose in renal impairment:

Creatinine Clearance (ml/min/1.73m²)	Infusion Rate (mg/kg/min)
5	0.20
10	0.23
20	0.28
30	0.33
40	0.38
50	0.43

S AVAILABLE FORMS/COST OF THERAPY
• Inj, Sol—IV: 1 mg/ml, 5 ml: **$31.26**
CONTRAINDICATIONS: Severe aortic stenosis, severe pulmonic stenosis, acute MI
PRECAUTIONS: Children, renal disease, hepatic disease; atrial flutter, fibrillation; outflow tract obstruction in hypertrophic subaortic stenosis, elderly
PREGNANCY AND LACTATION: Pregnancy category C; unknown if excreted into breast milk
SIDE EFFECTS/ADVERSE REACTIONS
CNS: Headache, tremor
CV: Chest pain, *dysrhythmias* (12%), hypotension
GI: Abdominal pain, anorexia, hepatotoxicity, jaundice, nausea, vomiting
HEME: **Thrombocytopenia**
METAB: Hypokalemia

SPECIAL CONSIDERATIONS
MONITORING PARAMETERS
• Fluid and electrolyte changes, renal function
• Improvement in cardiac output may increase diuresis, and K⁺ loss

minoxidil
(min-nox'i-dill)
Rx: *Oral:* Apo-Gain ✦, Loniten
Topical: Minoxigaine ✦
OTC: Rogaine, Rogaine Extra Strength for Men
Chemical Class: Piperidinopyrimidine derivative
Therapeutic Class: Antihypertensive (oral use); hair growth stimulant (topical use)

CLINICAL PHARMACOLOGY
Mechanism of Action: Relaxes arteriolar smooth muscle, causes vasodilation with reflex increase in heart rate, cardiac output; may increase cutaneous blood flow, stimulate hair follicles
Pharmocokinetics
PO: Onset 30 min, peak 2-3 hr, duration 24-48 hr, $t_{1/2}$ 4.2 hr; metabolized in liver, 97% renal excretion (metabolites); excreted in breast milk
TOP: Small amounts absorbed (0.3%-4.5%), absorption increased through inflamed skin; onset of action min 4 mo; growth peaks at 1 yr
INDICATIONS AND USES: Severe hypertension not responsive to other therapy, in conjunction with diuretic; topically to treat alopecia androgenetica (less effective in frontal hair loss)
DOSAGE
Adult and Adolescents
• PO 2.5-5 mg/day as single dose or divided bid not to exceed 100 mg/day, usual range 10-40 mg/day; double dose q3 days to appropriate response; for rapid control adjust q6h, monitor closely
• TOP 1 ml (2% sol) bid regardless of size of area, max 2 ml qd
Child <12 yr
• Initial dose PO 0.2 mg/kg/day (max 5 mg), effective range 0.25-1 mg/kg/day in 1 or 2 doses, max 50 mg/day
S AVAILABLE FORMS/COST OF THERAPY
• Tab, Uncoated—Oral: 2.5 mg, 100's: **$12.00-$47.25;** 10 mg, 100's: **$15.75-$182.80**
• Sol—Top: 2%, 60 ml: **$29.50**
CONTRAINDICATIONS: Acute MI, dissecting aortic aneurysm, pheochromocytoma (PO)
PRECAUTIONS: Children, renal disease, CAD, CHF (PO)
PREGNANCY AND LACTATION: Pregnancy category C; compatible with breast feeding
SIDE EFFECTS/ADVERSE REACTIONS
CV: Angina, **CHF,** edema, **pericardial effusion, pericarditis, pulmonary edema,** severe rebound hypertension, sodium and water retention, tachycardia, *T wave changes* (direction and magnitude, 60%)
GI: Nausea, vomiting
GU: Breast tenderness, gynecomastia
HEME: Decreased Hct (hemodilution), **leukopenia, thrombocytopenia**
SKIN: Hypertrichosis (80% of patients, resolves 1-6 months after discontinuation of drug), pruritus, rash, **Stevens-Johnson syndrome**
SKIN: Contact dermatitis, hypertrichosis; irritant
DRUG INTERACTIONS
Drugs
❷ *Guanethidine:* Orthostatic hypotension, may be severe
No known interactions with top sol

SPECIAL CONSIDERATIONS
Must be used in conjunction with diuretic (except dialysis patients) and β-blocker or other sympathetic nervous system depressant (to prevent reflex tachycardia)

---

italic = common side effects

bold italic = life-threatening reactions

PATIENT/FAMILY EDUCATION
• At least 4 mo of bid application necessary before evidence of hair growth with topical solution
• Continued treatment necessary to maintain or increase hair growth with topical solution

---

moexipril
(moe-ex'a-prile)
Rx: Univasc
Combinations
    Rx: with hydrochlorothiazide (Uniretic)
Chemical Class: Angiotensin-converting enzyme (ACE) inhibitor
Therapeutic Class: Antihypertensive; congestive heart failure agent; renal protectant

---

CLINICAL PHARMACOLOGY
Mechanism of Action: ACE inhibition suppresses the renin-angiotensin-aldosterone system, resulting in reduced peripheral arterial resistance; no change or an increase in cardiac output; increased renal blood flow, but no change in glomerular filtration rate; blood pressure reduction (standing and supine equally)
Pharmacokinetics
PO: Prodrug, requiring hepatic conversion to active metabolite (moexiprilat); bioavailability 13%; onset 1 hr, duration 24 hr; fecal excretion 50% (13% renal excretion); $t_{1/2}$ 2-10 hr
INDICATIONS AND USES: Hypertension, heart failure,* left ventricular dysfunction,* diabetic nephropathy*
DOSAGE
Adult
• Hypertension: Initial 7.5 mg PO 1 hr ac qd; maintenance 7.5-30 mg PO qd-bid
• Renal function impairment: CrCl <40 ml/min, 3.75 mg PO qd; max 15 mg/day
S AVAILABLE FORMS/COST OF THERAPY
• Tab, Uncoated—Oral: 7.5, 15 mg, 100's: **$49.69**
PRECAUTIONS: Hyperkalemia; surgery, anesthesia (hypotension); hypotension, renal artery stenosis, renal function impairment
PREGNANCY AND LACTATION: Pregnancy category C (1st trimester); category D (2nd and 3rd trimesters)
SIDE EFFECTS/ADVERSE REACTIONS
CNS: Dizziness, fatigue, headache, insomnia, peripheral neuropathy
CV: **CHF, dysrhythmia,** *hypotension,* Raynaud's syndrome
GI: Abdominal pain, aphthous ulcers, diarrhea, dysgeusia, gastric irritation, nausea, vomiting, weight loss
GU: Nephrotic syndrome, polyuria, proteinuria, renal insufficiency
HEME: **Agranulocytosis,** decreased hemoglobin, **neutropenia, pancytopenia, thrombocytopenia**
METAB: Electrolyte disturbance (hyperkalemia, hyponatremia)
RESP: Cough
SKIN: Alopecia, pemphigus, pruritus, rash, scalded-mouth sensation
DRUG INTERACTIONS
Drugs
❷ *Allopurinol:* Combination may predispose to hypersensitivity reactions
❸ *α-adrenergic blockers:* Exaggerated first dose hypotensive reactions when added to moexipril
❸ *Aspirin:* May reduce hemodynamic effects of moexipril; less likely at doses under 236 mg; less likely with nonacetylated salicylates

❸ *Cyclosporine:* Combination may cause renal insufficiency
❸ *Insulin:* Moexipril may enhance insulin sensitivity
❸ *Iron:* Moexipril may increase chance of systemic reaction to IV iron
❸ *Lithium:* Reduced lithium clearance
❸ *Loop diuretics:* Initiation of moexipril may cause hypotension and renal insufficiency in patients taking loop diuretics
❸ *NSAIDs:* May reduce hemodynamic effects of moexipril
❸ *Potassium-sparing diuretics:* Increased risk of hyperkalemia

SPECIAL CONSIDERATIONS
• Besides the once-daily dosing advantage of other long-acting ACE inhibitors, does not possess any characteristic to give it preference over any other ACE inhibitor; controlled comparisons are not available; low price may be major selling edge

---

moricizine
(mor-iss'i-zeen)
Rx: Ethmozine
Chemical Class: Phenothiazine derivative
Therapeutic Class: Antidysrhythmic (Class I)

CLINICAL PHARMACOLOGY
Mechanism of Action: Decreases rate of rise of action potential, prolongs refractory period, and shortens the action potential duration; depression of inward influx of sodium mediates these effects; slows atrial and AV nodal conduction; increase in resting blood pressure and heart rate; inhibits platelet aggregation; anticholinergic effects
Pharmacokinetics
PO: Peak 0.5-2.2 hr
Well absorbed; metabolized by the liver, metabolites are excreted in feces and urine; protein binding >90%; $t_{1/2}$ 1½-3½ hr
INDICATIONS AND USES: Symptomatic, life-threatening ventricular dysrhythmias
DOSAGE
Adult
• PO 600-900 mg/day in 2-3 divided doses; increase dosage in 150 mg increments at 3-day intervals up to 900 mg/day; decrease dose in patients with significant liver and renal dysfunction
S AVAILABLE FORMS/COST OF THERAPY
• Tab, Coated—Oral: 200 mg, 100's: **$96.91;** 250 mg, 100's: **$115.69;** 300 mg, 100's: **$131.72**
CONTRAINDICATIONS: 2nd-3rd degree AV block; right bundle branch block when associated with left hemiblock (bifascicular block) unless a pacemaker is present; cardiogenic shock
PRECAUTIONS: CHF, hypokalemia, hyperkalemia, sick sinus syndrome, children, impaired hepatic and renal function, cardiac dysfunction
PREGNANCY AND LACTATION: Pregnancy category B; secreted into breast milk (1 patient); potential for serious adverse effects exists
SIDE EFFECTS/ADVERSE REACTIONS
CNS: Depression, *dizziness,* euphoria, fatigue, headache, nervousness, perioral numbness, sleep disorders, tinnitus
CV: Bradycardia, chest pain, **CHF, dysrhythmias,** hypertension, **MI,** *palpitations,* syncope, thrombophlebitis
GI: Abdominal pain, diarrhea, *nausea,* vomiting
GU: Difficult urination, dysuria, incontinence, sexual dysfunction
RESP: **Apnea,** asthma, cough, *dyspnea,* hyperventilation, pharyngitis
MISC: Musculoskeletal pain, sweating

---

* = non FDA-approved use

DRUG INTERACTIONS
◪ *Cimetidine:* Increases serum moricizine concentrations
◪ *Theophylline:* Reduces serum theophylline levels by increasing clearance

SPECIAL CONSIDERATIONS
• Antidysrhythmic therapy has not been proven to be beneficial in terms of improving survival among patients with asymptomatic or mildly symptomatic ventricular dysrhythmias
• Studied in the CAST (Cardiac Arrhythmia Suppression Trial, I and II) with findings of excessive cardiac mortality and no benefit on long-term survival compared to placebo

---

morphine
(mor'feen)
Rx: Astramorph PF, Duramorph, Infumorph, Kadian, M-Eslon ✚, M.O.S.-Sulfate ✚, MS Contin, MSIR, Oramorph SR, RMS, Roxanol, Statex ✚
Chemical Class: Opiate derivative
Therapeutic Class: Narcotic analgesic
DEA Class: Schedule II

CLINICAL PHARMACOLOGY
Mechanism of Action: Altered processes affecting both the perception of pain and the emotional response to pain, at the spinal cord level, by interacting with opioid receptors (primarily μ-receptors)
Pharmacokinetics
PO: 60 mg = 10 IM morphine; duration of action: 8-12 hr (EXT REL preps); 4-5 hr (other oral dosage forms)
SC: Onset 10-30 min, peak analgesia 50-90 min, duration 4-5 hr
IM: Onset 10-30 min, peak analgesia 30-60, duration 4½ hr
IV: Peak analgesia 20 min
Metabolized by liver; 85% excreted by kidneys, 7%-10% biliary; $t_{1/2}$ 2½-3 hr
INDICATIONS AND USES: Severe pain; anesthesia (adjunct); diarrhea*; cough*; acute pulmonary edema*
DOSAGE
Adult
• *Chronic pain:* SC/IM 4-15 mg q4h prn; PO 5-30 mg q4h prn; EXT REL 15-60 mg q8-12h (base dose on 24-hr requirement of immediate-release morphine); Rec 10-20 mg q4h prn
• IV 4-15 mg diluted in 4-5 ml H_2O for inj, over 5 min
Child
• Analgesia: SC 0.1-0.2 mg/kg, not to exceed 15 mg
⑤ **AVAILABLE FORMS/COST OF THERAPY**
• Inj, Sol—Epidural, Intrathecal, IV: 0.5 mg/ml, 2 ml: **$7.68-$8.70;** 1 mg/ml, 2 ml (preservative free): **$8.30-$9.58**
• Inj, Sol—IM; IV; SC: 2 mg/ml, 1 ml: **$0.72-$1.10;** 4 mg/ml, 1 ml: **$0.71-$1.13;** 5 mg/ml, 30 ml: **$17.50;** 8 mg/ml, 1 ml: **$0.73-$1.16;** 10 mg/ml, 1 ml: **$0.78-$1.20;** 15 mg/ml, 1 ml: **$0.83-$1.70**
• Inj, Sol—IV: 25 mg/ml, 4 ml: **$9.44-$85.50;** 50 mg/ml, 10 ml: **$34.14-$286.75**
• Cap, Gel—Oral: 15 mg, 50's: **$14.45;** 20 mg, 60's: **$68.85;** 30 mg, 50's: **$26.97;** 50 mg, 60's: **$167.92;** 100 mg, 60's: **$298.34**
• Conc—Oral: 100 mg/5 ml, 120 ml: **$70.64**
• Sol—Oral: 10 mg/5 ml, 500 ml: **$20.10-$30.29;** 20 mg/5 ml, 500 ml: **$48.38-$51.08;** 20 mg/ml, 120 ml: **$40.00-$75.69**
• Supp—Rect: 5 mg, 12's: **$9.60-$14.35;** 10 mg, 12's: **$11.55-$16.95;** 20 mg, 12's: **$14.05-$20.56;** 30 mg, 12's: **$17.00-$28.71**
• Tab, Coated, SUS Action—Oral: 15 mg, 100's: **$64.71-$77.61;**

30 mg, 100's: **$122.98-$147.49;** 60 mg, 100's: **$239.97-$287.79;** 100 mg, 100's: **$367.51-$436.33;** 200 mg, 100's: **$799.00**
• Tab, Hypodermic—IM, IV: 30 mg, 100's: **$46.90**
• Tab, Hypodermic—IV, SC: 15 mg, 100's: **$27.95;** 10 mg, 100's: **$22.03**
• Tab, Uncoated—Oral: 15 mg, 100's: **$16.88-$25.36;** 30 mg, 100's: **$28.52-$43.05**
CONTRAINDICATIONS: Respiratory depression, hemorrhage, acute asthma attack, paralytic ileus, convulsive states (injection)
PRECAUTIONS: Addictive personality, elderly, hepatic disease, renal disease, child <18 yr, head injury, acute abdominal conditions, hypothyroidism, prostatic hypertrophy, Addison's disease
PREGNANCY AND LACTATION: Pregnancy category B; trace amounts enter breast milk; compatible with breast feeding
SIDE EFFECTS/ADVERSE REACTIONS
CNS: Addiction, confusion, *dizziness, drowsiness,* euphoria, headache, sedation
CV: Bradycardia, *hypotension,* palpitations
EENT: Blurred vision, diplopia, *miosis,* tinnitus
GI: Anorexia, biliary tract pressure, *constipation,* cramps, *nausea,* vomiting
GU: Urinary retention
RESP: ***Respiratory depression***
SKIN: Bruising, diaphoresis, flushing, pruritus, rash, urticaria
MISC: Histamine release (decreased blood pressure, fast heartbeat, increased sweating, redness or flushing of face, wheezing or troubled breathing)
DRUG INTERACTIONS
Drugs
◪ *Cimetidine:* Inhibition of narcotic hepatic metabolism, additive CNS effect
◪ *Rifampin:* May reduce narcotic concentrations and precipitate withdrawal
Labs
• *Increase:* Urine glucose, urine 17-ketosteroids

SPECIAL CONSIDERATIONS
• Treatment of overdose: Naloxone (Narcan) 0.2-0.8 mg IV
• Remains the strong analgesic of choice for acute, severe pain, acute MI pain, and the agent of choice for chronic cancer pain
• 200 mg EXT REL tablet for use only in opioid-tolerant patients
PATIENT/FAMILY EDUCATION
• Change position slowly to avoid orthostasis
• Avoid alcohol and other CNS depressants
• Physical dependency may result
• Do not chew or crush EXT REL preparations

---

nadolol
(nay-doe'loll)
Rx: Apo-Nadol, Corgard, Novo-Nadolol, Syn-Nadolol
Chemical Class: Nonselective β-adrenergic blocker
Therapeutic Class: Antihypertensive; antianginal

CLINICAL PHARMACOLOGY
Mechanism of Action: Competes with β-adrenergic agonists for available β-receptors in cardiac, bronchial, and vascular tissue; reduces heart rate, blood pressure and myocardial oxygen demand
Pharmacokinetics
PO: Onset variable, peak 3-4 hr, duration 17-24 hr, $t_{1/2}$ 16-20 hr; not metabolized; excreted in urine (unchanged)

---

italic = common side effects

bold italic = life-threatening reactions

INDICATIONS AND USES: Chronic stable angina pectoris; mild to moderate hypertension; prophylaxis of migraine headaches*
DOSAGE
Adult
• PO 40 mg qd, increase by 40-80 mg q3-7 days; maintenance 40-240 mg/day for angina, 40-320 mg/day for hypertension
⑤ AVAILABLE FORMS/COST OF THERAPY
• Tab, Uncoated—Oral: 20 mg, 100's: **$72.40-$101.58**; 40 mg, 100's: **$84.67-$119.09**; 80 mg, 100's: **$116.09-$163.29**; 120 mg, 100's: **$151.68-$212.82**; 160 mg, 100's: **$168.70-$236.70**
CONTRAINDICATIONS: Cardiogenic shock, 2nd or 3rd degree heart block, bronchospastic disease, sinus bradycardia, overt cardiac failure
PRECAUTIONS: Diabetes mellitus, renal disease, hyperthyroidism, peripheral vascular disease, myasthenia gravis, well-compensated heart failure
PREGNANCY AND LACTATION: Pregnancy category C; excreted into breast milk, milk concentrations 4-5 times higher than maternal serum, but infant would receive <10% of therapeutic adult dose; compatible with breast feeding
SIDE EFFECTS/ADVERSE REACTIONS
CNS: Depression, dizziness, fatigue, hallucinations, headache, lethargy, paresthesias
CV: AV block, *bradycardia,* chest pain, *CHF,* conduction disturbances, edema, flushing, *hypotension,* palpitations, peripheral ischemia, vasodilation
EENT: Sore throat
GI: Colitis, constipation, cramps, diarrhea, dry mouth, flatulence, hepatomegaly, increased transaminases, serum alkaline phosphatase; nausea, pancreatitis, taste distortion, vomiting
HEME: Agranulocytosis, thrombocytopenia
METAB: Hyperkalemia, hyperuricemia
RESP: Bronchospasm, cough, dyspnea, *laryngospasm,* nasal stuffiness, pharyngitis, respiratory dysfunction, wheezing
SKIN: Fever, pruritus, rash
DRUG INTERACTIONS
Drugs
⚅ *Adenosine:* Bradycardia aggravated
⚅ *Ampicillin:* Reduced nadolol bioavailability
⚅ *Antacids:* Reduced nadolol absorption
⚅ *Calcium channel blockers:* See dihydropyridine and verapamil
⚅ *Clonidine:* Exacerbation of rebound hypertension upon discontinuation of clonidine
⚅ *Dihydropyridines:* Additive hemodynamic effects; increased serum concentration of nadolol
⚅ *Dipyridamole:* Bradycardia aggravated
⚅ *Lidocaine:* Increased serum lidocaine concentrations possible
⚅ *Neostigmine:* Bradycardia aggravated
⚅ *NSAIDs:* Reduced antihypertensive effect of nadolol
⚅ *Physostigmine:* Bradycardia aggravated
⚅ *Prazosin:* First-dose response to prazosin may be enhanced by β-blockade
⚅ *Tacrine:* Bradycardia aggravated
❷ *Theophylline:* Antagonistic pharmacodynamic effects
⚅ *Verapamil:* Enhanced effects of both drugs, particularly AV node conduction slowing; reduced nadolol clearance

SPECIAL CONSIDERATIONS
• No unique advantage over less expensive β-blockers
PATIENT/FAMILY EDUCATION
• Do **not** discontinue abruptly

---

niacin (vitamin B₃; nicotinic acid)
(nye′a-sin)
Rx: Niacor, Niaspan, Nicolar;
OTC: Nia-Bid, Nia-C, Niacels, Nico-400, Nicotinex, Slo-Niacin
Chemical Class: B complex vitamin
Therapeutic Class: Vitamin; antilipemic

CLINICAL PHARMACOLOGY
Mechanism of Action: Necessary for lipid metabolism, tissue respiration, and glycogenolysis; lowers total serum cholesterol, low-density lipoprotein (LDL) cholesterol and triglyceride concentrations by inhibiting the synthesis of very-low-density lipoproteins (VLDL), which are precursors to the formation of cholesterol; raises high-density lipoprotein (HDL) cholesterol
Pharmacokinetics
PO: Readily absorbed from GI tract; peak 45 min; metabolized in liver, eliminated in urine (almost entirely as metabolites); $t_{1/2}$ 45 min
INDICATIONS AND USES: Vitamin deficiency (pellagra); types IIa, IIb, IV and V, hyperlipidemia as an adjunct to a low-cholesterol diet; to reduce risk of recurrent MI in patients with history of MI and hypercholesterolemia; reduction of atherosclerotic disease in patients with a history of CAD
DOSAGE
Adult
• *Recommended daily allowance PO:* Males 19-50 yr 19 mg/day; males >51 yr 15 mg/day; females 11-50 yr 15 mg/day; females >51 yr 13 mg/day
• *Pellagra:* PO 50-100 mg tid-qid; max 500 mg/day
• *Niacin deficiency:* PO 10-20 mg/day; max 100 mg/day
• *Hyperlipidemia:* PO 1.5-6 g/day divided bid-tid with or after meals (start at 100-250 mg/day and titrate gradually)
Child
• *Recommended daily allowance PO:* 0-0.5 yr 5 mg/day; 0.5-1 yr 6 mg/day; 1-3 yr 9 mg/day; 4-6 yr 12 mg/day; 7-10 yr 13 mg/day; males 11-14 yr 17 mg/day; males 15-18 yr 20 mg/day
• *Pellagra:* PO 50-100 mg tid
⑤ AVAILABLE FORMS/COST OF THERAPY
• Tab, Uncoated—Oral: 50 mg, 100's: **$1.15-$2.20**; 100 mg, 100's: **$1.20-$2.55**; 500 mg, 100's: **$2.25-$64.40**
• Cap, Gel, SUS Action—Oral: 125 mg, 100's: **$3.75-$5.70**; 250 mg, 100's: **$4.43-$5.94**; 400 mg, 100's: **$3.63-$6.98**; 500 mg, 100's: **$7.80**; 750 mg, 100's: **$7.05**
• Elixir—Oral: 50 mg/5 ml, 480 ml: **$8.25**
CONTRAINDICATIONS: Hepatic dysfunction, active peptic ulcer, severe hypotension, hemorrhage
PRECAUTIONS: Unstable CAD, gallbladder disease, history of jaundice or liver disease, history of peptic ulcer, history of arterial bleeding, gout, diabetes mellitus, tartrazine sensitivity
PREGNANCY AND LACTATION: Pregnancy category A (category C if used in doses greater than recommended daily allowance); actively excreted in human breast milk; recommended daily allowance during lactation is 18-20 mg
SIDE EFFECTS/ADVERSE REACTIONS
CNS: Transient headache
CV: Atrial fibrillation, hypotension, orthostasis
EENT: Cystoidmacular edema, toxic amblyopia
GI: Abdominal pain, activation of peptic ulcer, diarrhea, *GI distress, hepatotoxicity* (more common with sustained-release formulations), nausea, vomiting
METAB: Decreased glucose tolerance, hyperuricemia
MS: Myopathy, myositis, *rhabdomyolysis*

SKIN: Dry skin, keratosis nigricans, *pruritus, sensation of warmth, severe generalized flushing,* skin rash, tingling

DRUG INTERACTIONS

Drugs

🔟 *Lovastatin:* Isolated cases of myopathy and rhabdomyolysis have occurred, causality not established

Labs

• *Interference:* Plasma and urine catecholamines, urine glucose with Benedict's reagent

SPECIAL CONSIDERATIONS

• In 1 g doses: 10%-20% reduction of total plus LDL-cholesterol, 30%-70% reduction in triglycerides, and a 20%-35% increase in HDL-cholesterol

PATIENT/FAMILY EDUCATION

• Gradual dosage titration lessens flushing, adverse effects
• Avoid alcohol and hot beverages (increases flushing)
• Administer with meals and 2 glasses of water
• 125-350 mg of aspirin 20-30 min before dose may lessen flushing
• Do not miss any doses (flushing may return)

MONITORING PARAMETERS

• Liver function tests, blood glucose, uric acid regularly
• Fasting lipid profile q3-6 mo

---

nicardipine

(nye-card'i-peen)

Rx: Cardene, Cardene SR

Chemical Class: Dihydropyridine calcium channel blocker
Therapeutic Class: Antihypertensive; antianginal

CLINICAL PHARMACOLOGY

Mechanism of Action: Inhibits calcium ion influx across cell membrane in vascular smooth muscle and cardiac muscle; produces relaxation of coronary and peripheral vascular smooth muscle; reduces total peripheral resistance (afterload); increases myocardial oxygen delivery; negative inotropic activity; no effects on cardiac conduction system

Pharmacokinetics

PO: Onset 20 min, peak ½-2 hr; >95% bound to plasma proteins, significant 1st-pass effect (35% systemic bioavailability); kinetics nonlinear; excreted in urine (60%) and feces (35%); $t_{1/2}$ 2-4 hr

INDICATIONS AND USES: Chronic stable angina, hypertension, Raynaud's disease*

DOSAGE

Adult

• *Angina:* PO 20 mg tid, may increase after 3 days to 40 mg tid
• *Hypertension:* PO 20 mg tid, may increase to 40 mg tid; SR 30 mg bid, may increase to 60 mg bid; IV INF 5 mg/hr initially, may be increased by 2.5 mg/hr q5-15 min up to maximum of 15 mg/hr; following achievement of goal blood pressure, decrease inf rate to 3 mg/hr, then adjust rate as needed to maintain desired response

💲 AVAILABLE FORMS/COST OF THERAPY

• Cap—Oral: 20 mg, 100's: **$42.34;** 30 mg, 100's: **$67.32**
• Cap, Gel, SUS Action—Oral: 30 mg, 60's: **$39.68;** 45 mg, 60's: **$63.02;** 60 mg, 60's: **$75.47**
• Inj, Sol—IV: 25 mg/ampul, **$21.64**

CONTRAINDICATIONS: Advanced aortic stenosis
PRECAUTIONS: CHF, hypotension, hepatic insufficiency, renal function impairment, aortic stenosis, elderly, children

PREGNANCY AND LACTATION: Pregnancy category C; significant excretion into rat maternal milk

SIDE EFFECTS/ADVERSE REACTIONS

CNS: Anxiety, *asthenia,* depression, *dizziness,* fatigue, *headache,* insomnia, malaise, nervousness, paresthesia, somnolence, tremor
CV: Angina, bradycardia, **dysrhythmia,** hypotension, palpitations, peripheral edema, syncope, tachycardia
GI: Abdominal cramps, constipation, diarrhea, dry mouth, flatulence, gastric upset, nausea, vomiting
GU: Nocturia, polyuria
SKIN: Hair loss, pruritus, rash, urticaria
MISC: Cough, epistaxis, flushing, muscle cramps, nasal congestion, sexual dysfunction, shortness of breath, sweating, tinnitus, weight gain

DRUG INTERACTIONS

Drugs

🔟 *β-blockers:* Increased propranolol and metoprolol concentrations
🔟 *Calcium:* Reduced activity of nicardipine
🔟 *Cyclosporine, tacrolimus:* Increased blood cyclosporine concentrations
🔟 *Neuromuscular blocking agents:* Prolongation of neuromuscular blockade

---

nifedipine

(nye-fed'i-peen)

Rx: Adalat, Adalat PA ✹, Procardia; Sus Rel: Adalat CC, Adalat XC ✹, Procardia XL

Chemical Class: Dihydropyridine calcium channel blocker
Therapeutic Class: Antihypertensive; antianginal

CLINICAL PHARMACOLOGY

Mechanism of Action: Inhibits calcium ion influx across cell membrane in vascular smooth muscle and cardiac muscle; produces relaxation of coronary and peripheral vascular smooth muscle, reduces total peripheral resistance (afterload); increases myocardial oxygen delivery; negative inotropic activity; no effects on cardiac conduction system

Pharmacokinetics

PO: Peak 30 min, onset within 20 min (1-5 min if capsule bitten and swallowed)
SUS REL: Peak 6 hr
92%-98% bound to plasma proteins; metabolized by liver to inactive metabolites, excreted by kidneys; $t_{1/2}$ 2-5 hr

INDICATIONS AND USES: Vasospastic (Prinzmetal's or variant) angina, chronic stable angina, hypertension, prevention of migraine headache,* preterm labor,* hypertensive urgencies,* primary pulmonary hypertension,* esophageal disorders,* high altitude pulmonary edema*; Raynaud's disease*

DOSAGE

Adult

• PO 10 mg tid initially, usual range 10-20 mg tid; doses >120 mg/day are rarely necessary; PO XL 30-60 mg qd, titration to doses >120 mg/day is not recommended; PO CC 30 mg qd, titration to doses >90 mg/day not recommended

Child

• Hypertensive urgencies: PO 0.25-0.5 mg/kg/dose

💲 AVAILABLE FORMS/COST OF THERAPY

• Cap, Gel—Oral: 10 mg, 100's: **$8.81-$58.83;** 20 mg, 100's: **$17.48-$105.91**
• Tab, Coated, SUS Action—Oral: 30 mg, 100's: **$90.53-$119.61;** 60 mg, 100's: **$150.59-$207.01;** 90 mg, 100's: **$184.47-$214.35**

---

italic = common side effects

bold italic = life-threatening reactions

CONTRAINDICATIONS: Use of immediate-release preparations in patients with severe obstructive CAD or recent MI, hypertensive emergencies

PRECAUTIONS: CHF, hypotension, hepatic insufficiency, renal function impairment, aortic stenosis, elderly, children, recent β-blocker withdrawal

PREGNANCY AND LACTATION: Pregnancy category C; has been used for tocolysis and as an antihypertensive agent in pregnant women; compatible with breast feeding

SIDE EFFECTS/ADVERSE REACTIONS
(NOTE: Usually less frequent with extended-release preparations)
CNS: Anxiety, asthenia, depression, *dizziness,* fatigue, *headache,* insomnia, malaise, nervousness, paresthesia, somnolence, tremor
CV: Bradycardia, **dysrhythmia,** *hypotension,* palpitations, *peripheral edema,* syncope, tachycardia
GI: Abdominal cramps, constipation, diarrhea, dry mouth, flatulence, gastric upset, *nausea,* vomiting
GU: Nocturia, polyuria
SKIN: Hair loss, pruritus, rash, urticaria
MISC: Cough, epistaxis, flushing, muscle cramps, nasal congestion, sexual dysfunction, shortness of breath, sweating, tinnitus, weight gain

DRUG INTERACTIONS
Drugs
▣ *Barbiturates, rifampin, rifabutin:* Reduced plasma concentrations of nifedipine
▣ *β-blockers:* Enhanced effects of β-blockers, hypotension; increased metoprolol and propanolol concentrations
▣ *Calcium:* Reduced activity of nifedipine
▣ *Cimetidine, ranitidine, famotidine:* Increased nifedipine concentrations possible
▣ *Diltiazem:* Increased serum concentrations of nifedipine
▣ *Doxazosin:* Enhanced hypotensive effects
▣ *Food:* Increased absorption of Adalat CC
▣ *Grapefruit juice:* Increased serum nifedipine concentrations
▣ *Lansoprazole:* Increased nifedipine absorption
▣ *Magnesium:* Potential for transient hypotensive effect
▣ *Phenytoin:* Increased phenytoin concentration
▣ *Quinidine:* Reduced blood concentrations of quinidine
▣ *Vincristine:* Marked increase in vincristine half-life, clinical significance unknown

SPECIAL CONSIDERATIONS
• Given the seriousness of the reported adverse events and the lack of any clinical documentation attesting to a benefit, the use of nifedipine capsules for hypertensive urgencies or emergencies should be abandoned (*JAMA* 276:1328-1331,1996)
PATIENT/FAMILY EDUCATION
• Administer Adalat CC on an empty stomach
• Do not crush or chew sustained release dosage forms
• Empty Procardia XL tablets may appear in stool, this is no cause for concern

nimodipine
(nye-mode'i-peen)
Rx: Nimotop
Chemical Class: Dihydropyridine calcium channel blocker
Therapeutic Class: Cerebral vasodilator

CLINICAL PHARMACOLOGY
Mechanism of Action: Inhibits influx of extracellular calcium ions through voltage-dependent and receptor-operated slow calcium channels in the membranes of vascular smooth muscle; greater

effect on cerebral arteries; exact mechanism in patients with subarachnoid hemorrhage unknown, may be due to dilation of small cerebral resistance vessels, with resultant increase in collateral circulation, and/or direct effect involving prevention of calcium overload in neurons
Pharmacokinetics
PO: Peak 1 hr; >95% bound to plasma proteins; extensively metabolized in liver to inactive metabolites, excreted in urine (50%) and feces (32%); $t_{1/2}$ 1.7-9 hr
INDICATIONS AND USES: Recent subarachnoid hemorrhage, acute ischemic stroke,* prevention of migraine headache*
DOSAGE
Adult
• *Subarachnoid hemorrhage:* PO 60 mg q4h for 21 consecutive days beginning within 96 hr of occurrence of hemorrhage, reduce to 30 mg q4h in patients with hepatic failure; for patients unable to swallow oral capsules, the capsule may be punctured at both ends with an 18-gauge needle and the contents emptied directly into nasogastric tube, which is then flushed with 30 ml of normal saline
• *Prevention of migraine headache*:* PO 120 mg/day in divided doses; response may not be apparent for 1-2 mo
⑤ AVAILABLE FORMS/COST OF THERAPY
• Cap, Elastic—Oral: 30 mg, 100's: **$546.92**
PRECAUTIONS: Impaired hepatic, renal function; children <18 yr
PREGNANCY AND LACTATION: Pregnancy category C
SIDE EFFECTS/ADVERSE REACTIONS
CNS: Dizziness, headache, lightheadedness, mental depression
CV: ECG abnormalities, edema, flushing, hypotension, palpitations
GI: Constipation, hepatitis, jaundice, lower abdominal discomfort
HEME: Anemia, **thrombocytopenia**
MS: Muscle pain
RESP: Dyspnea
SKIN: Rash
DRUG INTERACTIONS
Drugs
▣ *Cimetidine:* Increased serum nimodipine concentrations
▣ *Omeprazole:* Increased serum nimodipine concentrations
▣ *Valproic acid:* Increased oral bioavailability of nimodipine

SPECIAL CONSIDERATIONS
MONITORING PARAMETERS
• Blood pressure

nisoldipine
(nye-sold'i-peen)
Rx: Sular
Chemical Class: Dihydropyridine calcium channel blocker
Therapeutic Class: Antihypertensive

CLINICAL PHARMACOLOGY
Mechanism of Action: Inhibits calcium ion influx across cell membrane in vascular smooth muscle and cardiac muscle; produces relaxation of coronary vascular smooth muscle, peripheral vascular smooth muscle; reduces total peripheral resistance (afterload); increases myocardial oxygen delivery
Pharmacokinetics
PO: Absolute bioavailability 5%; peak 6-12 hr; high-fat meal increases peak concentration by ~300%; highly metabolized in liver, excreted in urine; $t_{1/2}$ 7-12 hr
INDICATIONS AND USES: Hypertension

DOSAGE
Adult
• PO 20 mg qd; may increase by 10 mg/wk or longer intervals to maximum of 60 mg/day

$ AVAILABLE FORMS/COST OF THERAPY

• Tab, Coated—Oral: 10, 20, 30, 40 mg, 100's: **$82.00**

PRECAUTIONS: CHF, hypotension, following myocardial infarction, hepatic insufficiency, aortic stenosis, elderly, children

PREGNANCY AND LACTATION: Pregnancy category C

SIDE EFFECTS/ADVERSE REACTIONS

CNS: Anxiety, asthenia, depression, dizziness, fatigue, *headache,* insomnia, malaise, nervousness, paresthesia, somnolence, tremor

CV: Bradycardia, **dysrhythmia,** flushing, hypotension, palpitations, peripheral edema, syncope, tachycardia

EENT: Epistaxis, nasal congestion, sore throat, tinnitus

GI: Abdominal cramps, constipation, diarrhea, dry mouth, flatulence, gastric upset, nausea, vomiting

GU: Nocturia, polyuria, sexual dysfunction

MS: Muscle cramps

RESP: Cough, shortness of breath

SKIN: Hair loss, pruritus, sweating, urticaria

MISC: Weight gain

DRUG INTERACTIONS
Drugs
▪ *β-adrenergic blockers:* Increased propranolol concentration

▪ *Calcium:* Reduced activity of nisoldipine

▪ *Cimetidine, famotidine, nizatidine, omeprazole, ranitidine:* Increased nisoldipine concentrations possible

▪ *Food:* Increased absorption with high-fat meal or grapefruit juice

SPECIAL CONSIDERATIONS
• No significant advantages over other dihydropyridine calcium channel blockers

PATIENT/FAMILY EDUCATION

• Do not take with high-fat meal or grapefruit juice

---

nitroglycerin
(nye-troe-gli'ser-in)

Rx: (Translingual): Nitrolingual; (Sublingual): Nitrostat; (Buccal): Nitrogard; (Oral): Nitrocot, Nitroglyn, Nitrong, Nitro-Par, Nitro-Time; (Topical): Nitro-Bid, Nitrol; (Intravenous): Nitro-Bid IV, Nitrostat IV, Tridil; (Transdermal): Deponit, Minitran, Nitrodisc, Nitro-Dur, Transderm-Nitro

Chemical Class: Organic nitrate

Therapeutic Class: Antianginal

CLINICAL PHARMACOLOGY
Mechanism of Action: Reduces myocardial oxygen demand by reducing left ventricular preload (predominantly) and afterload because of venous (predominantly) and arterial dilation with more efficient redistribution of blood flow within the myocardium; dilates coronary arteries and improves collateral flow to ischemic regions

Pharmacokinetics
SL: Onset 1-3 min, peak 4-8 min, duration 30-60 min

LINGUAL SPRAY: Onset 2 min, peak 4-10 min, duration 30-60 min

BUCCAL: Onset 2-5 min, peak 4-10 min, duration 2 hr

PO: Onset 20-45 min, peak 45-120 min, duration 4-8 hr

TOP: Onset 15-60 min, peak 30-120 min, duration 2-12 hr

TRANSDERMAL: Onset 40-60 min, peak 60-180 min, duration 8-24 hr

IV: Onset immediate, peak immediate, duration 3-5 min

60% bound to plasma proteins, metabolized by liver to inorganic nitrate (extensive 1st-pass effect), eliminated in urine; $t_{1/2}$ 1-4 min

INDICATIONS AND USES: Acute angina (SL, translingual spray, buccal), angina prophylaxis (top, transdermal, translingual spray, buccal, oral), perioperative hypertension (IV), congestive heart failure associated with MI (IV), unresponsive angina pectoris (IV), acute MI (SL, top),* Raynaud's disease (top),* hypertensive crisis (IV)*

DOSAGE
Adult
• BUCCAL 1 mg q3-5h while awake initially, titrate dosage upward if angina occurs with tab in place

• PO 2.5-9 mg bid-qid, up to 26 mg qid

• IV 5 µg/min via continuous inf, increase by 5 µg/min q3-5 min to 20 µg/min; if no response, increase by 10 µg/min q3-5 min up to 200 µg/min

• TOP 1-2 inches q8h, up to 4-5 inches q4h

• TRANSDERMAL 0.2-0.4 mg/hr initially, titrate to 0.4-0.8 mg/hr; apply new patch daily; tolerance is minimized by removing patch for 10-12 hr/day

• SL 0.2-0.6 mg q5 min for max of 3 doses in 15 min; may also use prophylactically 5-10 min before activities that provoke angina attack

• TRANSLINGUAL 1-2 sprays under tongue q3-5 min for max of 3 doses in 15 min; may also use prophylactically 5-10 min before activities that provoke angina attack

Child
IV 0.25-0.5 µg/kg/min, titrate by 0.5-1 µg/kg/min q3-5 min prn; usual dose 1-3 µg/kg/min; max 20 µg/kg/min

$ AVAILABLE FORMS/COST OF THERAPY

• Aer Spray—Oral: 0.4 mg/spray, 14.49 g: **$24.82**

• Tab—SL: 0.15 mg, 100's: **$5.46;** 0.3 mg, 100's: **$6.77;** 0.4 mg, 100's: **$6.77;** 0.6 mg, 100's: **$6.77**

• Tab, Uncoated, SUS Action—Buccal: 1 mg, 100's: **$37.87;** 2 mg, 100's: **$40.09;** 3 mg, 100's: **$43.33**

• Tab, Coated, SUS Action—Oral: 2.6 mg, 100's: **$29.61-$60.35;** 6.5 mg, 100's: **$37.06-$43.49**

• Cap, Gel, SUS Action—Oral: 2.5 mg, 100's: **$5.55-$16.68;** 6.5 mg, 100's: **$6.45-$18.71;** 9 mg, 100's: **$8.25-$18.00**

• Oint—Percutaneous: 2%; 20, 30, 60 g: **$6.63-$16.33/60** g

• Disk—Percutaneous: 0.2 mg/hr 100's: **$173.93;** 0.3 mg/hr, 30's: **$55.00;** 0.4 mg/hr, 30's: **$57.80;** 100's: **$160.52**

• Film, CONT REL—Percutaneous: 0.1, 0.2, 0.3, 0.4, 0.5, 0.6, 0.8, 1.0 mg/hr 30's: **$39.18-$63.13**

• Inj, Sol—IV: 5 mg/ml, 10 ml: **$39.19-$69.13;** 0.1, 0.2, 0.4 mg/ml, 250 ml: **$16.01-$19.57**

CONTRAINDICATIONS: Severe anemia, closed-angle glaucoma, postural hypotension, early MI (SL), head trauma, cerebral hemorrhage, hypotension or uncorrected hypovolemia, inadequate cerebral circulation, increased intracranial pressure, constrictive pericarditis, pericardial tamponade (IV)

PRECAUTIONS: Early days of MI, hypertrophic cardiomyopathy; severe hepatic, renal disease; children, glaucoma, abrupt withdrawal, continuous delivery (tolerance develops rapidly, IV excepted)

PREGNANCY AND LACTATION: Pregnancy category C; use of SL for angina during pregnancy without fetal harm has been reported

SIDE EFFECTS/ADVERSE REACTIONS

CNS: Agitation, anxiety, apprehension, confusion, *dizziness,* dyscoordination, *headache,* hypoesthesia, hypokinesia, insomnia, nervousness, nightmares, restlessness, vertigo, weakness

---

italic = common side effects   **bold italic** = life-threatening reactions

CV: Atrial fibrillation, **collapse,** crescendo angina, **dysrhythmias,** palpitations, *postural hypotension,* premature ventricular contractions, rebound hypertension, retrosternal discomfort, syncope, tachycardia
EENT: Blurred vision
GI: Abdominal pain, diarrhea, dyspepsia, fecal incontinence, nausea, tenesmus, tooth disorder, vomiting
GU: Dysuria, impotence, urinary frequency
HEME: **Hemolytic anemia, methemoglobinemia**
MS: Arthralgia
SKIN: Allergic reactions (ointment), contact dermatitis (transdermal), crusty skin lesions, *cutaneous vasodilation with flushing,* **exfoliative dermatitis,** pallor, pruritus, rash, sweating
DRUG INTERACTIONS
Drugs
➋ *Ergot alkaloids:* Opposition to coronary vasodilatory effects of nitrates
▪ *Ethanol:* Additive vasodilation could cause hypotension
▪ *Metronidazole:* Ethanol contained in IV nitroglycerine preparations could cause disulfiram-like reaction in some patients
Labs
• *False increase:* Serum triglycerides

SPECIAL CONSIDERATIONS
• 10-12 hr drug-free intervals prevent development of tolerance
PATIENT/FAMILY EDUCATION
• Avoid alcohol
• Notify clinician if persistent headache occurs
• Take oral nitrates on empty stomach with full glass of water
• Keep tablets and capsules in original container, keep container closed tightly
• Dissolve SL tablets under tongue, lack of burning does not indicate loss of potency, use when seated, take at 1st sign of anginal attack, activate emergency response system if no relief after 3 tablets spaced 5 min apart
• Spray translingual spray onto or under tongue, do not inhale spray
• Place buccal tablets under upper lip or between cheek and gum, permit to dissolve slowly over 3-5 min, do not chew or swallow
• Spread thin layer of ointment on skin using applicator or dose-measuring papers, do not use fingers, do not rub or massage
• Apply transdermal systems to non-hairy area on upper torso, remove for 10-12 hr/day (usually hs)
MONITORING PARAMETERS
• Blood pressure, heart rate at peak effect times

---

nitroprusside
(nye-troe-pruss'ide)
Rx: Nitropress
Chemical Class: Cyanonitrosylferrate derivative
Therapeutic Class: Antihypertensive

CLINICAL PHARMACOLOGY
Mechanism of Action: Relaxes vascular smooth muscle and dilates peripheral arteries and veins; more active on veins than arteries; reduces left ventricular end-diastolic pressure and pulmonary capillary wedge pressure (preload); reduces systemic vascular resistance, systolic arterial pressure, and mean arterial pressure (afterload); dilates coronary arteries
Pharmacokinetics
IV: Onset immediate; rapidly metabolized by interaction with sulfhydryl groups in erythrocytes and tissues (cyanogen is pro-

duced and converted to thiocyanate in liver), eliminated via urine (metabolites); circulating $t_{1/2}$ 2 min
INDICATIONS AND USES: Hypertensive crisis, controlled hypotension during surgery, severe refractory congestive heart failure (in combination with dopamine),* acute MI*
DOSAGE
Adult
• IV INF 2 µg/kg/min initially, increase in increments of 2-4 µg/kg/min (up to 20 µg/kg/min), then in increments of 10-20 µg/kg/min; cyanide toxicity more likely when 500 µg/kg is administered by prolonged infusion (8 hr) of greater than 20 µg/kg/min
Child
• IV INF 1 µg/kg/min initially, increase in increments of 1 µg/kg/min at intervals of 20-60 min; do not exceed 10 µg/kg/min
$ **AVAILABLE FORMS/COST OF THERAPY**
• Inj, Lyphl-Sol—IV: 50 mg/vial, 1's: **$8.47**
CONTRAINDICATIONS: Decreased cerebral perfusion, arteriovenous shunt or coarctation of the aorta (i.e., compensatory hypertension), congenital (Leber's) optic atrophy, tobacco amblyopia
PRECAUTIONS: Hepatic disease, decreased renal function, prolonged infusion, elevated intracranial pressure, anemia, hypovolemia, poor surgical risks, hypothyroidism, hyponatremia
PREGNANCY AND LACTATION: Pregnancy category C
SIDE EFFECTS/ADVERSE REACTIONS
CNS: Apprehension, *dizziness, headache,* increased intracranial pressure
CV: Bradycardia, ECG changes, hypotension, palpitations, retrosternal discomfort, tachycardia
GI: Abdominal pain, ileus, nausea, retching
HEME: Decreased platelet aggregation, **methemoglobinemia**
METAB: Hypothyroidism
MS: Muscle twitching
SKIN: Diaphoresis, flushing, irritation at INF site, rash
MISC: **Thiocyanate or cyanide toxicity**
DRUG INTERACTIONS
Drugs
▪ *Clonidine:* Severe hypotensive reactions have been reported
▪ *Diltiazem:* Reduction in the dose of nitroprusside required to produce hypotension
▪ *Guanabenz, guanfacine:* Potential for severe hypotensive reactions

SPECIAL CONSIDERATIONS
MONITORING PARAMETERS
• Blood pressure, arterial blood gases, oxygen saturation, cyanide and thiocyanate concentrations, anion gap, lactate levels

---

norepinephrine
(nor-ep-i-nef'rin)
Rx: Levophed
Chemical Class: Catecholamine
Therapeutic Class: Vasopressor

CLINICAL PHARMACOLOGY
Mechanism of Action: Stimulates β₁-adrenergic receptors and β-adrenergic receptors causing increased myocardial contractility and heart rate as well as vasoconstriction; increases blood pressure and coronary artery blood flow; marked pressor effect primarily due to increased peripheral resistance

---

Pharmacokinetics
IV: Onset rapid, duration 1-2 min after INF discontinued; metabolized in liver and other tissues by monoamine oxidase (MAO) and catechol-*O*-methyltransferase (COMT) to inactive metabolites; pharmacologic action terminated mainly by uptake and metabolism in sympathetic nerve endings; excreted in urine (metabolites)
INDICATIONS AND USES: Acute hypotensive states, adjunct in treatment of cardiac arrest and profound hypotension
DOSAGE
Adult
• IV INF 8-12 µg/min; initiate at 4 µg/min and titrate to desired response
Child
• IV INF 0.05-0.1 µg/kg/min initially, titrate to desired effect
$ AVAILABLE FORMS/COST OF THERAPY
• Inj, Sol—IV: 0.1%, 4 ml: **$11.28-$15.12**
CONTRAINDICATIONS: Hypotension from blood volume deficits (except as an emergency measure until volume replacement can be completed), mesenteric or peripheral vascular thrombosis, cyclopropane and halothane anesthesia
PRECAUTIONS: Atherosclerosis, arteriosclerosis, diabetic endarteritis, Buerger's disease, elderly, extravasation (may cause necrosis and sloughing of surrounding tissue), sulfite sensitivity
PREGNANCY AND LACTATION: Pregnancy category D
SIDE EFFECTS/ADVERSE REACTIONS
CNS: Anxiety, *headache*
CV: Bradycardia, **cardiac dysrhythmias,** *chest pain,* hypertension, palpitations, tachycardia
EENT: Photophobia
GI: Nausea, vomiting
RESP: Respiratory distress
SKIN: Diaphoresis, gangrene, necrosis and sloughing following extravasation, pallor
MISC: Organ ischemia (due to vasoconstriction of renal and mesenteric arteries)
DRUG INTERACTIONS
Drugs
❷ *Amitriptyline, desipramine, imipramine, protriptyline:* Marked enhancement of pressor response to norepinephrine
❸ *Guanadrel, guanethidine:* Exaggerated pressor response to norepinephrine
❸ *MAOIs:* Slight increase in the pressor response to norepinephrine
❸ *Methyldopa:* Prolongation in the pressor response to norepinephrine

SPECIAL CONSIDERATIONS
• Antidote for extravasation ischemia: infiltrate with 10-15 ml of saline containing 5-10 mg of phentolamine
MONITORING PARAMETERS
• Blood pressure, heart rate, ECG, urine output, peripheral perfusion

penbutolol
(pen-bute'o-loll)
Rx: Levatol
Chemical Class: Nonselective β-adrenergic blocker
Therapeutic Class: Antihypertensive; antianginal

CLINICAL PHARMACOLOGY
Mechanism of Action: Competitive, nonselective, β-receptor antagonist; some intrinsic sympathomimetic activity; no membrane stabilizing activity; high lipid solubility

Pharmacokinetics
PO: Peak 1½-3 hr, duration >20 hr; absorption 100% bioavailability; metabolized by hepatic conjugation and oxidation; 80%-98% protein bound; metabolites excreted mainly in urine; $t_{1/2}$ 5 hr
INDICATIONS AND USES: Hypertension; angina pectoris*; MI*; migraine (prophylaxis)*; alcohol withdrawal syndrome*; aggressive behavior*; antipsychotic-induced akathisia*
DOSAGE
Adult
• Hypertension: 20 mg qd (flat dose-response curve)
$ AVAILABLE FORMS/COST OF THERAPY
• Tab, Uncoated—Oral: 20 mg, 100's: **$99.28**
CONTRAINDICATIONS: Cardiogenic shock, sinus bradycardia, 2nd and 3rd degree atrioventricular conduction block, asthma
PRECAUTIONS: Anesthesia and major surgery; diabetes mellitus; abrupt withdrawal with concurrent CAD or thyrotoxicosis
PREGNANCY AND LACTATION: Pregnancy category C
SIDE EFFECTS/ADVERSE REACTIONS
CNS: Dizziness, fatigue, headache, insomnia
CV: Bradycardia
GI: Diarrhea, dyspepsia, nausea
GU: Impotence
RESP: Cough, dyspnea
SKIN: Excessive sweating
DRUG INTERACTIONS
Drugs
❸ *Adenosine:* Bradycardia aggravated
❸ *Amiodarone:* Bradycardia, cardiac arrest, ventricular arrhythmia risk after initiation of penbutolol
❸ *Antacids.* Reduced penbutolol absorption
❸ *Calcium channel blockers:* See dihydropyridine calcium channel blockers and verapamil
❸ *Clonidine, guanabenz, guanfacine:* Exacerbation of rebound hypertension upon discontinuation of clonidine
❸ *Cocaine:* Cocaine-induced vasoconstriction potentiated; reduced coronary blood flow
❸ *Contrast media:* Increased risk of anaphylaxis
❸ *Digitalis:* Enhances bradycardia
❸ *Dihydropyridine, calcium channel blockers:* Additive pharmacodynamic effects
❸ *Dipyridamole:* Bradycardia aggravated
❸ *Epinephrine, isoproterenol, phenylephrine:* Potentiates pressor response; resultant hypertension and bradycardia
❸ *Flecainide:* Additive negative inotropic effects
❸ *Fluoxetine:* Increased β-blockade activity
❸ *Fluoroquinolones:* Reduced clearance of penbutolol
❸ *Insulin:* Altered response to hypoglycemia; increased blood glucose concentrations; impaired peripheral circulation
❸ *Lidocaine:* Increased serum lidocaine concentrations possible
❸ *Neostigmine:* Bradycardia aggravated
❸ *Neuroleptics:* Both drugs inhibit each other's metabolism; additive hypotension
❸ *NSAIDs:* Reduced antihypertensive effect of penbutolol
❸ *Physostigmine:* Bradycardia aggravated
❸ *Prazosin:* First-dose response to prazosin may be enhanced by β-blockade
❸ *Tacrine:* Bradycardia aggravated
❷ *Terbutaline:* Antagonized bronchodilating effects of terbutaline
❷ *Theophylline:* Antagonistic pharmacodynamic effects
❸ *Verapamil:* Enhanced effects of both drugs; particularly AV nodal conduction slowing; reduced penbutolol clearance

italic = common side effects   ***bold italic*** = life-threatening reactions

SPECIAL CONSIDERATIONS

• Exacerbation of ischemic heart disease following abrupt withdrawal due to hypersensitivity to catecholamines possible
Comparative trials indicate that penbutolol is as effective as propranolol and atenolol in the treatment of hypertension; may have fewer adverse CNS effects than propranolol

phenelzine
(fen'el-zeen)
Rx: Nardil
Chemical Class: Hydrazine derivative
Therapeutic Class: Monoamine oxidase (MAO) inhibitor antidepressant

CLINICAL PHARMACOLOGY
Mechanism of Action: MAOI resulting in increased endogenous concentrations of serotonin, norepinephrine, epinephrine, and dopamine in the CNS; chronic administration results in down regulation (desensitization) of α_2- or β-adrenergic and serotonin receptors, which may correlate with antidepressant activity
Pharmacokinetics
PO: Onset of action 4-8 wk, duration of MAO inhibition at least 10 days, peak serum concentration 2-4 hr, metabolized in liver, excreted in urine as metabolites and unchanged drug
INDICATIONS AND USES: Treatment-resistant depression, including patients characterized as atypical, nonendogenous, or neurotic
DOSAGE
Adult
• PO 15 mg tid initially, increase as tolerated to 60-90 mg/day; following achievement of maximal benefit, reduce dosage slowly over several weeks to lowest effective dose that maintains response
⑤ AVAILABLE FORMS/COST OF THERAPY
• Tab, Sugar Coated—Oral: 15 mg, 100's: **$42.05**
CONTRAINDICATIONS: Pheochromocytoma, congestive heart failure, liver disease, severe renal function impairment, cerebrovascular defect, cardiovascular disease, hypertension, history of headache, age >60 yr
PRECAUTIONS: Children <16 yr, hypotension, bipolar affective disorder, agitation, schizophrenia, hyperactivity, diabetes mellitus, seizure disorder, angina, hyperthyroidism, suicidal ideation
PREGNANCY AND LACTATION: Pregnancy category C
SIDE EFFECTS/ADVERSE REACTIONS
CNS: Agitation, akathisia, ataxia, chills, coma, confusion, *dizziness, drowsiness,* euphoria, fatigue, headache, hyperreflexia, hypomania, jitteriness, mania, memory impairment, muscle twitching, myoclonic movements, neuritis, overactivity, overstimulation, restlessness, *seizures,* sleep disturbance, tremors, vertigo, weakness
CV: **Dysrhythmias,** edema, **hypertension,** *orthostatic hypotension,* palpitations, tachycardia
EENT: Blurred vision, glaucoma, nystagmus
GI: Abdominal pain, anorexia, black tongue, constipation, diarrhea, dry mouth, elevated transaminases, hepatitis, nausea
GU: Dysuria, incontinence, sexual disturbance, urinary retention
HEME: **Agranulocytosis,** anemia, spider telangiectases, **thrombocytopenia**
METAB: Hypermetabolic syndrome, hypernatremia, SIADH-like syndrome
SKIN: Hyperhidrosis, photosensitivity, rash
MISC: Weight gain

DRUG INTERACTIONS
Drugs
▲ *Amphetamines, alcoholic beverages containing tyramine, metaraminol, phenylephrine, phenylpropanolamine, pseudoephedrine, tyramine:* Severe hypertensive reaction
❷ *Antidepressants, cyclic:* Excessive sympathetic response, mania, hyperpyrexia
⑤ *Barbiturates:* Prolonged effect of some barbiturates
▲ *Clomipramine:* Death
▲ *Dexfenfluramine, dextromethorphan, fenfluramine, meperidine:* Agitation, blood pressure changes, hyperpyrexia, convulsions
▲ *Fluoxetine, Sertraline:* Hypomania, confusion, hypertension, tremor
▲ *Food:* Foods containing large amounts of tyramine can result in hypertensive reactions
⑤ *Guanadrel, guanethidine:* May inhibit antihypertensive effects
⑤ *Levodopa:* Severe hypertensive reaction
❷ *Lithium:* Malignant hyperpyrexia
⑤ *Neuromuscular blocking agents:* Prolonged muscle relaxation caused by succinylcholine
⑤ *Reserpine:* Hypertensive reaction
⑤ *Sumatriptan:* Increased sumatriptan plasma concentrations
Labs
• *Aspartate aminotransferase:* Increased serum levels
• *Bilirubin:* False-positive increases in serum
• *Uric acid:* False-positive increases in serum

SPECIAL CONSIDERATIONS
PATIENT/FAMILY EDUCATION
• Avoid tyramine-containing foods, beverages, and OTC products containing decongestants or dextromethorphan and products such as diet aids
• May cause drowsiness, dizziness, blurred vision
• Use caution driving or performing other tasks requiring alertness
• Arise slowly from reclining position
• Therapeutic effect may require 4-8 wk

phenoxybenzamine
(fen-ox-ee-ben'za-meen)
Rx: Dibenzyline
Chemical Class: Haloalkylamine derivative
Therapeutic Class: Sympatholytic

CLINICAL PHARMACOLOGY
Mechanism of Action: Irreversible presynaptic and postsynaptic α-adrenergic receptor blocking agent; produces and maintains "chemical sympathectomy"; increases blood flow to skin, mucosa and abdominal viscera; lowers both supine and standing blood pressure
Pharmacokinetics
PO: Onset gradual over several hours, duration 3-4 days; metabolized via dealkylation, excreted in urine and bile; $t_{1/2}$ 24 hr
INDICATIONS AND USES: Pheochromocytoma (control of episodes of hypertension and sweating), micturition disorders (neurogenic bladder, functional outlet obstruction, partial prostatic obstruction),* peripheral vasospastic disorders*
DOSAGE
Adult
• PO 10 mg bid initially, increase dosage qod until optimal response obtained as judged by blood pressure; usual dosage range 20-40 mg bid-tid

* = non FDA-approved use

Child
• PO 1-2 mg/kg/day divided q6-8h
S AVAILABLE FORMS/COST OF THERAPY
• Cap, Gel—Oral: 10 mg, 100's: **$67.80**
CONTRAINDICATIONS: Conditions where a fall in blood pressure may be undesirable
PRECAUTIONS: Marked cerebral or coronary arteriosclerosis, renal damage, respiratory infection
PREGNANCY AND LACTATION: Pregnancy category C; indicated in hypertension secondary to pheochromocytoma during pregnancy, especially after 24 wk gestation when surgical intervention is associated with high rates of maternal and fetal mortality; no adverse fetal effects due to this treatment have been observed
SIDE EFFECTS/ADVERSE REACTIONS
CNS: Confusion, *dizziness,* drowsiness, sedation
CV: Palpitations, *postural hypotension, tachycardia*
EENT: Miosis, nasal congestion
GI: GI irritation, nausea, vomiting
GU: Inhibition of ejaculation
MISC: Fatigue

SPECIAL CONSIDERATIONS
PATIENT/FAMILY EDUCATION
• Avoid alcohol; avoid sudden changes in posture, dizziness may result
• Avoid cough, cold, or allergy medications containing sympathomimetics

phentolamine
(fen-tole'a-meen)
Rx: Regitine, Rogitine ♣
Chemical Class: α-adrenergic blocker
Therapeutic Class: Antihypertensive

CLINICAL PHARMACOLOGY
Mechanism of Action: Binds to α-adrenergic receptors, which causes vasodilation, decreased peripheral vascular resistance, decreased blood pressure
Pharmacokinetics
IV: Onset of action immediate, duration 10-15 min
IM: Onset 15-20 min, duration 3-4 hr
Metabolized in liver, excreted in urine (10% as unchanged drug)
INDICATIONS AND USES: Diagnosis of and treatment of hypertension associated with pheochromocytoma, treatment of dermal necrosis following extravasation of α-adrenergic drugs (norepinephrine, epinephrine, dobutamine, dopamine), hypertensive crises secondary to MAOI or sympathomimetic amine interactions and rebound hypertension on withdrawal of antihypertensives,* with papaverine as intracavernous injection for impotence*
DOSAGE
Adult
• *Diagnosis of pheochromocytoma:* IM/IV 5 mg
• *Hypertension, surgery for pheochromocytoma:* IM/IV 5 mg 1-2 hr before procedure, repeat q2-4h as needed
• *Drug extravasation:* Dilute 5-10 mg in 10 ml NS, infiltrate area with sol within 12 hr (blanching resolves within 1 hr if successful)
Child
• *Diagnosis of pheochromocytoma:* IM/IV 0.05-0.1 mg/kg/dose, max single dose 5 mg
• *Hypertension, surgery for pheochromocytoma:* IM/IV 0.05-0.1 mg/kg/dose 1-2 hr before procedure, repeat q2-4h as needed

• *Drug extravasation:* 0.1-0.2 mg/kg diluted in 10 ml NS infiltrated into area of extravasation within 12 hr
S AVAILABLE FORMS/COST OF THERAPY
• Inj, Conc, w/Buffer—IM, IV: 5 mg, 2 vials: **$58.53**
CONTRAINDICATIONS: Angina, MI
PRECAUTIONS: Peptic ulcer disease (may exacerbate)
PREGNANCY AND LACTATION: Pregnancy category C; unknown if excreted in breast milk
SIDE EFFECTS/ADVERSE REACTIONS
CNS: ***Cerebrovascular occlusion,*** dizziness, flushing, severe headache, weakness
CV: Angina, ***dysrhythmias,*** *hypotension,* ***MI, reflex tachycardia***
EENT: Nasal congestion
GI: Abdominal pain, diarrhea, dry mouth, nausea, vomiting
DRUG INTERACTIONS
Labs
• 5-hydroxyindoleacetic acid: Urine, falsely high colorimetric values

SPECIAL CONSIDERATIONS
• Urinary catecholamines preferred over phentolamine for screening for pheochromocytoma

pindolol
(pin'doe-loll)
Rx: Visken
Combinations
  Rx: with hydrochlorothiazide (Viskazide ♣)
Chemical Class: Nonselective β-adrenergic blocker with intrinsic sympathomimetic activity; isopropylamino-indole
Therapeutic Class: Antihypertensive; antianginal

CLINICAL PHARMACOLOGY
Mechanism of Action: Competitively blocks stimulation of β-adrenergic receptors (nonselectively); inhibits chronotropic, inotropic responses to β-adrenergic tone (decreases rate of SA node discharge, increases recovery time), slows conduction of AV node, decreases heart rate, which decreases O_2 consumption in myocardium; also decreases renin-aldosterone-angiotensin system; intrinsic sympathomimetic activity (ISA) manifests with smaller reduction in resting cardiac output and in the resting heart rate than are seen with drugs without ISA
Pharmacokinetics
PO: Peak effect 1-2 hr; 90%-100% absorption; 40% protein bound; 60%-65% metabolized by liver; $t_{1/2}$ 3-4 hr; 30%-45% excreted unchanged
INDICATIONS AND USES: Hypertension; angina*; anxiety*
DOSAGE
Adult
Hypertension: PO 5 mg bid, usual dose 15 mg/day (5 mg tid), may increase by 10 mg/day q3-4 wk to a max of 60 mg/day
S AVAILABLE FORMS/COST OF THERAPY
• Tab, Uncoated—Oral: 5 mg, 100's: **$23.25-$84.78;** 10 mg, 100's: **$33.75-$112.26**
CONTRAINDICATIONS: Cardiogenic shock; 2nd, 3rd degree heart block; severe bradycardia; overt cardiac failure; bronchial asthma
PRECAUTIONS: Major surgery, diabetes mellitus, renal disease, thyroid disease, COPD, well-compensated heart failure, nonallergic bronchospasm; abrupt withdrawal may precipitate CAD or sudden death; peripheral vascular disease, thyrotoxicosis

---

italic = common side effects

bold italic = life-threatening reactions

PREGNANCY AND LACTATION: Pregnancy category B; no reports available; other members of this class are excreted into milk, expect pindolol to do the same

SIDE EFFECTS/ADVERSE REACTIONS

CNS: Anxiety, *dizziness,* fatigue, hallucinations, *insomnia*
CV: AV block, bradycardia, chest pain, *CHF,* claudication, edema, hypotension, palpitation, tachycardia
EENT: Double vision, dry burning eyes, sore throat, *visual changes*
GI: Abdominal pain, diarrhea, *ischemic colitis, mesenteric arterial thrombosis,* nausea, vomiting
GU: Frequency, impotence
HEME: Agranulocytosis, purpura, thrombocytopenia
RESP: Bronchospasm, cough, *dyspnea,* rales
SKIN: Alopecia, pruritus, rash
MISC: Fever, joint pain, muscle pain

DRUG INTERACTIONS

Drugs
🔳 *Adenosine:* Bradycardia aggravated
🔳 *Antacids:* Reduced pindolol absorption
🔳 *Calcium channel blockers:* See dihydropyridine calcium channel blockers and verapamil
🔳 *Cimetidine:* Renal clearance reduced; AUC increased with cimetidine coadministration
🔳 *Clonidine, guanabenz, guanfacine:* Exacerbation of rebound hypertension upon discontinuation of clonidine
🔳 *Cocaine:* Cocaine-induced vasoconstriction potentiated; reduced coronary blood flow
🔳 *Contrast media:* Increased risk of anaphylaxis
🔳 *Digitalis:* Enhances bradycardia
🔳 *Dihydropyridine calcium channel blockers:* Additive pharmacodynamic effects
🔳 *Dipyridamole:* Bradycardia aggravated
🔳 *Epinephrine, isoproterenol, phenylephrine:* Potentiates pressor response; resultant hypertension and bradycardia
🔳 *Flecainide:* Additive negative inotropic effects
🔳 *Fluoxetine:* Increased β-blockade activity
🔳 *Fluoroquinolones:* Reduced clearance of pindolol
🔳 *Insulin:* Altered response to hypoglycemia; increased blood glucose concentrations; impair peripheral circulation
🔳 *Lidocaine:* Increased serum lidocaine concentrations possible
🔳 *Neostigmine:* Bradycardia aggravated
🔳 *Neuroleptics:* Both drugs inhibit each other's metabolism; additive hypotension
🔳 *NSAIDs:* Reduced antihypertensive effect of pindolol
🔳 *Physostigmine:* Bradycardia aggravated
🔳 *Prazosin:* First dose response to prazosin may be enhanced by β-blockade
🔳 *Tacrine:* Bradycardia aggravated
❷ *Terbutaline:* Antagonized bronchodilating effects of terbutaline
❷ *Theophylline:* Antagonistic pharmacodynamic effects
🔳 *Verapamil:* Enhanced effects of both drugs; particularly AV nodal conduction slowing; reduced pindolol clearance

Labs
• *Alkaline phosphatase:* Increased serum levels
• *Aspartate aminotransferase:* Decreased serum levels
• *Bilirubin:* Decreased serum level
• *Creatine kinase:* Decreased serum level

SPECIAL CONSIDERATIONS

• Abrupt discontinuation may precipitate angina; taper over 1-2 wk Effective antihypertensive and probably antianginal agent (though not approved for this indication), especially for patients who develop symptomatic bradycardia with β-blockade

pravastatin
(prav-i-sta'tin)
Rx: Pravachol
Chemical Class: HMG-CoA reductase inhibitor
Therapeutic Class: Antilipemic

CLINICAL PHARMACOLOGY

Mechanism of Action: Competitively inhibits 3-hydroxy-3-methylglutaryl-coenzyme A (HMG-CoA) reductase, which catalyzes the early rate-limiting step in cholesterol biosynthesis; increases HDL cholesterol, decreases LDL cholesterol; modestly decreases triglycerides

Pharmacokinetics
PO: Peak 1-1½ hr; absolute bioavailability 17%; 50% bound to plasma proteins; metabolized in liver, excreted in urine (20%) and feces (70%); $t_{1/2}$ 77 hr

INDICATIONS AND USES: Hypercholesterolemia (Types IIa and IIb)

DOSAGE

Adult
• PO 10-20 mg qhs, may increase to 40 mg qhs if needed

🔳 **AVAILABLE FORMS/COST OF THERAPY**
• Tab, Uncoated—Oral: 10 mg, 100's: **$168.79;** 20 mg, 90's: **$163.58;** 40 mg, 90's: **$299.08**

CONTRAINDICATIONS: Active liver disease, unexplained persistent elevated liver function tests

PRECAUTIONS: History of liver disease, renal function impairment, elderly, children <18 yr, alcoholism; risk factors predisposing to the development of renal failure secondary to rhabdomyolysis (severe acute infection, trauma, hypotension, uncontrolled seizure disorder, severe metabolic disorders, electrolyte imbalance)

PREGNANCY AND LACTATION: Pregnancy category X; small amounts excreted in breast milk; should probably not be used by women who are nursing

SIDE EFFECTS/ADVERSE REACTIONS

CNS: Dizziness, headache
CV: Chest pain
GI: Abdominal pain, anorexia, cholestatic jaundice, cirrhosis, constipation, fatty change in liver, flatulence, heartburn, hepatitis, increased serum transaminase levels, nausea, *pancreatitis,* vomiting
GU: Erectile dysfunction, loss of libido
MS: Arthralgia, localized pain, myalgia, myopathy, *rhabdomyolysis*
SKIN: Alopecia, photosensitivity, pruritus, rash
MISC: Fatigue, gynecomastia

DRUG INTERACTIONS

Drugs
❷ *Azole antifungals (fluconazole, itraconazole, ketoconazole, miconazole):* Increased plasma pravastatin levels via inhibition of metabolism with increased risk of rhabdomyolysis
🔳 *Cholestyramine:* Reduced bioavailability of pravastatin
🔳 *Clarithromycin:* Increased plasma pravastatin levels via inhibition of metabolism with increased risk of rhabdomyolysis
❷ *Clofibrate:* Small increased risk of myopathy with combination
🔳 *Colestipol:* Reduced bioavailability of pravastatin
🔳 *Danazol:* Increased plasma pravastatin levels via inhibition of metabolism with increased risk of rhabdomyolysis
🔳 *Erythromycin:* Increased pravastatin levels via inhibition of metabolism with increased risk of rhabdomyolysis
🔳 *Fluoxetine:* Increased pravastatin levels via inhibition of metabolism with increased risk of rhabdomyolysis
❷ *Gemfibrozil:* Small increased risk of myopathy with combination

▪ *Isradipine:* Isradipine may decrease pravastatin plasma concentrations

▪ *Nefazodone:* May inhibit hepatic metabolism of pravastatin with risk of rhabdomyolysis

▪ *Troleandomycin:* Increased pravastatin levels via inhibition of metabolism with increased risk of rhabdomyolysis

▪ *Warfarin:* Addition of pravastatin may increase hypoprothrombinemic response to warfarin via inhibition of metabolism (cytochrome P450 2C9)

SPECIAL CONSIDERATIONS

PATIENT/FAMILY EDUCATION
• Avoid prolonged exposure to sunlight and other UV light
• Promptly report any unexplained muscle pain, tenderness, or weakness, especially if accompanied by fever or malaise
• Strictly adhere to low cholesterol diet

MONITORING PARAMETERS
• ALT and AST at baseline, and at 12 weeks of therapy. If no change at 12 weeks, no further monitoring necessary (discontinue if elevations persist at >3 times upper limit of normal)
• CPK in any patient complaining of diffuse myalgia, muscle tenderness, or weakness
• Fasting lipid profile

---

prazosin
(pra′zoe-sin)
Rx: Minipress
Combinations
   Rx: with polythiazide (Minizide)
Chemical Class: Quinazoline derivative
Therapeutic Class: Antihypertensive; benign prostatic hypertrophy agent

---

CLINICAL PHARMACOLOGY
Mechanism of Action: Competitively inhibits postsynaptic α_1-adrenergic receptors; produces both arterial and venous dilation; reduces peripheral vascular resistance and blood pressure; blockade of α_1-adrenoceptors in bladder neck and prostate relaxes smooth muscle, improving urine flow rates in benign prostatic hypertrophy

Pharmacokinetics
PO: Oral bioavailability 48%-68%, peak 1-3 hr, duration of antihypertensive effect 10 hr; 92%-97% bound to plasma proteins; extensively metabolized to active metabolites, excreted in bile (90%) and urine (10%); $t_{1/2}$ 2-3 hr

INDICATIONS AND USES: Hypertension, benign prostatic hypertrophy,* Raynaud's vasospasm,* refractory congestive heart failure*

DOSAGE
Adult
• PO 1 mg bid-tid, give 1st dose at bedtime; increase as needed to 6-15 mg/day in divided doses; doses >20 mg/day usually do not increase efficacy

Child
• PO 0.5-7 mg tid

$ AVAILABLE FORMS/COST OF THERAPY
• Cap, Gel—Oral: 1 mg, 100's: **$6.24-$51.21;** 2 mg, 100's: **$7.20-$70.93;** 5 mg, 100's: **$11.93-$119.90**

CONTRAINDICATIONS: Hypersensitivity to quinazolines
PRECAUTIONS: Children, hepatic disease
PREGNANCY AND LACTATION: Pregnancy category C

SIDE EFFECTS/ADVERSE REACTIONS
CNS: Anxiety, asthenia, ataxia, depression, *dizziness,* fever, *headache,* hypertonia, insomnia, nervousness, paresthesia, somnolence
CV: Chest pain, dysrhythmia, edema, ***"1st-dose" syncope,*** flushing, palpitations, postural hypotension, tachycardia
EENT: Abnormal vision, tinnitus, vertigo
GI: Abdominal discomfort, constipation, diarrhea, dry mouth, flatulence, nausea, vomiting
GU: Incontinence, polyuria
MS: Arthralgia, myalgia
RESP: Dyspnea
SKIN: Pruritus, rash

DRUG INTERACTIONS
Drugs
▪ *ACE inhibitors:* Exaggerated first-dose response to prazosin
▪ *β-adrenergic blockers:* Exaggerated first-dose response to prazosin
▪ *NSAIDs:* Inhibits antihypertensive response to prazosin
▪ *Verapamil:* Reduces first pass metabolism of prazosin

SPECIAL CONSIDERATIONS

PATIENT/FAMILY EDUCATION
• Alert patients to the possibility of syncopal and orthostatic symptoms, especially with the 1st dose ("1st-dose syncope")
• Take initial dose at bedtime; arise slowly from reclining position

---

procainamide
(proe-kane′a-mide)
Rx: Procan SR, Pronestyl, Pronestyl-SR
Chemical Class: Procaine amide derivative
Therapeutic Class: Antidysrhythmic (Class IA)

CLINICAL PHARMACOLOGY
Mechanism of Action: Decreases myocardial excitability and conduction velocity; may depress myocardial contractility; increases threshold potential of ventricle, His-Purkinje system; prolongs effective refractory period and increases action potential duration in atrial and ventricular muscle; possesses anticholinergic properties, which may modify direct myocardial effects

Pharmacokinetics
IM: Onset 10-30 min, peak 15-60 min
PO: Peak 0.75-2.5 hr
15%-20% bound to plasma proteins; metabolized via acetylation in liver to N-acetyl procainamide (NAPA), which is a Class III antidysrhythmic; excreted in urine (25% as NAPA); $t_{1/2}$ 2.5-4.7 hr (NAPA 6-8 hr)

INDICATIONS AND USES: Life-threatening ventricular dysrhythmias, less severe but symptomatic ventricular dysrhythmias in select patients, maintenance of sinus rhythm following cardioversion in atrial fibrillation and/or flutter,* suppression of recurrent paroxysmal atrial fibrillation*

DOSAGE
Adult
• PO 250-500 mg q3-6h; PO SR 500-1000 mg q6h, usual dose 50 mg/kg/24 hr, max 4 g/24hr; IM 0.5-1 g q4-8h until PO therapy possible; IV 1 g INF over 25-30 min or 100-200 mg/day repeated q5 min as needed to total dose of 1 g as a loading dose, followed by continuous INF of 1-6 mg/min, titrate to patient response

---

italic = common side effects

bold italic = life-threatening reactions

Child
• PO 15-50 mg/kg/24 hr divided q3-6h, max 4 g/24 hr; IM 20-30 mg/kg/24 hr divided q4-6h, max 4 g/24 hr; IV 3-6 mg/kg INF over 5 min not to exceed 100 mg/day as a loading dose, then 20-80 µg/kg/min as a continuous INF, max 4 g/24 hr

Ⓢ AVAILABLE FORMS/COST OF THERAPY
• Cap, Gel—Oral: 250 mg, 100's: **$6.83-$53.93**; 375 mg, 100's: **$7.43-$74.79**; 500 mg, 100's: **$8.48-$97.10**
• Tab, Sugar Coated—Oral: 250 mg, 100's: **$12.70-$53.93**; 375 mg, 100's: **$74.79**; 500 mg, 100's: **$97.10**
• Tab, Coated, SUS Action—Oral: 250 mg, 100's: **$8.37-$25.99**; 500 mg, 100's: **$10.70-$63.72**; 750 mg, 100's: **$24.38-$94.60**; 1000 mg, 100's: **$121.04**
• Inj, Sol—IM, IV: 100 mg/ml, 10 ml: **$4.00-$36.44**; 500 mg/ml, 2 ml: **$4.00-$36.44**

CONTRAINDICATIONS: Complete heart block, lupus erythematosus, torsade de pointes

PRECAUTIONS: Following MI, 1st-degree AV block (unless ventricular rate controlled by pacemaker), asymptomatic premature ventricular contractions, digitalis intoxication, CHF, myasthenia gravis, renal insufficiency, children

PREGNANCY AND LACTATION: Pregnancy category C; compatible with breast feeding, however long-term effects in nursing infant unknown

SIDE EFFECTS/ADVERSE REACTIONS
CNS: Depression, *dizziness,* giddiness, hallucinations, headache, psychosis, weakness
CV: Hypotension, **2nd-degree heart block, ventricular arrhythmias** (more common with IV administration)
GI: Abdominal pain, anorexia, bitter taste, diarrhea, hepatomegaly, nausea, vomiting
HEME: **Agranulocytosis, hemolytic anemia (rare), neutropenia, thrombocytopenia**
SKIN: **Angioneurotic edema,** flushing, pruritus, rash, urticaria
MISC: *Lupus erythematosus-like syndrome* (arthralgia, pleural or abdominal pain, arthritis, pleural effusion, pericarditis, fever, chills, rash) in up to 30% on long-term therapy

DRUG INTERACTIONS
Drugs
🔳 *Amiodarone, cimetidine, trimethoprim:* Increased procainamide concentrations
🔳 *Cholinergic drugs:* Antagonism of cholinergic actions on skeletal muscle
🔳 *Procaine:* Interferes with procainamide concentration assay
Labs
• *False decrease:* Cholinesterase
• *False increase:* Potassium

SPECIAL CONSIDERATIONS

PATIENT/FAMILY EDUCATION
• Strict compliance to dosage schedule imperative
• Empty wax core from sustained release tablets may appear in stool; this is harmless

MONITORING PARAMETERS
• CBC with differential and platelets qwk for 1st 3 mo, periodically thereafter
• ECG: R/O overdosage if QRS widens >25% or QT prolongation occurs; reduce dosage if QRS widens >50%
• ANA titer increases may precede clinical symptoms of lupoid syndrome
• Serum creatinine, urea nitrogen
• Plasma procainamide concentration (therapeutic range 3-10 µg/ml; 10-30 µg/ml NAPA)

---

propafenone
(proe-pa-fen'one)
Rx: Rythmol
Chemical Class: 3-Phenylpropiophenone derivative
Therapeutic Class: Antidysrhythmic (Class IC)

CLINICAL PHARMACOLOGY
Mechanism of Action: Local anesthetic effects and direct stabilizing action on myocardial membranes; reduces upstroke velocity (Phase O) of the monophasic action potential; reduces fast inward current carried by sodium ions in Purkinje fibers, and to a lesser extent myocardial fibers; increases diastolic excitability threshold, prolongs effective refractory period, reduces spontaneous automaticity, and depresses triggered activity; weak β-blocking activity
Pharmacokinetics
PO: Bioavailability 3.4%-10.6%; metabolized in liver to 5-hydroxypropafenone and N-depropylpropafenone (active), excreted in urine; $t_{1/2}$ 2-10 hr in >90% of patients (10-32 hr in slow metabolizers)

INDICATIONS AND USES: Documented life-threatening ventricular dysrhythmias (e.g., sustained ventricular tachycardia), supraventricular tachycardias including atrial fibrillation and flutter,* dysrhythmias associated with Wolff-Parkinson-White syndrome*

DOSAGE
Adult
• PO 150 mg q8h initially; increase at 3-4 day intervals to 225 mg q8h and, if necessary, to 300 mg q8h; do not exceed 900 mg/day

Ⓢ AVAILABLE FORMS/COST OF THERAPY
• Tab, Coated—Oral: 150 mg, 100's: **$83.82-$88.00**; 225 mg, 100's: **$119.48-$125.41**; 300 mg, 100's: **$152.08-$159.68**

CONTRAINDICATIONS: Uncontrolled CHF, cardiogenic shock, disorders of impulse generation or conduction in the absence of an artificial pacemaker, bradycardia, marked hypotension, bronchospastic disorders, manifest electrolyte imbalance

PRECAUTIONS: Non-life-threatening dysrhythmias, recent MI, hepatic and renal function impairment, elderly, children

PREGNANCY AND LACTATION: Pregnancy category C

SIDE EFFECTS/ADVERSE REACTIONS
CNS: Anxiety, ataxia, *dizziness,* drowsiness, fatigue, headache, insomnia, tremor
CV: Angina, atrial fibrillation, *AV block,* bradycardia, bundle branch block, chest pain, **congestive heart failure** (due to negative ionotrope effects), edema, hypotension, *intraventricular conduction delay,* palpitations, premature ventricular contractions, **prodysrhythmia,** syncope, **ventricular tachycardia,** widened QRS complex
EENT: Blurred vision, *unusual taste*
GI: Abdominal pain, anorexia, *constipation,* diarrhea, dry mouth, dyspepsia, flatulence, liver abnormalities, *nausea, vomiting*
HEME: **Agranulocytosis, anemia, granulocytopenia,** increased bleeding time, **leukopenia,** positive ANA, purpura, **thrombocytopenia**
MS: Arthralgia, weakness
RESP: Dyspnea
SKIN: Diaphoresis, rash

DRUG INTERACTIONS
Drugs
🔳 *β-blockers:* Increased metoprolol or propranolol concentrations
🔳 *Cimetidine:* Increased propafenone concentrations
🔳 *Digitalis glycosides:* Increased serum digoxin concentrations

---

* = non FDA-approved use

▪ *Food:* Increased peak serum propafenone concentrations
▪ *Oral anticoagulants:* Increased serum warfarin concentrations, prolonged protime
▪ *Quinidine:* Increased propafenone concentrations but reduced concentrations of its active metabolite; net effect uncertain (toxicity vs reduced efficacy)
▪ *Rifampin, phenobarbital, rifabutin:* Reduced serum propafenone concentrations
▪ *Theophylline:* Increased plasma theophylline concentrations

SPECIAL CONSIDERATIONS

PATIENT/FAMILY EDUCATION
• Signs of overdosage include hypotension, excessive drowsiness, decreased heart rate, or abnormal heartbeat

MONITORING PARAMETERS
• ECG, consider dose reduction in patients with significant widening of the QRS complex or 2nd- or 3rd-degree AV block
• ANA, carefully evaluate abnormal ANA test, consider discontinuation if persistent or worsening ANA titers are detected

---

propranolol
(proe-pran'oh-lole)
Rx: Inderal, Inderal LA
Combinations
  Rx: with HCTZ (Inderide)
Chemical Class: Nonselective β-adrenergic blocker
Therapeutic Class: Antihypertensive; antianginal; antimigraine agent; antidysrhythmic (class II)

CLINICAL PHARMACOLOGY
Mechanism of Action: Competes with β-adrenergic agonists for available β_1- and β_2-receptor sites inhibiting the responses to β_1- and β_2-adrenergic stimulation; slows conduction of AV node; decreases blood pressure, heart rate, and myocardial contractility; decreases myocardial O_2 consumption
Pharmacokinetics
PO: Peak 60-90 min (L-A 6 hr), extensive 1st-pass effect
IV: Onset immediate
High lipid solubility; 90% bound to plasma proteins; metabolized in liver to active and inactive metabolites, excreted in urine; $t_{1/2}$ 4-6 hr (L-A 8-11 hr)
INDICATIONS AND USES: Hypertension, cardiac dysrhythmias, MI, hypertrophic subaortic stenosis, adjunctive therapy of pheochromocytoma, migraine prophylaxis, angina pectoris, essential tremor, alcohol withdrawal syndrome,* aggressive behavior,* antipsychotic-induced akathisia,* esophageal varices,* situational anxiety,* thyrotoxicosis symptoms,* performance anxiety*

DOSAGE
Adult
• *Hypertension:* PO 40 mg bid (L-A 80 mg qd) initially, usual range 120-240 mg/day divided bid-tid (L-A 120-160 mg qd), max 640 mg/day
• *Dysrhythmias:* PO 10-30 mg tid-qid; IV (reserve for life-threatening situations or dysrhythmias occurring during anesthesia) 0.5-3 mg, a 2nd dose may be administered after 2 min prn, additional doses at intervals no less than 4 hr until desired response obtained
• *Angina pectoris:* PO 10-20 mg tid-qid (L-A 80 mg qd) initially, usual range 160-240 mg/day divided tid-qid, maximum 320 mg/day
• *Hypertrophic subaortic stenosis:* PO 20-40 mg tid-qid (L-A 80-160 mg qd)

• *Pheochromocytoma:* PO 30 mg/day in divided doses (in conjunction with α-adrenergic blocking agent)
• *Migraine prophylaxis:* PO 80 mg/day in divided doses (L-A 80 mg qd) initially, increase to optimal prophylaxis, usual range 160-240 mg/day
• *MI:* PO 180-240 mg/day divided bid-qid beginning 5-21 days after MI
• *Essential tremor:* PO 40 mg bid initially, usual range 120-320 mg/day divided tid
Child
• *Dysrhythmias:* PO 0.5-1 mg/kg/day divided q6-8h, increase dose at 3-7 day intervals, usual range 2-4 mg/kg/day, max 16 mg/kg/day or 60 mg/day; IV 0.01-0.1 mg/kg slowly over 10 min, max 1 mg
• *Hypertension:* PO 0.5-1 mg/kg/day divided q6-12h, increase dose at 3-7 day intervals, usual range 1-5 mg/kg/day
• *Migraine prophylaxis:* PO 0.6-1.5 mg/kg/day in divided doses
$ **AVAILABLE FORMS/COST OF THERAPY**
• Tab, Uncoated—Oral: 10 mg, 100's: **$1.43-$37.15;** 20 mg, 100's: **$1.65-$50.39;** 40 mg, 100's: **$2.04-$64.06;** 60 mg, 100's: **$2.55-$82.70;** 80 mg, 100's: **$2.63-$91.79;** 90 mg, 100's: **$16.25-$23.16**
• Cap, Gel, SUS Action—Oral: 60 mg, 100's: **$53.40-$80.50;** 80 mg, 100's: **$63.75-$95.74;** 120 mg, 100's: **$80.25-$132.63;** 160 mg, 100's: **$106.73-$153.28**
• Sol—Oral: 20 mg/5 ml, 500 ml: **$31.50;** 40 mg/5 ml, 500 ml: **$45.01;** 80 mg/ml, 30 ml: **$30.48**
• Inj, Sol—IV: 1 mg/ml, 1 ml: **$4.31**
CONTRAINDICATIONS: Cardiogenic shock, 2nd or 3rd degree heart block, sinus bradycardia, CHF unless secondary to a tachydysrhythmia treatable with β-blockers, bronchial asthma or bronchospasm, severe COPD, cardiac failure
PRECAUTIONS: Major surgery, diabetes mellitus, renal disease, hepatic disease, thyroid disease, well-compensated heart failure, peripheral vascular disease, bradycardia, Down's syndrome
PREGNANCY AND LACTATION: Pregnancy category C; has been used during pregnancy for maternal and fetal indications without teratogenesis, but neonatal toxicity may occur; closely observe neonate during 1st 24-48 hr after birth for bradycardia, hypoglycemia, and other symptoms of β-blockade; compatible with breast feeding
SIDE EFFECTS/ADVERSE REACTIONS
CNS: Depression, *dizziness,* drowsiness, *fatigue,* hallucinations, insomnia, *lethargy,* memory loss, mental changes, strange dreams
CV: Bradycardia, **CHF,** cold extremities, postural hypotension, profound hypotension, ***2nd or 3rd degree heart block***
EENT: Dry, burning eyes; sore throat; visual disturbances
GI: Diarrhea, dry mouth, elevated LFTs, ***ischemic colitis, mesenteric arterial thrombosis,*** *nausea,* vomiting
GU: Impotence, sexual dysfunction
HEME: ***Agranulocytosis, thrombocytopenia***
METAB: Hyperglycemia, hyperlipidemia (increase TG, total cholesterol, LDL; decrease HDL), masked hypoglycemic response to insulin (sweating excepted)
RESP: ***Bronchospasm,*** dyspnea, wheezing
SKIN: Alopecia, pruritus, rash
DRUG INTERACTIONS
Drugs
▪ *Amiodarone:* Bradycardia, cardiac arrest, ventricular dysrhythmia shortly after initiation of β-blocker
▪ *Antidiabetics:* Masked symptoms of hypoglycemia, prolonged recovery of normoglycemia
▪ *Antipyrine:* Increased antipyrine concentrations
▪ *Barbiturates, rifampin:* Reduced concentrations of propranolol
▪ *β-agonists:* Antagonistic effects

---

italic = common side effects

bold italic = life-threatening reactions

◨ *Calcium channel blockers:* Increased concentrations of propranolol; increased bioavailability of nifedipine

◨ *Cimetidine, etintidine, fluoxetine, propoxyphene, propafenone, quinidine, quinolones:* Increased propranolol concentrations

◨ *Clonidine, guanabenz, guanfacine:* Exacerbation of hypertension upon withdrawal of clonidine

◨ *Cocaine:* Potentiation of cocaine-induced coronary vasospasm

◨ *Contrast media:* Increased risk anaphylaxis

◨ *Digitalis glycosides:* Increased digoxin concentrations

◨ *Epinephrine:* Enhanced pressor response to epinephrine

◨ *Flecainide:* Increased propranolol and flecainide concentrations; additive negative inotropic effects

◨ *Lidocaine:* Increased lidocaine concentrations

◨ *Local anesthetics:* Enhanced sympathomimetic side effects of epinephrine-containing local anesthetics

◨ *Neostigmine, physostigmine, tacrine:* Additive bradycardia

◨ *Neuroleptics:* Increased plasma concentrations of both drugs

◨ *NSAIDs:* Reduced hypotensive effect of propranolol

◨ *Phenylephrine:* Predisposition to acute hypertensive episodes

◨ *Prazosin, terazosin:* Enhanced 1st-dose response to prazosin

❷ *Theophylline:* Increased theophylline concentrations; antagonistic pharmacodynamic effects

Labs

• *False increase:* Bilirubin

SPECIAL CONSIDERATIONS

PATIENT/FAMILY EDUCATION

• Do not discontinue abruptly, may precipitate angina, sudden death; reduce over 1-2 wk

• Take pulse at home, notify clinician if less than 50 beats/min

• Avoid hazardous activities if dizziness, drowsiness, lightheadedness are present

• May mask the symptoms of hypoglycemia, except for sweating, in diabetic patients

MONITORING PARAMETERS

• Blood pressure, pulse

---

quinapril
(kwin'na-pril)

Rx: Accupril

Chemical Class: Angiotensin-converting enzyme (ACE) inhibitor

Therapeutic Class: Antihypertensive, CHF agent; renal protectant

---

CLINICAL PHARMACOLOGY

Mechanism of Action: Selectively suppresses renin-angiotensin-aldosterone system; inhibits ACE, preventing conversion of angiotensin I to angiotensin II; results in dilation of arterial, venous vessels

Pharmacokinetics

PO: Onset 1 hr, duration 24 hr; has little pharmacologic activity until metabolized to active metabolite (quinaprilat), excreted in urine (60%) and feces (37%); $t_{1/2}$ (quinaprilat) 2 hr

INDICATIONS AND USES: Hypertension, CHF, diabetic nephropathy*

DOSAGE

Adult

• *Hypertension:* PO 10 mg qd initially; adjust dose at 2 wk intervals according to blood pressure response; max 80 mg/day divided qd-bid

• *CHF:* PO 5 mg bid initially; adjust dose at weekly intervals to desired effect; usual range 20-40 mg/day divided bid; in renal impairment (CrCl 10-30 ml/min) initiate at 2.5 mg bid

◨ **AVAILABLE FORMS/COST OF THERAPY**

• Tab, Uncoated—Oral: 5 mg, 100's: **$90.91**; 10 mg, 100's: **$90.91**; 20 mg, 100's: **$90.91**; 40 mg, 100's: **$78.54**

PRECAUTIONS: Impaired renal and liver function, dialysis patients, hypovolemia, diuretic therapy, collagen-vascular diseases, congestive heart failure, elderly, bilateral renal artery stenosis

PREGNANCY AND LACTATION: Pregnancy category D; ACE inhibitors can cause fetal and neonatal morbidity and death when administered to pregnant women; when pregnancy is detected, discontinue ACE inhibitors as soon as possible

SIDE EFFECTS/ADVERSE REACTIONS

CNS: Dizziness, fatigue, *headache*

CV: Angina, palpitations, postural hypotension, syncope (especially with 1st dose)

GI: Abdominal pain, constipation, nausea, vomiting

GU: Decreased libido, impotence, increased BUN, creatinine

HEME: **Agranulocytosis, neutropenia, thrombocytopenia**

METAB: Hyperkalemia, hyponatremia, hypoglycemia

MS: Arthralgia, arthritis, myalgia

RESP: Asthma, bronchitis, cough

SKIN: Angioedema, pruritus, rash, sweating

DRUG INTERACTIONS

Drugs

❷ *Allopurinol:* Predisposition to hypersensitivity reactions

◨ *α-adrenergic blockers:* Exaggerated 1st dose hypotensive response

◨ *Aspirin:* Reduced hemodynamic effects; less likely with nonacetylated salicylates

◨ *Cyclosporine:* Renal insufficiency

◨ *Insulin:* Enhanced hypoglycemic response

◨ *Iron (parenteral):* Increased risk systemic reaction

◨ *Lithium:* Increased risk of serious lithium toxicity

◨ *Loop diuretics:* Initiation of ACE inhibitor therapy may cause hypotension and renal insufficiency

◨ *NSAIDs:* Inhibition of the antihypertensive response

◨ *Potassium, potassium-sparing diuretics:* Increased risk for hyperkalemia

SPECIAL CONSIDERATIONS

PATIENT/FAMILY EDUCATION

• Do not use salt substitutes containing potassium without consulting clinician

• Rise slowly to sitting or standing position to minimize orthostatic hypotension

• Notify clinician of mouth sores, sore throat, fever, swelling of hands or feet, irregular heartbeat, chest pain

• Dizziness, fainting, lightheadedness may occur during 1st few days of therapy

• May cause altered taste perception or cough; notify clinician if these persist

MONITORING PARAMETERS

• BUN, creatinine (watch for increased levels that may indicate acute renal failure)

• Potassium levels, although hyperkalemia is rare

---

quinidine
(kwin'i-deen)

Rx: Quinaglute Dura-Tabs, Quinalan, (gluconate); Cardioquin (polygalacturonate); Quinidex Extentabs, Quinora (sulfate)

Chemical Class: Dextrorotatory isomer of quinine
Therapeutic Class: Antidysrhythmic (Class IA); antimalarial

CLINICAL PHARMACOLOGY
Mechanism of Action: Decreases the rate of rise of diastolic (Phase 4) depolarization, thereby depressing automaticity in ectopic foci; slows depolarization, repolarization, and amplitude of the action potential leading to an increase in the refractoriness of atrial and ventricular tissue; exerts indirect anticholinergic effects through blockade of vagal innervation, which may facilitate conduction in the atrioventricular junction

Pharmacokinetics
PO: Peak 3-4 hr (gluconate), 1-1½ hr (sulfate), 6 hr (polygalacturonate); duration 6-8 hr (EXT REL tab 12 hr)
IM: Peak ½-1½ hr
80%-90% bound to plasma proteins; metabolized in liver, excreted in urine (10%-50% unchanged); $t_{1/2}$ 6 hr

INDICATIONS AND USES: *PO:* Premature ventricular contractions, ventricular tachycardia (when not associated with complete heart block), junctional (nodal) dysrhythmias, AV junctional premature complexes, paroxysmal junctional tachycardia, premature atrial contractions, paroxysmal atrial tachycardia, atrial flutter, atrial fibrillation (chronic and paroxysmal); *IM/IV* when PO therapy not feasible or when rapid therapeutic effect is required, life-threatening *Plasmodium falciparum* malaria

DOSAGE
Adult
• Give 200 mg test dose PO/IM several hr before full dosage to determine possibility of idiosyncratic reaction
• PO (sulfate) 100-600 mg q4-6h, initiate at 200 mg/dose and adjust dose to maintain desired therapeutic effect, max 3-4 g/d; SUS REL 300-600 mg q8-12h
• PO (gluconate) 324-972 mg q8-12h
• PO (polygalacturonate) 275 mg q8-12h
• IM 400 mg q4-6h
• IV 200-400 mg diluted and infused at a rate 10 mg/min
Child
• Give 2 mg/kg test dose PO/IM several hr before full dosage to determine possibility of idiosyncratic reaction
• PO (sulfate) 15-60 mg/kg/day divided into 4-5 doses or 6 mg/kg q4-6h; usual 30 mg/kg/day or 900 mg/m²/day given in 5 doses/day

$ AVAILABLE FORMS/COST OF THERAPY
• Tab, Uncoated—Oral (sulfate): 200 mg, 100's: **$7.50-$22.66**; 300 mg, 100's: **$13.50-$31.62**
• Tab, Coated, SUS Action—Oral (sulfate): 300 mg, 100's: **$64.85-$84.61**
• Tab, Uncoated—Oral (polygalacturonate): 275 mg, 100's: **$103.10**
• Tab, Uncoated, SUS Action—Oral (gluconate): 324 mg, 100's: **$17.25-$58.68**
• Inj, Sol—IM;IV (gluconate): 80 mg/ml, 10 ml: **$13.77**

CONTRAINDICATIONS: Digitalis intoxication manifested by AV condition disorders, complete AV block with an AV nodal or idioventricular pacemaker, left bundle branch block, or other severe intraventricular condition defects with marked QRS widening, ectopic impulses, and abnormal rhythms due to escape mechanisms, history of drug-induced torsade de pointes, history of long QT syndrome, myasthenia gravis

PRECAUTIONS: Treatment of atrial flutter without prior medication to control ventricular rate (e.g., digoxin, verapamil, diltiazem, β-blocker), marginally compensated cardiovascular disease, incomplete AV block, digitalis intoxication, hyperkalemia, renal, or hepatic insufficiency

PREGNANCY AND LACTATION: Pregnancy category C; use during pregnancy has been classified in reviews of cardiovascular drugs as relatively safe for the fetus; high doses can produce oxytocic properties and potential for abortion; excreted in breast milk; compatible with breast feeding

SIDE EFFECTS/ADVERSE REACTIONS
CNS: Apprehension, ataxia, confusion, delirium, dementia, depression, *dizziness,* excitement, fever, *headache,* vertigo
CV: Angioedema, arterial embolism, *bradycardia,* **complete AV block,** *hypotension,* prolonged QT interval, syncope, **torsade de pointes,** ventricular extrasystoles, ventricular flutter, **ventricular tachycardia and fibrillation,** widening of the QRS complex
EENT: Disturbed hearing (tinnitus, decreased auditory acuity), disturbed vision (mydriasis, blurred vision, disturbed color perception, photophobia, diplopia, night blindness, scotomata), optic neuritis, reduced visual field
GI: Abdominal pain, anorexia, *diarrhea,* esophagitis, hepatotoxicity, nausea, vomiting
HEME: **Acute hemolytic anemia, agranulocytosis,** leukocytosis, **neutropenia, thrombocytopenia,** thrombocytopenic purpura
MS: Arthralgia, increase in serum skeletal muscle creatine phosphokinase, myalgia
SKIN: Abnormalities of pigmentation, cutaneous flushing with intense pruritus, eczema, exfoliative eruptions, photosensitivity, psoriasis, purpura, rash, urticaria, vasculitis
MISC: Cinchonism (tinnitus, headache, nausea, visual changes), lupus nephritis, positive ANA, systemic lupus erythematosus

DRUG INTERACTIONS
Drugs
▪ *Acetazolamide, antacids, sodium bicarbonate:* Alkalinization of urine increases plasma quinidine concentrations
▪ *Amiloride:* Increased risk of arrhythmias in patients with ventricular tachycardia
▪ *Amiodarone, cimetidine, verapamil:* Increased plasma quinidine concentrations
▪ *Azole antifungals:* Inhibition of quinidine metabolism (CYP3A4), increased concentrations
▪ *Barbiturates, nifedipine, kaolinpectin, phenytoin, rifampin, rifabutin:* Decreased plasma quinidine concentrations
▪ *β-blockers:* Increased concentrations of metoprolol, propranolol, and timolol
▪ *Cholinergic agents:* Reduced therapeutic effects of cholinergic drugs
❷ *Codeine:* Inhibition of codeine to its active metabolite, diminished analgesia
▪ *Cyclic antidepressants:* Increased imipramine, nortriptyline and desipramine concentrations
▪ *Dextromethorphan:* Increased dextromethorphan concentrations, toxicity may result
▪ *Digitalis glycosides:* Increased digoxin and digitoxin concentrations, toxicity may result
▪ *Encainide:* Increased encainide serum concentrations in rapid encainide metabolizers
▪ *Haloperidol:* Increased haloperidol concentrations, toxicity
▪ *Macrolides:* Increased quinidine concentrations with erythromycin, troleandomycin, clarithromycin due to CYP34A inhibition
▪ *Mexiletine:* Increased mexiletine concentrations

italic = common side effects

bold italic = life-threatening reactions

🔳 *Neuromuscular blocking agents:* Enhanced effects of neuromuscular blocking agents

🔳 *Nifedipine:* Increased serum nifedipine concentrations

🔳 *Procainamide:* Marked increased procainamide concentrations

🔳 *Propafenone:* Increased propafenone concentrations and decreased concentrations of its active metabolite; net effect unknown

🔳 *Warfarin:* Enhanced anticoagulant response

Labs

• *False increase:* Urine 17-ketosteroids

SPECIAL CONSIDERATIONS

• 267 mg gluconate = 275 mg polygalacturonate = 200 mg sulfate

PATIENT/FAMILY EDUCATION

• Take with food to decrease GI upset

• Do not crush or chew sustained release tablets

MONITORING PARAMETERS

• Plasma quinidine concentration (therapeutic range 2-6 μg/ml)

• ECG

• Liver function tests during the 1st 4-8 weeks

• CBC periodically during prolonged therapy

---

ramipril
(ra-mi'pril)
Rx: Altace
Chemical Class: Angiotensin-converting enzyme (ACE) inhibitor
Therapeutic Class: Antihypertensive; CHF agent; renal protectant

CLINICAL PHARMACOLOGY

Mechanism of Action: Selectively suppresses renin-angiotensin-aldosterone system; inhibits ACE preventing the conversion of angiotensin I to angiotensin II; results in dilation of arterial, venous vessels

Pharmacokinetics

PO: Onset 1-2 hr, duration 24 hr; 73% bound to plasma proteins; has little pharmacologic activity until metabolized to active metabolite (ramiprilat), excreted in urine (60%) and feces (40%); $t_{1/2}$ (ramiprilat) 13-17 hr

INDICATIONS AND USES: Hypertension, congestive heart failure, diabetic nephropathy,* post MI, heart failure

DOSAGE

Adult

• *Hypertension:* PO 2.5 mg qd initially, adjust dose at 2 wk intervals according to blood pressure response, usual range 2.5-20 mg/day divided qd-bid; in renal impairment (CrCl <40 ml/min/1.73 m² initiate at 1.25 mg qd, max 5 mg/day)

• *Congestive heart failure:* PO 2.5 mg bid, titrate as tolerated to target dose of 5 mg bid; in renal impairment (CrCl <40 ml/min/1.73 m² initiate at 1.25 mg qd, max 2.5 mg bid)

🔳 **AVAILABLE FORMS/COST OF THERAPY**

• Cap, Gel—Oral: 1.25 mg, 100's: **$59.08;** 2.5 mg, 100's: **$69.31;** 5 mg, 100's: **$74.18;** 10 mg, 100's: **$86.00**

PRECAUTIONS: Impaired renal and liver function, dialysis patients, hypovolemia, diuretic therapy, collagen-vascular diseases, congestive heart failure, elderly, bilateral renal artery stenosis

PREGNANCY AND LACTATION: Pregnancy category D; ACE inhibitors can cause fetal and neonatal morbidity and death when administered to pregnant women; when pregnancy is detected, discontinue ACE inhibitors as soon as possible

SIDE EFFECTS/ADVERSE REACTIONS

CNS: Anxiety, dizziness, fatigue, *headache,* insomnia, paresthesia

CV: Angina, hypotension, palpitations, postural hypotension, syncope (especially with 1st dose)

GI: Abdominal pain, constipation, impaired taste sensation, nausea, pancreatitis, vomiting

GU: Decreased libido, impotence, renal insufficiency

HEME: **Agranulocytosis, neutropenia, thrombocytopenia**

METAB: Hyperkalemia, hyponatremia, hypoglycemia

MS: Arthralgia, arthritis, myalgia

RESP: Asthma, bronchitis, *cough,* dyspnea, sinusitis

SKIN: Angioedema, flushing, rash, sweating

DRUG INTERACTIONS

Drugs

❷ *Allopurinol:* Predisposition to hypersensitivity reactions

🔳 *α-adrenergic blockers:* Exaggerated 1st dose hypotensive response

🔳 *Aspirin:* Reduced hemodynamic effects; less likely with nonacetylated salicylates

🔳 *Cyclosporine:* Renal insufficiency

🔳 *Insulin:* Enhanced hypoglycemic response

🔳 *Iron (parenteral):* Increased risk of systemic reaction

🔳 *Lithium:* Increased risk of serious lithium toxicity

🔳 *Loop diuretics:* Initiation of ACE inhibitor therapy may cause hypotension and renal insufficiency

🔳 *NSAIDs:* Inhibition of the antihypertensive response to ACE inhibitors

🔳 *Potassium, potassium-sparing diuretics:* Increased risk for hyperkalemia

SPECIAL CONSIDERATIONS

PATIENT/FAMILY EDUCATION

• Do not use salt substitutes containing potassium without consulting clinician

• Rise slowly to sitting or standing position to minimize orthostatic hypotension

• Dizziness, fainting, lightheadedness may occur during 1st few days of therapy

• Capsules may be opened and contents sprinkled on small amount of applesauce or mixed in apple juice or water before consuming

MONITORING PARAMETERS

• BUN, creatinine (watch for increased levels that may indicate acute renal failure)

• Potassium levels, although hyperkalemia rarely occurs

---

reserpine
(re-ser'peen)
Rx: Serpasil ✦
Chemical Class: Rauwolfia alkaloid
Therapeutic Class: Antihypertensive; antipsychotic

CLINICAL PHARMACOLOGY

Mechanism of Action: Depletes stores of catecholamines and 5-hydroxytryptamine in many organs; depression of sympathetic nerve function results in decreased heart rate and lowering of arterial blood pressure; sedative and tranquilizing properties are thought to be related to depletion of catecholamines and 5-hydroxytryptamine from the brain

Pharmacokinetics

PO: Peak 3½ hr; slow onset of action, sustained duration of effect; 96% bound to plasma proteins; $t_{1/2}$ 33 hr

INDICATIONS AND USES: Hypertension, agitated psychotic states in patients unable to tolerate phenothiazines

---

* = non FDA-approved use

DOSAGE
Adult
• *Hypertension:* PO 0.5 mg qd for 1-2 wk, then 0.1-0.25 mg qd; higher doses increase incidence of mental depression and serious side effects
• *Psychotic states:* PO 0.5 mg qd, range 0.1-1 mg/day
Child
PO 20 µg/kg/day, max 0.25 mg/day
S AVAILABLE FORMS/COST OF THERAPY
• Tab, Uncoated—Oral: 0.1 mg, 100's: **$2.95-$5.50**; 0.25 mg, 100's: **$3.50-$7.65**
CONTRAINDICATIONS: Current depression or history of depression, active peptic ulcer, ulcerative colitis, patients receiving electroconvulsive therapy
PRECAUTIONS: History of peptic ulcer (increases GI motility and secretion), history of gallstones, renal function impairment, children
PREGNANCY AND LACTATION: Pregnancy category C; excreted into breast milk, no clinical reports of adverse effects in nursing infants have been located
SIDE EFFECTS/ADVERSE REACTIONS
CNS: Depression, *dizziness, drowsiness,* dull sensorium, *fatigue,* headache, *lethargy,* nervousness, nightmares, paradoxical anxiety, parkinsonian syndrome and other extrapyramidal tract symptoms (rare)
CV: Angina-like symptoms, *bradycardia, dysrhythmias* (particularly when used concurrently with digitalis or quinidine), edema, syncope
EENT: Conjunctival injection, deafness, epistaxis, glaucoma, nasal congestion, optic atrophy, uveitis
GI: Anorexia, diarrhea, dryness of mouth, hypersecretion, nausea, vomiting
GU: Decreased libido, dysuria, impotence
METAB: Breast engorgement, elevated prolactin, gynecomastia, pseudolactation, weight gain
MS: Muscular aches
RESP: Dyspnea
SKIN: Pruritus, purpura, rash
DRUG INTERACTIONS
Drugs
3 *Nonselective MAOIs:* Hypertensive reactions
Labs
• *False increase:* Serum bilirubin, urine creatinine
• *False positive:* Guaiacols spot test

SPECIAL CONSIDERATIONS
• Only remaining rauwolfia derivative available
PATIENT/FAMILY EDUCATION
• May cause drowsiness or dizziness, use caution driving or participating in other activities requiring alertness
• Therapeutic effect may take 2-3 wk

---

reteplase
(reh'te-place)
Rx: Retavase
Chemical Class: Tissue plasminogen activator
Therapeutic Class: Antithrombotic

CLINICAL PHARMACOLOGY
Mechanism of Action: Catalyzes the cleavage of endogenous plasminogen to generate plasmin; plasmin degrades the fibrin matrix of an offending thrombus—fibrinolysis

Pharmacokinetics
IV: Fibrinogen levels fall below 100 mg/dl 2 hr following double-bolus administration, mean fibrinogen level back to normal by 48 hr; coronary artery patency is usually achieved within 30-90 min; $t_{1/2}$ 13-16 min; cleared by liver and kidney
INDICATIONS AND USES: Acute myocardial infarction; lysis of coronary artery thrombi
DOSAGE
Adult
• *IV:* 10 + 10 U double-bolus injection, over 2 min, 30 min apart
S AVAILABLE FORMS/COST OF THERAPY
• Inj—Lyphl sol kit (2 × 10 U plus syringes, needles, etc.): **$2750**
CONTRAINDICATIONS: Active internal bleeding, history of cerebrovascular accident, recent intracranial or intraspinal surgery or trauma, intracranial neoplasm, arteriovenous malformation or aneurysm, known bleeding diathesis, severe uncontrolled hypertension
PRECAUTIONS: Recent major surgery, previous puncture of non-compressible vessels, cerebrovascular disease, recent gastrointestinal or genitourinary bleeding, recent trauma; hypertension: systolic BP ≥180 mm Hg and/or diastolic BP ≥110 mm Hg; high likelihood of left heart thrombus; acute pericarditis, subacute bacterial endocarditis, hemostatic defects including those secondary to severe hepatic or renal disease, severe hepatic or renal dysfunction, pregnancy, diabetic hemorrhagic retinopathy or other hemorrhagic ophthalmic conditions, septic thrombophlebitis, advanced age, patients currently receiving oral anticoagulants, any other condition in which bleeding constitutes a significant hazard
PREGNANCY AND LACTATION: Pregnancy category C
SIDE EFFECTS/ADVERSE REACTIONS
CV: **Cardiac tamponade, electromechanical dissociation, reinfarction**
HEME: **Bleeding**
SKIN: Allergic reactions
MISC: Fever
DRUG INTERACTIONS
Drugs
⦿ *Heparin, vitamin K antagonists, drugs that alter platelet function (i.e., aspirin, dipyridamole, and abciximab):* May increase the risk of bleeding

SPECIAL CONSIDERATIONS
• No other IV medications should be administered in the same line

---

selegiline
(seh-leg'ill-ene)
Rx: Carbex **✦**, Eldepryl
Chemical Class: Phenethylamine derivative
Therapeutic Class: Anti-Parkinson's agent

CLINICAL PHARMACOLOGY
Mechanism of Action: Inhibition of monoamine oxidase, type B, which blocks the catabolism of dopamine, increasing the net amount of dopamine available; other less well understood mechanisms also lead to an increase in dopaminergic activity
Pharmacokinetics: Rapidly absorbed, peak ½-2 hr; rapidly metabolized (active metabolites: N-desmethyldeprenyl, $t_{1/2}$ 2 hr; amphetamine, $t_{1/2}$ 17.7 hr, methamphetamine, $t_{1/2}$ 20 ½ hr); metabolites excreted in urine (45% in 48 hr)
INDICATIONS AND USES: Adjunct management of Parkinson's disease in patients being treated with levodopa/carbidopa who have had a poor response to therapy; early Parkinson's disease to delay progression*; atypical depression,* Alzheimer's disease*

---

italic = common side effects

bold italic = life-threatening reactions

DOSAGE
Adult
Parkinson's disease: PO 10 mg/day in divided doses 5 mg at breakfast and lunch; after 2-3 days, begin to reduce the dose of concurrent levodopa/carbidopa 10%-30%

S AVAILABLE FORMS/COST OF THERAPY
• Tab, Uncoated—Oral: 5 mg, 60's: **$134.60**

CONTRAINDICATIONS: Concurrent use with meperidine

PRECAUTIONS: Doses above 10 mg/day (doses in the 30-40 mg/day range are associated with nonselective monoamine oxidase inhibition)

PREGNANCY AND LACTATION: Pregnancy category C

SIDE EFFECTS/ADVERSE REACTIONS
CNS: Anxiety, apathy, back and leg pain, blepharospasm, chorea, confusion, delusions, dizziness, dystonic symptoms, grimacing, hallucinations, headache, increased apraxia, increased bradykinesia, increased tremors, involuntary movements, lethargy, migraine, mood changes, muscle cramps, nightmares, numbness, overstimulation, personality change, restlessness, sleep disturbances, tardive dyskinesia, tiredness, vertigo

CV: Angina pectoris, **dysrhythmia,** edema, hypertension, hypotension, orthostatic hypotension, palpitations, sinus bradycardia, syncope, tachycardia

EENT: Blurred vision, diplopia, dry mouth, tinnitus

GI: Abdominal pain, anorexia, constipation, diarrhea, dysphagia, heartburn, nausea, poor appetite, rectal bleeding, vomiting, weight loss

GU: Frequency, hesitation, nocturia, prostatic hypertrophy, retention, sexual dysfunction, slow urination

RESP: Asthma, shortness of breath

SKIN: Alopecia, facial hair, hematoma, increased sweating, photosensitivity, rash

DRUG INTERACTIONS
Drugs
❷ *Antidepressants, serotonin reuptake inhibitors (fluoxetine, fluvoxamine, paroxetine, sertraline):* Serious, sometimes fatal, reactions including hyperthermia, autonomic instability and mental status changes

❷ *Dexfenfluramine, fenfluramine:* Increased risk of serotonin syndrome

❷ *Dextroamphetamine:* Severe hypertension

❷ *Dextromethorphan:* Increased risk of serotonin syndrome

❸ *Guanadrel, guanethidine:* May inhibit the antihypertensive effects of antihypertensive agents

❸ *Insulin:* Excessive hypoglycemia may occur when MAOIs are administered to patients with diabetes

❸ *Levodopa:* May precipitate hypertensive crisis

⚠ *Methylphenidate:* Increased risk of hypertensive reactions

❸ *Moclobemide:* Increased pressor effects of tyramine; increased risk of adverse drug or food interactions

❷ *Narcotic analgesics (meperidine):* Stupor, muscular rigidity, severe agitation, elevated temperature, hallucinations, and death

❸ *Narcotic analgesics (morphine):* Stupor, muscular rigidity, severe agitation, elevated temperature, hallucinations, and death

⚠ *Reserpine:* Loss of antihypertensive effects

❸ *Succinylcholine:* Prolonged muscle relaxation caused by succinylcholine

⚠ *Sympathomimetics (metaraminol, phenylpropanolamine, pseudoephedrine):* Additive pressor response to sympathomimetic

❸ *Sympathomimetics (norepinephrine, phenylephrine):* Additive pressor response to sympathomimetic

Labs
• *False positive:* Urine ketones, urine glucose
• *False negative:* Urine glucose (glucose oxidase)
• *False increase:* Uric acid, urine protein

SPECIAL CONSIDERATIONS
• At low doses, irreversible type B MAOI; at higher doses is metabolized to amphetamine, inhibiting both A and B subtypes of MAO
• Several placebo-controlled studies have demonstrated a significant delay in the need to initiate levodopa therapy in patients who receive selegiline in the early phase of the disease
• May have significant benefit in slowing the onset of the debilitating consequences of Parkinson's disease

sibutramine
(sih-byoo'tra-meen)
Rx: Meridia
Chemical Class: Cyclobutanemethamine derivative
Therapeutic Class: Anorexiant
DEA Class: Schedule IV

CLINICAL PHARMACOLOGY
Mechanism of Action: Inhibits reuptake of norepinephrine, serotonin, and dopamine in the CNS

Pharmacokinetics
PO: Peak 1.2 hr, 77% absorption, extensive first pass metabolism in the liver; 97% bound to plasma proteins; metabolized in the liver by cytochrome P450(3A$_4$) to active desmethyl metabolites; excreted in urine (77%) and feces; t$_{1/2}$ 1.1 hr (14 and 16 hr for two active metabolites)

INDICATIONS AND USES: Management of obesity (initial body mass index ≥30 kg/m^2, or ≥27 kg/m^2 in the presence of other risk factors like hypertension, diabetes and dyslipidemia) in conjunction with a reduced calorie diet

DOSAGE
Adult
• PO 10 mg qd; may increase to 15 mg qd after 4 wk if inadequate results; safety and efficacy beyond 1 yr of therapy has not been determined

S AVAILABLE FORMS/COST OF THERAPY
• Cap—Oral: 5, 10 mg, 100's: **$290.00;** 15 mg, 100's: **$375.00**

CONTRAINDICATIONS: Patients receiving MAO inhibitors or other centrally acting appetite suppressants; anorexia nervosa

PRECAUTIONS: Hypertension, CAD, CHF, arrhythmia, stroke, narrow angle glaucoma, seizure disorders, gallstones, renal or hepatic dysfunction

PREGNANCY AND LACTATION: Pregnancy category C; excretion into breast milk unknown, not recommended in nursing mothers

SIDE EFFECTS/ADVERSE REACTIONS
CNS: Anxiety, depression, dizziness, emotional lability, *headache, insomnia,* nervousness, paresthesia, somnolence, stimulation

CV: Generalized edema, hypertension, migraine, palpitation, tachycardia, vasodilation

EENT: Ear disorder, ear pain, taste perversion

GI: Anorexia, constipation, dry mouth, dyspepsia, gastritis, increased appetite, nausea, rectal disorder, vomiting

GU: Dysmenorrhea, metrorrhagia

MS: Arthralgia, back pain, joint disorder, myalgia, tenosynovitis

RESP: Cough increase, laryngitis, pharyngitis, rhinitis, sinusitis

SKIN: Acne, rash, sweating

---

* = non FDA-approved use

MISC: Abdominal pain, asthenia, chest pain, flu syndrome, neck pain, thirst

DRUG INTERACTIONS

Drugs

❷ *MAO inhibitors:* Potential for the development of serotonin syndrome; at least 14 days should elapse between administration of MAO inhibitors and sibutramine

SPECIAL CONSIDERATIONS

• Primary pulmonary hypertension and cardiac valve disorders have been associated with other centrally acting weight loss agents that cause release of serotonin from nerve terminals; although sibutramine has not been associated with these effects in premarketing clinical studies, patients should be informed of the potential for these side effects and monitored closely for their occurrence

• Substantially increases blood pressure in some patients

• Maintenance of weight loss beyond 1 yr has not been studied

MONITORING PARAMETERS

• Regular blood pressure monitoring

---

simvastatin

(sim'va-sta-tin)

Rx: Zocor

Chemical Class: Lactone (inactive): HMG-CoA reductase inhibitor

Therapeutic Class: Antilipemic

CLINICAL PHARMACOLOGY

Mechanism of Action: Inhibits HMG-CoA reductase enzyme, which catalyzes the rate-limiting step in cholesterol biosynthesis (increases HDL-cholesterol mildly, dramatically decreases total cholesterol and LDL-cholesterol)

Pharmacokinetics

PO: Peak 1-2½ hr, 85% absorbed; extensive 1st-pass metabolism (active metabolites); 95% protein bound; excreted primarily in bile, feces (60%)

INDICATIONS AND USES: Reduction of elevated total and LDL cholesterol in patients with primary hypercholesterolemia (types IIa and IIb); reduction of morbidity and mortality in patients with coronary heart disease and hypercholesterolemia

DOSAGE

Adult

• PO 5-10 mg qd in PM initially, usual range 5-40 mg/day qd in PM, not to exceed 40 mg/day; dosage adjustments may be made in 4-wk intervals

⑤ **AVAILABLE FORMS/COST OF THERAPY**

• Tab, Plain Coated—Oral: 5 mg, 90's: **$106.84;** 10 mg, 90's: **$121.73;** 20 mg, 60's: **$212.34;** 40 mg, 60's: **$220.61**

CONTRAINDICATIONS: Active liver disease

PRECAUTIONS: Past liver disease, alcoholism, severe acute infections, trauma, hypotension, uncontrolled seizure disorders, severe metabolic disorders, electrolyte imbalances

PREGNANCY AND LACTATION: Pregnancy category X; breast milk excretion unknown; other drugs in this class are excreted in small amounts; manufacturer recommends against breast feeding

SIDE EFFECTS/ADVERSE REACTIONS

CNS: Dizziness, headache, insomnia, memory loss, peripheral neuropathy, tremor, vertigo

GI: Abdominal pain, constipation, diarrhea, dyspepsia, flatus, heartburn, liver dysfunction, nausea, ***pancreatitis,*** vomiting

GU: Erectile dysfunction, gynecomastia, loss of libido

HEME: ***Eosinophilia, hemolytic anemia, leukopenia, thrombocytopenia***

MS: Muscle cramps, myalgia, myositis, ***rhabdomyolysis***

SKIN: Alopecia, pruritus, rash, ***Stevens-Johnson syndrome***

DRUG INTERACTIONS

Drugs

❷ *Azole antifungals (fluconazole, itraconazole, ketoconazole, miconazole):* Increased simvastatin levels via inhibition of metabolism with increased risk of rhabdomyolysis

❸ *Cholestyramine, colestipol:* Reduced bioavailability of simvastatin

❸ *Danazol:* Inhibition of metabolism (CYP3A4) thought to yield increased simvastatin levels with increased risk of rhabdomyolysis

❷ *Fluoxetine:* Inhibits CYP3A4 hepatic metabolism with risk of rhabdomyolysis

❷ *Gemfibrozil:* Small increased risk of myopathy with combination

❸ *Isradipine:* Isradipine probably decreases simvastatin (like lovastatin) plasma concentrations minimally

❸ *Macrolide antibiotics (clarithromycin, erythromycin, troleandomycin):* Increased simvastatin levels via inhibition of metabolism with increased risk of rhabdomyolysis

❸ *Nefazodone:* Inhibit CYP3A4 hepatic metabolism (like lovastatin) with risk of rhabdomyolysis

❸ *Warfarin:* Addition of simvastatin may increase hypoprothrombinemic response to warfarin via inhibition of metabolism (CYP2C9)

SPECIAL CONSIDERATIONS

• Superior to fibrates, cholestyramine, and probucol in lowering total and LDL cholesterol levels

• No significant advantage over other lovastatin, pravastatin; base HMG-CoA selection on cost and availability

PATIENT/FAMILY EDUCATION

• Take with evening meal

---

sotalol

(soe'ta-lole)

Rx: Betapace, Linsotalol ✤, Sotacor ✤

Chemical Class: Nonselective β-adrenergic blocker

Therapeutic Class: Antidysrhythmic (Class II)

CLINICAL PHARMACOLOGY

Mechanism of Action: Nonselectively blocks β_1-(cardiac muscle) and β_2-receptors (bronchial and vascular musculature), inhibiting the chronotropic, inotropic, and vasodilator responses to β-adrenergic stimulation

Pharmacokinetics

PO: Onset 1-2 hr, peak effect 3-4 hr; $t_{1/2}$ 12 hr; excreted unchanged by kidney; low lipid solubility; not protein bound; absorption decreased 20%-30% by meals

INDICATIONS AND USES: Treatment of life-threatening ventricular dysrhythmias (e.g., sustained ventricular tachycardia); not recommended in less severe dysrhythmias

DOSAGE

• PO initial dose 80 mg bid; may increase to 240-320 mg/day adjusting dose q2-3d; some patients require doses up to 480-640 mg qd

• *Renal failure adjustment:* CrCl >60 ml/min administer q12h; CrCl 30-60 ml/min administer q24h; CrCl 10-30 ml/min administer q36-48h; individualize dose for CrCl <10 ml/min; increase dose after 5-6 doses prn

---

italic = common side effects

bold italic = life-threatening reactions

$ AVAILABLE FORMS/COST OF THERAPY
• Tab, Coated—Oral: 80 mg, 100's: **$177.66;** 120 mg, 100's: **$237.00;** 160 mg, 100's: **$296.22;** 240 mg, 100's: **$385.14**
CONTRAINDICATIONS: Uncompensated CHF, cardiogenic shock, bradycardia, heart block >1st degree, pulmonary edema, asthma, long QT syndrome
PRECAUTIONS: CHF, peripheral vascular disease, hypokalemia, hypomagnesemia, renal dysfunction, sick sinus syndrome
PREGNANCY AND LACTATION: Pregnancy category B; concentrated in breast milk (levels 3-5 times those of plasma); symptoms of β-blockade possible in infant, but considered compatible with breast feeding
SIDE EFFECTS/ADVERSE REACTIONS
CNS: Anxiety, confusion, depression, *dizziness,* drowsiness, *fatigue,* hallucinations, insomnia, nightmares, weakness
CV: Bradycardia, chest pain, **CHF,** hypotension, Raynaud's phenomena, **ventricular dysrhythmias including torsade de points**
GI: Constipation, diarrhea, nausea, stomach discomfort, vomiting
GU: Sexual dysfunction
HEME: **Agranulocytosis**
RESP: **Bronchospasm,** cough, dyspnea
DRUG INTERACTIONS
Drugs
🔳 *Adenosine:* Bradycardia aggravated
🔳 *Amiodarone:* Combination yielded bradycardia and hypotension in case reports
🔳 *Antacids:* Reduced sotalol absorption
🔳 *Calcium channel blockers:* See dihydropyridine calcium channel blockers and verapamil
🔳 *Cimetidine:* Renal clearance reduced; AUC increased with cimetidine coadministration
🔳 *Clonidine, guanabenz, guanfacine:* Exacerbation of rebound hypertension upon discontinuation of clonidine
🔳 *Cocaine:* Cocaine-induced vasoconstriction potentiated; reduced coronary blood flow
🔳 *Contrast media:* Increased risk of anaphylaxis
🔳 *Digitalis:* Enhances bradycardia
🔳 *Dihydropyridine calcium channel blockers:* Additive pharmacodynamic effects
🔳 *Dipyridamole:* Bradycardia aggravated
🔳 *Epinephrine, isoproterenol, phenylephrine:* Potentiates pressor response; resultant hypertension and bradycardia
🔳 *Flecainide:* Additive negative inotropic effects; case report of bradycardia, AV block, and cardiac arrest following switch from flecainide to sotalol
🔳 *Fluoxetine:* Increased β-blockade activity
🔳 *Fluoroquinolones:* Reduced clearance of sotalol
🔳 *Insulin:* Altered response to hypoglycemia; increased blood glucose concentrations; impaired peripheral circulation
🔳 *Lidocaine:* Increased serum lidocaine concentrations possible
🔳 *Neostigmine:* Bradycardia aggravated
🔳 *Neuroleptics:* Both drugs inhibit each other's metabolism; additive hypotension
🔳 *NSAIDs:* Reduced hemodynamic effects of sotalol
🔳 *Physostigmine:* Bradycardia aggravated
🔳 *Prazosin:* First-dose response to prazosin may be enhanced by β-blockade
🔳 *Tacrine:* Bradycardia aggravated
🅰 *Terbutaline:* Antagonized bronchodilating effects of terbutaline
🅰 *Theophylline:* Antagonistic pharmacodynamic effects
🔳 *Verapamil:* Enhanced effects of both drugs; particularly AV nodal conduction slowing; reduced sotalol clearance

Labs
• *Metanephrines total:* Falsely increases urine levels (may be double)

SPECIAL CONSIDERATIONS
PATIENT/FAMILY EDUCATION
• Do not discontinue abruptly
MONITORING PARAMETERS
• Because of prodysrhythmic risk, begin and increase drug in setting with cardiac rhythm monitoring
• QT intervals; discontinue or reduce dose if QT >550 msec
• Withdraw any previous antidysrhythmic therapy, allowing for at least 2-3 half lives
• After discontinuation of amiodarone, do not initiate sotalol until QT normalized

---

spironolactone
(speer-on-oh-lak'tone)
Rx: Aldactone, Novospiroton ✦
Chemical Class: Aldosterone antagonist
Therapeutic Class: Antihypertensive; potassium-sparing diuretic

CLINICAL PHARMACOLOGY
Mechanism of Action: Competes with aldosterone at receptor sites in distal tubule, resulting in excretion of sodium chloride, water, retention of potassium, phosphate; has antiandrogenic effect
Pharmacokinetics
PO: Onset 24-48 hr, peak 48-72 hr; >90% bound to plasma proteins; metabolized in liver, excreted in urine; crosses placenta; $t_{1/2}$ 1.4 hr
INDICATIONS AND USES: Edema, hypertension, diuretic-induced hypokalemia, primary hyperaldosteronism, nephrotic syndrome, cirrhosis of the liver with ascites, polycystic ovary disease,* female hirsutism*
DOSAGE
Adult
• *Edema or hypertension:* PO 25-200 mg/day in single or divided doses
• *Hypokalemia:* PO 25-100 mg/day in single or divided doses
• *Primary hyperaldosteronism diagnosis:* PO 400 mg/day for 4 days (short test) or 4 wk (long test), then 100-400 mg/day maintenance
• *Polycystic ovary disease or hirsutism:* PO 100-200 mg/day
Child
• Diuretic or antihypertensive or ascites: PO 1-3 mg/kg/day in single or divided doses
$ AVAILABLE FORMS/COST OF THERAPY
• Tab, Plain Coated—Oral: 25 mg, 100's: **$4.53-$38.64;** 50 mg, 100's: **$71.08;** 100 mg, 100's: **$119.29**
CONTRAINDICATIONS: Anuria, severe renal disease, hyperkalemia
PRECAUTIONS: Dehydration, hepatic disease, hyponatremia, renal insufficiency, patients receiving other potassium-sparing diuretics or potassium supplements, diabetic nephropathy, menstrual abnormalities, gynecomastia, acidosis, elderly
PREGNANCY AND LACTATION: Pregnancy category D; active metabolite excreted in breast milk; compatible with breast feeding
SIDE EFFECTS/ADVERSE REACTIONS
CNS: Ataxia, confusion, drowsiness, headache, lethargy
CV: Bradycardia, **CHF,** hypotension

GI: Anorexia, **bleeding,** constipation, cramps, *diarrhea,* gastritis, nausea, *vomiting*
GU: Amenorrhea, deepening voice, gynecomastia, hirsutism, impotence, irregular menses, postmenopausal bleeding
METAB: Hyperchloremic metabolic acidosis, hyperkalemia, hyponatremia
SKIN: Pruritus, rash, urticaria
DRUG INTERACTIONS
Drugs
🔳 *Ammonium chloride:* Combination may produce systemic acidosis
🔳 *Digoxin:* False or true increase in digoxin concentrations
🔳 *Disopyramide:* Increased potassium concentrations may enhance disopyramide effects on myocardial conduction
⚠ *Mitotane:* Spironolactone antagonizes the activity of mitotane
➋ *Potassium:* Increased risk of hyperkalemia
Labs
• *Corticosteroids:* Marked false increase in plasma corticosteroids
• *Cortisol:* Falsely increased fluorometric methods of measurement
• *Digoxin:* False increases in digoxin concentrations
• *17-Hydroxycorticosteroids:* False increases in urine measurements
• *17-Ketogenic steroids:* Falsely increases urine concentrations

SPECIAL CONSIDERATIONS
MONITORING PARAMETERS
• When used for diagnosis of primary hyperaldosteronism, positive results are: (long test) correction of hyperkalemia and hypertension; (short test) serum potassium increases during administration, but falls upon discontinuation

---

streptokinase
(strep-toe-kye'nase)
Rx: Kabikinase, Streptase
Chemical Class: Purified β-hemolytic streptococcus filtrate
Therapeutic Class: Thrombolytic

CLINICAL PHARMACOLOGY
Mechanism of Action: Activates conversion of plasminogen to plasmin; plasmin degrades fibrin clots, fibrinogen, other plasma proteins
Pharmacokinetics
IV/INTRACORONARY: Onset immediate; $t_{1/2}$ of streptokinase activator complex 23 min; mechanism of elimination unknown; no metabolites identified
INDICATIONS AND USES: Acute evolving transmural MI; pulmonary embolism; deep venous thrombosis, arterial thrombosis or embolism; arteriovenous cannulae occlusion not responsive to heparin flush
DOSAGE
Adult
• *Acute evolving transmural MI:* IV INF 1,500,000 IU diluted to a volume of 45 ml; administer over 1 hr; intracoronary (IC) dilute 250,000 IU vial to total volume of 125 ml, give 20,000 IU (10 ml) by bolus followed by 2000 IU/min for 60 min for total dose 140,000 IU
• *Thrombosis or embolism:* IV INF 250,000 IU over ½ hr; then 100,000 IU/hr for 72 hr for deep vein thrombosis or 100,000 IU/hr for 24 hr for pulmonary embolism or 100,000 IU/hr for 24-72 hr for arterial thrombosis or embolism
• *Arteriovenous cannula occlusion:* IV INF 250,000 IU/2 ml sol into each occluded limb of cannula slowly; clamp for 2 hr; aspirate contents; flush with saline sol and reconnect cannula

🅢 **AVAILABLE FORMS/COST OF THERAPY**
• Inj, Lyphl-Sol—Intracoronary; IV: 1,500,000 U/vial: **$511.75;** 750,000 U/vial: **$255.86;** 600,000 U/vial: **$160.00;** 250,000 U/vial: **$115.93**
CONTRAINDICATIONS: Active internal bleeding; recent (within 2 mo) CVA; intracranial or intraspinal surgery, intracranial neoplasm; severe uncontrolled hypertension
PRECAUTIONS: Recent (within 10 days) surgery, obstetric delivery, organ biopsy, trauma including CPR; high likelihood of left heart thrombus (e.g., mitral stenosis with atrial fibrillation); subacute bacterial endocarditis; hemostatic defects; age ≥75 yr; diabetic hemorrhagic retinopathy; septic thrombophlebitis or infected occluded AV cannula at seriously infected site; recent streptococcal infection; repeat administration (between 5 days and 12 mo of prior streptokinase)
PREGNANCY AND LACTATION: Pregnancy category C; no data available for breast feeding
SIDE EFFECTS/ADVERSE REACTIONS
CNS: Fever, headache
CV: Hypotension, **reperfusion dysrhythmias**
EENT: Periorbital edema
GI: Nausea, vomiting
HEME: Anemia, **bleeding (GI, GU, intracranial, retroperitoneal,** surface)
RESP: Altered respirations, **bronchospasm, noncardiogenic pulmonary edema,** shortness of breath
SKIN: Flushing, itching, phlebitis at IV INF site, rash, urticaria
MISC: Chills, sweating
DRUG INTERACTIONS
Labs
• *Fibrinogen:* False increase with certain methods
• *Lactate dehydrogenase isoenzymes:* False positive

---

sulfinpyrazone
(sul-fin-pyr'a-zone)
Rx: Anturan ✣, Anturane
Chemical Class: Pyrazolidine derivative
Therapeutic Class: Antigout agent; uricosuric

CLINICAL PHARMACOLOGY
Mechanism of Action: Inhibits tubular reabsorption of uric acid; also has antithrombotic and platelet inhibitory effects; lacks antiinflammatory and analgesic properties
Pharmacokinetics
PO: Well absorbed; 98%-99% bound to plasma proteins; 50% excreted in urine unchanged; $t_{1/2}$ 2.2-3 hr
INDICATIONS AND USES: Chronic and sulfathiazole/sulfacetamide/sulfabenzamide-intermittent gouty arthritis, prevention of recurrent MI (further study indicated),* prevention of systemic embolism in rheumatic mitral stenosis*
DOSAGE
Adult
• PO 200-400 mg/day in 2 divided doses initially, increase to 400-800 mg/day in 2 divided doses; use lowest dose that will control blood uric acid level
🅢 **AVAILABLE FORMS/COST OF THERAPY**
• Cap, Gel—Oral: 200 mg, 100's: **$16.43-$59.84**
• Tab, Uncoated—Oral: 100 mg, 100's: **$13.92-$37.17**
CONTRAINDICATIONS: Active peptic ulcer, symptoms of GI inflammation or ulceration, hypersensitivity to phenylbutazone or other pyrazoles, blood dyscrasias
PRECAUTIONS: Renal function impairment, healed peptic ulcer, dehydration, acute gout attack

---

italic = common side effects

bold italic = life-threatening reactions

PREGNANCY AND LACTATION: Pregnancy category C
SIDE EFFECTS/ADVERSE REACTIONS
GI: Aggravation or reactivation of peptic ulcer, *upper GI disturbances*
HEME: Agranulocytosis, aplastic anemia, anemia, leukopenia, thrombocytopenia
RESP: Bronchospasm (patients with aspirin-induced asthma)
SKIN: Rash
DRUG INTERACTIONS
Drugs
▪ *Antidiabetics:* Increased hypoglycemic effects
▪ *β-blockers:* Reduced hypotensive effects of β-blockers
● *Methotrexate:* Increased methotrexate levels with subsequent increased effect and potential toxicity
● *Oral anticoagulants:* Marked increases in hypoprothrombinemic response to oral anticoagulants
▪ *Salicylates:* Inhibited uricosuric effect of sulfinpyrazone
Labs
• *Cyclosporine:* Falsely decreased serum levels

SPECIAL CONSIDERATIONS
PATIENT/FAMILY EDUCATION
• Take with food, milk, or antacids to decrease stomach upset
• Avoid aspirin and other salicylate-containing products
• Drink plenty of fluids
MONITORING PARAMETERS
• Serum uric acid concentrations, renal function, CBC

---

terazosin
(ter-a′zoe-sin)
Rx: Hytrin
Chemical Class: Quinazoline derivative
Therapeutic Class: Antihypertensive; benign prostatic hypertrophy agent

CLINICAL PHARMACOLOGY
Mechanism of Action: Produces peripheral α_1-adrenergic blockade; reduces smooth muscle tone in prostate and bladder neck; reduces total peripheral resistance, lowering blood pressure
Pharmacokinetics
PO: Completely absorbed, peak 1 hr; 90%-94% bound to plasma proteins; $t_{1/2}$ 12 hr; excreted in urine (40%) and feces (60%), 70% as metabolites
INDICATIONS AND USES: Hypertension; benign prostatic hypertrophy (BPH)
DOSAGE
Adult
• *BPH:* PO 1 mg hs, increase to 2 mg, 5 mg, 10 mg/day (usual dose); not to exceed 20 mg/day; treatment at dose of 10 mg qd for 4-6 wk necessary to determine response
• *Hypertension:* PO 1 mg hs, increase to desired response; usual dose 1-5 mg qd, max 20 mg/day; measure BP at end of dosing interval to determine if bid dose needed
Ⓢ **AVAILABLE FORMS/COST OF THERAPY**
• Cap, Gel—Oral: 1, 2, 5, 10 mg, 100's: **$140.63**
PRECAUTIONS: Patients needing to perform hazardous tasks where syncope or dizziness could be dangerous
PREGNANCY AND LACTATION: Pregnancy category C; excretion into breast milk unknown
SIDE EFFECTS/ADVERSE REACTIONS
CNS: Depression, *dizziness, drowsiness,* fatigue, *headache,* paresthesia, syncope (especially 1st days of therapy), vertigo, weakness
CV: Edema, hypotension, palpitations, *postural hypotension*

EENT: Blurred vision, dry mouth, epistaxis, *nasal congestion,* red sclera, *sinusitis,* tinnitus
GI: Nausea
GU: Impotence, incontinence, urinary frequency
RESP: Dyspnea
MISC: Weight gain
DRUG INTERACTIONS
Drugs
▪ *Angiotensin-converting enzyme inhibitors (enalapril):* Potential for exaggerated first dose hypotensive episode when α-blockers added
▪ *Nonsteroidal antiinflammatory drugs (ibuprofen, indomethacin):* NSAIDs may inhibit antihypertensive effects
▪ *Propranolol:* Potential for exaggerated first dose hypotensive episode when α-blockers added

SPECIAL CONSIDERATIONS
• Marked lowering of BP with postural hypotension and syncope can occur ("1st-dose" effect), especially during 1st week of therapy and after increases in dose; incidence of postural hypotension 4%-5%
• Does not affect plasma PSA levels
• Prazosin may be equally effective but less expensive
PATIENT/FAMILY EDUCATION
• Always begin treatment at bedtime

---

ticlopidine
(tye-klo′pa-deen)
Rx: Ticlid
Chemical Class: Thienpyridine derivative
Therapeutic Class: Antiplatelet agent

CLINICAL PHARMACOLOGY
Mechanism of Action: Interferes with platelet membrane function by inhibiting adenosine diphosphate-induced platelet-fibrinogen binding and subsequent platelet-platelet interactions; time- and dose-dependent inhibition of platelet aggregation and release of platelet granule constituents; prolongation of bleeding time; effects on platelet function irreversible for the life of the platelet
Pharmacokinetics
PO: Peak 2 hr, rapidly absorbed (decreased 20% by meals); 98% bound to plasma proteins; extensively hepatically metabolized, excreted in urine (60%) and feces (23%); nonlinear (clearance decreases on repeated dosing); $t_{1/2}$ after a single 250 mg dose, 12.6 hr; with repeat dosing at 250 mg bid, $t_{1/2}$ rises to 4-5 days (steady state levels after approximately 14-21 days)
INDICATIONS AND USES: Reducing the risk of thrombotic stroke in aspirin intolerant patients or aspirin failures; prevention of thrombosis following intracoronary stent placement*
DOSAGE
Adult
• PO 250 mg bid with food
Ⓢ **AVAILABLE FORMS/COST OF THERAPY**
• Tab, Uncoated—Oral: 250 mg, 60's: **$91.32**
CONTRAINDICATIONS: Current blood dyscrasia (neutropenia, thrombocytopenia); hemostatic disorder or active pathologic bleeding (such as bleeding peptic ulcer or intracranial bleeding); patients with severe liver impairment
PRECAUTIONS: Past liver disease, renal disease, elderly, children, increased bleeding risk (trauma, surgery, or pathologic conditions, dental procedures)
PREGNANCY AND LACTATION: Pregnancy category B

---

* = non FDA-approved use

SIDE EFFECTS/ADVERSE REACTIONS

GI (40% have GI effects): Cholestatic jaundice, *diarrhea, GI discomfort,* hepatitis, increased cholesterol, LDL, VLDL, *nausea, vomiting*

HEME: **Agranulocytosis,** bleeding (epistaxis, hematuria, conjunctival hemorrhage, GI bleeding), **neutropenia, thrombocytopenia**

SKIN: Pruritus, rash

DRUG INTERACTIONS

Drugs

🔢 *Cyclosporine:* Potential for reduction in blood cyclosporine concentrations

🔢 *Phenytoin:* Potential for development of phenytoin toxicity, reduction in phenytoin dose may be necessary

🔢 *Theophylline:* Increased theophylline level via inhibition of metabolism, increased risk of toxicity

SPECIAL CONSIDERATIONS

• Due to the risk of life-threatening neutropenia or agranulocytosis and cost, ticlopidine should be reserved for patients intolerant to aspirin or who fail aspirin

MONITORING PARAMETERS

• CBC q2wk for 1st 3 mo of therapy, then periodically thereafter

---

timolol

(tim′oh-loll)

Rx: Oral: Blocadren,
Ophthalmic: Betimol, Timoptic, Timoptic-XE
Combinations
 Rx: with hydrochlorothiazide (Timolide 10-25)
Chemical Class: Nonselective, β-adrenergic blocker
Therapeutic Class: Antihypertensive; antiglaucoma agent

CLINICAL PHARMACOLOGY

Mechanism of Action: Ophth reduces intraocular pressure via reduction in production of aqueous humor; PO nonselective β-adrenergic receptor blocking agent, no significant intrinsic sympathomimetic, direct myocardial depressant, or local anesthetic activity, decreases positive chronotropic, positive inotropic, bronchodilator, and vasodilator responses to β-adrenergic receptor agonists

Pharmacokinetics

OPHTH: Onset 15-30 min, peak 1-2 hr, duration 24 hr

PO: Peak 2 hr

Rapidly and completely absorbed; excreted 30%-45% unchanged, 60%-65% metabolized by liver; $t_{1/2}$ 4 hr

INDICATIONS AND USES: OPHTH: ocular hypertension, chronic open-angle glaucoma; PO: hypertension, post-MI mortality reduction, migraine headache prophylaxis, sinus tachycardia,* persistent atrial extrasystoles,* tachydysrhythmias,* prophylaxis of angina pectoris*

DOSAGE

Adult

• *OPHTH* 1 gtt 0.25% sol in affected eye(s) bid, then 1 gtt qd for maintenance, may increase to 1 gtt 0.5% sol bid if needed

• *Hypertension:* PO 10 mg bid initially, usually maintenance 20-40 mg/day divided bid, not to exceed 60 mg/day

• *Post-MI prophylaxis:* PO 10 mg bid

• *Migraine:* 10 mg bid, up to 30 mg/day divided bid

💲 **AVAILABLE FORMS/COST OF THERAPY**

• Sol—Ophth: 0.25%, 2.5, 5, 10, 15 ml: **$21.87-$24.06**/10 ml; 0.5%, 2.5, 5, 10, 15 ml: **$25.94-$28.58**/10 ml

• Gel—Ophth: 0.25%, 2.5, 5, 7.5 ml: **$18.09**/5 ml; 0.5%, 2.5, 5, 7.5 ml: **$21.49**/5 ml

Tab, Uncoated—Oral: 5 mg, 100's: **$20.22-$42.74;** 10 mg, 100's: **$27.87-$57.26;** 20 mg, 100's: **$54.00-$97.48**

CONTRAINDICATIONS: Asthma, 2nd or 3rd degree heart block, sinus bradycardia, overt heart failure, congenital glaucoma (infants), severe COPD

PRECAUTIONS: Nonallergic bronchospasm, diabetes mellitus, pregnancy, children, myasthenia gravis

PREGNANCY AND LACTATION: Pregnancy category C; excreted into breast milk

SIDE EFFECTS/ADVERSE REACTIONS

CNS: Anxiety, confusion, depression, *dizziness,* fatigue, hallucinations, headache, insomnia, weakness

CV: Bradycardia, claudication, **CHF, dysrhythmias,** edema, **heart block, hypotension, syncope**

EENT: Conjunctivitis, *double vision,* dry burning eyes, eye irritation, keratitis, sore throat, *visual changes*

GI: Abdominal pain, anorexia, diarrhea, dyspepsia, **ischemic colitis, mesenteric arterial thrombosis,** nausea

GU: Frequency, impotence

HEME: **Agranulocytosis, purpura, thrombocytopenia**

METAB: Hyperglycemia, mask hypoglycemia

MS: Joint pain

RESP: **Bronchospasm,** cough, dyspnea, rales

SKIN: Alopecia, fever, pruritus, rash, urticaria

DRUG INTERACTIONS

Drugs

🔢 *Amiodarone:* Combined therapy may lead to bradycardia, cardiac arrest, or ventricular dysrhythmia

🔢 *Antidiabetics:* β-blockers increase blood glucose and impair peripheral circulation; altered response to hypoglycemia by prolonging the recovery of normoglycemia, causing hypertension, and blocking tachycardia

🔢 *Calcium channel blockers:* Additive hypotension (kinetic and dynamic)

🔢 *Clonidine:* Hypertension occurring upon withdrawal of clonidine may be exacerbated by timolol

🔢 *Disopyramide:* Additive negative inotropic cardiac effects

Epinephrine: Enhanced pressor response (hypertension and bradycardia)

🔢 *Isoproterenol:* Reduced isoproterenol efficacy in asthma

🔢 *Methyldopa:* Potential for development of hypertension in the presence of increased catecholamines

🔢 *Nonsteroidal antiinflammatory drugs:* Reduced antihypertensive effects of timolol

🔢 *Phenylephrine:* Potential for hypertensive episodes when administered together

🔢 *Prazosin:* First-dose response to prazosin may be enhanced by β-blockade

🔢 *Quinidine:* Increased timolol concentrations

🔢 *Tacrine:* Additive bradycardia

🔢 *Theophylline:* Antagonistic pharmacodynamic effects

SPECIAL CONSIDERATIONS

• Currently available β-blockers appear to be equally effective; cardioselective or combined α- and β-adrenergic blockade are less likely to cause undesirable effects and may be preferred

PATIENT/FAMILY EDUCATION

• Do not discontinue abruptly, taper over 2 wk; may precipitate angina

---

italic = common side effects

bold italic = life-threatening reactions

tirofiban hydrochloride
(ty-row-fye'-ban hy-dro-klor'-ide)
Rx: Aggrastat
Chemical Class: Platelet glycoprotein IIb/IIIa receptor antagonist
Therapeutic Class: Antiplatelet

CLINICAL PHARMACOLOGY
Mechanism of Action: Reversibly antagonizes fibrinogen binding to GP IIb/IIIa receptor, a platelet surface receptor, thus inhibiting platelet aggregation
Pharmacokinetics
IV: Greater than 90% inhibition is attained by end of 30-min infusion; $t_{1/2}$ ~2 hr; cleared by renal excretion 65%, 25% in feces; metabolism is limited; not highly bound to plasma protein
INDICATIONS AND USES: In combination with heparin, indicated for treatment of acute coronary syndrome, including those patients who are to be managed medically and those undergoing PTCA or artherectomy
DOSAGE
Adult
• *Aggrastat injection:* must first be diluted to same strength as Aggrastat Injection Premixed.
• *IV:* initial rate of 0.4 μg/kg/min for 30 min and then continued at 0.1 μg/kg/min. Patients with severe renal insufficiency (creatinine clearance <30 ml/min) should receive half usual rate of infusion. Infusion should be continued through angiography and for 12 to 24 hr after angioplasty or atherectomy
⑤ AVAILABLE FORMS/COST OF THERAPY
• IV: Injection for solution 250 μg/ml: **$420.00;** injection premixed containing tirofiban hydrochloride 50 μg/ml: **$700.00**
CONTRAINDICATIONS: Hypersensitivity to any component of product; active internal bleeding or history of bleeding diathesis within previous 30 days; history of intracranial hemorrhage, intracranial neoplasm, arteriovenous malformation or aneurysm; history of thrombocytopenia following prior exposure to tirofiban; history of stroke within 30 days or any history of hemorrhagic stroke; major surgical procedure or severe physical trauma within 30 days; history, symptoms, or findings suggestive of aortic dissection; severe hypertension (systolic blood pressure >180 mmHg or diastolic blood pressure >110 mmHg); concomitant use of another parenteral GP IIb/IIIa inhibitor; acute pericarditis
PRECAUTIONS: Bleeding precautions; minimize use of IM injections, urinary catheters, nasotracheal intubation, arterial and venous punctures, and nasogastric tubes due to risk of bleeding; severe renal insufficiency; platelet count <150,000/mm³
PREGNANCY AND LACTATION: Pregnancy category B; has been shown to cross placenta in animals; no harm to animal fetus in studies; should not be used in nursing mothers; may be present in human milk
SIDE EFFECTS/ADVERSE REACTIONS
CNS: Dizziness, headache
CV: Bradycardia, *dissection, coronary artery*
GI: Nausea
GU: Pelvic pain
HEME: **Bleeding, intracranial bleeding, thrombocytopenia**
MS: Leg pain
SKIN: Sweating
MISC: Edema, swelling, vasovagal reaction, fever
DRUG INTERACTIONS
Drugs
❷ *Anticoagulants:* Increase in bleeding time, use caution
❷ *Aspirin:* Increase in bleeding time, use caution
❷ *Clopidogrel:* Increase in bleeding time, use caution
❷ *Dipyridamole:* Increase in bleeding time, use caution

❷ *Heparin:* Increase in bleeding time, use caution
❷ *Levothyroxine:* Increase in tirofiban clearance, clinical significance is unknown
❷ *NSAIDs:* Increase in bleeding time, use caution
❷ *Omeprazole:* Increase in tirofiban clearance, clinical significance is unknown
❷ *Ticlopidine:* Increase in bleeding time, use caution

SPECIAL CONSIDERATIONS
• Shown to decrease rate of combined end point of death, new MI, or refractory ischemia/repeat cardiac procedure
• Special care of femoral artery access site is required
MONITORING PARAMETERS
• Bleeding is most common drug-related adverse effect reported. Monitor platelet counts, Hgb, Hct before treatment, within 6 hr after loading infusion, and at least daily thereafter during therapy; if thrombocytopenia develops, discontinue tirofiban and heparin

tocainide
(toe-kay'nide)
Rx: Tonocard
Chemical Class: Lidocaine derivative
Therapeutic Class: Antidysrhythmic (Class IB)

CLINICAL PHARMACOLOGY
Mechanism of Action: Decreases sodium and potassium, resulting in decreased excitability of myocardial cells
Pharmacokinetics
PO: Peak ½-2 hr; oral bioavailability 100%; metabolized by liver (negligible 1st-pass metabolism), excreted in urine; $t_{1/2}$ 10-17 hr
INDICATIONS AND USES: Life-threatening ventricular dysrhythmias (i.e., sustained ventricular tachycardia)
DOSAGE
Adult
• PO initial 400 mg q8h; usual maintenance dose 1200 to 1800 mg/day divided tid
⑤ AVAILABLE FORMS/COST OF THERAPY
• Tab, Plain Coated—Oral: 400 mg, 100's: **$80.42;** 600 mg, 100's: **$102.50**
CONTRAINDICATIONS: Hypersensitivity to amides, severe heart block (2nd or 3rd degree)
PRECAUTIONS: Children, renal disease, liver disease, CHF, respiratory depression, myasthenia gravis, blood dyscrasias
PREGNANCY AND LACTATION: Pregnancy category C
SIDE EFFECTS/ADVERSE REACTIONS
CNS: Confusion, dizziness, headache, involuntary movement, irritability, paresthesias, psychosis, restlessness, *seizures,* tremors
CV: Angina, bradycardia, *cardiovascular collapse,* chest pain, *CHF, heart block,* hypotension, *prodysrhythmic effect,* PVCs, tachycardia
EENT: Blurred vision, hearing loss, tinnitus
GI: Anorexia, diarrhea, hepatitis, nausea, vomiting
HEME: **Agranulocytosis, blood dyscrasias, hypoplastic anemia, leukopenia, thrombocytopenia**
MS: Lupus-like illness, positive ANA
SKIN: Edema, rash, swelling, urticaria
DRUG INTERACTIONS
Drugs
❶ *Antacids:* Antacids which increase urinary pH may increase tocainide serum concentrations
❶ *Rifampin:* Reduction of serum tocainide concentrations

SPECIAL CONSIDERATIONS
• Can be considered oral lidocaine; antidysrhythmic drugs have not been shown to improve survival in patients with ventricular

---

* = non FDA-approved use

dysrhythmias; class I antidysrhythmic drugs (e.g., tocainide) have increased the risk of death when used in patients with non-life-threatening dysrhythmias

MONITORING PARAMETERS
• Blood concentrations (therapeutic concentrations 4-10 μg/ml)

---

tolazoline
(toe-laz′a-leen)
Rx: Priscoline
Chemical Class: Imidoline derivative
Therapeutic Class: Peripheral vasodilator

CLINICAL PHARMACOLOGY
Mechanism of Action: Peripheral vasodilation occurs by direct relaxation of vascular smooth muscle; also has weak α-adrenergic blocking properties
Pharmacokinetics
IM/SC: Peak 30-60 min, duration 3-4 hr; excreted in urine; $t_{1/2}$ 3-10 hr
INDICATIONS AND USES: Persistent pulmonary hypertension of newborn; hypoxic pulmonary hypertension,* arterial trauma,* clonidine overdose,* cor pulmonale,* lumbar puncture headache,* peripheral vascular disease,* spasmodic torticollis*
DOSAGE
Newborn
• IV 1-2 mg/kg via scalp vein followed by IV INF 1-2 mg/kg/hr
⑤ AVAILABLE FORMS/COST OF THERAPY
• Inj, Repository—IV: 25 mg/ml, 4 ml: **$12.95**
PRECAUTIONS: Active peptic ulcer, mitral stenosis
PREGNANCY AND LACTATION: Pregnancy category C
SIDE EFFECTS/ADVERSE REACTIONS
CV: ***Cardiovascular collapse, dysrhythmias,*** edema, hypertension, *orthostatic hypotension,* tachycardia
GI: Diarrhea, ***GI hemorrhage,*** hepatitis, nausea, peptic ulcer, vomiting
GU: Hematuria, oliguria
HEME: ***Leukopenia, thrombocytopenia***
RESP: ***Pulmonary hemorrhage***
SKIN: Chills, *flushing,* increased pilomotor activity, rash, sweating, tingling
DRUG INTERACTIONS
Drugs
▣ Epinephrine, norepinephrine, phenylephrine: Decrease blood pressure response; rebound hypertension

---

torsemide
(tor′se-mide)
Rx: Demadex
Chemical Class: Pyridine-sulfonamide derivative
Therapeutic Class: Loop diuretic

CLINICAL PHARMACOLOGY
Mechanism of Action: Inhibits the $Na^+/K^+/Cl^-$ carrier system in the thick ascending portion of the loop of Henle where it increases urinary excretion of Na, Cl, and water, but does not significantly alter glomerular filtration rate, renal plasma flow, or acid-base balance
Pharmacokinetics
IV: Onset 10 min, peak 1 hr
PO: Onset 1 hr, peak 1-2 hr
Bioavailability 80%; minimal 1st-pass metabolism; volume of distribution 12-15 L (doubled in CHF, renal failure); cleared via hepatic metabolism (80%) and renal excretion (20%); $t_{1/2}$ 3½ hr
INDICATIONS AND USES: Edema associated with CHF, hepatic cirrhosis and chronic renal failure; hypertension
DOSAGE
Adult
NOTE: Because of high bioavailability, IV and PO doses are interchangeable
• *CHF, chronic renal failure:* PO/IV 10-20 mg qd, titrate upward to response (usually doubling) to max 200 mg/day
• *Cirrhosis:* PO/IV 5-10 mg qd (usually with aldosterone antagonist or potassium-sparing diuretic), titrate upward to response (usually by doubling) to max 40 mg/day
• *Hypertension:* 5-10 mg qd
⑤ AVAILABLE FORMS/COST OF THERAPY
• Inj, Sol—IV: 10 mg/ml, 2 ml: **$3.85**
• Tab, Uncoated—Oral: 5 mg, 100's: $48.56; 10 mg, 100's: **$53.81;** 20 mg, 100's: **$62.86;** 100 mg, 100's: **$233.04**
CONTRAINDICATIONS: Anuria
PRECAUTIONS: Dehydration, hepatic cirrhosis and ascites, impaired renal function, electrolyte imbalance
PREGNANCY AND LACTATION: Pregnancy category B
SIDE EFFECTS/ADVERSE REACTIONS
CNS: Asthenia, dizziness, *headache (7%),* insomnia, nervousness
CV: Atrial fibrillation, chest pain, ***ventricular tachycardia***
GI: Constipation, diarrhea, dyspepsia, edema
METAB: Hypocalcemia, hypokalemia, hypomagnesemia, increases in BUN, creatinine, uric acid, glucose, total cholesterol
MS: Arthralgia, myalgia
RESP: Cough, rhinitis
SKIN: Rash
DRUG INTERACTIONS
Drugs
▣ *ACE inhibitors:* Initiation of ACE inhibitor in the presence of intensive diuretic therapy may result in precipitous fall in blood pressure; ACE inhibitors may induce renal insufficiency in the presence of diuretic-induced sodium depletion
▣ *Bile acid-binding resins:* Reduced bioavailability and diuretic response of torsemide
▣ *Digitalis glycosides:* Diuretic-induced hypokalemia may increase risk of digitalis toxicity
▣ *Fluoxetine:* Case reports of sudden death in 2 patients taking fluoxetine and a similar drug, furosemide; causal relationship not established
▣ *NSAIDs:* Reduced diuretic and antihypertensive efficacy of torsemide

SPECIAL CONSIDERATIONS
• Offers potential advantages over other loop diuretics, including a longer duration of action and fewer adverse electrolyte and metabolic effects; available data not extensive or convincing enough at present to recommend replacement of standard loop diuretic (furosemide); considered alternative in refractory patients

---

italic = common side effects

bold italic = life-threatening reactions

trandolapril
(tran-dole'a-pril)
Rx: Mavik
Combinations
   Rx: with verapamil (Tarka)
Chemical Class: Angiotensin-converting enzyme (ACE) inhibitor
Therapeutic Class: Antihypertensive

CLINICAL PHARMACOLOGY
Mechanism of Action: Selectively suppresses renin-angiotensin-aldosterone system; inhibits ACE, preventing the conversion of angiotensin I to angiotensin II; results in dilation of arterial, venous vessels
Pharmacokinetics
PO: Trandolapril is a prodrug that is deesterified in the liver to its active metabolite, trandolaprilat; peak 1 hr (4-10 hr trandolaprilat); 80% bound to plasma proteins; eliminated in urine (30%) and feces (66%); $t_{1/2}$ of trandolaprilat 10 hr
INDICATIONS AND USES: Hypertension, CHF,* diabetic nephropathy*
DOSAGE
Adult
• PO 1 mg qd (non-black patients) or 2 mg qd (black patients); increase at 1-wk intervals as needed to maximum dose of 8 mg/day (doses >4 mg/day may be divided bid); in renal impairment (CrCl <30 ml/min), hepatic impairment, or in patients receiving diuretics, initiate therapy with 0.5 mg qd
$ AVAILABLE FORMS/COST OF THERAPY
• Tab—Oral: 1 mg, 2 mg, 4 mg, 100's: **$60.00**
CONTRAINDICATIONS: History of angioedema with previous ACE inhibitor therapy
PRECAUTIONS: Impaired renal or hepatic function, hypovolemia, diuretic therapy, collagen-vascular diseases, CHF, elderly, bilateral renal artery stenosis
PREGNANCY AND LACTATION: Pregnancy category C (1st trimester), category D (2nd and 3rd trimesters); ACE inhibitors can cause fetal and neonatal morbidity and death when administered to pregnant women; when pregnancy is detected, discontinue ACE inhibitors as soon as possible
SIDE EFFECTS/ADVERSE REACTIONS
CNS: Anxiety, *dizziness, fatigue, headache,* insomnia, paresthesia
CV: Angina, hypotension, palpitations, postural hypotension, syncope (especially with 1st dose)
GI: Abdominal pain, constipation, melena, nausea, vomiting
GU: Decreased libido, impotence, increased BUN, creatinine; urinary tract infection
HEME: **Agranulocytosis, neutropenia**
METAB: Hyperkalemia, hyponatremia
MS: Arthralgia, arthritis, myalgia
RESP: Asthma, bronchitis, *cough,* dyspnea, sinusitis
SKIN: Angioedema, flushing, rash, sweating
DRUG INTERACTIONS
Drugs
■ *Lithium:* Increased risk of serious lithium toxicity
■ *Loop diuretics:* Initiation of ACE inhibitor therapy in the presence of intensive diuretic therapy results in a precipitous fall in blood pressure in some patients; ACE inhibitors may induce renal insufficiency in the presence of diuretic-induced sodium depletion
■ *NSAIDs:* Inhibition of the antihypertensive response to ACE inhibitors
■ *Potassium-sparing diuretics:* Increased risk for hyperkalemia

SPECIAL CONSIDERATIONS
• No clear-cut advantage over other ACE inhibitors; choice should be made on cost and availability
PATIENT/FAMILY EDUCATION
• Do not use salt substitutes containing potassium without consulting clinician
• Persistent dry cough may occur and usually does not subside unless medication is stopped; notify clinician if this effect occurs
MONITORING PARAMETERS
• BUN, creatinine (watch for increased levels that may indicate acute renal failure); potassium levels, although hyperkalemia rarely occurs

tranylcypromine
(tran-ill-sip'roe-meen)
Rx: Parnate
Chemical Class: Nonhydrazine
Therapeutic Class: Monoamine oxidase inhibitor (MAOI) antidepressant

CLINICAL PHARMACOLOGY
Mechanism of Action: Increases concentrations of endogenous epinephrine, norepinephrine, serotonin, dopamine in storage sites in CNS by inhibition of monoamine oxidase
Pharmacokinetics
PO: Onset 10 days, well absorbed; metabolized by liver, excreted by kidneys (within 24 hr); monoamine oxidase activity is recovered in 3-5 days (possibly up to 10 days) after withdrawal
INDICATIONS AND USES: Atypical depression; bulimia*; panic disorder with agoraphobia*
DOSAGE
Adult
• PO 10 mg bid; may increase to 30 mg/day after 2 wk; max 60 mg/day
$ AVAILABLE FORMS/COST OF THERAPY
• Tab, Plain Coated—Oral: 10 mg, 100's: **$50.25**
CONTRAINDICATIONS: Hypertension, CHF, severe hepatic disease, pheochromocytoma, severe renal disease, severe cardiac disease, cerebrovascular defects
PRECAUTIONS: Suicidal patients, convulsive disorders, severe depression, schizophrenia, hyperactivity, diabetes mellitus
PREGNANCY AND LACTATION: Pregnancy category C
SIDE EFFECTS/ADVERSE REACTIONS
CNS: Anxiety, confusion, *dizziness, drowsiness,* fatigue, headache, hyperreflexia, insomnia, mania, stimulation, tremors, weakness, weight gain
CV: **Dysrhythmias,** *hypertension,* **hypertensive crisis,** *orthostatic hypotension*
EENT: Blurred vision
GI: *Anorexia,* constipation, diarrhea, dry mouth, nausea, vomiting, weight gain
GU: Change in libido, urinary frequency
HEME: Anemia
METAB: Syndrome of inappropriate antidiuretic hormone release-like syndrome
SKIN: Flushing, increased perspiration, rash
DRUG INTERACTIONS
Drugs
▲ *Amphetamines, ephedrine, metaraminol, phenylephrine, phenylpropanolamine, pseudoephedrine, tyramine-containing foods:* Severe hypertensive reactions
■ *Antidiabetics:* Prolonged hypoglycemia
■ *Barbiturates:* Prolonged effect of barbiturates

---

* = non FDA-approved use

▲ *Clomipramine, fluoxetine, fluvoxamine, paroxetine, sertraline:* Severe or fatal reactions, serotonin related
▲ *Ethanol:* Hypertensive response with alcoholic beverages containing tyramine
▪ *Guanethidine:* Inhibited antihypertensive response to guanethidine
▪ *Levodopa:* Hypertensive response; carbidopa minimizes the reaction
● *Lithium:* Hyperpyrexia with phenelzine
▲ *Meperidine:* Serotonin accumulation—agitation, blood pressure elevations, hyperpyrexia, seizures
▪ *Norepinephrine:* Increased pressor response to norepinephrine
▪ *Reserpine:* Severe hypertensive reactions
▲ *Sumatriptan:* Increased sumatriptan concentrations, possible toxicity

SPECIAL CONSIDERATIONS
• Irreversible nonselective MAOI effective for typical and atypical depression; equal efficacy to other MAOIs with quicker onset of action, and an amphetamine-like activity with a higher potential for abuse; no anticholinergic or cardiac effects
PATIENT/FAMILY EDUCATION
• Therapeutic effects may take 1-4 wk
• Avoid alcohol ingestion, CNS depressants, OTC medications (cold, weight loss, hay fever, cough syrup)
• Prodromal signs of hypertensive crisis are increased headache, palpitations; discontinue drug immediately
• Do not discontinue medication abruptly after long-term use
• Avoid high-tyramine foods (aged cheese, sour cream, beer, wine, pickled products, liver, raisins, bananas, figs, avocados, meat tenderizers, chocolate, yogurt)

---

triamterene
(trye-am′ter-een)
Rx: Dyrenium
Combinations
   Rx: with hydrochlorothiazide (Dyazide, Maxzide)
Chemical Class: Pteridine derivative
Therapeutic Class: Potassium-sparing diuretic

CLINICAL PHARMACOLOGY
Mechanism of Action: Inhibits reabsorption of sodium ions in exchange for potassium and hydrogen ions at the distal renal tubule; degree of natriuresis and diuresis produced by inhibition of the exchange mechanism is limited
Pharmacokinetics
PO: Onset 2-4 hr, peak 3 hr, duration 7-9 hr; primarily metabolized to sulfate conjugate of hydroxytriamterene (active), 21% excreted in urine unchanged; $t_{1/2}$ 1½-2 hr
INDICATIONS AND USES: Edema associated with CHF, cirrhosis of the liver, and the nephrotic syndrome; steroid-induced edema, idiopathic edema, and edema due to secondary hyperaldosteronism; may be used alone or with other diuretics either for its added diuretic effect or its potassium-conserving potential
DOSAGE
Adult
• PO 100 mg bid pc; do not exceed 300 mg/day; when combined with other diuretics or antihypertensives, decrease total daily dosage initially and adjust to patient's needs
Child
• PO 2-4 mg/kg/day in 1-2 divided doses; max 6 mg/kg/day or 300 mg/day

---

▪ **AVAILABLE FORMS/COST OF THERAPY**
• Cap, Gel—Oral: 50 mg, 100's: **$37.10**; 100 mg, 100's: **$46.60**
CONTRAINDICATIONS: Anuria, severe or progressive kidney disease or dysfunction (with possible exception of nephrosis), severe hepatic disease, preexisting elevated serum potassium, patients receiving spironolactone or amiloride
PRECAUTIONS: Diabetes, renal function impairment, hepatic function impairment, children, electrolyte imbalance, renal stones, predisposition to gouty arthritis
PREGNANCY AND LACTATION: Pregnancy category D (category B according to manufacturer); many investigators consider diuretics contraindicated in pregnancy, except for patients with heart disease; may decrease placental perfusion; excreted in cow's milk, no human data
SIDE EFFECTS/ADVERSE REACTIONS
CNS: Dizziness, headache
GI: Diarrhea, dry mouth, jaundice, liver enzyme abnormalities, *nausea,* vomiting
GU: Elevated BUN and creatinine, has been found in renal stones, ***interstitial nephritis***
HEME: Megaloblastic anemia, ***thrombocytopenia***
METAB: Electrolyte imbalance, hyperkalemia, hypokalemia
SKIN: Photosensitivity, rash
MISC: Fatigue, weakness
DRUG INTERACTIONS
Drugs
▪ *ACE inhibitors:* Hyperkalemia in predisposed patients
▪ *Amantadine:* Increased toxicity of amantadine
▪ *NSAIDs:* Acute renal failure with indomethacin and possibly other NSAIDs
● *Potassium:* Hyperkalemia in predisposed patients
Labs
• *False increase:* Serum digoxin concentrations
• *Interference:* Urinary catecholamines

SPECIAL CONSIDERATIONS
PATIENT/FAMILY EDUCATION
• Take with meals
• Avoid prolonged exposure to sunlight
• Take single daily doses in AM
MONITORING PARAMETERS
• ECG if hyperkalemia suspected
• Serum potassium, BUN, serum creatinine
• Liver function tests

---

urokinase
(yoor-oh-kine′ase)
Rx: Abbokinase, Abbokinase Open-Cath (not for systemic administration)
Chemical Class: Renal enzyme
Therapeutic Class: Thrombolytic

CLINICAL PHARMACOLOGY
Mechanism of Action: Promotes thrombolysis by directly converting plasminogen to plasmin
Pharmacokinetics: Onset of fibrinolysis is rapid, duration 4 hr; cleared by liver, small amount excreted in urine and bile; unknown if crosses placenta or if excreted in breast milk; $t_{1/2}$ 10-20 min
INDICATIONS AND USES: Venous thrombosis, pulmonary embolism, arterial thrombosis, arterial embolism, arteriovenous cannula occlusion, lysis of coronary artery thrombi after MI, thrombotic stroke*

---

italic = common side effects

bold italic = life-threatening reactions

DOSAGE

Adult and Child

• *Pulmonary embolism and arterial or venous thrombosis:* IV 4400 IU/kg over 10 min followed by 4400 IU/kg/hr for 12 hr; after thrombin time has decreased to less than twice normal control value (approx 3-4 hr), begin heparin (no loading dose)

• *Venous catheter occlusion:* Instill into catheter a volume of urokinase (5000 IU/ml) equal to the internal volume of catheter over 1-2 min; aspirate from catheter 1-4 hr later, flush catheter with saline, may repeat with 10,000 U/ml sol if not cleared

• *Coronary artery thrombosis (adult):* Intracoronary (following IV heparin bolus of 2500 to 10,000 units) 6000 IU/min for up to 2 hr (average dose 500,000 IU); repeat angiography q15min until artery maximally opened; continuing heparin therapy recommended

⑤ AVAILABLE FORMS/COST OF THERAPY

• Inj, Lyphl-Sol—IV: 5000 U/ml, 1 ml: **$56.26** (not for systemic administration); 9000 U/vial: **$98.13** (not for systemic administration); 250,000 U/vial: **$433.31**

CONTRAINDICATIONS: (Systemic therapy only, no contraindications to use for declotting catheter); active bleeding, intraspinal surgery, CNS neoplasms; ulcerative colitis, enteritis; coagulation defects, rheumatic valvular disease; cerebral embolism, thrombosis, hemorrhage within 2 mo; intraarterial diagnostic procedure, surgery, or trauma within 10 days; severe hypertension

PRECAUTIONS: Moderate hypertension, recent lumbar puncture, patients receiving IM medications, renal disease, hepatic disease, childbirth within 10 days, diabetic retinopathy, age >75 yr

PREGNANCY AND LACTATION: Pregnancy category B; no data available on breast feeding

SIDE EFFECTS/ADVERSE REACTIONS

CV: **MI,** tachycardia, transient hypertension or hypotension
GI: Nausea, vomiting
HEME: **Internal bleeding (GI, GU, vaginal, IM, retroperitoneal or intracranial sites),** surface bleeding
METAB: Acidosis
RESP: **Bronchospasm,** dyspnea, hypoxemia
SKIN: Rash
MISC: Chills, fever

DRUG INTERACTIONS

Drugs

🖪 *Anticoagulants and antiplatelet agents:* Bleeding complications

SPECIAL CONSIDERATIONS

MONITORING PARAMETERS

• Before therapy check coagulation tests such as PT, aPTT, thrombin time, fibrinogen, and fibrin degradation products, Hct, platelet count, bleeding time (some sources recommend not administering urokinase if 15 min)

• Proceed with therapy before results known in therapy for acute coronary artery occlusion

• During therapy, continue to monitor coagulation tests and/or tests of fibrinolytic activity; results do not reliably predict efficacy or risk of bleeding

• Treat bleeding with cryoprecipitate or fresh frozen plasma

---

valsartan ·
(val-sar'tan)
Rx: Diovan
Chemical Class: Angiotensin II receptor antagonist
Therapeutic Class: Antihypertensive

CLINICAL PHARMACOLOGY

Mechanism of Action: Vasoconstrictor and aldosterone-secreting effects of angiotensin II selectively blocked at the angiotensin (AT_1) receptor in vascular smooth muscle and adrenal gland; independent of angiotensin II synthesis

Pharmacokinetics

PO: Peak 2-4 hr, duration 24 hr; steady state maximal reduction in blood pressure 2-4 wk; bioavailability approx 25%; food decreases exposure significantly; elimination as unchanged drug in feces (83%) and urine (13%); $t_{1/2}$ 6 hr

INDICATIONS AND USES: Hypertension; CHF*

DOSAGE

Adult

• *Hypertension:* PO 80-320 mg qd

⑤ AVAILABLE FORMS/COST OF THERAPY

• Caps—Oral: 80 mg, 100's: **$114.00**; 160 mg, 100's: **$114.00**

PRECAUTIONS: Renal insufficiency, hepatic insufficiency

PREGNANCY AND LACTATION: Pregnancy category C (1st trimester); category D (2nd and 3rd trimesters)

SIDE EFFECTS/ADVERSE REACTIONS

CNS: Dizziness, headaches
CV: Palpitations
GI: Abdominal pain, constipation, diarrhea, dyspepsia, flatulence, liver function test abnormalities
GU: Impotence
METAB: Hyperkalemia
MS: Back pain, muscle cramps, myalgia
RESP: Cough, dyspnea, pharyngitis, rhinitis, sinusitis
SKIN: Pruritus and rash
MISC: Anemia, fatigue

SPECIAL CONSIDERATIONS

• Second angiotensin II antihypertensive agent to market

---

verapamil
(ver-ap'a-mill)
Rx: Calan, Calan SR, Covera HS, Isoptin, Isoptin SR, Verelan
Combinations
Rx: with trandolapril (Tarka)
Chemical Class: Phenylalkylamine; calcium channel blocker
Therapeutic Class: Antihypertensive; antianginal; antidysrhythmic (Class IV)

CLINICAL PHARMACOLOGY

Mechanism of Action: Inhibits calcium ion influx across cell membrane during cardiac depolarization; produces relaxation of coronary vascular smooth muscle; dilates coronary arteries; decreases SA and AV node conduction; dilates peripheral arteries

Pharmacokinetics

IV: Onset 3 min, peak 3-5 min, duration 10-20 min
PO: Onset variable (30 min for non-sustained-release preparations), peak 1-2.2 hr, duration 17-24 hr, 90% absorption; extensive 1st-pass metabolism; bioavailability 20%-35%; 83%-90% protein bound; metabolized by liver to norverapamil (20% activity of verapamil), excreted in urine (96% as metabolites); $t_{1/2}$ (biphasic) 4 min, 3-7 hr (terminal)

---

* = non FDA-approved use

INDICATIONS AND USES: Chronic stable angina pectoris, vasospastic angina, unstable angina, dysrhythmias (atrial flutter, atrial fibrillation, paroxysmal supraventricular tachycardia [PSVT]), hypertension, prophylaxis of migraine headaches*
DOSAGE
Adult
• *Angina:* PO initial 80-120 mg tid; titrate to 480 mg/day based on response (adjust dose weekly)
• *Dysrhythmias (atrial fibrillation/digitalized):* PO 240-320 mg/day in tid or qid dosage
• *Dysrhythmias (supraventricular tachycardia):* IV bolus initial 5-10 mg over 2 min; repeat dose 10 mg, 30 min after 1st if ineffective
• *Hypertension:* PO 80 mg bid initially, increase as need to 480 mg/d divided bid; SUS REL 180-240 mg qd initially, increase as need up to 360 mg/day
Child 0-1 yr
• *Dysrhythmias (PSVT):* IV bolus 0.1-0.2 mg/kg over >2 min with ECG monitoring; repeat if necessary in 30 min
Child 1-15 yr
• *Dysrhythmias (PSVT):* IV bolus 0.1-0.3 mg/kg over >2 min; repeat in 30 min; not to exceed 10 mg in a single dose
$ AVAILABLE FORMS/COST OF THERAPY
• Inj, Sol—IV: 2.5 mg/ml, 2 ml: **$2.35-$12.99**
• Tab, Coated, SUS REL—Oral: 180 mg, 100's: **$38.25-$118.50;** 240 mg, 100's: **$38.25-$146.40;** 360 mg, 100's: **$190.00**
• Tab, Plain Coated—Oral: 40 mg, 100's: **$21.45-$33.17;** 80 mg, 100's: **$5.18-$47.72;** 120 mg, 100's: **$8.25-$64.52**
CONTRAINDICATIONS: Sick sinus syndrome, 2nd or 3rd degree heart block, hypotension less than 90 mm Hg systolic, cardiogenic shock, severe CHF
PRECAUTIONS: CHF, hypotension, hepatic injury, children, renal disease, concomitant IV β-blocker therapy, cirrhosis, Duchenne's muscular dystrophy
PREGNANCY AND LACTATION: Pregnancy category C; excreted in breast milk (approx 25% of maternal serum); compatible with breast feeding
SIDE EFFECTS/ADVERSE REACTIONS
CNS: Asthenia, dizziness, headache, lightheadedness
CV: **AV block,** bradycardia, **CHF,** edema, hypotension, palpitations
GI: Constipation, nausea
GU: Nocturia, polyuria
SKIN: Rash
DRUG INTERACTIONS
Drugs
▪ *Amiodarone:* Cardiotoxicity with bradycardia and decreased cardiac output
▪ *Barbiturates:* Reduced plasma concentrations of verapamil
▪ *Benzodiazepines:* Marked increase in midazolam concentrations, increased sedation likely to result
▪ *β-blockers:* β-blocker serum concentrations increased (atenolol, metoprolol, propranolol); increased risk of bradycardia or hypotension
▪ *Calcium:* Inhibited activity of verapamil
❷ *Carbamazepine:* Increased carbamazepine toxicity when verapamil added to chronic anticonvulsant regimens; reduced metabolism
▪ *Cimetidine:* Increased verapamil concentrations and effect by cimetidine
▪ *Cyclosporine, tacrolimus:* Increased concentrations of these drugs, nephrotoxicity possible
▪ *Diclofenac:* Reduced verapamil concentrations
▪ *Digitalis glycosides:* Increased digoxin concentrations by approximately 70%

▪ *Doxazosin, prazosin, terazosin:* Enhanced hypotensive effects
▪ *Doxorubicin:* Increased doxorubicin concentrations
▪ *Encainide:* Increased encainide concentrations
▪ *Ethanol:* Increased ethanol concentrations, prolonged and increased levels of intoxication
▪ *Imipramine:* Increased imipramine concentrations
▪ *Lithium:* Potential for neurotoxicity
▪ *Neuromuscular blocking agents:* Prolonged neuromuscular blockade
▪ *Quinidine:* Quinidine toxicity via inhibition of metabolism
▪ *Rifampin, rifabutin:* Induced metabolism; reduced verapamil concentrations
▪ *Theophylline:* Verapamil inhibits metabolism, increases theophylline levels

SPECIAL CONSIDERATIONS
• Dihydropyridine calcium channel blockers preferred over verapamil and diltiazem in patients with sinus bradycardia, conduction disturbances, and for combination with a β-blocker
• Differentiate PSVT from narrow complex ventricular tachycardia before IV administration; failure to do so has resulted in fatalities

warfarin
(war'far-in)
Rx: Coumadin, Warfilone
Chemical Class: Coumarin derivative
Therapeutic Class: Oral anticoagulant

CLINICAL PHARMACOLOGY
Mechanism of Action: Interferes with synthesis of vitamin K–dependent coagulation factors, causing sequential depression of factors VII, IX, X, and II activity in a dose-dependent manner; has no direct effect on established thrombus, but prevents further extension of formed clot
Pharmacokinetics
PO: Rapidly and completely absorbed, peak activity 1½-3 days, duration 2-5 days; 97%-99% bound to plasma proteins; metabolized by hepatic microsomal enzymes, excreted in urine and feces (inactive metabolites); $t_{1/2}$ 36 hr
INDICATIONS AND USES: Prophylaxis and treatment of venous thrombosis, pulmonary embolism, atrial fibrillation with embolism, thromboembolic complications associated with cardiac valve replacement and death, recurrent MI, and systemic embolism after MI; recurrent transient ischemic attack,* hypercoagulable states*
DOSAGE
Adult
• PO initiate with 5 mg qd for 2-4 days; adjust dosage according to INR determinations; make dose adjustments in 5%-20% increments based on weekly dose of warfarin usual maintenance dose 2-10 mg qd based on INR determinations
Child
• PO 0.1 mg/kg/day with a range of 0.05-0.34 mg/kg/day; adjust dosage according to INR determinations; consistent anticoagulation may be difficult to maintain in children <5 yr
$ AVAILABLE FORMS/COSTS OF THERAPY
• Sol, Inj—IV; 5 mg, **$18.03**
• Tab, Uncoated—Oral: 1 mg, 100's: **$50.87-$54.42;** 2 mg, 100's: **$53.08-$56.82;** 2.5 mg, 100's: **$58.56-$75.76;** 3 mg, 100's: **$58.70;** 4 mg, 100's: **$55.13-$58.98;** 5 mg, 100's: **$55.51-$59.40;** 6 mg, 100's: **$87.48;** 7.5 mg, 100's: **$81.43-$87.82;** 10 mg, 100's: **$90.36**

italic = common side effects

bold italic = life-threatening reactions

CONTRAINDICATIONS: Active bleeding, hemorrhagic blood dyscrasias; hemorrhagic tendencies, history of bleeding diathesis, recent cerebral hemorrhage; active ulceration of the GI tract; ulcerative colitis; open traumatic or surgical wounds; recent or contemplated brain, eye, spinal cord surgery, or prostatectomy; regional or lumbar block anesthesia; bacterial endocarditis; pericarditis; visceral carcinoma; severe or malignant hypertension; eclampsia or preeclampsia; threatened abortion; emaciation; pregnancy; history of warfarin-induced necrosis

PRECAUTIONS: Trauma, infection, renal insufficiency, hypertension, vasculitis, indwelling catheters, severe diabetes, active tuberculosis, postpartum, protein C deficiency, hepatic insufficiency, elderly, children, hyperthyroidism, hypothyroidism, CHF, breastfeeding, polyarteritis, diverticulitis, antibiotic therapy, malnutrition

PREGNANCY AND LACTATION: Pregnancy category X; use in 1st trimester carries significant risk to the fetus; exposure in the 6th-9th wk of gestation may produce a pattern of defects termed the fetal warfarin syndrome with an incidence up to 25% in some series; compatible with breast feeding for normal, full-term infants

SIDE EFFECTS/ADVERSE REACTIONS

GI: Anorexia, cholestatic jaundice, **hepatotoxicity,** mouth ulcers, nausea, paralytic ileus, sore mouth, vomiting

GU: Albuminuria, anuria, red-orange urine, **renal tubular necrosis**

HEME: **Hemorrhage, leukopenia**

SKIN: Alopecia, dermatitis, **exfoliative dermatitis, necrosis or gangrene of skin and other tissues,** urticaria

MISC: Systemic cholesterol microembolization ("purple toes" syndrome)

DRUG INTERACTIONS

Drugs

 Acetaminophen: Repeated doses of acetaminophen may increase the hypoprothrombinemic response to warfarin

 Allopurinol, amiodarone, ciprofloxacin, clarithromycin, erythromycin, fluconazole, fluorouracil, flu-vastatin, fluvoxamine, glucagon, isoniazid, itraconazole, ketoconazole, lovastatin, miconazole, nalidixic acid, neomycin (oral), norfloxacin, ofloxacin, propafenone, propoxyphene, quinidine, sertraline, sulfonamides, sulfonylureas, thyroid hormones, triclofos, troleandomycin, vitamin E, zafirlukast: Enhanced hypoprothrombinemic response to warfarin

 Aminoglutethimide, carbamazepine, cyclophosphamide, ethchlorvynol, griseofulvin, mercaptopurine, methimazole, mitotane, nafcillin, propylthiouracil, vitamin K: Reduced hypoprothrombinemic response to warfarin

 Aspirin: Increased risk of bleeding complications

 Azathioprine, chloramphenicol, cimetidine, clofibrate, co-trimoxazole, danazole, dextrothyroxine, disulfiram, gemfibrozil, metronidazole, sulfinpyrazone, testosterone derivatives: Enhanced hypoprothrombinemic response to warfarin

 Barbiturates, glutethimide, rifampin: Reduced hypoprothrombinemic response to warfarin

 Bile acid-binding resins: Variable effect on hypoprothrombinemic effect of warfarin

 Cephalosporins: Enhanced hypoprothrombinemic response to warfarin with moxalactam, cefoperazone, cefamandole, cefotetan, and cefmetazole

 Chloral hydrate: Transient increase in hypoprothrombinemic response to warfarin

 Ethanol: Enhanced hypoprothrombinemic response to warfarin with acute ethanol intoxication

 Heparin: Prolonged activated partial thromboplastin time in patients receiving heparin; prolonged prothrombin times in patients receiving warfarin

 NSAIDs: Increased risk of bleeding in anticoagulated patients

 Oral contraceptives: Increase or decrease in anticoagulent response; increased risk of thromboembolic disorders

 Phenytoin: Transient increase in hypoprothrombinemic response to warfarin with initiation of phenytoin therapy, followed within 1-2 wk by inhibition of hypoprothrombinemic response to warfarin

 Salicylates: Increased risk of bleeding in anticoagulated patients; enhanced hypoprothrombinemic response to warfarin with large salicylate doses

Labs

• *Interference:* May cause orange-red discoloration of urine, which may interfere with some lab tests

SPECIAL CONSIDERATIONS

• Avoid use of initial doses >5 mg

• INR during 1st 5 days of therapy does not correlate with degree of anticoagulation

• Anticoagulant effect of warfarin may be reversed by administration of vitamin K or fresh frozen plasma; should only use in situations where INR is severely elevated >10, or when patient is actively bleeding

PATIENT/FAMILY EDUCATION

• Strict adherence to prescribed dosage schedule is necessary

• Avoid alcohol, salicylates, and drastic changes in dietary habits

• Do not change from one brand to another without consulting clinician

MONITORING PARAMETERS

• INR q4-6 wk once stabilized; more frequently if INR out of range

---

* = non FDA-approved use

Index

A

A wave, 41
  cannon, 42
  diastolic heart failure and, 281
  giant, 42
Abciximab, 190t
Abdomen in physical examination, 43
Abdominal aortic aneurysm; *see* Aortic
  aneurysm, abdominal
Abdominal-jugular test, 41
Abortion, cardiac indications for, 447
Abuse, drug, 497-499, 498
Accelerated idioventricular ventricular
  rhythm, 183
  reperfusion and, 183
Accessory pathway arrhythmia, 304
Acebutolol, 151t
Activities of daily living, 500-501
Adenosine
  perfusion scanning and, 100t
  pregnancy and, 448t
Adenosine receptor, 4
Adjunctive therapy for heart failure, 271-
  272
Adrenergic nervous system, 261
Adrenocortical deficiency, 420t
Adriamycin-induced cardiomyopathy, 291
African-American patient, hypertension in,
  374-375
Age
  arrhythmias and, 503
  atherosclerosis and, 116t
  cardiovascular effects of, 500, 501t
  congestive heart failure and, 502-503
  coronary artery disease and, 500-502
  diastolic heart failure and, 282
  hyperlipidemia and, 505
  hypertension and, 504-505, 504t
  reperfusion and, 185
  valvular disease and, 503
Airplane travel, Eisenmenger's syndrome
  and, 357
Airway disease
  antihypertensive drugs in, 376
  chest pain with, 136t
Alcohol
  atherosclerosis and, 119
  hypertension and, 365
Alcoholism, 471-474, 472t, 473t, 474t,
  475t
  CAGE questions about, 473t, 498
  cardiovascular system effects of, 472-473
  clinical features of, 473
  dilated cardiomyopathy with, 290-291
  epidemiology of, 471-472
  management of, 473-474
  treatment of, 497

Algorithm
  for noncardiac surgery, *508*
  perioperative cardiac complications and,
    510t
Allergy
  cardiac catheterization and, 111t
  catheterization and, 112
Alpha-adrenergic blocking agent
  diabetes mellitus and, 416t
  for hypertension, 370t
Alphamethyldopa in pregnancy, 448t
Ambulatory blood pressure monitoring, 363
Ambulatory monitoring in atrial fibrillation,
  298-299
American College of Cardiology, 287
American Heart Association, 287
Amiloride for hypertension, 369t
Aminoglycoside antibiotic in pregnancy,
  448t
Amiodarone
  atrial fibrillation and, 301t
  cardiopulmonary resuscitation and, 535
  heart failure and, 271
  pregnancy and, 448t
  to prevent sudden death, 206, 208
Amlodipine
  angina and, 154t
  heart failure and, 270
Amoxicillin for endocarditis prophylaxis,
  257t
Ampicillin for endocarditis prophylaxis,
  257t
Amrinone in heart failure, 271
Amyloid heart disease, 294
Analgesia, postoperative, 517
Ancillary study
  for heart failure, 265t
  types of, 74
Anemia with endocarditis, 249
Anesthesia for noncardiac surgery, 513-517,
  514t, 515t, 516t, 517t
Aneurysm
  aortic; *see* Aortic aneurysm
  pseudoaneurysm, 205
Angina pectoris, 135-167
  chronic stable, 136t, 140-159
    clinical course of, 157
    clinical features of, 144
    epidemiology of, 140
    follow-up for, 157-159
    laboratory studies of, 144-146, *146*
    management of, 146-157, 148t,
      149t-152t, 154t-158t
    pathophysiology of, *140*, 140-144, *141*,
      143
  clinical features of, 135, 137

Angina pectoris—cont'd
  diabetes mellitus and, 417
  electrocardiographic changes with, 65t
  epidemiology, 135
  in female patient, 450
  hypothyroidism and, 420
  laboratory studies for, 137-139, 138t
  management of, 139-140
  Prinzmetal's variant, 163-165
  silent ischemia and, 165
  ST segment depression in, 63
  syndrome X and, 165
  unstable, 136t, 159-163, 159t, *160*, 161t
    reperfusion after myocardial infarction
      and, 184
Angiocardiography, radionuclide, 101-102, 101t
Angiography
  angina and, 145
  carotid artery disease and, 401
  cor pulmonale and, 406
  coronary, 105
    peripheral arterial disease and, 387
  coronary artery disease and, 155t
  gender differences in, 452
  magnetic resonance
    carotid artery disease and, 401, 402t
    peripheral arterial disease and, 82-83
  myocardial infarction and, 191-192
    reperfusion after, 183, 191
  peripheral arterial disease and, 386-387
  pulmonary, 409-410
  stroke and, 401
  syncope and, 328t
  unstable angina and, 161-162
Angioplasty
  myocardial infarction and, 192
  percutaneous transluminal coronary,
    156-157, 157t, 158t
  Prinzmetal's angina and, 164
  surgery *versus*, 107t, 155-157
Angiosarcoma, 429
Angiotensin blocking agent, diabetes mellitus and, 416t
Angiotensin II receptor blocker
  heart failure and, 269-270
  for hypertension, 371t, 372t
Angiotensin-aldosterone system, 261
Angiotensin-converting enzyme inhibitor
  diabetes mellitus and, 416, 416t
  heart failure and, 264, 266-267, 266t,
    269-270
    diastolic, 285t
    in elderly, 502
    with systolic dysfunction, 266t
  for hypertension, 366, 371t, 372t, 373
    diabetes mellitus and, 375-376

Page numbers in *italic* indicate illustrations; page numbers followed
by *t* indicate tables.

Angiotensin-converting enzyme inhibitor—cont'd
for hypertension—cont'd
renal insufficiency and, 375-376
ischemia after myocardial infarction and, 209t
mitral regurgitation and, 224
myocardial infarction and, 177, 178t
congestive heart failure and, 199
to prevent sudden death after, 208
Anisoylated plasminogen streptokinase activator complex, 187-188
Ankle brachial index, 385-386
peripheral arterial disease and, 80-81
Ankylosing spondylitis, 423-424
Anomalous pulmonary venous return, 487t
Anorexia in heart failure, 38
Anorexiant drug, 470-471
Anterior myocardial infarction, 172
diastolic and systolic contours in, 198
hypotension and, 196t
Anterolateral myocardial infarction, 174
Antiarrhythmic agent
heart failure and, 271-272
pregnancy and, 448t
Antibiotic
endocarditis and, 253-254, 255, 257t
peripheral vascular disease and, 459
pregnancy and, 446, 447t, 448t
wound infection and, 458
Antibody
cytoplasmic, 423
endocarditis and, 249
Anticoagulation
angina and, 147-148
atrial fibrillation and, 300
cardiac catheterization and, 111t
heart failure and, 272
myocardial infarction and, 177-178, 203t
noncardiac surgery and, 512-513, 513t
pregnancy and, 449t
pulmonary embolism and, 410
reperfusion contraindicated with, 187
strategies for, 3-4
unstable angina and, 162
Anticonvulsant, 496
Antidepressant, tricyclic, 494, 495
Antihypertensive agent
bradyarrhythmia caused by, 323
diabetes mellitus and, 416, 416t
in elderly patient, 505
Antiinflammatory drug in pericarditis, 202
Antioxidant in atherosclerosis, 130-131
Antiplatelet therapy; see also Aspirin
angina and, 147-148
unstable, 162
atherosclerosis and, 119
myocardial infarction and, 203t
strategies for, 3-4
thrombolysis and, 188-189
Antipsychotic drug, 497
Antithrombotic therapy, reperfusion and, 189-190
Anxiety, 491-493
Aorta
coarctation of
congenital, 351-352
continuous murmur of, 53t
radiography of, 79
occlusive disease of, 382
trauma to, 382-383, 533t
Aortic aneurysm
abdominal, 378-379
clinical features of, 378

Aortic aneurysm—cont'd
diagnosis of, 378-379, 379t
epidemiology of, 378
management of, 379
pathophysiology of, 378
testing for, 84
trash foot with, 390
cardiomyopathy versus, 293
familial, 486t
radiography of, 79
rupture of, continuous murmur of, 53t
testing for, 84
thoracic, 379-380, 380t
Aortic balloon valvuloplasty, 502
Aortic disease, echocardiography for, 94
Aortic dissection, 380-382, 381
chest pain with, 136t
transthoracic echocardiography for, 94
Aortic pressure
catheterization and, 104, 104
systolic, 110
Aortic regurgitation, 235-238
catheterization evaluation of, 109t
clinical features of, 232t, 237
echocardiographic assessment of, 90t
etiology of, 235
first heart sound and, 45
management of, 237-238
murmur of, 49t, 52
pathophysiology of, 235, 236, 237
pregnancy and, 444
Aortic stenosis, 230-235
cardioembolism and, 437
catheterization evaluation of, 109t
clinical features of, 231, 232, 232t, 233
echocardiographic assessment of, 90t, 91
epidemiology of, 230
management of, 233-235, 233-235
murmur of, 48, 49t, 50
pathophysiology of, 230-231, 231
pregnancy and, 444
supravalvular, 487t
Aortic valve, bicuspid, 487t
Aortitis, 382
Apical pulse, 43-44
Apnea, sleep
cardiomyopathy with, 290
hypertension and, 365
obesity and, 467-468
apo B 100, familial defective, 486t
Arbutamine, 100t
Arrhythmia
accessory pathway, 304
atrial, 296-305; see also Atrial entries
bradyarrhythmia, 320-325; see also Bradyarrhythmia
disability and, 520-521
echocardiography for, 95
in elderly, 503
heart failure and, 271-272
myocardial infarction and, 171
as complication of, 199-201
sudden death caused by, 206
pregnancy and, 446
reperfusion causing, 183
stroke and, 435-436
syncope caused by, 326
ventricular, 307-319; see also Ventricular entries
Arterial dilator, diastolic heart failure and, 284
Arterial disease
coronary; see Coronary artery disease
peripheral, 384-392

Arterial disease—cont'd
peripheral—cont'd
diagnostic testing for, 80-83
echocardiography in, 80
Arterial insufficiency
atherosclerosis and, 118-119
infection and, 459
Arterial pressure line, 538-539
Arterial pulse, abnormal patterns of, 37t
Arteriography, 82
Arteriovenous fistula, 53t
Arteriovenous hemofiltration, continuous, 271
Arteritis, temporal, 425
Artery, renal, stenosis of, 364
Arthritis, rheumatoid, 423
Artifact in nuclear cardiology, 98
Aspirin
angina and, 147-148
cardiac catheterization and, 111t
ischemia after myocardial infarction and, 209t
myocardial infarction and, 175, 178t
for pericarditis, 202
peripheral arterial disease and, 387
pregnancy and, 449t
stroke and, 393t
thrombolysis and, 189
ASPSAC, reperfusion and, 187-188
Assist device
cardiac, 543
left ventricular, 541
heart failure and, 273
Ataxia, Friedreich's, 435
Atenolol
angina and, 151t
heart failure and, diastolic, 285t
Atherosclerosis, 115-134
antihypertensive agent with, 367, 372
clinical features of, 118-119
dyslipidemia and, 121-134; see also Dyslipidemia
in elderly patient, 116t
endothelial cells and, 5-6
laboratory tests for, 80
pathogenesis of, 124
pathophysiology of, 118, 118t
renal disease and, 478-480
risk factors for, 115, 116t, 117-118, 117t, 130-131
Atrial abnormality, electrocardiographic, 57-58, 57t
Atrial arrhythmia; see also Atrial entries, below
fibrillation and flutter, 296-302, 297, 298, 299t
pacemaker for, 337
pathophysiology of, 298
tachycardia, 302-305, 303, 304, 306
Atrial automatic ectopic tachycardia, 305
Atrial fibrillation
cardiac surgery and, 544
cardioembolism and, 437
mitral stenosis and, 220
noncardiac surgery and, 512
Atrial flutter, 296-302
clinical features of, 297
epidemiology of, 296
laboratory studies for, 297-299, 298, 299t
management of, 299-302, 301t
mitral stenosis and, 220
myocardial infarction and, 201
noncardiac surgery and, 512
pathophysiology of, 296-297, 297

Atrial myxoma, 428
  echocardiography and, 94
  heart sounds with, 48
Atrial natriuretic peptide, 4
Atrial pressure
  coarctation of aorta and, 351
  left, catheterization and, 108-109
Atrial septal defect
  congenital, 347, *348*, 349
  incomplete right bundle branch block
    and, 58, *61*
  radiography of, 79
Atrial tachycardia
  automatic ectopic, 305
  cardiomyopathy from, 305-306, *306*
  myocardial infarction and, 201
  paroxysmal supraventricular, 302-305,
    303, 304
  sinus, 302
Atrioventricular block, pacemaker for, 332t
Atrioventricular dissociation, 42
Atrioventricular node
  beta-adrenergic blocking agent and, 152
  heart block and, 320-321, 321t, *322*
Atrioventricular node heart block, infranodal
  versus, 334
Atrioventricular node reentrant tachycardia,
    302
Atrium; *see also* Atrial *entries*
  echocardiography of, *88*
  myxoma of, 428
  on radiograph, 78
Austin Flint murmur, 49t, 52
Autoimmune disease
  aortitis and, 382
  endocarditis and, 252
Automatic ectopic tachycardia, 305
Automatic external defibrillator, 318
Automatic implantable cardiac defibrillator,
    disability and, 520-521
Automaticity
  atrial arrhythmia and, 296
  ventricular tachycardia and, 311
Autonomic receptor, 4
Autoregulation of coronary blood flow, 141
Azithromycin, endocarditis prophylaxis
    with, 257t

B

Bacteremia
  after procedures, 246t
  endocarditis and, 248-249, 251
  nosocomial, 457
    treatment of, 458
  procedures causing, 255
Bacterial endocarditis; *see* Endocarditis
Balloon pump, intraaortic
  cardiogenic shock and, 195
  intensive care unit and, *540,* 540-541
  right ventricular infarct syndrome and,
    198
Balloon valvotomy
  aortic, 234
  mitral, 221
Balloon valvuloplasty, aortic, in elderly, 502
Baroreceptor, syncope and, 325
Baroreflex failure, 365
Battery, pacemaker, 335
Bayesian analysis, 71, 72
Beat; *see* Heart beat
Becker muscular dystrophy, 433, 434t, 485t
Behavior counseling in obesity, 469-471,
    470t

Benzodiazepine
  alcohol withdrawal and, 474
  for depression, 496
Beta-adrenergic blocking agent
  angina and, 149-153, 151t
    Prinzmetal's, 164
    unstable, 162
  diabetes mellitus and, 416t
  heart failure and, 268-269, 269t
    diastolic, 284, 285t
    for hypertension, 370t, 372t
  hyperthyroidism and, 419
  myocardial infarction and, 175-176, 176t,
    178t
    ischemia and, 209t
    to prevent ischemia and, 210
    reperfusion and, 190
    sudden death prevention with, 206,
    208
  noncardiac surgery and, 511
  pregnancy and, 449t
Beta-carotene, atherosclerosis and, 130
Bicarbonate, cardiopulmonary resuscitation
    and, 535
Bicuspid aortic valve, 487t
Bifascicular block, 58
  pacemaker for, 332t
Bile acid resin, 131
Biliary disease, chest pain with, 136t
Biology, molecular
  cardiovascular disease and, 485-488
  coronary artery disease and, 6-7
Biopsy
  cor pulmonale and, 407
  endomyocardial, 431, 461
  reperfusion contraindicated after, 187
Bipolar pacemaker lead, 335
Bisferiens pulse, 37t
Bisoprolol
  angina and, 151t
  heart failure and, 269t
Biventricular hypertrophy, 349
Black patient, hypertension in, 374-375
Blalock-Taussig shunt, 351
Bleeding, reperfusion and, 185-186, 187
Blood cell count
  chest pain and, 137
  hypertension and, 363
  myocardial infarction and, 171-172
Blood culture in endocarditis, 248
Blood flow
  pulmonary, in Eisenmenger's syndrome,
    354
  stable angina and, 141
Blood gases in pulmonary embolism, 409
Blood pressure
  aortic dissection and, 382
  hypertension and, 359-377; *see also* Hy-
    pertension
  in physical examination, 36-38
  stroke and, 401
  syncope and, 327
Blue sclera, 39t
Blue toe syndrome, 390
Borderline hypertension, 360-361
Brachial index, ankle, 80-81
Bradyarrhythmia, 320-325
  carotid sinus syncope and, 324
  clinical features of, 322
  heart block and, 324-325
  laboratory evaluation of, *322,* 322-323,
    323
  management of, 323-324

Bradyarrhythmia—cont'd
  myocardial infarction and, 201
  pathophysiology of, 321-322
  sick sinus syndrome causing, 324
  sinoatrial node syndromes causing, 320-
    321, 321t
Bradycardia, definition of, 56
Brain natriuretic peptide, 4
Breathing, Kussmaul, 38
Bretylium, 535
Broken pacemaker lead, 341
Bronchospasm
  beta-adrenergic blocking agent and, 152
  chest pain with, 136t
Bronchospastic lung disease, 376
Bruce protocol for treadmill testing, 69
Bucindolol, 269t
Buerger's disease, 390
Bumetanide
  heart failure and, 268t
  for hypertension, 369t
  palliative therapy and, 551, 551t
Bundle branch block
  left
    electrocardiography of, 58, *60*
    myocardial infarction and, 174
    pacemaker for, 331
    stress testing and, 74
  right
    electrocardiography of, 58, *59, 61*
    myocardial infarction and, 174, *174*
    pacemaker for, 331
Bundle of His in heart block, *325*
Bypass, heart-lung, 542
Bypass graft, coronary artery, 545-546
  cardioembolism and, 439
  diabetes mellitus and, 417
  disability and, 519-520
  in female patient, 452
  indications of, 156t

C

Cachexia, cardiac, 38
CAGE questions about alcoholism, 473t,
    498
Calcification, 78-79
Calcium
  hypertension and, 363
  hypocalcemia and, 420t
Calcium-channel blocker
  angina and, 152, 154t
  diabetes mellitus and, 416t
  heart failure and, 270
    diastolic, 284
  for hypertension, 371t, 372t
  myocardial infarction and, 176-179
  pregnancy and, 449t
  unstable angina and, 162
Candida albicans
  endocarditis and, 250t
  endocarditis caused by, 251
Canine therapy, myocardial infarction and,
    215
Cannon A wave, 42
Captopril
  diastolic heart failure and, 285t
  pregnancy and, 448t
Carbon dioxide, 38
Cardiac cachexia, 38
Cardiac catheterization, 103-112; *see also*
    Catheterization, cardiac
Cardiac denervation syndrome in diabetes,
    417

Cardiac examination, 43-53
  apical pulse, 43-44
  heart sounds in, *44, 44-49, 44t, 45, 46t,*
    47
  murmurs and, 48, 49t-50t, 50-53
    continuous, 52-53, 53t
    diastolic, 52
    systolic, 48, 49t-50t, 50-52
  pericardial friction rub and, 53
Cardiac malposition, 353-354
Cardiac mass, 94
Cardiac muscle, thrombolysis saving, 181
Cardiac rhythm; *see* Electrocardiography;
    Rhythm, cardiac
Cardiac surgery; *see* Surgery
Cardiac tamponade, *343,* 343-344
  as emergency, 529-531
Cardiac-assist device, 543
Cardioembolism, 392, 393, 436-439; *see also*
    Embolism; Embolus
  echocardiography for, 94-95
Cardiogenic pulmonary edema, 531-532
Cardiogenic shock, 194-196, 195t, 196t
Cardiology, nuclear, 97-102; *see also* Nuclear
    imaging
Cardiomyopathy
  atrial tachycardia causing, 305-306, *306*
  classification of, 289t
  diabetes mellitus and, 417
  diastolic heart failure and, 286
  dilated, 288-293
    cardioembolism and, 438
    causes of, 290
    clinical features of, 288-289
    diabetic, 292
    epidemiology of, 288
    heredity in, 289
    infection causing, 292
    obesity and, 290
    other cardiomyopathies *versus,* 292-293
    pacemaker for, 333t
    pathophysiology of, 288
    peripartum, 292
    sleep apnea with, 290
    tachyarrhythmias in, 291
    thiamine deficiency and, 289-290
    toxins causing, 290-291
    ventricular tachycardia and, 315-316
    X-linked, 485t
  hypertrophic, 295
    diastolic heart failure with, 286
    dilated *versus,* 292-293
    genetic, 484t
    murmur of, 50-51
    pacemaker for, 333t
    pregnancy and, 445
    ventricular tachycardia and, 315-316
  mitochondrial, 484t
  myocarditis and, 461
  obesity and, 465
  pericarditis *versus,* 285-286
  peripartum, 445
  restrictive, 293-295
  tachycardia-induced, 305-306
  ventricular tachycardia and, 315-316
Cardiomyoplasty, 272-273
Cardioplegia, 542-543
Cardiopulmonary resuscitation, 533-535
  reperfusion contraindicated after, 187
Cardiovascular receptor, 4
  adenosine, 4
  cardiac natriuretic peptides and, 4

Cardiovascular studies for syncope,
    327-328
Cardioversion
  atrial fibrillation and, 300-301, 301t
  heart failure and, 272
  pacemaker and, 340
  ventricular tachycardia and, 314-315
Carotid artery
  asymptomatic disease of, 401-402, 402t
  endarterectomy of, 393t
  stroke and, 396t
  testing for disease of, 84
Carotid sinus syncope, 324
Carotid sinus syndrome, 333t, 335
Carteolol, 151t
Carvedilol
  angina and, 151t
  heart failure and, 269t
Catecholamine
  cardiogenic shock and, 195
  dilated cardiomyopathy and, 291
Catheterization
  cardiac, 103-113
    aortic regurgitation and, 237-238
    aortic stenosis and, 233
    chest pain and, 139
    cor pulmonale and, 406-407
    for coronary artery disease, 103-107,
      104, 105, 107t
    diastolic heart failure and, 281
    general care for, 109-110, 111t, 112
    mitral regurgitation and, 224
    mitral stenosis and, *218,* 220
    risks of, 103
    tricuspid regurgitation and, 241
    tricuspid stenosis and, 242
    for valvular disease, 107-109, 109t, *110*
  pulmonary artery, 539, *539*
Catheter-related infection, 457
c7E3, 4
Cefazolin for endocarditis prophylaxis,
    257t
Cell, endothelial, 5-6
Cellular response-to-injury hypothesis, 118,
    118t
Cellular telephone, pacemaker and, 340
Central cyanosis, 40t
Cephalothin in pregnancy, 448t
Cerebral edema, 398
Cerebral thromboembolus, 438
Cerebrospinal fluid in stroke, 397t
Cerebrovascular disease
  carotid artery, 401-402, 402t
  stroke, 392-401; *see also* Stroke
  syncope with, 327
Chamber, cardiac; *see also* Atrium; Ventricular
    entries; Atrial *entries;* Ventricle *entries*
  echocardiography of, *88*
  on radiograph, 77-78
Chelation for atherosclerosis, 119
Chemistry panel for chest pain, 137
Chemotherapy
  complications of, 431-432
  dilated cardiomyopathy caused by, 291
Chest pain
  angina pectoris causing, 135-167; *see also*
    Angina pectoris
  echocardiography for, 86-87, 89
  mitral valve prolapse and, 227-228
  reperfusion after myocardial infarction
    and, 184-185
  syndromes with, 136t

Chest pain—cont'd
  of uncertain etiology
    clinical features of, 135, 137
    epidemiology, 135
    laboratory studies for, 137-139, 138t
    management of, 139-140
Chest x-ray; *see* Radiographic evaluation
Cheyne Stokes respiration, 38
Child, pacemaker in, 341
Chimeric-7E3, 4
Chlamydia pneumoniae, 116t
Chlorothiazide, 268t
Chlorpromazine, 497
Chlorthalidone
  heart failure and, 268t
  for hypertension, 369t
Cholesterol; *see also* Dyslipidemia
  diet and, 125
  reverse transport of, *129*
Cholestyramine, 131
Chronic decompensated mitral regurgita-
    tion, 223
Cigarette smoking as risk factor; *see* Smoking
Circulation
  biology of
    anticoagulation and antiplatelet agents
      and, 3-4
    cardiovascular and autonomic receptors
      and, 4
    endothelial cell function and, 5-6
    gene therapy and, 6-7
    lipoprotein risk factors and, 4-5
  collateral, angina and, 143, *143*
CK-MB, 171, 172t
Claudication, 385-387, *386*
Click
  ejection, pulmonic stenosis and, 51
  systolic, 48
Clindamycin for endocarditis prophylaxis,
    257t
Clonidine
  for hypertension, 369t
  pregnancy and, 448t
Clopidogrel
  peripheral arterial disease and, 387-388
  stroke and, 393t
Clubbing
  cyanosis and, 38
  significance of, 40t
Coagulation disorder, reperfusion con-
    traindicated in, 187
Coarctation of aorta
  congenital, 351-352
  continuous murmur of, 53t
  radiography of, 79
Cocaine abuse, 497-498
Colestipol, 131
Collateral circulation, angina and, 143 143
Commotio cordis, 532-533
Compensated mitral regurgitation, 223
Complete blood count
  chest pain and, 137
  hypertension and, 363
  stroke and, 396t
Computed tomography
  abdominal aortic aneurysm and, 378-379,
    379t
  aortic trauma and, 383
  chest pain and, 139
  endocarditis and, 249
  pulmonary embolism and, 410
  stroke and, 395, 396t, 398, 399